ADOLESCENT HEALTH CARE
A Practical Guide
THIRD EDITION

ADOLESCENT HEALTH CARE
A Practical Guide
THIRD EDITION

Lawrence S. Neinstein, MD
Associate Professor of Pediatrics and Medicine
University of Southern California School of Medicine
Executive Director
USC University Park Health Center
Los Angeles, California

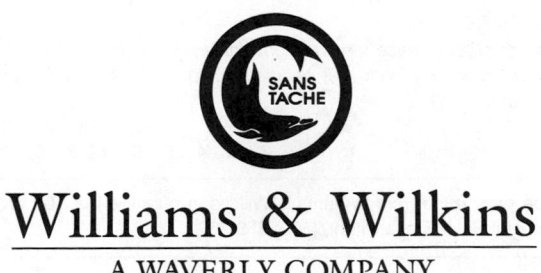

Williams & Wilkins
A WAVERLY COMPANY

BALTIMORE • PHILADELPHIA • LONDON • PARIS • BANGKOK
BUENOS AIRES • HONG KONG • MUNICH • SYDNEY • TOKYO • WROCLAW

Editor: Kathleen Courtney Millet
Production Coordinator: Raymond E. Reter
Cover Designer: Wilma E. Rosenberger
Production Service: Joy Moore, Cracom Corporation, St. Louis
Designer: Judy Schmitt, Cracom Corporation, St. Louis
Illustration Planner: Jeanne Gulledge, Cracom Corporation, St. Louis
Typesetter: Cracom Corporation, St. Louis
Printer and Binder: Port City Press, Baltimore

351 West Camden Street
Baltimore, Maryland 21201-2436 USA

Rose Tree Corporate Center
1400 North Providence Road
Building II, Suite 5025
Media, Pennsylvania 19063-2043 USA

Visit Williams & Wilkins on the Internet: http://www.wwilkins.com

Accurate indications, adverse reactions and dosage schedules for drugs are provided in this book, but it is possible that they may change. The reader is urged to review the package information data of the manufacturers of the medications mentioned.

Printed in the United States of America

First Edition 1984
Second Edition 1991

Library of Congress Cataloging-in-Publication Data

Neinstein, Lawrence S.
    Adolescent health care : a practical guide / Lawrence S.
  Neinstein. — 3rd ed.
        p.   cm.
    Includes bibliographical references and index.
    ISBN 0-683-06375-8
    1. Adolescent medicine—Handbooks, manuals, etc.   I. Title.
    [DNLM: 1. Adolescent Medicine—handbooks.   WS 39 N414a 1996]
  RJ550.N45   1996
  616'.00835—dc20
  DNLM/DLC
  for Library of Congress   95-47009
                                                                           CIP

The publishers have made every effort to trace the copyright holders for borrowed material. If they have inadvertently overlooked any, they will be pleased to make the necessary arrangements at the first opportunity.

                                              97 98 99 00
                                        2 3 4 5 6 7 8 9 10

Reprints of chapters may be purchased from Williams & Wilkins in quantities of 100 or more. Call Isabella Wise, Special Sales Department, (800) 358-3583.

To my incredible family,
my wife, Debra,
and my children,
Yael, Aaron, and David,
and to my parents,
Shirley and Alvin
and
Roz and Ben

Foreword

In the 35 years since the emergence of adolescent medicine as an established field of health care, clinicians, investigators, and the public alike have begun to recognize and understand the unique nature of adolescence and the variety of very special problems that develop during the course of the teenage years. Indeed, many of the conditions that have their origins during the adolescent period are identified with and even represent the stressors seen in today's larger culture and society.

Thus, in many ways adolescents mirror both the very best and worst of the 20th century. And yet, nearly 100 years age, G. Stanley Hall noted the important role of adolescence as a period of change, evolution, and the unique opportunity to add new dimensions to human growth and development. Rather than treat adolescence as a disease, we have come to recognize the need for a broad, developmental perspective of adolescence in which the vast majority of young people learn essential lessons for living the rest of their lives. Frequently, in our attempts to reconcile the phenomenon of adolescence in our own minds, we forget that young people do survive and become mature, productive adults.

With learning comes vulnerability. Much of what has been written about adolescence and the present drug, violence, and HIV epidemics focuses on the causality of adolescent risk behaviors and perceptions of vulnerability and invulnerability. Risk-taking activities associated with learning about independence, identity, and personality formation; preparing for intimacy and mature adult behavior; establishing skills necessary for the workplace; and indeed, learning "survival" skills in order to live in today's world are the cornerstones of adolescent development.

Even though teens rely heavily on their peers and less so on parental support, they still need adult acceptance, information, understanding, and not infrequently, advocacy on their behalf. They obtain help from other adult relatives, teachers, health providers, counselors, parents of friends, and other adults who are able to recognize needs and interpret acting-out, destructive behaviors that can lead to real life crises and tragedy.

Thus, successful interventions with adolescents are based, for the most part, on an understanding of this unique period of life, an ability to perceive the special needs of the adolescent (and their parents as well), effective communication skills, and a certain awareness of the "adolescent" that resides in each and every one of us who have managed to make it through our own adolescent adventures and growth process.

Health providers add still another dimension to successful intervention. As physicians, nurses, social workers, psychologists, and other health workers, we bring knowledge of the interrelation between medical conditions and the teenager's environment; special skills for management and treatment of diseases; tools for disease prevention, health promotion, and education; and an understanding of the necessary interdisciplinary nature of adolescent health-care services and programs. This expertise by health professionals does not minimize the importance of the broader abilities necessary to relate to adolescents mentioned earlier; rather, medicine and the medical encounter offer an unusual opportunity to intervene effectively with this age group.

With this very much in mind, the third edition of *Adolescent Health Care: A Practical Guide* builds on the two earlier editions by Larry Neinstein and adds a group of coauthors with expertise in adolescent health care. The updated 82 chapters and accompanying new reference material in this widely acclaimed book bring a very workable format for day-to-day use by the health professional.

Among the extensively revised chapters included in this third edition, Abigail English authors a chapter on legal issues, Anita Nelson coauthors several chapters on contraception, Fran Kaufman coauthors several chapters on growth and development and endocrinology issues, Marvin Belzer coauthors an updated chapter on HIV infections during adolescence, Richard MacKenzie coauthors chapters on eating disorders and high-risk behavior, Arno Hohn coauthors a chapter on hypertension, Marc Jacobsen and Michael Kohn coauthor a chapter on hyperlipidemia, and Howard Schubiner and Arthur Robin coauthor a chapter on attention deficit disorders. New chapters have also been added about youth violence by Curren Warf and noninflammatory rheumatism by Bram Bernstein.

Most importantly, the easy outline format is maintained in this new edition. *Adolescent Health Care* emphasizes practical and concise approaches to adolescent and young adult health care, provides a clear understanding of the disease process, defines the most likely differential diagnoses, and describes current treatment and procedures. Larry Neinstein builds on his own real-life experiences as a clinician-educator with a clarity of purpose and vision of the scientific basis and human understanding necessary for management of the adolescent and young adult patient. In this regard, his more than two decades of practice in adolescent and young adult medicine as Associate Director of Adolescent Medicine at Childrens Hospital of Los Angeles assures that this new edition will be an important reference for anyone working in the field.

DALE C. GARELL, MD
Professor of Pediatrics
University of Southern California School of Medicine
Vice President of Pediatrics and Academic Affairs
Childrens Hospital of Los Angeles

Preface

As a health professional for over 20 years, I have been glad to see that the interest in the health care of adolescents and young adults has continued to increase to the point that a need for a third edition of this book has arisen. Besides the continued interest in the primary care specialties of pediatrics, internal medicine, and family medicine, there is a new board subspecialty in adolescent medicine. The American Board of Pediatrics and the American Board of Internal Medicine are now requiring extensive training in adolescent health in their training programs. Groups such as the Society for Adolescent Medicine and the American College Health Association are maturing into important advocacy and educational organizations for adolescents and young adults. The individuals who care for youths are a wonderful mixture of multiple specialties and disciplines that stretch from physicians, physician assistants, nurse practitioners, psychologists, social workers, health educators, nurses, nutritionists, teachers, and many more.

I again want to thank all of the health-care providers who have provided me with such wonderful feedback on the second edition. The second edition has been used worldwide and was translated into Spanish, providing an additional resource for practitioners.

The availability of information and the rapidity with which it changes has continued to increase in the 1990s. Thus it is important to address these changes in this third edition. Many users of this book have continually provided me with feedback regarding this book's usefulness in the provision of primary care to adolescents and young adults. The book has been used extensively in teaching situations and in clinical care protocol development. I have tried to maintain the practical aspects of this book in the third edition while adding new information. This was facilitated by increasing coauthorship with experts on many of the chapters and expanding the scope. Continuing from the second edition, many chapters have been extensively rewritten, such as those on hyperlipidemia, the office visit, health screening, nutrition, legal issues, hypertension, sports medicine, HIV infections, oral contraceptives, emergency contraceptives, long-acting progestins, HPV, management of drug abuse, school problems, and many others. In addition, chapters on violence in adolescents and noninflammatory rheumatism have been added.

I have continued to strive to make all the chapters practical and easy to read, allowing the user to rapidly extract information. My intent is to have this book provide enough information to thoroughly and appropriately, but concisely, evaluate and work-up the common and less common problems that occur in this age group. I also have aimed to have the book serve as a source for additional references and resources. Thus, tables, statistics, references, and resources have been extensively updated and revised to reflect the ever-changing information in health care and in this age group. In addition, the appendices have been expanded and updated to offer additional resource information.

During this year, I have moved professionally into the area of college health as well as continuing my work in adolescent health. I dedicate this edition to those health professionals all over the world who care for adolescents and young adults. Hopefully, this edition will continue to serve as a source of information for you who care for and teach about individuals in this critical period of life. As always, your feedback on this edition is welcome so that I can continue to make this practical guide as practical and useful as possible.

Preface to First Edition

Adolescent Health Care: A Practical Guide is written for those health-care professionals involved in the care of adolescents, including pediatricians, family practitioners, internists, gynecologists, housestaff, nurses, nurse practitioners, and others. The list is long because the challenge of adolescent medicine crosses the specialty boundaries of medicine as well as the lines separating the medical, psychological, and social areas of health care.

This volume is designed for day-to-day office use. Topics are reviewed in a format that outlines and highlights subjects for easy reference. Selection of subject areas was discussed with housestaff and other experts in adolescent medicine and primary care medicine in order to assure that pertinent areas of interest were not overlooked. In this connection, many subspeciality concerns have been excluded, as they were felt to be better examined in internal medicine or pediatric texts.

Normal growth and psychosocial development of adolescents is discussed first in the book, in order to provide a framework in which to consider abnormalities. Among the chapters featured, for example, are those on problems unique to adolescence (i.e., gynecomastia); problems exacerbated by adolescence (i.e., suicide, school problems); and problems with unique considerations during adolescence (i.e., thyroid disease, chest pain). In addition, because of the high prevalence of teenage sexual activity, sexually transmissible diseases, and drug use, extensive sections of the book have been devoted to these areas. To assist the health-care practitioner in treating adolescents, other chapters concentrate on developing rapport with teens, legal issues associated with teenage care, and psychosocial problems in teens. Useful doctor's office and hospital materials are furthermore included, such as questionnaires for initial interviews, history and physical examination forms, and patient handouts on contraception. The book's numerous tables provide statistics on the adolescent age group in areas such as morbidity, mortality, hypertension, and hyperlipidemia. These have been drawn from many sources and endeavor to provide the practitioner with age-relevant statistics. Last, to assist the practitioner in finding available community resources, an extensive Appendix has been added.

Working with adolescents is exciting, challenging, and sometimes difficult and frustrating. Adolescence is a time of rapid growth and development of mind and body, presenting difficulties in adjustment for the teenager, the family, and the physician. It is also a time of high risk for many problems such as suicide and sexually transmissible diseases, as well as being a critical period for detecting chronic illnesses and risk factors for cardiovascular disease. Moreover, it is an ideal time to educate adolescents about how to best care for their bodies. This book is dedicated to helping the health-care professional meet these challenges.

Acknowledgments

The effort of many are required to put forth a book such as this. I am indebted to two mentors who inspired me in my work with adolescents, young adults, and college students. I am deeply indebted to the late Adie Klotz, MD, my friend, teacher, and inspiration, who helped me to realize the need and excitement of working with young people. I want to thank Richard G. MacKenzie, MD, who has also helped to guide me in the path of the excitement of working with adolescents and young adults. He has always encouraged me in the directions I have taken and has further contributed to this edition by coauthoring several chapters.

I want to acknowledge the contributions of Eric Cohen, MD, who sadly died this past year. Eric was a friend and colleague throughout my professional career in adolescent medicine. He was a wonderful clinician, teacher, and person who provided much guidance to adolescents, young adults, and young professionals over many years. Eric was one of the creators of the HEADSS psychosocial profile and did much to further the importance of going beyond the chief complaint when providing health care. Eric was also a coauthor of several chapters in this book. His kindness and spirit will be missed in the USC community, the youth community, and the adolescent medicine community.

I want to express my appreciation to the many experts who served as coauthors on many of the chapters in this book. Their knowledge and experience have helped to improve this edition. I personally want to thank them for their time and effort and timely response to my sometimes sudden requests for rapid reviews of material.

I must express my appreciation to the numerous fellows in adolescent medicine and house officers at Childrens Hospital of Los Angeles who helped me to continue to refine this edition. I also thank the wonderful staff of the Division of Adolescent Medicine at Childrens Hospital of Los Angeles who have always taught me so much about adolescent medicine. Many other physicians, nurses, nurse practitioners, and other health-care professionals have also given me their assessments and helpful comments in the development of this third edition.

Special thanks go to several individuals at USC who have helped in the manuscript preparation. Cathy Perez at Childrens Hospital who helped with resource information and manuscript development. Lucy Vergara at the USC University Park Health Center who was always there to assist in communicating with Williams & Wilkins and preparing the manuscript. Doreen Keogh for her efforts with references from the library at Childrens Hospital of Los Angeles.

There are many individuals at Williams & Wilkins who deserve recognition in the development of this edition. Katey Millet has been with this work since its inception at Urban & Schwarzenberg. She has once again served as editor-in-chief and helped me with the transition to Williams & Wilkins. I also want to thank Ray Reter for his help in the production of this book. Joy Moore and the staff at Cracom Corporation have helped extensively with copyediting and other production details. I thank Joy for her hard work and close communication.

There are also individuals very close to me who deserve special recognition. My parents have continued to provide emotional support through the difficult process of another edition and life in general. They also have shown me what appropriate, loving, and involved parenting can mean during one's adolescence and life. Without their guidance, I would not have had the skills and ability to complete this book. A second set of parents, my in-laws, have also provided incredible support during the past 25 years and during the writing of this edition. Loving thanks to all four of you.

Last, and most important, I must thank my loving wife, Debbie, and my children, Yael, Aaron, and David. Debbie has continued to support me despite far, far too many late nights spent "banging" away at my computer. Tolerating my absences through these three editions has been difficult at times. Yael, Aaron, and David provide me incredible support in their wonderful examples of what a healthy late adolescent, middle adolescent, and early adolescent, respectively, can be all about. With the second edition, a computer invaded our home. With this edition, two new computers and a notebook computer invaded our home. I love all of you and thank you for your understanding, support, and encouragement with this third edition.

Contributors

MARTIN M. ANDERSON, MD, MPH
Associate Professor of Pediatrics
Director, Adolescent Medicine Program
University of California, Los Angeles, School of
Medicine
Los Angeles, California

MARVIN E. BELZER, MD
Assistant Professor of Clinical Pediatrics and
Medicine
Division of Adolescent Medicine
University of Southern California School of
Medicine
Childrens Hospital of Los Angeles
Los Angeles, California

BRAM BERNSTEIN, MD
Professor of Clinical Pediatrics
University of Southern California School of
Medicine
Head, Division of Rheumatology
Childrens Hospital Los Angeles
Los Angeles, California

ERIC COHEN, MD*
Associate Clinical Professor of Pediatrics and
Family Practice
University of Southern California School of
Medicine
Los Angeles, California

ABIGAIL ENGLISH, JD
Project Director, Adolescent Health Care Project
National Center for Youth Law
Chapel Hill, North Carolina

BRUCE S. HEISCHOBER, MD
Assistant Professor of Emergency Medicine and
Adolescent Medicine
Loma Linda University School of Medicine
Attending Physician, Adolescent Medicine
Loma Linda University-Children's Hospital
Loma Linda, California

*Deceased.

ALBERT HERGENROEDER, MD
Associate Professor of Pediatrics
Chief, Adolescent Medicine and Sports
Medicine Section
Baylor College of Medicine
Houston, Texas

KAREN S. HIMEBAUGH, MD
Assistant Clinical Professor of Obstetrics and
Gynecology
University of California, Los Angeles, School of
Medicine
Los Angeles, California

ARNO R. HOHN, MD
Professor of Pediatrics
University of Southern California School of
Medicine
Head, Division of Cardiology
Childrens Hospital of Los Angeles
Los Angeles, California

MARC S. JACOBSEN, MD
Associate Professor of Pediatrics
Albert Einstein College of Medicine
Bronx, New York
Attending Physician, Division of Adolescent
Medicine
Director, Center for Atherosclerosis
Prevention
New Hyde Park, New York

MARIA A. JULIANI, PHD
Clinical Assistant Professor of Pediatrics
University of Southern California School of
Medicine
Coordinator, Psychological Services
Division of Adolescent Medicine
Childrens Hospital of Los Angeles
Los Angeles, California

FRANCINE RATNER KAUFMAN, MD
Associate Professor of Pediatrics
University of Southern California School of
 Medicine
Director, Comprehensive Childhood Diabetes
 Center
Childrens Hospital of Los Angeles
Los Angeles, California

MICHAEL R. KOHN, MD
Fellow, Adolescent Medicine
Schneider Children's Hospital
Long Island Jewish Medical Center
New Hyde Park, New York

PAUL S. KURTIN, MD
Vice President
Quality and Resource Management
Childrens Hospital and Health Center
San Diego, California

RICHARD MACKENZIE, MD
Associate Professor of Pediatrics
University of Southern California School of
 Medicine
Director, Division of Adolescent Medicine
Childrens Hospital of Los Angeles
Los Angeles, California

WILBERT H. MASON, JR., MD, MPH
Professor of Clinical Pediatrics
Department of Pediatrics/Division of Infectious
 Diseases
University of Southern California School of
 Medicine
Attending Physician
Childrens Hospital of Los Angeles
Los Angeles, California

WENDY G. MITCHELL, MD
Professor of Neurology and Pediatrics
University of Southern California School of
 Medicine
Attending Physician, Child Neurology
Childrens Hospital of Los Angeles
Los Angeles, California

LAWRENCE S. NEINSTEIN, MD
Associate Professor of Pediatrics and Medicine
University of Southern California School of
 Medicine
Executive Director
USC University Park Health Center
Los Angeles, California

ANITA NELSON, MD
Associate Professor of Obstetrics and
 Gynecology
University of California, Los Angeles, School of
 Medicine
Los Angeles, California
Medical Director, Women's Health Care Clinic
Research Training Program
Harbor-UCLA Medical Center
Torrance, California

ANITA S. PAKULA, MD
Clinical Instructor of Dermatology
University of California, Los Angeles, School of
 Medicine
Los Angeles, California

DREW PINSKY, MD
Program Medical Director
Department of Chemical Dependency
Las Encinas Hospital
Pasadena, California

SUSAN J. RABINOVITZ, RN, MPH
Associate Director Programs
Division of Adolescent Medicine
Childrens Hospital of Los Angeles
Los Angeles, California

ARTHUR L. ROBIN, MD
Professor of Psychiatry and Pediatrics
Wayne State University School of Medicine
Detroit, Michigan

LINDA E. SCHACK, MD
Clinical Assistant Professor of Family Medicine
 and Pediatrics
University of Southern California School of
 Medicine
Los Angeles, California

ARLENE SCHNEIR, MPH
Coordinator, Risk Reduction Program
Division of Adolescent Medicine
Childrens Hospital of Los Angeles
Los Angeles, California

HOWARD SCHUBINER, MD
Associate Professor of Pediatrics and Internal
 Medicine
Wayne State University School of Medicine
Division of Adolescent Medicine
Children's Hospital of Michigan
Detroit, Michigan

JOAN SHAPIRO, PHD
Consultant
Department of Pediatrics
Childrens Hospital of Los Angeles
Los Angeles, California

ROBERT E. STANTON, MD
Professor of Clinical Pediatrics
University of Southern California School of
 Medicine
Attending Cardiologist
Childrens Hospital of Los Angeles
Los Angeles, California

DEBORAH C. STEWART, MD
Associate Professor of Clinical Pediatrics
Division of General Pediatrics
University of California, Irvine, School of
 Medicine
Medical Director, Child Abuse Services Team
 (CAST)
Orange, California
Medical Director, Child Protection Center
Long Beach, California

DIANE TANAKA, MD
Assistant Clinical Professor of Pediatrics
University of California, Los Angeles, School of
 Medicine
Los Angeles, California

DAN W. THOMAS, MD
Associate Professor of Pediatrics
University of Southern California School of
 Medicine
Head, Division of Gastroenterology
Childrens Hospital of Los Angeles
Los Angeles, California

DALE J. TOWNSEND, MD
Pediatric Orthopaedics
Kaiser Hayward Medical Center
The Permanente Medical Group
Kaiser Permanente
Hayward, California

CURREN WARF, MD
Medical Director
High Risk Youth Program
Attending Physician, Division of Adolescent
 Medicine
Childrens Hospital of Los Angeles
Los Angeles, California

LONNIE K. ZELTZER, MD
Professor of Pediatrics
Director, Pediatric Pain Program
University of California, Los Angeles, School of
 Medicine
Los Angeles, California

Contents

SECTION I

General Considerations in Adolescent Health Care

SECTION II

Endocrine Problems

SECTION III

Cardiovascular Problems

SECTION IV

Orthopaedic Problems and Sports Medicine

SECTION V

Dermatological Disorders

SECTION VI

Neurological Disorders

SECTION VII

Genitourinary Disorders

SECTION VIII

Infectious Diseases

SECTION IX

Eating Disorders

SECTION X

Miscellaneous Medical Disorders

SECTION XI

Sexuality and Family Planning

SECTION XII

Adolescent Gynecology

SECTION XIII

Sexually Transmitted Diseases

SECTION XIV

Drug Use and Abuse

SECTION XV

Psychosocial Problems and Concerns

SECTION XVI

Appendices

General Considerations in Adolescent Health Care

CHAPTER 1

Normal Physical Growth and Development

Lawrence S. Neinstein and Francine Ratner Kaufman

Adolescence marks a time of dramatic physical and psychosocial changes, usually beginning and ending in the second decade of life. The physical changes vary widely in both amount and duration from individual to individual. Health-care providers must understand these changes and be able to appreciate differences between normal variations and abnormalities in growth and pubertal development. This chapter provides an overview of normal adolescent growth and development.

ENDOCRINE CHANGES DURING PUBERTY

Initiation of Puberty

Puberty is not an isolated event but represents a transitional period on the continuum between the juvenile state and adulthood. The exact components of this sequence are still obscure, although much has been revealed in the past few years. The hypothalamic-pituitary-gonadal axis starts functioning during fetal life, and it is only repression by the central nervous system (CNS) that prevents puberty during the first decade of life.

Fetus   Gonadotropin-releasing hormone (GnRH), luteinizing hormone (LH), follicle-stimulating hormone (FSH), estrogen, and testosterone (in the male fetus) are detectable in the fetus by 10 weeks of gestation, and the hormone levels rise between 10 and 20 weeks. LH is secreted in a pulsatile manner as a result of intermittent GnRH stimulation. FSH and LH levels are lower in males secondary to elevated serum testosterone levels. During the fetal period, the hypothalamus is imprinted to that of a male (tonic center) or that of a female (tonic and cyclic center). This may be the result of testosterone or local brain estrogen levels. After week 20, gonadotropins decrease, owing to a maturation of the CNS and an increase in hypothalamic sensitivity.

Infancy and Prepuberty   At birth, after the fall in placental sex-steroid levels, the concentrations of serum LH and FSH rise to midpubertal levels for several months. Serum testosterone levels in male infants and serum estradiol levels in female infants also rise. This pattern is consistent with a mature differentiated hypothalamic-pituitary unit. For a short time, the hypothalamic-pituitary-gonadal control mechanisms function similarly to an adult. This short period can provide a window of opportunity to study the hypothalamic-pituitary-gonadal axis as it might appear years later during puberty. However, by 9 months to 1 year of age in the male and by 2 years of age in the female, gonadotropins and gonadal steroids fall to prepu-

3

bertal levels and remain so until puberty. Although the period between age 4 and approximately age 10 in the female is characterized by low levels of gonadotropins and ovarian steroids, the ovaries are fully developed and capable of being stimulated by gonadotropins.

Puberty   The exact trigger of puberty is unknown; however, it is known that puberty is associated with three distinct changes in the hypothalamic-pituitary unit, as follows:

1. A nocturnal sleep-related augmentation of pulsatile LH secretion begins as a result of the increase in the pulsatile release of GnRH (Marshall and Kelch, 1986).
2. The sensitivity of the hypothalamus and the pituitary to estradiol and testosterone decreases so that the gonadotropins, LH and FSH, begin to increase. This is probably the result of sequential maturation of the CNS.
3. In the female, a positive feedback system develops. Critical levels of estrogen trigger a large release of GnRH, stimulating LH to initiate ovulation.

Gonadotropic Changes

The gonadotropins, LH and FSH, rise during puberty in both males and females (Fig. 1.1). LH tends to increase steadily through puberty, while FSH tends to plateau at sexual maturity rating 3 (SMR 3, discussed later in this chapter).

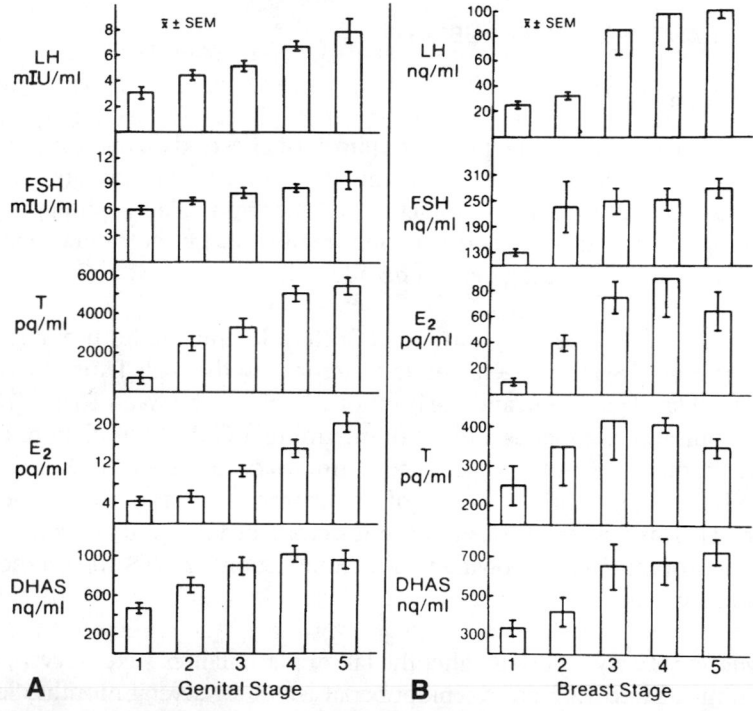

FIGURE 1.1.   **A,** Blood concentrations of gonadotropins and sex steroids in males during puberty. **B,** Blood concentrations of gonadotropins and sex steroids in females during puberty. *DHAS,* dehydroepiandrosterone-sulfate; E_2, estradiol; *FSH,* follicle-stimulating hormone; *LH,* luteinizing hormone; *T,* testosterone. (From Barnes HV. Recognizing normal and abnormal physical growth and development during puberty. In: Moss AV, ed. Pediatrics update: Reviews for physicians. New York: Elsevier-North Holland, 1979.)

Sex Hormone Changes

All the following hormones increase during puberty:

Estrone (E_1)
Estradiol (E_2)
Progesterone (P)
17-Hydroxyprogesterone (17-HP)
Testosterone (T)
5α-Dihydrotestosterone (DHT)
Androstenedione (A)
Dehydroepiandrosterone (DHA)
Dehydroepiandrosterone-sulfate (DHEA-S)

The increases in estradiol, testosterone, and DHEA-S are outlined in Figure 1.1.

Adrenal Gland Changes

The increased secretion of sex steroids from the adrenal gland in the prepubertal and pubertal periods is independent of hypothalamic-pituitary-gonadal changes. The two events are temporally related in that the onset of adrenarche occurs about 2 years before the increase in gonadal sex steroids. However, studies in children with adrenal insufficiency indicate that adrenal androgens are not necessary for pubertal development or the adolescent growth spurt.

The major androgens secreted by the adrenal gland are DHA, DHEA-S, and androstenedione. These also contribute to circulating estrone and testosterone by extraglandular conversion. DHA and DHEA-S increase progressively from about age 7 to age 13–15.

Other Hormonal Changes

Thyroid Hormone and Glucagon   Thyroid hormone and glucagon do not change significantly during normal puberty.

Insulin   Insulin secretion increases approximately 30% during puberty, secondary to a decreased sensitivity to insulin in adolescents as compared to prepubertal children (Bloch et al., 1987).

Growth Hormone and Somatomedins

1. Somatomedins include insulin-like growth factors I and II (IGF-I and IGF-II).
2. IGF-I and IGF-II are a class of peptide hormones that are growth-promoting hormones.
3. IGF-I and IGF-II promote growth, are under human growth hormone (hGH) stimulation, have some insulin-like activity, and bind to insulin receptors and to separate receptors.
4. IGF-I and IGF-II are generated in the liver and under negative feedback by hGH.
5. IGF-I and IGF-II are stimulated by insulin, prolactin, thyroid hormone, and hGH and inhibited by glucocorticoids, malnutrition, and chronic renal failure.
6. IGF levels are usually concordant with hGH (i.e., both low in hypopituitarism and high in acromegaly). Can be discordant with normal hGH and low IGF levels in Laron-type dwarfism, renal failure, and glucocorticoid excess.
7. IGF-I and IGF-II are mainly bound to IGF binding protein-3 (IGFBP-3).

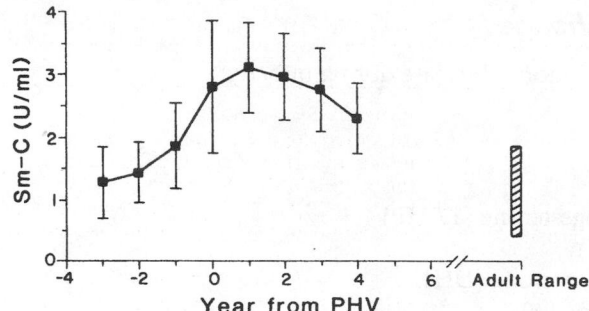

FIGURE 1.2. Relationship of plasma concentrations of IGF-I/somatomedin-C (*Sm-C*) to peak height velocity (*PHV*) during adolescent development. Shown is plasma concentration of IGF-I/somatomedin-C (mean ± 1 SD) in boys and girls followed longitudinally in relation to years from attainment of PHV. (From Cara JF, Rosenfield RL, Furlanetto RW. A longitudinal study of the relationship of plasma somatomedin-C concentration to the pubertal growth spurt. Am J Dis Child 1987;141: 562–564. Copyright 1987, American Medical Association.)

Both growth hormone levels and IGF-I levels seem to rise during puberty (Albertsson-Wikland et al., 1994; Argente et al., 1993). Albertsson-Wikland et al. (1994) evaluated 24-hour growth hormone profiles in 208 healthy children and adolescents. Mean secretion rates were comparable in prepubertal boys and girls. Secretion rates increased during puberty, occurring earlier in girls (SMR 2–4) than boys (SMR 4). Rates decreased to prepubertal values at SMR 5. Plasma IGF-I levels also increase during adolescence above adult levels (Juul et al., 1994; Rosenfield et al., 1983). Juul et al. (1994) found that mean serum IGF-I levels rose slowly in prepubertal children from 80–200 μg/L with a steep increase during puberty to about 500 μg/L. After puberty, levels fell throughout adulthood to levels of 100 μg/L at age 80. The maximal IGF-I was at age 14.5 in girls and about 1 year later in boys. Argente et al. (1993) also found a rise during puberty of IGF-I peaking 2 years earlier in girls than in boys. Thus, the increase is most marked during mid and late puberty and correlates best with pubertal stage, bone age, and time from peak height velocity (PHV) (Fig. 1.2). In females the elevation is correlated with rising estradiol levels in a biphasic manner. Low levels of estradiol stimulate IGF-I, while higher levels of estradiol probably suppress IGF-I. Serum IGF-II levels remain stable throughout puberty. IGFBP-3 also increases during puberty. IGFBP-3 can be measured and correlates with growth hormone and IGF concentrations. Growth hormone–releasing hormone (GHRH) levels have been found to rise during puberty and to correlate with pubertal stage. GHRH may have a role in the pubertal growth spurt (Argente et al., 1986).

Hormonal Actions

A thorough knowledge of the physiological roles of certain hormones is important to understanding pubertal changes and possible variations and abnormalities. Table 1.1 lists these hormones and their functions.

Control of Gonadotropin Secretion in Adults

Stimulus for gonadotropin secretion in adults comes from the CNS by intermittent secretion of GnRH from the hypothalamus to the pituitary. GnRH is secreted in a pulsatile fashion, which is critical for the pulsatile secretion of gonadotropins. The frequency and amplitude of

TABLE 1.1.   Primary Action of Major Hormones of Puberty

Hormone	Sex	Action
FSH	Male	Stimulates gametogenesis.
	Female	Stimulates development of primary ovarian follicles.
		Stimulates activation of enzymes in ovarian granulosa cells to increase estrogen production.
LH	Male	Stimulates testicular Leydig's cells to produce testosterone.
	Female	Stimulates ovarian theca cells to produce androgens and the corpus luteum to synthesize progesterone.
		Midcycle surge induces ovulation.
Estradiol	Male	Increases rate of epiphyseal fusion.
	Female	Stimulates breast development.
		Low level enhances linear growth, while a high level increases the rate of epiphyseal fusion.
		Triggers midcycle surge of LH.
		Stimulates development of labia, vagina, uterus, and ducts of the breasts.
		Stimulates development of a proliferative endometrium in the uterus.
		Increases fat mass of the body.
Testosterone	Male	Accelerates linear growth.
		Increases rate of epiphyseal fusion.
		Stimulates development of the penis, scrotum, prostate, and the seminal vesicles.
		Stimulates growth of pubic, facial, and axillary hair.
		Increases larynx size and thus deepens the voice.
		Stimulates sebaceous gland secretion of oil.
		Increases libido.
		Increases muscle mass.
		Increases red blood cell mass.
	Female	Accelerates linear growth.
		Stimulates growth of pubic and axillary hair.
Progesterone	Female	Converts a proliferative uterine endometrium to a secretory endometrium.
		Stimulates lobuloalveolar breast development.
Adrenal androgens	Male and female	Stimulates pubic hair and linear growth.

the GnRH pulse are critical to the secretion of gonadotropins, as increasing or decreasing the frequency of pulses from 1 pulse/hr can inhibit gonadotropin secretion. The control of GnRH secretion is not well understood and is probably under the influence of a variety of neurotransmitters such as catecholamines (dopamine and norepinephrine), serotonin, and endogenous opioid peptides (endorphins and enkephalins). The drive for the pulsating nature of GnRH probably resides within the hypothalamus. Sex steroids generally have a negative influence on the production of gonadotropins. This negative feedback may occur at the level of the hypothalamus or pituitary, or both. In females, at estradiol levels of about 200 pg/mL or greater, a positive feedback effect results in a surge of gonadotropin secretion and ovulation.

PHYSICAL GROWTH DURING PUBERTY

Physiology of Growth

Growth involves an interaction between the body's endocrine and skeletal systems. Many of the body's hormones influence growth, such as growth hormone, thyroxine, insulin, and corticosteroids (all of which influence growth rate) and parathyroid hormone, 1,25-dihydroxy-vitamin D, and calcitonin (all of which affect skeletal mineralization).

The key hormone in growth is hGH. Pituitary secretion of this hormone is regulated by growth hormone-releasing factor (GHRF) and somatostatin. Growth hormone secretion is increased by GHRF and decreased by somatostatin. GHRF is released in a pulsatile fashion, with maximum rates at the onset of slow wave sleep. There is negative feedback of hGH secretion via hGH itself and the somatomedins.

The effects of growth hormone are primarily modulated through the somatomedins, hormones now more commonly referred to as IGFs. The two major types are IGF-I, which is identical to somatomedin-C, and IGF-II. As the term implies, these hormones have qualitative biological effects that are similar to insulin. The major mechanism for growth appears to be through hGH's stimulating IGF-I, which affects bone growth. Serum levels of IGF-I increase with age and pubertal development. However, levels vary widely from individual to individual.

The maturation of bones appears to be under the major influence of thyroid hormones, adrenal androgens, and gonadal sex steroids. Excess secretion of these hormones causes advanced bone maturation, and at the time of puberty, deficiency causes delay. At puberty, both sex steroids and growth hormone participate in the pubertal growth spurt. The ending of the growth spurt is secondary to epiphyseal closure, due to the action of the sex steroids.

The adolescent health-care provider must understand the numerous physical changes that occur during puberty.

Growth Spurt

An increase in physical size is a universally recognized event of puberty.

Height Growth

1. Average normal growth velocities before puberty include the following:

1st year of life	25 cm/yr
2nd year	10 cm/yr
3rd year	8 cm/yr
4th year	7 cm/yr
5th–10th years	5–6 cm/yr

2. Height velocity increases again during puberty and peaks during the adolescent growth spurt.
3. Pubertal growth accounts for 20–25% of final adult height, a total averaging 23–28 cm in females and 26–28 cm in males.
4. The average growth spurt lasts 24–36 months.
5. The growth spurt is highly variable from adolescent to adolescent. Growth during the year of PHV in the normal female averages 9 cm/yr and varies normally from 5.4 cm to 11.2 cm. In the normal male, the PHV averages 10.3 cm/yr and varies normally from 5.8 cm to 13.1 cm. Typical individual curves showing velocity of growth in boys and girls are demonstrated in Figure 1.3. (Normal growth velocity curves derived from longitudinal studies in England by Tanner and Whitehouse in 1976 are available from Castlemead Publications, Swains Mill, 4A Crane Mead, Ware, Hertfordshire, SG12 9PY, England. Also available are newer curves for North American children, including colored curves for early and late maturers. These can be obtained from Serono Inc., 280 Pond Street, Randolph, MA 02368, or direct from Castlemead Publications.) (See Figs. 1.22 through 1.25.)
6. Males on average are 12–13 cm taller than females primarily because of the 2-year delay in bone closure as compared to females. This accounts for about a 10-cm difference between the two sexes; in addition, males also have 2–3 cm more of growth during their growth spurt.

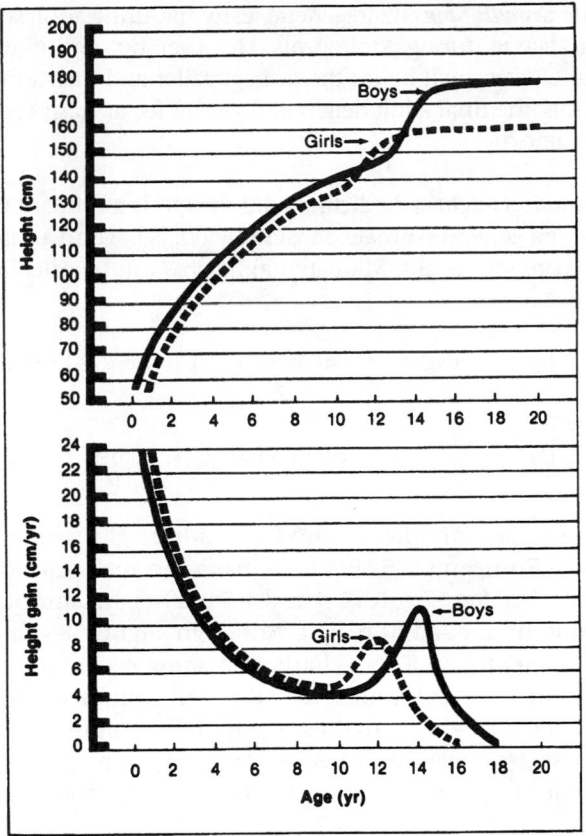

FIGURE 1.3. Typical individual velocity curves for height in boys and girls. Height-attained growth curve (*top*), and growth velocity curve for height (*bottom*). (From Hill DE, Fiser RH. Chronic disease and short stature. Postgrad Med 1977;62.)

Weight Growth

1. Weight velocity increases and peaks during the adolescent growth spurt.
2. Pubertal weight gain accounts for about 50% of an individual's ideal adult body weight.
3. The onset of accelerated weight gain and the peak weight velocity (PWV) attained are highly variable. For example, the normal weight gain during the year of PWV can vary from 4.6 kg to 10.6 kg in the female and from 5.7 kg to 13.2 kg in the male. (Normal weight velocity curves are also available from Castlemead Publications at the address given on the previous page.)

Differences in Growth Spurts between Males and Females

1. PHV occurs about 18–24 months earlier in the female than in the male.
2. PHV in females averages 2 cm/yr less than in males.
3. PWV coincides with PHV in males, but PWV occurs 6–9 months after PHV in females.

Seasonal Variations in Velocity Curves   Growth velocities vary during the year but generally increase the fastest during the spring and summer. For this reason, growth velocities should be calculated over a 6- to 12-month period.

Early versus Late Growth Spurts   In general, early-maturing adolescents will have a larger PHV and PWV than late-maturing adolescents. However, by starting the growth spurt later, the late-maturing adolescent will be on the average taller and heavier when he or she starts the growth spurt. Thus, the final adult height and weight for an early- or a late-maturing adolescent may be the same.

Prediction of Mature Height   Predicting adult height is a difficult task. Several methods can be used to provide a general estimate. Most individuals have an adult height that is within 2 inches of the midparental height. Midparental heights can be calculated by the following formulas:

For girls:

$$\frac{(\text{father's height} - 13 \text{ cm or } 5 \text{ inches}) + \text{mother's height}}{2}$$

For boys:

$$\frac{(\text{father's height} + 13 \text{ cm or } 5 \text{ inches}) + \text{mother's height}}{2}$$

Table 1.2 demonstrates another method of adult height prediction using tables designed by Bayley and Pinneau (1952) that are based on the use of current height, skeletal age, and chronological age. Figures 1.4 and 1.5 use height, chronological age, and sexual maturity rating to predict adult height. Although slightly less accurate, this method does not require a skeletal age. These charts also show corrected height percentiles for different levels of pubertal development. In addition, computer programs have become available to predict adult height. With these computer programs, basic information, such as parental heights, skeletal age, and whether menses have begun, is given; then the program calculates adult height using several methodologies, including that of Bayley and Pinneau.

Pubertal Changes in Body Composition

Lean Body Mass

1. Females: The lean body mass decreases from about 80% of body weight in early puberty to about 75% at maturity. The lean body mass increases in total amount but decreases in percentage because adipose mass increases at a greater rate.
2. Males: The lean body mass increases from about 80–85% to about 90% at maturity. This primarily reflects increased muscle mass from circulating androgens.

Adipose Mass   The percentage of body fat increases in females during puberty and decreases in adolescent males (Table 1.3).

Pelvic Remodeling in Females   During puberty the female pelvis widens more rapidly than it increases in the anteroposterior dimension. The forepart of the pelvis also widens and becomes more rounded.

Skeletal Mass   Bone mass changes parallel the alterations in lean body mass. The skeletal structure also undergoes epiphyseal maturation under the influence of estradiol and testosterone. Skeletal maturation, or bone age, can be determined by comparing a radiograph of an adolescent's hand, wrist, or knee to standards of maturation in a normal population.

TABLE 1.2. Prediction of Adult Height Using Skeletal Age

Directions: 1. Obtain skeletal age by wrist and hand radiograph using the standards of Greulich and Pyle (1959).
2. Find x for equation in table under skeletal age, using:
    Row A if skeletal age is within 1 year of chronological age;
    Row B if skeletal age is 1–2 years below chronological age; and
    Row C if skeletal age is 1–2 years advanced beyond chronological age.
3. Sole equation:

$$\text{adult height} = \frac{\text{present height}}{x}$$

	Skeletal Age									
	9–0	9–3	9–6	9–9	10–0	10–3	10–6	10–9	11–0	11–3
Males										
A.	.752	.761	.769	.777	.784	.791	.795	.800	.804	.812
B.	.786	.794	.800	.807	.812	.816	.819	.821	.823	.827
C.	.720	.728	.734	.741	.747	.753	.758	.763	.767	.776
Females										
A.	.827	.836	.844	.853	.862	.874	.884	.896	.906	.910
B.	.841	.851	.858	.866	.874	.884	.896	.907	.918	.922
C.	.790	.800	.809	.819	.828	.841	.856	.870	.883	.887

	Skeletal Age									
	11–6	11–9	12–0	12–3	12–6	12–9	13–0	13–3	13–6	13–9
Males										
A.	.818	.827	.834	.843	.853	.863	.876	.890	.902	.914
B.	.832	.839	.845	.852	.860	.869	.880	.890	.902	.914
C.	.786	.800	.809	.818	.828	.839	.850	.863	.875	.890
Females										
A.	.914	.918	.922	.932	.941	.950	.958	.967	.974	.978
B.	.926	.929	.932	.942	.949	.957	.964	.971	.977	.981
C.	.891	.897	.901	.913	.924	.935	.945	.955	.963	.968

	Skeletal Age									
	14–0	14–3	14–6	14–9	15–0	15–3	15–6	15–9	16–0	16–3
Males										
A.	.927	.938	.948	.958	.968	.973	.976	.980	.982	.985
B.	.927	.938	.948	.958	.968	.973	.976	.980	.982	.985
C.	.905	.918	.930	.943	.958	.967	.971	.976	.980	.983
Females										
A.	.980	.983	.986	.988	.990	.991	.993	.994	.996	.996
B.	.983	.986	.989	.992	.994	.995	.996	.997	.998	.999
C.	.972	.977	.980	.983	.986	.988	.990	.992	.993	.994

	Skeletal Age									
	16–6	16–9	17–0	17–3	17–6	17–9	18–0	18–3	18–6	
Males										
A.	.987	.989	.991	.993	.994	.995	.996	.998	1.0	
B.	.987	.989	.991	—	—	—	—	—	—	
C.	.985	.988	.990	—	—	—	—	—	—	
Females										
A.	.997	.998	.999	.999	1.0	—	—	—	—	
B.	.999	.999	1.0	—	—	—	—	—	—	
C.	.995	.997	.998	.999	.999	—	—	—	—	

From Freidman I, Goldberg E. Reference materials for the practice of adolescent medicine. Pediatr Clin North Am 1980; 27:193.

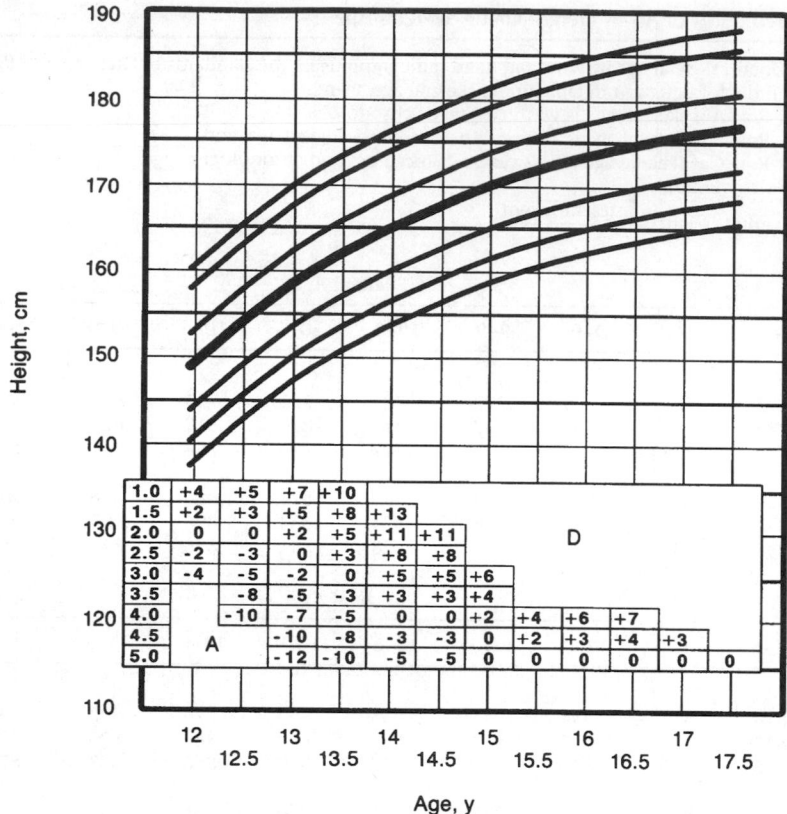

FIGURE 1.4.   Growth curve and correction table for male adolescents. Mean height (*bold line*) and distribution (95th, 90th, 75th, 25th, 10th, and 5th percentile lines) for adolescents maturing at modal rate. Correction table below curves shows mean difference in height between subjects of same age at different stages of puberty (*indicated by left column*). To obtain a height percentile adjusted for rate of pubertal maturation, first average Tanner (1962) stages for pubic hair and genitalia to form sexual maturity index score and then determine correction factor for patient's age from correction table. Add (or, if correction factor is negative, subtract) correction factor to (from) measured height and plot adjusted height onto curves. To estimate final adult height, extrapolate adjusted height percentile to adulthood. For example, if teen is 15 years of age, 165 cm tall, and Tanner 4, correction factor would be +2, which would yield height percentile of between the 25th and 50th and adult height of about 173 cm. (From Wilson DM, Draemer HC, Ritter PL, et al. Growth curves and adult height estimation for adolescents. Am J Dis Child 1987;141:565–570. Copyright 1987, American Medical Association.)

Bone age is one index of physiological maturation, providing an idea of the proportion of total growth accomplished. For example, if an adolescent is 15 years old and has a bone age of 12, there will be more potential growth than if the same adolescent's bone age were 15. The use of skeletal age is discussed further in Chapter 8.

Internal Organs   The growth of the brain, heart, liver, and kidneys during puberty is less than that of muscle and bone. Thus, the percentage of body weight represented by the brain, heart, liver, and kidney decreases from about 10% to about 5% at maturity.

Erythrocyte Mass   The change in erythrocyte mass is outlined in Figure 1.6. The increase in males is secondary to increasing levels of circulating androgens.

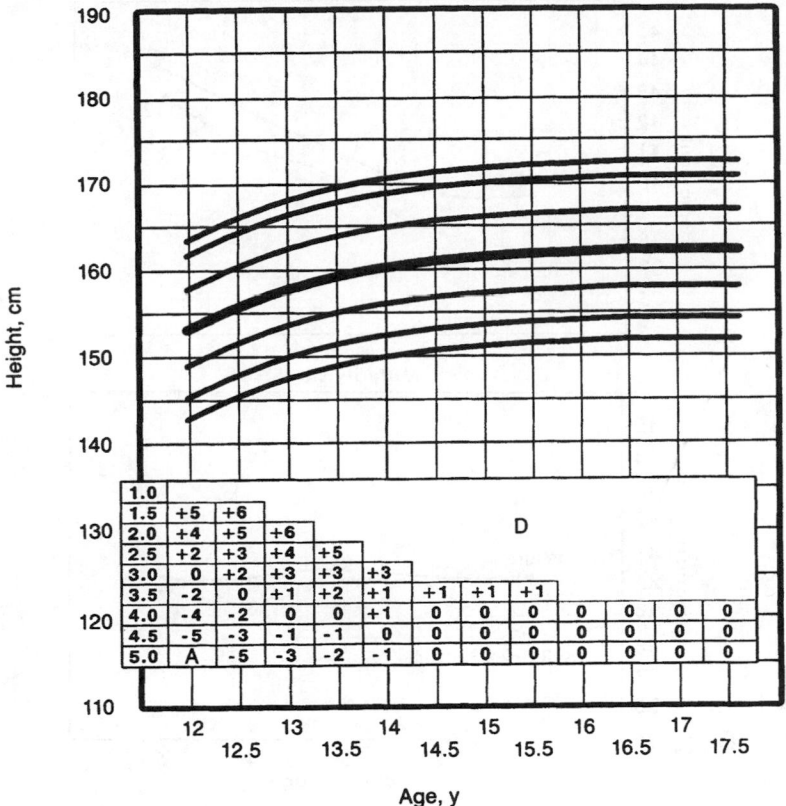

FIGURE 1.5. Growth curve and correction table for female adolescents. Mean height (*bold line*) and distribution (95th, 90th, 75th, 25th, 10th, and 5th percentile lines) for adolescents maturing at modal rate. Correction table below curves shows mean difference in height between subjects of same age at different stages of puberty (*indicated by left column*). To obtain a height percentile adjusted for rate of pubertal maturation, first average Tanner (1962) stages for pubic hair and breasts to form sexual maturity index score and then determine correction factor for patient's age from correction table. Add (or, if correction factor is negative, subtract) correction factor to (from) measured height and plot adjusted height on to curves. To estimate final adult height, extrapolate adjusted height percentile to adulthood. (From Wilson DM, Draemer HC, Ritter PL, et al. Growth curves and adult height estimation for adolescents. Am J Dis Child 1987;141:565–570. Copyright 1987, American Medical Association.)

TABLE 1.3. Percentage of Body Fat during Puberty

Stage of Puberty	% Body Fat
Female	
1	15.7
2	18.9
3	21.6
4	26.7
Male	
1	14.3
2	11.2

Percentage of body fat remains unchanged in stages 3, 4, and 5.

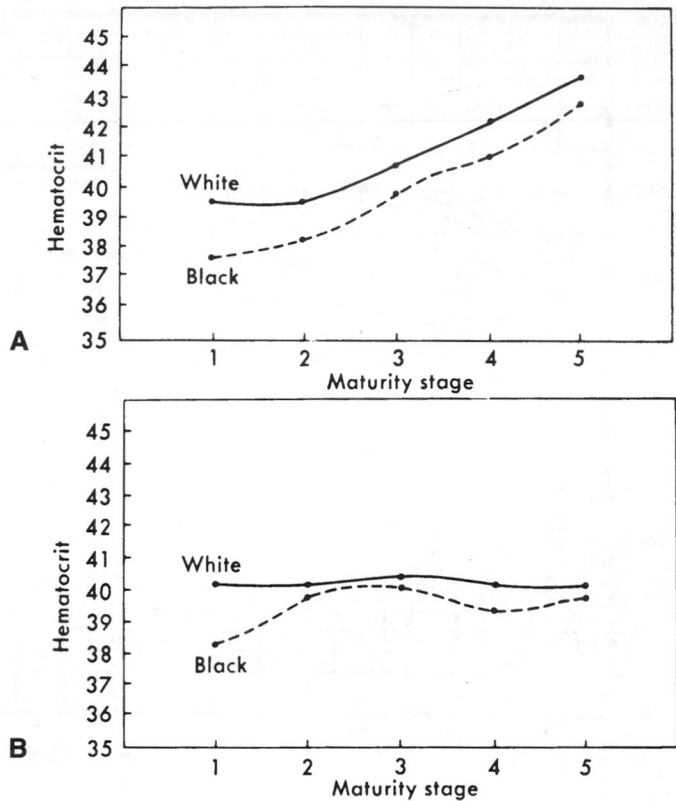

Figure 1.6. Hematocrit values for African-American and white boys (**A**) and girls (**B**) during puberty. (From W.A. Daniel, Hematocrit: Maturity relationship in adolescence. Reproduced by permission of Pediatrics vol. 52, page 388, copyright 1973.)

Biochemical Changes

The biochemical changes that occur during puberty reflect the underlying skeletal growth. For example, serum alkaline phosphatase levels change depending on maturation level (Table 1.4). The levels tend to increase until midpuberty, at which point they decrease until adult levels are attained.

Serum ferritin levels also change during adolescence. About one-third of body iron is stored in cells as ferritin or hemosiderin. Ferritin is a macromolecule composed of a protein shell in which can be stored up to 4500 atoms of iron. Plasma ferritin in healthy persons sensitively reflects total-body iron stores. The test for plasma ferritin is useful because it is as sensitive as serum iron and total iron-binding capacity (TIBC) but is more specific, detecting iron deficiency at very early stages. During childhood and early adolescence, the median plasma ferritin concentration rises from 10 ng/mL to 45 ng/mL in both males and females. During adolescence, the values in males and females diverge. With the male growth spurt, the median level rises to 90 ng/mL and remains there. In the female the level stays between 25 ng/mL and 30 ng/mL during the reproductive years as a result of losses during menstruation and pregnancy. Figure 1.7 reviews the changes in body mass, height, weight, and testosterone levels during puberty.

TABLE 1.4. Serum Alkaline Phosphatase Level

Sexual Maturity Rating	Male	Female
1	74 ± 21 IU	79 ± 16
2	89 ± 29	93 ± 21
3	116 ± 41	84 ± 41
4	103 ± 43	39 ± 21
5	70 ± 39	32 ± 12

Adapted from Bennett DL, Ward MS, Daniel WA. The relationship of serum alkaline phosphatase concentrations to sexual maturity ratings in adolescents. J Pediatr 1976;88:633–636.

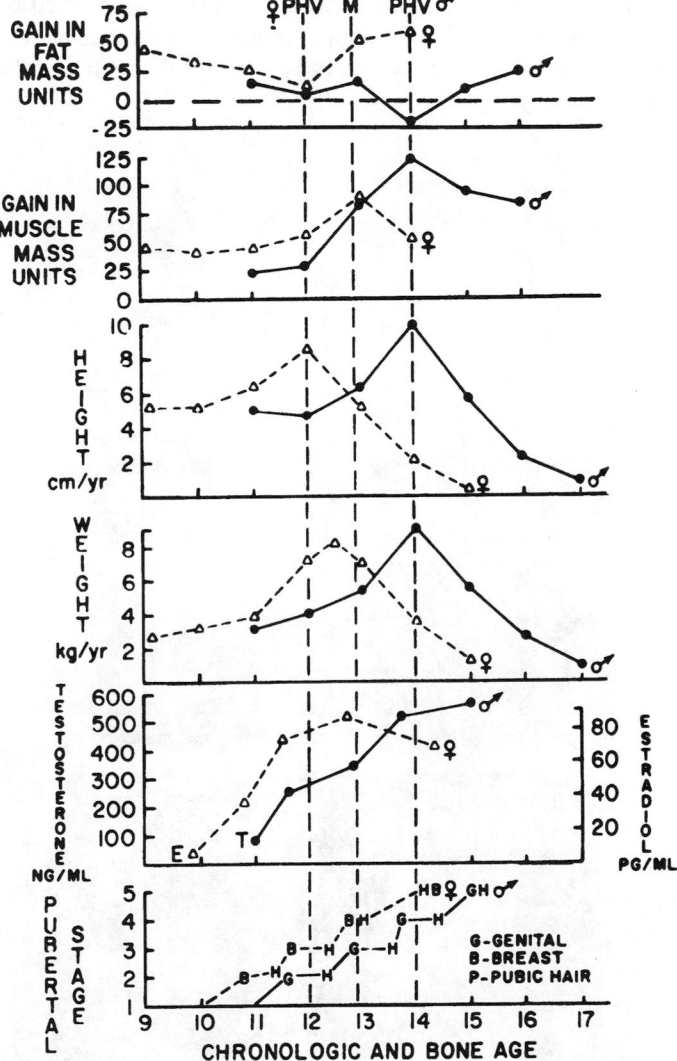

FIGURE 1.7. Correlations between major events of puberty in the average male and female. (From Barnes HV. Adolescent medicine. In: Harvey AM, ed. The principles and practice of medicine. 19th ed. New York: Appleton-Century-Crofts, 1976.)

Secondary Sexual Development During Puberty

The secondary sexual characteristics (pubic hair, breast development, and testes and penile development) are major changes occurring in the adolescent period. In addition to being able to recognize normal from abnormal sexual development, health-care professionals must be equipped to answer, and feel comfortable dealing with, the multitude of questions that may arise from adolescents and their parents, not only regarding sexual maturation but issues of sexuality as well.

Sexual Maturity Ratings

To classify more specifically the level of pubertal maturation and more accurately determine normality, a sexual maturity scale is essential. According to the scale developed by Tanner (1962), sexual maturity ratings (SMRs) are divided into five classes based on pubic hair and breasts in females and pubic hair and genitalia in males. These stages are described next and are shown both in photographs and drawings in Figures 1.8 through 1.14 (some individuals find drawings easier to interpret).

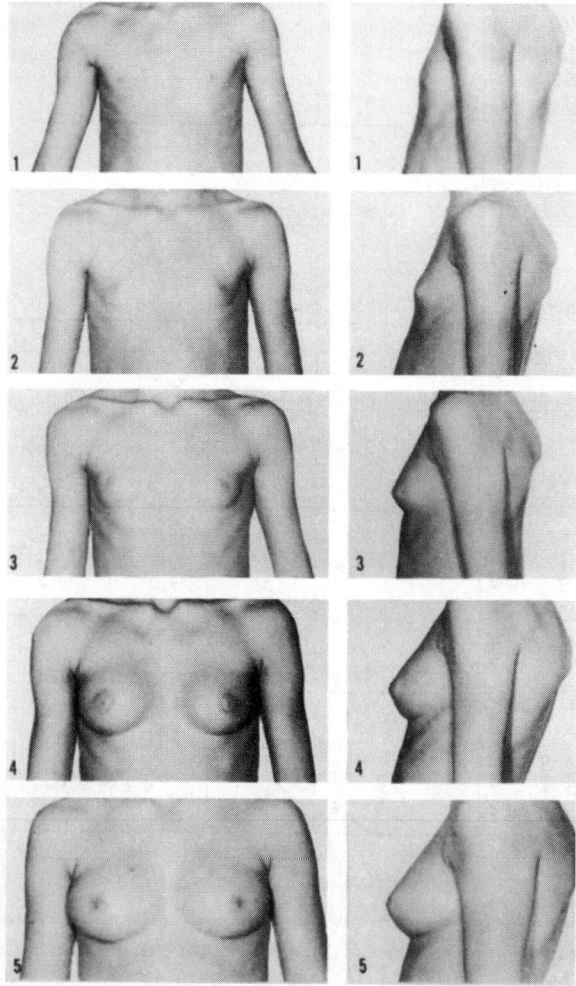

Figure 1.8. Stages of breast development. (Reproduced, by permission, from J.M. Tanner, M.D., University of London, Institute of Child Health.)

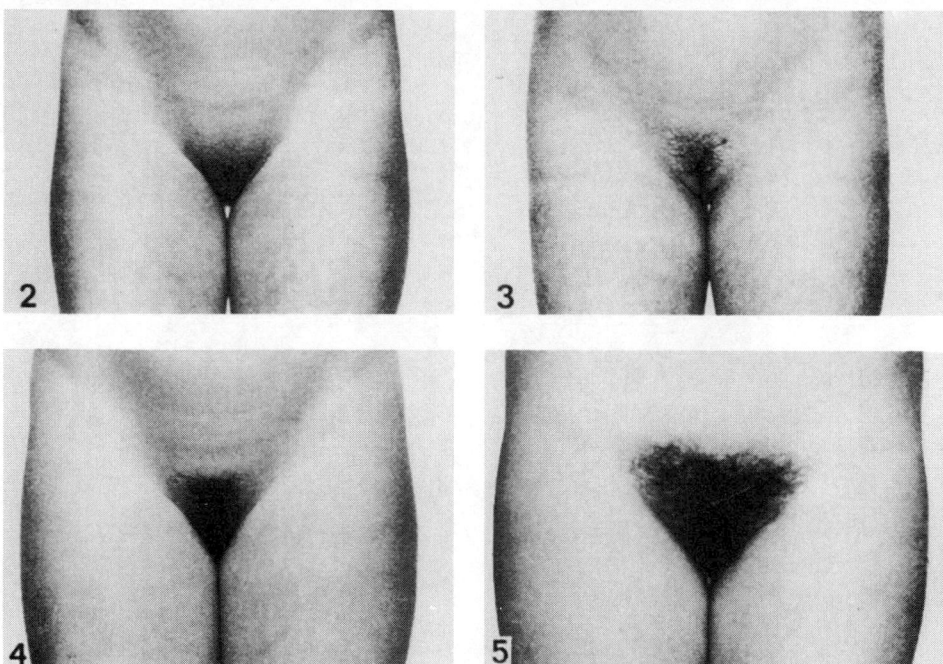

FIGURE 1.9.   Stages of female pubic hair development. (Reproduced, by permission, from J.M. Tanner, M.D., University of London, Institute of Child Health.)

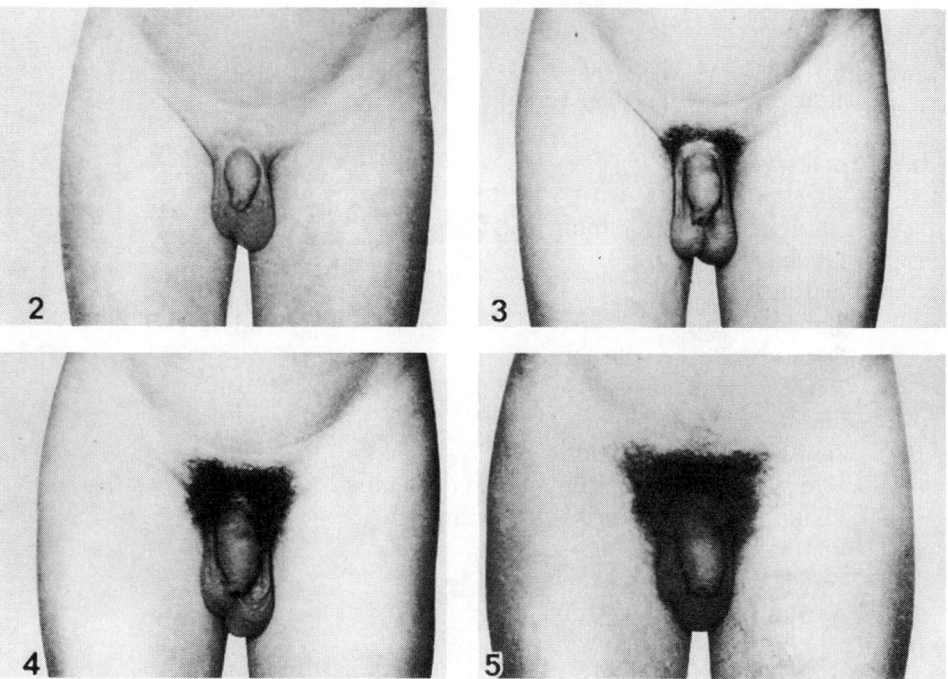

FIGURE 1.10.   Stages of male pubic hair development. (Reproduced, by permission, from J.M. Tanner, M.D., University of London, Institute of Child Health.)

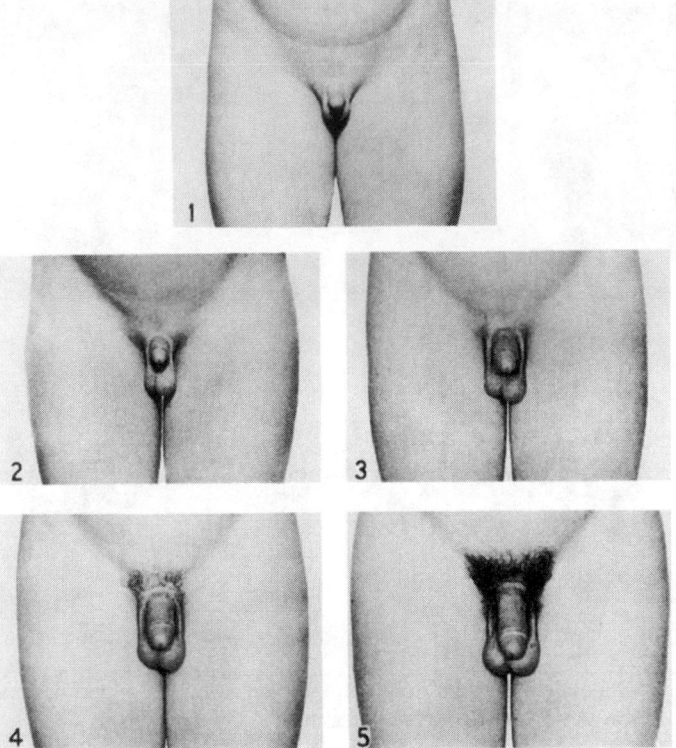

FIGURE 1.11.   Stages of male genital development. (Reproduced, by permission, from J.M. Tanner, M.D., University of London, Institute of Child Health.)

1. Males
    a. Genital stage 1 (G1): Prepubertal
        — Testes: Volume less than 1.5 mL
        — Phallus: Childlike
    b. Genital stage 2 (G2)
        — Testes: Volume 1.6–6 mL
        — Scrotum: Reddened, thinner, and larger
        — Phallus: No change
    c. Genital stage 3 (G3)
        — Testes: Volume 6–12 mL
        — Scrotum: Greater enlargement
        — Phallus: Increased length
    d. Genital stage 4 (G4)
        — Testes: Volume 12–20 mL
        — Scrotum: Further enlargement and darkening
        — Phallus: Increased length and circumference
    e. Genital stage 5 (G5)
        — Testes: Volume more than 20 mL
        — Scrotum and phallus: Adult
2. Females
    a. Breast stage 1 (B1)
        — Breast: Prepubertal; no glandular tissue
        — Areola and papilla: Areola conforms to general chest line

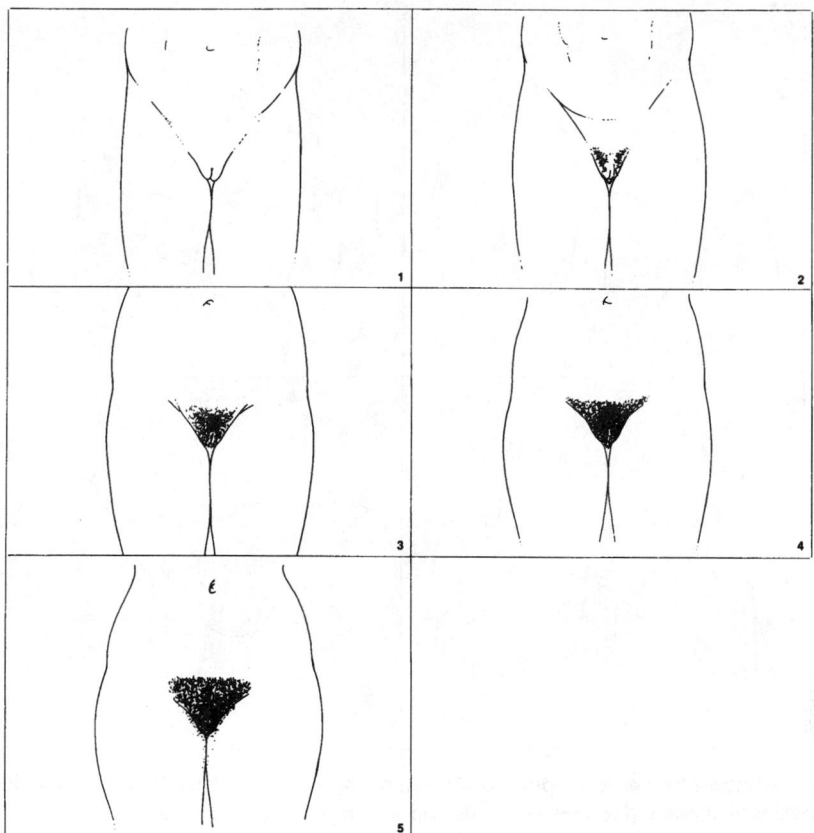

FIGURE 1.12.   Female pubic hair development. *Sex maturity rating 1:* Prepubertal. No pubic hair. *Sex maturity rating 2:* Straight hair is extending along the labia and, between ratings 2 and 3, begins on the pubis. *Sex maturity rating 3:* Pubic hair has increased in quantity, is darker, and is present in the typical female triangle but in smaller quantity. *Sex maturity rating 4:* Pubic hair is more dense, curled, and adult in distribution but is less abundant. *Sex maturity rating 5:* Abundant, adult-type pattern; hair may extend onto the medial aspect of the thighs. (From Daniel WA, Paulshock BZ. A physician's guide to sexual maturity rating. Patient Care May 30, 1979. Illustration by Paul Singh-Roy.)

 b. Breast stage 2 (B2)
  — Breast: Breast bud; small amount of glandular tissue
  — Areola: Areola widens
 c. Breast stage 3 (B3)
  — Breast: Larger and more elevation; extends beyond areolar parameter
  — Areola and papilla: Areola continues to enlarge but remains in contour with the breast
 d. Breast stage 4 (B4)
  — Breast: Larger and more elevation
  — Areola and papilla: Areola and papilla form a mound projecting from the breast contour
 e. Breast stage 5 (B5)
  — Breast: Adult (size variable)
  — Areola and papilla: Areola and breast in same plane, with papilla projecting above areola

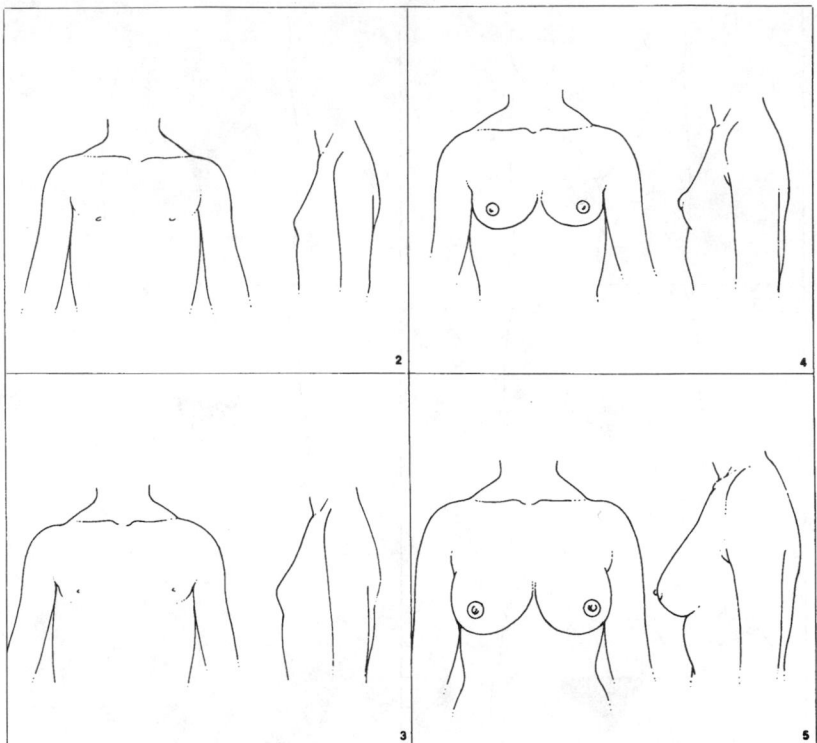

FIGURE 1.13. Female breast development. *Sex maturity rating 1 (not shown):* Prepubertal. Elevations of papilla only. *Sex maturity rating 2:* Breast buds appear. Areola is slightly widened and projects as small mound. *Sex maturity rating 3:* Enlargement of the entire breast with no protrusion of the papilla or of the nipple. *Sex maturity rating 4:* Enlargement of the breast and projection of areola and papilla as a secondary mound. *Sex maturity rating 5:* Adult configuration of the breast with protrusion of the nipple. Areola no longer projects separately from remainder of breast. (From Daniel WA, Paulshock BZ. A physician's guide to sexual maturity rating. Patient Care May 30, 1979. Illustration by Paul Singh-Roy.)

3. Male and female: pubic hair
    a. Pubic hair stage 1 (PH1)
       — None
    b. Public hair stage 2 (PH2)
       — Small amount of long, slightly pigmented, downy hair along the base of the scrotum and phallus in the male or the labia majora in females; vellus hair versus sexual type hair (PH3)
    c. Pubic hair stage 3 (PH3)
       — Moderate amount of more curly, pigmented, and coarser hair, extending more laterally
    d. Pubic hair stage 4 (PH4)
       — Hair that resembles adult hair in coarseness and curliness but does not extend to medial surface of thighs
    e. Pubic hair stage 5 (PH5)
       — Adult type and quantity, extending to medial surface of thighs

Importance of Sexual Maturity Ratings Certainly, height, weight, and age are important in evaluating an individual. However, during adolescence these three factors do not

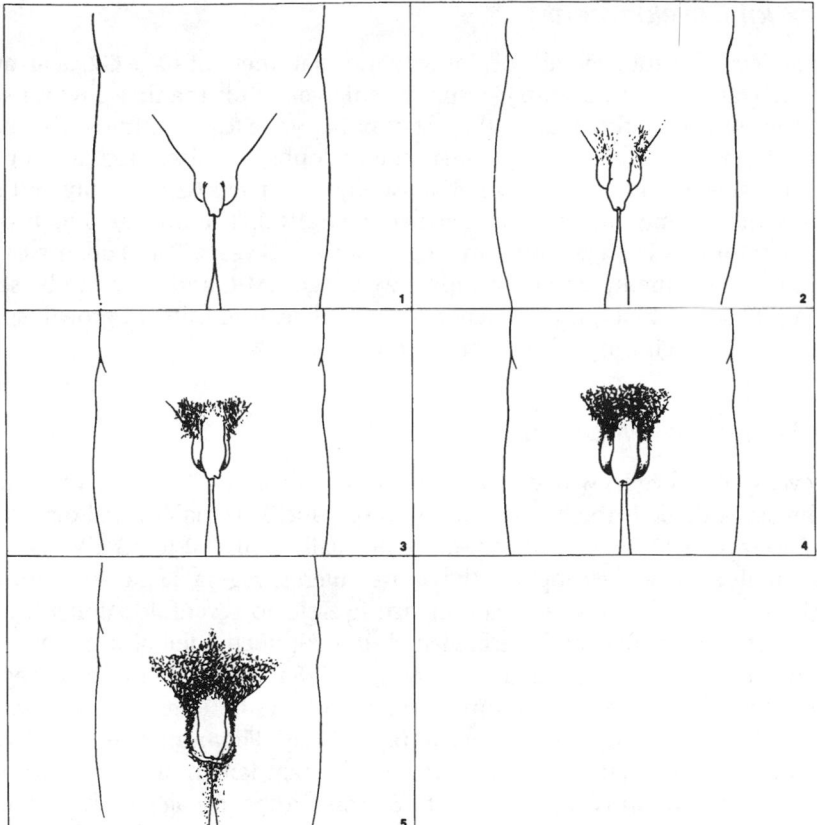

FIGURE 1.14.   Male genital and pubic hair development. Ratings for pubic hair and for genital development can differ in a typical boy at any given time, as pubic hair and genitalia do not necessarily develop at the same rate. *Sex maturity rating 1:* Prepubertal. No pubic hair. Genitalia unchanged from early childhood. *Sex maturity rating 2:* Light, downy hair develops laterally and later becomes dark. Penis and testes may be slightly larger. Scrotum becomes more textured. *Sex maturity rating 3:* Pubic hair has extended across the pubis. Testes and scrotum are further enlarged. Penis is larger, especially in length. *Sex maturity rating 4:* More abundant pubic hair with curling. Genitalia resemble those of an adult. Glans has become larger and broader. Scrotum is darker. *Sex maturity rating 5:* Adult quantity and pattern of pubic hair, with hair present along the inner borders of the thighs. The testes and the scrotum are adult in their size. (From Daniel WA, Paulshock BZ. A physician's guide to sexual maturity rating. Patient Care May 30, 1979. Illustration by Paul Singh-Roy.)

provide enough information; growth during adolescence is so variable that age is a poor reference point from which to gauge change. Thus, the SMR is essential in evaluating an adolescent.

The SMR should be recorded at the initial general physical examination and yearly thereafter. Such a record can provide critical information in identifying abnormal puberty or in reassuring the adolescent that he or she is normal. SMRs are also a helpful reference in evaluating the following items:

Hematocrit (see Fig. 1.6 and Table 1.8)
Alkaline phosphatase (see Table 1.4)
Menarche
Ejaculation

Male Sexual Development

Male sexual development generally begins with the attainment of stage G2, at an average age of 11.6 years (range 9.5–13.5 years). Testicular enlargement is the first physical sign of puberty in about 98% of males. During the rest of puberty the testes, epididymis, and prostate increase in size sevenfold, and the phallus usually doubles in size. Ejaculation usually has occurred in males during SMR 3. SMR 4 is usually associated with fertility, but sperm are usually present in some quantities of ejaculate by SMR 3. The average length of time for completion of puberty is 3 years but can range from 2 to 5 years. The sequence of events for an average male and the interrelationship between age, SMR, and PHV can be seen in Figures 1.15A and 1.16. The typical sequence is adrenarche, beginning of growth spurt, testicular development, beginning of pubic hair, PHV.

Female Sexual Development

Female development begins with either the attainment of stage B2 or PH2. In the majority of females, breast budding is the first physical sign of puberty. Female sexual development occurs at an average of 11.2 years but can range normally from 9.0 to 13.4 years. During puberty, the female's breasts develop and the ovaries, uterus, vagina, labia, and clitoris increase in size. The uterus and ovaries increase in size fivefold to sevenfold. Winer-Muram et al. (1989) evaluated the ovaries and uterine length in peripubertal females. The uterine length increased from a mean of 3.3 ± 1.3 cm^3 in girls aged 7–8 to 6.98 ± 1 cm^3 in girls aged 15–16. The corpus-to-cervix ratio increased from 1.1 ± 0.4:1 to 1.33 ± 0.2:1 cm^3. Ovarian size increased from 1.9 ± 0.7 cm^3 (age 7–8) to 3.5 ± 0.4 cm^3 (age 15–16). Fifty-nine of the 75 girls had multiple ovarian cysts ranging from 3 to 10 mm^3. The average length of time for completion of puberty is 4 years but can range from 1.5 to 8 years. In the average adolescent female, the growth spurt starts about 1 year before breast development. This is followed by an average of 1.1 years until PHV and then followed in an average of 1 year by menarche. Menarche occurs in 19% of adolescents during PH3 and in 56% during PH4. Figures 1.15B and 1.17 show the interrelationships between age, SMR, and growth velocities.

Zacharias and Rand (1983) have examined adolescent growth in height in contemporary American girls and have found the following:

	Mean	*Standard Deviation (SD)*
Height spurt takeoff	8.69 years of age	1.58
Age at PHV	11.63 years of age	1.21
Completion of PHV	13.10 years of age	1.12
Duration of spurt	4.43 years of age	1.21
Height gained	27.23 cm	7.08

The height at PHV was 91% of adult height, and the spurt contributed to 16.75% of adult height. There is little or no correlation between adult height and either age of onset of growth spurt, age of PHV, velocity at peak, or pubertal height gain. However, there is a correlation between adult height and the height at onset of growth spurt or height at PHV.

PHV occurs later in males in relationship to sexual development than in females (Fig. 1.15).

Variations of Pubertal Development

The age of pubertal onset, the duration between SMRs, and the growth of adolescents are highly variable. To provide adequate care to the adolescent, the health practitioner must appreciate these normal variations. The accompanying group of figures and tables, as listed

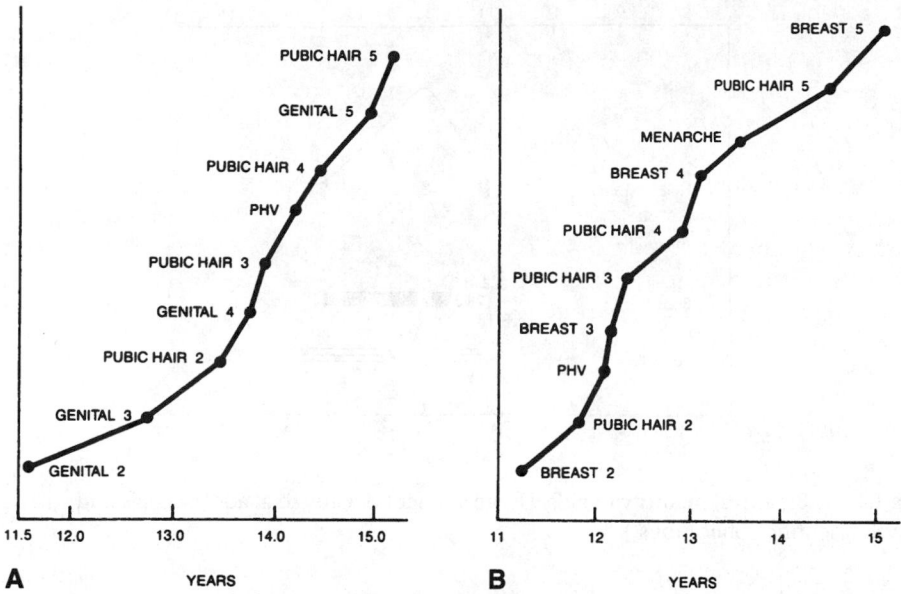

FIGURE 1.15. A, Sequence and mean ages of pubertal events in males. B, Sequence and mean ages of pubertal events in females. (From Root AW. Endocrinology of puberty. J Pediatr 1973;83.)

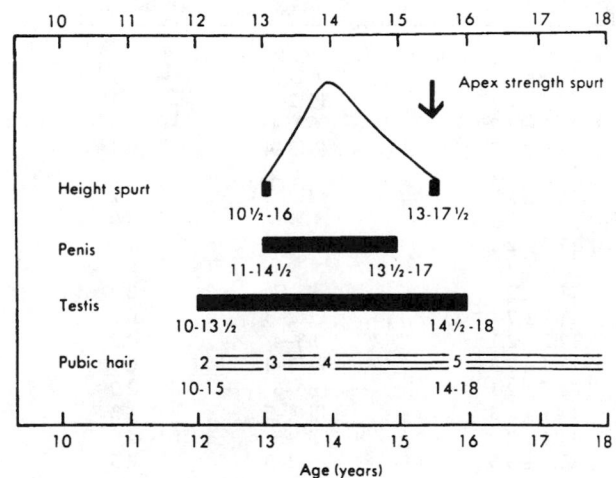

FIGURE 1.16. Biological maturity in boys. (From Tanner JM. Growth at adolescence. 2nd ed. © 1962 by Blackwell Scientific Publications.)

next, outlines useful normal limits for male and female growth and development. Table 1.5 is especially helpful in determining normality of development. Specific information provided by the figures and tables is as follows:

Figures 1.18 through 1.21 are normal growth charts.

Figures 1.22 through 1.25 are height and height velocity curves for American adolescents, with consideration for those with early, average, and late maturation.

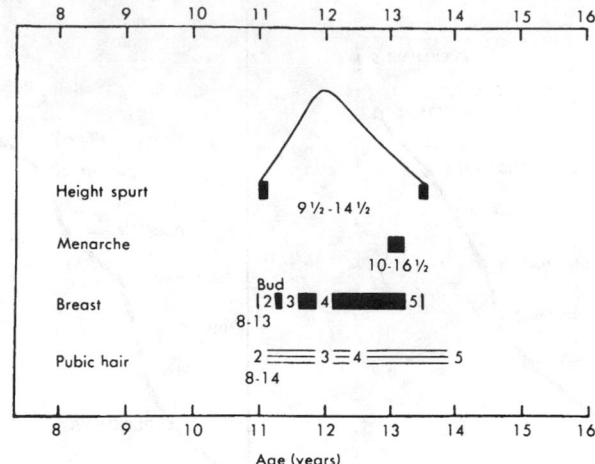

FIGURE 1.17. Biological maturity in girls. (From Tanner JM. Growth at adolescence. 2nd ed. © 1962 by Blackwell Scientific Publications.)

TABLE 1.5. Means and Normal Variation in the Timing of Adolescent Secondary Sexual Development

Stage	Mean Age of Onset ± 2 SD (yr)	Stage	Mean	5th	95th
			Time between Stages (yr)		
				Percentile	
Males					
G2	11.6 ± 2.1	G2–3	1.1	0.4	2.2
G3	12.9 ± 2.1	PH2–3	0.5	0.1	1.0
PH2	13.4 ± 2.2[a]	G3–4	0.8	0.2	1.6
G4	13.8 ± 2.0	PH3–4	0.4	0.3	0.5
PH3	13.9 ± 2.1	G4–5	1.0	0.4	1.9
PH4	14.4 ± 2.2	PH4–5	0.7	0.2	1.5
G5	14.9 ± 2.2	G2–5	3.0	1.9	4.7
PH5	15.2 ± 2.1	PH2–5	1.6	0.8	2.7
Females					
B2	11.2 ± 2.2	B2–3	0.9	0.2	1.0
PH2	11.7 ± 2.4	PH2–3	0.6	0.2	1.3
B3	12.2 ± 2.1	B3–4	0.9	0.1	2.2
PH3	12.4 ± 2.2	PH3–4	0.5	0.2	0.9
PH4	12.9 ± 2.1	B4–5	2.0	0.1	6.8
B4	13.1 ± 2.3	PH4–5	1.3	0.6	2.4
PH5	14.4 ± 2.2	B2–5	4.0	1.5	9.0
B5	15.3 ± 3.5	PH2–5	2.5	1.4	3.1

From Barnes HV. Physical growth and development during puberty. Med Clin North Am 1975;59:1305.
[a]Mean is probably too high due to experimental method.

Table 1.5 lists normal variation of timing of secondary sexual development.
Table 1.6 lists male genital size by age.
Table 1.7 lists testicular volumes by SMRs.
Table 1.8 lists hematocrit values by SMRs and race.
Table 1.9 lists serum gonadotropins by pubertal stage in males.
Table 1.10 lists serum gonadotropins by pubertal stage in females.
Table 1.11 lists serum concentrations of sex steroids by SMR.

Text continued on page 33.

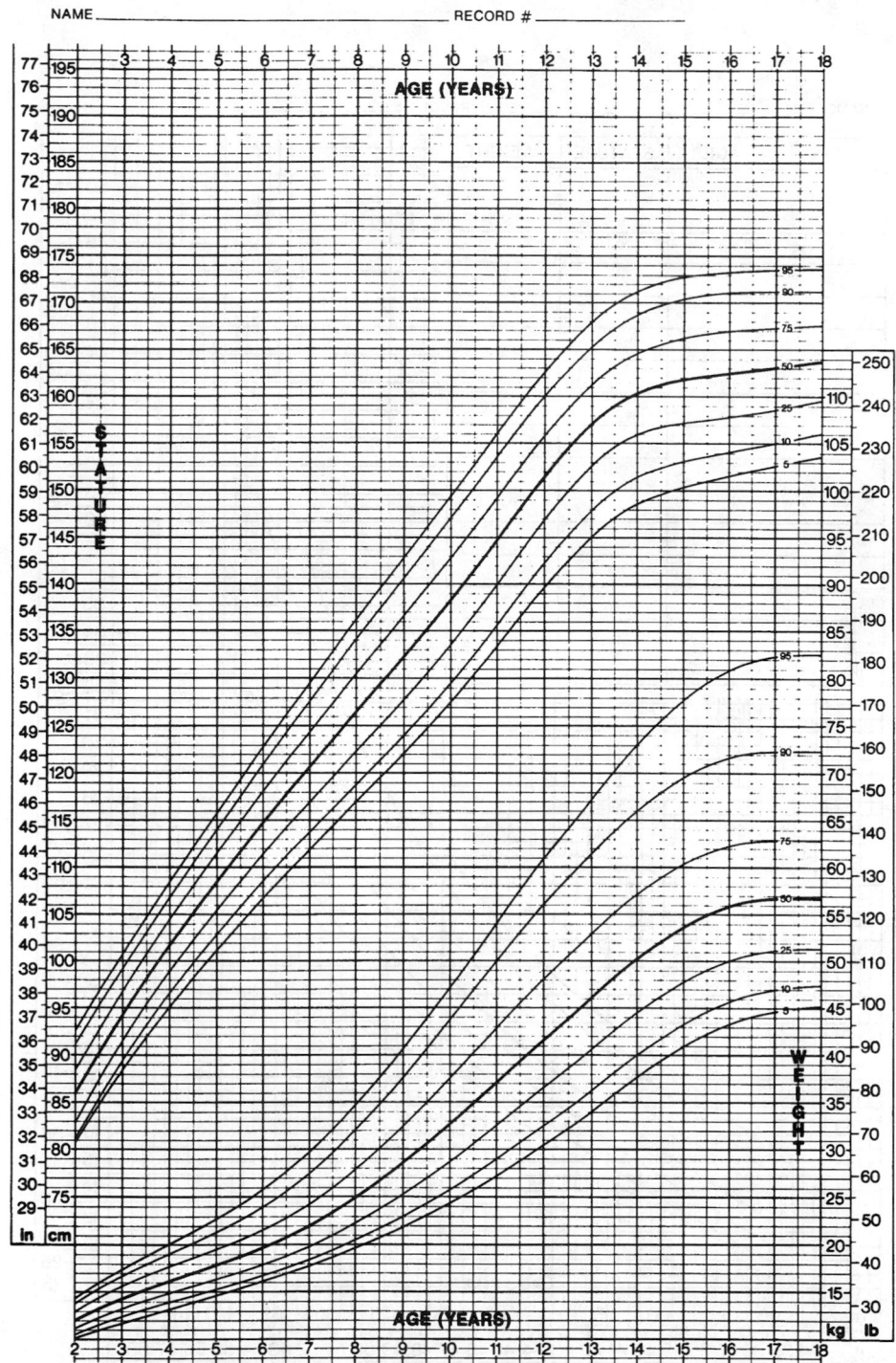

NAME _____   RECORD # _____

FIGURE 1.18.   Normal physical growth of girls, 2–18 years of age. National Center for Health Statistics percentiles. (From National Center for Health Statistics, NCHS growth charts, 1976, Monthly Vital Statistics Report. 25(3), Suppl. (HRA) 76–1120. Rockville, Maryland: National Center for Health Statistics, 1976.)

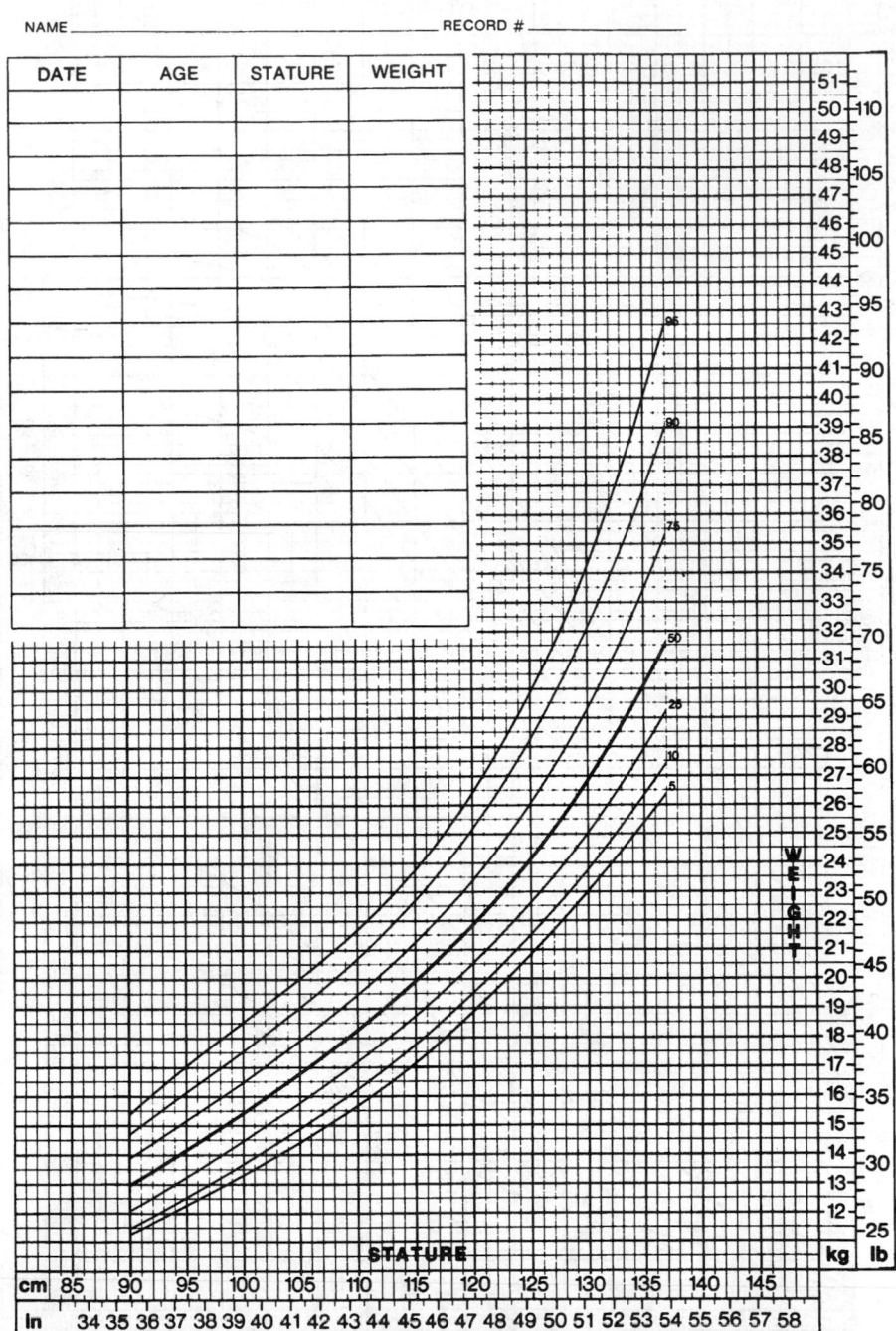

FIGURE 1.19. Normal prepubescent physical growth of girls. National Center for Health Statistics percentiles. (From National Center for Health Statistics, NCHS growth charts, 1976, Monthly Vital Statistics Report. 25(3), Suppl. (HRA) 76–1120. Rockville, Maryland: National Center for Health Statistics, 1976.)

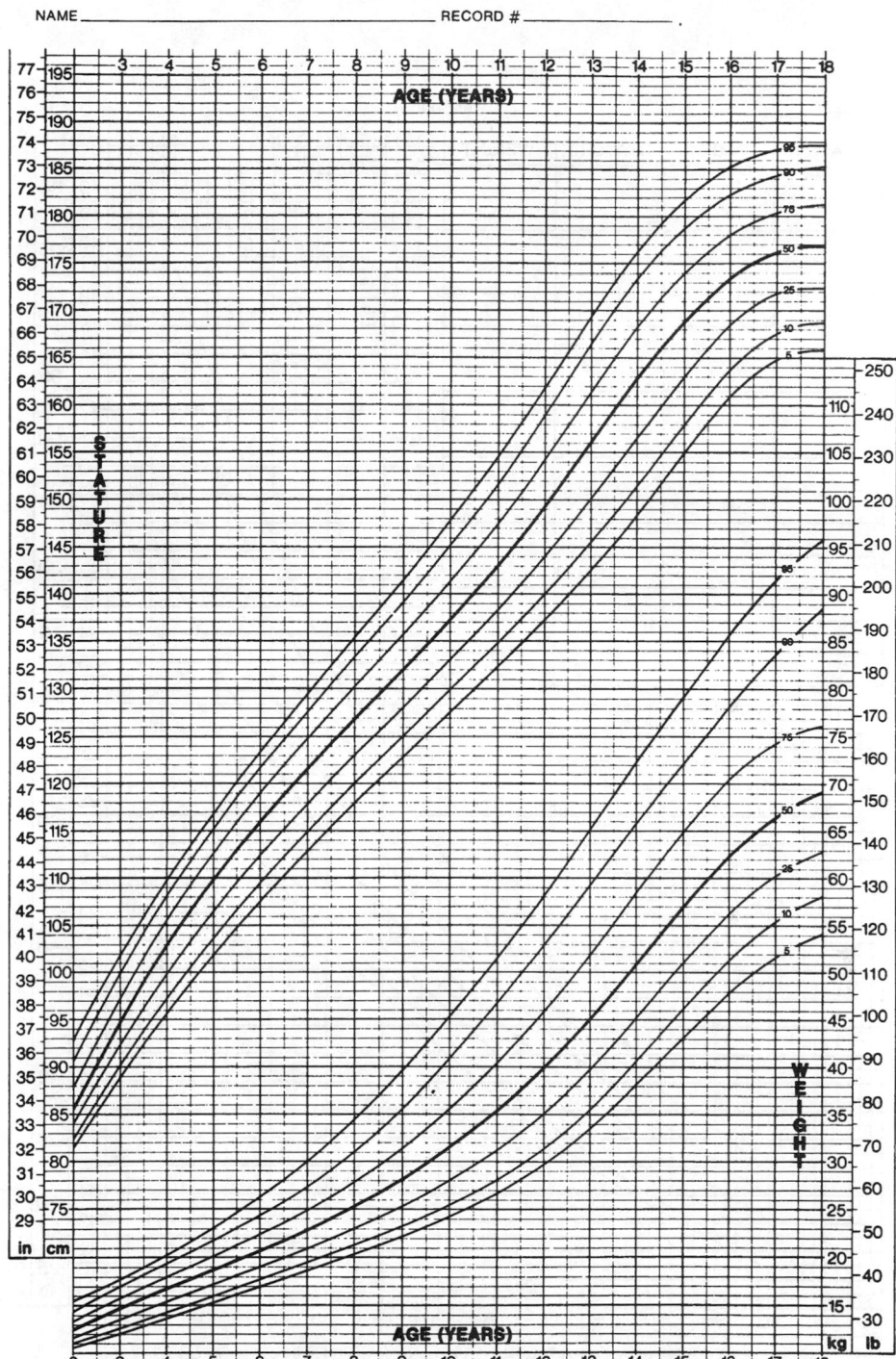

FIGURE 1.20.   Normal physical growth of boys, 2–18 years of age. National Center for Health Statistics percentiles. (From National Center for Health Statistics, NCHS growth charts, 1976, Monthly Vital Statistics Report. 25(3), Suppl. (HRA) 76–1120. Rockville, Maryland: National Center for Health Statistics, 1976.)

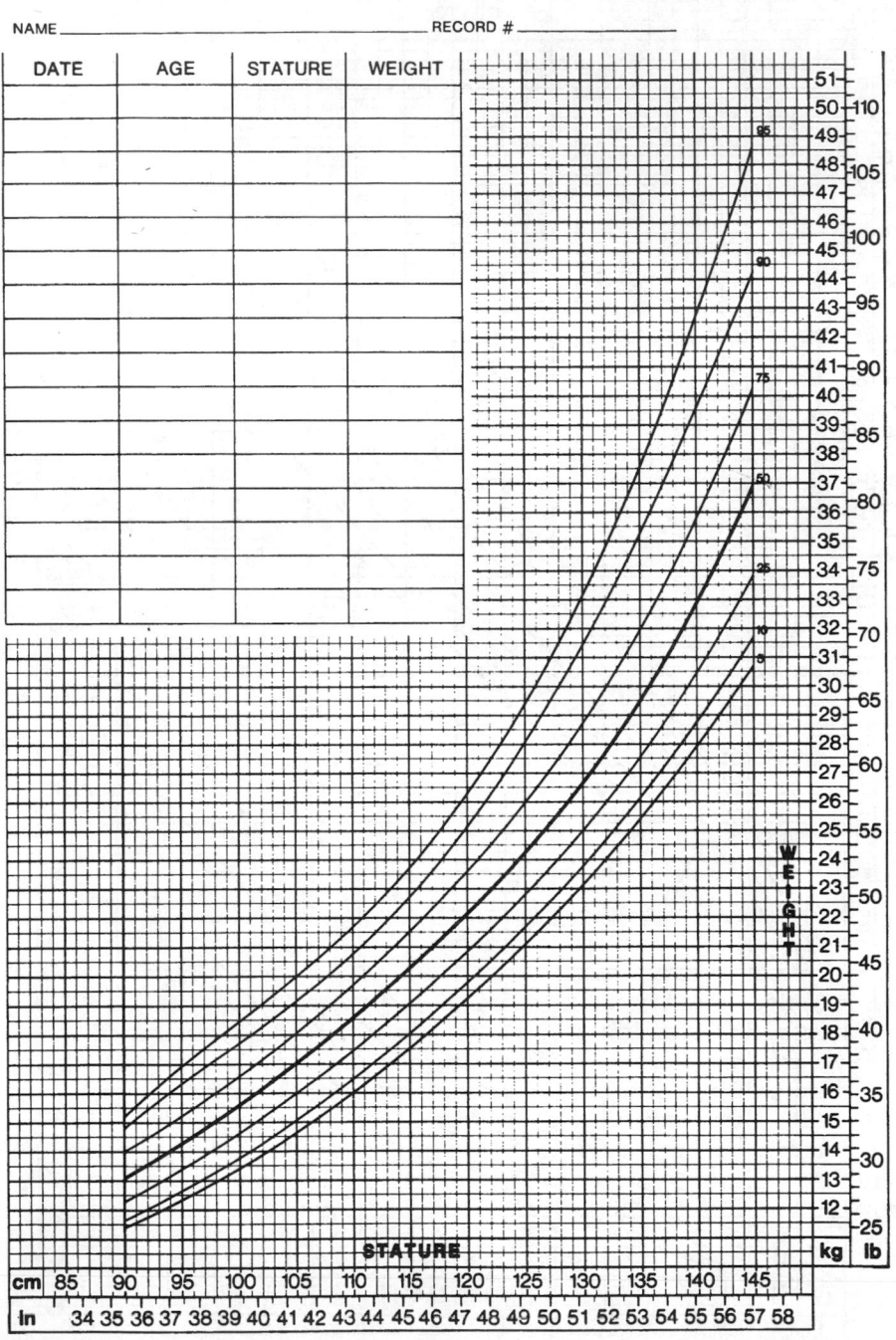

FIGURE 1.21. Normal prepubescent physical growth of boys. National Center for Health Statistics percentiles. (From National Center for Health Statistics, NCHS growth charts, 1976, Monthly Vital Statistics Report. 25(3), Suppl. (HRA) 76–1120. Rockville, Maryland: National Center for Health Statistics, 1976.)

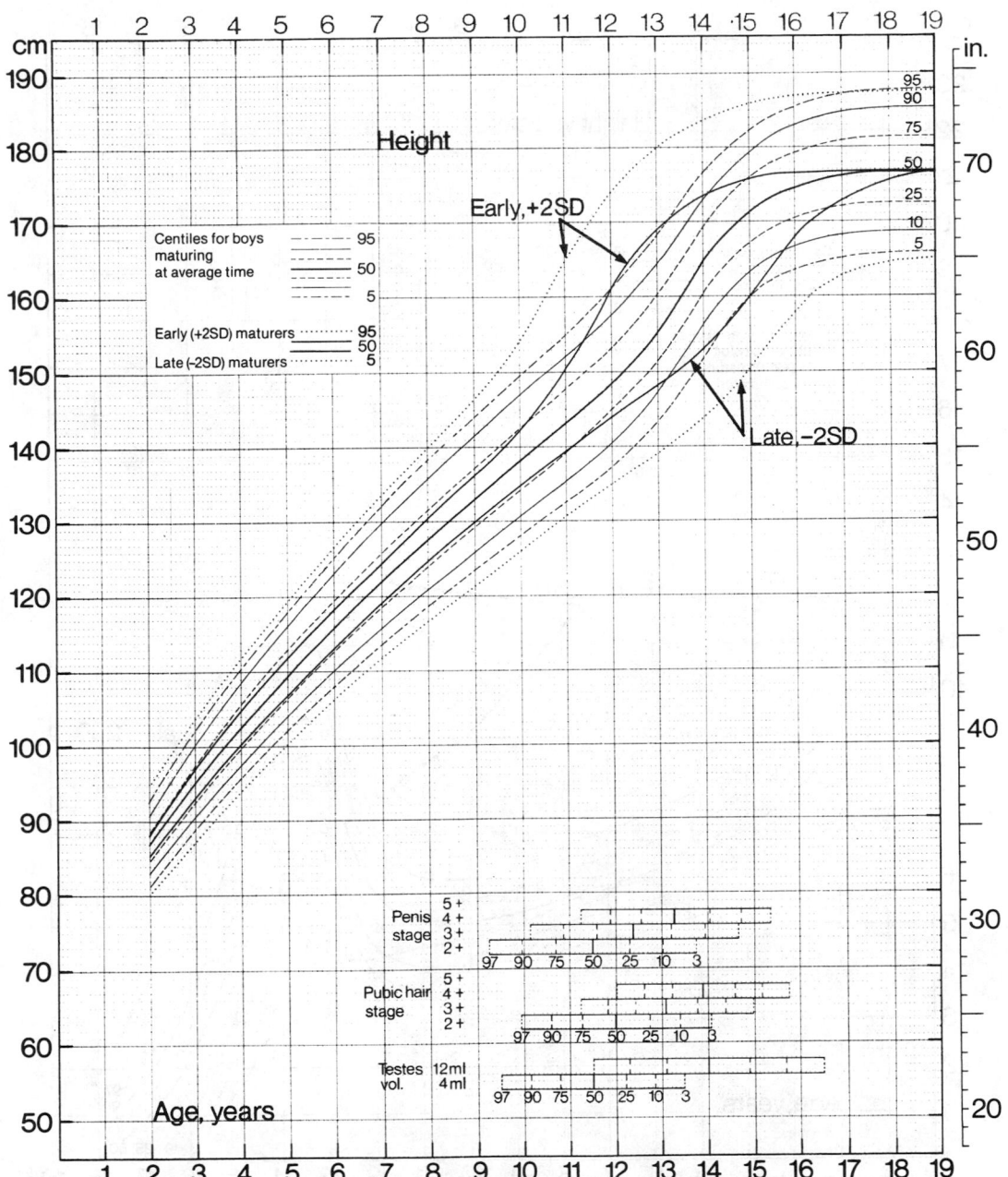

FIGURE 1.22.   Height attained for American boys. (From Tanner JM, Davies PW. Clinical longitudinal standards for height and height velocity for North American children. J Pediatr 1985;107:317.)

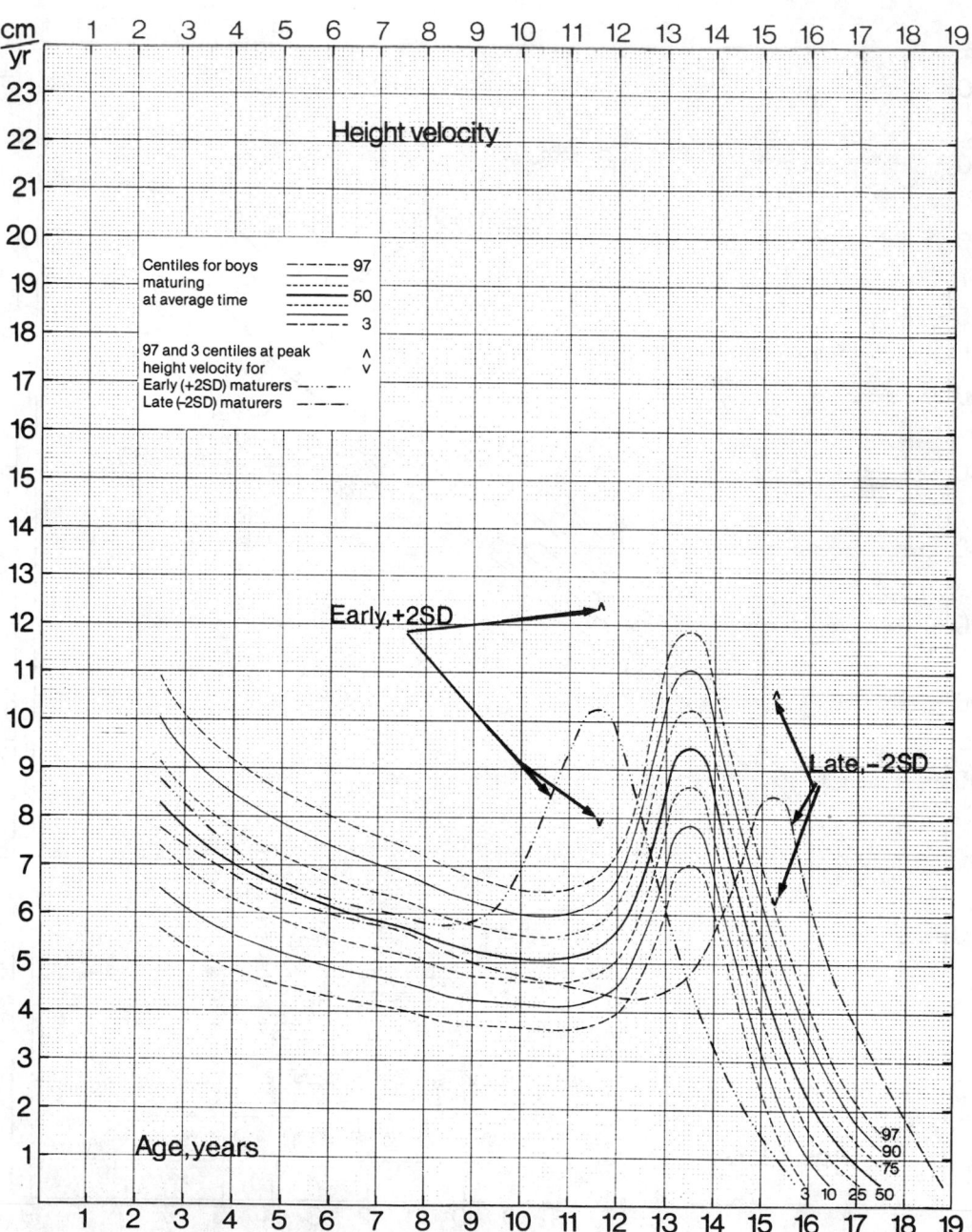

Figure 1.23.   Height velocity for American boys. (From Tanner JM, Davies PW. Clinical longitudinal standards for height and height velocity for North American children. J Pediatr 1985;107:317.)

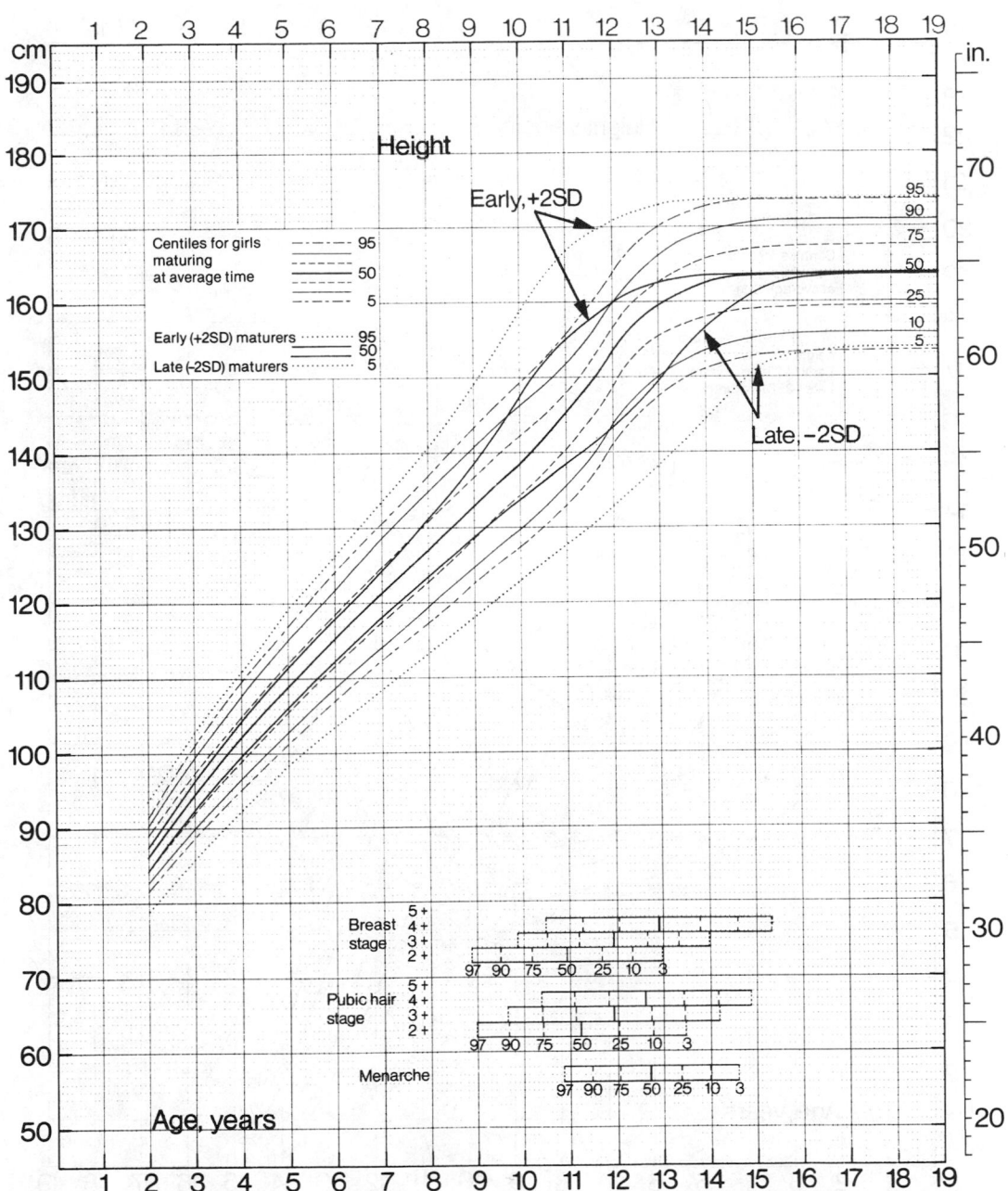

FIGURE 1.24.   Height attained for American girls. (From Tanner JM, Davies PW. Clinical longitudinal standards for height and height velocity for North American children. J Pediatr 1985;107:317.)

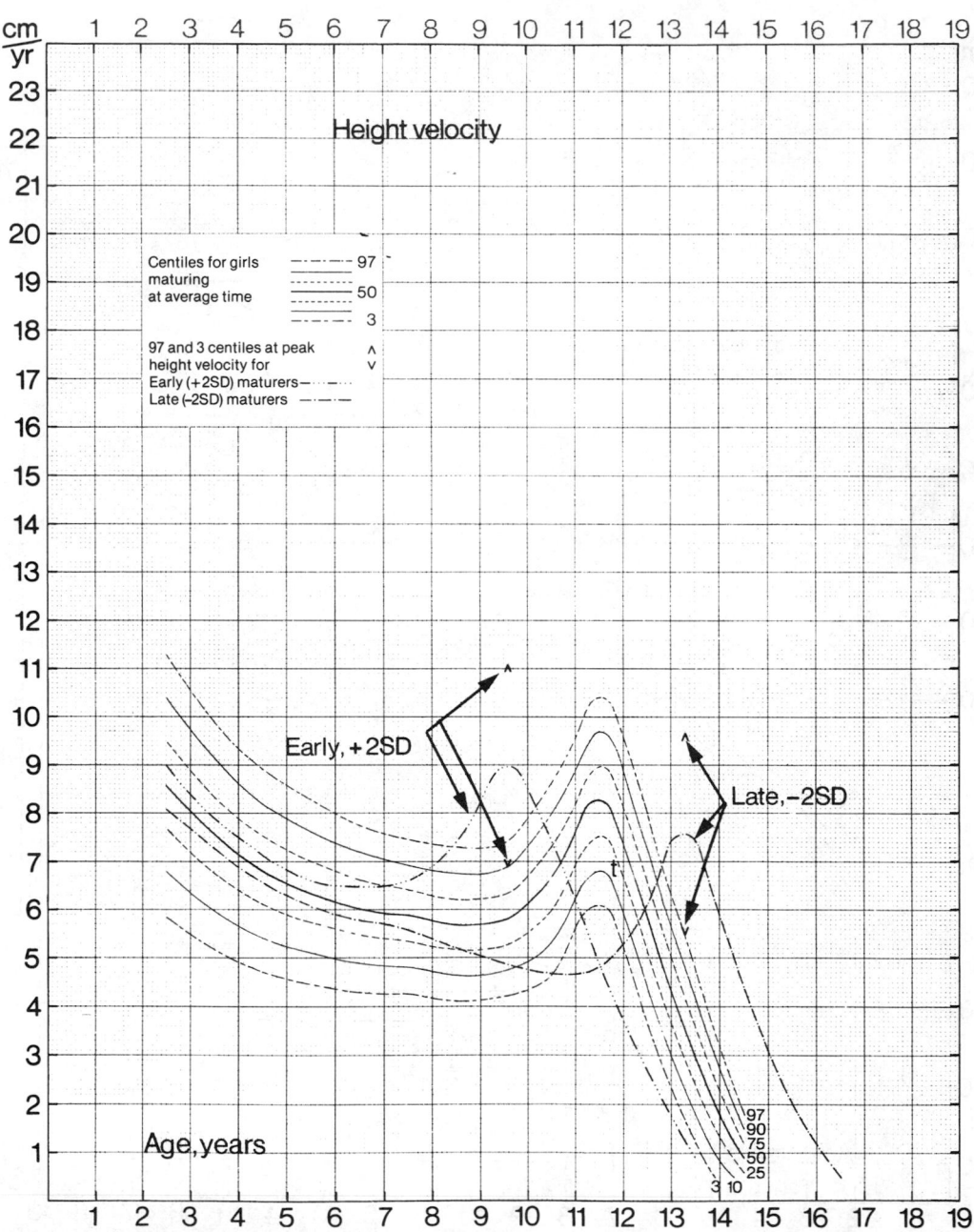

Figure 1.25.   Height velocity for American girls. (From Tanner JM, Davies PW. Clinical longitudinal standards for height and height velocity for North American children. J Pediatr 1985;107:317.)

TABLE 1.6.   Male Genital Size by Age

Age (yr)	Testicular Volume (mL)		Phallus Length (cm)	
	Mean	Range[a]	Mean	Range[a]
10	1.3	1–3	6.4	4–8
11	1.8	1–3	6.7	4–8
12	4.0	1–6	7.0	5–10
13	7.0	3–11	7.8	5–12
14	10.8	5–16	9.7	6–14
15	12.8	7–18	11.2	8–15
16	14.4	9–18	12.3	10–15
17	17.6	11–19	13.0	10–16
18	18.2	13–23	13.2	11–17

From Barnes HV. Recognizing normal and abnormal physical growth and development during puberty. In: Moss AV, ed. Pediatrics update: Reviews for physicians. New York: Elsevier-North Holland, 1979.
[a]Acceptable normal ranges.

TABLE 1.7.   Testicular Volume by Sexual Maturity Rating

Sex Maturity Rating	Volume (cm³)			
	Left Testis		Right Testis	
	Mean	SD	Mean	SD
1	4.8	2.8	5.2	3.9
2	6.4	3.2	7.1	3.9
3	14.6	6.5	14.8	6.1
4	19.8	6.2	20.4	6.8
5	28.3	8.5	30.2	9.6

Adapted from Daniel WA Jr., Feinstein RA, Howard-Peebles P, Baxley WD. Testicular volumes of adolescents. J Pediatr 1982; 101:1010.
[a]Mean of genital and pubic hair ratings.

TABLE 1.8.   Changes in Hematocrit Values by Pubertal Stage and Race

Stage	1		2		3		4		5	
	African-American	White	African-American	White	African-American	White	African-American	White	African-American	White
Males										
Mean (%)	37.7	39.5	38.4	39.8	39.7	40.9	41.1	42.3	42.7	43.8
SD (%)	2.5	2.4	2.5	3.0	2.4	2.6	2.7	2.5	3.1	2.7
Females										
Mean (%)	37.3	39.1	38.9	39.2	39.0	39.6	38.4	39.2	38.7	39.2
SD (%)	2.6	3.0	3.2	2.1	3.7	2.6	3.5	2.4	2.8	3.0

From Friedman IM, Goldberg E. Reference materials for the practice of adolescent medicine. Pediatr Clin North Am 1980; 27:193.

Spermarche

Spermarche, the onset of sperm emission, implies the establishment of spermatogenesis. Spermarche appears to be an early pubertal event, although there is wide variation in adolescents. Spermarche occurs at a median age of 13.4 (range 11.7–15.3), with an average testicular volume of 11.5 and a median SMR of 2.5. It precedes PHV in most adolescents and may occur with little or no evidence of pubic hair development (Hirsch et al., 1985; Nielsen et al., 1986). Guizar-Vazquez et al. (1992) found that spermarche occurred at a mean time of G2 and PH1.

Table 1.9. Serum Gonadotropins by Pubertal Stage in Males

Pubertal Stage[a]	FSH (IU/L) Mean (Range)	LH (IU/L) Mean (Range)	T (ng/dL) Mean ± SD (Range)
1	4.5 (2.5–7.0)	3.9 (2.5–5.8)	10 ± 1
2	5.9 (3.0–9.0)	6.8 (4.0–12.0)	85 ± 5
3	8.1 (2.5–14.0)	8.5 (6.0–11.0)	121 ± 17
4	8.5 (3.5–15.0)	9.5 (4.0–15.5)	493 ± 42
5	8.0 (2.9–14.3)	11.5 (4.4–19.0)	605 (260–1000)

From Friedman IM, Goldberg E. Reference materials for the practice of adolescent medicine. Pediatr Clin North Am 1980; 27:193.
[a]Ratings of genital stages.

Table 1.10. Serum Gonadotropins by Pubertal Stage in Females

	FSH (IU/L) Mean (Range)	LH (IU/L) Mean (Range)
Pubertal stage		
1	4.2 (3.1–5.7)	2.9 (2.0–7.5)
2	5.5 (4.6–7.1)	3.9 (2.5–11.5)
3	8.0 (5.0–12.0)	8.4 (2.5–14.0)
4	8.0 (3.5–13.0)	11.3 (3.0–29.0)
Phase of menstrual cycle		
Follicular	12.3 (10.4–14.2)	18.9 (15.2–22.6)
Midcycle peak	18.8 (14.3–22.8)	80.3 (62.4–98.2)
Luteal	7.4 (6.6–8.3)	14.2 (11.9–16.5)

From Friedman IM, Goldberg E. Reference materials for the practice of adolescent medicine. Pediatr Clin North Am 1980; 27:193.

Menarche

Menarche is one of the major development landmarks of female puberty and usually occurs in a fairly consistent position (SMR 3 or SMR 4) in pubertal development. The relationship between menarche and age, PHV, and body composition is described next.

Menarche in Relationship to Age and Physical Growth

On the average, menarche occurs in American girls at 12 years, 4 months (it varies normally from 9 to 17 years of age), 3.3 years after the start of the growth spurt and 1.11 years after PHV. The age of menarche has gradually decreased during the last century, as illustrated in Figure 1.26. Recent studies indicate this trend may be ceasing. Menarche always occurs after the PHV has been attained. Growth after menarche is limited. A 1972 study by Roche and Davila (1972) indicates that between menarche and the attainment of adult stature, girls gain 4.3 cm at the 10th percentile, 7.4 cm at the 50th percentile, and 10.6 cm at the 90th percentile.

The age of menarche depends on such factors as race, socioeconomic status, heredity, nutrition, and culture. It occurs later at higher altitudes, in rural areas, and in larger families.

Menarche in Relationship to Body Composition

Menarche may be dependent on body composition. Frisch and Revelle (1970) estimate that at menarche the mean adipose mass is 11.5 kg and the percent body fat is 24%. The height

TABLE 1.11.   Serum Concentrations (ng/dL) of Sex Steroids by Sexual Maturity Rating

	Sexual Maturity Rating				
	1	2	3	4	5
Male					
Estrone					
Mean	2	3	3	4	3
Range	1–6	1–7	1–7	2–7	1–7
Estradiol					
Mean	2	1	2	4	3
Range	<1–3.5	<1–4	<1–3	1–6	1–5
Progesterone					
Mean	30	36	40	40	35
17-Hydroxyprogesterone					
Range	30–36	34–40	52–62	78–93	—
Testosterone					
Mean	10	18	52	170	350
Range	3–110	2–300	27–910	92–840	200–1000
Dihydrotestosterone					
Mean	3	4	13	26	13
Range	2–20	2–28	6–36	5–51	1–76
Androstenedione					
Mean	54	49	85	69	90
Range	13–79	17–81	48–122	40–111	50–200
Dehydroepiandrosterone					
Mean	192	300	396	396	450
Range	2–326	50–558	119–592	178–645	180–700
Female					
Estrone					
Mean	4	5	7	12	3
Range	1–8	1–9	1–11	1–19	2–8
Estradiol					
Mean	2	3	13	16	8
Range	<1–3	<1–6	<1–27	1–30	1–40
Progesterone					
Range	10–13	16	16–23	30–161	29–75[a]
17-Hydroxyprogesterone					
Range	32–38	38–52	55–69	101–127	11–80[a]
Testosterone					
Mean	11	19	28	48	38
Range	2–18	14–65	19–80	20–85	20–85
Dihydrotestosterone					
Range	2–16	3–24	9–25	9–32	—
Androstenedione					
Mean	35	72	103	176	141
Range	10–100	38–106	40–150	40–210	58–224
Dehydroepiandrosterone					
Mean	133	326	427	498	741
Range	19–300	45–1600	125–1700	153–1620	389–109

From McAnarney ER, Kreipe RE, Orr DP, Comerci GD, eds. Textbook of adolescent medicine. Philadelphia: WB Saunders, 1992:1181. Adapted from Copeland KC, Brookman RR, Rauh JL. Assessment of pubertal development. Columbus, Ohio: Ross Laboratories, 1986. (Ranges derived from several studies.)
[a]Follicular phase.

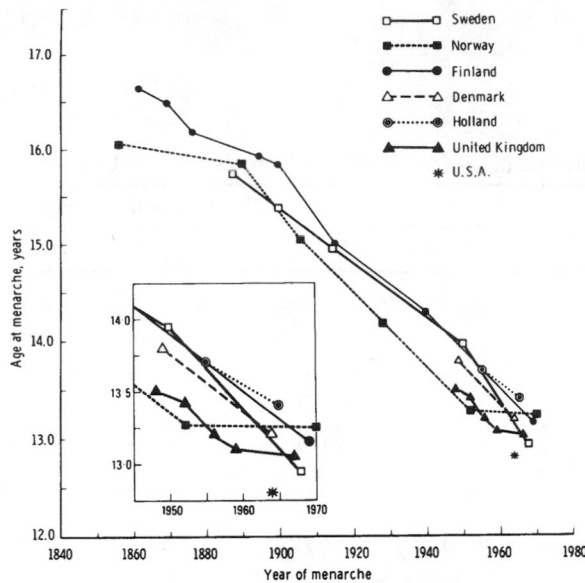

Figure 1.26. Secular trend in age in menarche. (Reproduced, by permission from J.M. Tanner, Fetus into man. © 1978 by Harvard University Press, Cambridge, Mass.)

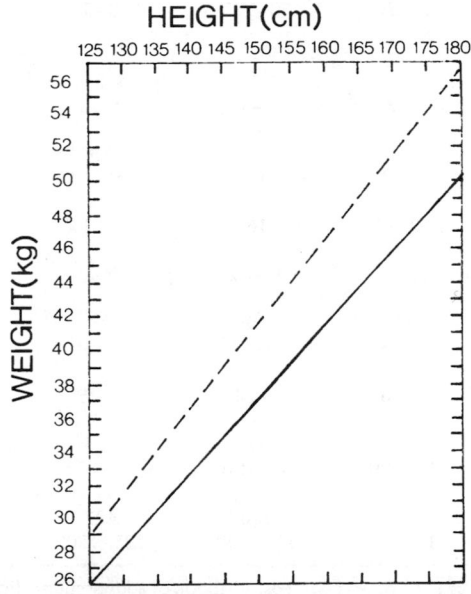

Figure 1.27. The weight for height at which menarche is likely to occur (*solid line*) and the weight for height at which regular ovulatory menstrual periods are likely to be maintained (*dashed line*). (From Frisch RE, McArthur JW. Menstrual cycles: fatness as a determinant of minimum weight for height necessary for their maintenance or onset. Science 1974;185:949. © 1974 by American Association for the Advancement of Science.)

and weight of an adolescent in relationship to menarche and ovulatory cycles is outlined in Figure 1.27.

CONCERN ABOUT GROWTH AND DEVELOPMENT

This chapter has discussed most of the features of normal adolescent growth and development. As essential as it is for the health-care provider to have a firm grasp of the facts of normal growth and development, a clear understanding and feeling for what these changes mean to the adolescent are also critically important. As their bodies change, adolescents develop tremendous concern about whether their bodies are right or will be right. The great variation in timing of puberty, with resultant differences in the physical maturity of similar-aged adolescents, serves to heighten teenagers' worries. Practitioners must be adept at detecting the adolescent's concerns about height, weight, pubic hair growth, or phallus size, for example, even though these concerns may not be stated overtly in the initial complaint.

The health-care provider can better empathize with the adolescent by thinking through the answers to the following questions about the health practitioner's own adolescence:

1. When I was 14 years old, my physical appearance could best be described as:
2. My greatest concern about my body was:
3. My medical problems during adolescence were:
4. One of my greatest misconceptions about the anatomy or physiology of the opposite sex was:
5. (Females) My feeling about my first period was:
6. (Males) My feelings about wet dreams were:

SUMMARY

The changes of puberty are a marvel of nature and a testimony to the intricacies and wonders of the human hormonal system. The health-care provider must understand these changes and the wide variations of normalcy. He or she must also be able to sense the profound effect these changes have on the adolescent and be prepared to be a source of information, reassurance, and help if abnormalities are detected.

BIBLIOGRAPHY

Albertsson-Wikland K, Rosberg S, Karlberg J, et al. Analysis of 24-hour growth hormone profiles in healthy boys and girls of normal stature: relation to puberty. J Clin Endocrinol Metab 1994;78:1195.

Argente J, Barrios V, Pozo J, et al. Normative data for insulin-like growth factors (IGFs), IGF-binding proteins, and growth hormone-binding protein in a healthy Spanish pediatric population: age and sex-related changes. J Clin Endocrinol Metab 1993;77:1522.

Argente J, Evain-Brion D, Munoz-villa A, et al. Relationship of plasma growth hormone-releasing hormone levels to pubertal changes. J Clin Endocrinol Metab 1986;63:680.

Barnes HV. Physical growth and development during puberty. Med Clin North Am 1975;59:1305.

Barnes HV. Recognizing normal and abnormal physical growth and development during puberty. In: Moss AV, ed. Pediatrics update: reviews for physicians. New York: Elsevier-North Holland Publishing, 1979: 103–129.

Bloch CA, Clemons P, Sperling MA. Puberty decreases insulin sensitivity. J Pediatr 1987;11:481.

Bramswig JH, Fasse M, Holthoff ML, et al. Adult height in boys and girls with untreated short stature and constitutional delay of growth and puberty: accuracy of five different methods of height prediction. J Pediatr 1990;117:886.

Brook CGD, Stanhope R, Hindmarsh P, et al. The control of the onset of puberty. Acta Endocrinol 1986; 113(suppl):202.

Cameron N. Assessment of growth and maturation during adolescence. Horm Res 1993;39(suppl 3):9.

Cara JF. Growth hormone in adolescence: normal and abnormal. Endocr Metab Clin North Am 1993;22:533.

Cara JF, Rosenfield RL, Furlanetto RW. A longitudinal study of the relationship of plasma somatomedin-C concentration to the pubertal growth spurt. Am J Dis Child 1987;141:562.

Daniel WA, Paulshock BZ. A physician's guide to sexual maturity rating. Patient Care: 1979;May 30:122.

Daniel WA Jr, Feinstein RA, Howard-Peebles P, et al. Testicular volumes of adolescents. J Pediatr 1982; 101:1010.

Friedman IM, Goldberg E. Reference materials for the practice of adolescent medicine [Appendix from Symposium on Adolescent Medicine]. Pediatr Clin North Am 1980;27:193.

Frisch RE. A method of prediction of age of menarche from height and weight at ages 9–13 years. Pediatrics 1974;53:384.

Frisch RE, Nagel JS. Prediction of adult height of girls from age of menarche and height at menarche. J Pediatr 1974;85:838.

Frisch RE, Revelle R. Height and weight at menarche and a hypothesis of critical body weights and adolescent events. Science 1970;169:397.

Garcia-Baltazar J, Figueroa-Perea JG, Reyes-Zapata H, et al. The reproductive characteristics of adolescents and young adults in Mexico City. Salud Publica Mex 1993;35:682.

Greulich WW, Pyle SI. Radiographic atlas of skeletal development of the hand and wrist. 2nd ed. Stanford, California, and London: Stanford University Press and Oxford University Press, 1959.

Grumback MM. The neuroendocrinology of puberty, Hosp Pract 1980;15:51.

Guizar-Vazquez JJ, Rosales-Lopez A, Ortiz-Jalomo R, et al. Age of onset of spermaturia (spermarche) in 669 Mexican children and its relation to secondary sexual characteristics and height. Bol Med Hosp Infant Mex 1992;49:12.

Harlan WR, Crillo GP, Cornoni-Huntley J, et al. Secondary sex characteristics of boys 12 to 17 years of age: the U.S. Health Examination Survey. J Pediatr 1979;95:293.

Harlan WR, Harlan EA, Grillo GR. Secondary sex characteristics of girls 12–17 years of age: the U.S. Health Examination Survey. J Pediatr 1980;96:1074.

Hirsch M, Lunenfeld B, Moden M, et al. Spermarche: the age of onset of sperm emission. J Adolesc Health Care 1985;6:35.

Hope GM, Dyment PG. The relationship of serum alkaline phosphatase levels to stages of pubic hair development. Cleve Clin Q 1975;42:313.

Juul A, Bang P, Hertel NT, et al. Serum insulin-like growth factor-I in 1030 healthy children, adolescents and adults: relation to age, sex, stage of puberty, testicular size, and body mass index. J Clin Endocrinol Metab 1994;78:744.

Kletter GB, Padmanabhan V, Brown MB, et al. Serum bioactive gonadotropins during male puberty: a longitudinal study. J Clin Endocrinol Metab 1993;76: 432.

Kletzky OA, Lobo RA. Reproductive neuroendocrinology. In: Mishell DR Jr, Davajan V, eds. Infertility, contraception, and reproductive endocrinology. 2nd ed. Oradell, New Jersey: Medical Economics Books, 1986.

Lee PA. Pubertal neuroendocrine maturation: early differentiation and stages of development. Adolesc Pediatr Gynecol 1988;1:3.

Marshall JC, Kelch RP. Gonadotropin-releasing hormone: role of pulsatile secretion in the regulation of reproduction. N Engl J Med 1986;315:1459.

Marshall WA, Tanner JM. Variations in the pattern of pubertal changes in girls. Arch Dis Child 1969;44: 291.

Marshall WA, Tanner JM. Variations in the pattern of pubertal changes in boys. Arch Dis Child 1970; 45:13.

Martha PM Jr, Rogol AD, Carlsson LM. A longitudinal assessment of hormonal and physical alterations during normal puberty in boys. I. Serum growth hormone-binding protein. J Clin Endocrinol Metab 1993;77:452.

Martorell R, Mendoza FS, Castillo RO. Genetic and environmental determinants of growth in Mexican-Americans. Pediatrics 1989;84:864.

National Center for Health Statistics. NCHS growth charts, 1976. Monthly Vital Statistics Report 25(3), Suppl. (HRA) 76–1120. Rockville, Maryland: National Center for Health Statistics, 1976.

Nielsen CT, Skakkebaek NE, Richardson DW, et al. Onset of the release of spermatozoa (spermarche) in boys in relation to age, testicular growth, pubic hair, and height. J Clin Endocrinol Metab 1986; 62:532.

Roche AF, Davila GH. Late adolescent growth in stature. Pediatrics 1972;50:874.

Rohn RD. Papilla (nipple) development during female puberty. J Adolesc Health Care 1982;3:217.

Rohn RD. Papilla (nipple) development in puberty: the adolescent male. J Adolesc Health Care 1985;6:429.

Root AW. I: normal sexual maturation. J Pediatr 1973; 83:1.

Rosenfield RI, Furlanetto R, Bock D. Relationship of somatomedin-C concentrations to pubertal changes. J Pediatr 1983;103:723.

Roy S, Brenner PF. Puberty. In: Mishell DR Jr, Davajan V, eds. Infertility, contraception and reproductive endocrinology. 2nd ed. Oradell, New Jersey: Medical Economics Books, 1986.

Tanner JM. Growth at adolescence. 2nd ed. Springfield, Illinois: Charles C Thomas, 1962.

Tanner JM, Davies PW. Clinical longitudinal standards for height and height velocity for North American Children. J Pediatr 1985;107:317.

Tanner JM, Landt KW, Cameron N, et al. Prediction of adult height from height and bone age in childhood: a new system of equations (TW Mark II) based on a sample including very tall and very short children. Arch Dis Child 1983;58:767.

Tanner JM, Whitehouse RH, Cameron N, et al. Assessment of skeletal maturity and prediction of adult height. 2nd ed. London: Academic Press, 1983.

Valberg LS. Plasma ferritin concentrations: their significance and relevance to patient care. Can Med Assoc J 1980;122:1240.

Vaughan VC. On the utility of growth curves. JAMA 1992;267:975.

Wilson DM, Draemer HC, Ritter PL, et al. Growth curves and adult height estimation for adolescents. Am J Dis Child 1987;141:565.

Winer-Muram HT, Emerson DE, Muram D, et al. The sonographic features of the peripubertal ovaries. Adolesc Pediatr Gynecol 1989;2:160.

Yip R, Scanlon K, Trowbridge F. Improving growth status of Asian refugee children in the United States. JAMA 1992;267:937.

Zacharias L, Rand WM. Adolescent growth in height and its relation to menarche in contemporary American girls. Ann Hum Biol 1983;10:209.

Zacharias L, Wurtman RJ, Schatzoff M. Sexual maturation in contemporary American girls. Am J Obstet Gynecol 1970;108:833.

CHAPTER 2
Psychosocial Development in Normal Adolescents

Lawrence S. Neinstein, Maria A. Juliani, and Joan Shapiro

No brief manual can hope to illuminate fully the complicated psychosocial developmental process of adolescence. This chapter offers an elementary framework from which to approach the study of this developmental process and discusses ways to enhance interactions between health-care providers and adolescents.

Although in terms of physical development adolescence can be described as the period of life beginning with the appearance of secondary sexual characteristics and terminating with the cessation of somatic growth, in modern Western culture the behavioral aspects of this period have become equally important. Adolescence is, in fact, a biopsychosocial process that may start before the onset of puberty and last well beyond the termination of growth. The events and problems that arise during this period are often perplexing to parents, health-care professionals, and adolescents. It is a time in which, for example, the previously obedient, calm child may turn moody and rebellious.

It is vital that health professionals who furnish comprehensive care for adolescents understand the adolescent psychosocial developmental process. Such an understanding is not only beneficial in routine adolescent health care but can help adolescents and their families through problem periods involving, for example, failure in school, depression, suicidal tendencies, and out-of-control behavior. This chapter examines the phases and tasks of normal adolescent psychosocial growth and development, beginning with some general comments about the process of adolescence.

THE PROCESS OF ADOLESCENCE

It is important, first, to keep in mind that no outline of psychosocial development can describe adequately every adolescent. Adolescents are not a homogeneous group but display wide variability in biological and emotional growth. Each adolescent responds to life's demands and opportunities in a unique and personal way. In addition, in recent years more attention has been given to the influence of the media in the emotional and psychological aspects of adolescent development.

Second, the transition from childhood to adulthood does not occur by a continuous, uniform synchronous process. In fact, biological, social, emotional, and intellectual growth may by totally asynchronous. In addition, growth may be accented by frequent periods of regression. It must be remembered that all of life, from birth to death, is a constant process of change and that adolescence is not the only difficult period.

Third, whereas adolescence has been described as a period of extreme instability or "normal psychosis," most adolescents survive with no lasting difficulties, and many are unperturbed by the process. In actuality, about 80% of adolescents cope well with the developmental process. Of these 80%, about 30% have an easy continual growth process, 40% have periods of stress intermingled with periods of calm, and 30% have tumultuous development marked by bouts of intense storm and stress. In a national survey, approximately 90% of 16-year-old boys and girls reported that they got along well with their mothers, while 75% reported getting along well with their fathers (Rutter, 1980). Only about one in five families reported difficult parent/child relationships. Adolescent girls in normal families reported that on average they have a minor conflict with their parents every $1^1/_2$ days, while adolescent boys reported a conflict every 4 days (Montemayor, 1982). In 75% of these conflicts, the incident was between the adolescent and their mother. Mother-daughter conflicts lasted an average of 15 minutes and conflicts with sons lasted about 6 minutes.

Phases and Tasks of Adolescence

Adolescence can be conceptualized by dividing the process into three psychosocial developmental phases:

1. Early adolescence: Approximate ages 10–13, or middle school years
2. Middle adolescence: Approximate ages 14–17, or high school years
3. Late adolescence: Approximate ages 17–21, or college or 4 years of work after high school

These stages overlap among different adolescents. By the end of adolescence most individuals have been emancipated from parents and other adults and have attained a psychosexual identity and sufficient resources from education, family, and community to begin to support themselves in an emotionally, socially, and financially satisfying way. In addition, they have learned how to appropriately gain support from other individuals when needed.

Several tasks characterize the development of the adolescent and are discussed in the next several sections in conjunction with the various phases of adolescence. These tasks include:

1. Achieving independence from parents
2. Adopting peer codes and lifestyles
3. Assigning increased importance to body image and acceptance of one's body image
4. Establishing sexual, ego, vocational, and moral identities

EARLY ADOLESCENCE (APPROXIMATE AGES 10–13)

Early adolescent psychosocial development is heralded by rapid physical changes with the onset of puberty. These physical changes engender self-centeredness and initiate the adolescent's struggle for independence. The onset of puberty is earlier by 1–2 years for girls than for boys, along with the concomitant psychosocial and emotional changes.

Independence-Dependence Struggle

Early adolescence is characterized by the beginning of the shift from dependence on parents to independent behavior. Common events at this time include:

1. Less interest in parental activities and more reluctance to accept advice or criticism
2. An emotional void created by separation from parents, without the presence of an alternative support group, which can create behavioral problems often manifested as a decrease in school performance
3. Wide mood and behavior swings

Body Image Concerns

Rapid physical changes lead the adolescent to be increasingly preoccupied with body image and the question of, "Am I normal?" The early adolescent's concern with body image is characterized by four factors:

1. Preoccupation with self
2. Uncertainty about appearance and attractiveness
3. Frequent comparison of own body with those of other adolescents
4. Increased interest in sexual anatomy and physiology, including anxieties and questions regarding menstruation, wet dreams, masturbation, and breast and penis size

Peer Group Involvement

With the beginning of movement away from the family, the adolescent becomes more dependent on friends as a source of comfort. The early adolescent's peer group involvement is characterized by:

1. Solitary friendships with a member of the same sex: This idealized friendship can become intense (boys, for example, may become comrades-in-arms with sworn pacts and allegiances, and young teenage girls may develop deep crushes on men as well as women)
2. Strongly emotional, tender feelings toward peers, which may lead to homosexual feelings, fears, and relationships
3. Peer contact primarily with the same sex, with some contact of the opposite sex made in groups of friends

Identity Development

At the same time that rapid physical changes are occurring, the adolescent's cognitive abilities are improving markedly. In Piaget's (1969) cognitive theory, this corresponds to the evolution from concrete thinking (concrete operational thoughts) to abstract thinking (formal operational thoughts). During this time, the adolescent is expected to achieve academically and to prepare for the future. This period of identity development is characterized by:

1. Increased ability to reason abstractly: This ability is usually turned inward, leading to increased self-interest and fantasy. For example, the young adolescent may feel himself or herself constantly "onstage."
2. Frequent daydreaming, which is not only normal but an important component in identity development
3. Setting unrealistic or idealistic (depending on the individual) vocational goals (for example, rock star, airplane pilot, or truck driver)
4. Testing authority, which is common behavior in adolescents as they attempt to better define themselves and which frequently causes tension between the adolescent and his or her family or teachers
5. A need for greater privacy, with diary or journal writing often becoming highly important
6. Emergence of sexual feelings often relieved through masturbation or the telling of dirty jokes
7. Development of the adolescent's own value system, leading to additional challenges to family and others
8. Lack of impulse control, which can result in dangerous risk-taking behavior

9. Tendency to magnify one's personal situation (although adolescents often feel that they are continually onstage, they may also be convinced that they are alone and that their problems are unique)

MIDDLE ADOLESCENCE (APPROXIMATE AGES 14–16)

Middle adolescence is characterized by an increased scope and intensity of feelings, as well as by the rise in importance of peer group values.

Independence-Dependence Struggle

Conflicts become more prevalent as the adolescent exhibits less interest in parents and devotes more of his or her time to peers.

Body Image Concerns

Most middle adolescents, having experienced the majority of their pubertal changes, are less preoccupied with these changes. Although there is greater acceptance and comfort with the body, much time is spent trying to make it more attractive. Clothes and makeup may become all-important.

Peer Group Involvement

At no other time than middle adolescence is the powerful role of peer groups more evident. Characteristics of this involvement include:

1. Intense involvement by the adolescent in his or her peer subculture
2. Conformity by the adolescent with peer values, codes, and dress, in an attempt to further separate from family
3. Increased involvement in heterosexual relations, manifested by dating activity, sexual experimentation, and intercourse
4. Involvement with clubs, team sports, gangs, and other groups

Despite the fact that this group of adolescents is susceptible to peer pressure, peer pressure can be overrated. Adolescents' reactions to peer pressure are extremely varied, and peer pressures can also involve a desire to excel academically, in sports, or in other positive activities.

Identity Development

The abilities to abstract and to reason continue to increase in middle adolescence, along with a new sense of individuality. The middle adolescent's ego development is characterized by:

1. Increased scope and openness of feelings, with a new ability to examine the feelings of others
2. Increased intellectual ability and creativity
3. Less idealistic vocational aspirations (adolescents with average and below-average intellectual abilities often realize their limitations at this time and may consequently experience lowered self-esteem and depression)
4. A feeling of omnipotence and immortality, leading to risk-taking behavior, which is certainly a factor in the high rate of accidents, suicides, drug use, pregnancies, and sexually transmitted diseases that become prevalent at this stage

Late Adolescence (Approximate Ages 17–21)

Late adolescence is the last phase of the adolescent's struggle for identity and separation. If all has proceeded fairly well in early and middle adolescence, including the presence of a supportive family and peer group, the adolescent will be well on his or her way to handling the tasks and responsibilities of adulthood. If the previously mentioned tasks have not been completed, however, then problems such as depression, suicidal tendencies, or other emotional disorders may develop with the increasing independence and responsibilities of young adulthood.

Independence-Dependence Struggle

For most, late adolescence is a time of reduced restlessness and of increased integration. The adolescent has become a separate entity from his family and now may better appreciate the importance of his parents' values, to the point of allowing their help as partners; thus, parental advice may once again be sought and accepted. It is not, however, uncommon for some adolescents to be hesitant to accept the responsibilities of adulthood and to remain dependent on family and peers.

Body Image Concerns

The late adolescent has completed pubertal development and growth and is typically unconcerned with this process, unless an abnormality has occurred.

Peer Group Involvement

Peer group values become less important to late adolescents as they become more comfortable with their own values and identity. Much time is spent in a relationship with one person. Such relationships involve less exploitation and experimentation and more sharing, with the selection of a partner based more on mutual understanding and enjoyment than on peer acceptance.

Identity Development

The ego development of the late adolescent is characterized by:

1. The development of a rational and realistic conscience
2. The development of a sense of perspective, with the abilities to delay, to compromise, and to set limits
3. The development of practical vocational goals and the beginning of financial independence
4. Further refinement of moral, religious, and sexual values

Conclusion

No individual's adolescence exactly fits the description of phases and tasks in this chapter. However, most adolescents follow the general pattern as outlined. An understanding of this general pattern helps health-care providers evaluate an adolescent's behavior. Table 2.1 summarizes the developmental tasks for each phase of adolescence.

TABLE 2.1. Psychosocial Development of Adolescents

Task	Early Adolescence	Middle Adolescence	Late Adolescence
Independence	Less interest in parental activities Wide mood swings	Peak of parental conflicts	Reacceptance of parental advice and values
Body image	Preoccupation with self and pubertal changes Uncertainty about appearance	General acceptance of body Concern over making body more attractive	Acceptance of pubertal changes
Peers	Intense relationships with same-sex friend	Peek of peer involvement Conformity with peer values Increased sexual activity and experimentation	Peer group less important More time spent in sharing intimate relationships
Identity	Increased cognition Increased fantasy world Idealistic vocational goals Increased need for privacy Lack of impulse control	Increased scope of feelings Increased intellectual ability Feeling of omnipotence Risk-taking behavior	Practical, realistic vocational goals Refinement of moral, religious, and sexual values Ability to compromise and to set limits

BIBLIOGRAPHY

Brown RT. Assessing adolescent development. Pediatr Ann 1978;7:16.

Coleman JC. Understanding adolescence today: a review. Children Society 1993;7:137.

Hill JP. Understanding early adolescence: a framework. Carrboro, North Carolina: Center for Early Adolescence, 1980.

Hill P. Recent advances in selected aspects of adolescent development. J Child Psychol Psychiatry 1993;34:69.

Lipsitz JS. Sexual development of young adolescents. Chapel Hill: University of North Carolina, Center for Early Adolescence, 1980.

Litt IF. The interaction of pubertal and psychosocial development during adolescence. Pediatr Rev 1991;12:249.

Lohner T. Adolescent psychosocial growth and development. Prim Care: Adolesc Med 1987;14:13.

Mehr M. The psychosocial and psychosexual unfolding of adolescence. Semin Fam Med 1981;2:155.

Montemayor R. The relationships between parent-adolescent conflict and the amount of time adolescents spend alone and with parent and peers. Child Dev 1982;53:1512.

Nottelmann E, Susman EJ, Inoff-Germain G, et al. Developmental processes in early adolescence: relationships between adolescent adjustment problems and chronologic age, pubertal stage, and puberty related serum hormone levels. J Pediatr 1987;110:473.

Piaget J. The intellectual development of the adolescent. In: Caplan G, and Lebovici S, eds. Adolescence: Psychological perspectives. New York: Basic Books, 1969.

Remschmidt H. Psychosocial milestones in normal puberty and adolescence. Horm Res 1994;41(suppl 2):19.

Rutter M. Changing youth in a changing society. Cambridge, Massachusetts: Harvard University Press, 1980.

Sider RC, Kreider SD. Coping with adolescent patients. Med Clin North Am 1977;61:839.

Slap GB. Normal physiological and psychosocial growth in the adolescent. J Adolesc Health Care 1986;7:139.

Steinberg LD. Understanding families with young adolescents. Carrboro, North Carolina: Center for Early Adolescence, 1980.

CHAPTER 3

The Office Visit, Interview Techniques, and Recommendations to Parents

The personality of the physician and his philosophy of medical care are considered to be most important in the medical care of adolescents. [The physician] should be mature and open-minded. He should be genuinely interested in teenagers as persons first, then in their problems, and also in their parents. He should not only like teenagers but must also feel at ease with them. He should be able to communicate well with his patients and their parents.

Committee on Care of Adolescents in Private Practice
of the Society for Adolescent Medicine

Providing care to adolescents in a sensitive, flexible, and developmentally oriented manner requires interest, time, and experience on the part of practitioners. No book can adequately teach the art of relating to patients or adolescents; it is a skill that is ultimately perfected through practice. A good medical interview with adolescents is important, as it allows the practitioner not only to collect information but to set the tone for future interactions. This chapter contains general guidelines for establishing better rapport with adolescents, as well as suggested interviewing techniques. At the end of the chapter there are also some suggestions for parents in communicating better with their teen.

GENERAL GUIDELINES FOR THE OFFICE VISIT

Liking the Adolescent

To provide effective care and establish rapport with the adolescent, the health-care provider must like adolescents. If the practitioner dislikes or is extremely uncomfortable with teenagers, it is best to refer them elsewhere.

Meeting the Adolescent and Family: The First Session

It is important for the practitioner to introduce himself or herself to the family and to the adolescent as the adolescent's physician. Either of two basic approaches may be used to start the interview:

1. Family together: Some health-care providers prefer to see the family together first. This approach can yield a great deal of information in the first few minutes regarding family dynamics. For example, if the adolescent is asked why he or she wants to be seen and the

mother quickly answers for the adolescent, a sense about the adolescent-mother relationship is gained. When the family is seen together, it is helpful to have the teen introduce the family members to the practitioner. This gives the adolescent the message that the practitioner is primarily interested in him or her. Following this part of the interview, the adolescent should be interviewed alone.

2. Adolescent alone: Another basic approach is to start the interview by interviewing the adolescent alone. Some health-care providers favor this approach in the belief that it quickly helps to establish rapport and a sense of trust. However, it is important to inform the adolescent that some input regarding the patient's past history will be required from the parent during the initial interview. At this point, the family may be brought in to continue the interview. Whichever method is used, the adolescent should be the primary information source.

Office Setup

1. Space: Adolescents prefer their own waiting area in a pediatrician's office. They do not like to be treated as a young child. It is helpful if the waiting room has materials such as magazines appropriate for adolescents and health education items. If the office is used for other age groups, one examination room should be set aside for use with teens. The examination table should be facing away from the door.

   The office should have enough room to accommodate the family, as well as the adolescent. It is preferable not to interview the adolescent and family in the examination room on the first comprehensive visit. The desk in the office should be oriented so that the health-care provider sits beside the desk, not behind it. Placing a large desk between the adolescent and oneself can create an artificial barrier.

2. Appointments: Usually, initial comprehensive visits for an adolescent should be scheduled to last 1 hour. If the practitioner is pressed for time, doing the history at the first visit and the physical examination on another day is a reasonable approach. Most follow-up appointments should be scheduled for after-school hours. At the end of the first visit, the decision should be made with the teen and the family as to whether the adolescent will make future visits on his or her own.

3. Billing: The issue of fee payment should be discussed early. This can even be done when the first appointment is made. The area of confidentiality can become somewhat muddled when the parents are paying for services. The adolescent must realize that an insurance payment may result in parents finding out about visits and the diagnosis.

   Ideally, a mutual agreement is reached with the adolescent and parents in this area. Alternatives include:
   a. Confidential billing (if the insurance company allows) so that the parents are not aware of the exact nature of the visits
   b. Having the adolescent pay for his or her own bills on a flexible installment plan and reduced fees
   c. Having the adolescent obtain Medicaid funds for conditions such as pregnancy, family planning, and substance abuse
   d. Referral to a clinic that can provide free confidential care

4. Availability of books: It is helpful to place books or pamphlets in the waiting room or office on topics such as puberty, sexually transmitted diseases, and contraception. The presence of such books helps the adolescent to feel that it is "OK" to talk about these subjects.

5. Avoiding interruptions: Constant interruptions or phone calls during the interview tend to decrease rapport. The office staff should hold all nonemergency questions or phone calls until after the interview.

6. Note taking: The practitioner should take as few notes as possible during the interview. When note taking is necessary, the practitioner should first request the teen's permission.

Establishing Rapport

Establishing rapport with an adolescent, especially with a nonverbal or hostile teenager, can be difficult. Helpful suggestions include:

1. Begin the interview by introducing yourself to the teen and parents or guardians. It is helpful to shake the hand of the adolescent.
2. Begin by chatting informally about friends, school, or hobbies. Not only does this decrease tension, but it enables the practitioner to gain important insights into the adolescent's personality, mood, and thought content.
3. Let the adolescent talk for a while, even if he or she meanders.
4. Treat the adolescent's comments as seriously as you would an adult's. The teenager should feel you are treating him or her as a person, not as a child or patient.
5. Start with nonthreatening health questions, such as a review of systems, especially if the adolescent is highly tense or suspicious.
6. Explore with the adolescent the issues that concern him or her. These issues may differ radically from concerns expressed by the parent.

Ensuring Confidentiality

It is important to establish a sense of confidentiality with the adolescent. The limits of this confidentiality may vary depending on the type of medical practice and current laws of a particular state, and the adolescent should be aware of these limits. For example, it should be explained that discussions will be kept confidential unless a problem becomes a threat to the adolescent or to others or unless the adolescent is consulted first. Regarding the presence of parents, adolescents are often more willing to discuss topics with their parents in the safer environment of the physician's office. Many parents will naturally be concerned about being separated from their teen during the interview process. One approach is to explain to the parents early the philosophy of your practice in a statement like the following: "As we are proceeding in gathering information about John, I would like to tell you both how I work with adolescents. After I finish talking with all of you together, I am going to speak with John alone for a few minutes. Then I will take him to the examination room for a physical examination. When this is done, I will call you back to go over the findings and my recommendations. During this time, I may discuss some matters that John would prefer I keep in confidence. It has been my philosophy to respect that confidence. Certainly, if there were any serious problem that were a threat to John's life or health I would inform you. Now, before we break as a group, are there any other concerns that you have about John that we have not discussed?"

Avoiding Surrogate Parent Role

Rather than being a surrogate parent, the health-care provider should function as an extra-parental adult. The emphasis should be on listening, advising, and guiding, using as non-judgmental an approach as possible.

Avoiding an Adolescent Role

The adolescent is looking for a practitioner who can be a sensitive and mature resource, not someone who is "one of the gang" and who dresses and talks like an adolescent.

Sidestepping Power Struggles

It is difficult to force adolescents into action. In other words, no one is better at being an adolescent than an adolescent. Do not try, therefore, to beat adolescents at their own game. Teenagers respond better if they can arrive at their own conclusions.

Acting as an Advocate

The adolescent encounters any number of adults who are unsupportive and who stress the adolescent's negative attributes. Try to emphasize an adolescent's positive characteristics and abilities. Keep in mind, however, that supporting the adolescent in "down" times is not the same as supporting inappropriate behavior.

Importance of Listening

Listening can often be the key to developing rapport with an adolescent. However, listening can be difficult, as thoughts usually wander or focus on the next response. The health-care provider should practice his or her listening skills to give full attention to the adolescent's statements and feelings. Good listening skills include:

Stay focused on what the teen is telling you.
Ask questions that help move the conversation along.
Be cautious in giving advice before asked.
Try and understand the teen's perspective.

Instilling Responsibility

Adolescents should be made aware that they are responsible for their own care. The more responsibility that adolescents take for their personal progress, the fewer problems that occur with compliance. Adolescents have a great ability to instill guilt in health-care providers. The practitioner can feel overwhelmed with the burden of changing the adolescent's life and habits. This burden should be shifted onto the adolescent.

Displaying Interest and Concern

The adolescent must be able to feel the health-care provider's interest and concern. Shrugging off concerns as unimportant is a sure way to alienate the adolescent.

Family and Parents

Although the adolescent may be the primary patient, the parents cannot be overlooked. Parents' input and insight are crucial, for in a real sense the family is the patient. To ignore the family's involvement in an adolescent's problem can often prolong the problem. Families must be consulted for the following reasons:

1. To elucidate past medical history and present concerns
2. To understand family dynamics and structure
3. To alleviate the parents' sense of rejection or guilt
4. To help bring about changes in the family unit and in the adolescent

Nonverbal Cues

Much can be learned by observing the adolescent's body language such as hand movements, manner of sitting, eye movements, or eyes slightly brimming with tears when certain subjects are discussed.

Process versus Content

Although inappropriate behavior should not be condoned, the health-care provider must explore the reasons behind the action. For example, shoplifting may occur secondary to peer pressure, family, or school problems.

Hidden Agenda

Adolescents will often present with chief complaints that are unrepresentative of their true concerns. An adolescent presenting with mild acne or pelvic pain may in actuality be afraid she is pregnant. An adolescent male with chest pains may be concerned about gynecomastia. Gentle but persistent exploration of the adolescent's concerns is often necessary before the true chief complaint is evident.

Developmentally Oriented Approach

In the course of interviewing and evaluating the adolescent, the health-care provider should be conscious of the adolescent's developmental process and tasks. The areas of sex, school performance, family, peer group, identity, and future should all be explored. Evaluative expectations should be based on the stage of emotional development the adolescent has attained. Early or middle adolescents, for example, certainly cannot be expected to think and behave as logically as adults. Below are sample questions regarding various adolescent tasks:

1. Body image: Do you have any questions or problems with the physical changes you are experiencing? Do you like yourself as you are? What would you change? Many teens have questions about periods, wet dreams, or changes in breasts or pubic hair. Do you?
2. Peer relationships: Who is your best friend? How many close friends do you have? What kinds of activities do you participate in? What do you do for fun?
3. Independence: Do you get along with your parents? Over what issues do family arguments occur? Is your privacy respected at home?
4. Identity: Are you satisfied with the way things are going for you? If you could change certain aspects of your life, what would you do and why? Are you working now?
5. Sexuality: Are you dating? Do you have a particular girlfriend/boyfriend with whom you are serious? Do you have questions or concerns about sexual activities, contraception, sexually transmitted diseases, or pregnancy?

Another approach that the author and colleagues have taken at the Teenage Health Center at Childrens Hospital of Los Angeles to obtain psychosocial/developmental information has been the HEADSS interview, covering the topics of *Home, Education, Activities, Drugs, Sex* (activity, orientation, and sexual abuse), and *Suicide*. An advantage of this approach is that the practitioner moves from less personal questions to more personal and potentially threatening questions, as follows:

Home Where is the teen living? Who lives with the teen? How is the teen getting along with parents and siblings? Are there any recent moves? Has the teen ever run away or been incarcerated? The practitioner should not begin with a statement such as "Tell me about your parents," as this question assumes that the teen has two living parents.

Education   Is the teen in school? What is the teen good and bad at in school? What classes are particularly interesting or boring? What grade average does the teen maintain? Has the teen repeated or failed any classes? Has the teen received any suspensions? How is the teen getting along with teachers? What goals does the teen have when he or she finishes school? If the teen is older or out of school, the practitioner should ask about employment. The practitioner should avoid asking "How is school?" as this will lead to an "OK" answer.

Activities   What does the teen do after school? What does the teen do to have fun and with whom? Does the teen participate in any sports activities? Church activities? What reading does the teen do? What music does the teen like? Does the teen have or use a car, and does the teen use seat belts? What are the teen's hobbies? Does the teen have friends? A best friend? How much time does the teen spend watching TV or playing video games? Do not start with a question like "Do you have any activities or hobbies?" as this results in a yes or no response.

Drugs   What types of drugs are used by the teen's peers? What types of drugs are used by family members? What types of drugs does the teen use and what amount and frequency? Does the teen use intravenous drugs? What is the source of income to pay for these drugs? The manner in which these questions are asked can significantly alter the responses. Consider the following examples.

MD 1:   Do you ever use drugs?
Teen: No!

That probably would end the questioning on drug use.

MD 2:   I know that drugs are fairly common on school campuses. What drugs are common on your campus?
Teen: Oh, I don't know, maybe pot and crack.
MD 2:   It is not uncommon for some teens to try some of these drugs. Have any of your friends tried them?
Teen: Some of them.
MD 2:   How do you handle the situation when your friends are using drugs? Do you ever try?
Teen: Yeah, once in a while. I really have only tried pot, and that was only twice.
MD 2:   The two most common drugs that I have seen teens use are often not thought of as drugs. These are alcohol and cigarettes. How much alcohol do you drink in a week?
Teen: Oh, I usually don't drink during the week, but on weekends I really get blasted almost every Friday and Saturday night.

Sexuality   Is the teen dating? What are the degree and types of sexual experience? Is the teen involved with another individual in a sexual relationship? Does the teen prefer sex with the same, opposite, or both sex(es)? Has the teen had sexual intercourse? How old was the teen in his or her first sexual encounter? How many partners does the teen have? Is there a concern about masturbation? Has the teen had a sexually transmitted disease, and what are the teen's knowledge base and concerns about sexually transmitted diseases? Does the teen use contraception and with what frequency? Does the teen use condoms and with what frequency? Is there a history of pregnancy or abortion? Does the teen enjoy sexual activity? Sexuality is another area where the style of questioning can dramatically alter the response. Consider the following examples.

MD 1:	Are you sexually active?
Teen:	No.
MD 1:	Tell me about your boyfriend or girlfriend.
Teen:	I don't have one.

In this instance, the teen may not even know what "sexually active" means or think that this implies a certain frequency of sexual intercourse. In addition, asking only about heterosexual relations may close the opportunity to find out about homosexual concerns or behavior.

MD 2:	Jane, I mentioned that I may be asking you some questions that were personal but very important to your health. Again, this is information that I will be keeping confidential. The area I want to discuss has to do with relationships. Are you going out with anyone right now?
Teen:	Yes.
MD 2:	What is this person's first name?
Teen:	Bill.
MD 2:	As you know, there are many teens who are sexually active. By that I mean that they have had sexual intercourse. There are also many teens who have chosen not to have sexual intercourse. How have you handled this part of your relationship with Bill or with other boys you have dated?
Teen:	I have not had sex with Bill yet, although we are thinking about it. I did have sex once about 6 months ago at a party.

Suicide   Has the teen had any prior suicide attempts? Does the teen have any current suicidal ideation? It is very appropriate to ask direct questions about suicidal ideation such as "Have you ever thought about killing yourself?" or "Have you ever tried?" or "Would you kill yourself?" or "Do you have a plan?" Direct questions do not precipitate suicidal action and are the best way to obtain such information.

Sexual Abuse or Physical Abuse   In any teen with significant problems in any of the previously mentioned areas, it is crucial to ask about abuse. This includes individuals with runaway behavior, significant family dysfunction, change in school grades, lack of friends, substance abuse, early onset of sexual activity, or history of suicide attempts.

Questions regarding sexual orientation and sexual abuse are particularly sensitive for the adolescent. These questions need to be introduced with an explanation of why the questions are being asked. Refer to Chapters 41 and 81 for further discussion of adolescent homosexuality and adolescent sexual abuse, respectively.

Physical Examination

The physical examination provides an excellent opportunity to educate the adolescent about his or her changing body. For example, the adolescent female may be taught to perform routine breast examinations, or the young adolescent male may be reassured about genital development. The adolescent may, in addition, raise concerns not mentioned during the initial interview. The true chief complaint may, in fact, be revealed during the physical examination.

Another issue of concern has been the question of who should be present during the physical examination. In general, the adolescent is examined without the presence of the guardian or parent. However, some adolescents prefer to have their parent present. The teen could be asked first, whether they prefer their parent in the room during the examination. Particularly, the younger adolescent or the developmentally delayed adolescent may wish to have a parent or guardian with them.

A chaperon should be used by male physicians during the breast and genital examination of female adolescents. Theoretically, the same concept would hold for a female examiner during a male's genital examination. However, this has usually not occurred in clinical practice.

Closure

At the close of the initial or follow-up visit, the health-care provider should address the following:

1. Provide a brief summary of the proposed diagnosis and treatment, addressed primarily to the adolescent.
2. Discuss any other resources available to the adolescent.
3. Allow the adolescent time to discuss any final questions or concerns.
4. Schedule any follow-up appointments.
5. Inform the adolescent that the health-care provider is available at other times. The adolescent should feel free to make follow-up appointments or telephone calls either for medical or emotional reasons.

INTERVIEWING

The following is a list of suggestions to assist the practitioner during the interview.

1. Shake hands with the adolescent first.
2. Ask questions in context.
3. Avoid lecturing and admonishing.
4. Bring the adolescent into the present. If the adolescent is focusing on his or her homework or on yesterday's date with a girlfriend or boyfriend, the interviewer is unlikely to gather much useful information.
5. Focus initial history taking on the presenting complaints/problems.
6. Identify who has the problem (i.e., is this the teen's concern or the parents').
7. Take a neutral stance.
8. The less the interviewer says is usually the better.
9. Be attentive.
10. Avoid writing during the interview, especially during sensitive questions.
11. When asking direct questions:
    a. Use less personal questions before more personal questions.
    b. Use open-ended questions.
12. Talk in terms that an adolescent will understand.
13. Do not misinterpret an adolescent's response.
14. Criticize the activity, not the adolescent.
15. Highlight the positive.
16. Assess your own ability to listen. A practitioner's difficulty in listening may be related to his or her own resentments or opinions of the adolescent's behavior.

Listed next are recommended interviewing techniques. Some aspects of interviewing, such as the initial introduction and establishing of rapport, were mentioned earlier in the general guidelines.

Open-Ended Questions

The use of open-ended questions such as "Tell me more about it" or "What does your pain prevent you from doing?" or "What was that like for you?" often facilitate communication more than the use of direct questions such as "Did that make you feel bad?"

Reflection Responses

The reflection response mirrors the adolescent's feelings. Consider the following example.

MD: How do you like school?
Teen: I hate it.
MD: You hate it?
Teen: Yeah, my teachers always. . . .

Restatement and Summation

Stopping to restate the adolescent's feelings or to summarize the interview may often help to clarify the problem or encourage the adolescent to make additional comments. An example might be "Let me see if I understand. You really like Jim, but you do not want to have sexual intercourse with him. However, you feel if you say no, he will stop liking you and drop you for someone else."

Clarification

Asking the adolescent to clarify a statement or feeling may help to crystallize the problem. For example, the practitioner's asking "What did you mean by that?" can also be useful in clarifying colloquial jargon. For example:

Teen: My friend and I like to go scaming. We do it most every weekend.
MD: Scaming? Help me out with that one? What does that mean?

Not only does such a question open up communication, but it makes the teen feel like an authority on a subject and that the practitioner is human too and does not know everything.

Insight Questions

Some questions may give the health-care practitioner better insight into the adolescent:

What do you do well?
If you had one wish, what would it be?
When are you the happiest?
What do you do when you're angry?
What do you see yourself doing in 1(5) year(s)?
What do your mother and father do when you're not there?
What do you do when you are not in school?

Reassuring Statements

The use of reassuring statements dealing with embarrassing subjects may often facilitate discussion. For example: "Almost all boys your age masturbate or play with themselves, and this is quite normal. I wonder if you like to do this sometimes?"

Support and Empathy

A noncriticizing response that recognizes and acknowledges the adolescent's feelings is often helpful during the interview. Examples of this type of response are: "I can really understand how bad that must have felt" or "That really must have made you feel sad" or "I'm impressed that you have taken care of yourself so well, despite all the problems that you've had."

Special Interview Problems

1. Garrulous adolescent: The overtalkative adolescent can sometimes be directed with a statement like: "I can see you like talking about _____. Why?"
2. Quiet adolescent: With the quiet adolescent, trying to get him or her to talk about anything, whether school, sports, or television, can often help to break the silence.
3. Anxious adolescent: The use of reassuring statements is frequently effective, such as "It is often difficult to talk about _____."

Interview Structure

The interview may meander, but it should have structure, including a beginning, middle, and end:

1. Beginning: The beginning of the interview should include introductions, attempts to put the adolescent at ease, and an explanation of what will be happening and why.
2. Middle: The middle part of the interview should move into defining the adolescent's problems and feelings.
3. End: The end of the interview should include informing the adolescent about the results of the examination and about what will happen next. Time should be provided for the adolescent to ask questions.

As stated at the beginning of the chapter, developing interviewing skills requires practice and interest on the part of the examiner. Reviewing one's interviews through the use of video equipment is an excellent technique for improving skills. Such techniques are of special value for physicians, who rarely undergo observation in their training. Appropriate consent from both teen and parent or guardian should be obtained.

Alternative techniques such as written questionnaires and computer surveys can also be used in conjunction with the verbal interview to obtain information about the adolescent.

Written Questionnaires Several questionnaires are employed in the Teenage Health Center at Childrens Hospital of Los Angeles and are found in Chapter 4 in this volume. Another is described by Cavanaugh (1986).

Computer Surveys The computer can be a nonthreatening format to some adolescents. Paperny has developed interactional questionnaires for teens on areas such as psychosocial risk profile, adolescent pregnancy, and family planning. These are available by writing David Paperny, Teen Health Computer Programs, 2516 Pacific Heights Road, Honolulu, HI 96813-1027.

Family Considerations

As noted earlier, the family is, in many respects, the patient. To fully understand the adolescent or to effect change requires interviewing and often working with the family. The dynamics of the family and the relationships between the different subsystems (spouse, parent/child, or sibling) should be understood. Not all health-care providers want to or should provide family therapy. But any health-care provider wishing to provide comprehensive care to adolescents must feel comfortable interviewing and working with families. Some excellent references for dealing with families are:

> *Families and Family Therapy* by S. Minuchin (Cambridge, Massachusetts: Harvard University Press, 1978)
>
> *Family Therapy Techniques* by S. Minuchin (Cambridge, Massachusetts: Harvard University Press, 1981)
>
> *Leaving Home: The Therapy for Disturbed Young People* by J. Haley (New York: McGraw-Hill, 1980)
>
> *Parents and Adolescents: Living Together. Part 2: Family Problem Solving* by M. Forgatch and G. Patterson (Eugene, Oregon: Castalia Publishing, 1989)
>
> *Problem Solving Therapy: New Strategies for Effective Family Therapy* by J. Haley (San Francisco: Jossey-Bass, 1976)
>
> *Psychosomatic Families* by S. Minuchin (Cambridge, Massachusetts: Harvard University Press, 1978)
>
> *Techniques of Family Therapy* by J. Haley and L. Hoffman (New York: Basic Books, 1967)
>
> *The Family Is the Patient: An Approach to Behavioral Pediatrics for the Clinician* by B. W. Allmond (St. Louis: C. V. Mosby, 1979)

Internal Considerations

Although the health-care provider should be careful not to project feelings about his or her own adolescence onto a teenager being treated, remembering one's own adolescence can help the professional to empathize with teenagers. Try immersing yourself in adolescent feelings and experiences by asking yourself:

> What did I look like at 13 years old? 15 years old? 18 years old?
> What things embarrassed me the most?
> What physical problems worried me the most?
> What was my first sexual experience like?
> What things did I enjoy most during those years?
> Who was my best friend? What did we do together?
> What things started arguments between my parents and me?
> How did I feel about my parents and my siblings?
> How much did I confide in my parents?
> What was my first date like?
> What did I like most about school? What did I like the least?
> What dreams did I have for the future?

RECOMMENDATIONS TO PARENTS OF ADOLESCENTS

Parents often ask health-care providers for suggestions of reference books or of methods for coping better with adolescents. Helpful methods for parents might begin with the previously stated recommendations for health-care providers, as discussed above.

General Guidelines

1. Listen to the teenager.
2. Treat his or her comments seriously.
3. Avoid power struggles.
4. Be flexible.
5. Show interest and concern in the adolescent's activities.
7. Spend time together and time alone together.
8. Show trust in the teenager.
9. Make resources available to the adolescent.
10. Strive for a good combination in the family between working together, playing together, and loving. Playing together and having fun together is an important part of establishing good parental-teen relationships.

Challenges of Teen Years

Parents should be aware that while most adolescents do well and go through adolescence without too much distress, it can be a challenging time period. These challenges include:

1. Parents must adapt to change in relationship with their teen, as teen's peers become an increasingly important influence and as the teen seeks increasing independence.
2. Parents must limit testing and experimentation by teens: Teens may experiment with many different types of behaviors including sex, drinking, and using other drugs. However, parents should remember that despite how teens may act, the vast majority of teens accept their parents' basic values. In one study, over 75% of adolescents even reported accepting their parents discipline practice (Rutter, 1980). Teen experimentation does not mean that teens reject their parents' basic values.
3. Parents must not overreact to rejection of one or both parents by the teen for a time period.

Daydreaming

Parents worry about teenagers wasting time and daydreaming. However, parents should be reassured that this is a normal part of the adolescent developmental process.

Communication

The practitioner should encourage parents to avoid barriers to communication, including:

1. Comparison with other teenagers
2. Lecturing or moralizing
3. Minimizing a problem
4. Excessive talking
5. Taking over an adolescent's problem
6. Taking everything too seriously
7. Overreacting, especially reaching conclusions based only on appearance, dress, or language
8. Phrases such as:
   a. The trouble with you is. . . .
   b. How could you do this to me?
   c. Is that all? I thought it was something important.
   d. In my day. . . .

    e. You're wrong.
    f. How could you feel like that?
    g. That's a dumb thing to say.
    h. Don't bother me now.
    i. You're stupid . . . crazy . . . incompetent.

9. The "shoulds": My child should be what I want him to be, he should satisfy my needs, or she should always feel loving.

The practitioner should encourage the parents to stress positive aspects of communication:

1. Empathize with the adolescent.
2. Stress the positive attributes of the adolescent. Adolescents get enough negative feedback. A dose of positive feedback and reinforcement when they do good work, such as follow through on their chores, can go a long way in positive communication.
3. Deliver clear messages.
4. Respect each other's privacy.
5. Keep a sense of humor.
6. Resolve conflicts together. Decisions that occur in the home about the adolescent should involve the adolescent's input. This can take place in the form of weekly family meetings. In this way, the adolescent is much more likely to carry through with the decisions. Family meetings or brainstorming sessions can be a helpful way to resolve conflicts. During brainstorming sessions to resolve conflicts parents should:
    a. Involve all family members in the process.
    b. Come up with at least five possible solutions.
    c. Write down all possible suggestions even if they seem outrageous.
    d. Avoid criticisms.
    e. Employ some humor when possible.
    f. Take a break if the session becomes too argumentative.
    g. Discuss the pros and cons of the most viable alternative ideas.
    h. After writing down several possible suggestions, try to agree on one solution or a solution that combines two different suggestions. Parents may also wish to ask other families how they solved similar problems and situations.

    A good resource on family problem solving is found in *Parents and Adolescents: Living Together. Part 2: Family Problem Solving* by M. Forgatch and G. Patterson (Eugene, Oregon: Castalia Publishing, 1989).

7. Involve teens in topics they like. When several hundred youths were asked what they wished to discuss with their parents, the top eight topics included:
    a. Family matters: Discussions about decisions that affected the whole family or themselves like allowance, curfew, and rules
    b. Controversial issues locally or nationally
    c. Emotional issues
    d. The "whys" of life
    e. The future
    f. Current affairs
    g. Personal interests of the teen
    h. Parents' life histories

Limit Setting

Adolescents need firm, fair, and explicit limits. Again, involvement of the adolescent in the limit-setting process is beneficial.

House Rules   Some families work better together if there is a set of "house rules." These prescribe the expectations for behaviors and guidelines for the family to live together as a group. Well-defined house rules can become quite important during the adolescent years. Having these rules discussed and written down can avoid conflicts over what behaviors are acceptable. If there is a particular problem in following a rule, then the parents may want to implement associated consequences if the rule is broken. However, the rules should be fair, consistent, and involve input from the teen. Teens may be eager to participate in the establishment of such rules when they find out that they might include a rule such as "no one will enter someone else's room without knocking first." Rules are mainly needed for teen or family member behaviors that are a problem. There should probably be a maximum of about 5–10 rules. Here is a sample set of house rules adapted from Patterson and Forgatch (1987):

1. Dinner will be at about 6 PM and everyone is expected to be home and ready to eat at that time.
2. Family members are expected to speak courteously to each other.
3. Before opening someone's door, knock and wait for an answer.
4. If you make a mess, you clean it up.
5. Going out on school nights must be discussed in advance. Schoolwork must be caught up beforehand.
6. Parties must be prearranged, and an adult must be present at the party.
7. Without an adult present, only teens of the same sex are allowed in the home.
8. Curfew on weekdays is 10:30 PM and midnight on weekends.
9. The car must be returned when borrowed, with the same amount of gas that it had previously.

These are just samples and should be changed to meet each families needs, expectations, and values.

Requests That Work   A key to making requests that work is limiting their number. Trained observers have found that normal mothers make 17 requests per hour and that mothers from problem families average over 27 requests per hour. Lobitz and Johnson (1975) found that when parents were asked to increase the number of requests they made to their children, the rate of problem behaviors and noncompliance doubled. Key components in making useful requests from teens include:

1. Decreasing or limiting the number of requests
2. Well-timed requests: Timing of requests or other feedback to adolescents is critical. Poorly timed requests (i.e., while teen is doing homework, on the phone, or in a bad mood) are surely met with anger, refusal, or rebellion.
3. Making requests in a polite and pleasant manner
4. Making requests one at a time: Dumping three or four requests on a teen at once is another behavior sure to trigger noncompliance and anger from the teen.
5. Using statements rather than questions in making a request
   a. Question approach:
      Parent: John, how would you like to take out the garbage tonight?
      John: No Dad, I'm busy with homework tonight.
   b. Statement approach:
      Parent: John, please take out the garbage now, it is your turn.
      John: I'm busy Dad.
      Parent: John, take out the garbage.
6. Make requests specific: For example, if giving the teen a time to be home from a movie, it should be a specific time, not "early."

In a study of compliance to parental requests, Patterson and Forgatch (1987) found that the average rate of compliance from normal children with requests from mothers was 57% and from fathers 47%. So parents should expect at least a 50–60% rate of compliance.

Practitioners can refer parents to numerous books and articles, a sampling of which is listed in Appendix I of this book.

BIBLIOGRAPHY

American College of Physicians. Health care needs of the adolescent. [Position paper]. Ann Intern Med 1989;110:930.

Boggio N, Cohall AT. Evaluating the adolescent: the search for the hidden agenda. Emerg Med 1990;January 30:18.

Cavanaugh RM Jr. Obtaining a personal and confidential history from adolescents: an opportunity for prevention. J Adolesc Health Care 1986;7:118.

Coupey SM. Medical interviews with adolescents. Med Aspects Human Sex 1984;18:65.

Felice ME, Friedman SB. Behavioral considerations in the health care of adolescents. Pediatr Clin North Am 1982;29:399.

Fishman HC. Treating troubled adolescents: a family therapy approach. New York: Basic Books, 1988.

Forgatch M, Patterson G. Parents and adolescents: living together. Part 2: family problem solving. Eugene, Oregon: Castalia Publishing, 1989.

Goldenring JM, Cohen E. Getting into adolescent heads. Contemp Pediatr 1988;5:75.

Greydanus DE. American Academy of Pediatrics: caring for your adolescent. Ages 12 to 21. New York: Bantam, 1991.

Johnson RL, Tanner NM. Approaching the adolescent patient. In: Hofmann AD, Greydanus DE, eds. Adolescent medicine. 2nd ed. Norwalk, Connecticut: Appleton & Lange, 1989.

Latta RJ, Lee PD. Counseling adolescents in office practice. J Curr Adolesc Med 1981;3:15.

Lobitz WC, Johnson SM. Parental manipulation of the behavior of normal and deviant children. Child Dev 1975;46:719.

MacKenzie RG. Workshop: interviewing the adolescent. Presented at meeting of American Academy of Pediatrics, New Orleans, Oct. 31, 1987.

MacKenzie RG. Approach to the adolescent in the clinical setting. Med Clin North Am 1990;74:1085.

Patterson G, Forgatch M. Parents and adolescents: living together. Part 1: the basics. Eugene, Oregon: Castalia Publishing, 1987.

Rutter M. Changing youth in a changing society. Cambridge, Massachusetts: Harvard University Press, 1980.

Sider RC, Kreider SD. Coping with adolescent patients. Med Clin North Am 1977;61:839.

CHAPTER 4
Health Screening and Evaluation

Lawrence S. Neinstein and Howard H. Schubiner

The goals of health screening for the adolescent are to promote optimal physical, mental, emotional, and social growth and development. Visits to a health-care provider should reinforce positive health behavior patterns while discouraging negative behaviors in areas such as exercise, nutrition, sexuality, driving, smoking, and relationships. Although there is a low incidence of serious medical problems during adolescence, numerous issues and concerns emerge involving physical development, sexuality, peers, family, school, and drug use. The adolescent period is also an excellent time for health professionals to practice preventive medicine by instilling positive health values.

Much discussion has centered on what constitutes appropriate, cost-effective health-screening procedures for various age groups. At present, there is no consensus regarding the recommended frequency of health screening in any age group. However, several organizations have intensively investigated the appropriateness of various screening techniques in different age groups.

The U.S. Preventive Services Task Force has come out with recommendations on periodic health examination based on age, pregnancy, and health risk. These recommendations (Tables 4.1 and 4.2) include preventive services that have been examined by the Task Force and have been found to be effective in preventing morbidity or mortality. The recommendations are not a complete list of all preventive services that should be offered during the periodic health examination. Three expert panels have evaluated the full range of preventive services for adults ages 18 and over. These include the Canadian Task Force on Periodic Health Examination, the U.S. Preventive Services Task Force, and the American College of Physicians. The recommendations of these expert panels that pertain to young nonpregnant adults are listed in Table 4.3 and reviewed in a comprehensive, comparison fashion by Sox (1994) and Hayward et al. (1991).

The most recent guidelines for health screening in adolescents are the American Medical Association's (AMA's) guidelines for adolescent preventive services (GAPS). GAPS is a comprehensive package of recommendations for primary care providers on how to deliver care to adolescents. The GAPS recommendations were developed by the AMA's Division of Adolescent Health with the assistance of a national scientific advisory board. The methods used to develop GAPS was established by the AMA and the Institute of Medicine. The American Academy of Pediatrics has also reviewed preventive care for adolescents and children as part of the Bright Futures project. Both of these projects suggest annual preventive visits for adolescents. The GAPS recommendations suggest additional counseling for parents twice during adolescence, and comprehensive physical examinations are recommended at three visits during the ages of 11–21. The GAPS recommendations are listed in Figure 4.1 and Table 4.4. A detailed review of the recommendations can be found in the book *AMA Guidelines for Adolescent Preventive Services (GAPS): Recommendations and Rationale* (Baltimore: Williams & Wilkins, 1994). During the next several years procedures on how to implement the GAPS recom-

TABLE 4.1. U.S. Preventive Services Task Force Recommendations on Periodic Health Examination for Ages 11–24[a]

Leading causes of death	
Motor vehicle/other unintentional injuries	
Homicide	
Suicide	
Malignant neoplasms	
Heart diseases	

Interventions for the General Population

Screening
  Height, weight
  Blood pressure[b]
  Papanicolaou (Pap) test[c] (females)
  Chlamydia screen[d] (females <20 yr)
  Rubella serology or vaccination history[e] (females >12 yr)
  Assess for problem drinking
Counseling
  Injury prevention
    Lap and shoulder belts
    Bicycle, motorcycle, or all-terrain vehicle helmets[f]
    Smoke detector[f]
    Safe storage or removal of firearms[f]
  Substance use
    Avoid tobacco use
    Avoid underage drinking, illicit drug use[f]
    Avoid alcohol/drug use while driving, swimming, boating, etc.[f]
  Sexual behavior
    STD prevention: abstinence[f]; avoid high-risk behavior[f]; condoms/female barrier with spermicide[f]
    Unintended pregnancy: contraception

Diet and exercise
  Limit fat, cholesterol; maintain caloric balance; emphasize grains, fruits, vegetables
  Adequate calcium intake (females)
  Regular physical activity[f]
Dental health
  Regular visits to dental care provider[f]
  Floss, brush with fluoride toothpaste daily[f]
Immunizations
  Tetanus-diphtheria (Td) boosters (11–16 yr)
  Hepatitis B[g]
  MMR (11–12 yr)[h]
  Varicella (11–12 yr)[i]
  Rubella[e] (females >12 yr)
Chemoprophylaxis
  Multivitamin with folic acid (females planning or capable of pregnancy)

From U.S. Preventive Services Task Force. Guide to clinical preventative services. 2nd ed. Baltimore: Williams & Wilkins, 1996:1vi–1vii.

[a]MMR, measles, mumps, rubella; PPD, purified protein derivative; RPR, rapid plasma reagin; VDRL, Venereal Disease Research Laboratory test.

[b]Periodic blood pressure for persons aged ≥21 yr.

[c]If sexually active at present or in the past: q≤3yr. If sexual history is unreliable, begin Pap tests at age 18 yr.

[d]If sexually active.

[e]Serologic testing, documented vaccination history, and routine vaccination against rubella (preferably with MMR) are equally acceptable alternatives.

[f]The ability of clinician couseling to influence this behavior is unproven.

[g]If not previously immunized: current visit, 1 and 6 months later.

[h]If no previous second dose of MMR.

[i]If susceptible to chickenpox.

mendations will be further refined. This will require educational interventions at the medical school, residency, and postgraduate training level. It will also require intensive discussions with managed care programs to discuss coverage for these recommendations.

School health assessments have become a larger issue with the growing availability of school-based and school-linked clinics. The American Academy of Pediatrics has reviewed key elements of comprehensive health examinations relating to school health (Committee on School Health, 1991). Practitioners are also referred to a report entitled:

> *Physicians in Partnership with Schools: A Guide to Policies and Programs*, School Health Committee, California Chapter 2, American Academy of Pediatrics, P.O. Box 2134, Inglewood, CA 90305

Text continued on page 75.

TABLE 4.1.   *continued*

Interventions for High-Risk Populations	
Population	*Potential Interventions[j]*
High-risk sexual behavior	RPR/VDRL (HR1); screen for gonorrhea (female) (HR2), HIV (HR3), chlamydia (female) (HR4); hepatitis A vaccine (HR5)
Injection or street drug use	RPR/VDRL (HR1); HIV screen (HR3); hepatitis A vaccine (HR5); PPD (HR6); advice to reduce infection risk (HR7)
TB contacts; immigrants; low income	PPD (HR6)
Native Americans and Alaska Natives	Hepatitis A vaccine (HR5); PPD (HR6); pneumococcal vaccine (HR8)
Travelers to developing countries	Hepatitis A vaccine (HR5)
Certain chronic medical conditions	PPD (HR6); pneumococcal vaccine (HR8); influenza vaccine (HR9)
Settings where adolescents and young adults congregate	Second MMR (HR10)
Susceptible to varicella, measles, mumps	Varicella vaccine (HR11); MMR (HR12)
Blood transfusion between 1975–1985	HIV screen (HR3)
Institutionalized persons; health care/lab workers	Hepatitis A vaccine (HR5); PPD (HR6); influenza vaccine (HR9)
Family history of skin cancer; nevi; fair skin, eyes, hair	Avoid excess and midday sun, use protective clothing[f] (HR13)
Prior pregnancy with neural tube defect	Folic acid 4.0 mg (HR14)
Inadequate water fluoridation	Daily fluoride supplement (HR15)

[j]High-risk definitions:

HR1: Persons who exchange sex for money or drugs, and their sex partners; persons with other sexually transmitted diseases (STDs) (including HIV); and sexual contacts of persons with active syphilis. Clinicians should also consider local epidemiology.

HR2: Females who have: two or more sex partners in the last year; a sex partner with multiple sexual contacts; exchanged sex for money or drugs; or a history of repeated episodes of gonorrhea. Clinicians should also consider local epidemiology.

HR3: Males who had sex with males after 1975; past or present injection drug use; persons who exchange sex for money or drugs, and their sex partners; injection drug-using, bisexual, or HIV-positive sex partner currently or in the past; blood transfusion during 1978–1985; persons seeking treatment for STDs. Clinicians should also consider local epidemiology.

HR4: Sexually active females with multiple risk factors including: history of prior STD; new or multiple sex partners; age under 25; nonuse or inconsistent use of barrier contraceptives; cervical ectopy. Clinicians should consider local epidemiology of the disease in identifying other high-risk groups.

HR5: Persons living in, traveling to, or working in areas where the disease is endemic and where periodic outbreaks occur (e.g., countries with high or intermediate endemicity; certain Alaska Native, Pacific Island, Native American, and religious communities); men who have sex with men; injection or street drug users. Vaccine may be considered for institutionalized persons and workers in these institutions, military personnel, and day-care, hospital, and laboratory workers. Clinicians should also consider local epidemiology.

HR6: HIV positive, close contacts of persons with known or suspected TB, health-care workers, persons with medical risk factors associated with TB, immigrants from countries with high TB prevalence, medically underserved low-income populations (including homeless), alcoholics, injection drug users, and residents of long-term facilities.

HR7: Persons who continue to inject drugs.

HR8: Immunocompetent persons with certain medical conditions, including chronic cardiac or pulmonary disease, diabetes mellitus, and anatomic asplenia. Immunocompetent persons who live in high-risk environments or social settings (e.g., certain Native American and Alaska Native populations).

HR9: Annual vaccination of: residents of chronic care facilities; persons with chronic cardiopulmonary disorders, metabolic diseases (including diabetes mellitus), hemoglobinopathies, immunosuppression, or renal dysfunction; and health-care providers for high-risk patients.

HR10: Adolescents and young adults in settings where such individuals congregate (e.g., high schools and colleges), if they have not previously received a second dose.

HR11: Healthy persons aged ≥13 yr without a history of chickenpox or previous immunization. Consider serologic testing for presumed susceptible persons aged ≥13 yr.

HR12: Persons born after 1956 who lack evidence of immunity to measles or mumps (e.g., documented receipt of live vaccine on or after the first birthday, laboratory evidence of immunity, or a history of physician-diagnosed measles or mumps).

HR13: Persons with a family or personal history of skin cancer, a large number of moles, atypical moles, poor tanning ability, or light skin, hair, and eye color.

HR14: Women with prior pregnancy affected by neural tube defect who are planning pregnancy.

HR15: Persons aged <17 yr living in areas with inadequate water fluoridation (<0.6 ppm).

TABLE 4.2.   U.S. Preventive Services Task Force Recommendations on Periodic Health Examination for Pregnant Women[a]

Interventions for the General Population	Interventions for High-Risk Populations	
	Population	*Potential Interventions[f]*
Screening		
First visit		
Blood pressure	High-risk sexual behavior	Screen for chlamydia (1st
Hemoglobin/hematocrit		visit) (HR1), gonorrhea
Hepatitis B surface antigen		(1st visit) (HR2), HIV
RPR/VDRL		(1st visit) (HR3); HBsAg
Chlamydia screen (<25 yr)		(3rd trimester) (HR4);
Rubella serology or vaccination history		RPR/VDRL (3rd
D(Rh) typing, antibody screen		trimester) (HR5)
Offer CVS (<13 wk)[b] or amniocentesis	Blood transfusion	HIV screen (1st visit) (HR3)
(15–18 wk)[b] (age ≥35 yr)	1978–1985	
Offer hemoglobinopathy screening	Injection drug use	HIV screen (HR3); HBsAg
Assess for problem or risk drinking		(3rd trimester) (HR4);
Offer HIV screening[c]		advice to reduce
Follow-up visits		infection risk (HR6)
Blood pressure	Unsensitized D-negative	D(Rh) antibody testing
Urine culture (12–16 wk)	women	(24–28 wk) (HR7)
Offer amniocentesis (15–18 wk)[b]	Risk factors for Down	Offer CVS[b] (1st trimester),
(age ≥35 yr)	syndrome	amniocentesis[b] (15–18
Offer multiple marker testing[b] (15–18 wk)		wk) (HR8)
Offer serum α-fetoprotein[b] (16–18 wk)	Prior pregnancy with	Offer amniocentesis[b]
Counseling	neural tube defect	(15–18 wk), folic acid
Tobacco cessation; effects of passive smoking		4.0 mg[d] (HR9)
Alcohol or other drug use		
Nutrition, including adequate calcium intake		
Encourage breastfeeding		
Lap and shoulder belts		
Infant safety car seats		
STD prevention: avoid high-risk sexual		
behavior[d]; use condoms[d]		
Chemoprophylaxis		
Multivitamin with folic acid[e]		

From U.S. Preventive Services Task Force. Guide to clinical preventative services. 2nd ed. Baltimore: Williams & Wilkins, 1996:1xii–1xiii.

[a]See Table 4.1 for other preventive services recommended for women of this age group.

[b]Women with access to counseling and follow-up services, reliable standardized laboratories, skilled high-resolution ultrasound, and, for those receiving serum marker testing, amniocentesis capabilities.

[c]Universal screening is recommended for areas (states, counties, or cities) with an increased prevalence of HIV infection among pregnant women. In low-prevalence areas, the choice between universal and targeted screening may depend on other considerations.

[d]The ability of clinician counseling to influence this behavior is unproven.

[e]Beginning at least 1 month before conception and continuing through the first trimester.

[f]High-risk definitions:

  HR1: Women with history of STD or new or multiple sex partners. Clinicians should also consider local epidemiology. Chlamydia screen should be repeated in 3rd trimester if at continued risk.

  HR2: Women under age 25 with two or more sex partners in the last year, or whose sex partner has multiple sexual contacts; women who exchange sex for money or drugs; and women with a history of repeated episodes of gonorrhea. Clinicians should also consider local epidemiology. Gonorrhea screen should be repeated in the 3rd trimester if at continued risk.

  HR3: In areas where universal screening is not performed due to low prevalence of HIV infection, pregnant women with the following individual risk factors should be screened: past or present injection drug use; women who exchange sex for money or drugs; injection drug-using, bisexual, or HIV-positive sex partner currently or in the past; blood transfusion during 1978–1985; persons seeking treatment for STDs.

  HR4: Women who are initially HBsAg negative who are at high risk due to injection drug use, suspected exposure to hepatitis B during pregnancy, multiple sex partners.

  HR5: Women who exchange sex for money or drugs, women with other STDs (including HIV), and sexual contacts of persons with active syphilis. Clinicians should also consider local epidemiology.

  HR6: Women who continue to inject drugs.

  HR7: Unsensitized D-negative women.

  HR8: Prior pregnancy affected by Down syndrome, advanced maternal age (≥35 yr), known carriage of chromosome rearrangement.

  HR9: Women with previous pregnancy affected by neural tube defect.

TABLE 4.3. Preventive Care Guidelines for Asymptomatic, Low-Risk Young Adults: Recommendations from Various North American Health Organizations

Area/Vaccine or Drug/Topic	American College of Physicians	Canadian Task Force on Periodic Health Examination	U.S. Preventive Services Task Force
Height and weight			
General	Not considered	(C) No recommendation	MF 18+ q1–3yr
Selective	Not considered	(B) MF 18+ if one or more woman of low socioeconomic status, food faddist, adolescent woman, native Indian or Inuit	No recommendation
Blood pressure measurement			
General	18+ MF q1–2yr and at every visit for other reasons	(A) MF 25+ q5yr and at every visit for other reasons	MF 18+ q2yr and at every visit for other reasons
Selective	MF 18+ q1yr if diastolic blood pressure is 85–89 mm Hg MF 18+ at least q1yr if one or more: previous hypertension DM, known CAD or other cardiovascular disease, moderate or extreme obesity, African-American race, history of hypertension in parents or siblings	(A) No recommendation	MF 18+ every year if diastolic blood pressure is 85–89 mm Hg
Assessment of depression and suicidal intent			
General	None for young adults	(D) Recommendation against	Recommendation against
Selective	No recommendation	(C) MF 18+ for suicide risk if one or more: evidence of psychiatric disorder, substance abuse, family history of suicide attempt	MF 18+ for suicide risk if one or more: adolescent, young adult, personal or family history of depression, chronic illness living alone, recent bereavement or separation or unemployment, sleep disturbance, multiple somatic complaints, drug or alcohol abuse
Assessment of visual impairment			
General	Not considered	(C) No recommendation	MF 18–39 Recommendation against
Selective	Not considered	(C) No recommendation	No recommendation
Assessment of hearing impairment			
General	Not considered	(B) MF 18+ by history	None for young adult
Selective	Not considered	MF 18+ by history if one or more: exposure to jet engines or other noisy machinery, farm equipment amplified music, gunfire, snowmobiles, or model airplanes for more than 2 hr several times per week	MF 19+ if regularly exposed to excessive noise

Adapted from Hayward RSA, Steinbert EP, Ford DE, et al. Preventive care guidelines: 1991. Ann Intern Med 1991;114:758–783.
Strength of Recommendations
Classification:
A: Good evidence supports the recommendation that the intervention be included.
B: Fair evidence supports the recommendation that the intervention be included.
C: Poor evidence supports the inclusion or exclusion of the intervention, but recommendations may be made on other grounds.
D: Fair evidence supports the recommendation that the intervention be excluded from consideration.
E: Good evidence supports the recommendation that the intervention be excluded from consideration.
CAD, coronary artery disease; CSF, cerebrospinal fluid; DM, diabetes mellitus; F, female; HDL, high-density lipoprotein; HIV, human immunodeficiency virus; IBW, ideal body weight; IV, intravenous; M, male; PVD, peripheral vascular disease; STD, sexually transmitted disease; TB, tuberculosis. *Table continued on following page.*

Table 4.3. *continued*

Area/Vaccine or Drug/Topic	American College of Physicians	Canadian Task Force on Periodic Health Examination	U.S. Preventive Services Task Force
Examination of oral cavity to detect oral cancer			
General	Not considered	(C) Not for young adults	Recommendation against
Selective	Not considered	(C) MF 18+ if tobacco use	MF 18+ if one or more: tobacco use, excessive alcohol exposure, suspicious lesions detected through self-examination
Thyroid palpation			
General	Not considered	Not considered	No recommendation
Selective	Not considered	Not considered	MF 18+ if personal history of upper body radiation
Complete skin examination			
General	Not considered	(D) Recommendation against	Recommendation against
Selective	Not considered	(B) MF 18+ if one or more: outdoor occupation, contact with polycyclic aromatic hydrocarbons	MF 18+ if one or more: increased sun exposure, personal or family history of skin cancer, dysplastic nevi or congenital nevi
Breast examination by clinician			
General	None for young adult	None for young adult	None for young adult
Selective	F 18+ q1yr if personal history of breast cancer	F 35+ q1yr if family history of premenopausal breast cancer in a first-degree relative or otherwise at high risk	(C) F 35+ q1yr if family history of premenopausal breast cancer in a first-degree relative
Pelvic examination by bimanual palpation			
General	Not considered	Not considered	Recommendation against unless doing gynecologic examination for other reasons
Selective	Not considered	Not considered	No recommendation
Testicular examination			
General	Not considered	(C) No recommendation	No recommendation
Selective	Not considered	M 18+ if one or more: cryptorchidism, ambiguous sex, testicular atrophy	M 19–39 if one or more: cryptorchidism, orchiopexy, testicular atrophy
Digital rectal examination for prostate cancer			
General	Not considered	(C) No recommendation	No recommendation
Selective	Not considered	No recommendation	No recommendation
Laboratory test recommendations			
Hemoglobin measurement for iron deficiency anemia			
General	Recommendation against	(C) Recommendation against	Recommendation against
Selective	F 18+ if recent immigrant from underdeveloped country	F 18–64 if of low socioeconomic status	No recommendation
Urine analysis			
General	Recommendation against screening for bacteriuria	(D) Recommendation against screening for bacteriuria or for bladder cancer	(C) None for young adults
Selective	Recommendation against	(B) MF 18+ urine cytology to screen bladder cancer in smokers and persons occupationally exposed to bladder carcinogens	(C) MF 18+ to screen for bacteriuria if diabetic

TABLE 4.3. *continued*

Area/Vaccine or Drug/Topic	American College of Physicians	Canadian Task Force on Periodic Health Examination	U.S. Preventive Services Task Force
Fasting plasma glucose			
General	Recommendation against	(D) Recommendation against	Recommendation against
Selective	F 18+ if intends to become pregnant and has risk factors for DM as listed below MF 18+ if one or more: DM in first-degree relative, age >50 yr, weight >25% over IBW, personal history of gestational DM, membership in ethnic group with high prevalence of DM	(B) MF 18+ if one or more: family history of DM, hyperglycemia associated with pregnancy, evidence of early occlusive vascular disease	MF 18+ if one or more: family history of DM, marked obesity, personal history of gestational DM
Nonfasting cholesterol			
General	MF 18+ q5yr	(C) M 30–59	(C) MF 18+ q5yr
Selective	MF 18+ more frequently if one or more: smoker, family history of hypercholesterolemia or premature cardiovascular in a parent or sibling, use of lipid-altering drugs, hypertension, CAD, or secondary cause of hyperlipidemia such as DM	No recommendation	MF 18+ more frequently if one or more: previous abnormal cholesterol, male, early CAD in a first-degree relative smoker, hypertension, HDL <35 mg/dL, DM, previous stroke or PVD, severe obesity
Thyroid function testing			
General	Recommendation against	(D) Recommendation against screening for hyperthyroidism (C) Recommendation against screening for hypothyroidism	Recommendation against
Selective	None for young adults	None for young adults	None for young adults
HIV serology			
General	Recommendation against	Not considered	(C) Recommendation against
Selective	MF 18+ if one or more: member of a high-risk group by virtue of sexual or drug-taking behavior, woman of child-bearing age with any risks for HIV infection, received blood transfusion between 1978 and 1985, person planning marriage who may be at increased risk	Not considered	(C) MF 18+ if one or more: recently acquired STD, homosexual or bisexual man or partner of same, IV drug abuser, prostitute, has multiple sexual contacts or partner of same, received blood transfusion between 1978 and 1985, long-term resident of high-prevalence area

Table continued on following page.

TABLE 4.3. *continued*

Area/Vaccine or Drug/Topic	American College of Physicians	Canadian Task Force on Periodic Health Examination	U.S. Preventive Services Task Force
Syphilis serology			
General	Recommendation against	(D) Recommendation against	Recommendation against
Selective	MF 18+ if one or more: sexual contact of known case; member of a high-risk group, such as homosexuals; resident of area of high prevalence	(A) MF 18+ if multiple sexual partners	(B) MF 18+ if one or more: sexual contact of proved case, prostitute, has multiple sexual partners, resident of area of high prevalence
Resting electrocardiogram			
General	MF 18–65 recommendation against	(C) Recommendation against	Recommendation against
Selective	MF 18+ no recommendation if one or more cardiac risk factor(s) present	No recommendation	M 18+ if a cardiac event would endanger public safety
Tuberculin skin testing (PPD)			
General	Not considered	(E) Recommendation against	Recommendation against
Selective	Not considered	(A) MF 18+ if exposed to TB at home or work or living in community with high infection rate	MF 18+ if one or more: exposed to TB case in the home, clinics or shelters for the homeless, substance abuse treatment centers, dialysis units, correctional institutions, recent immigrants or refugees from high prevalence areas; migrant workers; HIV or renal failure; immunosuppressive drugs, including steroids
Chest radiograph to detect lung cancer All three groups recommend against in smokers and nonsmokers			
Mammography			
General	All three groups only recommend after the age of 50		
Selective	F 18+ q1yr if personal history of breast cancer	F 35+ q1yr if at high risk	F 35+ q1yr if family history of premenopausal breast cancer in a first-degree relative
Pap smear			
General	F 20–65 q3yr	(B) F 18–35 q3yr	F 18–65 q1–3yr
Selective	F 20–65 q2yr if at increased risk after consideration of risk factors	(B) F 18+ q1yr if one or both: early onset of sexual activity, multiple sexual partners	F 18+ more frequently if one or more: early onset of sexual activity, multiple sexual partners, low socioeconomic status
Gonorrhea culture			
General	Not considered	(D) Recommendation against	Recommendation against
Selective	Not considered	(A) MF 18+ if multiple sexual partners	(A) MF 18–64 if one or more: prostitute, multiple sexual partners, sexual contact with proved cases, history of repeated STDs

TABLE 4.3.   *continued*

Area/Vaccine or Drug/Topic	American College of Physicians	Canadian Task Force on Periodic Health Examination	U.S. Preventive Services Task Force
Chlamydia testing			
General	Not considered	(D) Recommendation against	Recommendation against
Selective	Not considered	(C) MF 18+ if in high-risk group such as partners of persons with nongono-coccal urethritis	MF 18–64 if one or more: attending STD clinic or other health setting that sees high-risk patients, multiple sexual partners, partner with multiple sexual contacts, partner of persons with positive culture
Stool examination for occult blood			
General	Not for young adults	MF 18–39 recommendation against	(C) No recommendation
Selective	Not for young adults	Not for young adults	Not for young adults
Adult immunizations			
Hepatitis B (inactivated virus vaccine)			
General	Recommendation against	Recommendation against	Recommendation against
Selective	MF 18+ initial series if at increased risk for occupational, environ-mental, social, or fam-ily exposure, intimate family contact with infected persons, resi-dent of institutions for the mentally retarded, prison inmate, home-less person, homosex-ual or bisexual man, person with multiple STDs or partner of same, intimate contact with persons from endemic areas, early renal disease or hemo-philia, health-care worker, IV drug abuser	(A) MF 18+ initial series if one or more: dialysis, blood product exposure, health-care personnel, institutionalized mentally retarded person, IV drug abuser, homosexual, contact with patients with disease or carriers	(A) MF 18+ initial series if one or more: homosexual man, IV drug user, blood product recipient, health-care worker with blood product exposure
Inactivated influenza vaccine			
General	Not for young adult	(E) MF 18–64 recommenda-tion against	Not for young adults
Selective	MF 18–64 q1yr if one or more: resident of long-term care facility, health-care occupa-tion, chronic cardio-pulmonary disorder or other chronic disease requiring regular med-ical care (HIV-infected patient, organ trans-plant recipient, alco-holic, cancer patient), person providing care to high-risk persons, or resident of area with increased risk for exposure	(A) MF 18+ q1yr if chronic debilitating disease	(A) MF 18+ q1yr if one or more: resident of long-term care facility, chronic cardiopulmonary disease, hemoglobinopathy, diabetes, metabolic disease, renal dysfunction, immunosuppression; health-care provider for high-risk patients

Table continued on following page.

Table 4.3. *continued*

Area/Vaccine or Drug/Topic	American College of Physicians	Canadian Task Force on Periodic Health Examination	U.S. Preventive Services Task Force
Measles live virus vaccine (most use MMR)			
General	No recommendation	Not considered	No recommendation
Selective	MF 18+ two doses if born after 1956 and without documentation of receipt of live vaccine, physician-diagnosed measles, or laboratory evidence of immunity; revaccinate if college student or health-care worker and previously given only one dose of vaccine or killed measles vaccine	Not considered	MF 18+ once if born after 1956 and no proof of immunity, documentation of receipt of live vaccine or physician-documented measles
Pneumococcal polysaccharide 23-valent vaccine			
General	Not for young adults	Not for young adults	Not for young adults
Selective	MF 18–64 once if one or more: chronic cardiac or pulmonary disease, asplenia chronic liver disease, alcoholism, DM, chronic renal failure, hematologic malignancy, chemotherapy organ transplant recipient, HIV infection, CSF leak	(A) MF 18+ once if one or more: sickle cell anemia, asplenia	MF 18+ once if one or more: chronic cardiac or pulmonary disease, sickle cell disease, the nephrotic syndrome, Hodgkin's disease, asplenia, DM, alcoholism, cirrhosis, renal disease, immunosuppression, HIV infection
Rubella live virus vaccine			
General	Recommendation against by all three groups		
Selective	MF 18+ once if lacking documentation of receipt of live vaccine on or after first birthday, particularly women of child-bearing age and young adults studying or working in educational, health-care, or military institutions	(A) F 18–44 once if lacking proof of immunity and agreeing not to become pregnant for 3 months	(A) F 18 to menopause once if lacking proof of vaccination or serologic evidence of immunity and agreeing not to become pregnant for 3 months
Tetanus-diphtheria toxoid			
General	MF 18+ q10yr	(A) MF 18+ q10yr	(A) MF 18+ q10yr
Selective	No recommendation	No recommendation	No recommendation
Healthy lifestyles and preventive counseling recommendations			
Caloric balance	MF 18+ provide guidelines for a healthful, well-balanced diet and encourage behavior modification to reduce and obesity	Not considered	MF 18+ provide diet and exercise advice to all persons to achieve and maintain desirable weight by keeping caloric intake balanced with energy expenditures

TABLE 4.3. *continued*

Area/Vaccine or Drug/Topic	American College of Physicians	Canadian Task Force on Periodic Health Examination	U.S. Preventive Services Task Force
Fat, cholesterol	MF 18+ advise to reduce intake of calories from fat to 25–30% or less of total calorie intake	Not considered	MF 18+ give dietary guidance on how to reduce total fat intake to less than 30% of total calories, saturated fat consumption to less than 10% of total calories, and dietary cholesterol to less than 300 mg/day
Fiber	MF 18+ advise to eat more high-fiber foods such as whole grain cereals, legumes, vegetables, and fruits	Not considered	MF 18+ encourage patients to eat a variety of foods with emphasis on whole grain products, cereals, vegetables, and fruits
Sodium	MF 18+ advise to limit consumption of salt-cured, smoked, and nitrite-preserved foods	Not considered	MF 18+ advise patients to eat foods low in sodium and to limit salt added to food in preparation or consumption
Calcium		(C) F 18+ maintain liberal intake of natural and supplemental calcium	F 18+ counsel about methods to ensure adequate calcium intake
Iron		F 18–44 selective counseling for women of low socio-economic status, food faddists	F 18–64 all menstruating women, counsel about adequate iron intake
Physical activity and exercise			
Physical activity		No recommendation for young adults	MF 18+ provide all patients with information on the role of regular physical activity in disease prevention and assist in selecting appropriate type of exerciser
Cancer Surveillance			
Skin self-examination		Not considered	No recommendation
Breast self-examination	F 20+ every month	F 18–40 no recommendation	(C) No recommendation
	(American Cancer Society: F 20+ every month)		
Testes self-examination		(C) No recommendation	No recommendation
	(American Cancer Society: M 18+ every month)		
Sexual practices			
STDs		Not considered	(B) MF 18+ use of barrier methods to reduce risk of STD (C) MF 18-64 counsel about STD transmission, partner selection, condom use, avoiding anal intercourse
HIV		Not considered	(A) MF 18+ teach blood, needle, sexual behavior precautions for same high-risk groups for whom HIV testing is indicated
Unintended pregnancy		(B) F 18+ prevent unwanted pregnancy by asking teen-agers about sexual activity and recommending appropriate contraception	MF 18–64 counsel about unintended pregnancy and contraceptive options

Table continued on following page.

TABLE 4.3.   *continued*

Area/Vaccine or Drug/Topic	American College of Physicians	Canadian Task Force on Periodic Health Examination	U.S. Preventive Services Task Force
Substance abuse			
Tobacco	MF 18+ actively counsel patients to quit smoking	(A) MF 18+ counsel to prevent tobacco use; emphasize if one or more: ocp use, DM hypertension, high cholesterol level; asbestos, uranium, silica, grain exposure	(A) MF 18+ repeated smoking cessation messages from multiple sources over an extended period of time; primary prevention messages to nonsmoking adolescents
Alcohol	MF 18+ patient education and counseling about the appropriate use of alcohol	(B) MF 18–64 case finding to identify problem drinking, followed by counseling	MF 18+ counsel to limit alcohol consumption, to stop alcohol consumption during pregnancy, not to drive after drinking
Intravenous street drugs	MF 18+ patient education and counseling about licit and illicit drugs	Not considered	MF 18–64 counsel IV drug users about dangers of psychoactive drug use, encourage cessation of drug use, alert to risks of using unsterilized needles
Injury prevention			
Motor vehicle accident	MF 18+ counsel patients to use seat belts	(C) MF 18–64 ask and teach about seat belt safety; control underlying medical conditions that increase risks associated with driving	(C) MF 18+ advise about seat belt use, alcohol or drug-related risks with driving, general road safety, motorcycle helmet use
Back injuries		Not considered	MF 18–64 teach injury prevention if one or more: previous back injury, high-risk body configuration, current or planned high-risk activities
Fire injuries		(C) Encourage safety in home and community	MF 18+ encourage smoke detector installation and maintenance and discuss danger of smoking near bed or upholstery
Violence		Not considered	M 19–39 teach dangers of hand weapons and violent behavior; keep firearms in child-resistant containers
Promoting dental health			
Dental hygiene		(A) MF 18–74 q1yr, encourage daily oral hygiene, dental visits	(A) MF 18+ q1yr (plaque) (C) MF 18+ q1yr (caries), encourage regular tooth brushing, flossing, dental visits
Stress and bereavement			
Functional assessment	Not considered	(C) MF 18–64 elicit history of marital and sexual problems	MF 18+ remain alert for symptoms of abnormal bereavement, depression, physical abuse, and suicide risk in persons with recent bereavement, divorce, separation, unemployment, alcohol or other substance abuse, depression, living alone or serious medical illness

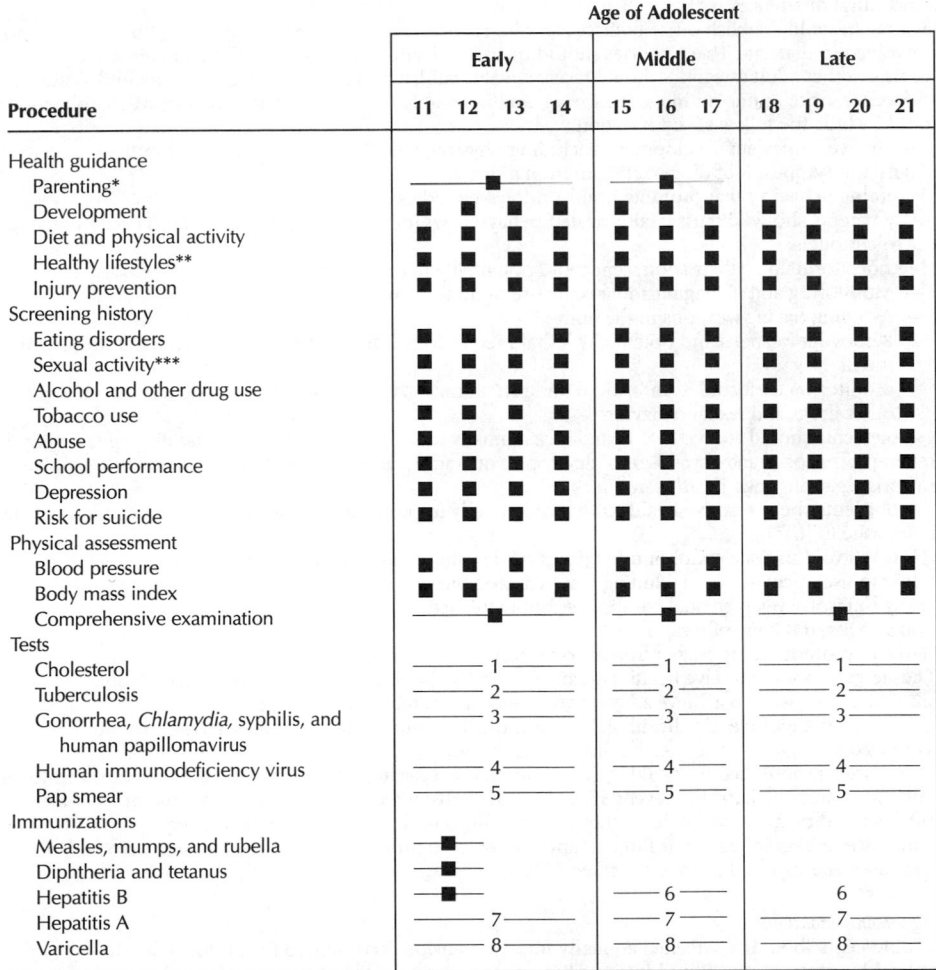

Procedure	Age of Adolescent										
	Early				Middle			Late			
	11	12	13	14	15	16	17	18	19	20	21
Health guidance											
Parenting*		■			■						
Development	■	■	■	■	■	■	■	■	■	■	■
Diet and physical activity	■	■	■	■	■	■	■	■	■	■	■
Healthy lifestyles**	■	■	■	■	■	■	■	■	■	■	■
Injury prevention	■	■	■	■	■	■	■	■	■	■	■
Screening history											
Eating disorders	■	■	■	■	■	■	■	■	■	■	■
Sexual activity***	■	■	■	■	■	■	■	■	■	■	■
Alcohol and other drug use	■	■	■	■	■	■	■	■	■	■	■
Tobacco use	■	■	■	■	■	■	■	■	■	■	■
Abuse	■	■	■	■	■	■	■	■	■	■	■
School performance	■	■	■	■	■	■	■	■	■	■	■
Depression	■	■	■	■	■	■	■	■	■	■	■
Risk for suicide	■	■	■	■	■	■	■	■	■	■	■
Physical assessment											
Blood pressure	■	■	■	■	■	■	■	■	■	■	■
Body mass index	■	■	■	■	■	■	■	■	■	■	■
Comprehensive examination			■			■			■		
Tests											
Cholesterol			1			1			1		
Tuberculosis			2			2			2		
Gonorrhea, *Chlamydia*, syphilis, and human papillomavirus			3			3			3		
Human immunodeficiency virus			4			4			4		
Pap smear			5			5			5		
Immunizations											
Measles, mumps, and rubella	■										
Diphtheria and tetanus	■										
Hepatitis B	■					6			6		
Hepatitis A			7			7			7		
Varicella			8			8			8		

1. Screening test performed once if family history is positive for early cardiovascular disease or hyperlipidemia.
2. Screen if positive for exposure to active TB or lives/works in high-risk situation (e.g., homeless shelter, health care facility).
3. Screen at least annually if sexually active.
4. Screen if high risk for infection.
5. Screen annually if sexually active or if 18 years or older.

6. Vaccinate if high risk for hepatitis B infection.
7. Vaccinate if at risk for hepatitis A infection.
8. Vaccinate if no reliable history of chicken pox.
* A parent health guidance visit is recommended during early and middle adolescence.
** Includes counseling regarding sexual behavior and avoidance of tobacco, alcohol, and other drug use.
*** Includes history of unintended pregnancy and sexually transmitted disease.

FIGURE 4.1. Recommended frequency of GAPS preventive services. (From GAPS Executive Committee, Department of Adolescent Health. American Medical Association guidelines for adolescent preventive services, recommendations monograph. Chicago: American Medical Association, 1995:2.)

TABLE 4.4.   GAPS Recommendations

1. From ages 11–21, all adolescents should have an annual preventive services visit.
   a. These visits should address both biomedical and psychosocial aspects.
   b. Complete physical examinations should be done during three of these preventive visits.
      One each during early (11–14), middle (15–17), and late (18–21) adolescence
2. Preventive services should be age and developmentally appropriate and should be sensitive to individual and sociocultural differences.
3. Physicians should establish office policies regarding confidential care for adolescents and how parents will be involved in that care. These policies should be made clear to adolescents and their parents.
4. Parents or other adult caregivers should receive health guidance at least once during their child's early adolescence, once during middle adolescence, and preferably once during late adolescence. Health guidance should include the following information:
   a. Normative adolescent development, including physical, sexual, and emotional development
   b. Signs and symptoms of disease and emotional distress
   c. Parenting behaviors that promote healthy adolescent adjustment
   d. Why parents should discuss health-related behaviors with their adolescents, plan family activities, and act as role models
   e. Methods for helping their adolescent avoid potentially harmful behaviors:
      — Monitoring and managing adolescents use of motor vehicles
      — Avoiding having weapons in the home
      — Removing weapons and potentially lethal medications from the homes of adolescents with suicidal intent
      — Monitoring their adolescent's social and recreational activities for the use of tobacco, alcohol, and other drugs and sexual behavior
5. All adolescents should receive health guidance annually to promote a better understanding of their physical growth, psychosocial and psychosexual development, and the importance of becoming actively involved in decisions regarding their health care.
6. All adolescents should receive health guidance annually to promote the reduction of injuries. Counseling includes the following:
   a. How to avoid use of alcohol or other drugs while using motor or recreational vehicles
   b. How to use safety devices, including seat belts and bicycle helmets
   c. How to resolve interpersonal conflicts without violence
   d. How to avoid the use of weapons
   e. How to promote appropriate physical conditioning before exercise
7. All adolescents should receive health guidance annually about dietary habits, including the benefits of a healthy diet, and ways to achieve a healthy diet and safe weight management.
8. All adolescents should receive health guidance annually about the benefits of exercise and should be encouraged to engage in safe exercise on a regular basis.
9. All adolescents should receive health guidance annually regarding responsible sexual behaviors, including abstinence. Latex condoms to prevent STDs, including HIV infection, and appropriate methods of birth control should be made available, as should instructions on how to use them effectively.
10. All adolescents should receive health guidance annually to promote avoidance of tobacco, alcohol, other abusable substances, and anabolic steroids.

Screening recommendations
11. All adolescents should be screened annually for hypertension according to the protocol developed by the National Heart, Lung, and Blood Institute Second Task Force on Blood Pressure Control in Children.
12. Selected adolescents should be screened to determine their risk of developing hyperlipidemia and adult coronary heart disease, following the protocol developed by the Expert Panel on Blood Cholesterol Levels in Children and Adolescents.
13. All adolescents should be screened annually for eating disorders and obesity by determining weight and stature, and asking about body image and dieting patterns.
14. All adolescents should be asked annually about their use of tobacco products, including cigarettes and smokeless tobacco.
15. All adolescents should be asked annually about their use of alcohol and other abusable substances and about their use of over-the-counter or prescription drugs for nonmedical purposes, including anabolic steroids.
    a. Adolescents whose substance use endangers their health should receive counseling and mental health treatment, as appropriate.
    b. Adolescents who use anabolic steroids should be counseled to stop.
    c. The use of urine toxicology for the routine screening of adolescents is not recommended.

Adapted from GAPS Executive Committee, Department of Adolescent Health. American Medical Association guidelines for adolescent preventive services. Chicago: AMA, 1992.

TABLE 4.4. *continued*

16. All adolescents should be asked annually about involvement in sexual behaviors that may result in unintended pregnancy and STDs, including HIV infections.
    a. Sexually active adolescents should be asked about their use and motivation to use condoms and contraceptive methods, their sexual orientation, the number of sexual partners they have had in the past 6 months, if they have exchanged sex for money or drugs, and their history of prior pregnancy or STDs.
    b. Adolescents at risk for pregnancy, STDs, or sexual exploitation should be counseled on how to reduce this risk.
17. Sexually active adolescents should be screened for STDs. STD screening includes the following:
    a. Cervical culture (females) or urine leukocyte esterase analysis (males) to screen for gonorrhea
    b. An immunologic test of cervical fluid (female) or urine leukocyte esterase analysis (male) to screen for genital *Chlamydia*
    c. A serologic test for syphilis if individual has lived in an area endemic for syphilis, has had other STDs, has had more than one sexual partner within the last 6 months, has exchanged sex for drugs or money, or is a male who has engaged in sex with other male(s)
    d. Evaluation for human papilloma virus by visual inspection (males and females) and by Pap test.
    The frequency of screening for STDs depends on the sexual practices of the individual and the history of previous STDs.
18. Adolescents at risk for HIV infection should be offered confidential HIV screening with the ELISA and confirmatory test. Testing should be performed only after informed consent is obtained from the adolescent and should be performed in conjunction with both pretest and posttest counseling.
19. Female adolescents who are sexually active or any female 18 or older should be screened annually for cervical cancer by use of a Pap test.
20. All adolescents should be asked annually about behaviors or emotions that indicate recurrent or severe depression or risk of suicide.
21. All adolescents should be asked annually about a history of emotional, physical, and sexual abuse.
22. All adolescents should be asked annually about learning or school problems.
23. Adolescents should receive a tuberculin skin test if they have been exposed to active tuberculosis, have lived in a homeless shelter, have been incarcerated, have lived in or come from an area with a high prevalence of tuberculosis, or currently work in a health-care setting.

Recommendations for immunizations
24. All adolescents should receive prophylactic immunizations according to the guidelines established by the federally convened Advisory Committee on Immunization Practices.
    a. Adolescents should receive a bivalent dT vaccine 10 years after their previous DPT vaccination.
    b. All adolescents should receive a second trivalent MMR vaccination, unless there is documentation of two vaccinations earlier during childhood. An MMR should not be given to adolescents who are pregnant.
    c. Susceptible adolescents who engage in high-risk behaviors should be vaccinated against hepatitis B virus. Widespread use of the hepatitis B vaccine is encouraged because risk factors are often not easily identifiable among adolescents. Universal hepatitis B vaccination should be implemented in communities where IV drug use, adolescent pregnancy, or STD infections are common.

Certain developmental traits and health behaviors of adolescents make the availability of certain services such as reproductive health services, sexually transmitted disease treatment, and mental health and substance abuse counseling and treatment extremely critical. Guidelines for health screening is only part of the issue. To serve adolescents appropriately, preventive and treatment services must be available in a wide range of health care settings. These include physicians offices, health maintenance organizations (HMOs), community-based adolescent health and family planning and public health clinics, and school-based and school-linked health clinics. Coverage for these services will continue to become a larger issue with the expansion of managed health-care systems. National standards such as those discussed in this chapter (GAPS) may help to increase the possibility that insurers will cover adolescent preventive services. However, provision of comprehensive preventive and treatment services to adolescents nationwide is a lofty goal requiring further integration of services across multiple access points, including public, private, school, and community settings.

General Suggestions for Evaluation

Because the adolescent is no longer a child but is not yet an adult, the pediatrician, internist, or family practitioner may be a bit uneasy during the evaluation. The following considerations are important to keep in mind and should make the screening evaluation process more comfortable for both the teenager and practitioner.

1. Much of the history should be obtained directly from the teenager, with the parents out of the room.
2. A sense of confidentiality should be established so that the teenager feels comfortable with the physician and trusts him or her enough to discuss delicate subjects. In sensitive areas, the examiner should try to approach the teen from a direct, but empathetic and nonjudgmental, stance.
3. Creating an appropriate atmosphere for screening and evaluation includes minimizing interruptions, avoiding phone calls, and avoiding thumbing through charts.
4. In addition to the time spent alone with the adolescent, some time should be reserved to talk alone with the parent(s) and to talk with the family as a unit.
5. There should be adequate time left at the end of the evaluation to summarize the session and for questions from the adolescent.
6. The physical examination provides a perfect chance to discuss concerns that the adolescent might have about a particular area. An opportunity to discuss self-examination techniques for the breasts and testes for older adolescents can occur as part of the physical examination.
7. There should be an opportunity to discuss risk-taking behaviors such as use of drugs or alcohol, drinking and driving, and legal difficulties.

Health-Screening Forms

There is considerable debate as to whether a personal interview or a screening form allows for more rapid securing of confidential material. The answer is probably best left to the discretion of the individual practitioner or health center. At the end of this chapter are several sample health questionnaires for adolescents. Figure 4.2 is a short questionnaire for teens. Included with this questionnaire is the Family APGAR developed by Smilkstein (1984) at the Department of Family Medicine, University of Washington. The Family APGAR is a short screening questionnaire designed to examine satisfaction with the variables of adaptation, partnership, growth, affection, and resolve in the respondent's family. These five questions are rated on a 0–2 scale with a 0–10 total score (2 = almost always, 1 = some of the time, 0 = hardly ever). The Family APGAR has been validated by correlating it with both a previously validated instrument (Pless Satterwhite Family Function Index) and therapist-assessed family function. Mean Family APGAR scores from various groups include:

College students	7.6
Psychiatric outpatients	5.8
Family medicine patients	8.2

Adolescent clinic patients (Shapiro et al., 1987):

Total	6.0
Teens living at home	6.5
Teens living in residential placement	4.0
Teens with suicidal ideation	2.6
Teens with family problems identified on interview	3.8

Figure 4.3 is a more comprehensive teen health form. Figure 4.4 is a short form for parents, and Figure 4.5 is a more comprehensive form for parents. Figure 4.6 is a comprehensive history and physical examination form. These forms are intended only as guidelines for practitioners or clinics interested in developing their own forms. Schubiner et al. (1994) has also developed the SAFE TIMES Questionnaire, which has been shown to be effective in the identification of problem areas in adolescents. Other example forms are available from the Ohio Academy of Family Physicians, 4074 North High Street, Columbus, OH 43214. In addition to screening forms, Paperny has developed a set of interactive computerized programs for teens on areas such as psychosocial risk profile, adolescent pregnancy, and family planning. These are available by writing:

David Paperny, Teen Health Computer Programs, 2516 Pacific Heights Road, Honolulu, HI 96813-1027.

Interactive videos that both identify risks and provide health educational information are under development. The remainder of the chapter discusses specific aspects of screening and evaluation.

Date: _____

These are some questions that many people think about, but have a hard time asking. Perhaps it would be easier for you to just check (✓) anything that you would be interested in asking or finding out. You may leave any question or the whole form blank if you wish. This form will not become part of your permanent hospital record.

1. Do you think something could be wrong with your:

____Height	____Ears	____Heart
____Weight	____Nose	____Stomach (pain, vomiting)
____Head	____Mouth, teeth	____Skin (rash, acne)
____Eyes	____Neck	____Sexual organs
____Back	____Chest, breasts	____Arms/legs/hands/feet
____Appearance (looks)	____Mind (thinking)	____Lungs/breathing

2. Do you have any questions about:

____Menstrual periods	____Dating	____Diets/foods
____Having children	____Masturbation	____Dying
____Pregnancy	____Rape/sexual abuse	____Habits
____Sex	____Jobs	____Smoking
____Birth control	____Drugs/alcohol	____Your future
____Sexually transmitted diseases (HIV/herpes/ warts/gonorrhea)	____Exercise ____Homosexuality	____Other

3. Do you have any problems with:

____Friends	____Others at school	____Controlling temper
____No friends	____Grades at school	____Nothing to do
____Brothers/sisters	____Teachers	____Thoughts about killing
____Parents/family	____Ability to learn	yourself
____Family members or friends who drink too much alcohol	____Privacy ____Eating ____Sleeping	____Feeling unsafe ____Depression ____Drugs/alcohol
____Weight	____Gangs	

FIGURE 4.2. Short screening questionnaire for teenagers, developed at the Childrens Hospital of Los Angeles. Family APGAR from Smilkstein G. The family APGAR: a proposal for a family function test and its use by physicians. J Fam Pract 1984;6:1231. *Figure continued on following page.*

4. Would you like to see someone at the Teenage Health Center to discuss any personal concerns (relationships, family, school, drugs, alcohol, sexuality, etc.)? Yes ____ No ____

5. Do you like yourself? (circle one number)

5	4	3	2	1
Yes, a lot	Usually	Sometimes	Not a lot	Almost never

6. Do you think you are healthy? (circle one)

Yes	Usually	Sometimes	Usually not	No

7. Other questions or problems you want to discuss:

8. For each sentence, please check (✓) one of the answers that best fits the way you feel.

	Almost Always	Some of the Time	Hardly Ever
I am satisfied with the help that I receive from members of my family when something is troubling me.	____	____	____
I am satisfied with the way members of my family discuss items of common interest and share problem solving with me.	____	____	____
I find that members of my family accept my wishes to take on new activities or make changes.	____	____	____
I am satisfied with the way members of my family express affection and respond to my feelings such as anger, sorrow, and love.	____	____	____
I am satisfied with the way members of my family and I share time together.	____	____	____

Please use this space if you wish to comment or explain any of the above.

FIGURE 4.2. *continued*

HISTORY

The history is the most important aspect of the screening evaluation. Essential areas include family history, past medical history, review of systems, psychosocial history, and current medical problems.

Past Medical History

Past medical history should be obtained from both the parents and the adolescent, including the following:

1. Childhood infections and illnesses
2. Prior hospitalizations and surgery
3. Prior accidents
4. Allergies
5. Prescription and over-the-counter medications
6. Disabilities
7. Immunization history
8. Developmental history
   a. Prenatal, perinatal, and infancy history
   b. History of problems with walking, talking, eating, or learning
   c. Peer relations
   d. School functioning

Name_____   Date_____

A. GENERAL INFORMATION

1. Full Name _____   2. Sex: Male _____ Female _____
3. Address _____
4. Name you would like to be called _____
5. Home phone_____   6. When were you born? _____
   month day year
7. If it is necessary to contact you about an appointment or tests, may we:
   Call you? yes ____ no ____ (if yes, no message will be left unless you wish us to)
                              ____ leave message
   Write you? yes ____ no ____
8. In case of an emergency, whom should we call?
   Name_____   Phone _____
9. Is this clinic the main place you go for health care? yes ____ no ____
10. What other places do you go for health care or counseling? This is very important be-
    cause it may be necessary to check records at other places to find out about diseases you
    have had, medicines prescribed, or tests that have been done in the past. It can save you
    time and money and be useful in helping you with current or future problems. *We will
    not get this information unless you sign a permission slip.*
    Private doctor or clinic (name)_____
    _____
11. When did you last have (please give approximate dates):
    A dental exam? _____
    An eye exam?_____
    A physical exam?_____
12. Is there anything about your health that worries you? (please specify)

B. PRESENT HEALTH CONCERNS

13. On a scale of one to ten, how would you rate your general health?
    1   2   3   4   5   6   7   8   9   10
    awful   great
14. Do any of these common concerns apply to you? Check those that do:

____Trouble falling asleep	____Skin problems
____Waking up in the night	____Worried about parents
____Being tired during the day	____Trouble with school or teachers
____Wetting the bed	____Troubled about future plans
____Headaches	____Feeling down or depressed
____Stomachaches	____Problems with periods
____Dizzy spells	____Worried about a place to live
____Leg pains	____Worried about sex or pregnancy
____Worried about my height or weight	____Other (explain) _____

15. As you probably know, drugs change your body chemistry. If certain drugs are taken to-
    gether they can have a bad reaction; they can cancel each other out or can produce vi-
    olent or dangerous changes in your body. It's important to know what you are currently
    taking so we can avoid giving you any drugs that might have a bad reaction. Are you tak-
    ing any drugs that were prescribed by a doctor? no ____ yes ____
16. If yes, what drugs and for what problem? _____
    _____

FIGURE 4.3.   Comprehensive screening questionnaire for teenagers, used by the Adolescent Health Program, University of Minnesota. (From Blum R, ed, Adolescent health care. New York: Academic Press,
1982.)   *Figure continues through page 83.*

17. What about using any other drugs—either street drugs or nonprescription drugs? Check those that apply (of course, all information that you give will be private and will be shared with no one outside the clinic):
    ____Aspirin   ____Water pills
    ____Laxatives   ____Midol
    ____Pain pills   ____Diet pills
    ____No Doz   ____Marijuana
    ____Sleeping pills   ____Speed
    ____Cold pills   ____Methadone
    ____Cigarettes   ____Heroin
    ____Alcohol (beer, wine, liquor)   ____Other (specify) _____

18. Is your drug taking something you would like to talk about with someone at the clinic? no ____ yes ____

19. Allergies are also important to know about. Especially important are those that cause you major problems. Have you ever had an allergic reaction to anything such as drugs, food, animals, or plants? An allergic reaction could mean sneezing, breaking out in a rash, itching, or having trouble breathing.
    no ____ yes ____ What things caused it? _____

20. Sex is often an important part of people's lives. Though it's very private and sometimes embarrassing, we hope you will share some information with us so we can better help meet your personal needs, concerns, and questions. This information, of course, like the rest of your history and exam, is strictly confidential. If you are having sex, what kind(s) of birth control methods do you and your partner now use?
    ____Not having sex   ____Condoms (rubbers)
    ____None   ____Diaphragm
    ____Withdrawal   ____I.U.D. (intrauterine device)
    ____Rhythm   ____Pill
    ____Foam   ____Other (explain) _____

21. Have you used other birth control methods in the past? no ____ yes ____ If you have, what did you use and why did you stop using it?_____
    _____

22. Do you have pain or bleeding associated with intercourse? no ____ yes ____

23. Do you have any questions about sex or birth control that you would like to talk about with someone at the clinic? no ____ yes ____

24. Have you ever been sexually mistreated by a member of your family? no ____ yes ____
    By someone else? no ____ yes ____

25. Is this something you would like to talk about with someone at the clinic? no ____ yes ____

C. GENERAL HEALTH

26. If you could have three wishes come true, what would they be?
    1._____
    2._____
    3._____

27. Have any of the following *recently happened* to you or a member of your immediate family?
    ____Marriage   ____Given birth   ____Death
    ____Divorce   ____Loss of job   ____Moved away from home

28. On a scale of one to ten, how well is your life going so far?
    1 2 3 4 5 6 7 8 9 10
    terrible   terrific

29. What would you like to change about your life?

30. Who do you talk to when things are not going well? _____

31. Are you employed and, if so, where? _____

Figure 4.3. *continued*

32. Are you exposed to any chemicals or loud noises on your job? no ____ yes ____
    If so, what?_____

33. Do you go to school? no ____ yes ____ Where?_____

34. What do you like *best* about school or work?

35. What do you like *least* about school or work?

36. Now, think for a few minutes about this list of general health habits. Are there any things you would like to change? If YES, please check the appropriate space:
    Would like to change

____Nutrition or diet	____Using drugs
____Exercise	____Getting along better with my family
____Smoking	____Doing better in school
____Drinking	____Sexuality
____Sleeping	____Finding a job
____Relaxation (handling stress)	____Learning specific skills (swimming,
____Wearing a seat belt or motorcycle helmet	first aid, driving safely)
____Making or keeping friends	____Other (explain) _____

37. How do you think we at the clinic can help you with the changes you wish to make?

D. FAMILY HEALTH

38. Some problems tend to run in families. It's important for you to know if you might be at extra risk for certain problems. That way you might be able to stop or prevent a problem from happening to you.
    Is there anyone in your family whose health worries you? no ____ yes ____
    If yes, who and why? _____

39. As far as you know, does anyone in your family have diabetes, high blood pressure, heart disease, cancer, kidney disease, or any birth defects? yes ____ no ____
    If yes:

Which relative (for example, aunt, grandfather, etc.)	What problems?
_____	_____
_____	_____
_____	_____
_____	_____

40. Are both your mother and father alive? yes ____ no ____ If no, please explain:
    _____

41. How many brothers and sisters do you have? brothers ____ sisters ____

42. How old are they? _____

43. Who lives at home with you? (for example, brothers, sisters, parents, grandparents, friends, others): _____
    _____

44. While we're on the subject of family, what would you like to change about your family?

45. What would you like to keep the same?

46. What kinds of things do you and your family argue about the most?

47. Do you feel you are physically mistreated (hit or beaten) by a member of your family?
    yes ____ no ____

48. Is this something you would like to talk about with someone at the clinic? yes ____ no ____

FIGURE 4.3. *continued*

E. PAST HEALTH HISTORY

49. Have you ever:
   a. Stayed overnight in the hospital? no _____ yes _____
      For what?_____ When?_____
   b. Had an operation or abortion? no _____ yes _____
      What kind?_____ When?_____
   c. Had any serious injuries (concussions, broken bones, etc.)? no _____ yes _____
      What kind?_____ When?_____

50. As you were growing up, you probably had some childhood diseases or possibly other problems. Please check those that you remember having had (or now have).

   _____Measles   _____Vaginal or pelvic infections
   _____Mumps   _____Dizzy spells
   _____Chickenpox   _____Breathing problems
   _____German measles (rubella)   _____Bladder or kidney problems (urine infections)
   _____Rheumatic fever   _____Heart problems or high blood pressure
   _____Diabetes   _____Stomach problems
   _____Cancer   _____Trouble seeing or hearing
   _____Seizures   _____Venereal disease
   _____Headaches   _____Other _____
   _____Hepatitis   _____

51. Immunizations protect us from illness. Which of the following shots have you had? (If you don't know, please check with your family.)

                                         Date of last shot
      Tetanus   _____
      Rubella (German measles)   _____

Figure 4.3. *continued*

Family History

Most family history information is obtained from the parents, including the following:

1. Age and health status of family members
2. History of chronic illnesses in the family such as diabetes, cancer, heart disease, hypertension, stroke, mental illness, and alcoholism
3. Vocational status of parents

Psychosocial History

The psychosocial history is obtained primarily from the adolescent while interviewing him or her alone. Some material will also be gathered from the parents or from interviews of the family together. Obtaining much of this information is dependent on establishing rapport between the practitioner and adolescent. Dealing first with the presenting complaint or medical issues will allow time for the adolescent to feel at ease before psychosocial issues are discussed. Psychosocial history includes:

1. Family function: Present family members, intactness of the family, and relationships between the adolescent and other family members
2. School functioning: Grade average, school enjoyment and adjustment, and preferred subjects
3. Peer relations: Relationships with the same and opposite sex, dating patterns, and sexual activity

---

F. FOR WOMEN ONLY

52. Have you started having menstrual periods? no _____ yes _____
53. If yes: How old were you when you had your first period? _____ years
    About how many days between periods? _____ days
    How long does your period usually last? _____ days
    Do you ever miss periods? no _____ yes _____
    Date of your last period:_____
54. Do you have any of the following with your period?

	a lot	some	none
Bleeding in the middle of the month	_____	_____	_____
Tension	_____	_____	_____
Dizziness	_____	_____	_____
Headaches	_____	_____	_____
Period too long or too short	_____	_____	_____
Weight gain	_____	_____	_____
Breast tenderness	_____	_____	_____
Discharge	_____	_____	_____
Cramps	_____	_____	_____
Vomiting	_____	_____	_____

55. Do you know how to examine your breasts for lumps? no _____ yes _____
56. When was the last time you examined them? _____
57. Have you ever noticed a breast lump? no _____ yes _____
58. D.E.S. (diethylstilbestrol) is a hormone that used to be given to women to prevent problems in pregnancy. Did your mother take D.E.S. while she was pregnant with you? yes _____ no _____ don't know _____. If you don't know, it's important to ask her. If she did take it, you may have an increased risk of certain health problems, such as vaginal cancer.
59. Have you ever been pregnant? no _____ yes _____
    If yes, how many times? _____ What was your decision regarding pregnancy?
    _____
    _____

FIGURE 4.3.   *continued*

4. Vocational plans
5. Interests: Hobbies and free-time activities
6. Emotions: Feelings of sadness, loneliness, depression, or suicidal thoughts

At the Teenage Health Center at the Childrens Hospital of Los Angeles, the psychosocial history has been summarized using the acronym HEADSS (*H*ome, *E*ducation, *A*ctivities [including peers], *D*rugs, *S*exuality, and *S*uicide). (See Chapter 3 for further discussion.)

REVIEW OF SYSTEMS

The review of systems covers the following areas:

1. Vision: Trouble reading or watching television, glasses
2. Hearing: Infections, trouble hearing, earaches
3. Dental: Prior care, pain, concerns (e.g., braces)
4. Head: Headaches, dizziness
5. Nose and throat: Frequent colds or sore throats
6. Skin: Acne, moles, rashes, warts

Your child's:

Date _____

Date of Birth _____

Name _____   Age _____

Place a check (✓) by any condition below that is a problem for your child or about which you have a question.

____Headache	____Bed-wetting
____Fainting, dizziness	____Vaginal irritation, discharge
____Vision problem	____Muscle, joint complaint
____Eye pain, redness	____Skin (rash, sores, acne)
____Hearing problem	____Fatigue, tiredness
____Ear pain, drainage	____Sleep difficulties, excess
____Nasal congestion	____Mood (nervous, depressed, other)
____Tooth or gum problem	____Behavior problem
____Tongue, mouth, lips	____Use of prescribed medications
____Throat, swallowing	____Use of nonprescription medications
____Neck lump, pain	____Menstruation
____Chest pain	____Sexual concerns (includes venereal
____Breast lump, pain, discharge	disease, masturbation, contraception, etc.)
____Breathing difficulty, cough	____Future planning
____Heart problem, murmur	____Other problems or questions not listed
____Stomach pain, upset	on this form: (describe)
____Weight, appetite problem	_____
____Diet	_____
____Diarrhea, constipation	_____
____Urine trouble, pain	

Figure 4.4.   Short screening questionnaire for parents of teenagers, developed at the Teenage Health Center, Childrens Hospital of Los Angeles.

7. Cardiovascular: Shortness of breath, chest pain, palpitations, sports endurance, frequency of exercise
8. Respiratory: Cough, smoking, tuberculosis, asthma
9. Gastrointestinal: Abdominal pain, diarrhea, vomiting, bleeding
10. Genitourinary: Dysuria, bed-wetting, frequency, bleeding
11. Musculoskeletal: Joint pains or swelling
12. Central nervous system: Convulsions, fainting
13. Dietary habits: Recall of dietary content of past day or "typical" day
14. Menstrual: Menarche, frequency of menses, duration, pain
15. Sexual: Sexual activity, contraception, pregnancy, abortions, sexually transmitted diseases
16. Drugs: Drug use, type, and frequency

Physical Examination

The physical examination is another major segment in the screening evaluation of the adolescent. The examination allows the examiner to detect unnoticed diseases, discuss health concerns, observe the state of pubertal growth, and instruct the adolescent in methods of self-examination. The examination should be performed with the adolescent's concerns for privacy in mind. The reason for the examination should also be explained to the adolescent. Chief aspects of the physical examination (Fig. 4.6) in the adolescent are discussed in the subsections following.

QUESTIONNAIRE FOR PARENTS OR GUARDIANS

This questionnaire is designed to help the medical staff of this clinic gain a full understanding of your child's medical problems and social development. Please fill out this form as accurately as possible. Your answers are considered privileged and confidential information. If any questions arise in regard to filling out any portion of this questionnaire, please leave those spaces blank until you speak with your doctor.

Date of first visit _____

Patient's name _____

                (last)   (middle)   (first)

Date of birth_____ Telephone # _____

         (day) (month) (year)   (home)

Questionnaire answered by _____ (mother)

                                  _____ (father)

                                  _____ (other; specify)

I. Past History

Has your son or daughter ever had any of the following problems?

1. Measles   1. Yes ____ No ____ ? ____ Age ____
2. Mumps   2. Yes ____ No ____ ? ____ Age ____
3. German measles (rubella or three-day measles)   3. Yes ____ No ____ ? ____ Age ____
4. Chickenpox   4. Yes ____ No ____ ? ____ Age ____
5. Rheumatic fever   5. Yes ____ No ____ ? ____ Age ____
6. Arthritis (red, painful joints)   6. Yes ____ No ____ ? ____ Age ____
7. Unusual bleeding problems or easy bruising   7. Yes ____ No ____ ? ____ Age ____
8. TB (tuberculosis)   8. Yes ____ No ____ ? ____ Age ____
9. Convulsions (fits)   9. Yes ____ No ____ ? ____ Age ____

Has your son or daughter ever had:

1. Any other serious illnesses?   1. Yes ____ No ____ Specify _____
2. Any surgery?   2. Yes ____ No ____ Specify _____
3. Any reason to be hospitalized?   3. Yes ____ No ____ Specify _____

II. Allergic History

Has your son or daughter ever had a problem with:

1. Asthma   1. Yes ____ No ____ ? ____ Age ____
2. Hay fever   2. Yes ____ No ____ ? ____ Age ____
3. Hives   3. Yes ____ No ____ ? ____ Age ____
4. An allergic reaction to penicillin or to any other medication?   4. Yes ____ No ____ ? ____ Age ____

III. Development and Perinatal History

1. Is your son or daughter adopted?   1. Yes ____ No ____
    Comment_____
    _____

2. If so, is he or she aware of the adoption?   2. Yes ____ No ____ ? ____
    Comment_____
    _____

3. During this pregnancy, did the child's mother have any problems with nausea, vomiting, high blood pressure, protein in the urine, swelling of the feet, or excessive weight gain? If so, which one(s)?   3. Yes ____ No ____ ? ____
    Comment_____
    _____

FIGURE 4.5. Comprehensive questionnaire for parents of teenagers, developed at the Teenage Health Center, Childrens Hospital of Los Angeles. *Figure continues through page 89.*

4. Did the child's mother experience any vaginal bleeding during this pregnancy prior to the delivery?

4. Yes _____ No _____ ? _____
    Comment _____
    _____

5. Did the child's mother take any medications during the pregnancy? If so, which medications?

5. Yes _____ No _____ ? _____
    Comment _____
    _____

6. Were forceps used during the delivery?

6. Yes _____ No _____ ? _____
    Comment _____
    _____

7. Did the child leave the hospital at the same time the mother was released?

7. Yes _____ No _____ ? _____
    Comment _____
    _____

8. Were there any problems with your son's or daughter's health immediately following the birth?

8. Yes _____ No _____ ? _____
    Comment _____
    _____

9. Was you child breast-fed or bottle-fed?

9. Breast-fed _____ Bottle-fed _____
    How long? _____

10. Were there any problems with toilet training?

10. Yes _____ No _____ ? _____
    Comment _____
    _____

11. Did your son or daughter have any difficulty learning to read or write?

11. Yes _____ No _____ ? _____
    Comment _____
    _____

12. Have there been problems with bed-wetting or difficulty maintaining control of bowel function?

12. Yes _____ No _____ ? _____
    Comment _____
    _____

13. At what age did your child walk alone?
14. At what age did your child speak words?
15. At what age did your child speak phrases?

IV. **Family History**
    Has anyone in the family had (include aunts, uncles, and grandparents):

1. Allergies

1. Yes _____ No _____
    Comment _____
    _____

2. Tuberculosis

2. Yes _____ No _____ ? _____
    Comment _____
    _____

3. Diabetes

3. Yes _____ No _____ ? _____
    Comment _____
    _____

4. Severe headaches

4. Yes _____ No _____ ? _____
    Comment _____
    _____

5. Convulsions (fits)

5. Yes _____ No _____ ? _____
    Comment _____
    _____

6. Emotional problems

6. Yes _____ No _____ ? _____
    Comment _____
    _____

7. Arthritis (red, painful joints)

7. Yes _____ No _____ ? _____
    Comment _____
    _____

Figure 4.5.   *continued*

8. Heart disease

8. Yes _____ No _____ ? _____
   Comment _____
   _____

9. Early death

9. Yes _____ No _____ ? _____
   Comment _____
   _____

10. Hypertension (high blood pressure)

10. Yes _____ No _____ ? _____
    Comment _____
    _____

11. Eczema

11. Yes _____ No _____ ? _____
    Comment _____
    _____

12. Mental retardation

12. Yes _____ No _____ ? _____
    Comment _____
    _____

13. Cancer

13. Yes _____ No _____ ? _____
    Comment _____
    _____

14. Hay fever or hives

14. Yes _____ No _____ ? _____
    Comment _____
    _____

15. Are there any present illnesses in your immediate family?

15. Yes _____ No _____ ? _____
    Comment _____
    _____

16. Have there been any recent tragic or upsetting events in the immediate family life that may have affected your son or daughter?

16. Yes _____ No _____ ? _____
    Comment _____
    _____

V. Immunizations
Has your son or daughter had:
1. DPT

1. Yes _____ No _____ ? _____
   Comment _____
   _____

2. Polio
   a. Oral (by mouth)

2.
   Yes _____ No _____ ? _____
   Date _____

   b. Vaccine (needle)

   Yes _____ No _____ ? _____
   Date _____

3. Measles, mumps, or German measles vaccine

3. Yes _____ No _____ ? _____
   Date _____

VI. Social History
1. Does your son or daughter perform satisfactorily at school?

1. Yes _____ No _____
   Comment _____
   _____

2. Does your son or daughter comply with rules?

2. Yes _____ No _____ ? _____
   Comment _____
   _____

3. Does your son or daughter get along well with members of his or her own sex?

3. Yes _____ No _____ ? _____
   Comment _____
   _____

FIGURE 4.5. *continued*

4. Does your son or daughter usually follow the rules at home?

4. Yes ____ No ____ ? ____
Comment _____
_____

5. Does your son or daughter usually obey the law?

5. Yes ____ No ____ ? ____
Comment _____
_____

6. Are you employed at the present time? Occupation?

6. Yes ____ No ____ ? ____
Comment _____
_____

7. Is your spouse employed at the present time? Occupation?

7. Yes ____ No ____ ? ____
Comment _____
_____

8. Does your child have his or her own bedroom? If not, who does he or she share it with?

8. Yes ____ No ____ ? ____
Comment _____
_____

9. Has your son or daughter ever been to a child guidance clinic or mental health clinic?

9. Yes ____ No ____ ? ____
Comment _____
_____

10. Has your son or daughter ever been hospitalized for an emotional problem(s)? If so, what hospital? When? How long?

10. Yes ____ No ____ ? ____
Comment _____
_____

11. Is your son or daughter receiving counseling at the present time? If yes, through what agency?

11. Yes ____ No ____ ? ____
Comment _____
_____

12. Is your son or daughter currently on probation?

12. Yes ____ No ____ ? ____
Comment _____
_____

13. Does your son or daughter have difficulty getting along with his or her father?

13. Yes ____ No ____ ? ____
Comment _____
_____

14. Does your son or daughter have difficulty getting along with his or her mother?

14. Yes ____ No ____ ? ____
Comment _____
_____

15. Are you a single parent? If so, when and how did this come about?

15. Yes ____ No ____ ? ____
Comment _____
_____

16. Does your son or daughter have a drug problem?

16. Yes ____ No ____ ? ____
Comment _____
_____

17. Does your son or daughter have difficulty getting to sleep?

17. Yes ____ No ____ ? ____
Comment _____
_____

VII. Present Problem

_____
_____
_____
_____
_____
_____
_____

FIGURE 4.5. *continued*

VIII. Family Composition

Name	Age	Height	Weight	Education	Occupation	Health Problems	Living in Home

FIGURE 4.5. *continued*

Height, Weight, Vital Signs   The following should be checked:

1. Height
2. Weight
3. Blood pressure
4. Pulse

The height and weight allow for serial observation of the adolescent's growth and for the detection of obesity. Blood pressure should be recorded with the appropriately sized cuff. If there is an elevation, the recording should be rechecked on at least three separate visits.

Sexual Maturity Rating   The sexual maturity rating (SMR) (see Chapter 1) allows for adequate assessment of appropriate growth and for evaluation of areas such as hemoglobin, stature, and menarche that are more dependent on SMR than age.

Skin   Check for evidence of acne, scabies, warts, fungal infections, and other lesions.

Teeth and Gums   Teeth and gums present frequent problems in the adolescent age group. Check for evidence of dental caries or gum infections. Regular checkups with a dentist should be encouraged.

Neck   Check for thyromegaly or adenopathy.

Cardiopulmonary   Check for heart murmurs or clicks.

Abdomen   Check for evidence of hepatosplenomegaly, tenderness, and masses.

Musculoskeletal   Check for scoliosis.

Breast   Examine for masses or gynecomastia.

Genitalia (Male)   Examine the testicles; check for hernia. Rectal examination is not routinely indicated as a screening procedure in the adolescent male.

Neurological   Test reflexes and coordination.

Childrens Hospital
Los Angeles
DIVISION OF ADOLESCENT MEDICINE
Initial History and Physical Examination

Date: Age: Referred by:
Problems: (patient)   Problems: (parents)

History:

PAST HISTORY:

Birth (prenatal, postnatal, delivery problems):

Growth and development:

Medical conditions/Past illnesses:

Accident and injuries:

Surgery:

Hospitalizations:

Psychological:

Medications:

ALLERGIES:

Figure 4.6.   Comprehensive teenage history and physical examination form, developed at Childrens Hospital of Los Angeles.

IMMUNIZATIONS:

	Initial Series (year)	Booster (year)	
DPT	_____	_____	Other:
DT	_____	_____	
Polio	_____	_____	
Mumps	_____	_____	
Measles	_____	_____	
Rubella	_____	_____	
MMR	_____	_____	
Hepatitis B vaccine	_____	_____	

TB skin test (date, type, result) _____

PSYCHOSOCIAL HISTORY (Use HEADSS Format)

> **Do not photocopy or release without proper authorization, which includes complying with laws regarding minors' medical release of information.**

Home:

Education:

Eating behaviors:

Activities (including work, peers, gangs, sports, TV, exercise, etc.):

Drug/alcohol/tobacco history:

Sexual history (including abuse):

Suicidal ideation, attempts and affect:

Other:

FIGURE 4.6.   *continued (Figure continues through page 94.)*

Review of Systems:	Comments	NL	ABNL
Growth and development			
Weight change			
Head and neck			
Eye			
Ear/hearing			
Nose and throat			
Teeth/orthodontia			
Breasts			
Respiratory			
Cardiovascular			
Gastrointestinal			
Genitourinary			
Dermatologic			
Musculoskeletal			
Hematologic			
Neurologic			

STDs:
Contraception:

GYNECOLOGIC

Menarche (age):

Menses: LNMP:
                Length of cycle:
                Duration of menses:
                Dysmenorrhea (grade 0–IV)

Pain or bleeding between periods?

Vaginal discharge?

Pregnancy?   G.   P.   Ab.^{S} Ab.^{T}

FIGURE 4.6.   *continued*

Pelvic Examination   A pelvic examination is indicated if the adolescent female requests it or for females with one of the following:

1. Pelvic pain
2. Vaginal discharge
3. History of sexual intercourse
4. Severe menstrual disorders

An annual pelvic examination is recommended for sexually active females.

Visual Screening   Among 12- to 17-year-old adolescents, about 25% have visual acuity of 20/40 or less. This often develops during early adolescence. Adolescents should have a visual screening on initial evaluation and every 2–3 years thereafter. This can be done with a

PHYSICAL EXAMINATION: Date: Sex: M   F

Height: Pulse: Temperature:

Weight: Respiratory rate: Blood pressure:

Visual acuity: R: /   L: /

0 = No examination ✓ = NL		ABNL	Comments
General			
Hair			
Skin			
Lymph nodes			
Head			
Eyes			
Ears			
Nose			
Throat			
Teeth and gums			
Neck and thyroid			
Chest and lungs			
Breasts			
Heart			
Pulses			
Abdomen			
Male			
SMR P.H. I II III IV V			
Gent. I II III IV V			
Penis			
Testes			
Hernia			
Rectal			

FIGURE 4.6.   *continued*

standard Snellen's chart or a similar test. To pass a line the adolescent should view the chart with one eye covered and be able to read one-half or more of the line correctly. Referral should be made for vision less than 20/30 in either or both eyes.

Hearing Screening   Every adolescent should have at least one hearing screening test performed during the adolescent years. It is important that this test be performed in a quiet room to allow for detection of subtle defects that may be contributing to a learning problem. Screening examinations are usually conducted at frequencies of 1000 Hz, 2000 Hz, and 4000 Hz at 20 dB. Referral for more comprehensive hearing testing is indicated if there is a failure to hear 1000 Hz or 2000 Hz at 20 dB or 4000 Hz at 25 dB. The more comprehensive threshold test evaluates for the lowest intensity of sound heard at frequencies of 250 Hz, 1000 Hz, 2000 Hz, and 4000 Hz. Evaluation is indicated with a threshold of 25 dB at two or more frequencies or 35 dB for any frequency.

0 = No examination ✓ = NL		ABNL	Comments
Female			
SMR P.H. I II III IV V			
Breast I II III IV V			
External genitalia			
Vagina			
Cervix			
Uterus			
Adnexa			
Rectal			
Wet mount/KOH			
Back (?Scoliosis)			
Extremities			
Neurologic			
Cranial nerves			
Motor			
Sensory			
Coordination			
Reflexes			
Other			
Psychologic status			
Audiogram			

PROBLEM LIST/ASSESSMENT:
    1. WAC

PLAN: (circle)
    1. Return appointment_____
    2. PPD
    3. CBC
    4. Urinalysis
    5. GC culture/DNA
    6. Chlamydia culture/DNA
    7. Pap smear
    8. Sickle cell prep
    9. Wet mount/KOH
    10. VDRL/RPR
    11. Immunizations_____
    12. Consultations_____
    13.
    14.
    15.

Examined By: _____

Attending Physician:_____

Figure 4.6.   *continued*

LABORATORY TESTS

Laboratory tests should be kept to a minimum in the asymptomatic adolescent. Suggested screening tests include the following.

Hemoglobin or Hematocrit

During adolescence there is a significant prevalence of iron deficiency anemia due to rapid growth, poor nutritional habits, and menstrual losses. A screening hemoglobin or hematocrit is recommended at the first encounter with the adolescent or at the end of puberty or both. While the normal levels remain stable for females throughout adolescence, the normal levels in males are dependent on age and, more importantly, on SMR. Lower levels of the normal hematocrit in white males range from 35.6% at SMR 1 to 40.6% at SMR 5, while the range in African-American males is from 34.9% (SMR 1) to 39.3% (SMR 5).

Urinalysis

A routine urinalysis, including a dipstick test for glucose and protein and a microscopic evaluation, is recommended at the first encounter with the adolescent or at the end of puberty or both. A culture is indicated if abnormal pyuria is noted.

Sickle Cell Screening

Screening for sickle cell anemia is recommended at the first visit with African-American adolescents.

Rubella Titer

This test can be performed before rubella immunization in pubertal females. The test is not mandatory and should not impede effective immunization programs.

Sexually Active Adolescents

Suggested tests for sexually active teenagers include:

1. Females: Annual Pap smear, cervical gonorrhea and chlamydia culture or nonculture test, syphilis serology, and vaginal wet mount are recommended.
2. Males: Leukocyte esterase test on first 15 mL of random urine and annual syphilis serology are recommended. In high risk populations annual urethral culture for gonorrhea and chlamydia screening can be considered.
3. Homosexual males: Annual syphilis serology, gonorrhea cultures (urethral, rectal, and pharyngeal), chlamydia screening, and hepatitis B screening (surface antigen and antibody) are recommended. Homosexual males with negative surface antigen and antibody tests should receive hepatitis B vaccine.

Tuberculin Testing

A purified protein derivative (PPD) test (Mantoux test) should be administered on the first encounter with the adolescent (if the adolescent has not had a positive tuberculosis [TB] test) and repeated thereafter, depending on the recommendations of the local health department (in high-risk areas, this is usually yearly). Recommendations from the Centers for Disease Control and Prevention (CDC) on interpretation of the PPD results include:

1. An induration of more than or equal to 5 mm is classified as positive in the following:
   a. Persons who have human immunodeficiency virus (HIV) infection or risk factors of HIV infection but unknown HIV status
   b. Persons who have had recent close contact with persons who have active TB
   c. Persons who have fibrotic chest radiographs (consistent with healed TB).
2. An induration of more than or equal to 10 mm is classified as positive in all persons who do not meet any of the criteria above but who have other risk factors for TB, including:
   a. High-risk groups
      — Injecting drug users known to be HIV seronegative
      — Persons who have other medical conditions that reportedly increase the risk of progressing from latent TB infection to active TB (e.g., silicosis, gastrectomy or jejunoileal bypass; being 10% or more below ideal body weight; chronic renal failure with renal dialysis; diabetes mellitus; high-dose corticosteroid or other immunosuppressive therapy; some hematologic disorders, including malignancies such as leukemias and lymphomas; and other malignancies)
      — Children less than 4 years of age.
   b. High-prevalence groups
      — Persons born in countries in Asia, Africa, the Caribbean, and Latin America that have high prevalence of TB
      — Persons from medically underserved, low-income populations
      — Residents of long-term care facilities (e.g., correctional institutions and nursing homes)
      — Persons from high-risk populations in their communities, as determined by local public health authorities
3. An induration of more than or equal to 15 mm is classified as positive in persons who do not meet any of the above criteria.
4. Recent converters are defined on the basis of both size of induration and age of the person being tested:
   a. More than or equal to 10 mm increase within a 2-year period is classified as a recent conversion for persons less than 35 years of age
   b. More than or equal to 15 mm increase within a 2-year period is classified as a recent conversion for persons more than or equal to 35 years of age

Liver Function Tests

Liver function tests are not a routine screening test but should be obtained as indicated by the drug or alcohol history.

Cholesterol and Fasting Triglyceride Testing

Cholesterol and fasting triglyceride tests are indicated in adolescents with heart disease, hypertension, diabetes mellitus, or a family history of heart disease or hyperlipidemia. Intervention is indicated for individuals with a total cholesterol level of more than 180–200 mg/dL. Some authorities advocate at least one screening cholesterol during adolescence. Targeted screening in adolescents misses one-third to one-half of those teens with an elevated cholesterol. However, the recommended intervention for most adolescents with mild-to-moderate hyperlipidemia is a low-fat diet, which can be taught to all adolescents.

Human Immunodeficiency Virus Antibody Testing

Routine screening for antibody to HIV is a controversial matter. Individuals at risk should be considered for HIV testing after a discussion regarding the benefits and possible negative consequences of the results (see Chapter 31). Individuals with one sexually transmitted disease should be screened for others.

IMMUNIZATIONS

Obtaining the immunization history and completing the proper immunizations is an increasingly important area in adolescent care for several reasons. First, a high prevalence of common childhood diseases occurs during adolescence and the young adult years. In 1994, 51% of measles, 30% of mumps, and 21% of rubella cases were in individuals ages 10–24. Approximately 13.8% of varicella cases in which the age was reported occurred in youth aged 10–24. Approximately 20% of adolescents are susceptible to diphtheria, tetanus, and pertussis; 15% to measles; 15% to mumps; and 20–30% to rubella. This is secondary to lack of prior immunization; partial immunization; the use of older, inadequate vaccines; or in some cases, vaccine failure. Second, with increasing immunization rates, especially among the young, and with decreasing disease incidences, the unimmunized population is less exposed to diseases. Thus, there is an enlarging unimmunized, susceptible population. Another problem in the adolescent population is the lack of records or of documentation of prior immunizations. Physicians should be aware that new vaccines such as varicella are becoming available and thus recommendations can change.

For fax information from the CDC on immunizations, call 404-332-4565. Detailed information on vaccinations is available at this number both by fax and voice. For international traveling questions, the hotline number is 404-332-4559.

Diphtheria, Tetanus, Pertussis

1. Pertussis vaccination is not recommended after age 7, owing to the low prevalence of serious infections and the high incidence of serious side effects.
2. Boosters of adult tetanus and diphtheria toxoids (Td) are recommended routinely every 10 years after the initial series. The time for this first booster usually occurs during adolescence. (Recommendations for tetanus immunization are listed in the immunization schedule later in this chapter.) Side effects include local reactions of erythema and induration, occasional Arthus hypersensitivity (reaction), and rarely systemic reactions such as urticaria and anaphylaxis.
3. The diphtheria booster should be given along with the routine tetanus boosters every 10 years after the initial series.

Measles

Measles has been decreasing dramatically in the United States, with 441,703 cases in 1960; 47,351 in 1970; 13,506 in 1980; 2933 in 1988; and 312 in 1993. There was an increase to 963 in 1994, but the number dropped to 288 in 1995. While the potential still exists for epidemics on college campuses, reported cases are low at present secondary to cyclical changes in measles incidence, increases in measles vaccination coverage among preschool-aged children, and increased use of a second shot of vaccine among school- and college-aged youth. Because of the low incidence of measles, cases should be confirmed by serology.

Because of the problem of waning immunity, it is now recommended to give children and adolescents a second vaccination either at primary school or junior high school entry. If this is missed, it should be given whenever the teen presents for health care. This is also recommended for young adults entering college or other postsecondary institutions if they have not previously received two doses. All students born during or after 1957 who enter institutions of post–high school education should have documentation of receiving two doses of measles vaccine (preferably as measles-mumps-rubella [MMR] vaccine) and one dose of rubella vaccine or other evidence of measles and rubella immunity.

The following are recommended vaccination procedures for measles:

1. Vaccinate adolescents if there is no evidence of prior immunization after 1 year of age with live measles virus vaccine, physician-diagnosed measles, or laboratory-confirmed immunity (routine serology is not recommended).
2. Individuals vaccinated before 1968 should be revaccinated with live vaccine because these patients were usually vaccinated with killed measles vaccine and are at increased risk of developing atypical measles (fever, pneumonitis, and atypical rash) if exposed to the wild virus. However, their titer response to revaccination is questionable.
3. The following outlines procedures for unvaccinated adolescents with exposure to live virus:
   a. If within 3–5 days' exposure, give measles vaccine.
   b. If after 5 days' exposure, give immune serum globulin 0.25 mL/kg, followed by measles vaccine 8–12 weeks later.
4. The American Academy of Pediatrics and the Advisory Committee on Immunization Practices recommend, if feasible, a second measles (or MMR) vaccine to adolescents and young adults who have received only one initial vaccine.

Mumps

The number of cases of mumps has declined dramatically from 59,647 cases in 1975, 8576 in 1980, 2982 in 1985, 1537 in 1994, and 840 in 1995. Approximately 65% of mumps now occurs between 10–19 years of age, with about 20% or more of adolescents developing orchitis. A live mumps virus vaccine was developed in 1967. The vaccine has few side effects, and over 90% of susceptible patients develop protective, long-lasting antibodies.

1. Susceptible adolescents should receive a single dose of mumps vaccine alone or with measles or rubella. Susceptible adolescents include those without physician-diagnosed mumps or laboratory evidence of immunity (tests for immunity are unnecessary, as revaccination is safe), as well as individuals lacking documented live mumps virus vaccination at age 12 months or more.
2. Avoid vaccination in adolescents who are pregnant, have a severe febrile illness, have an immunodeficiency, are receiving immunosuppressive therapy, or have leukemia or lymphoma.
3. Exposed, susceptible adolescents should be immunized with the vaccine to prevent future infection, as there is a chance that the adolescent was not infected from the current exposure. There is no evidence of efficacy of immune globulin.

Rubella

The number of cases of rubella has continued a marked decline, with 46,975 cases in 1966; 16,652 in 1975; 3904 in 1980; 630 in 1985; 221 in 1988; and 200 in 1995. While the number in 1994 was low, this represented a 30% increase over the record low number of cases reported in 1992. Colleges can be high-risk areas for rubella transmission. As such, proof of rubella and measles immunity should be required for attendance for male and female students. All students born during or after 1957 who enter institutions of post–high school education should have documentation of receiving two doses of measles vaccine (preferably as MMR) and at least one dose of rubella vaccine or other evidence of measles and rubella immunity. The diagnosis of acute rubella should be confirmed serologically with either the presence of IgM antibody or a significant rise in IgG.

Pregnancy   The U.S. Public Health Service recommends that females of childbearing age be asked if they are pregnant. If they say no, they should be advised of the theoretical risk of vaccination to the fetus and instructed to avoid pregnancy for 3 months. They then should be immunized. When time and cost are not prohibitive, adolescent females can be tested serologically before vaccination. However, this should no longer be considered mandatory and should not interfere with immunization programs. Clinical diagnosis should not be re- lied on as evidence of rubella infection. In 1979, a new vaccine, RA 27/3 (Meruvax II), was introduced that leads to higher titers and has fewer side effects. A review of rubella vaccina- tion for the period 1971–1989 following 321 known rubella-susceptible pregnant women vaccinated with live rubella vaccine within 3 months before or 3 months after conception shows that none of the infants had malformations compatible with congenital rubella infec- tion. The estimated risk with 95% confidence limits is from 0% to 1.2% with an observed risk of zero. Certainly if there is any question that the adolescent might be pregnant, the vac- cination should be withheld until this question is resolved.

Males   Males without evidence of prior vaccination should also be vaccinated to de- crease the prevalence of susceptible individuals in the population and thus the risk to preg- nant females.

Immunocompromised Adolescents   Replication of vaccine viruses can be enhanced in per- sons with immune deficiency diseases and in persons with immunosuppression, as occurs with leukemia, lymphoma, and generalized malignancy or resulting from treatment with alkylating agents, antimetabolites, radiation, or large doses of corticosteroids. Thus, such per- sons (except those with HIV infection) should not receive live rubella virus vaccine. Asymp- tomatic HIV-infected persons in need of an MMR vaccination should receive it. MMR should also be considered for all symptomatic HIV-infected adolescents and young adults, including those with the diagnosis of acquired immunodeficiency syndrome (AIDS). At present, infor- mation available on MMR vaccination among asymptomatic and symptomatic HIV-infected individuals has not demonstrated serious or unusually adverse events. Adolescents with leukemia in remission can be vaccinated, as well as those who have had short-term (<2 weeks), low-to-moderate-dose systemic corticosteroid therapy, topical steroid therapy, or in- tra-articular injections.

Vaccinations should not be given to adolescents with a severe febrile illness but should not be postponed because of a mild illness, such as an upper respiratory infection. A history of anaphylactic reactions to egg ingestion must only be considered if measles or mumps anti- gens are included with the rubella vaccine. Anaphylactic reactions to neomycin are also a con- traindication to vaccination, as the vaccine contains trace amounts of neomycin.

Polio

At present there are two safe and effective vaccines: live virus trivalent oral polio vaccine (OPV) and killed virus trivalent inactivated polio vaccine (IPV). The relative merits of each are still being disputed. OPV has increased risks in adults, so it is not recommended for in- dividuals over the age of 18; in these patients the use of IPV is recommended, if indicated. There is also a possible small risk to susceptible adults who come in contact with adolescents who receive OPV. Currently in the United States most health-care facilities accept this small risk. Alternatives include giving the parents IPV 2 months before OPV is given to the adoles- cent or giving the whole family IPV. A more potent inactivated polio vaccine (Poliovax) has been licensed. Indications for this vaccine are similar to IPV. Neither IPV nor OPV should be given to pregnant females. IPV is recommended for persons with a compromised immune system and their household contacts.

Varicella

Varicella, chickenpox, had a live-attenuated vaccination approved in 1995 for use in children, adolescents and adults. There were over 151,000 cases reported of varicella in 1994 with an estimated 3.7 million cases in the United States per year. The vaccine is marketed under the name Varivax and is about 70–90% effective in preventing varicella. Varicella causes about 100 deaths per year and results in more than 9000 hospitalizations. The estimate from the CDC is that about $384 million could be saved annually with vaccine usage. The American Academy of Pediatrics recommends universal use of the vaccine in early childhood and for healthy adolescents and adults without a reliable chickenpox history. Some authorities recommend obtaining varicella serology prior to vaccination in an adolescent who has no history of chickenpox. Varivax is a live attenuated vaccine. It is not recommended for children under the age of 1, pregnant women, people hypersensitive to gelatin or other vaccine components, those with a history of anaphylactoid reaction to neomycin or those with active febrile infection. The vaccine should also be avoided in those with malignant neoplasms, those receiving immunosuppressive therapy, or those with acquired or primary immunodeficiency. About 5–10% of those vaccinated may develop a rash, which can be contagious. A single dose is advised for children 12 and younger, and two injections 4–8 weeks apart for those 13 and older. The vaccine can be administered with measles, mumps, and rubella vaccines. The vaccine almost always either prevents the disease or results in a milder form of the disease. Adverse reactions include redness, hardness and swelling at the injection site, fatigue, malaise, and nausea.

Hepatitis B Vaccine

The vaccines used today in the United States include two recombinant vaccines (Recombivax-HB and Engerix-B). The Advisory Committee on Immunization Practices recommends the three-dose hepatitis B vaccine series for adolescents aged 11–12 who have not been previously immunized. If all adolescents and young adults are not immunized, then the following individuals should be vaccinated:

1. Persons with lifestyle risk
   a. Heterosexual partners with multiple partners (more than one partner in preceding 6 months) or any sexually transmitted disease
   b. Homosexual and bisexual men
   c. Injecting drug users
2. Persons with occupational risk
   a. Special patient groups such as recipients of hemodialysis treatment and clotting factor concentrates
   b. Environmental risk factors
      — Household and sexual contacts of carriers
      — Adoptees from countries of high hepatitis B endemicity
      — Populations with high endemicity of hepatitis B infection such as Alaskan Natives, Pacific Islanders, and refugees from endemic areas
      — Clients and staff of institutions for mentally retarded individuals
      — Inmates of long-term correctional facilities
      — Certain international travelers
      — Other contacts of hepatitis B carriers: Persons in casual contact with carriers in settings such as schools and offices are at minimal risk of hepatitis B infection and vaccine is not routinely recommended

The vaccine when given in a three-dose series induces protective antibodies (anti-HBs) in over 90% of healthy adults and more than 95% of infants, children, and adolescents from birth through 19 years of age. See Chapter 30 for vaccination details.

Influenza

Influenza continues to cause major outbreaks of illness, usually beginning in December and January. If the vaccine is used, it should be given starting in September. Most influenza vaccines contain three virus strains (two type A and one type B), representing the strains most commonly found worldwide and thought to be the most likely to cause infections in the coming year. The vaccine is recommended for the following:

1. High-risk individuals
   a. Individuals with chronic illnesses, particularly those involving their respiratory or cardiovascular system, including asthma
   b. Residents of long-term care facilities
2. Health-care practitioners who have extensive contact with high-risk patients or providers of care at long-term care facilities
3. Children or adolescents receiving long-term aspirin therapy and who are therefore at risk for Reye's syndrome following an influenza illness
4. Persons infected with HIV
5. Any adolescent or young adult who wishes to lower his or her risk of acquiring an influenza infection

The vaccine contains only noninfective material. Side effects include local redness and induration; systemic effects include fever, malaise, and myalgias. There is no evidence of a paralytic illness like Guillain-Barré syndrome occurring with vaccines used after 1976, and a large study in adults (Margolis, 1990) found no significant difference in side effects between those who were vaccinated and those given a placebo.

Amantadine Prophylaxis   Amantadine is 70–90% effective in preventing illness in individuals infected with type A influenza but is *not* effective against type B. Administered within 24–48 hours after the onset of symptoms, amantadine can reduce the severity and duration of the disease. The drug should be used in high-risk individuals who have either not been immunized or were immunized too late. It is also useful in immunosuppressed adolescents who may not respond to the vaccine. Amantadine can also be used in healthy adolescents to reduce the severity of type A influenza. In very high-risk individuals the drug should be continued throughout the flu season.

Prophylactic Dose   100–200 mg/day; 100 mg is probably as effective as 200 mg and is associated with fewer side effects.

Treatment Dose   100–200 mg/day

Uncommon Vaccinations during Adolescence

Pneumococcal Vaccine   Pneumococcal vaccine is indicated in individuals with a chronic illness, particularly of the cardiovascular or pulmonary system. It is also indicated in those who are at increased risk of pneumococcal disease, including patient's with nephrotic syndrome, sickle cell disease, asplenia or functional asplenia, HIV infection, and B-cell immune deficiency and patients at risk for meningitis. The duration of immunity is unclear; some centers recommend reimmunization with pneumococcal vaccine (Pneumovax 23) 3–5 years after primary immunization in especially high-risk patients.

Haemophilus influenzae *Type B*   *H. influenzae* type B vaccine is indicated for those adolescents not previously immunized who are at risk because of splenic dysfunction or other at-risk conditions. A single dose of 0.5 mL is recommended.

Immunization Schedule for Adolescents

Diphtheria/Tetanus

1. Completely immunized adolescents should be given adult Td, one dose 10 years after the last booster and every 10 years thereafter.
   a. For minor, clean wounds: Booster only if none in the last 10 years
   b. For other wounds: Booster if none in the past 5 years
   c. For tetanus-prone wounds (such as deep puncture wounds): Booster dose and human tetanus immunoglobulin, 250 units; use separate syringes and separate injection sites.
2. No prior immunization or incomplete immunization:
   a. Td adult type: Two doses 6–8 weeks apart with a booster in 8–12 months
   b. For minor, clean wounds: Td dose followed by a complete series
   c. Other wounds: Td and human tetanus immune globulin, 250 units, using separate syringes and separate sites

Pertussis

1. No routine vaccination after age 7
2. In high-risk exposure: 0.2 mL pertussis vaccine and erythromycin 1 g/day for 10 days

Measles   Administer a single dose of live attenuated vaccine for any of the following:

1. Only one documented prior live vaccine
2. Vaccination given before the age of 12 months
3. Vaccination given with killed vaccine

If no prior vaccination or documented disease, give two doses of MMR 6–8 weeks apart.

Mumps   A single dose is advisable at any age for either of the following reasons:

1. No physician-documented mumps
2. No documented prior vaccination after 12 months of age

Rubella   A single dose is advisable at any age if no proof of documented prior vaccination after 12 months of age can be found. Two doses of MMR 6–8 weeks apart are preferred for those adolescents with no prior rubella vaccinations or no documented positive serology for rubella. Caution should be used in postmenarcheal females to avoid vaccination within 3 months of a pregnancy.

Polio

1. In adolescents who have been completely immunized, further vaccination is not required unless the adolescent is at risk for high exposure. In such adolescents a booster of OPV or IPV is recommended.

2. In adolescents who have had partial or no prior immunization, OPV should be administered, two doses, 8 weeks apart, with a booster in 8–12 months. In youths over 18 residing in the United States, routine polio immunization is not necessary, as the exposure risk is small. If there is an exposure risk, a full series of IPV injections, including three injections 4–8 weeks apart and a fourth 6–12 months after the third, should be given.

Hepatitis B Vaccine   The most common schedule to immunize susceptible adolescents is three doses given at time 0, then 1 month and 6 months after the first. Adolescents should receive the injection in the deltoid muscle. The administration of hepatitis B vaccine does not interfere with the simultaneous administration of other vaccines. The recommendations vary by product and age and are given in detail in Chapter 30.

Sample Schedule for Unimmunized Adolescents

1. First visit: Td #1, OPV #1, PPD (if no history of positive PPD in the past), MMR #1
2. Two months later: Td #2, OPV #2, MMR #2
3. Six to 12 months after Td #2: OPV: Td #3, OPV #3
4. Td every 10 years

The three-dose hepatitis vaccine series is also recommended for adolescents and young adults at risk. Teens not previously immunized for varicella or who lack a reliable history of chickenpox should be vaccinated by 13 years of age, if possible. Children under age 13 should receive a single 0.5 mL dose; persons aged 13 and older should receive two 0.5 doses 4–8 weeks apart.

1. Any and all of these vaccines can be given simultaneously, at separate anatomic sites.
2. If a delay occurs between doses, regardless of length, the series can continue without restarting.
3. Intervals between doses should not be less than those indicated earlier.

Possible Allergies or Contraindications

1. Measles, rubella (MR), Influenza: Anaphylactic reaction can occur to those allergic to eggs.
2. MR, OPV: Anaphylactic reaction to neomycin can occur to those with systemic allergy to neomycin.
3. OPV, IPV: Anaphylactic reaction to streptomycin can occur to those allergic to streptomycin.
4. Hepatitis B: Anaphylactic allergy to yeast can occur to those allergic to yeast.
5. Almost all inactivated vaccines: Anaphylactic allergy to thimerosal (a preservative used in vaccines and contact lens cleaning solution) can occur to those allergic to thimerosal.

Pregnancy   Do not give MMR. Give OPV only if at high risk for exposure

Immune Globulin or Blood Transfusion within Past 3 Months   Do not give MMR until after 3 months unless exposure risk is high.

Immunodeficiency or Immunosuppression   Do not give MMR or OPV. Also do not give OPV if any other household member is immunodeficient or immunosuppressed. See below for HIV-infected youth.

HIV-infected Youth

Vaccine	Asymptomatic	Symptomatic
Td	Yes	Yes
OPV	No	No
IPV	Yes	Yes
MMR	Yes	Yes, consider
Hepatitis B	Yes	Yes
Pneumococcal	Yes	Yes
Influenza	Optional	Yes

Vaccination during Illness   The Immunization Practices Advisory Committee of the U.S. Public Health Service states that "minor illnesses such as mild upper respiratory infections (URI) with or without low-grade fever are not contraindications for vaccination." Inappropriately avoiding vaccination because of a mild acute illness has contributed to many missed opportunities for giving vaccinations to children and adolescents.

Vaccination during Pregnancy   Because of a theoretical risk to the developing fetus, live, attenuated virus vaccines are not routinely given to pregnant females or to those likely to become pregnant within 3 months of receiving the vaccine. There is no convincing evidence of risk to the fetus after immunization of pregnant women with inactivated virus vaccines, bacterial vaccines, or toxoids. This includes tetanus and diphtheria toxoid. There is also no risk to the fetus from passive immunization of pregnant women with immune globulin. Since measles, mumps, and rubella vaccine viruses are not transmitted from individuals receiving them, children of pregnant women may receive these vaccines. Although live polio virus is shed from children recently immunized with OPV, this vaccine can be given to children of pregnant women.

Erroneous Contraindications Against Vaccination (from the Advisory Committee on Immunization Practices)

1. A reaction of a previous dose of diphtheria and tetanus toxoids and pertussis (DTP) vaccine with only soreness, redness, or swelling
2. Mild acute illness with low-grade fever
3. Current antimicrobial therapy
4. Pregnancy in the mother or another household contact
5. Recent exposure to an infectious disease
6. Breast-feeding
7. A history of nonspecific allergies
8. Allergy to penicillin or other antimicrobials except anaphylactic reactions to neomycin or streptomycin
9. Allergies to duck meat or duck feathers
10. A family history of seizures in children who require vaccination

Informed Consent   Since October 1, 1994 all health-care providers who administer MMR, polio, DTP, and Td vaccines have been required to distribute vaccine information sheets (VIS) every time a patient is vaccinated. The clinic or office should either obtain a signature of the patient, parent, or teen's legal representative to acknowledge receipt of the VIS or make a notation on the medical record, indicating VISs were provided. Some health districts' forms include the following on a single sheet:

1. Consent for vaccination and notification that individual received VIS
2. Immunization type, date of administration, injection site

3. Manufacturer and lot number of vaccine
4. Name and address of the health-care provider administering the vaccine

VISs are available from local public health departments or local immunization projects. These come as camera-ready copies and allow for the addition of local identification information.

PREVENTIVE CARE FOR ADOLESCENTS

The recommendations of the American Academy of Pediatrics, the U.S. Preventive Services Task Force, and the AMA regarding preventive health visits for adolescents have been discussed previously in this chapter. Many different mechanisms have been employed to obtain this information:

1. Interviews (see Chapter 3)
2. Health screening questionnaires (see Chapter 3 and this chapter)
3. Computerized screening programs

Priority health behavior goals for adolescents include:

1. Using seat belts
2. Not drinking or using drugs and driving
3. Using condoms if sexually active
4. Not smoking
5. Eating a low-fat diet
6. Getting regular aerobic exercise

These are the most effective and achievable lifetime behaviors to reduce the years of potential life lost because of major killers, including motor vehicle accidents, AIDS, cardiovascular disease, and cancer.

Two mnemonics, SAFE TEENS and SAFE TIMES (Schubiner, 1989), have been suggested for important preventive care areas for adolescents.

SAFE TEENS	*SAFE TIMES*
S: Sexuality	S: Sexuality
A: Accidents	A: Affect (depression)
F: Firearms/homicides	Abuse of alcohol, drugs, tobacco
E: Emotions/suicide	F: Family problems/conflicts
T: Toxins	E: Self-examination
E: Environment (school, home, friends)	T: Timing of development (adjustment, height, weight)
E: Exercise	I: Immunizations
N: Nutrition	M: Meals (nutrition, cholesterol, exercise)
S: Shots/immunizations	E: Education/employment
	S: Safety (injuries, seat belts, weapons, fights)

Preventive Health Interventions

The practice of medicine is often more of an art than a science. Only by experience can a practitioner develop a style that "works" for them. Most clinicians working with adolescent patients feel comfortable in screening for psychosocial morbidity and assessing the level of risk in an individual. However, the next steps, that is, how to deliver health education and the development of brief office interventions, are not as often delineated. Some precepts from behavioral medicine are important in designing office interventions. Health education should be targeted to a specific need of the patient. The patient should agree with the physician on what behaviors must be changed and how to change them. Barriers to the proposed change should be explored, and specific reinforcement should be included. This can only occur if the clinician works with the patient rather than lecturing to the patient. The GAPS project has attempted to develop a standardized method of assessment and intervention that includes these health education concepts yet is practical for office practice.

The GAPS guidelines were outlined earlier in the chapter. An outline of the GAPS method of assessment and intervention follows. A new publication by the AMA, *GAPS: Clinical Evaluation and Management Handbook*, includes fully developed algorithms for each of the GAPS recommendations. The handbook is available from: American Medical Association, Department of Adolescent Health, 515 N. State St., Chicago, IL 60610.

G: Gather Initial Information Screen for problems using simple trigger questions such as "Have you been feeling down and blue?" or "Do you usually wear seat belts while riding in a car?" If the screen is negative (no risk identified), offer some simple information or reinforcement of the positive behavior.

If the screen is positive, proceed to the next level.

A: Assess Further Assess for the level of risk in the specific topic area. Identify how serious the problem is by asking about the patient's level of involvement and assessing the patient's age level of maturity, the availability of family and other support, and the consequences for the patient's health and functional tasks (i.e., school, peer relationships).

If the patient is at low risk, give reinforcement or information about the issue.

If the patient is at high risk, he or she probably needs an in-depth evaluation or referral that may be beyond the bounds of an office visit.

If the patient is at medium risk, he or she could receive the following intervention (if the physician feels comfortable with the topic area).

P: Problem Identification, Pros and Cons, Plan The three parts in this section are to work with the patient toward an agreement on the problem, to help the patient decide if he or she wants to make a change, and to develop a plan for that change. The goal is to be "patient centered" in your approach, i.e., help the patient decide what is in his or her best interest, rather than forcing the patient to accept your own view of the behavior.

Problem identification is an attempt to define the problem in terms the patient accepts. For example, questions such as "You seem to be down and blue, is that something that is a problem for you right now?" or "Do you think it would be better for you if you used condoms?" may help the patient further define the problem. If agreement on problem definition is reached, proceed to the next step. If the patient does not agree that there is a problem with a specified behavior, do not push the issue but give some simple information and set up some guidelines for when you think the problem would merit more discussion/intervention. For example, a question such as "You clearly don't think that this is a problem area, but when would you consider it one?" would assist in setting boundaries that define the problem. Finally, if the problem is too significant to put off, refer the individual for further assistance.

In the pros and cons step, guide the adolescent to weigh the pros and cons of making a certain change. The adolescent may find several reasons to make or not make the change in behavior. This step is only needed if there is some ambivalence toward the proposed change.

During plan development find out what the adolescent is willing to do. Again, the decision should be in the adolescent's hands. If the adolescent is only willing to try using a condom once, that could become the plan. However, most adolescents are willing to make significant changes, such as always wearing seat belts or not drinking alcohol, for a specified time period, usually a few weeks or months. Try to avoid sweeping changes that are unrealistic, like avoiding alcohol use for the rest of their lives. Make sure the plan is concrete and fully defined.

S: Self-Efficacy, Gathering Support, Solving Barriers, Shaking on a Contract   Self-efficacy is assessed by asking if the adolescent thinks he or she will be able to carry out the proposed plan. If the adolescent is ambivalent, you may need to modify an overly ambitious plan.

Gathering support is an important step because it allows the adolescent to identify people who can help them in their plan. Hopefully, the adolescent will be able to call on resources such as trusted adults or close friends. At times the adolescent may want help in contacting these people to help explain certain situations.

Solving barriers is the term used to determine what barriers the adolescent can foresee and to work with the adolescent to develop strategies to overcome them. For example, if the adolescent will have difficulty not drinking at a party, he or she must have a plan for how to deal with that. It is usually best if the adolescent comes up with his or her own solutions, but sometimes the adolescent will welcome suggestions or options he or she might not have considered.

"Shaking on a contract" is a crucial step. It serves as a reinforcer to the proposed plan and implies some commitment on the adolescent's part. Written contracts can also be used. It is important to specify the action you agree to and the time frame in which the action is to be taken. Make sure that the adolescent feels comfortable with the plan and understands it. If you are able to involve another party into the contract, such as a friend or parent, there is likely to be better compliance.

Follow-up is critical and should be arranged (in some form, either a visit or telephone contact) in the time frame agreed to in the contract.

SUMMARY

G: Gather initial information (screen)
— If negative, reinforce the positive behavior
— If positive, go to next step
A: Assess further (determine level of risk)
— If low, reinforce, offer help if ever needed
— If high, plan an immediate intervention (refer)
— If moderate, go to the next step
P: Problem identification (agree on the problem)
— Pros and cons (Is the patient interested in making a change?)
— Plan (Develop a plan. What is the patient willing to do?)
S: Self-efficacy (Does the patient think he or she can make the change?)
— Gathering support (Who can help?)
— Solve barriers (Find solutions to potential barriers to the change.)
— Shake on a contract (commitment to a specific action over a specific time frame)

BIBLIOGRAPHY

American College of Physicians, Health and Public Policy Committee. Pneumococcal vaccine. Ann Intern Med 1986;104:118.

American Medical Association: AMA guidelines for adolescent preventive services (GAPS): recommendations and rationale. Baltimore: Williams & Wilkins, 1994.

Amin NM. Adult immunizations. Am Fam Physician 1986;33:89.

Amren DP, Mayer TR. National immunization policy-making. Postgrad Med 1985;77:93.

Blum RW, Runyan C. The comprehensive health history and physical examination. In: Blum RW, ed.

Adolescent health care. New York: Academic Press, 1982.

Breslow L, Somers AR. The lifetime health monitoring program: a practical approach to preventive medicine. N Engl J Med 1977;206:601.

Centers for Disease Control. Rubella prevention: recommendation of the Immunization Practices Advisory Committee. Ann Intern Med 1984;101:505.

Centers for Disease Control. Diphtheria, tetanus, and pertussis: guidelines for vaccine prophylaxis and other preventive measures. Ann Intern Med 1985; 103:896.

Centers for Disease Control. Rubella and congenital rubella syndrome United States, 1984–1985.

Morbidity and Mortality Weekly Report 1986;35:129.

Centers for Disease Control. Rubella vaccination during pregnancy United States, 1971–1985. MMWR 1986;35:275.

Centers for Disease Control. Update: measles Canada, 1986. MMWR 1986;35:331.

Centers for Disease Control. Immunization practices in colleges United States. MMWR 1987;36:209.

Centers for Disease Control. Measles United States, 1987. MMWR 1988;37:527.

Centers for Disease Control. Measles prevention: supplementary statement. MMWR 1989;38:11.

Centers for Disease Control. Measles Los Angeles County, California, 1988. MMWR 1989;38:49.

Centers for Disease Control. Mumps United States, 1985–1988. MMWR 1989;38:101.

Centers for Disease Control. Mumps prevention. MMWR 1989;38:388.

Centers for Disease Control. Summary cases of specified notifiable diseases, United States. MMWR 1989; 37:802.

Centers for Disease Control. Rubella prevention: recommendations of the Immunization Practices Advisory Committee. MMWR 1990;39(No. RR-15):1.

Centers for Disease Control. Increase in rubella and congenital rubella syndrome—United States, 1988–1990. MMWR 1991;40:93.

Centers for Disease Control. Measles—United States, first 26 weeks, 1993. MMWR 1993;42:813.

Centers for Disease Control. Absence of reported measles—United States, November 1993. MMWR 1993;42:925.

Centers for Disease Control. Summary of notifiable diseases, United States, 1994. MMWR 1994;43(53):1–98.

Centers for Disease Control. Rubella and congenital rubella syndrome—United States, January 1, 1991–May 7, 1994. MMWR 1994;43:391.

Centers for Disease Control. Recommended childhood immunization schedule—United States, January 1995. MMWR 1995;43:959.

Centers for Disease Control. Mumps surveillance—United States, 1988–1993. MMWR 1995;44(SS-3):1.

Cherry JD. The "new" epidemiology of measles and rubella. Hosp Pract 1980;15:49.

Committee on Infectious Diseases, 1987–1988. Red book, 1988. Elk Grove Village, Illinois: American Academy of Pediatrics, 1988.

Committee on Practice and Ambulatory Medicine, American Academy of Pediatrics. Vision screening and eye examination in children. Pediatrics 1986;77: 918.

Committee on School Health: School health assessments. Pediatrics 1991;88:649.

Cross AW. Health screening in schools [Parts 1 and 2]. J Pediatr 1985;107:487 and 653.

Eisele CJ. Rubella susceptibility in women of childbearing age. J Obstet Gynecol Neonatal Nurs 1993;22: 260.

Fitzgerald TM, Glotzer DE. Vaccine information pamphlets: more information than parents want? Pediatrics 1995;95:331.

Frame PS. Health maintenance in clinical practice: strategies and barriers. Am Fam Physician 1992;45: 1192.

Fulginiti VA. The problems of poliovirus immunization. Hosp Pract 1980;15:61.

Fulginiti VA, Comerci GD. Immunization for adolescents. Paediatrician 1981;10:191.

Gardner P, Schaffner W. Immunization of adults. N Engl J Med 1993;17:1252.

Gershon AA, LaRussa P, Hardy I, et al. Varicella vaccine: the American experience. J Infect Dis 1992;166:S63.

Gilchrist VJ. Preventive health care for the adolescent. Am Fam Physician 1991;43:869.

Gillum JE, Garrison MW, Crossley KB, et al. Hemophilus influenzae, pneumococcal, and meningococcal infections, rabies, and hepatitis. Postgrad Med 1989;85:199.

Gillum JE, Garrison MW, Crossley KB, et al. Polio, diphtheria, tetanus, pertussis, measles, mumps, rubella, and influenza. Postgrad Med 1989;85:183.

Hayward RSA, Steinbert EP, Ford DE, et al. Preventive care guidelines, 1991. Ann Intern Med 1991;114: 785.

Hersch BS, Fine PEM, Kent WK, et al. Mumps outbreak in a highly vaccinated population. J Pediatr 1991; 119:187.

Hess GH, ed. Immunization guidelines. Kansas City, Missouri: American Academy of Family Physicians, 1988.

Klein JO, ed. Report of the Committee on Infectious Disease. Evanston, Illinois: American Academy of Pediatrics, 1982.

Klein JD, Slap GB, Elster AB, et al. Adolescents and access to health care. Bull N Y Acad Med 1993;70:219.

Kollar LM, Rosentahl SL, Biro FM. Hepatitis B vaccine series compliance in adolescents. Pediatr Infect Dis J 1994;13:1006.

Lerman Y, Riskin-Mashiach S, Cohen D, et al. Immunity to measles in young adults in Israel. Infection 1993;21:154.

Lieu TA, Cochi SL, Black SB, et al. Cost-effectiveness of a routine varicella vaccination program for U.S. children. JAMA 1994;271:375.

Lindegren ML, Fehrs LJ, Hadler SC, et al. Update: rubella and congenital rubella syndrome, 1980–1990. Epidemiol Rev 1991;13:341.

Marcuse EK. Changing views on vaccination for "childhood" diseases. Consultant November 1981;271.

Margolis KL, Nichal KL, Poland GA. Frequency of adverse reactions to influenza vaccine in the elderly: a randomized placebo-controlled trial. JAMA 1990; 264:1139.

Marks A, Cohen MI. Health screening and assessment of adolescents. Pediatr Ann 1978;7:596.

Marks AM, Fisher M. Health assessment and screening during adolescence. Pediatrics 1987;80(suppl):135S.

Medical Practice Committee, American College of Physicians. Periodic health examination: a guide for designing individualized preventive health care in the asymptomatic patient. Ann Intern Med 1981;95:729.

Mumps vaccine: recommendation of the Immunization Practices Advisory Committee. Ann Intern Med 1980;92:803.

Mumps vaccine: updated recommendation. Clin Pediatr 1980;19:712.

National Vaccine Advisory Committee. The measles epidemic: the problems, barriers, and recommendations. JAMA 1991;266:1547.

Peter G. Measles immunization: recommendations, challenges, and more information. JAMA 1991;265:2111.

Peter G. Childhood immunizations. N Engl J Med 1992; 327:1794.

Plotkin SA. Rabies vaccination in the 1980s. Hosp Pract 1980;15:65.

Schubiner HH. Preventive health screening in adolescent patients. Prim Care 1989;16:211.

Schubiner H, Eggly S. Strategies for health education for adolescent patients: a preliminary investigation. J Adolesc Health 1995;17:37.

Schubiner H, Tzelepis A, Wright K, et al. The clinical utility of the SAFE TIMES questionnaire. J Adolesc Health 1994;15:374.

Shapiro J, Neinstein LS, Rabinovitz S. The family APGAR: use of a simple family-function screening test with adolescents. Fam Sys Med 1987;5:220.

Smilkstein G. The family APGAR: a proposal for a family function test and its use by physicians. J Fam Pract 1984;6:1231.

Sox HC Jr. Preventive health services in adults. N Engl J Med 1994;330:1589.

Strebel PM, Sutter RW, Cochi SL, et al. Epidemiology of poliomyelitis in the United States: one decade after the last reported case of indigenous wild virus-associated disease. Clin Infect Dis 1992;14:568.

Thompson RS, Taplin SH, McAfee TA, et al. Primary and secondary prevention services in clinical practice. Twenty years' experience in development, implementation, and evaluation. JAMA 1995;273: 1130.

US Department of Health, Education and Welfare. Adolescent health care: a guide for BCHS-supported programs and projects, Millar HEC, ed. DHEW Pub. #NO(HSA)79-5234. Washington, DC: US Government Printing Office, 1980.

US Preventive Services Task Force. The periodic health examination: age-specific charts. Am Fam Physician 1990;41:189.

US Public Health Service: Implementing preventive care. Am Fam Physician 1994;50:103.

Varicella vaccine. Med Lett 1995;37:55.

Zimmerman RK, Clover RD. Adult immunizations—a practical approach for clinicians: part I. Am Fam Physician 1995;51:859.

Zimmerman RK, Clover RD. Adult immunizations—a practical approach for clinicians: part II. Am Fam Physician 1995;51:1139.

CHAPTER 5
Vital Statistics and Injuries

This chapter summarizes important vital statistics on the mortality, morbidity, and demographics of the adolescent population in the United States.

MORTALITY

Although the adolescent period is generally considered a healthy time of life, considerable morbidity and mortality do occur. Owing to the fact that data supplied by the National Center for Health Statistics for the adolescent years break down into the 5- to 14-year-old age group and the 15- to 24-year-old age group, it is more difficult to evaluate data for different phases of adolescence. Significant mortality data during adolescence include:

1. Unintentional injuries are the fourth leading cause of death in the United States for the total population but the leading cause of death among 12- to 24-year-olds. The leading cause of death from unintentional injuries are motor vehicle crashes.
2. Adolescent males have twice the mortality rate of adolescent females.
3. Over 80% of deaths of persons 15–24 years old are secondary to violent causes, including accidents, suicides, and homicides.
4. The leading cause of death was the same for the white and African-American populations for all age groups except 15–24 and 25–44 years. The leading cause of death for the white population in ages 15–24 and 25–44 was accidents and adverse effects. For the African-American population homicide and legal intervention was the leading cause of death among the 15- to 24-year-old population, and human immunodeficiency virus (HIV) infection was the leading cause for those aged 25–44. Homicide and legal intervention consistently ranked higher for the Hispanic population than for the non-Hispanic white population for all age groups between 15–24 and 45–64 years. In addition, HIV infection for the Hispanic population aged 1–14, 15–24, 25–44, and 45–64 consistently ranked higher than that for the non-Hispanic white population for these same age groups. Leading causes of death comparing Hispanic, white non-Hispanic, African-American, Asian, and American Indian populations are reported in Tables 5.1 and 5.2.
5. Between 1985 and 1991 the age-adjusted homicide rate increased 31% to 10.9 deaths per 100,000 population, reversing a downward trend seen in the first half of the decade. The largest increase in homicide rate was in the 15- to 24-year-old African-American male population for whom the homicide rate more than doubled to 159 deaths per 100,000 youth in 1991. This was nine times the rate for white males. The homicide rate for young Hispanic males was about 3.5 times the rate for white males. There has been a downward trend since 1992 in the general population from 10.5 per 100,000 in 1993 to 9.7 per 100,000 in 1994.
6. Firearm deaths have been reported since 1992. In 1994 in the United States there were 39,720 deaths from firearm injuries, including those related to accidents, suicides, and homicides. Most of the firearm deaths were related to suicides and homicides. Among

TABLE 5.1. Leading Causes of Death among 15- to 24-Year-Olds for Hispanic, White Non-Hispanic, and African-American Youth: United States, 1992

Hispanic	Number	White Non-Hispanic	Number	African-American	Number
Homicide	1732	Accidents and adverse	9528	Homicide	4652
Accidents and adverse effects	1624	effects		Accidents and adverse effects	1684
		Suicide	2154		
Suicide	425	Homicide	1412	Suicide	536
Malignant neoplasms	216	Malignant neoplasms	1195	Diseases of heart	305
Human immuno-deficiency virus	91	Diseases of heart	529	Human immuno-deficiency virus	286
		Congenital anomalies	315		
Diseases of heart	83	Human immuno-deficiency virus	193	Malignant neoplasms	276
Congenital anomalies	44			Anemias	86
Cerebrovascular diseases	27	Pneumonia and influenza	134	Chronic obstructive pulmonary diseases	80
Pneumonia and influenza	24	Cerebrovascular diseases	117	Congenital anomalies	70
Complications of pregnancy, childbirth	20	Chronic obstructive pulmonary disease	90	Pneumonia and influenza	57

Adapted from Centers for Disease Control and Prevention/National Center for Health Statistics. Advance report of final mortality statistics, 1992. Monthly Vital Statistics Report December 8, 1994;43:(6, suppl).

TABLE 5.2. Death Rates for Selected Causes for Persons 1–14 and 15–24 Years of Age by Race: United States, 1989–1991 (Deaths per 100,000 Population)

Cause of Death	White	African-American	Asian	American Indian	Hispanic
1–14 years					
All causes	28.4	48.3	22.7	37.3	30.2
Unintentional injuries	12.0	18.3	8.2	19.3	12.4
Homicide	1.2	5.2	1.4	2.4	2.2
Cancer	3.3	3.1	2.7	2.1	3.4
Congenital anomalies	2.6	3.4	2.3	2.9	2.8
All other causes	9.3	18.2	8.2	10.6	9.5
15–24 years					
All causes	89.3	161.9	50.1	142.0	103.3
Unintentional injuries	45.8	34.7	21.0	73.3	43.4
Motor vehicle accidents	36.1	21.7	16.1	51.9	32.9
Homicide	9.6	77.9	8.8	17.9	30.5
Suicide	13.8	9.1	8.3	26.3	9.9
All other causes	20.1	40.2	12.1	24.5	19.5

Adapted from National Center for Health Statistics. Health, United States, 1993 [DHHS publication (PHS) 94–1232]. Hyattsville, Maryland: US Government Printing Office, 1994.

these deaths, 60% occurred among white males, 23% among African-American males, 10% among white females, and 3.9% among African-American females. The largest number was in the 15- to 24- and 25- to 34-year-old age groups. Between 1985 and 1991 the age-adjusted death rate for firearm injuries increased 19%. During this period the firearm death rate for African-American males aged 15–24 increased more than 2.5 times to 162 deaths per 100,000, or about five times that rate in white males.

7. Excluding violent causes of death, cancer is the number one cause of adolescent mortality.
8. HIV has become one of the 10 leading causes of death in all ages between 1 and 65. HIV infection ranked seventh for ages 1–4, seventh for ages 5–14, sixth for ages 15–24, second for ages 25–44, and eighth for ages 45–64.

The following are national estimates of some of the risks of adolescents as the year 2000 approaches (Scales, 1988):

Table 5.3.   Death Rates of Adolescents Due to All Causes, according to Race, Sex, and Age in the United States for Selected Years 1950–1992 (Rate per 100,000)

Race, Sex, and Age Group (yr)	Year						
	1950	1960	1970	1975	1980	1987	1992
White male							
10–14	67.1	51.6	48.5	43.3	37.4	32.8	28.2
15–19	130.5	125.2	147.1	144.5	142.7	116.3	106.0
20–24	173.0	166.9	199.0	189.5	190.9	156.9	135.4
White female							
10–14	41.3	30.8	27.9	24.4	21.9	17.9	17.2
15–19	62.3	50.3	57.8	52.4	53.7	48.7	43.3
20–24	79.8	60.4	65.7	59.8	57.3	49.5	44.3
African-American male							
10–14	94.8	79.2	63.8	57.1	45.4	46.1	44.9
15–19	216.0	165.5	230.9	167.4	134.5	144.2	218.4
20–24	366.9	271.8	448.8	357.3	294.5	266.9	321.0
African-American female							
10–14	66.6	44.1	40.1	31.7	27.7	22.7	25.4
15–19	172.7	81.3	86.2	65.8	50.3	49.0	50.5
20–24	251.3	138.1	144.1	115.1	91.8	86.2	84.3
Total							
10–14	58.1	44.0	40.6	35.7	30.8	26.9	24.6
15–19	108.6	92.2	110.3	101.5	97.9	84.6	84.3
20–24	146.0	123.6	148.0	138.2	132.7	113.2	105.7

Adapted from National Center for Health Statistics. Health, United States, 1981 and 1993 [DHHS publication (PHS) 94–1232]. Hyattsville, Maryland: US Government Printing Office, 1994, and Kochanek KD, Hudson BL. Advance report of final mortality statistics, 1992, Monthly Vital Statistics Report December 8, 1994;43(6, suppl).

- Every 31 seconds, a teen becomes pregnant, with 40% of today's teens becoming pregnant at least once during adolescence.
- Every 2 minutes, a teen gives birth.
- Every 78 seconds, a teen attempts suicide.
- Every 20 minutes, a teen is killed in an accident.
- Every 90 minutes, one teen is murdered and another commits suicide.
- By age 18, one in eight teens will run away from home at least once.

Table 5.3 summarizes the death rates of adolescents from 1950 to 1992 by race, sex, and age. Table 5.4 summarizes the common causes of mortality for children and adolescents from 1950 to 1992. Tables 5.5 and 5.6 summarize recent mortality numbers and rates of the top causes of death in adolescents by sex and race.

Cancer

The fourth leading cause of death among adolescents is cancer. During adolescence there is an increase in the incidence and mortality from lymphomas, Hodgkin's disease, and bone and genital tumors. Leukemia is the number one cause of death from malignancies in the 15- to 24-year-old age group, while lymphomas are the most prevalent malignancy. Tables 5.7 and 5.8 give mortality and incidence rates, respectively, of tumors during childhood, adolescence, and young adulthood.

Injuries

Injuries are the major health problem of adolescents and the leading cause of death in this age group. Nonfatal injuries are also extremely common.

TABLE 5.4. Mortality Rates for Common Causes of Death among Children and Adolescents, 1950–1992, in the United States (Rate per 100,000)

Cause and Age Group (yr)	1950	1960	1970	1980	1985	1987	1992	(Number in 1992)
Accidents, all								
5–14	20.1	26.0	20.1	15.0	12.5	12.3	9.3	3,388
15–24	48.2	58.4	68.7	61.7	48.4	48.9	37.8	13,662
Motor vehicle accidents								
5–14	8.8	7.9	10.2	7.9	6.8	7.0	5.2	1,904
15–24	34.4	38.0	47.2	44.8	36.1	37.8	28.5	10,305
Homicide								
5–14	0.5	0.5	0.9	1.2	1.2	1.2	1.6	587
15–24	6.3	5.9	11.7	15.6	12.1	14.0	22.2	8,019
Suicide								
5–14	0.2	0.3	0.3	0.4	0.8	0.7	0.9	314
15–24	4.5	5.2	8.8	12.3	12.9	12.9	13.0	4,693
Malignant neoplasms								
5–14	6.7	6.8	6.0	4.3	3.5	3.3	3.0	1,105
15–24	8.6	8.3	8.3	6.3	5.4	5.1	5.0	1,809
HIV								
5–14	—	—	—	—	—	—	0.6	104
15–24	—	—	—	—	—	—	3.4	578
Cardiac								
5–14	2.1	1.3	0.8	0.9	0.9	1.2	0.8	284
15–24	6.8	4.0	3.0	2.9	2.8	3.6	2.7	968
Congenital anomalies								
5–14	2.4	3.6	2.2	1.6	1.4	1.3	1.2	448
15–24	1.8	2.7	2.1	1.4	1.2	1.3	1.2	450
Pneumonia and influenza								
5–14	3.2	2.6	1.6	0.6	0.4	0.3	0.3	104
15–24	3.2	3.0	2.4	0.8	0.6	0.7	0.6	229
Cerebrovascular								
5–14	0.5	0.7	0.7	0.3	0.2	0.2	0.2	64
15–24	1.6	1.8	1.6	1.0	0.8	0.6	0.5	197
Total								
5–14	60.1	46.6	41.3	30.6	26.3	25.6	22.5	8,193
15–24	128.1	106.3	127.7	115.4	95.9	99.4	95.6	34,548

Adapted from National Center for Health Statistics. Health, United States, 1989 and 1993 [DHHS publication (PHS) 94–1232]. Hyattsville, Maryland: US Government Printing Office, 1994, and Kochanek KD, Hudson BL. Advance report of final mortality statistics, 1992. Monthly Vital Statistics Report December 8, 1994;43(6, suppl).

- Injuries are the leading cause of death between the ages of 1 and 44 in the United States.
- Unintentional injuries, suicide, and homicide cause 80% of the deaths in the adolescent age group. Among adolescents, unintentional injuries cause about 48% of the deaths in the 10- to 14-year-old age group and 57% in the 15- to 19-year-old age group. Intentional injuries comprise about 8% and 21%, respectively.
- Deaths are only a small part of a problem that encompasses millions of nonfatal injuries. For every adolescent injury resulting in death, there are an estimated 41 injuries that involve hospitalization and 1100 injuries that are treated in an emergency room. Even more are treated by private physicians, clinics, and school personnel and at home.
- The 15- to 24-year-old age group has the highest costs related to injury of any rate group in the United States.

One problem in evaluating injury statistics is that data collection often uses different age groupings to classify subjects. There is also no mandatory national reporting system for accidents or injuries. Useful data are available from:

TABLE 5.5.   Deaths from Selected Causes, by 5-Year Age Groups, Sex, and Race: United States, 1990

Cause of Death; Sex	Age Range (yr)				
	5–9	10–14	15–19	20–24	25–29
All causes	3,995	4,441	15,711	21,022	26,579
Male	2,363	2,764	11,671	16,202	19,794
Female	1,632	1,677	4,040	4,820	6,785
White	2,949	3,323	11,678	15,230	19,018
Male	1,750	2,070	8,515	11,693	14,309
Female	1,199	1,253	3,163	3,537	4,709
African-American	876	963	3,467	5,119	6,838
Male	512	601	2,737	3,994	4,949
Female	364	362	730	1,125	1,889
Accidents	1,771	1,879	7,561	8,680	8,264
Male	1,129	1,289	5,558	6,912	6,452
Female	642	590	2,003	1,768	1,812
White	1,290	1,457	6,470	7,357	6,828
African-American	397	348	805	1,023	1,152
Motor vehicle accidents	970	1,089	5,918	6,689	5,606
Male	595	665	4,172	5,189	4,254
Female	375	424	1,746	1,500	1,352
White	736	893	5,187	5,745	4,686
African-American	186	155	524	707	710
Suicides	6	258	1,979	2,890	3,192
Male	4	191	1,656	2,504	2,667
Female	2	67	323	386	525
White	4	219	1,701	2,481	2,731
African-American	2	29	183	282	357
Homicides and legal intervention	156	356	3,042	4,312	4,180
Male	70	229	2,571	3,651	3,392
Female	86	127	471	661	788
White	88	179	1,170	1,795	1,864
African-American	62	170	1,794	2,407	2,237
Neoplasias	603	569	759	1,060	1,897
Leukemia	187	195	274	261	309
Lymphatic	31	50	99	194	355
Male	324	297	441	637	1,025
Female	245	228	318	423	872
White	464	433	606	864	1,526
African-American	82	72	122	170	321
Major cardiovascular diseases	162	239	440	784	1,515
Male	86	129	289	469	918
Female	76	110	151	315	597
White	124	170	312	508	1,032
African-American	30	60	117	255	436
Congenital anomalies	286	182	224	267	236
Pneumonia and influenza	76	58	85	146	477
Chronic obstructive pulmonary diseases	34	81	82	133	167
Asthma	28	74	76	107	130
Cerebrovascular disease	33	40	74	160	334
Anemias	28	23	47	77	84
Diabetes mellitus	7	17	29	86	224
Complications of pregnancy	0	0	40	67	84
Septicemia	32	14	28	56	100
Nephritis	9	11	17	40	75
Meningitis	23	14	14	15	29
Chronic liver disease	3	4	10	34	196
Intestinal obstruction	17	10	7	15	17
Appendicitis	6	7	5	6	5
Ulcer of stomach and duodenum	2	2	3	8	24

Adapted from National Center for Health Statistics. Vital statistics of the United States, 1990, Volume II: Mortality, Part B. Hyattsville, Maryland: DHHS Public Health Service, 1994.

TABLE 5.6. Death Rates from the 10 Leading Causes of Death in 15- to 24-Year-Olds by Race and Sex: United States, 1992 (Deaths per 100,000)

	Death Rate				
	All Races, Both Sexes	All Races, Males	All Races, Females	Both Sexes, White	Both Sexes, African-American
Accidents and adverse effects	37.8	55.5	19.3	39.4	31.6
Homicide and legal intervention	22.2	37.3	6.4	10.9	86.7
					(154.4, males)
Suicide	13.0	21.9	3.7	13.5	10.0
Malignant neoplasms	5.0	5.9	4.1	5.0	5.2
Diseases of heart	2.7	3.4	1.9	2.2	5.7
Human immunodeficiency virus	1.6	2.3	0.9	1.0	5.4
Congenital anomalies	1.2	1.5	1.0	1.3	1.3
Pneumonia and influenza	0.6	0.7	0.6	0.6	1.1
Complications of pregnancy			0.6		
Cerebrovascular diseases	0.5	0.6		0.5	
Chronic obstructive pulmonary diseases	0.5	0.6	0.5	0.4	1.5
Anemias					
All other causes	10.4	12.2	8.3	9.0	1.6

Adapted from Kochanek KD, Hudson BL. Advance report of final mortality statistics, 1992. Monthly Vital Statistics Report December 8, 1994;43(6, suppl).

- National Electronic Injury Surveillance System (NEISS) of the U.S. Consumer Product Safety Commission (data from a sample of nationwide hospitals)
- Fatal Accident Reporting System (FARS) of the U.S. Department of Transportation's National Highway Traffic Safety Commission
- National Poison Control Data Network
- National Health Interview Survey (NHIS) conducted by the National Center for Health Statistics
- Individual research studies

Epidemiology

1. Injuries are the major health problem of adolescents, causing 80% of the deaths in teenagers and young adults. The leading causes of unintentional injuries are motor vehicle accidents, motorcycle accidents, and drowning. Unintentional injuries claim more lives than all other causes of death combined in 10- to 19-year-olds.
2. Injuries are the leading cause of loss of productive years of life.
3. For adolescents, from one-third to one-half of injuries occur at school or work, with another one-third to one-half occurring at or near home.
4. Age: According to a Massachusetts study, the adolescent age group had the highest injury rate of all age groups, 2,718/10,000 per year. Of these, 96.5% are treated and released, 3.4% are admitted, and 0.1% die. The top causes of injuries were motor vehicle accidents, falls, striking objects, and sports. The incidence of the leading cause of accidental death, motor vehicle accidents, peaks at age 19, with a large spike between ages 14 and 19, and falls dramatically after age 20.
5. Gender: Overall rates of injury death for 10- to 19-year-old males exceed those for females by as much as 9.9:1 and for motor vehicle occupants in the 15–19 age group 2.4:1. Overall, four out of five injury victims are male.
6. Race: Rates for Native Americans exceed those for African-Americans and whites by almost 100%. Homicide rates are particularly high for African-American adolescents,

TABLE 5.7. Mortality Related to Leading Cancer Sites in Children and Adolescents by Age, Sex, and Race (Death Rate per 100,000): United States, 1984–1988

Age Group (yr)	Site	Mortality Rate				
		Total	Males	Females	White	African-American
5–9	Total	3.5	4.0	3.0	3.6	3.2
	Leukemias	1.4	1.7	1.1	1.5	1.1
	Brain and CNS	0.9	1.0	0.9	1.0	0.9
	Other endocrine	0.3	0.4	0.3	0.3	0.3
	Non-Hodgkin's disease	0.2	0.3	0.1	0.2	0.1
	Kidney and renal pelvis	0.2	0.1	0.2	0.2	0.2
10–14	Total	3.3	3.6	2.9	3.3	3.2
	Leukemias	1.3	1.5	1.1	1.4	1.2
	Brain and CNS	0.7	0.8	0.6	0.7	0.7
	Bone and joints	0.3	0.3	0.3	0.3	0.3
	Non-Hodgkin's disease	0.2	0.4	0.1	0.3	0.2
	Hodgkin's disease	0.1	0.1	0.1	0.1	0.1
15–19	Total	4.6	5.4	3.7	4.6	4.5
	Leukemias	1.4	1.8	1.1	1.5	1.3
	Brain and CNS	0.7	0.8	0.6	0.7	0.6
	Bone and joints	0.6	0.7	0.4	0.6	0.4
	Non-Hodgkin's disease	0.4	0.6	0.3	0.4	0.4
	Hodgkin's disease	0.3	0.3	0.2	0.2	0.3
	Ovary	0.1	—	0.2	0.0	0.1
	Testis	0.1	0.0	—	0.1	0.0
20–24	Total	5.9	7.2	4.7	5.9	6.5
	Leukemias	1.4	1.7	1.0	1.4	1.4
	Brain and CNS	0.6	0.7	0.5	0.6	0.6
	Non-Hodgkin's disease	0.6	0.7	0.4	0.6	0.6
	Hodgkin's disease	0.6	0.7	0.5	0.6	0.4
	Bone and joints	0.4	0.6	0.2	0.4	0.4
	Testis	0.3	0.5	—	0.3	0.1
	Melanoma of skin	0.2	0.3	0.2	0.3	0.0
	Colon	0.2	0.2	0.1	0.1	0.4
	Ovary	0.1	—	0.2	0.1	0.1
	Breast	0.1	0.0	0.4	0.1	0.2
25–29	Total	9.1	9.8	8.4	8.9	10.7
	Leukemias	1.3	1.6	1.1	1.3	1.6
	Brain and CNS	1.0	1.1	0.8	1.0	0.5
	Non-Hodgkin's disease	0.8	1.2	0.5	0.7	1.0
	Hodgkin's disease	0.7	0.9	0.5	0.8	0.5
	Melanoma of skin	0.6	0.7	0.5	0.7	0.1
	Breast	0.6	0.0	1.2	0.6	1.0
	Colon	0.5	0.5	0.4	0.4	0.8
	Cervix	0.4	—	0.9	0.4	0.7
	Testis	0.3	0.7	—	0.4	0.1
	Lung	0.3	0.3	0.2	0.2	0.5
	Bone and joints	0.2	0.3	0.1	0.2	0.1
	Ovary	0.2	—	0.4	0.2	0.2

Adapted from Ries LAG, Hjanky BF, Miller BA, et al. Cancer statistics review 1973, 1973–1988 [NIH publication 91-2789]. Bethesda, Maryland: National Cancer Institute, 1991.

while suicide rates are higher for both whites and Native Americans than for African-Americans.

7. Social economic status: Poverty areas have higher rates of fires, homicides, unintentional shootings, drowning, and motor vehicle accidents.
8. Nonfatal injuries: Fraser et al. (1995) examined the incidence of nonfatal injuries in a nationally representative sample of adolescents under the age of 18 (1988 Child Health

TABLE 5.8. Incidence Rates of Leading Cancer Sites in Children and Adolescents by Age, Sex, and Race (Rate per 100,000): United States, 1991

Age Group (yr)	Site	Mortality Rate				
		Total	Males	Females	White	African-American
5–9	Total	10.8	11.7	9.8	10.7	12.2
	Leukemias	3.6	3.8	3.4	3.4	5.0
	Brain and CNS	3.4	3.5	3.0	3.5	3.2
	Bone and joints	0.9	0.5	1.3	0.8	0.9
	Non-Hodgkin's disease	0.8	1.4	0.2	1.0	—
	Soft tissue	0.8	0.8	0.7	0.6	0.9
	Kidney and renal pelvis	0.7	0.8	0.6	0.7	0.5
	Hodgkin's disease	0.3	0.6	—	0.2	0.9
10–14	Total	12.7	12.7	12.7	13.3	10.6
	Brain and CNS	3.2	3.5	2.9	3.1	2.8
	Leukemias	2.3	2.3	2.3	2.6	1.4
	Bone and joints	1.6	1.0	2.1	1.8	1.4
	Hodgkin's disease	1.4	0.8	2.0	1.5	0.9
	Non-Hodgkin's disease	1.0	1.6	0.2	1.1	0.9
	Soft tissue	0.5	0.6	0.7	0.5	—
	Melanoma of skin	0.4	0.3	0.4	0.5	—
	Thyroid	0.3	0.1	0.5	0.4	—
	Ovary	0.3	—	0.6	0.2	0.5
	Digestive system	0.2	0.2	0.2	0.2	0.5
	Oral cavity	0.1	0.2	—	0.2	—
15–19	Total	19.3	21.5	17.0	20.4	13.5
	Hodgkin's disease	3.8	4.2	3.4	4.3	3.3
	Leukemias	2.5	2.9	2.2	2.7	1.4
	Testis	1.9	3.7	—	2.3	—
	Non-Hodgkin's disease	1.7	2.2	1.0	1.8	1.4
	Brain and CNS	1.6	2.2	0.9	1.7	0.9
	Bone and joints	1.3	2.0	0.5	1.2	0.9
	Melanoma of skin	1.3	0.9	1.7	1.6	—
	Thyroid	1.1	0.2	2.1	1.2	0.5
	Soft tissue	1.0	0.7	1.2	0.8	0.9
	Ovary	1.0	—	1.9	0.8	1.9
	Oral cavity	0.6	0.7	0.4	0.7	0.5
20–24	Total	32.2	29.9	34.5	34.6	18.5
	Hodgkin's disease	4.9	4.5	5.4	6.1	1.3
	Thyroid	4.2	1.4	7.0	4.4	2.6
	Melanoma of skin	3.8	2.4	5.1	4.3	—
	Testis	3.5	6.9	—	3.8	0.9
	Brain and CNS	2.4	2.0	2.7	2.8	0.9
	Non-Hodgkin's disease	2.1	2.3	1.9	2.0	2.6
	Leukemias	1.9	2.5	1.1	2.0	0.9
	Ovary	1.3	—	2.7	1.4	0.4
	Digestive	1.3	1.7	1.0	1.2	1.3
	Soft tissue	1.0	1.3	0.8	1.2	0.4
	Cervix	1.0	—	1.9	0.9	1.3
	Bone and joints	1.0	1.0	1.0	0.9	0.9
	Breast	0.6	—	1.1	0.5	1.3
	Oral cavity	0.4	0.4	0.5	0.6	—
25–29	Total	58.1	59.7	56.4	59.8	40.6
	Melanoma of skin	7.0	6.1	7.9	7.8	—
	Testis	6.6	13.2	—	7.4	—
	Breast	5.2	—	7.8	3.3	6.6
	Non-Hodgkin's lymphoma	5.1	7.5	2.7	4.8	7.0
	Hodgkin's disease	5.0	5.5	4.5	5.7	3.3
	Thyroid	4.8	2.0	7.6	5.4	0.4
	Cervix	3.5	—	7.1	3.3	4.5
	Brain and CNS	3.2	3.8	2.7	3.5	2.5
	Digestive	2.5	2.7	2.3	2.3	1.6
	Leukemia	1.9	2.1	1.7	1.6	2.9

National Cancer Institute, unpublished data.

117

TABLE 5.9.   Accidental Deaths by Age and Type, 1993, and Unintentional-Injury Death Rates, United States for 15- to 24-Year-Olds, 1903–1993

Age	All Types	Motor Vehicle	Drowning	Fires, Burns	Firearms	Falls	Ingestion	Poison
5–14	3,660	2,011	455	382	203	69	30	56
15–24	15,278	11,664	907	256	542	233	46	561

Adapted from National Safety Council. Accident facts, 1994. Chicago: National Safety Council, 1994.

TABLE 5.10.   Accidental Death Rates among Youth: United States, 1903–1993

Year	Total by Age		Motor Vehicle by Age	
	5–14	15–24	5–14	15–24
1903	46.8	65.0		
1910	39.1	65.3		
1920	44.9	55.5	14.6	8.7
1930	36.9	62.3	14.7	27.4
1940	28.8	53.5	11.5	28.7
1950	22.6	55.0	8.8	34.5
1960	19.1	55.6	7.9	37.7
1970	20.1	68.0	10.2	46.7
1980	15.0	61.7	7.9	44.8
1985	12.4	47.5	6.5	35.6
1986	12.1	51.5	6.8	39.7
1993	9.7	38.2	5.4	29.1

Adapted from National Safety Council. Accident facts, 1994. Chicago: National Safety Council, 1994.

Supplement of the National Health Interview Survey, Fraser, 1995). The incidence of nonfatal accidents, injuries, and poisonings was 16.6/100, resulting in 3.2 mean number of bed days, 4.1 mean number of school absence days, and 20.1% with limited activity due to the injury. The incidence was highest in older adolescents 14–17 (18.1/100), males (20.3/100), whites (19.5/100), and midwestern U.S. residents (18.1/100). The most frequent injuries were cuts (59.6/1000), sprains (51.3/1000), and broken bones (43.3/1000).

9. Accidental death rates by age and type are outlined in Table 5.9 and trends during this century in Table 5.10.

Factors Contributing to Adolescent Injuries

Factors contributing to high injury rates in adolescents often relate to the discrepancies between an adolescent's physical development and his or her cognitive and emotional development. Differences also exist between the adolescent's developmental state and the environment in which the teen must function. Several characteristics of the adolescent can exacerbate this problem:

- Experimentation with risky behaviors or situations
- Challenge of authority or rules
- Desire for peer approval and a tendency to follow peer activities or suggestions

Placing these characteristics into an environment in which alcohol and drugs are readily available and adding fast cars lead to a significant risk for injury and death.

Automobile Injuries

Automobile injuries are the leading cause of morbidity and mortality in those 1–44 years of age. The transportation environment is the most dangerous milieu for the adolescent, whether as a motor vehicle occupant, motorcyclist, bicyclist, or pedestrian.

- Automobile injuries cause more than 50% of the deaths of those aged 16–19.
- The death rate per mile driven is highest in those aged 16–19. In 1991 alone, motor vehicle crashes killed 6730 youths ages 15–20.
- The 15- to 24-year-old age group comprises 14.7% of the licensed drivers but 26.9% of the fatal motor vehicle crashes and 28.4% of all drivers in accidents. The highest fatality rate per driver was in drivers aged 16. See Table 5.11 for accident rates by age. Overall, males had 27 fatalities per one billion miles driven compared to 17 for females. Females have higher involvement rates for all accidents with rates of 101 per ten million miles driven compared to 87 for males.
- Adolescent drivers not only have high mortality rates but are also responsible for a high death rate in passengers. The majority of adolescent passengers killed are driven by other adolescents.
- Most fatal motor vehicle injuries in adolescents occur in the evening and early morning hours, especially on weekends. (Adolescents do 20% of their driving at night, but more than half of the crash fatalities are during nighttime hours.)

TABLE 5.11.   Age of Drivers, Total Number, and Number in Accidents: United States, 1993[a]

| | Licensed Drivers | | Drivers in Accidents | | | | Per Number of Drivers | |
| | | | Fatal | | All | | | |
Age Group	Number	%	Number	%	Number	%	Fatal[b]	All[c]
Total	178,878,000	100.0	53,900	100.0	21,100,000	100.0	32	12
Under 16	47,000	([d])	400	0.7	100,000	0.5	([e])	([e])
16	1,431,000	0.8	1,100	2.0	570,000	2.7	77	40
17	2,126,000	1.2	1,400	2.6	680,000	3.2	66	32
18	2,521,000	1.4	1,700	3.2	730,000	3.5	67	29
19	2,764,000	1.6	1,800	3.3	700,000	3.3	65	25
19 and under	8,889,000	5.1	6,400	11.8	2,780,000	13.2	72	31
20	2,984,000	1.7	1,500	2.8	640,000	3.0	50	21
21	3,338,000	1.9	1,700	3.2	650,000	3.1	51	19
22	3,532,000	2.0	1,800	3.3	670,000	3.2	51	19
23	3,538,000	2.0	1,600	3.0	640,000	3.0	45	18
24	3,483,000	2.0	1,500	2.8	610,000	2.9	43	18
20–24	16,875,000	9.6	8,100	15.1	3,210,000	15.2	48	19
25–34	40,423,000	23.0	13,500	25.0	5,500,000	26.1	33	14
35–44	38,650,000	22.0	10,400	19.3	4,160,000	19.7	27	11
45–54	27,026,000	15.4	5,900	10.9	2,380,000	11.3	22	9
55–64	19,494,000	11.1	3,800	7.1	1,420,000	6.7	19	7
65–74	16,861,000	9.6	3,000	5.6	1,080,000	4.9	18	6
75 and over	7,661,000	4.4	2,800	5.2	620,000	2.9	37	8

Adapted from National Safety Council. Accident facts, 1994. Chicago: National Safety Council, 1994.
[a]Drivers in accidents based on reports from 20 state traffic authorities. Number of licensed drivers by age from the Federal Highway Administration. Procedures for estimating the number of accidents were changed for the 1990 edition and are not comparable to those in previous editions.
[b]Drivers in fatal accidents per 100,000 licensed drivers in each age group.
[c]Drivers in all accidents per 100 licensed drivers in each age group.
[d]Less than 0.05.
[e]Rates for drivers under age 16 are substantially overstated due to the high proportion of unlicensed drivers involved.

- The frequency of motor vehicle injuries varies by age and sex. Per passenger mile, the highest rates are among those aged 16–24. From age 10 on, the fatality rates are higher for males than females. In those aged 16–24, death rates of males are more than double those of females. White males have the highest motor vehicle–related death rate.
- Ages at peak death rate: Motor vehicle–related death rates for males peak at 71/100 million miles at age 17. Motor vehicle–related death rates for females peak at age 19 with a rate of 30/100 million miles.
- Death rates increase for motor vehicle occupants, motorcyclists, and pedestrians until age 20. For bicyclists the rates peak between 11 and 15 years of age, and for motorcyclists between 17 and 22 years of age.

Risk Factors   Seventy-one percent of crashes are estimated to be due to driver error and not to vehicular or environmental factors.

1. Precrash factors
   a. Use of alcohol: About 50% of fatally injured drivers have blood alcohol levels of 0.10% or higher (legal limit in most states). Twenty-five percent of adolescent drivers in fatal daytime multivehicle crashes have a high blood alcohol content, as do nearly 75% of adolescent drivers in fatal nighttime single-vehicle accidents. The rate of alcohol-related fatal crashes per unit of travel is highest among drivers aged 16–19. Younger drivers also seem to be more adversely affected at lower blood alcohol levels than do older drivers. In addition, alcohol may also increase the risks of injury in the crash phase by reducing the tolerance of body tissues to trauma. Loiselle et al. (1993) compared 134 adolescents admitted to a pediatric trauma service compared to teens admitted for asthma. Of the trauma–related admissions, 34% of the teens had positive tests for alcohol or drugs of abuse. The number of positive tests in the asthmatic teens was only 2% (1/49). The most commonly detected drugs were alcohol (eight), benzodiazepines (eight), cocaine (five), and cannabinoids (four). There was also a much higher rate of positive toxicology screening tests among adolescents with an intentional versus unintentional mechanism of injury (21 of 71 versus 1 of 63).
   b. Other drugs: While not as many studies are available on other drugs as compared to alcohol, other drugs also seem to play a factor. An analysis of 440 fatally injured male drivers between 15 and 34 years of age in California detected the presence of alcohol in 70%, marijuana in 37%, cocaine in 11%, and diazepam in 4%.
   c. Morbidity: Drivers with chronic medical conditions such as diabetes, epilepsy, alcoholism, cardiovascular disease, and mental illness may experience higher crash rates.
2. Crash phase risk factors: Occupant restraints: Estimates of effectiveness of occupant restraints vary but range between 40% and 60%. In order, increasing effectiveness rates go to lap belts, air bags, automatic belts, lap or shoulder belts, air bags with lap belts, and air bags with lap or shoulder belts. In 1970, 77% of persons killed in motor vehicle crashes were not wearing seat belts. Adolescents have the highest proportion of belt nonuse (83%) of any age group involved in fatal motor vehicle crashes.

Nonautomobile Injuries

Motorcycle

- Fifty percent of motorcycle fatalities are among those aged 15–24.
- Incidence of nonfatal injuries peaks for motorcycle injuries at age 18.
- Odds of death while driving a motorcycle are about 1 in 50 per person per year.

Drowning   The second leading cause of nonintentional injuries and deaths in adolescents is drowning.

- Sex: More common in males by a ratio of 12:1 in boat-related accidents and 5:1 in non-boat-related accidents.
- Age: Rate of drowning peaks at age 18.
- Time: Increased prevalence on Saturdays and Sundays and during May through August.
- Forty percent to 50% of drowning in adolescents are associated with the use of alcohol.
- Site: In adolescents, most drownings are in natural bodies of freshwater such as lakes, rivers, streams, and ponds rather than the ocean or a swimming pool, where younger children are usually hurt.
- Boating: A total of 800 deaths and 3560 injuries in recreational boating accidents were reported to the Coast Guard in 1993. The age group 20–29 had more deaths while boating than any other age group.

Firearms   Firearms are the third leading cause of unintentional death in this age group.

- Adolescents and young adults have the highest rate of unintentional firearm-related fatalities, with males ages 15–19 having the highest risk.
- Firearm deaths have increased 19% from 1985 to 1991.
- The overwhelming percentage of deaths from firearms occurs in males (over 80%).
- More than half the fatalities occur in and around the home, generally while a gun is being cleaned or played with.
- Many adolescents in rural and urban areas either own or have close access to a gun.
- As many as 90% of firearm deaths are either related to suicide or homicide (Table 5.12).

Bicycle Accidents

- Deaths from bicycle accidents have increased over twofold in the past 30 years, as a result of the large increase in individuals involved in bicycling.
- Head injuries account for 62% of bicycle-related deaths, for 33% of bicycle-related emergency department visits, and for 67% of bicycle-related hospital admissions. Bicycle-related injuries and deaths cost society about $8 billion each year. However, only approximately 18% of bicyclists wear helmets all or most of the time.
- Bicycle injuries are greatest among those under the age of 15 (about 70%), peaking between ages 10 and 14. Over 40% of all deaths from bicycle-related head injury were among persons less than 15 years of age.
- Among those over 14 years of age, as many as 65% with brain injury were intoxicated at the time of riding. Eighty percent of the deaths and injuries were associated with riders who had violated a bicycling rule.
- Bicycle injuries are now up to over 1 million per year in the United States.

Skateboard Injuries   Skateboard injuries have fluctuated widely. In 1974 there were only 3200 reported injuries. With the sudden popularity of skateboarding, this increased to over 140,000 in 1977, peaking in 1978 with an estimated 350,000. Since that time, there has been a decline in skateboard use, with injuries falling to fewer than 20,000 per year.

All-Terrain Vehicles   In 1986 about 86,000 injuries occurred with all-terrain vehicles. Two-thirds of the injuries were to those less than 25 years of age and 40% to individuals less than 16 years of age. Sales of three-wheeled vehicles are now prohibited. Four-wheel vehicles

Table 5.12. Firearm Mortality among Children, Youth, and Young Adults, 1–34 Years Old: United States, 1991

[Death rate per 100,000 population. Deaths classified according to the ninth revision of the *International Classification of Diseases*]

Item	Under 5 Years	5–9 Years	10–14 Years	15–19 Years	20–24 Years	25–29 Years	30–34 Years
Male							
Total							
White	0.5	0.5	4.6	29.1	34.6	29.0	26.0
African-American	1.4	1.5	11.5	140.5	184.3	129.4	94.8
Accidents							
White	0.1	0.3	1.6	2.9	1.6	1.0	0.8
African-American	0.2	0.6	2.0	6.3	4.7	2.2	1.2
Suicide							
White	(*a*)	(*a*)	1.5	13.6	17.7	15.3	14.9
African-American	(*a*)	(*a*)	1.1	9.0	14.4	13.4	10.5
Homicide							
White	0.3	0.3	1.4	11.8	14.9	12.3	10.1
African-American	1.1	0.9	8.2	123.6	164.4	113.4	82.9
Female							
Total							
White	0.4	0.3	1.0	4.6	5.1	4.9	5.5
African-American	1.5	0.5	3.0	12.7	17.7	16.5	13.9
Accidents							
White	0.1	0.1	0.1	0.2	0.2	0.1	0.1
African-American	0.4	0.1	0.2	0.2	(*a*)	0.1	0.1
Suicide							
White	(*a*)	(*a*)	0.4	2.1	2.0	2.4	2.8
African-American	(*a*)	(*a*)	0.1	0.8	0.7	1.9	0.7
Homicide							
White	0.3	0.2	0.5	2.2	2.7	2.3	2.4
African-American	1.1	0.4	2.7	11.2	16.8	14.4	13.1
Accidents							
White	0.1	0.1	0.1	0.2	0.2	0.1	0.1
African-American	0.4	0.1	0.2	0.2	(*a*)	0.1	0.1

Adapted from Statistical abstract of the United States 1994. 114th ed. Washington, DC: US Department of Commerce, 1994.
[a]Not applicable.

are still sold and have the potential for serious injury if the driver is not well trained and careful. The use of alcohol also increases the likelihood of accidents and injuries.

Poisonings Most unintentional poisonings occur in the home, with a sex ratio of 2:1, male to female. Poisonings often involve drugs, medications, mushrooms, shellfish, and carbon monoxide. Drugs are the most common cause of fatalities, with aspirin, sedatives, hypnotics, psychotherapeutics, and amphetamines comprising the largest groups. Alcohol and motor vehicle exhaust are another large group. It is often difficult to distinguish unintentional poisoning from intentional overdose, particularly in individuals older than 10.

School Environment and Sports Since adolescents spend much of their day in school, it would be expected that many of the injuries to them would occur at school. In fact one-third to one-half of their injuries do occur in school. However, most such injuries are minor, with males injured more commonly than females. Falls are the most common cause of injury in secondary schools and usually cause contusions, abrasions, or local swelling. Also frequent are strains, sprains, and dislocations, especially of the upper extremity. Injuries typically occur in the classroom, in school shops and laboratories, on the playground, or in organized sports.

Sports Injuries

- More injuries occur during practice than during competition.
- Injuries are much more common in grades 10–12 than 7–9.

A study in Canada by Feldman et al. (1983) of school sports injuries found the following:

Incidence per Level of School (per 100 Students per Year)

K–2	4.1
3–5	6.2
6–8	7.2
9–13	5.3

- School-related sports injuries increase until about age 17 and then decrease.
- The ratio of male-to-female injuries is higher in the 9th grade (3.7:1) but declines to 0.5 in the 12th grade.
- The highest number of injuries to females occurs in softball and gymnastics, while football and wrestling cause the most injuries in males. Football has the highest prevalence of serious injuries, with 260 deaths between 1973 and 1980 in high school and college football players.

Other sports with high injury rates include wrestling, softball, gymnastics, basketball, soccer, track, and baseball. Injury rates (adapted from Paulson, 1988) include:

Injuries per 100 Participants

Football	80
Wrestling	11–75
Softball	44
Gymnastics	40 (females) 28 (males)
Track (cross country)	35 (females) 29 (males)
Basketball	31 (males)
Soccer	30
Baseball	18 (males)

Football Fatalities   There were four fatalities related to football in 1993 compared to one in 1992. Three of the four were associated with high school football, one with college football, and all involved head injuries. There were also nine indirect fatalities caused by systemic failure as a result of exertion while participating in football activities. Eight of these were associated with high school football.

Home Environment   As a location for injury, the home environment declines in adolescence to 27% overall (22% in males and 39% in females). The leading causes of death at home are poisons, fires, burns, and firearms.

Intentional Injuries

Suicide   Suicide has changed from a problem of primarily older persons to one that affects primarily adolescents and young adults. Suicide rates in youth remained stable between 1900 and 1955 and then began to rise dramatically. The rates rose in the 15- to 24-year-old age group from 4.5 per 100,000 in 1950 to 13.0 per 100,000 in 1992. Most of the increase has been secondary to an increase in the suicide rates of white males. Close to 60% of suicides involved firearms. The actual numbers of suicides may be much greater than recorded, as suicides are commonly underreported on death certificates.

Homicide   Homicide has emerged as a major health problem in the United States, particularly for young African-American males. Homicide remains the number two cause of death in the 15- to 24-year-old population and the number one cause of death in adolescent and young adult African-American males aged 15–24. The homicide rate for African-American males ages 15–24 has increased dramatically to 159 per 100,000 in 1992 from 72 per 100,000 in 1982. Homicide death rates have also remained high for the Hispanic population in the 15–24 age group.

Recovery from Injuries: Consideration in the Adolescent

The recovery process from a serious injury, particularly a head injury, can be difficult and is even more challenging when confounded by the adolescent developmental process. Problems include:

1. Lack of knowledge in the medical field regarding the process of recovery from trauma
2. Difficulty in distinguishing between developmental issues of adolescents and problems secondary to the injury, such as irritability or poor judgment
3. Family expectations that may fail to adjust to changes resulting from the injury
4. Mental changes including impaired judgment, decreased attention span, irritability, short-term memory loss, and memory deficits

Prevention of Injuries

The following are important considerations for the health-care practitioner, parent of a teen, or school or camp instructor in prevention of common injuries.

Motor Vehicle Accidents

1. Implement nighttime curfews: New York and Pennsylvania have experienced a greater than 60% reduction in fatalities among 16-year-olds by enforcing a nighttime curfew on driving for this age group. Preusser et al. (1993) found that 47 cities with curfews had a 34% reduction in fatal injuries for 13- to 17-year-olds compared to 77 cities without curfews.
2. Delay age of licensure to 17.
3. Raise the drinking age to 21.
4. Implement mandatory seat belt laws: A study comparing injuries with and without seat belts found that those using seat belts had a 60% decrease in severity index, a 65% decrease in the need for hospitalizations, and a 66% decrease in hospital-related expenses.
5. Equip cars with air bags as standard equipment.
6. Implement mandatory motorcycle helmet laws.
7. Implement severe penalties for use of alcohol and driving.
8. Adolescents should be taught never to ride with a driver who has been drinking or taking drugs. In 1982 the state of Tennessee increased the penalties for driving under the influence (DUI) and in 1984 increased the legal drinking age to 21. Motor vehicle accidents decreased 33% for those 15–18 years of age.

Drowning

1. Encourage swimming lessons.
2. Advise never to swim alone.
3. Advise against hyperventilation for long dives.
4. Stress the dangers of drinking while swimming or boating.

Fires and Burns   Implement guidelines to follow in case of fire in the house.

Skateboards Advise on the use of a helmet, padding, and slip-resistant shoes.

Bicycles

1. Review traffic rules.
2. Advise on the use of appropriate size bike.
3. Advise against night riding.
4. Advise against double riding and stunt riding.
5. Advise on the use of a protective helmet: Bicycle helmets should be worn by all persons (i.e., bicycle operators and passengers) at any age when bicycling. These helmets should meet the standards of American National Standard Institute (ANSI), the Snell Memorial Foundation, or American Standard Testing Materials (ASTM).
6. Implement mandatory bicycle helmet usage: It is estimated that increasing bicycle helmet usage to 100% would decrease about 500 fatal and 151,400 nonfatal bicycle-related head injuries per year.

Motorcycle

1. Discourage use of motorcycles, particularly by persons under age 18.
2. Encourage mandatory helmet legislation.
3. Advise against drinking and driving.
4. Advise on the use of a helmet, above-ankle boots, and heavy gloves.

Sports Injuries

1. Arrange for prior medical clearance before participation is allowed.
2. Teach sports skills prior to participation.
3. Enforcement of proper rules by qualified officials is important.
4. Advise on the use of protective equipment.
5. Encourage proper training and conditioning of the athlete.
6. Encourage proper sites for the sports and only play the game if conditions are acceptable.
7. Provide prompt first aid if injury occurs.
8. Arrange team composition based on body size and skills, not just chronological age.

Homicides Strategies to prevent homicides have been actively investigated in recent years. Interventions to reduce homicide rates include:

1. Encourage advocacy to pass gun control legislation. Dolins and Christoffel (1994) provide a basic framework for developing an advocacy plan for community practitioners.
2. Provide conflict resolution skills among adolescents. This has been used successfully in several communities.
3. Encourage parents to remove guns from the home or if present to keep guns unloaded and locked up.
4. Advise parents to limit viewing of gun violence in the media.

MORBIDITY

Although the mortality rates of adolescents are low compared to adults, there is significant morbidity among teens. Table 5.13 lists the morbidity of selected diseases in adolescents during 1993, and Table 5.14 lists acute conditions in adolescents as reported in the 1991 National Health Interview Survey. Several surveys of adolescent visits are available. These data are summarized below:

TABLE 5.13. Morbidity of Selected Notifiable Diseases in Adolescents in the United States, 1994

Disease	Age Group (yr)				Total (All Ages)
	10–14	15–19	20–24	25–29	
Acquired immunodeficiency syndrome	146	324	2,604	10,162	78,279
Hepatitis A	2,492	2,036	2,770	2,981	26,796
Hepatitis B	165	807	1,618	1,940	12,517
Hepatitis, non-A, non-B	21	70	172	420	4,470
Gonorrhea	8,508	123,079	121,084	60,204	413,647
Lyme	831	632	473	640	13,043
Measles	128	255	112	43	963
Mumps	271	128	59	61	1,537
Rubella	4	11	32	33	227
Syphilis	118	2,234	4,067	3,814	20,638
Toxic shock syndrome	20	25	19	22	192
Tuberculosis	272	544	1,281	1,808	24,361
Varicella	771	256	207	218	151,219

Adapted from Centers for Disease Control and Prevention. Summary of notifiable diseases, United States, 1994. MMWR 1994;43(53):1.

TABLE 5.14. Number of Acute Conditions per 100 Persons per Year, by Age and Type of Condition: United States, 1991

Type of Acute Condition	All Ages	5–17	18–24
All acute conditions	191.8	270.2	194.6
Respiratory conditions	100.6	150.1	106.3
Influenza	52.1	78.6	58.1
Common cold	28.6	38.7	34.1
Other acute upper respiratory infections	11.7	21.9	8.0
Acute bronchitis	4.5	6.7	3.8
Pneumonia	1.7	1.4	1.0
Other respiratory conditions	2.0	2.8	1.3
Injuries	24.0	29.6	32.2
Fractures and dislocations	3.0	5.0	3.7
Sprains and strains	5.4	5.9	7.3
Open wounds and lacerations	4.7	6.9	7.6
Contusions	4.7	5.4	7.4
Other current injuries	6.1	6.3	6.1
Infective and parasitic diseases	18.5	38.4	14.0
Common childhood diseases	1.8	4.7	0.3
Intestinal virus	4.0	8.4	3.1
Viral infections	6.1	10.0	5.3
Other	6.5	15.3	5.4
Digestive system conditions	6.6	9.1	5.3
Dental conditions	1.4	1.2	0.8
Indigestion, nausea, and vomiting	2.9	6.1	3.2
Other digestive conditions	2.4	1.8	1.3
Selected other acute conditions	30.1	34.3	25.0
Eye conditions	1.2	1.0	0.8
Acute ear infections	10.3	14.3	2.7
Other ear conditions	1.7	2.9	0.2
Acute urinary conditions	3.5	1.7	4.2
Menstruation disorders	0.6	0.7	1.5
Other disorders of female genital tract	1.1	—	1.8
Delivery and conditions of pregnancy	1.6	0.2	6.5
Skin conditions	1.9	2.6	1.6
Acute musculoskeletal conditions	4.0	2.7	3.2
Headache, excluding migraine	1.3	2.9	1.2
Fever	2.9	5.3	1.3

Adapted from National Center for Health Statistics. Vital and health statistics: current estimates from the National Health Interview Survey, 1991 [CDC Series 10 #184 DHHS publication 93–1512]. Hyattsville, Maryland: US Government Printing Office, 1992.

1. Neinstein (unpublished data, 1987): Teenage Health Center, Childrens Hospital of Los Angeles

   Gynecological, 30.2%
   Psychosocial, 28.2%
   Dermatological, 7.8%
   Gastrointestinal, 5.3%
   Infectious diseases, 4.4%
   Neurological, 3.5%
   Allergy, 3.1%
   Endocrinological, 3.1%
   Genitourinary, 2.3%
   Ears, nose, and throat, 1.7%
   Orthopaedic, 1.6%
   Hematological, 1.5%
   Genetic, 1.3%
   Trauma, 0.9%
   Cardiac, 0.9%
   Rheumatological, 0.4%

2. The 10 most frequent principal reasons and diagnoses from the National Ambulatory Medical Care Survey, 1989, are listed in Table 5.15.
3. Distribution of office visits by selected diagnostic and therapeutic services from the National Ambulatory Medical Care Survey, 1989, is listed in Table 5.16.

TABLE 5.15.   Number and Percent Distribution of Office Visits by 10 Most Frequent Principal Reasons and Principal Diagnoses for Ages 15–24: United States, 1989

	Number of Visits in Thousands	Percent Distribution of All Visits	Cumulative Percent
Principle reason for visit			
All visits	137,502	100.0	
Routine prenatal examination	7,115	10.6	
Symptoms referable to throat	3,055	4.6	
Acne or pimples	2,214	3.3	
General medical examination	1,950	2.9	
Physical examination required for employment	1,834	2.7	
Stomach pain, cramps, and spasm	1,748	2.6	
Cough	1,712	2.6	
Knee symptoms	1,318	2.0	
Headache, pain in head	1,288	1.9	
Postoperative visit	1,096	1.6	
Principle diagnosis			
All principal diagnoses	66,868	100.0	
Normal pregnancy	7,042	10.5	10.5
General medical examination	3,709	5.5	16.0
Diseases of sebaceous glands	2,952	4.4	20.4
Acute upper respiratory infections	1,384	2.1	22.5
Sprains and strains of other and unspecified parts of back	1,236	1.8	24.3
Other diseases due to viruses and chlamydiae	1,221	1.8	26.1
Allergic rhinitis	1,219	1.8	27.9
Acute tonsillitis	1,152	1.7	29.6
Acute pharyngitis	1,127	1.7	31.3
Chronic sinusitis	996	1.5	32.8

Adapted from National Center for Health Statistics. Vital and health statistics: National Ambulatory Medical Care Survey: 1989 summary: series 13: data from the National Health Survey [110, DHHS publication 92-1771]. Hyattsville, Maryland: US Government Printing Office, 1992.

TABLE 5.16. Number and Percent Distribution of Office Visits by Selected Diagnostic and Therapeutic Services according to Patient's Age and Sex: United States, 1989

Selected Visit Characteristics	Number of Visits in Thousands	Percent Distribution of All Visits	Age Group (yr)		
			Under 15	15–24	25–44
			Number of visits in thousands		
All visits	692,702	—	137,502	66,868	192,593
			Percent distribution		
Total	—	100.0	100.0	100.0	100.0
Diagnostic/screening services[a]					
None	265,834	38.4	64.6	36.8	35.4
Pap test	32,766	4.7	0.1[b]	7.6	9.3
Pelvic examination	51,965	7.5	0.2[b]	14.8	15.1
Breast palpation[c]	37,929	5.5	0.1[b]	7.0	9.6
Mammogram[c]	10,655	1.5	0.0[b]	0.2[b]	1.9
Visual acuity	45,192	6.5	4.2	4.3	4.2
Blood pressure check	241,899	34.9	7.4	37.7	40.3
Urinalysis	87,716	12.7	6.1	18.4	18.0
Chest x-ray examination	18,419	2.7	1.4	1.3	2.1
Digital rectal examination[c]	25,071	3.6	0.3[b]	2.9	4.8
Proctoscopy or sigmoidoscopy	3,134	0.5	0.0[b]	0.1[b]	0.3
Stool blood examination[c]	15,576	2.2	0.3[b]	0.9	2.1
Oral glucose tolerance[c]	3,056	0.4	0.0[b]	0.5[b]	0.6
Cholesterol measure[c]	24,828	3.6	0.6	1.3	3.2
HIV serology[d]	1,013	0.1	0.0[b]	0.2[b]	0.2[b]
Other blood test	88,210	12.7	6.9	9.7	11.5
Other	176,242	25.4	22.9	27.9	24.8
Counseling/advice[a,c]					
None	435,792	62.9	62.6	65.5	62.9
Weight reduction	43,853	6.3	0.9	2.5	6.3
Cholesterol reduction	21,533	3.1	0.2[b]	0.5[b]	1.7
Smoking cessation	15,109	2.2	0.3[b]	2.1	2.5
HIV transmission	1,044	0.2	0.1[b]	0.3[b]	0.3
Breast self-examination	15,779	2.3	0.1[b]	2.6	3.8
Other	193,272	27.9	36.2	28.7	27.2
Nonmedication therapy[a]					
None	558,986	80.7	88.2	81.2	76.2
Psychotherapy	22,182	3.2	0.9	2.8	5.6
Corrective lenses	8,572	1.2	0.6	0.7[b]	0.9
Ambulatory surgery	13,095	1.9	0.7	2.2	2.2
Physiotherapy	16,204	2.3	0.3[b]	2.4	3.5
Other	78,797	11.4	9.5	11.7	12.9
Number of new or continued drugs ordered or provided by physician per visit					
None	275,913	39.8	37.0	44.4	44.8
One	230,077	33.2	40.6	34.3	33.1
Two	108,720	15.7	17.1	14.6	14.3
Three–five	77,992	11.2	5.3	6.8	7.9
Disposition[a]					
No follow-up planned	66,377	9.6	17.9	12.7	9.0
Return at specified time	424,583	61.3	45.0	55.4	60.5
Return if needed	160,282	23.1	32.0	25.4	23.7
Telephone follow-up planned	24,962	3.6	3.6	3.5	3.8
Referred to other physician	20,071	2.9	1.8	3.0	3.1
Returned to referring physician	6,138	0.9	0.5	0.4[b]	0.7
Admit to hospital	7,163	1.0	0.5	0.7[b]	0.9
Other	15,536	2.2	1.3	2.3	2.4

Adapted from National Center for Health Statistics. Vital and health statistics: National Ambulatory Medical Care Survey: 1989 summary: series 13: data from the National Health Survey [110, DHHS publication 92–1771]. Hyattsville, Maryland: US Government Printing Office, 1992.

[a]Total may exceed total number of visits because more than one category may be reported per visit.
[b]Not enough numbers to be standard of reliability or precision.
[c]Category is new in the 1989 National Ambulatory Medical Care Survey (NAMCS).
[d]HIV, human immunodeficiency virus.

128

The National Health Survey

The National Health Survey, a comprehensive governmental survey of the health of a representative sample (approximately 7000) of noninstitutionalized youths aged 12–17, was conducted in the United States from 1966 to 1970 by the National Center for Health Statistics (1974–1975, Series II). Some of the results of this survey are below.

Hearing

1. Some degree of hearing handicap was indicated in 1.5% of youths (i.e., mean thresholds of 15 dB or higher at frequencies of 500–2000 Hz). However, this did not include youths residing in special schools for hearing impaired persons or in other institutions.
2. Hearing levels for girls were generally lower than for boys.
3. Some abnormality of the eardrum was indicated in 15.2% of youths. Although the youths with abnormal eardrums had worse hearing than youths with normal eardrums, their hearing was still within normal limits.

Eyes

1. Twelve percent had moderate-to-severe eye-muscle imbalance in the lateral plane.
2. Forty-three percent were unable to read at the 20/20 level (48% for females and 39% for males).
3. Thirty-four percent wore glasses or contact lenses.
4. One out of 12 had one or more significant eye abnormalities, with the most prevalent problems being tropia and strabismus.

Dental   The youths examined had an average of 6.2 teeth each that were missing (0.7), decayed (1.7), or filled (3.8).

Skin

1. Acne was the most common skin problem and occurred in 72.3% of the sample.
2. Other skin problems included fungal infections (1.5%), eczema (0.9%), and psoriasis (0.3%).

National Adolescent Student Health Survey and Youth Risk Behavior Survey

The National Adolescent Student Health Survey (NASHS; Centers for Disease Control, 1989) was the first national survey since the 1960s to assess the extent to which adolescent students in the United States may be at risk for several significant health problems. The survey involved 11,419 8th and 10th grade students in a national probability sample of 217 schools in 20 states.

The Youth Risk Behavior Survey (YRBS) is a component of the Centers for Disease Control and Prevention's (CDC's) Youth Risk Behavior Surveillance System (YRBBS), which has measured the prevalence of priority health-risk behaviors among adolescents since 1990. It has been conducted among high school students in grades 9–12 in public and private schools in all 50 states and the District of Columbia in 1990, 1991, and 1993. The YRBS yields longitudinal information about the prevalence of selected self-reported health-risk behaviors. The 1992 National Health Interview Survey (NHIS) included a representative sample of 120,000 civilians in the United States in 49,000 households. The YRBS was also used in a follow-up

Table 5.17.   Percentage of Persons Aged 12–21 Years Who Engaged in Selected Health-Risk Behaviors, by Age Group: United States, Youth Risk Behavior Survey, 1992

Behavior	Age Group (yr)			
	12–13	14–17	18–21	Total
Used safety belts[a]	31.6	33.5	36.1	34.2
Used motorcycle helmets[b]	48.4	41.6	44.7	44.1
Rode with a drinking driver[c]	11.3	21.7	34.5	25.0
Participated in a physical fight[d]	49.0	43.8	29.4	38.8
Carried a weapon[e]	12.6	17.1	13.6	14.8
Lifetime cigarette use[f]	29.9	58.0	76.9	60.4
Current cigarette use[g]	7.7	25.4	37.6	27.0
Current smokeless tobacco use[h]	2.7	8.8	8.5	7.5
Lifetime alcohol use[i]	28.0	65.6	86.7	67.3
Current episodic heavy drinking[j]	4.3	21.0	39.7	25.6
Lifetime marijuana use[k]	3.4	20.4	45.8	27.5
Lifetime cocaine use[l]	0.4	2.5	11.4	5.8
Ever injected drugs[m]	0.1	0.9	1.2	0.9
Ever had sexual intercourse	([n])	43.4	81.7	63.0
Sexual intercourse with 4 or more sex partners	([n])	13.3	41.3	27.6
Used condom during most recent sexual intercourse[o]	([n])	58.5	36.9	43.5
Used birth controls pills during most recent sexual intercourse[o]	([n])	18.2	34.8	29.7
Ate fruits and vegetables[p]	17.0	13.4	10.9	13.1
Ate foods typically high in fat[q]	32.9	34.2	27.7	31.3
Engaged in moderate physical activity[r]	34.8	27.4	21.2	26.3

Adapted from Centers for Disease Control and Prevention. Health risk behaviors among persons aged 12–21 years— United States, 1992. MMWR 1994;43:231.

[a]Safety belts used "always" when riding in a car or truck as a passenger.

[b]Helmets used "always" among respondents who rode motorcycles.

[c]Rode at least once during the 30 days preceding the survey in a car or other vehicle driven by someone who had been drinking alcohol.

[d]Fought at least once during the 12 months preceding the survey.

[e]Carried a gun, knife, or club at least 1 day during the 30 days preceding the survey.

[f]Ever tried cigarette smoking, even one or two puffs.

[g]Smoked cigarettes on 1 or more of the 30 days preceding the survey.

[h]Used chewing tobacco or snuff on 1 or more of the 30 days preceding the survey.

[i]Ever drank alcohol.

[j]Drank five or more drinks of alcohol on at least one occasion during the 30 days preceding the survey.

[k]Ever used marijuana.

[l]Ever used cocaine.

[m]Respondents were classified as injecting-drug users only if they:
  1. Reported injecting-drug use not prescribed by a physician and
  2. Answered one or more to any of these questions: "During your life, how many times have you used any form of co-caine including powder, crack, or freebase?"; "During your life, how many times have you used any other type of il-legal drug such as LSD, PCP, ecstasy, mushrooms, speed, ice, heroin, or pills without a doctor's prescription?"; or "During your life, how many times have you taken steroid pills or shots without a doctor's prescription?"

[n]Respondents aged 12–13 years were not asked this question.

[o]Among respondents who had had sexual intercourse during the 3 months preceding the survey.

[p]Ate five or more servings of fruits and vegetables (e.g., fruit, fruit juice, green salad, and cooked vegetables) the day pre-ceding the survey.

[q]Ate no more than two servings of foods typically high in fat (e.g., hamburger, hot dogs, or sausage; french fries or potato chips; and cookies, doughnuts, pie, or cake) the day preceding the survey.

[r]Walked or rode a bicycle at least 30 minutes at a time on 5 or more of the 7 days preceding the survey.

survey to the NHIS using a representative sample of youth aged 12–21 years during April 1992–March 1993. This survey was completed by 10,645 respondents, including 2195 individuals ages 12–13, 4126 individuals ages 14–17, and 4324 individuals ages 18–21. The 1991 YRBS included 12,272 high school youth in grades 9–12, and the 1993 sample included 16,296 high school youth. No YRBS was conducted for high school students in 1992.

Significant findings from the NASHS 1989, the YRBS 1991, and the YRBS and NHIS 1992 (Tables 5.17, 5.18, and 5.19) are listed below:

1. Unintentional injuries: Fifty-six percent of students had not used a seat belt the last time they rode in a car, truck, or van. Forty-four percent of the 10th graders and 32% of the 8th graders had been in a car during the past month with a driver who had used alcohol or other drugs before driving (NASHS, 1989). Persons aged 12–13 were significantly less likely than those aged 18–21 to have reported "always" using safety belts when riding as a passenger in a car (YRBS and NHIS, 1992). Those persons riding in the past 30 days with a driver who had been drinking alcohol increased with each age group from 11.3% in 12- to 13-year-olds to 21.7% in 14- to 17-year-olds and 34.5% in 18- to 21-year-olds (YRBS and NHIS, 1992).
2. Fighting and violence: Fifty percent of boys and 34% of girls had been in at least one physical fight during the past year (YRBS, 1991). Over 40% of the boys and 11% of the girls reported carrying a weapon at least once in the preceding 30 days (YRBS, 1991). The percentage of adolescents and young adults who reported physical fighting during the 12 months before the survey decreased with each age group (YRBS and NHIS, 1992). Thirteen percent of high school students reported being physically attacked during the past year while at school or on a school bus, and 16% reported being attacked outside of school (NASHS, 1989).
3. Suicide: Twenty-one percent of the boys and 37% of the girls reported seriously considering committing suicide at some time; 24.9% of the females and 12.5% of the males had made suicide plans; and 10.7% of the females and 3.9% of the males had attempted suicide (YRBS, 1991).
4. Tobacco, alcoholic beverages, and drugs: Sixty-five percent of 9th graders and 74.5% of 12th graders reported trying tobacco (YRBS, 1991). Twenty-three percent of 9th graders and 30.1% of 10th graders reported being current smokers (YRBS, 1991). Individuals ages 18–21 were three times more likely than 12- to 13-year-olds in the YRBS and NHIS 1992 survey to have used alcohol in their lifetime (86.7% versus 28.0%), nine times more likely to report current heavy drinking (39.7% versus 4.3%), 13 times more likely

TABLE 5.18. Percentage of High School Students Who Reported Selected Sexual Risk Behaviors, by Year: United States, Youth Risk Behavior Survey (YRBS), 1990, 1991, 1993

Behavior	1990	1991	1993
Ever had sexual intercourse	54.2	54.1	53.0
Sexual intercourse with 4 or more sex partners	19.0	18.7	18.8
Had sexual intercourse during the 3 months preceding the survey	39.4	37.5	37.6
Used alcohol or drugs before last sexual intercourse	NA	11.8	11.0
Used condom during most recent sexual intercourse	NA	46.2	52.8
Used birth controls pills during most recent sexual intercourse	14.6	17.8	18.4

Adapted from Centers for Disease Control and Prevention. Trends in sexual risk behavior among high school students—United States, 1990, 1991, 1993. MMWR 1995;44:124.
NA, data not available.

TABLE 5.19.   Percentage of Persons Aged 12–19 Years Who Engaged in Selected Health-Risk Behaviors, by School Enrollment Status: United States, Youth Risk Behavior Survey, National Health Interview Survey, 1992

	School Enrollment Status	
Behavior	In-School	Out-of-School
Used safety belts[a]	33.2	23.2
Used motorcycle helmets[b]	43.7	45.6
Rode with a drinking driver[c]	18.9	28.4
Participated in a physical fight[d]	44.2	51.0
Carried a weapon[e]	15.5	22.9
Lifetime cigarette use[f]	50.9	57.7
Current cigarette use[g]	20.4	33.7
Current smokeless tobacco use[h]	6.8	8.4
Lifetime alcohol use[i]	55.2	62.9
Current episodic heavy drinking[j]	17.1	21.8
Lifetime marijuana use[k]	15.9	7.1
Lifetime cocaine use[l]	2.1	7.1
Ever injected drugs[m]	0.8	3.9
Ever had sexual intercourse	45.4	70.1
Sexual intercourse with 4 or more sex partners[n]	14.0	36.4
Used condom during most recent sexual intercourse[o]	59.8	50.2
Ate fruits and vegetables[p]	14.5	10.1
Ate foods typically high in fat[q]	65.7	70.0
Engaged in moderate physical activity[r]	29.2	31.1

Adapted from Centers for Disease Control and Prevention. Health risk behaviors among adolescents who do and do not attend school—United States, 1992. MMWR 1994;43:129.

[a]Safety belts used "always" when riding in a car or truck as a passenger.

[b]Helmets used "always" among respondents who rode motorcycles.

[c]Rode at least once during the 30 days preceding the survey in a car or other vehicle driven by someone who had been drinking alcohol.

[d]Fought at least once during the 12 months preceding the survey.

[e]Carried a gun, knife, or club at least 1 day during the 30 days preceding the survey.

[f]Ever tried cigarette smoking, even one or two puffs.

[g]Smoked cigarettes on 1 or more of the 30 days preceding the survey.

[h]Used chewing tobacco or snuff on 1 or more of the 30 days preceding the survey.

[i]Ever drank alcohol.

[j]Drank five or more drinks of alcohol on at least one occasion during the 30 days preceding the survey.

[k]Ever used marijuana.

[l]Ever used cocaine.

[m]Respondents were classified as injecting-drug users only if they:
  1. Reported injecting-drug use not prescribed by a physician and
  2. Answered one or more to any of these questions: "During your life, how many times have you used any form of cocaine including powder, crack, or freebase?"; "During your life, how many times have you used any other type of illegal drug such as LSD, PCP, ecstasy, mushrooms, speed, ice, heroin, or pills without a doctor's prescription?"; or "During your life, how many times have you taken steroid pills or shots without a doctor's prescription?"

[n]Respondents aged 12–13 years were not asked this question.

[o]Among respondents who had had sexual intercourse during the 3 months preceding the survey.

[p]Ate five or more servings of fruits and vegetables (e.g., fruit, fruit juice, green salad, and cooked vegetables) the day preceding the survey.

[q]Ate no more than two servings of foods typically high in fat (e.g., hamburger, hot dogs, or sausage; french fries or potato chips; and cookies, doughnuts, pie, or cake) the day preceding the survey.

[r]Walked or rode a bicycle at least 30 minutes at a time on 5 or more of the 7 days preceding the survey.

to have used marijuana during their lifetimes (45.8% versus 3.4%), and 28 times more likely to have used cocaine during their lifetime (11.4% versus 0.4%). Intravenous drug use varied from 1.2% in the 18- to 21-year-olds to 0.9% in the 14- to 17-year-olds to 0.1% in the 12- to 13-year-olds (YRBS and NHIS, 1992).

5. Sexual activity: Persons aged 18–21 were much more likely to have reported sexual intercourse (81.7%) or to have had four or more sex partners in the past (41.3%) compared to 14- to 17-year-olds (43.3% and 13.3%) (YRBS and NHIS, 1992). The trends in sexual behaviors in the 1990, 1991, and 1993 YRBS are reviewed in Table 5.18.

6. AIDS: Forty-seven percent of students believed that donating blood increases the risk of HIV, and 51% felt that washing after sex might decrease the chance of getting an HIV infection. Most understood the risk associated with sexual intercourse and intravenous drug use (NASHS, 1989).

7. Nutrition and eating habits: Thirty-two percent of the boys and 48% of the girls reported eating breakfast two or less days during the past week. Sixty-one percent of girls and 28% of boys reported dieting during the past year, with 16% using diet pills, 12% vomiting, and 8% using laxatives (NASHS, 1989). Consumption of five or more servings of fruits and vegetables during the day before the survey decreased as age group increased (12- to 13-year-olds, 17.0%; 14- to 17-year-olds, 13.4%; and 18- to 21-year-olds, 10.9%) (YRBS and NHIS, 1992).

8. Health products and services: Forty-three percent of students knew from reading a cereal box label which ingredient was present in the largest amount (NASHS, 1989).

9. Physical activity: Participation in moderate physical activity decreased with increasing age group (YRBS and NHIS, 1992).

10. School status (in school versus out of school) was a large predictor of high risk behaviors (Table 5.19).

TABLE 5.20.   Actual and Projected Number of Adolescents in the United States (in Thousands)

Actual	5–9 yr		10–14 yr		15–19 yr	
	Number	%	Number	%	Number	%
1970	19,969	9.8	20,804	10.2	19,084	9.4
1980	16,601	7.4	18,241	8.1	21,157	9.3
1990	18,591	7.3	16,793	6.9	16,968	7.2
1992	18,359	7.2	18,100	7.1	17,882	6.7

Note: The adolescent group aged 10–14 should crest in the year 2000, with the group aged 15–19 cresting in population in 2025.

Projected (Middle Projection)	5–13 yr		14–17 yr		18–24 yr	
	Number	%	Number	%	Number	%
1995	34,140	13.0	14,519	5.4	25,281	10.1
2000	35,869	13.2	15,519	5.7	25,306	9.4
2005	34,869	12.8	16,564	5.9	27,309	9.8
2010	32,100	12.1	16,542	5.8	29,005	10.1
2020	31,272	11.9	14,404	5.3	26,764	9.3
2030	31,773	11.9	14,792	5.4	25,260	9.1
2040	30,299	11.6	14,537	5.3	26,092	9.3
2050	30,174	11.7	13,986	5.3	24,920	9.1

Adapted from Council on Long Range Planning and Development in cooperation with the American Academy of Pediatrics. The future of pediatrics: implications of the changing environment of medicine. JAMA 1987;258:240, and Statistical abstract of the United States 1994. 114th ed. Washington, DC: US Department of Commerce, 1994.

Some of the National Health Objectives as measured by the Youth Risk Behavior Surveillance System from the Public Health Service in Healthy People 2000 include:

1. Physical activity: Increase to at least 30% the proportion of people aged 6 and older who engage regularly in light-to-moderate physical activity for at least 30 minutes per day.
2. Drugs
   a. Reduce the initiation of cigarette smoking by children and youth so that no more than 15% have become regular smokers by age 20.
   b. Reduce smokeless tobacco use by males aged 12–24 to a prevalence of no more than 4%.
   c. Increase by at least 1 year the average age of first use of cigarettes from 11.6, alcohol from 13.1, and marijuana from 13.4 by adolescents aged 12–17.
   d. Reduce the proportion of young people who have used alcohol in the past month to 12.6%, marijuana to 3.2%, and cocaine to 0.6%.
   e. Reduce the proportion of high school seniors and college students engaging in recent occasions of heavy drinking of alcoholic beverages to no more than 28% of high school seniors and 32% of college students.
   f. Reduce to no more than 3% the proportion of male high school seniors who use anabolic steroids.

TABLE 5.21. Children Under 18 Years Old, by Presence of Parents: United States, 1970–1993

(As of March, excludes persons under 18 years old who maintained households of family groups.)

Race, Hispanic Origin, Year	Number (in Thousands)	Both Parents	Percent Living With:					Father Only	Neither Parent
			Mother Only						
			Total	Divorced	Married, Spouse Absent	Never Married (Single)	Wid-owed		
All races[a]									
1970	69,162	85	11	3	5	1	2	1	3
1980	63,427	77	18	8	6	3	2	2	4
1985	62,475	74	21	9	5	6	2	3	3
1990	64,137	73	22	8	5	7	2	3	3
1993	66,893	71	23	9	6	8	1	3	3
White									
1970	58,790	90	8	3	3	Z	2	1	2
1980	52,242	83	14	7	4	1	2	2	2
1985	50,836	80	16	8	4	2	1	2	2
1990	51,390	79	16	8	4	3	1	3	2
1993	53,075	77	17	8	4	4	1	3	2
African-American									
1970	9,422	59	30	5	16	4	4	2	10
1980	9,375	42	44	11	16	13	4	2	12
1985	9,479	40	51	11	12	25	3	3	7
1990	10,018	38	51	10	12	27	2	4	8
1993	10,660	36	54	10	12	31	1	3	7
Hispanic[b]									
1970	4,006[c]	78	NA	NA	NA	NA	NA	NA	NA
1980	5,459	75	20	6	8	4	2	2	4
1985	6,057	68	27	7	11	7	2	2	3
1990	7,174	67	27	7	10	8	2	3	3
1993	7,776	65	28	7	8	11	1	4	4

From Statistical abstract of the United States 1994. 114th ed. Washington, DC: US Department of Commerce, 1994.
NA, not available.
Z, less than 0.5%.
[a]Includes other races not shown separately.
[b]Hispanic persons may be any race.
[c]All persons under 18 years old.

TABLE 5.22. Number of Office Visits and Percentage Distribution, by Medical Specialty: United States, 1989

	Age Group (yr)		
Physician Specialty	Under 15	15–24	25–44
	Number of visits in thousands		
All visits	137,502	66,868	192,593
General and family practice	32,604	22,988	58,963
Pediatrics	81,781	4,266	808
Internal medicine	1,253	5,008	19,352
Obstetrics and gynecology	246	12,128	38,284
Ophthalmology	2,201	1,464	5,843
Orthopaedic surgery	3,426	4,936	12,227
Dermatology	2,365	4,193	8,144
General surgery	1,047	1,715	6,702
Psychiatry	862	1,597	8,654
Otolaryngology	3,254	1,486	4,324
Cardiovascular disease	21	234	995
Urological surgery	551	363	2,300
Neurology	282	550	2,316
Other	7,609	5,941	23,679
	Percent distribution of visits		
All visits	100.0	100.0	100.0
Any practitioner	19.8	9.7	27.8
General and family practice	23.7	34.4	30.6
Pediatrics	59.5	6.4	0.4
Internal medicine	0.9	7.5	10.0
Obstetrics and gynecology	0.2	18.1	19.9
Ophthalmology	1.6	2.2	3.0
Orthopaedic surgery	2.5	7.4	6.3
Dermatology	1.7	6.3	4.2
General surgery	0.8	2.6	3.5
Psychiatry	0.6	2.4	4.5
Otolaryngology	2.4	2.2	2.2
Cardiovascular disease	0.0	0.4	0.5
Urological surgery	0.4	0.5	1.2
Neurology	0.2	0.8	1.2
Other	5.5	8.9	12.3
	Visit rate per 100 persons[a]		
All visits	255.3	188.1	244.4
Any practitioner	2.6	1.9	2.4
General and family practice	60.5	64.7	74.8
Pediatrics	151.9	12.0	1.0
Internal medicine	2.3	14.1	24.6
Obstetrics and gynecology	0.5	34.1	48.6
Ophthalmology	4.1	4.1	7.4
Orthopaedic surgery	6.4	13.9	15.5
Dermatology	4.4	11.8	10.3
General surgery	1.9	4.8	8.5
Psychiatry	1.6	4.5	11.0
Otolaryngology	6.0	4.2	5.5
Cardiovascular disease	0.0	0.7	1.3
Urological surgery	1.0	1.0	2.9
Neurology	0.5	1.5	2.9
Other	14.1	16.7	30.1

Adapted from National Center for Health Statistics. Vital and health statistics: National Ambulatory Medical Care Survey: 1989 summary: series 13: data from the National Health Survey [110, DHHS publication 92–1771]. Hyattsville, Maryland: US Government Printing Office, 1992.
[a]Visit rates are based on US Bureau of the Census national estimates of the civilian, noninstitutionalized US population for July 1, 1989.

TABLE 5.23.   Health Insurance Coverage Status by Selected Characteristics: United States, 1994

	Total Persons (in Millions)	Private Coverage (%)	Government (%)	Not Covered (%)
Under 18	67.1	69.3	21.6	12.4
18–24	24.3	59.5	11.1	28.9
25–34	41.9	68.8	8.6	20.9

Adapted from Statistical abstract of the United States 1994. 114th ed. Washington, DC: US Department of Commerce, 1994.

3. Sexual activity
   a. Reduce the proportion of adolescents who have engaged in sexual intercourse to no more than 15% by age 15 and no more than 40% by age 17.
   b. Increase to at least 90% the proportion of sexually active, unmarried people aged 19 and younger who use contraception, especially combined method contraception that both effectively prevents pregnancy and provides barrier protection against disease.
   c. Increase to at least 50% the proportion of sexually active, unmarried people who used a condom at last sexual intercourse (60% for young women aged 15–19 and 75% for young men aged 15–19).
4. Suicide: Reduce by 15% the incidence of injurious suicide attempts among adolescents aged 14–17.
5. Violence
   a. Reduce by 20% the incidence of physical fighting among adolescents aged 14–17.
   b. Reduce by 20% the incidence of weapon carrying by adolescents aged 14–17.
6. Safety
   a. Increase use of occupant protection systems such as safety belts and inflatable safety restraints to at least 85% of motor vehicle occupants.
   b. Increase use of helmets to at least 80% of motorcyclists and at least 50% of bicyclists.

DEMOGRAPHICS

Although the adolescent population is declining (as demonstrated in Table 5.20), it is estimated that when zero growth is reached, the 14- to 24-year-old age group will always be at least 14.2% of the population. Table 5.20 reviews recent population trends in adolescents. Table 5.21 includes family composition by presence of parents, 1970–1993.

TRENDS IN OFFICE-BASED AMBULATORY CARE

For all age groups since 1975, the total number of ambulatory care office visits increased by 22%. However, the overall visit rate has been stable since 1975 at about 2.7 visits per person per year. In general, females, whites, and older persons have higher visit rates than males, African-Americans and other races, and younger persons. For 1985 and 1989, visit rates for persons aged 15–24 were the lowest of any age group. Most of the decline in visits in this age group appear to be secondary to a decrease in female visit rates and may be due to a decrease in the visit rate for prenatal care. Between 1975 and 1989 the percentage of visits to generalists decreased and visits to medical and surgical specialists increased. In 1975, 41.3% of all office visits were made to general and family practice physicians, compared with only 30.5% in 1985 and 20.8% in 1989. However, with the current strong emphasis on primary and managed care, this is already changing. Table 5.22 reviews the number of office visits by medical specialty. Adolescents between the ages of 18 and 24 have the highest likelihood of being uninsured; Table 5.23 reviews health insurance coverage by age.

BIBLIOGRAPHY

Baker SP, Whitfield RA, O'Neill B. Geographic variations in mortality from motor vehicle crashes. N Engl J Med 1987;316:1384.

Bass JL, Gallagher SS, Mehta KA. Injuries to adolescents and young adults. Pediatr Clin North Am 1985; 32:31.

Biometry Branch, Division of Cancer Prevention and Control, National Cancer Institute, SEER Program. Cancer incidence and mortality in United States, 1973–1981 [NIH publication 85–1837]. Bethesda, Maryland: US Department of Health and Human Services, 1984.

Brent DA, Perper JA, Allman CJ. Alcohol, firearms, and suicide among youth. JAMA 1987;257:3369.

Centers for Disease Control. Homicide among young black males. MMWR 1985;34:629.

Centers for Disease Control. Public Health surveillance of 1990 injury control objectives for the nation. MMWR 1988;37(SS-1):5–12.

Centers for Disease Control. Results from the National Adolescent Student Health Survey. MMWR 1989; 38:147.

Centers for Disease Control and Prevention. Health risk behaviors among adolescents who do and do not attend school—United States, 1992. MMWR 1994;43:129.

Centers for Disease Control and Prevention. Health risk behaviors among persons aged 12–21 years—United States, 1992. MMWR 1994;43:231.

Centers for Disease Control and Prevention. Trends in sexual risk behavior among high school students—United States, 1990, 1991, 1993. MMWR 1995;44: 124.

Centers for Disease Control and Prevention. Injury-control recommendations: bicycle helmets. MMWR 1995;44:1.

Chorba TL, Reinfurt D, Hulka BS. Efficacy of mandatory seat-belt use legislation: the North Carolina experience from 1983–1987. JAMA 1988;260:3593.

Christoffel KK. Child and adolescent injury in the United States: how occupational injuries fit in. Am J Ind Med 1993;24:301.

Christoffel KK, Christoffel T. Handguns as a pediatric problem. Pediatr Emerg Care 1986;2:75.

Council on Long Range Planning and Development in cooperation with the American Academy of Pediatrics. The future of pediatrics: implications of the changing environment of medicine. JAMA 1987; 258:240.

Current estimates from the National Health Interview Survey, 1991: vital and health statistics [CDC Series 10 #184 DHHS 93–1512]. Hyattsville, Maryland: US Government Printing Office, 1991.

Decker MD, Graitcer PL, Schaffner W. Reduction in motor vehicle fatalities associated with an increase in the minimum drinking age. JAMA 1988;260:3604.

Division of Injury Epidemiology and Control, Centers for Disease Control. Bicycle-related injuries: data from the National Electronic Injury Surveillance System. JAMA 1987;257:3334.

Dolins JC, Christoffel KK. Reducing violent injuries: priorities for pediatrician advocacy. Pediatrics 1994; 94:638.

Feldman W, Woodward CA, Hodgson C, et al. Prospective study of school injuries: incidence, types, related factors, and initial management. Can Med Assoc J 1983;129:1279.

Flisher AJ, Ziervogel CF, Chalton DO, et al. Risk-taking behavior of Cape Peninsula high-school students. Part VI. Road-related behavior. S Afr Med J 1993;83: 486.

Fraser JJ Jr. Nonfatal injuries in adolescents: United States, 1988 [Abstract]. J Adolesc Health 1995;16: 146.

Gallagher SS, Finison K, Guyer R. The incidence of injuries among 87,000 Massachusetts children and adolescents: results of the 1980–81 Statewide Childhood Injury Prevention Program Surveillance System. Am J Public Health 1984;74:1340.

Gould JH, DeJong AR. Injuries to children involving home exercise equipment. Arch Pediatr Adolesc Med 1994;148:1107.

Greensher J. Non-automotive vehicle injuries in adolescents. Pediatr Ann 1988;17:114.

Halperin SF, Bass JL, Mehta KA, et al. Unintentional injuries among adolescents and young adults: a review and analysis. J Adolesc Health Care 1983;4:275.

Hingson R, Merrigan D, Heeren T. Effects of Massachusetts raising its legal drinking age from 18 to 20 on deaths from teenage homicide, suicide, and nontraffic accidents. Pediatr Clin North Am 1985;32:221.

Hoekelman RA, Pless IB. Decline in mortality among young Americans during the 20th century: prospects for reaching national mortality reduction goals for 1990. Pediatrics 1988;82:582.

International Association of Cancer Registries and International Agency for Research on Cancer. Cancer incidence in five continents, vol 5 [IARC scientific publication 88]. Lyon, France: International Association for Research on Cancer, 1987.

Jacobson MS, Rubenstein EM, Bohannon WE, et al. Follow-up of adolescent trauma victims: a new model of care. Pediatrics 1986;77:236.

Jordan EA, Duggan AK, Hardy JB. Injuries in children of adolescent mothers: home safety education associated with decreased injury risk. Pediatrics 1993;91:481.

Kann L, Wareen W, Collins JL, et al. Results from the national school-based 1991 Youth Risk Behavior Survey and progress toward achieving related health objectives for the nation. Public Health Rep 1993;108:47.

Kochanek KD, Hudson BL. Advance report of final mortality statistics, 1992. Monthly Vital Statistics Report December 8, 1994;43(6)(suppl).

Loiselle JM, Baker MD, Templeton JM Jr, et al. Substance abuse in adolescent trauma. Ann Emerg Med 1993;22:1530.

Macknin ML, Medendorp SV. Association between bicycle helmet legislation, bicycle safety education, and the use of bicycle helmets in children. Arch Pediatr Adolesc Med 1994;148:255.

Munoz E. Economic costs of trauma, United States, 1982. J Trauma 1984;24:237.

National Academy of Sciences. Injury in America. Washington DC: National Academy Press, 1985.

National Center for Health Statistics. Advance report of final mortality statistics, 1992. Monthly Vital Statistics Report 1994;43.

National Center for Health Statistics. Vital statistics of the United States, 1990, Volume II. Mortality, Part B. Hyattsville, Maryland: DHHS Public Health Service, 1994.

National Center for Health Statistics. Vital and health statistics: National Ambulatory Medical Care Survey: 1989 summary: series 13: data from the National Health Survey [110, DHHS publication 92-1771]. Hyattsville, Maryland: US Government Printing Office, 1992.

National Center for Health Statistics. Vital and health statistics: current estimates from the National Health Interview Survey, 1991 [DHHS publication 93-1512]. Hyattsville, Maryland: US Government Printing Office, 1992.

National Center for Health Statistics. Health, United States, 1993 [DHHS publication (PHS) 94-1232]. Hyattsville, Maryland: US Government Printing Office, 1994.

National Safety Council. Accident facts, 1994. Chicago: National Safety Council, 1994.

O'Carroll PW, Harel Y, Waxweiler RJ. Measuring adolescent behaviors related to intentional injuries. Public Health Rep 1993;108(suppl 1):15.

Orlowski JP. Adolescent drowning: swimming, boating, diving, and scuba accidents. Pediatr Ann 1988;17:125.

Orsay EM, Turnbull TL, Dunne M, et al. Prospective study of the effect of safety belts on morbidity and health care costs in motor-vehicle accidents. JAMA 1988;260:3598.

Paulson JA. The epidemiology of injuries in adolescents. Pediatr Ann 1988;17:84.

Polen MR, Friedman GD. Automobile injury: selected risk factors and prevention in the health care setting. JAMA 1988;259:77.

Preusser DF, Zador PL, Williams AF. The effect of city curfew ordinances on teenage motor vehicle fatalities. Accid Anal Prev 1993;25:641.

Prothrow-Stith D, Spivak H. The violence prevention project: a public health approach. Science, Technology, and Human Values 1987;12:3.

Public Health Service: Healthy people 2000: national health promotion and disease prevention objectives [DHHS publication (PHS) 91-50212]. Washington DC: Public Health Service, 1990.

Ries LAG, Hjanky BF, Miller BA, et al. Cancer statistics review 1973, 1973-1988 [NIH publication 91-2789]. Bethesda, Maryland: National Cancer Institute, 1991.

Rivara FP. Motor vehicle injuries during adolescence. Pediatr Ann 1988;17:107.

Robertson LS. Motor vehicles. Pediatr Clin North Am 1985;32:87.

Runyan C, Kotch JB, Margolis LH, et al. Childhood injuries in North Carolina: a statewide analysis of hospitalizations and deaths. Am J Public Health 1985;75:1429.

Scales P. Helping adolescents create their futures. Family Life Educator 1988;Fall:4.

Schor EL. Unintentional injuries: patterns within families. Am J Dis Child 1987;141:1280.

Selbst SM, Alexander D, Ruddy R. Bicycle related injuries. Am J Dis Child 1987;141:140.

Statistical abstract of the United States 1994. 114th ed. Washington, DC: US Department of Commerce, 1994.

Stevens WS, Rodgers BM, Newman BM. Pediatric trauma associated with all terrain vehicles. J Pediatr 1986;109:25.

Torg JS, Begso JJ, Sennett B. The National Football Head and Neck Injury Registry: 14 year report on cervical quadriplegia (1971-1984). Clin Sports Med 1987;6:61.

US Bureau of the Census. Statistical abstract of the United States, 1988. 108th ed. Washington DC: US Bureau of the Census, 1987.

Waxweiler RJ, Harel Y, O'Carroll PW. Measuring adolescent behaviors related to unintentional injuries. Pub Health Rep 1993;108(suppl 1):11.

Webster DW, Wilson ME. Gun violence among youth and the pediatrician's role in primary prevention. Pediatrics 1994;94:617.

Weiss BD. Bicycle helmet use by children. Pediatrics 1986;77:677.

Wilson MH, Shock S. Preventing motor vehicle-occupant and pedestrian injuries in children and adolescents. Curr Opin Pediatr 1993;5:284.

Wintemute GJ, Kraus JF, Teret SP, et al. Drowning in childhood and adolescence: a population based study. Am J Public Health 1987;77:830.

CHAPTER 6

Nutrition

Lawrence S. Neinstein and Linda E. Schack

Nutrition is an essential component of total adolescent health care. Two important changes occurring during adolescence can cause a crisis in the teenager's nutritional needs. First, growth in height, weight, and body components is greater and more rapid than at any time since infancy. Second, an adolescent's eating habits may change from regular meals prepared at home to irregular meals, skipped meals, and nutrition-poor snacks and fast-food meals. Adolescents have been found to have the highest prevalence of any age group of an unsatisfactory nutritional status. Practitioners should assess nutritional status and provide appropriate nutritional counseling as part of health supervision visits. The Food Guide Pyramid is a helpful educational tool that can be used to assist teenagers in improving their diets.

POTENTIAL NUTRITIONAL PROBLEMS

Risk Factors

1. *Increased nutritional needs* during adolescence relate to the following factors:
   a. Adolescents gain 50% of their adult weight.
   b. Adolescents gain 20% of their adult height.
   c. Adolescents gain 50% of their adult skeletal mass.
   d. Caloric and protein requirements are maximal.
2. The *increased physical activity* of adolescents makes proper nutrition essential.
3. *Poor eating habits* contribute to nutritional problems:
   a. Missed meals are common.
   b. High-sugar snacks of low nutritional value are popular.
   c. Peer pressure leads to erratic eating behavior.
   d. The adolescent's family may exhibit poor eating habits, and meal preparation may be inadequate.
   e. Many meals are obtained from vending machines or fast-food restaurants.
      Table 6.1 lists the fat and sodium content of popular fast foods and ice cream snacks. Note that many of these foods approach or exceed 50% of their calories from fat.
4. *Special considerations or stresses:*
   a. Sports
   b. Menstruation
   c. Teenage pregnancy
   d. Substance abuse
   e. Special diets (i.e., vegetarian)

TABLE 6.1. Fat and Sodium Contents of Popular Fast Foods

	Serving Size (g)	Calories	Cholesterol (mg)	Sodium (mg)	% of Calories from Fat
Hamburgers					
Jumbo Jack (Jack in the Box)	229	560	65	700	52
Big Mac (McDonald's)	215	490	90	890	49
Whopper (Burger King)	270	630	90	850	56
Famous Star (Carl's Jr.)	244	610	50	890	56
Sandwiches					
Arby's Roast Beef	155	383	43	936	42
Filet-o-Fish (McDonald's)	141	370	50	730	43
Fish Supreme (Jack in the Box)	245	590	60	1170	49
Other					
Large fries (McDonald's)	122	400	0	200	50
Kentucky Fried Chicken drumstick and thigh	143	390	180	780	54
Taco (Taco Bell)	78	180	32	276	56
Domino's thin crust pizza (1/3 of 12" cheese pizza)	141	364	26	1012	38
16 oz chocolate shake (McDonald's)	480 ml	350	25	240	17
Ice Cream Desserts					
Dove Bar					67
Häagen-Dazs					57
Ice Cream					48
Ice Milk					27
Frozen Yogurt					17
Sherbet					8

Sample Alternative Meals	Total Fat (g)	% of Calories from Fat	% of Saturated Fat	Cholesterol (g)
Regular McDonald's				
Quarterpounder	21	45	18	86
French fries	22	49	11	0
Chocolate chip cookies	16	42	14	4
Total Fat	59			90
Alternative				
McLean Deluxe	10	29	12	37
Small Fries	12	49	11	0
Shake	2	5	2	10
Total Fat	24			47

All these factors contribute to the findings of both the Food and Drug Administration's Ten State Nutritional Survey in the 1960s (U.S. Department of Health, 1972) and the National Health and Nutrition Examination Survey during 1971–1974 (National Center for Health Statistics, 1979) that the highest prevalence of unsatisfactory nutritional status occurs in the adolescent age group. Of particular note were deficiencies of calcium, iron, riboflavin, thiamine, and vitamins A and C.

Associated Difficulties

1. Iron deficiency: 5–8% prevalence during adolescence
2. Obesity: 11–15% prevalence during adolescence
3. Dental caries: Increased by high-sugar snacks
4. Deficiencies in protein, minerals, and vitamins during pregnancy

DIETARY ASSESSMENT

Assessing the dietary status of an adolescent should form part of the comprehensive health evaluation. This becomes even more important if a nutritional deficit is suspected, if a chronic illness is present, or if the teenager is pregnant. Nutritional assessment can include dietary, anthropometric, clinical, and laboratory data.

Dietary Data

Dietary information can be obtained from a food record kept by the teenager, a dietary history obtained from a nutritionist, a 24-hour recall, or a diet questionnaire. Figure 6.1 is an

---

DIET QUESTIONNAIRE

1. Do you drink milk? Yes _____ No _____
   If yes, whole milk _____
              2% low-fat milk _____
              skim milk_____

2. Please indicate which of the following foods you eat and how often:

	Never or hardly ever (less than once a week)	Sometimes (not daily but at least once a week)	Every day or nearly every day
Cheese, yogurt, ice cream	_____	_____	_____
Eggs	_____	_____	_____
Dried beans, peas, peanut butter	_____	_____	_____
Bread, rice, pasta, grits, cereal, tortillas, potatoes	_____	_____	_____
Fruits or fruit juices	_____	_____	_____
Vegetables	_____	_____	_____

3. If you eat fruits or drink fruit juices every day or nearly every day, which ones do you eat or drink most often?_____

   _____

4. If you eat vegetables every day or nearly every day, which ones do you eat most often?

   _____

5. Do you usually eat anything between meals? If yes, name the two or three snacks that you have most often:_____

   _____

6. Do you take vitamins or iron? Yes _____ No _____
   If yes, how often? _____
   What kind?_____

7. Are you on a special diet? Yes _____ No _____
   If yes, what is the reason?
      Allergy—specify type of diet: _____

      _____

      Weight reduction—specify: _____

      _____

      Other—specify reason for diet and type of diet:_____

      _____

FIGURE 6.1.   Diet questionnaire for adolescents. (Adapted from Fomon S. Nutritional disorders of children: prevention, screening, and follow-up [DHEW Publication [HSE] 78–5104]. Rockville, Maryland: US Department of Health, Education, and Welfare, Health Services Administration, 1976.)

example of a diet questionnaire for adolescents. If a questionnaire is not used, the adolescent can be screened with questions such as:

1. "Do you feel that your weight is too much, too little, or about right?"
2. "Have you recently lost or gained weight, or have you stayed the same?"
3. "Are there any foods that you have eliminated from your diet?"
4. "How many meals do you usually eat in a day?"
5. "Tell me everything you have eaten in the last 24 hours."
6. "Are you on a diet?"
7. "What is the most you have ever weighed, and what would you like to weigh?"

Anthropometric Measurements

1. Weight—A short-term measurement of nutrition: Use balance beam scale and have teen remove shoes and heavy clothing. Weight-for-age charts are available as part of the growth charts published by the National Center for Health Statistics (NCHS) (see Figs. 1.18 and 1.20). An estimate of ideal weight in postpubertal adolescents of medium build is
   a. Males: 5 feet = 106 pounds plus 6 pounds for each additional inch.
   b. Females: 5 feet = 100 pounds plus 5 pounds for each additional inch.
2. Height—A long-term indicator of nutrition: Stadiometer is most accurate. Have teen remove shoes and stand with heels touching wall. Height-for-age charts are also available on NCHS growth charts.
3. Weight-for-height—A good indicator of obesity in preadolescents: These data are available only on NCHS growth charts for preadolescents. However, weight/height-for-age charts are included in Chapter 32 for adolescents ages 12–17.
4. BMI: The Expert Committee on Clinical Guidelines for Overweight in Adolescent Preventive Services (Himes and Dietz, 1994) recommends screening adolescents by using the body mass index (BMI). BMI = weight (kg) divided by the square of the height (m) or BMI = weight in kg/(height in m)^2. A BMI exceeding the 85th percentile (120% of normative values) is considered the definition of obesity. Values in adolescents are listed in Table 6.2.
5. Skin fold measurements—Helpful in evaluating the adipose tissue component and degree of obesity: Formulas for calculating percent body fat with skin fold measurements are included in Chapter 32.

Tᴀʙʟᴇ 6.2. Percentile Values of Body Mass Index, National Health and Nutrition Examination Survey: United States 1971–1974[a]

Age (yr)	Male (Percentile)			Female (Percentile)		
	5th	50th	95th	5th	50th	95th
10	14.2	16.6	22.2	14.3	17.1	24.2
11	14.6	17.2	23.5	14.6	17.8	25.7
12	15.1	17.8	24.8	15.0	18.3	26.8
13	15.6	18.4	25.8	15.4	18.9	27.9
14	16.1	19.1	26.8	15.7	19.4	28.6
15	16.6	19.7	27.7	16.1	19.9	29.4
16	17.2	20.5	28.4	16.4	20.2	30.0
17	17.7	21.2	29.0	16.9	20.7	30.5
18	18.3	21.9	29.7	17.2	21.1	31.0
19	19.0	22.5	30.1	17.5	21.4	31.3

Adapted from Hammer LD, Kraemer HC, Wilson DC, et al. Standardized percentile curves of body-mass index for children and adolescents. Am J Dis Child 1991; 145:260.
[a]BMI (body mass index) = wt (kg)/ht^2 (m)

TABLE 6.3.   Midarm Circumference Measurements in Adolescents

Age (yr)	Standard (cm)		90% Standard (cm)	
	Male	Female	Male	Female
13	23.0	23.0	20.7	20.7
14	24.3	24.0	21.9	21.6
15	25.3	24.5	22.7	22.0
16	26.2	24.9	23.6	22.4
17	27.5	25.0	24.7	22.5
18–19	29.2	26.0	26.3	23.4

Adapted from Alton IR. Nutritional needs and assessment of adolescents. In Blum, RW, ed. Adolescent health care. New York: Academic Press, 1982.

6. Midarm circumference measurement—Evaluates muscle and adipose tissue and is a good indicator of nutritional status: Midarm circumference should be measured on the nondominant arm at a midpoint between the tip of the olecranon process and the tip of the acromion, with the arm relaxed at the side. The measurement should be taken without compressing the arm. Values less than 90% of standard indicate nutritional depletion. Table 6.3 shows standard midarm circumference measurements for adolescents.

Clinical Evaluation

Clinical evaluation includes examination of skin, eyes, lips, tongue, teeth, gums, hair, and nails. The following is a list of clinical findings and possible nutritional causes.

1. Skin
   a. Pallor: Iron deficiency
   b. Follicular hyperkeratosis: Vitamin A deficiency or excess
   c. Xanthoma: Hyperlipidemia
   d. Petechiae: Vitamin C deficiency
2. Eyes
   a. Night blindness: Vitamin A deficiency
   b. Angular palpebritis: Riboflavin, niacin deficiencies
3. Lips
   a. Angular stomatitis, cheilosis: Riboflavin, niacin deficiencies
4. Tongue
   a. Glossitis: Niacin, folic acid, vitamin B_{12}, or vitamin B_6 deficiencies
   b. Papillary atrophy: Riboflavin, niacin, folic acid, vitamin B_{12}, or iron deficiencies
   c. Loss of taste: Zinc deficiency
5. Gums soft, spongy, or bleeding: Vitamin C deficiency
6. Excessive dental caries: Diet high in refined sugar
7. Hair dry, dull, and brittle: Protein-calorie malnutrition
8. Nails
   a. Brittle nails with frayed borders: Malnutrition, iron deficiency, or calcium deficiency
   b. Concave or eggshell nails (free edge curved sharply outward): Vitamin A deficiency
9. Other signs of general malnutrition
   a. Muscle wasting
   b. Delayed sexual maturation
   c. Amenorrhea
   d. Hepatomegaly

Laboratory Tests

Laboratory tests helpful in assessing nutritional status include hemoglobin, hematocrit, ferritin, serum protein, and albumin.

Nutritional Requirements

Recommended dietary allowances (RDA) for adolescents are reviewed in Table 6.4. These are based on the recommendations of the Food and Nutrition Board, National Academy of Sciences (1989).

Energy Requirements

Energy requirements are determined by basal metabolic rate, growth needs, and level of activity. Energy is provided by fat (which supplies 9 kcal/g), carbohydrates (4 kcal/g), and protein (4 kcal/g). Alcohol (7 kcal/g) can also be a significant source of calories. Diets in teenagers should probably contain no more than 30% of calories from fat. Suggested caloric intakes are listed in the RDA table, but these will vary widely according to body size and activity level.

Protein

Protein requirements increase during adolescence by about 10 g/day to 1 g/kg in males and 0.8 g/kg in females. Most teenagers' diets exceed the RDA for protein.

TABLE 6.4.   Recommended Dietary Allowances for Adolescents

| | Male (yr) | | | Female (yr) | | | | | |
| | | | | | | | | Lactating | |
Category	11–14	15–18	19–24	11–14	15–18	19–24	Pregnancy	1st 6 months	2nd 6 months
Weight (kg)	45	66	72	46	55	58			
Height (cm)	157	176	177	157	163	164			
Energy (cal)	2500	3000	2900	2200	2200	2200	+300	+500	+500
Protein (g)	45	59	58	46	44	46	60	65	62
Vitamins									
Vitamin A (IU)	1000	1000	1000	800	800	800	800	1300	1200
Vitamin D (IU)	10	10	10	10	10	10	10	10	10
Vitamin E (IU)	10	10	10	8	8	8	10	12	11
Vitamin K (µg)	45	65	70	45	55	60	65	65	65
Vitamin C (mg)	50	60	60	45	60	60	70	95	90
Thiamine (mg)	1.3	1.5	1.5	1.1	1.1	1.1	1.5	1.6	1.6
Riboflavin (mg)	1.5	1.8	1.7	1.3	1.3	1.3	1.6	1.8	1.7
Niacin (mg)	17	20	19	15	15	15	17	20	20
Vitamin B_6 (mg)	1.7	2.0	2.0	1.4	1.5	1.6	2.2	2.1	2.1
Folacin (µg)	150	200	200	150	180	180	400	280	260
Vitamin B_{12} (µg)	2.0	2.0	2.0	2.0	2.0	2.0	2.2	2.1	2.6
Minerals									
Calcium (mg)	1200	1200	1200	1200	1200	1200	1200	1200	1200
Phosphorus (mg)	1200	1200	1200	1200	1200	1200	1200	1200	1200
Magnesium (mg)	270	400	350	280	300	280	320	355	340
Iron (mg)	12	12	10	15	15	15	30	15	15
Zinc (mg)	15	15	15	12	12	12	15	19	16
Iodine (µg)	150	150	150	150	150	150	175	200	200
Selenium (µg)	40	50	70	45	50	55	65	75	75

Adapted from Food and Nutrition Board, Commission on Life Sciences, National Research Council. Recommended dietary allowances. 10th ed. Washington DC: National Academy Press, 1989.

Minerals

1. Iron: There is an increased need for iron in both males and females during adolescence, in males because of the increase in muscle mass and blood volume and in females due to menstrual losses. High-iron foods include lean red meats, spinach, green vegetables, and fortified cereal. Nonheme iron, which is present in plant sources, is less bioavailable, but its absorption can be enhanced by concurrent intake of vitamin C.
2. Calcium: Skeletal growth causes an increased need for calcium, of about 400 mg/day, during adolescence. Many adolescents have inadequate calcium intakes, possibly in part due to the substitution of carbonated beverages for milk. In addition to dairy products, calcium is found in tofu, sardines, and dark-green leafy vegetables.
3. Zinc: Daily needs increase from 10 mg to 15 mg during adolescence. Zinc is needed for adequate growth, sexual maturation, and wound healing. Good food sources of zinc include lean meats, seafood, eggs, and milk.

Vitamins

Vitamin requirements increase during adolescence, especially for vitamin B_{12}; folate; vitamins D, A, C, and E; thiamine; niacin; and riboflavin. Supplements of antioxidant vitamins (A, C, E, and β-carotene) have been shown to probably reduce the risk of cardiovascular disease and certain cancers, but there is no current recommendation to prescribe these routinely.

GUIDELINES FOR NUTRITIONAL THERAPY

General Recommendations

1. Stress with the adolescent the effects of dietary changes on current lifestyle: Appearance, muscle development for sports, feeling energetic, etc.
2. Use the Food Guide Pyramid (Fig. 6.2) to recommend the appropriate number of daily servings from each food group.
3. Encourage teenagers to be aware of the comparative nutritional values of fast foods and to read food labels (Fig. 6.3).
4. Suggest that teenagers exercise at least 3 days a week, for a minimum of 20 minutes.
5. Simplify good nutrition concepts by recommending the following to adolescents and their families:
   a. Eat a variety of foods.
   b. Maintain a healthy weight.
   c. Choose foods low in saturated fat and cholesterol.
      — Broil or bake instead of fry foods.
      — Select leaner cuts of meats.
      — Substitute low-fat or nonfat milk for whole-milk dairy products.
      — Use more polyunsaturated fats.
   d. Eat more fruits, vegetables, and grains.
   e. Use sugar and salt sparingly.
      — Avoid presweetened cereals and products.
      — Keep sugar bowl and salt shaker off the table.
      — Drink fruit juices instead of soft drinks.
      — Decrease intake of candy, cookies, and pie.
      — Avoid salty and smoked meats.

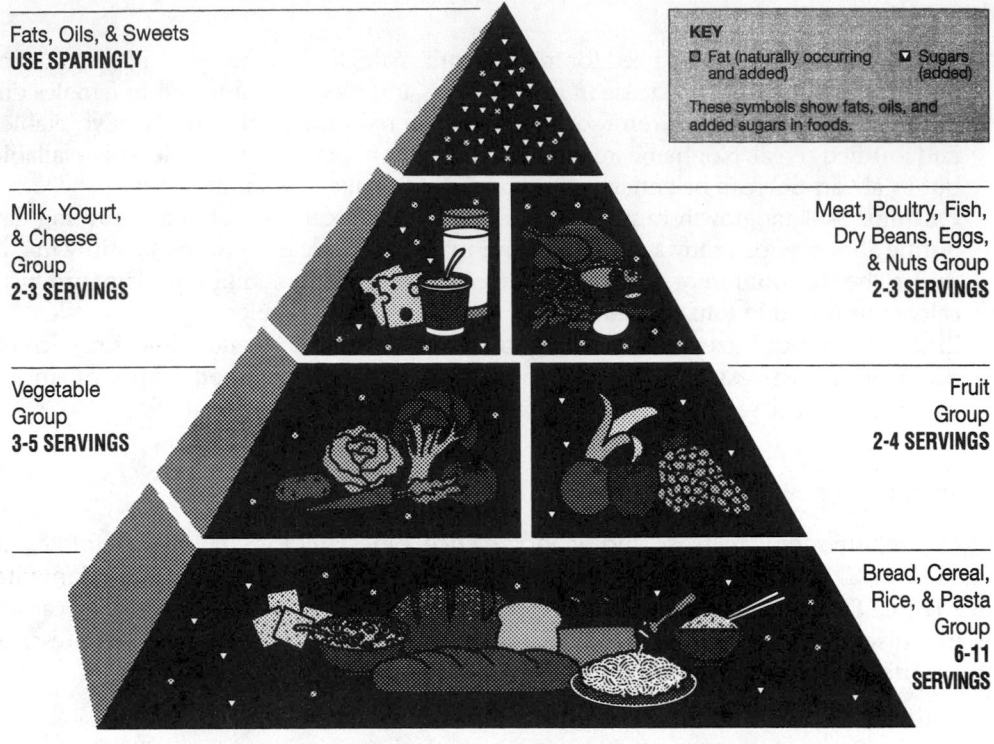

How to Use The Daily Food Guide

What counts as one serving?

Breads, Cereals, Rice, and Pasta
1 slice of bread
1/2 cup of cooked rice or pasta
1/2 cup of cooked cereal
1 ounce of ready-to-eat cereal

Vegetables
1/2 cup of chopped raw or
  cooked vegetables
1 cup of leafy raw vegetables

Fruits
1 piece of fruit or melon wedge
3/4 cup of juice
1/2 cup of canned fruit
1/4 cup of dried fruit

Milk, Yogurt, and Cheese
1 cup of milk or yogurt
1-1/2 to 2 ounces of cheese

**Meat, Poultry, Fish, Dry Beans,
Eggs, and Nuts**
2-1/2 to 3 ounces of cooked lean
  meat, poultry, or fish
Count 1/2 cup of cooked beans,
  or 1 egg, or 2 tablespoons of
  peanut butter as 1 ounce of lean
  meat (about 1/3 serving)

Fats, Oils, and Sweets
LIMIT CALORIES FROM THESE
especially if you need to lose weight

The amount you eat may be
more than one serving. For
example, a dinner portion of
spaghetti would count as two
or three servings of pasta.

FIGURE 6.2.   Food guide pyramid; a guide to daily food choices. (From Focus on food labeling, FDA Consumer Special Report. Rockville, Maryland: US Food and Drug Administration, 1993. Black-and-white reproducibles suitable for producing office handout material may be ordered from the US Food and Drug Administration (HFI–40), 5600 Fishers Lane, Rockville, MD 20856; 301-443-3220.)

Special Conditions

1. Vegetarian diets: Adolescents may be vegetarian for reasons of health or because of eco-logical, economic, religious, or philosophical beliefs. Teens who are vegetarians should be supported and encouraged, as their diets are likely to be more healthful than that of

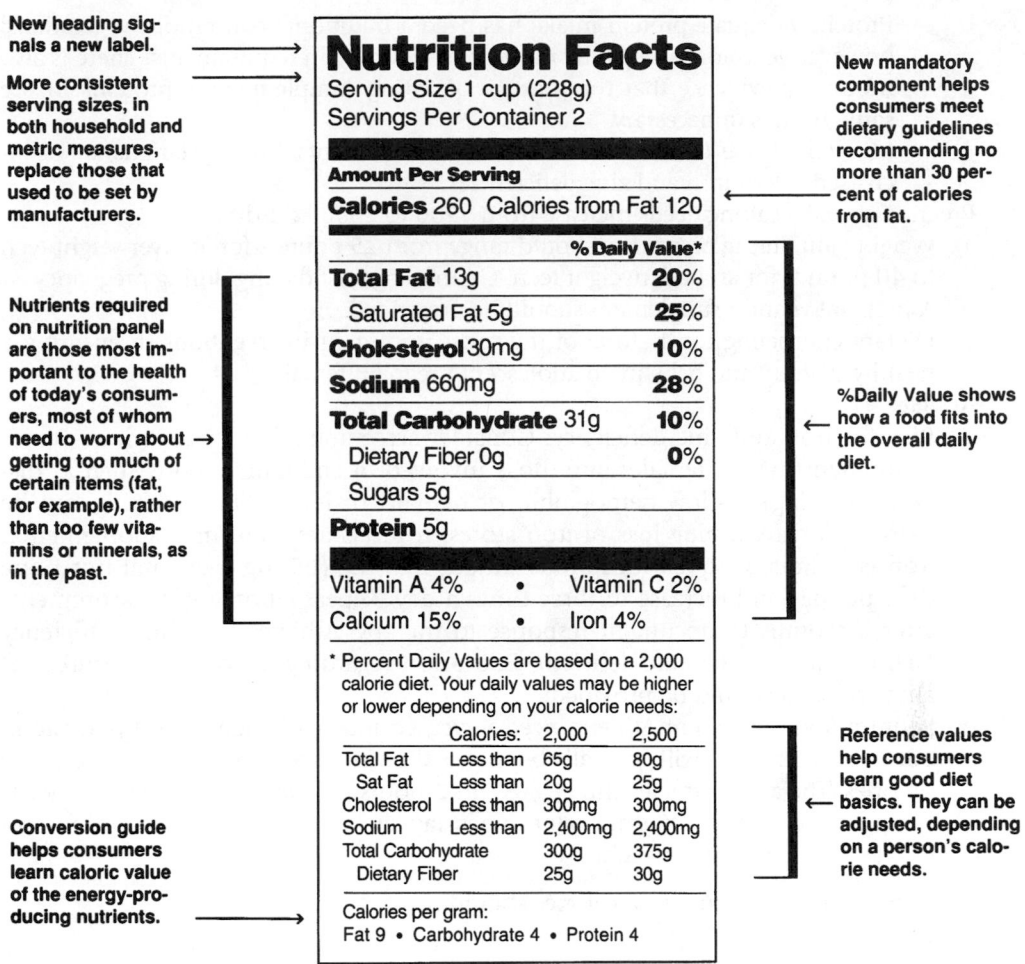

New heading signals a new label.

More consistent serving sizes, in both household and metric measures, replace those that used to be set by manufacturers.

Nutrients required on nutrition panel are those most important to the health of today's consumers, most of whom need to worry about getting too much of certain items (fat, for example), rather than too few vitamins or minerals, as in the past.

Conversion guide helps consumers learn caloric value of the energy-producing nutrients.

New mandatory component helps consumers meet dietary guidelines recommending no more than 30 percent of calories from fat.

%Daily Value shows how a food fits into the overall daily diet.

Reference values help consumers learn good diet basics. They can be adjusted, depending on a person's calorie needs.

Nutrition Facts
Serving Size 1 cup (228g)
Servings Per Container 2

Amount Per Serving

Calories 260   Calories from Fat 120

	% Daily Value*
Total Fat 13g	**20**%
Saturated Fat 5g	**25**%
Cholesterol 30mg	**10**%
Sodium 660mg	**28**%
Total Carbohydrate 31g	**10**%
Dietary Fiber 0g	**0**%
Sugars 5g	
Protein 5g	

Vitamin A 4%	•	Vitamin C 2%
Calcium 15%	•	Iron 4%

* Percent Daily Values are based on a 2,000 calorie diet. Your daily values may be higher or lower depending on your calorie needs:

	Calories:	2,000	2,500
Total Fat	Less than	65g	80g
Sat Fat	Less than	20g	25g
Cholesterol	Less than	300mg	300mg
Sodium	Less than	2,400mg	2,400mg
Total Carbohydrate		300g	375g
Dietary Fiber		25g	30g

Calories per gram:
Fat 9 • Carbohydrate 4 • Protein 4

FIGURE 6.3. Nutrition label. (From US Department of Agriculture and US Department of Health and Human Services. [DHHS publication (FDA) 93–2262].)

the typical adolescent. Nutritional counseling may be of benefit to ensure adequate intakes of vitamins and minerals and to determine the need for supplements.

a. Types of vegetarians
   — *Semivegetarians* eat milk products and limited seafood and poultry but no red meat.
   — *Lactovegetarians* consume milk products but no eggs, meat, fish, or poultry.
   — *Ovolactovegetarians* consume milk products and eggs but no meat, fish, or poultry.
   — *Ovovegetarians* consume eggs but no milk products, meat, fish, or poultry.
   — *Vegans* consume vegetable foods only and no foods of animal origin (i.e., no eggs, milk products, meat, fish, or poultry).

b. Supplemental needs of vegetarians
   — Vitamins: Semivegetarians, lactovegeterians, and ovolactovegetarians have no need for supplements if attention is paid to dietary composition. Ovovegetarians and vegans may need supplemental riboflavin and vitamins D and B_{12}.

— Protein: Adequate protein intake has been a traditional concern for vegetarians; however, vegetarians generally meet or exceed protein requirements. There is also mounting evidence that the practice of eating complementary proteins in the same meal is unnecessary.

— Minerals: There is no uniform need for supplements, but vegetarians are at increased risk of iron and zinc deficiencies.

2. Pregnancy: Daily caloric needs increase from 2200 to 2500 kcal/day.
   a. Weight gain during pregnancy should range from 25 pounds for an overweight teen to 40 pounds for an underweight teen. Counsel against dieting during pregnancy.
   b. A prenatal vitamin supplement should be prescribed.
   c. Dietary counseling can be one of the most important interventions in ensuring a healthy delivery and baby in an adolescent pregnant female.

3. Athletes
   a. Risk for iron and zinc deficiency: Consider screening adolescent athletes (especially menstruating females and those involved in endurance sports such as distance running) for low hemoglobin or hematocrit levels. Serum ferritin can be helpful in determining loss of iron stores. If levels are abnormal, supplemental iron is indicated. Start with ferrous sulfate, 325 mg (65 mg elemental iron) one time per day and increase to three times a day. Repeat laboratory measurements after 2 months to document response to therapy. Athletes with iron deficiency anemia may also be zinc deficient. Education regarding good dietary sources of zinc and iron should be provided.
   b. Sodium and potassium: Athletes need increased intake of sodium and potassium, but this requirement will generally be met as they increase their calorie intake.
   c. Calories: The active athlete who engages in 2 hours per day of heavy exercise needs approximately 800–1700 extra calories per day above the recommended minimum for age, sex, height, and weight.

   Approximate distribution of calories should be:
   Protein: 15%
   Fat: 25%
   Carbohydrate: 60%

   d. Hydration: Attention must be given to hydration before and during activity:
      — The athlete should drink 10–16 ounces of cold water 1–2 hours before exercise.
      — Repeat 20–30 minutes before exercise.
      — Drink 4–6 ounces cold water every 10–15 minutes during exercise.
      — Cold fluids are preferable because gastric emptying is more rapid.
      — Plain water can be used for exercise periods under 2 hours.
      — Sports drinks may be used to provide carbohydrates for longer events. Fructose-containing solutions should be avoided, as fructose is less well absorbed than sucrose or glucose and can cause gastrointestinal upset.
   e. Weight restrictions: Avoid any major weight restrictions during the adolescent growth spurt. Alterations in diet to cause rapid weight gain or loss should be discouraged. Eating disorders are prevalent among female athletes, especially those involved in running, swimming, diving, gymnastics, and dance. Therefore, carefully question all female athletes regarding body image, desired weight, and amenorrhea. Anorexia nervosa should be considered in an athlete with secondary amenorrhea.
   f. Carbohydrate loading: This technique has been used to increase muscle glycogen stores in endurance sports such as distance running. It involves an initial depletion of carbohydrate achieved by vigorous workouts, followed by several days of a low-car-

bohydrate diet and then a loading period just before competition. For some athletes the low-carbohydrate period can adversely affect training. Modifications of the classic technique are being developed to address this issue. For optimal performance, advise athletes to eat a high-carbohydrate, low-fat meal 3–6 hours before an event. Foods high in carbohydrates should also be eaten after competition to replace glycogen stores.

BIBLIOGRAPHY

Alton IR. Nutritional needs and assessment of adolescents. In: Blum RW, ed. Adolescent health care. New York: Academic Press, 1982.

Canadian Paediatric Society Nutrition Committee. Adolescent nutrition, 1. Introduction and summary [Part 1 of 6]. Canad Med Assoc J 1983;129:419.

Coleman E. Sports drink update. Sports Nutrition 1988;1:190.

Committee on Nutrition. Pediatric nutrition handbook, 2nd ed. Elk Grove Village, Illinois: American Academy of Pediatrics, 1985.

Coyle EF. Carbohydrates and athletic performance. Sports Nutrition 1988;1:195.

Dunger DB, Preece MA. Growth and nutrient requirements at adolescence. In: Grand RJ, Sutphen JL, Dietz WH Jr, eds. Pediatric nutrition: theory and practice. Boston: Butterworths, 1987.

Dwyer J. Diets for children and adolescents that meet the dietary goals. Am J Dis Child 1980;134:1077.

Food and Nutrition Board, Commission on Life Sciences, National Research Council. Recommended dietary allowances, 10th ed. Washington DC: National Academy Press, 1989.

Forbes GB. Nutrition and growth. In: McAnarney ER, Kreipe RE, Orr DP, et al., eds. Textbook of adolescent medicine. Philadelphia: WB Saunders, 1992.

Hammer LD, Kraemer HC, Wilson DC, et al. Standardized percentile curves of body-mass index for children and adolescents. Am J Dis Child 1991;145:260.

Himes JH, Dietz WH. Guidelines for overweight in adolescent preventive services recommendations from an expert committee. The Expert Committee on Clinical Guidelines for Overweight in Adolescent Preventive Services. Am J Clin Nutr 1994;59:307.

Lifshitz F, Tarim O, Smith MM. Nutrition in adolescence. Endocrinol Metab Clin North Am 1993;22:673.

Loosli AR. Reversing sports-related iron and zinc deficiencies. Phys Sportsmed 1993;21:70.

Marion DD, King JC. Nutritional concerns during adolescence. Pediatr Clin North Am 1980;27:125.

Mellin L. Shapedown: weight management program for adolescents. San Francisco: Balboa Publishing, 1980.

National Center for Health Statistics: Caloric and selected nutrient values for persons 1–74 years of age: first Health and Nutrition Examination Survey 1971–1974 [Vital and Health Statistics Series 11, 209, DHEW publication (PHS) 79–1657]. Hyattsville, Maryland: National Center for Health Statistics, 1979.

Probart CK, Bird PJ, Parker KA. Diet and athletic performance. Med Clin North Am 1993;77:757.

Rees JM, Worthington-Roberts B. Position of the American Dietetic Association: nutrition care for pregnant adolescents. J Am Diet Assoc 1994;94:449.

Reynolds RD. Vitamin supplements: current controversies. J Am Coll Nutr 1994;13:118.

Squire DL. Heat illness: fluid and electrolyte issues for pediatric and adolescent athletes. Pediatr Clin North Am 1990;37:1085.

Steen SN. Nutrition for young athletes: special considerations. Sports Med 1994;17:152.

US Department of Agriculture, US Department of Health and Human Services. Nutrition and your health: dietary guidelines for Americans [Home and Garden bulletin 232]. Washington DC: US Government Printing Office, 1985; revised 1990.

US Department of Health, Education, and Welfare. Ten State Nutrition Survey, 1968–1970, Highlights. Washington DC: US Department of Health, Education, and Welfare, Health Services and Mental Health Administration, Center for Disease Control, US Government Printing Office, 1972.

US Department of Health, Education, and Welfare. Adolescent health care: a guide for BCHS-supported programs and projects. Millar HEC, ed. [DHEW publication (HSA) 79–5234]. Washington DC: US Government Printing Office, 1979.

US Food and Drug Administration. FDA Consumer Special Issue on Food Labeling [S/N 017-017-012-00360-5]. Washington DC: US Government Printing Office, 1993.

White R, Frank E. Health effects and prevalence of vegetarianism. West J Med 1994;160:465.

CHAPTER 7

Understanding Legal Aspects of Care

Abigail English

Whenever a health-care practitioner treats an adolescent, it is important for the practitioner to have a clear understanding of the legal framework within which care is to be provided. Because many adolescents are minors—under the age of 18—their legal status differs from that of adults. Therefore, the laws related to their health care have distinct aspects based on their age and legal status. The issues that arise most frequently in providing health care to adolescents who are minors fall into three specific areas:

1. Consent: Who is authorized to give consent and whose consent is required?
2. Confidentiality: Who has the right to control the release of confidential information about the care, including medical records, and who has the right to receive such information?
3. Payment: Who is financially liable for payment and is there a source of insurance coverage or public funding available that the adolescent can access?

THE LEGAL FRAMEWORK

Over the past three decades the legal framework that applies to the delivery of adolescent health care has evolved in several significant ways. First, the courts have recognized that minors, as well as adults, have constitutional rights, although there has been considerable controversy concerning the scope of those rights. Second, a growing number of states are enacting statutes to authorize minors to give their own consent for health care. Third, the financing of health care services for all age groups and income levels is undergoing major change, at an increasingly rapid pace, which has had and will continue to have a significant impact on adolescents' access to health care.

Constitutional Issues

Beginning with *In re Gault* in 1967, in which the United States Supreme Court stated that "neither the Fourteenth Amendment nor the Due Process Clause is for adults alone," the Court has held repeatedly that minors have constitutional rights. The *Gault* decision, which accorded minors certain procedural rights when they are charged by the state with juvenile delinquency offenses, was followed by others recognizing that minors also had rights of free speech under the First Amendment (*Tinker v. Des Moines Independent School District*, 1969) and that they had privacy rights as well (*Planned Parenthood of Central Missouri v. Danforth*, 1976; *Carey v. Population Services International*, 1977). Although the Supreme Court subsequently rendered decisions that were more equivocal about the scope of minors' constitutional rights, the basic principles articulated in the early cases still stand.

The area of most frequent constitutional litigation—and to some degree the greatest controversy—has been the rights of minors with respect to reproductive health care, particularly abortion. The *Carey* case clearly established that the right of privacy protects minors' access to contraceptives, while the history of constitutional litigation with respect to abortion has been more complex. Following the decision in *Danforth*, which held that parents do not have an arbitrary veto power with respect to the abortion decisions of their minor daughters, the Supreme Court decided several additional cases—beginning with *Bellotti v. Baird* in 1979 and culminating most recently with *Planned Parenthood of Southeastern Pennsylvania v. Casey* in 1992—addressing parental notification and consent issues related to abortion. The import of these cases has been that while a state may enact a mandatory parental involvement requirement for minors' abortions it must also, at minimum, establish an alternative procedure, usually known as a "judicial bypass." In the bypass proceeding a minor must be permitted, without parental involvement, to seek a court order authorizing an abortion: if she is mature enough to give an informed consent, the court must allow her to make her own decision and, if she is not mature, the court must determine whether an abortion would be in her best interest. Many, but not all, states have enacted such parental involvement or judicial bypass statutes, some of which have been enjoined by the courts.

State and Federal Statutes

Although the constitutional litigation concerning minors' rights in the health-care arena has attracted significant attention, most of the specific legal provisions that affect adolescents' access to health care are contained in state and federal statutes or "common law" decisions of the state courts. These provisions cover a broad range of issues related to consent, confidentiality, and payment and are critical in defining the parameters of what practitioners in the adolescent health field are legally permitted and required to do. Thus, practitioners providing services to adolescents must develop a familiarity not only with the general constitutional principles that have evolved in recent decades but also with federal statutes and with the state statutes that apply in their own states.

CONSENT

The law generally requires the consent of a parent before medical care can be provided to a minor. There are, however, numerous exceptions to this requirement. In many situations someone other than a biologic parent—such as a foster parent, a juvenile court, a social worker, or probation officer—may be able to give consent in the place of the parent. Moreover, in emergency situations care may be provided without prior consent to safeguard the life and health of the minor. Most significant for the adolescent health-care practitioner, however, are the legal provisions that authorize minors themselves to give consent for their care. These provisions are typically based on either the status of the minor or the services sought. (See the appendix at the end of this chapter, which sets forth some of these provisions.)

All states have enacted one or more provisions that authorize minors to consent to certain services. These services most frequently include pregnancy related care; abortion; diagnosis and treatment for sexually transmitted diseases (STDs), human immunodeficiency virus (HIV), or acquired immunodeficiency syndrome (AIDS), and reportable or contagious diseases; examination and treatment related to sexual assault; counseling and treatment for drug or alcohol problems; and mental health treatment, especially outpatient care. Some of these statutes contain age limits, which most frequently fall between age 12 and age 15.

Similarly, all states have enacted one or more provisions that authorize minors who have attained a specific status to give consent for their own health care. Pursuant to these provisions, the following groups of minors may be authorized to do so: emancipated minors; those who are living apart from their parents; married minors; minors who are the parents of a child; high school graduates; and minors who have attained a certain age. Moreover, in a few states explicit statutes authorize minors who are "mature minors" to consent for care. Few states have enacted all of these provisions; thus, practitioners are advised to consult their local state laws.

The Mature Minor Doctrine and Informed Consent

Even in the absence of a specific statute, however, "mature minors" may have the legal capacity to give consent for their own care. The mature minor doctrine emerged from court decisions, primarily state court decisions, addressing the circumstances in which a physician could be held liable in damages for providing care to a minor without parental consent. Pursuant to the doctrine there is little likelihood that a practitioner will incur liability for failure to obtain parental consent in situations in which the minor is an older adolescent (typically at least age 15) who is capable of giving an informed consent and in which the care is not high risk, is for the minor's benefit, and is within the mainstream of established medical opinion. In fact, during the past few decades diligent searches have found no reported decisions holding a physician liable in such circumstances solely on the basis of failure to obtain parental consent when nonnegligent care was provided to a mature minor who had given informed consent. The basic criteria for determining whether a patient is capable of giving an informed consent are that the patient must be able to understand the risks and benefits of any proposed treatment or procedure and its alternatives and must be able to make a voluntary choice among the alternatives. These criteria apply to minors, as well as adults.

Privacy and Confidentiality

There are numerous reasons why it is important to maintain confidentiality in the delivery of health-care services to adolescents. Possibly the most important is to encourage adolescents to seek necessary care, but additional reasons include supporting adolescents' growing sense of privacy and autonomy and protecting them from the humiliation and discrimination that could result from disclosure of confidential information.

The confidentiality obligation has numerous sources in law and policy. They include the federal and state constitutions; federal statutes and regulations (such as those that pertain to Medicaid, family planning programs, federal drug and alcohol programs, maternal and child health programs, or community and migrant health centers); state statutes and regulations (such as medical confidentiality statutes, medical records statutes, privilege statutes, professional licensing statutes, or funding statutes); court decisions; and professional ethical standards.

Because these varied provisions sometimes conflict, or are less than clear in their application to minors, it is important that practitioners have some general guidelines to follow—

or questions to ask—in developing their understanding of how to handle confidential information. Confidentiality protections are rarely, if ever, absolute, so it is important for practitioners to understand what may be disclosed (based on their discretion and professional judgment), what must be disclosed, and what may not be disclosed. In reaching this understanding, a few of the most relevant questions include the following:

- What information is confidential (since it is confidential information that is protected against disclosure)?
- What information is not confidential (since such information is not protected)?
- What exceptions are there in the confidentiality requirements?
- What information can be released with consent?
- What other mechanisms allow for discretionary disclosure?
- What mandates exist for reporting or disclosing confidential information?

In general, even confidential information may be disclosed as long as authorization is obtained from the patient or another appropriate person. Often, when minors have the legal right to consent to their own care, they also have the right to control disclosure of confidential information about that care. This is not always the case, however, since there are a number of circumstances in which disclosure over the objection of the minor might be required: for example, if a specific legal provision requires disclosure to parents; a mandatory reporting obligation applies, as in the case of suspected physical or sexual abuse; or the minor poses a severe danger to himself or others.

When the minor does not have the legal right to consent to care or to control disclosure, the release of confidential information must generally be authorized by the minor's parent or the person (or entity) with legal custody or guardianship. Even when this is necessary, however, it is still advisable—from an ethical perspective—for the practitioner to seek the agreement of the minor to disclose confidential information and certainly, at minimum, to advise the minor at the outset of treatment of any limits to confidentiality. Fortunately, in many circumstances issues of confidentiality and disclosure can be resolved by discussion and informal agreement between a physician, the adolescent patient, and the parents without reference to legal requirements.

PAYMENT

There is an integral relationship among the legal provisions that pertain to consent, confidentiality, and payment in the delivery of health-care services to adolescents. To the extent that an adolescent does not have available a source of free care or access to insurance coverage, provisions that purport to enable adolescents to give their own consent for care and to obtain it on a confidential basis do not actually guarantee access. It may seem implicit that if a minor is authorized to consent to care, it is the minor rather than the parent who is responsible for payment and, in fact, some state statutes explicitly so provide. In reality, however, few if any adolescents are able to pay for health care. Consequently, any legal provisions that make available to them free care or insurance coverage—such as eligibility requirements for Medicaid or policies that enable them to obtain confidential services from a managed care plan in which their family is enrolled—are critical in ensuring their access to care.

Adolescents are uninsured and underinsured—by either private or public insurance (i.e., Medicaid)—to a greater extent than other groups in the population. This is particularly true for adolescents in low-income families. Moreover, even when adolescents are covered by public or private insurance, they may be unable to access that coverage without the involvement of their parents. Thus, more than other age groups, they may be dependent on care that is provided at no cost or based on a sliding fee scale through federal- and state-funded programs. Although the legal framework for financing of health-care services is undergoing dramatic changes in general and not only for adolescents, it is nevertheless essential that practitioners familiarize themselves with all potential options whereby adolescent health services can be paid for, including the available sources of public and private funding. It is only through a comprehensive understanding by practitioners of the legal framework for adolescent health services, including the relationships among consent, confidentiality, and payment issues, that adolescents' access to the health care they need can be assured.

BIBLIOGRAPHY

Bellotti v. Baird, 443 US 622 (1979).

Carey v. Population Services International, 431 US 678 (1977).

Council on Scientific Affairs, American Medical Association. Confidential health services for adolescents. JAMA 1993;269:1420.

Crosby MC, English A. Mandatory parental involvement/judicial bypass laws: do they promote adolescents' health? J Adolesc Health 1991;12:143.

English A. Treating adolescents: legal and ethical considerations. Med Clin North Am 1990;74:1097.

English A, Matthews M, Extavour K, et al. State minor consent statutes: a summary. Cincinnati: Center for Continuing Education in Adolescent Health, Children's Hospital Medical Center, 1995.

Gans J. A policy compendium on confidential health services for adolescents. Chicago: American Medical Association, 1993.

Holder A. Legal issues in pediatric and adolescent med-

icine. New Haven, Connecticut: Yale University Press, 1985.

In re Gault, 387 US 1 (1967).

Morrissey JM, Hoffman AD, Thrope JC. Consent and confidentiality in the health care of children and adolescents: a legal guide. New York: The Free Press, 1986.

Paradise E, Horowitz R. Runaway and homeless youth: a survey of state law. Washington, DC: American Bar Association Center on Children and the Law, 1994.

Planned Parenthood of Central Missouri v. Danforth, 428 US 52 (1976).

Planned Parenthood of Southeastern Pennsylvania v. Casey, 505 US 833 (1992).

Soler MI, Shotton AC, Bell JR. Glass walls: confidentiality provisions and interagency collaborations. San Francisco: Youth Law Center, 1993.

Tinker v. Des Moines Independent School District, 393 US 503 (1969).

APPENDIX[a]

HOW THE STUDY WAS CONDUCTED

The Alan Guttmacher Institute (AGI) compiled information on state statutes relating to an unmarried and unemancipated minor's authority to consent to contraceptive services, prenatal care and delivery services, services in connection with sexually transmitted diseases (STDs) and human immunodeficiency virus (HIV) infection, drug and alcohol abuse treatment, mental health care, general nonemergency medical care, abortion, and in the case of a minor parent, medical care for her child. We used three sources: J. Gittler, M. Quigley-Rick, and M. J. Saks, *Adolescent Health Care Decision Making: The Law and Pub-*

---

[a]Reproduced with permission of the Alan Guttmacher Institute from Donovan P. Our daughters' decisions: the conflict in state law on abortion and other issues. New York: The Institute, 1992.

lic Policy, Carnegie Council on Adolescent Development, Washington, D.C., 1990; J. M. Morrissey, A. D. Hofmann, and J. C. Thrope, *Consent and Confidentiality in the Health Care of Children and Adolescents: A Legal Guide,* Free Press, New York, 1986; and AGI's files of state laws and its *State Reproductive Health Monitor: Legislative Proposals and Actions.* Data on the age at which minors may marry without parental consent and drop out of school was collected from M. Guggenheim and A. Sussman, *The Rights of Young People,* Bantam, New York, 1985.

We then wrote a summary of the relevant laws and age limits for each state (see Appendix Table 1, p. 156) and sent this to the state's attorney general with a request for confirmation of the accuracy and currency of the information or for needed changes and the most recent statutory citation. In addition, we asked the attorneys general whether state law allowed a minor parent to consent to the adoption of her child and, if so, to provide the statute and the statutory citation.

The attorneys general of 30 states and the corporation counsel of the District of Columbia responded to our request for information. The accuracy and currency of our information for the remaining 20 states was checked through the bound volumes of state statutes and, in a few instances, through Westlaw, a computerized database of state laws; Audrey Samers, an associate in the law firm of Fried, Frank, Harris, Shriver & Jacobson, conducted this check.

Information on the age of majority was compiled by Anne Martin of the AGI, through a telephone survey of state attorneys general conducted in August and September of 1991. For the few states that would not respond to our request for this information, the age of majority was obtained through research of state statutes.

To the best of our knowledge, the information in this report is accurate as of January 1, 1991. In some instances, we have included more recent information.

APPENDIX TABLE 1. Laws Affecting an Unmarried, Unemancipated Minor's Right to Make Decisions about Medical Care, Abortion, and Other Important Issues, 50 States and the District of Columbia

State	Age of Majority	Contraceptive Services	Prenatal Care and Delivery Services	STD/VD Services	Medical Care	
					HIV Testing and Treatment	Treatment for Drug and Alcohol Abuse
Alabama	19	NL	MC	MC[4,5]	NL	MC
Alaska	18	MC	MC	MC	NL	NL
Arizona	18	NL	NL	MC	NL	MC[4]
Arkansas	18	MC	MC[14]	MC	NL	NL
California	18	MC	MC	MC[4]	MC[4,18]	MC[4]
Colorado	18	MC	NL	MC	MC	MC
Connecticut	18	NL	NL	MC	NL	MC
Delaware	18	MC[4]	MC[4,14]	MC	MC[4,18]	MC[4,25]
Washington, DC	18	MC	MC	MC	NL	MC
Florida	18	MC[28,29]	MC[15]	MC	MC	MC
Georgia	18	MC	MC	MC[5]	NL	MC[5]
Hawaii	18	MC[5,14,22,33]	MC[5,14,22,33]	MC[5,22,33]	NL	MC[5,34]
Idaho	18	MC	NL	MC[22,35]	NL	MC
Illinois	18	MC[29]	MC[15]	MC[4]	NL	MC[4,39]
Indiana	18	NL	NL	MC	NL	MC
Iowa	18	NL	NL	MC	MC	MC
Kansas	18	MC[44]	MC[45]	MC[5]	NL	MC[46]
Kentucky	18	MC	MC	MC	NL	MC

NA, not applicable; NL, no law found; MC, minor may consent; MD, minor may decide; PC, parental consent required; PN, parental notice required.

1. Includes only parental consent and notification laws that are currently being enforced. These laws include a judicial bypass except where indicated.
2. States with no law relating specifically to unmarried and unemancipated minors may have a law authorizing married and emancipated minors or teenagers over the age of majority to consent to general medical care that, by implication, requires unmarried and unemancipated minors to have parental consent.
3. In addition to the consent of the minor mother, some states require consent of the unwed father if he can be located or if paternity has been established, but others do not require the father to be informed of adoption proceedings.
4. Minor must be 12 or older; in Arizona, applies to a minor seeking treatment for drug abuse but not for alcohol abuse.
5. Physician may notify parents; in Maryland, the law prohibits disclosure of information about an abortion; in Georgia, notification provision applies to treatment for drug abuse only.
6. Law does not distinguish between outpatient and inpatient services; it was therefore assumed that a minor may consent to both.
7. Minor must be 14 or older, a high school graduate, married, pregnant or parent.
8. Minor must be 16 or older; in Vermont, minor under 16 may drop out of school after completing 10th grade.
9. Minor must be represented by an attorney.
10. Minor may consent if she has a child.
11. Law makes not distinction between minor and adult parents, and it was therefore assumed that the consent of a minor parent is sufficient.
12. Enforcement of a law requiring parental consent or judicial bypass in enjoined.
13. Minor may drop out at age 14 if employed and, in the District of Columbia, after completing eighth grade.
14. Law excludes abortion.
15. Law includes surgery; in Massachusetts, law excludes psychosurgery.
16. Minor may consent if mature enough to understand the nature and consequences of the proposed treatment.
17. Both parents must be notified unless one parent is not readily available; in Minnesota, a "diligent" effort must be made to locate both parents (see: Minn. Stat., sect. 144.343(2)-(6)); in Arkansas, a "reasonably diligent effort" must be made (see Ark. Code Ann., sect. 20-16-801 et seq.).
18. Law applies to testing only.
19. Law applies to a minor who is mature enough to participate "intelligently" in treatment or counseling and would present a danger to himself or herself or others, or is an alleged victim of incest or child abuse; parents shall be involved unless health professional thinks involvement would be inappropriate.
20. State law does not allow a minor to drop out of school before graduation.
21. Minor must be 15 or older.
22. Minor must be 14 or older.
23. Minor under 16 must receive intensive counseling from physician or other qualified professional, who must discuss the possibility of involving the minor's parents.
24. Minor parent must have court-appointed guardian (guardian ad litem).
25. Law applies to treatment for alcohol abuse only.

Mental Health Services		General Non-emergency Medical Care[2]	Abortion Services[1]	Decisions on Minor's Own Behalf		Decisions on Behalf of Minor's Child	
Outpatient	Inpatient			Dropping Out of School	Getting Married	Medical Care for Child	Placing Child for Adoption[3]
MC[6,7]	MC[6,7]	MC[7]	PC	MD[8]	PC	MC	MC[9]
NL	NL	MC[10]	NL	MD[8]	PC	MC	MC[11]
NL	NL	NL	NL[12]	MD[8,13]	PC	NL	MC
NL	NL	MC[15,16]	PN[17]	MD[8]	PC	MC	MC[11]
MC[4,19]	NL	NL	NL[12]	NA[20]	PC	NL	MC
MC[5,21]	MC[5,21]	NL	NL	MD[8]	PC	MC	MC
NL	MC[22]	NL	MC[23]	MD[8,13]	PC	MC	MC[24]
NL	NL	NL	NL[26]	MD[8]	MD[27]	MC	MC
MC[6]	MC[6]	NL	MC	MD[8,13]	PC	MC	MC
MC[4,30]	MC[30,31]	NL	NL[12]	MD[8]	MD[27]	MC	MC[11]
NL	MC[4,32]	NL	PN	MD[8]	MD[27]	MC	MC
NL	NL	NL	NL[26]	NA[20]	PC	NL	MC
NL	PN[36]	MC[37]	PN[17,38]	MD[8]	PC	MC	MC
MC[4,5,40]	PN[36]	MC[15,41]	NL[42]	MD[8]	PC	MC	MC
NL	NL	NL	PC	MD[31]	PC	NL	MC[43]
NL	NL	NL	NL	MD[8,13]	PC	NL	MC[11]
NL	PN[36]	MC[8,15,47]	NL	MD[8]	PC	MC	MC
MC[8]	MC[8]	MC[10]	NL[12]	NA[20]	MD[48]	MC	MC[24]

26. Law authorizing a minor to consent to prenatal care and delivery services excludes abortion; however, this condition imposes a blanket prohibition on abortion without parental consent and therefore appears to be unconstitutional under Supreme Court decisions.
27. Minor who is pregnant or has a child may marry without parental consent; in Florida, a judge must authorize a marriage in such circumstances; in Maryland, the minor must be at least 16.
28. Law excludes sterilization.
29. Minor may consent if she is pregnant or a parent, or if a doctor believes she may suffer a health hazard if services are not provided. Illinois law also authorizes minor to consent if referred by a physician or Planned Parenthood clinic; Maine law does not apply to pregnant minors.
30. Law requires hearing to determine voluntariness.
31. Minor must be 17 or older.
32. Minor may consent to observation and diagnosis only; parental consent needed for treatment.
33. Law excludes surgical procedures.
34. Minor may consent to counseling services only.
35. Minor may consent to diagnosis and treatment of contagious, infectious, and reportable diseases.
36. Minor may consent, but parent must be notified upon minor's admission. In Illinois and Tennessee, minor must be 16 years old to consent to admission; in Idaho, Kansas and Pennsylvania, 14 years; in Washington, 13 years.
37. The state's medical consent statute permits "any person of ordinary intelligence and awareness" to consent to hospital, medical, surgical or dental care (see: Idaho Code, sect. 39-4302). However, a later section of the law appears to give parents the authority to consent for a minor child (sect. 39-4303). According to the attorney general's office, the agency "frequently" interprets the law as authorizing minors to consent. (R. Hardin, deputy attorney general, personal communication to P. Donovan, AGI, Oct. 22, 1990.)
38. Law does not include judicial bypass.
39. "Reasonable" efforts must be made to involve minor's family in treatment for drug abuse; physician must notify parents within three months of initiation of treatment for alcohol abuse (see: Ill. Rev. Stat., ch. 111, pars. 4504, 4505).
40. Minor may consent to five outpatient sessions.
41. Minor may consent if she is pregnant.
42. Enforcement of a law requiring parental notice or judicial bypass in enjoined.
43. Minor may consent unless court determines that it is in the best interests of the child being adopted to require the consent of a minor parent's parent.
44. State law permits family planning services to be provided to "any person who is over 18 years of age and who is married or who has been referred . . . by a person licensed to practice medicine and surgery." (See: Kan. Stat. Ann., sect. 23-501 [1981].) According to the Kansas attorney general, a city or county would not be subject "to any liability for providing contraceptive services to minors [without parental consent] that does not exist with respect to providing such services to adults." (See: letter from Attorney General Robert T. Stephan to Thomas R. Powell, city attorney, and Henry H. Blase, county counselor, Wichita, Kans., Dec. 6, 1989; and Attorney General Opinion No. 87-66.)
45. Minor may consent when parent is not "available." The statute does not define available. (See: Kan. Stat. Ann., sect. 38-123 [1981].)
46. Law applies to treatment for drug abuse only.

Table continued on following page.

Appendix Table 1. *continued*

State	Age of Majority	Contraceptive Services	Prenatal Care and Delivery Services	STD/VD Services	HIV Testing and Treatment	Treatment for Drug and Alcohol Abuse
					Medical Care	
Louisiana	18	NL	NL	MC[5]	NL	MC[5,46]
Maine	18	MC[29]	NL	MC[5]	MC[18]	MC[5]
Maryland	18	MC[5,28]	MC[5]	MC[5]	NL	MC[5]
Massachusetts	18	NL	MC[14]	MC	NL	MC[4,46,53]
Michigan	18	NL	MC	MC[5,15]	MC[5,15]	MC[5,15]
Minnesota	18	NL	MC[5]	MC[5]	NL	MC[5]
Mississippi	21[58]	MC[59]	MC[15]	MC	NL	MC[5,21]
Missouri	18	NL	MC[5,14,15]	MC[5,15]	NL	MC[5,61]
Montana	18	MC[5]	MC[5,15]	MC[5,15]	NL	MC[5,15]
Nebraska	19	NL	NL	MC	NL	MC
Nevada	18	NL	NL	MC	NL	MC[46]
New Hampshire	18	NL	NL	MC[22]	NL	MC[4,46]
New Jersey	18	NL	MC[5,15]	MC[5,15]	NL	MC[5,66]
New Mexico	18	MC	NL[67]	MC	MC[18]	MC[46]
New York	18	MC	MC[70]	MC	MC[18]	MC[25]
North Carolina	18	MC[14,28]	MC[14,28]	MC	NL	MC
North Dakota	18	NL	NL	MC[22]	NL	MC[22]
Ohio	18	NL	NL	MC	MC[18]	MC
Oklahoma	18	MC[73]	MC	MC	NL	MC
Oregon	18	MC[5,75]	NL	MC	NL	MC[22,46]

47. Minor may consent if parent is not "immediately available." (See: Kan. Stat. Ann., sect. 38-123b [1981].)
48. A pregnant minor may marry without parental consent, but with court approval.
49. Minor who believes he or she is afflicted by an "illness or disease" may consent to treatment. (See: La. Rev. Stat. Ann., sect. 40:1095[1977].)
50. Judge may authorize marriage of minor of any age without parental consent "when there is a compelling reason." (See: La. Rev. Stat. Ann., sect. 9:212(Supp. 1991).)
51. Minor must have the consent of parent or other adult family member, or use the judicial bypass, or be counseled by the attending physician or a counselor, who can be a psychiatrist, psychologist, social worker, ordained clergyman, physician's assistant, nurse practitioner, guidance counselor, or nurse.
52. Law requires notification of one parent with no bypass. However, a physician may waive notification if the minor does not live with a parent; if the doctor determines that the minor is mature enough to give informed consent or that notification may lead to physical or emotional abuse of the minor, or otherwise be contrary to her best interests; or if reasonable effort to give notice was unsuccessful. The statute is not being enforced, pending a statewide referendum on the law in November 1992.
53. Minor may consent if found drug-dependent by two doctors; bars consent to methadone maintenance therapy and treatment with antipsychotic medication.
54. Both parents must consent. If parents are divorced, only the custodial parent must consent; in Massachusetts, the same is true if one parent is "unavailable." (See Mass. Gen. Laws c. 112, s. 12F.)
55. Law excludes abortion referral services and chemotherapy; minor may consent to 12 sessions or to services over a period of four months.
56. Minor must have the consent of parent, guardian or court-appointed guardian.
57. Age will change to 18 in the year 2000.
58. General age of consent to medical care is 18; however, any minor who is mature enough to understand the nature and consequences of the proposed medical or surgical treatment may consent.
59. Minor may consent if referred by a doctor, clergyman, family planning agency, school, or state agency.
60. Females 15 or older and males 17 or older may marry without parental consent; however, parents must be notified if either party is under age 21.
61. Law includes surgical care and hospital admission.
62. Minor parent may also consent to medical care for any child in his or her legal custody.
63. Minor must have completed eighth grade.
64. Anther statute bars a minor from entering into contracts, so attorney general's office reported that parental consent is usually required. (S. Nelson, Montana Juvenile Justice Bureau, personal communication to P. Donovan, AGI, Dec. 2, 1990.)
65. Court may require consent of minor parent's parent.
66. Parents must be notified if minor is admitted to a facility for alcohol abuse.
67. Minor may consent to testing and examination to confirm pregnancy.
68. Any minor may consent to counseling or psychotherapy; a minor 14 or older may consent to psychotropic (mind-affecting) medication or behavior modification program unless the parent objects.

| Mental Health Services | | General Non-emergency Medical Care[2] | Abortion Services[1] | Decisions on Minor's Own Behalf | | Decisions on Behalf of Minor's Child | |
| | | | | Dropping Out of School | Getting Married | Medical Care for Child | Placing Child for Adoption[3] |
Outpatient	Inpatient						
NL	MC[8]	MC[5,15,49]	PC	MD[31]	MD[50]	MC	MC[11]
MC[5,6]	MC[5,6]	NL	MC[51]	MD[31]	PC	NL	MC[11]
MC[5,6,8]	MC[5,6,8]	MC[5,10]	NL[52]	MD[8]	MD[27]	MC	MC[11]
MC[8]	MC[8]	MC[10,14,15,28,41]	PC[54]	MD[8]	PC	MC	MC[11]
MC[22,55]	NL	NL	PC	MD[8]	PC	MC	PC[56]
NL	MC[8]	MC[10]	PN[17]	MD[8,57]	PC	MC	PC
NL	NL	MC[15,58]	NL[12]	MD[31]	MD[60]	MC	MC
NL	NL	MC[10]	PC	MD[8]	PC	MC[62]	MC
MC[8]	MC[8]	MC[5,10,15]	NL	MD[8,63]	PC	MC[5]	MC[64]
NL	NL	NL	PN	MD[8]	MD[31]	NL	MC[11]
NL	MC	MC[10,16,28]	NL[42]	MD[31]	PC	MC	MC
NL	NL	MC[16]	NL	MD[8]	PC	NL	MC[65]
NL	NL	NL	NL	MD[8]	PC	MC	MC
MC[68]	PC	NL	NL	MD[8,69]	PC	NL	MC
MC	MC[8]	MC[10]	NL	MD[8,71]	PC	MC	MC
MC	NL	NL	NL[26]	MD[31]	PC	NL	MC
NL	NL	NL	PC[54]	MD[8]	PC	NL	MC
MC[22,72]	NL	NL	PN	NA[20]	PC	NL	MC
NL	NL	MC[10]	NL	NA[20]	MD[74]	MC	MC[8]
MC[22]	NL	MC[5,15,21]	NL	MD[76]	PC	NL	MC[11]

69. Minor may drop out if authorized by local school board.
70. Law refers to prenatal care; includes medical and hospital services.
71. Minor must be 17 in New York City.
72. Law excludes use of medications; covers period of 30 days or six sessions, after which parent must consent to further treatment.
73. Minor may consent if she has ever been pregnant.
74. Minor may marry without parental consent if she has given birth to an illegitimate child or is pregnant and the marriage has been authorized by a court.
75. A minor 15 or older may consent to sterilization if "all less drastic alternative contraceptive methods . . . have proved unworkable or inapplicable or are medically counter-indicated." (See: Or. Rev. Stat., sect. 436.205(c)[1989].)
76. Minor may drop out at age 16 if employed.
77. Minor 16 or older may consent to any legal health services except operations.
78. Consent may be given by grandparent.
79. Minor 16–18 may petition court for permission to marry, but must be represented by a court-appointed guardian to speak for or against the petition, and the parents must be notified. The court may authorize the marriage if it determines it to be in the minor's best interest.
80. Parents must be notified if minor needs immediate hospitalization.
81. Minor may consent to outpatient services only.
82. Attorney general says statutory history of law authorizing a minor to consent to services in connection with birth control, pregnancy and family planning indicates that the law is intended to encompass abortion. (C. S. Nance, assistant attorney general, personal communication to J. I. Rosoff, AGI, Aug. 28, 1990.)
83. According to attorney general, since nothing in the Code of Virginia defines the age at which a person is capable of giving consent, "it would appear that a minor parent may provide consent to medical care for his or her child." (Ibid.)
84. Mature minor is authorized to consent under *State versus Koome*, 84 Wn. 2d 901, 530 P.2d 260 (1975).
85. Minor must be 13 or older.
86. Minor may drop out at age 15 if employed or if school superintendent determines that minor is proficient in grades 1–9.
87. State law bars minor from consenting to sterilization.
88. Notification (or use of judicial bypass) can be waived if second physician determines that minor is mature enough to give consent or that notice would not be in her best interests.
89. Minor may consent unless court concludes minor's age precludes informed consent.
90. Abortion provider must "strongly encourage" minor "to consult" her parents or another family member or appropriate person. Every provider must have a policy on parental involvement that includes information on the availability of services to assist the minor in involving her parents. (See: Wis. Stat. Ann., sect. 146.78(5).)
91. State-supported family planning services may be provided to "any person who may benefit from these services." (See: Wyo. Stat., sect. 42-5-101(a).

Table continued on following page.

APPENDIX TABLE 1. *continued*

State	Age of Majority	Contraceptive Services	Prenatal Care and Delivery Services	STD/VD Services	Medical Care	
					HIV Testing and Treatment	Treatment for Drug and Alcohol Abuse
Pennsylvania	18	NL	MC	MC	NL	MC
Rhode Island	18	NL	NL	MC	MC[18]	MC
South Carolina	18	NL[77]	NL[77]	NL[77]	NL[77]	MC
South Dakota	18	NL	NL	MC	NL	MC
Tennessee	18	MC	MC	MC	NL	MC[5,46]
Texas	18	NL	MC[14,15]	MC[15]	NL	MC
Utah	18	NL	MC	MC	NL	NL
Vermont	18	NL	NL	MC[4,80]	NL	MC[4,80]
Virginia	18	MC[28]	MC[28]	MC	NL	MC[81]
Washington	18	NL[84]	NL[84]	MC[22]	NL	MC[22,81]
West Virginia	18	NL[87]	NL	MC	NL	MC
Wisconsin	18	NL	NL	MC	NL	MC[4]
Wyoming	19	MC[91]	NL	MC	NL	NL

Mental Health Services		General Non-emergency Medical Care[2]	Abortion Services[1]	Decisions on Minor's Own Behalf		Decisions on Behalf of Minor's Child	
Outpatient	Inpatient			Dropping Out of School	Getting Married	Medical Care for Child	Placing Child for Adoption[3]
NL	PN[36]	MC[73]	NL[12]	MD[31]	PC	MC	PN
NL	NL	NL	PC	MD[8]	PC	MC	PC
NL[77]	MC[8]	MC[8,77]	PC[78]	MD[8]	PC	MC	MC
NL	NL	NL	NL	MD[8]	PC	NL	MC[11]
MC[8]	PN[36]	NL	NL[12]	MD[8]	PC	NL	MC
MC	MC[8]	NL	NL[26]	MD[31]	MD[79]	NL	MC[11]
NL	MC[8]	NL	PN[17,38]	NA[20]	PC	MC	MC
NL	MC[22]	NL	NL	MD[8]	PC	NL	MC
MC	NL	NL	NL[82]	NA[20]	PC	NL[83]	MC
MC[85]	PN[36]	NL	NL[84]	MD[86]	PC	NL	MC[24]
NL	NL	NL	PN[88]	MD[8]	PC	NL	MC[89]
NL	NL	NL	MC[90]	MD[8]	PC	NL	MC[11]
NL	NL	NL	PC	MD[8]	PC	NL	MC

SECTION II

Endocrine Problems

CHAPTER 8

Abnormal Growth and Development

Lawrence S. Neinstein and Francine Ratner Kaufman

Chapter 1 described the numerous and varied normal physical changes of adolescence. Sometimes, however, an adolescent's growth falls outside the range of normal. For example, the adolescent may be too short, too tall, or possibly not as sexually developed as his or her peers. These are areas of enormous concern to the adolescent and to his or her family, and the health-care provider, consequently, must have a clear understanding of how to manage these problems.

DELAYED PUBERTY

Definition

In general, two standard deviations (SD) above and below the mean are used to define the range of normal variability. An adolescent who falls above or below these limits deserves a careful evaluation for hypothalamic, pituitary, or gonadal dysfunction, or undiagnosed chronic illness. Table 1.5, in Chapter 1, is helpful in determining guidelines for evaluation. Further guidelines are listed next.

Male Guidelines   A male may be considered to have delayed puberty if:

1. Genital (G) stage 1 persists beyond age 13.7 years, or pubic hair (PH) stage 1 persists beyond 15.1 years of age.
2. More than 5 years have elapsed from initiation to completion of genital growth.
3. The following sexual maturity ratings (SMRs) persist past the listed guidelines:

   G2 > 2.2 years   PH2 > 1.0 year
   G3 > 1.6 years   PH3 > 0.5 year
   G4 > 1.9 years   PH4 > 1.5 years

Female Guidelines   An adolescent female may be considered to have delayed maturation if:

1. Breast (B) stage 1 persists beyond age 13.4, or pubic hair stage 1 persists beyond 14.1 years, or there is failure to menstruate beyond 16 years of age.
2. More than 5 years have elapsed between initiation of breast growth and menarche.
3. The following sexual maturity ratings persist past the listed guidelines:

B2 > 1.0 year   PH2 > 1.3 years
B3 > 2.2 years   PH3 > 0.9 year
B4 > 6.8 years   PH4 > 2.4 years

Differential Diagnosis

The differential diagnosis of delayed puberty can be divided between those processes associated with short stature and those associated with normal stature.

Pubertal Delay without Short Stature

1. Constitutional delay of puberty
2. Acquired gonadotropin deficiency
   a. Tumors: Craniopharyngioma, hypothalamic glioma, astrocytoma, pituitary adenomas
   b. Trauma
   c. Infections: Viral encephalitis, tuberculosis
   d. Histiocytosis X
   e. Sarcoidosis
3. Isolated gonadotropin deficiency
   a. Kallmann's syndrome
   b. Other disorders with luteinizing hormone (LH) and follicle-stimulating hormone (FSH) deficiency
4. Acquired gonadal disorders
   a. Infections: Gonorrhea, tuberculosis, viral
   b. Trauma
   c. Postsurgical removal
   d. Postradiation, chemotherapy
5. Congenital gonadal disorders
   a. Klinefelter's syndrome
   b. Anorchism
   c. Pure gonadal dysgenesis
   d. Enzyme defects in androgen and estrogen production
6. Androgen receptor defects
   a. Testicular feminization
   b. Reifenstein's syndrome
7. Chronic diseases
   a. Congenital or acquired heart disease
   b. Asthma
   c. Inflammatory bowel disease
   d. Juvenile rheumatoid arthritis
   e. Systemic lupus erythematosus
   f. Anorexia nervosa
   g. Hyperthyroidism
   h. Galactosemia (in girls)

Pubertal Delay with Short Stature

1. Constitutional delay of puberty and normal variant short stature
2. Panhypopituitarism
   a. Congenital
   b. Acquired

    — Infectious: Viral, tuberculosis
    — Posttraumatic
    — Tumors
    — Sarcoidosis
    — Histiocytosis

3. Congenital syndromes
   a. Turner's: Female
   b. Noonan's: Male or female
   c. Mixed gonadal dysgenesis
   d. Prader-Labhart-Willi
   e. Laurence-Moon-Biedl
   f. Alström's
4. Glucocorticoid excess
5. Chronic diseases
   a. Chronic heart disease
   b. Asthma
   c. Inflammatory bowel disease
   d. Juvenile rheumatoid arthritis
   e. Tuberculosis
   f. Chronic renal failure
   g. Renal tubular acidosis
   h. Sickle cell anemia
   i. Hypothyroidism
   j. Diabetes mellitus
   k. Systemic lupus erythematosus
   l. Anorexia nervosa
   m. Cystic fibrosis
   n. Infection with human immunodeficiency virus (HIV)

Evaluation of Delayed Puberty

The vast majority of adolescents with delayed maturation have constitutional delay of puberty. However, this diagnosis is made by excluding other causes. Following is a discussion of the evaluation of the adolescent with delayed puberty, including criteria for a provisional diagnosis of constitutional delay of puberty.

History

1. Growth record: This is important in determining the timing and form of any deviations from the norm. Examples of growth charts in various disease states are provided in Figures 8.1 through 8.7.
2. Family history: Obtaining the family history will determine whether there is a history of late puberty in other family members. The heights of parents, siblings, and grandparents should be ascertained, as well as the age at menarche of the mother and the adolescent's sisters. Also helpful are questions such as: Was the father small as a teenager in relation to his classmates? At what age did he start to shave? The majority of patients (>60%) with constitutional delay of puberty have a positive family history.
3. Review of systems: This helps to rule out any chronic systemic illness.
4. Nutritional history and eating habits: This helps to discount a problem of chronic malnutrition.

Text continued on page 175.

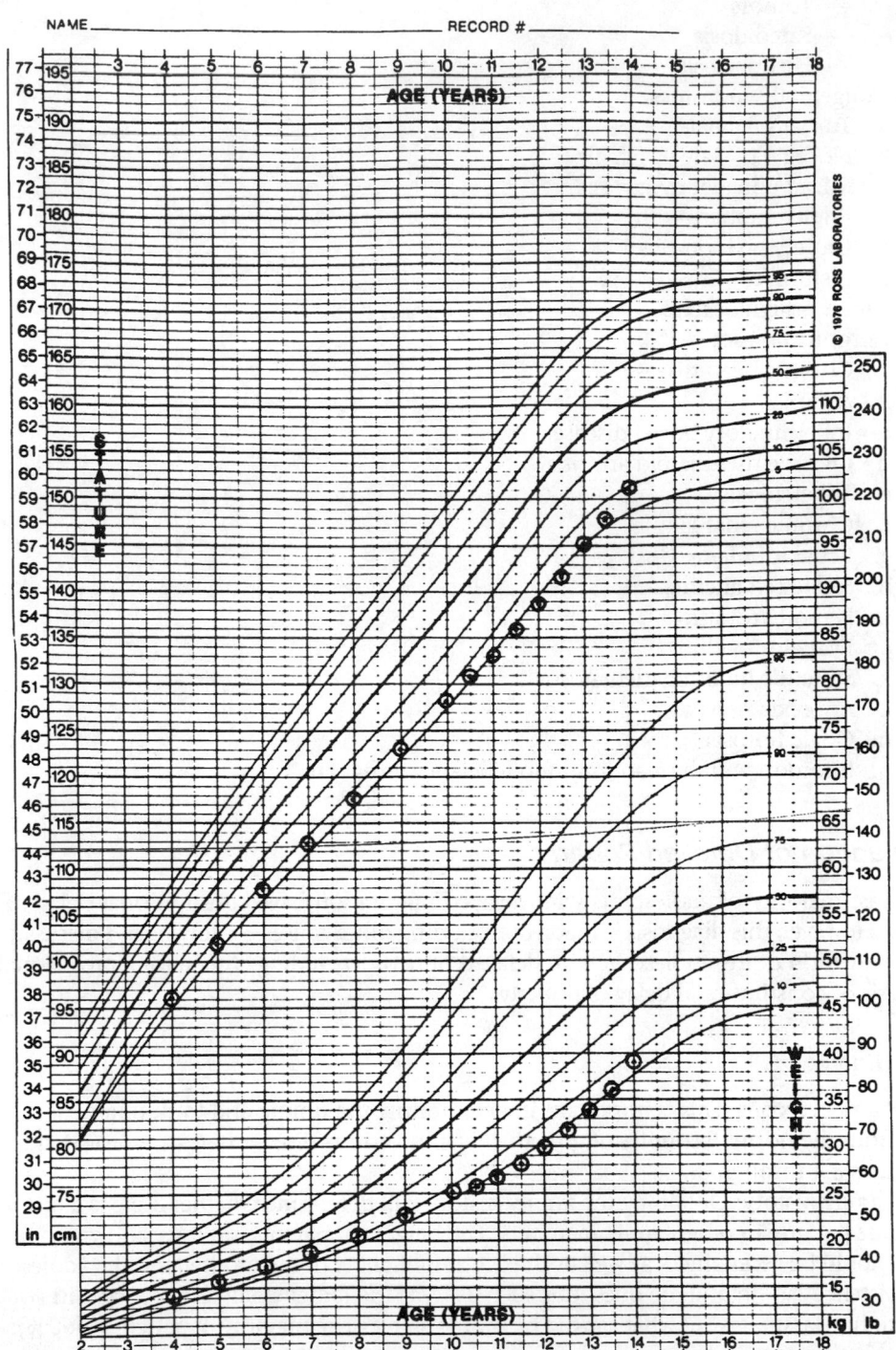

FIGURE 8.1. Constitutional delay of puberty in girls, 2 to 18 years of age (National Center for Health Statistics percentiles). (Adapted from National Center for Health Statistics, NCHS growth charts, 1976, Monthly Vital Statistics Report 25[3], suppl [HRA] 76–1120. Rockville, Maryland: Health Resources Administration, June 1976. © 1976 by Ross Laboratories.)

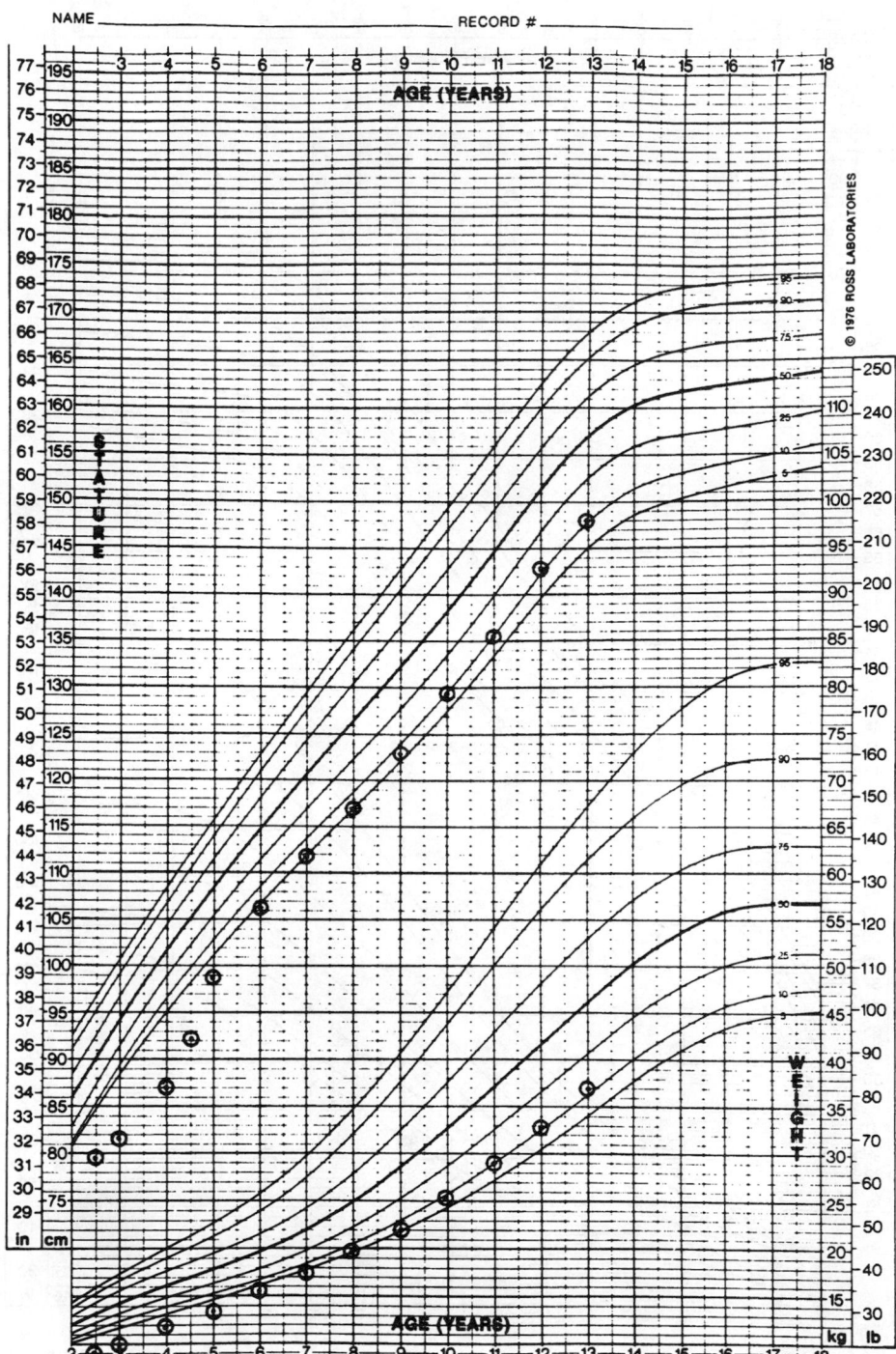

FIGURE 8.2.   Catch-up growth in girls, 2 to 18 years of age, with prematurity or deprivation states (National Center for Health Statistics percentiles). (Adapted from National Center for Health Statistics, NCHS growth charts, 1976, Monthly Vital Statistics Report 25[3], suppl [HRA] 76–1120. Rockville, Maryland: Health Resources Administration, June 1976. © 1976 by Ross Laboratories.)

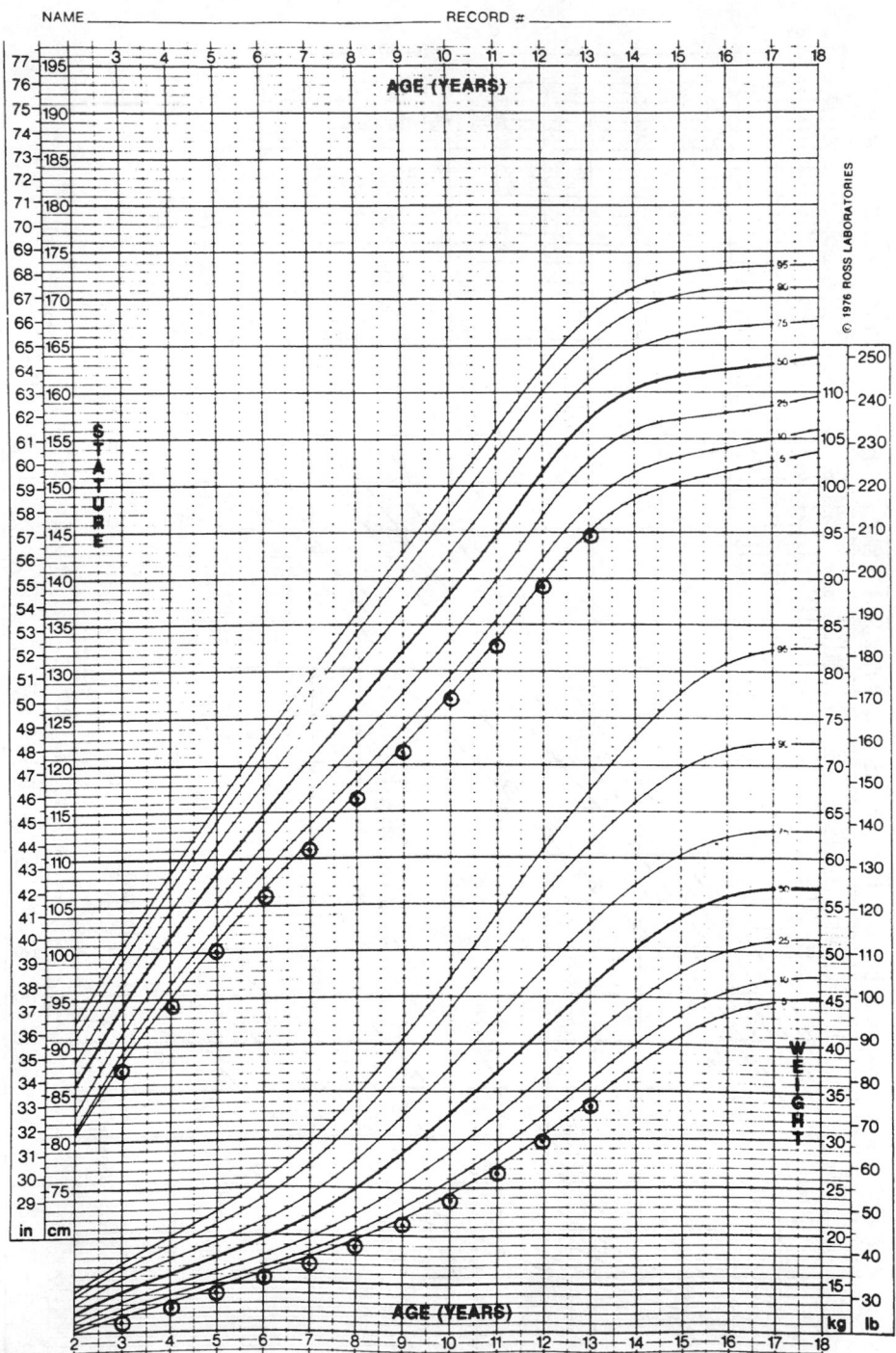

FIGURE 8.3. Low height and low weight in girls, 2 to 18 years of age, with familial short stature, primordial short stature, or constitutional delay of puberty (National Center for Health Statistics percentiles). (Adapted from National Center for Health Statistics, NCHS growth charts, 1976, Monthly Vital Statistics Report 25[3], suppl [HRA] 76–1120. Rockville, Maryland: Health Resources Administration, June 1976. © 1976 by Ross Laboratories.)

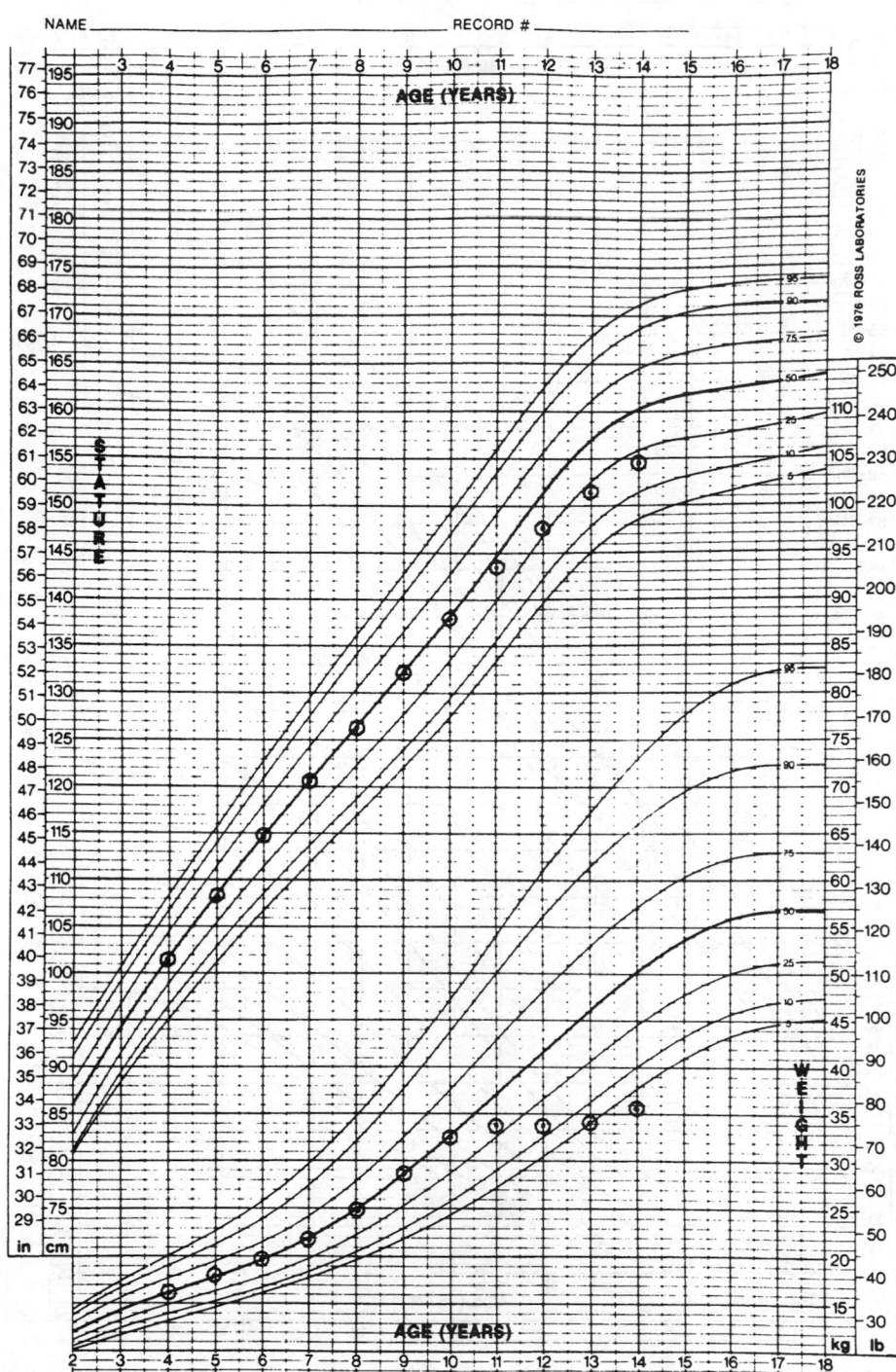

FIGURE 8.4.   Decreased height and markedly decreased weight in girls, 2 to 18 years of age, with chronic illness states (National Center for Health Statistics percentiles). (Adapted from National Center for Health Statistics, NCHS growth charts, 1976, Monthly Vital Statistics Report 25[3], suppl [HRA] 76–1120. Rockville, Maryland: Health Resources Administration, June 1976. © 1976 by Ross Laboratories.)

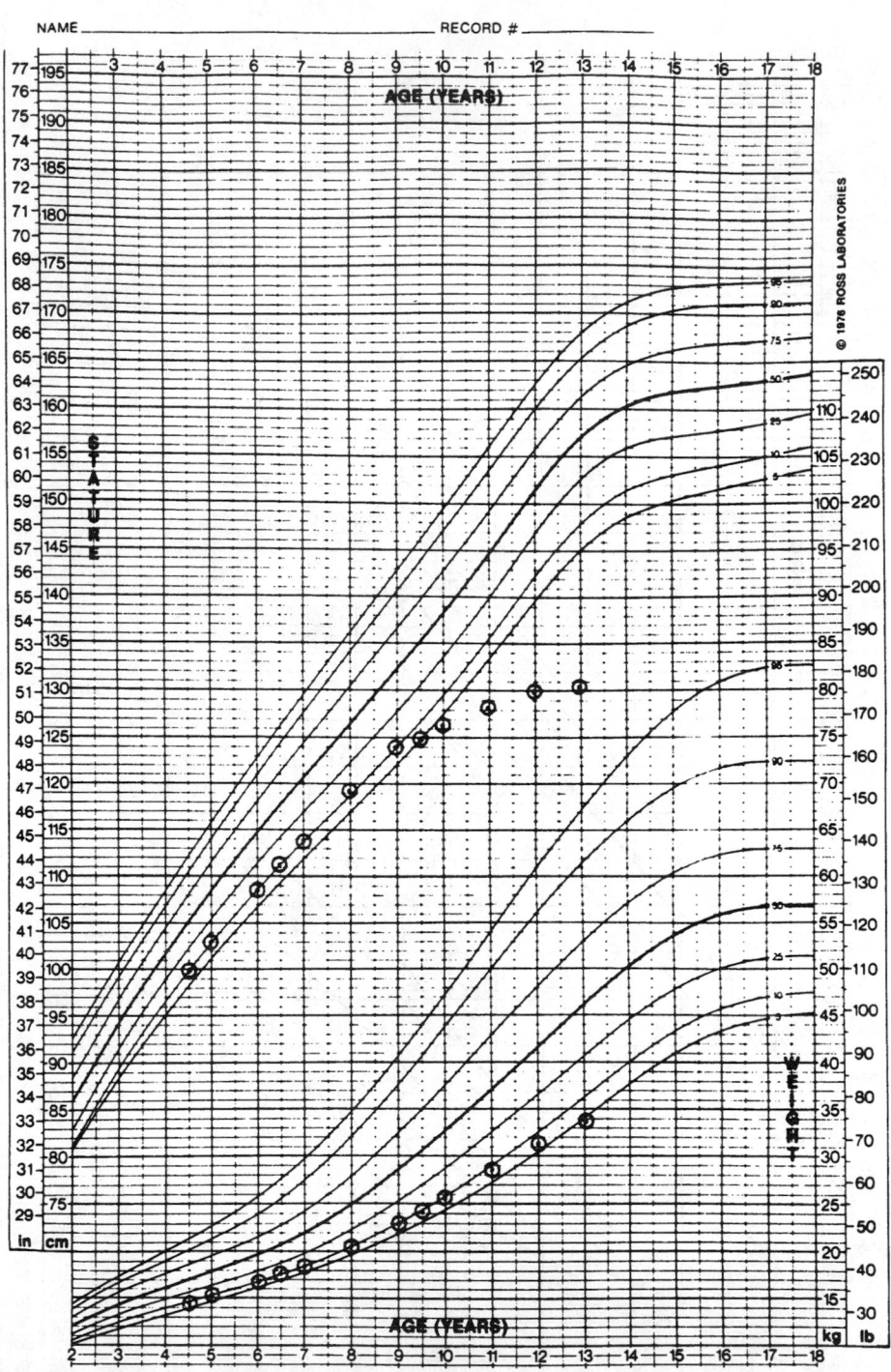

FIGURE 8.5. Markedly decreased height and decreased weight in girls, 2 to 18 years of age, with hypopituitary states, metabolic disorders such as rickets, or hypothyroidism (National Center for Health Statistics percentiles). (Adapted from National Center for Health Statistics, NCHS growth charts, 1976, Monthly Vital Statistics Report 25[3], suppl [HRA] 76–1120. Rockville, Maryland: Health Resources Administration, June 1976. © 1976 by Ross Laboratories.)

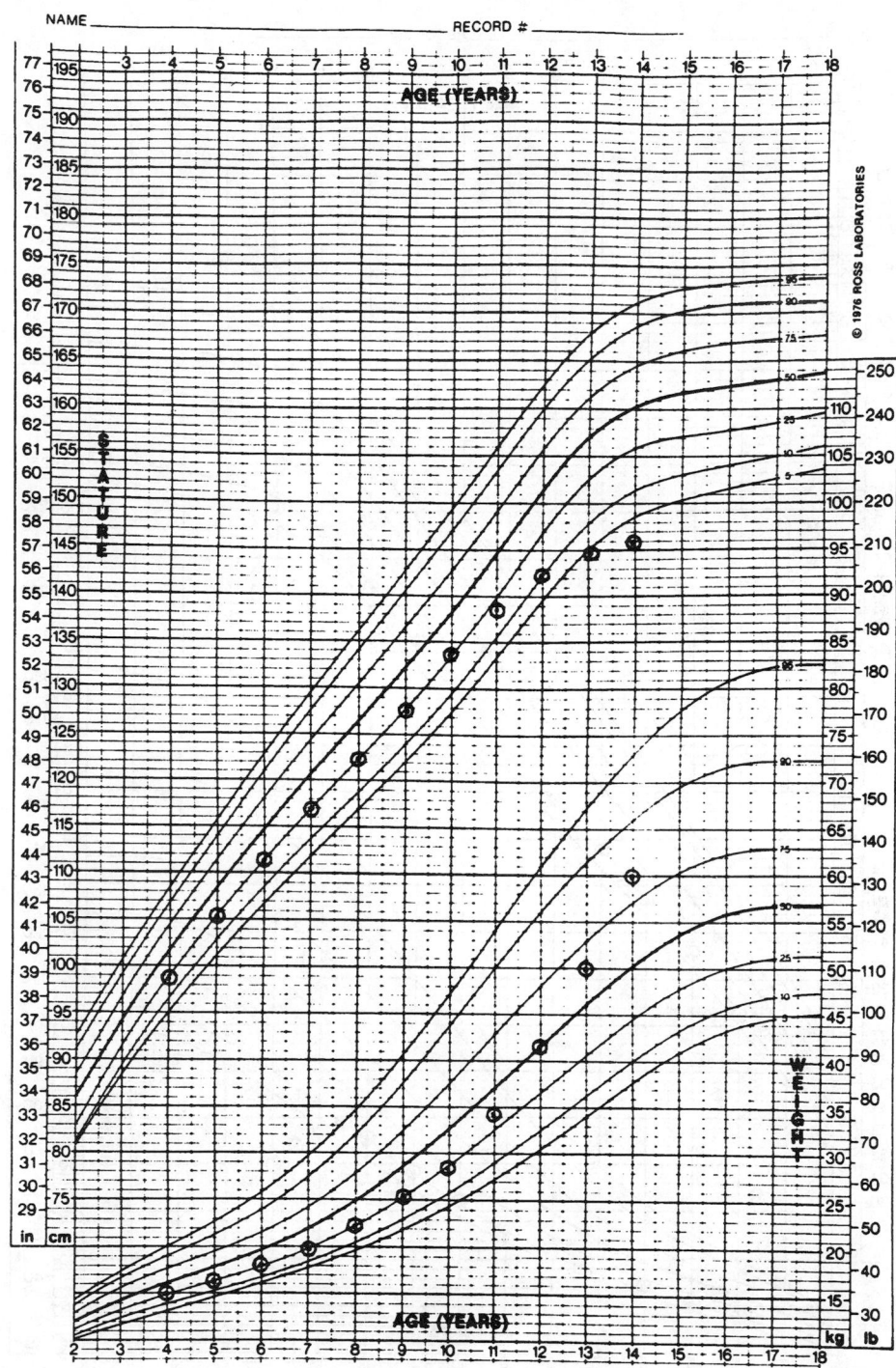

FIGURE 8.6. Decreased height and increased weight in girls, 2 to 18 years of age, with Cushing's syndrome and hypothyroidism (National Center for Health Statistics percentiles). (Adapted from National Center for Health Statistics, NCHS growth charts, 1976, Monthly Vital Statistics Report 25[3], suppl [HRA] 76–1120. Rockville, Maryland: Health Resources Administration, June 1976. © 1976 by Ross Laboratories.)

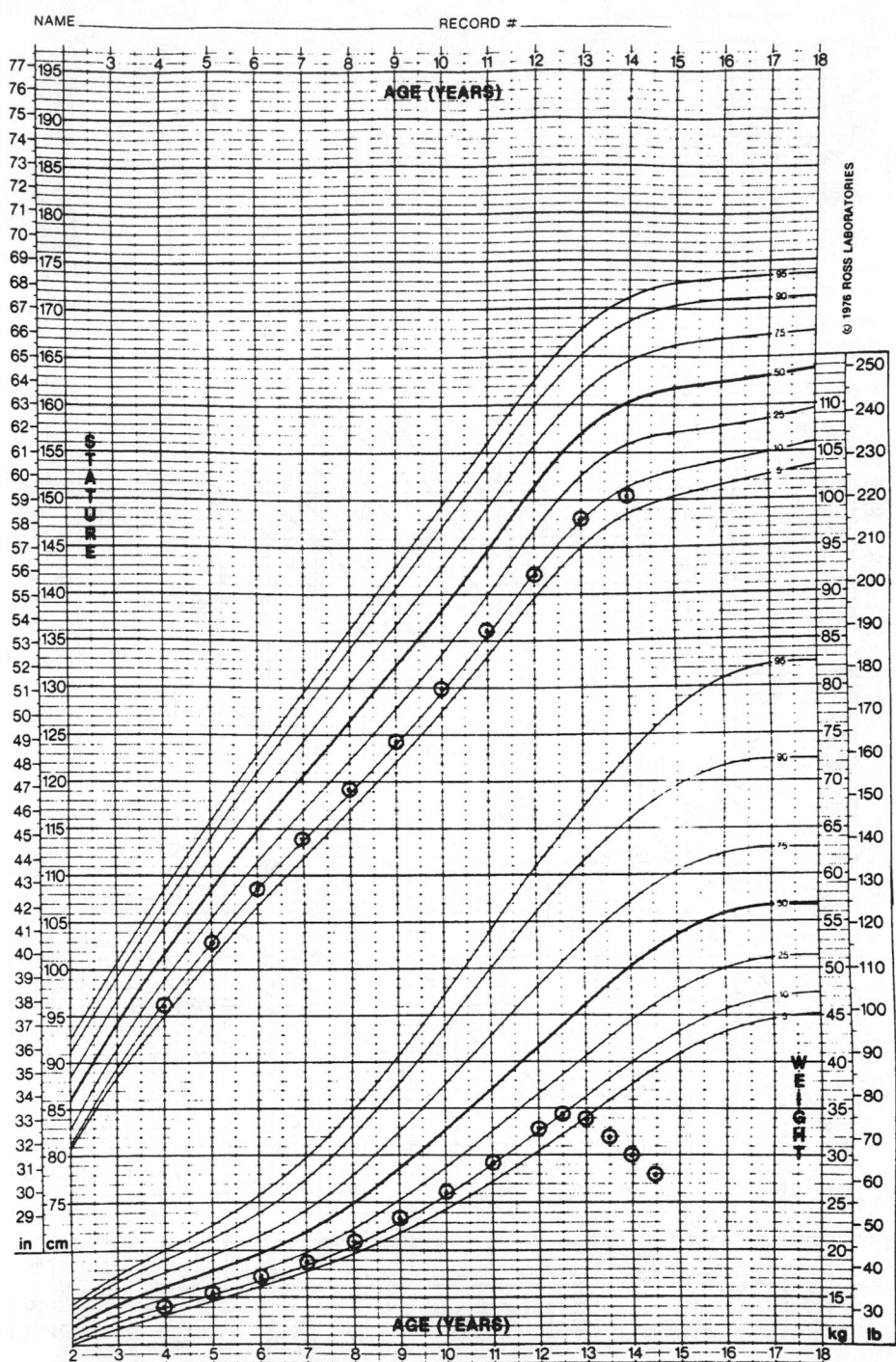

FIGURE 8.7.   Markedly decreased weight in girls, 2 to 18 years of age, with anorexia nervosa (National Center for Health Statistics percentiles). (Adapted from National Center for Health Statistics, NCHS growth charts, 1976, Monthly Vital Statistics Report 25[3], suppl [HRA] 76–1120. Rockville, Maryland: Health Resources Administration, June 1976. © 1976 by Ross Laboratories.)

Physical Examination   A complete physical examination is indicated for the adolescent with delayed puberty, but the following areas are of particular importance:

1. Nutritional status
2. Body measurements, including height, weight, arm span, and upper/lower (U/L) body-segment ratios
   a. U/L ratio: Determined by measuring the height from the top of the head to the symphysis pubis and dividing by the height from the symphysis pubis to the floor. Normally the ratio is 1.7 at birth, 1 at age 10 years, and 0.9–1.0 in adulthood. Adult African-American individuals tend to have longer limbs, so the U/L ratio is closer to 0.85–0.9. There are no standards in Asian and American Indian populations, but these individuals tend to have shorter limbs and therefore would tend to have a higher normal U/L ratio than white populations.
   b. Hypothyroidism: The U/L ratio will remain greater than 1. Most patients with a chondrodysplasia will also have an abnormally high U/L ratio.
   c. Hypogonadism: The U/L ratio will be close to 0.9 or less. A normal ratio will be found in growth hormone deficiency, constitutional delay of puberty, and chronic illness states.
3. Sexual maturity rating: It is critically important to evaluate the SMR to determine whether puberty has started, as well as for longitudinal follow-up.
4. Thyroid: Check for evidence of goiter. Absence of goiter can be seen with hypothyroidism.
5. Chest: Check for evidence of chronic pulmonary disease.
6. Heart: Check for evidence of congenital heart disease.
7. Abdomen: Check for evidence of liver or spleen enlargement as a sign of a chronic systemic disorder.
8. Pelvic examination: An external vaginal examination should be performed on all females, and if amenorrhea is a problem, a complete pelvic examination is indicated.
9. Neurological examination: This will help to eliminate from consideration any intracranial pathology. Ophthalmoscopic and visual-fields examination is done to rule out abnormalities of the optic nerves and to look for evidence of intracranial hypertension.

Laboratory Tests

1. Complete blood cell count: Check for evidence of anemia or leukocytosis.
2. Urinalysis: Check for evidence of renal disease.
3. Sedimentation rate: Check for evidence of a chronic systemic disease.
4. A serum chemistry profile should include measurements of glucose, creatinine, calcium, phosphorus, serum albumin, protein, and liver function tests.
5. Bone age: Determination of bone age is an essential part of the evaluation for delayed puberty. Delayed bone age will be seen in adolescents with hypopituitarism, hypothyroidism, chronic illness, and constitutional delay of puberty. Normal or delayed bone age may be seen in patients with Turner's syndrome. Bone age is also helpful when used in conjunction with height age and chronological age. Height age is determined by locating the corresponding age at which the patient's height would be equal to the 50th percentile. Table 8.1 describes typical relationships between bone age, height age, and chronological age for various causes of delayed puberty and/or short stature.
6. Lateral skull x-ray study: Check for sella turcica changes.
7. Hormone levels: Check adjusted thyroxine (T_4) level and thyroid-stimulating hormone (TSH) level.

TABLE 8.1.   Typical Relationships between Bone Age, Height Age, and Chronological Age for Causes of Delayed Puberty and/or Short Stature

Cause of Delayed Puberty or Short Stature	Relationship between Bone Age (BA), Chronological Age (CA), and Height Age (HA)
Genetic	$HA < BA = CA$
Skeletal dysplasia	$HA \leq BA < CA$ or $BA < HA < CA$
Constitutional	$HA = BA < CA$
Hypopituitarism	$HA \leq BA < CA$
Hypothyroidism	$BA < HA < CA$
Hypogonadism	$BA \leq HA < CA$

Additional Tests   Other tests are necessary in some evaluations, especially if the diagnosis of constitutional delay of puberty is in doubt. These tests could include:

1. Karyotype: A karyotype is particularly useful in ruling out Turner's syndrome in the short female.
2. Upper gastrointestinal tract series, small-bowel follow-through, and barium enema series: These tests are indicated if history or laboratory findings suggest inflammatory bowel disease.
3. Gonadotropin levels: High levels suggest gonadal failure, whereas low levels suggest hypothalamic pituitary failure. FSH levels elevated for the degree of pubertal development after 9 years of age can be seen in patients with Turner's syndrome and can be used as a screening test before obtaining a karyotype.
4. Comparison of a total urine LH secretion during sleep and a matched time period while awake: Puberty has begun if a nocturnal increase in LH secretion is present. Early-morning plasma testosterone levels can also be a predictor of imminent pubertal development in clinically prepubertal boys (Wu et al., 1993).
5. Growth-hormone measurements: Because a single fasting level is insufficient to diagnose growth-hormone (GH) deficiency, stimulation tests are necessary. Listed below are several commonly used tests. A normal response is a GH level in excess of 7–10 ng/mL after stimulation. GH deficiency has been classically defined as a lack of an increase in serum GH to 7 ng/mL or more in response to two pharmacologic stimulation tests in a child growing at a subnormal rate. Of these tests, the combination of either the L-Dopa or propranolol test and the clonidine test is probably the best outpatient screen, and the insulin tolerance test and the arginine infusion test are probably the most reliable.
   a. Sleep: Test GH level 1–2 hours after onset of sleep.
   b. Exercise: Test GH level before and after 15 minutes of vigorous stair climbing.
   c. Glucagon: Test GH levels before and at 30-minute intervals for 3 hours after glucagon, 1 mg, is given intramuscularly (IM) or subcutaneously.
   d. Insulin: Test GH levels before and at 15-minute intervals for 1 hour after regular insulin, 0.1 unit/kg body weight, is given intravenously (IV). This test requires constant monitoring for severe hypoglycemia, and intravenously administered glucose should be readily available to terminate the test if necessary.
   e. L-Dopa with or without propranolol: After an overnight fast, administer L-Dopa, 500 mg, plus propranolol, 0.75 mg/kg (up to 40 mg). Serum is drawn for determination of GH levels 60 minutes and 90 minutes later.
   f. Arginine infusion: L-Arginine monohydrochloride, 0.5 g/kg (up to a maximum of 30 g), is given intravenously for a 30-minute period. GH is measured at 0, 15, 30, 50, 90,

and 120 minutes after the start of the arginine infusion. This test is an excellent confirmatory test.

    g. Clonidine: A dose of 0.1–0.15 mg/m^2 can be given orally, and GH is measured at 0, 30, 60, and 90 minutes.

    h. Secretion rates of human growth hormone (hGH) for a 12- to 24-hour period: Current data suggest that some individuals have poor growth because of an abnormal secretion in the number and/or amplitude of GH pulses. This type of evaluation for a neurosecretory defect is currently performed primarily in conjunction with a research protocol.

    i. Sexual maturity rating: If the subject has not achieved an SMR of 4 or 5, consideration of estrogen priming before GH testing should be made (Marin et al., 1994).

6. Somatomedin-C or insulin-like growth factor I (IGF-I): Somatomedins are a family of insulin-like peptide growth factors. They are influenced by GH secretion and act to increase the growth of skeletal tissues. Somatomedin-C levels reflect GH activity but can be influenced by a variety of other factors and conditions, including malnutrition, liver disease, or renal impairment. The correlation with growth is not exact. For example, a teen may grow normally but have a low somatomedin-C level. Only a high-normal IGF-I concentration excludes GH deficiency. Other factors, such as the IGF binding proteins (e.g., IGFBP-3) that transport IgF in the serum, can also be measured as a reflection of GH and IGF-I sufficiency.

    a. Normal levels (IGF-I): Levels vary with age. They are lowest during infancy and increase throughout childhood to peak values during puberty. When somatomedin-C/IgF levels are interpreted, they should be compared to age-related norms or to bone age, if either is markedly different from chronological age.

    b. Low levels: Levels of GH can be low in patients with GH deficiency, malnutrition, chronic illness states, hypothyroidism, resistance to endogenous GH, and errors in GH structure.

7. Gonadotropin-releasing hormone (GnRH) stimulation test: This test can help determine whether the adolescent has normal pituitary function for his or her pubertal stage. Serum LH and FSH levels are measured before and every 30 minutes for 3 hours after infusion of 100 µg of GnRH. In primary gonadal failure, LH and FSH levels will increase after infusion, whereas in pituitary failure there is little increase. In constitutional delay of puberty, the LH and FSH response is small but consistent with bone age and pubertal stage. Simultaneous measurement of gonadal steroid production (testosterone or estradiol) at the beginning and end of the GnRH stimulation test will help to interpret the gonadotropin levels. This test is not reliable for differentiating constitutional delay from hypogonadotropic hypogonadism before a bone age of about 12 years. For girls, an accurate indication of pubertal entrance is a peak LH/peak FSH ratio greater than 0.66, whereas for boys the most accurate indication of the beginning of puberty is a spontaneous nighttime LH level of greater than 12 IU/L (Oerter et al., 1990).

8. Human chorionic gonadotropin (hCG) test: For this test, chorionic gonadotropin (Pregnyl) is given by four IM injections of 5000 IU/m^2 each on days 1, 3, 8, and 10. Serum testosterone levels are determined before the first injection and on day 15. A stimulated level of testosterone less than 10 nm/L, or 300 ng/dL, is suggestive of hypogonadotropic hypogonadism.

Constitutional Delay of Puberty   About 90–95% of delayed puberty is constitutional delay of puberty. This diagnosis is made by excluding the other causes, as discussed. However, using the guidelines in Table 8.2, suggested by Barnes (1979), one can confidently make a provisional diagnosis. When such an adolescent's predicted adult height is below the third

TABLE 8.2. Criteria for Provisional Diagnosis of Constitutional Delay of Puberty

Required features
  Detailed negative review of systems
  Evidence of appropriate nutrition
  Linear growth of at least 3.7 cm/yr
  Normal findings on physical examination, including genital anatomy, sense of smell, and U/L body segment ratio
  Normal CBC, sedimentation rate, urinalysis results, adjusted T_4 concentration, and noncastrate levels of serum LH and FSH
  Normal sella turcica by x-ray study
  Bone age delayed 1.5–4.0 years compared with chronological age
Supportive features
  Family history of constitutional delay of puberty
  Height between 3rd and 25th percentiles for chronological age

Adapted from Barnes HV. Recognizing normal and abnormal growth and development during puberty. In: Moss AV, ed. Pediatrics update: reviews for physicians. New York: Elsevier–North Holland Publishing, 1979:103.

percentile (<64 inches for males and <59 inches for females), the teenager is often labeled as having idiopathic or genetic short stature.

Basic Considerations In an evaluation of any adolescent with delay of puberty, four basic questions should be kept in mind:

1. Is there evidence of any disorder outside the genital reproductive system that could contribute to growth failure?
2. To what extent has skeletal maturation progressed?
3. Is there evidence of interruption in either gonadal or hypothalamic-pituitary function?
4. Is the chromosomal sex consistent with the genital sex of the patient?

Clues to Diagnosis

1. Gonadotropin deficiency
   a. Low serum FSH and LH levels, particularly if bone age is more than 13 years
   b. Low response to GnRH if pituitary failure is present
   c. In males: Low testosterone response to hCG (Dunkel et al., 1985a, 1985b)
   d. Abnormal sella turcica
   e. History of neurological symptoms, central nervous system (CNS) infections, or disease
   f. Possible absence of sense of smell (Kallmann's syndrome)
2. Gonadal disorder
   a. History of genital radiation, surgery, infection, or trauma
   b. Castrate levels of FSH and LH
   c. Abnormal karyotype, such as 46,XY in a phenotypic female
   d. Low U/L segment ratio
   e. Arm span may exceed height by more than 2 inches
   f. Gynecomastia in a male
   g. Small testes in males with genetic hypogonadal disorders: Testes rarely exceed 6 cm^3 in volume
3. Turner's syndrome: Excluding constitutional delay of puberty, one of the more common causes of maturation delay is Turner's syndrome. The patient may have a 45,XO karyotype or a mosaic karyotype such as 45,XO/46,XX. Turner's syndrome patients usually have some of the following characteristics:
   a. Short stature
   b. Streak gonads

    c. Absent pubertal growth spurt
    d. Poor development of secondary sexual characteristics, with less breast development than pubic hair development
    e. Lymphedema
    f. Cubitus valgus
    g. Webbing of the neck
    h. Low hairline
    i. Shield-shaped chest
    j. Coarctation of the aorta
    k. Horseshoe kidneys
    l. Short fourth metacarpal
    m. Multiple pigmented nevi
    n. Normal vagina, cervix, and uterus
    o. Poor space-form perception
4. Chronic illness
    a. Abnormal findings on review of systems or physical examination
    b. Falling off height and weight curves at onset of disease
    c. Abnormal complete blood cell count (CBC), sedimentation rate, urinalysis results, or chemistry panel results

Management of Maturational Delay

Most adolescents with maturational delay will have constitutional delay of puberty. These patients and their families will need constant support and reassurance that puberty and growth will occur. Follow-up is necessary, to be certain that any other abnormality was not overlooked and that puberty does begin. If severe psychological problems arise because of differences in physical size or sexual maturation of the adolescent compared with his or her peers, hormonal therapy can be tried briefly (up to 6 months). Teenagers who most commonly complain about delayed puberty are male adolescents. In male adolescents, oxandrolone, 0.05–0.25 mg/kg per day, can be tried, or testosterone enanthate can be given at doses of 44–200 mg/m^2 per month IM for 3 to 6 months. The effects of hormonal intervention have been examined by Zachmann and Prader (1970), Hopwood et al. (1979), Rosenfeld et al. (1982), Wilson et al. (1988), Rosenfield et al. (1986), Richman and Kirsch (1988), Soliman et al. (1995). These studies confirm an increase in growth velocities without excessive bone age advancement. Low doses of testosterone seem to be effective in stimulating virilization and growth without significant loss of height potential (Adan et al., 1994). Any suppression of the hypothalamic-pituitary-gonadal axis during treatment seems reversible after treatment is stopped. If androgen therapy is used, the risk of liver damage and of possible attenuation of mature height should be discussed with the adolescent and his family. Finkelstein et al. (1992) reported that adult men with a history of constitutionally delayed puberty have a decreased radial and spinal bone mineral density. This suggests that the timing of sexual maturation may be an important determinant of peak bone mineral density.

    Most other causes of delayed puberty are irreversible. Thus the health-care provider must be prepared to help the adolescent with long-term follow-up and psychological support. Many areas will need to be dealt with, such as:

1. Identification of the problem
2. Potential for growth and sexual maturation
3. Sexual identity
4. Reproductive potential

Health practitioners need to be honest in explaining to the adolescent what they believe he or she can comprehend. At the same time, telling a phenotypic female, for example, that she has male chromosomes is probably not advisable and is liable to add sexual-identity confusion to an age already fraught with uncertainties. In this instance, the term "abnormal chromosome" is preferable.

Turner's Syndrome and Gonadal Dysgenesis

1. If shortness is marked, one can begin with small amounts of androgens: oxandrolone, 0.075–0.25 mg/kg per day, or fluoxymesterone, 2.0 mg/day. Androgens have the following disadvantages:
   a. Potential for hepatic toxic effects
   b. Potential for mild androgenic characteristics
   c. Delay of treatment with estrogen and thus delay of inducement of female secondary sexual characteristics

   Although Turner's syndrome has been treated in the past with low doses of anabolic androgens, studies on final adult height have not shown a significant increase with this therapy. Anabolic steroids as the sole therapy for this condition are therefore no longer recommended.

   Ross et al. (1983) reported on the potential benefit of low doses of estrogen to improve linear growth in patients with Turner's syndrome. Martinez et al. (1987) confirmed the ability of ethinyl estradiol to increase growth velocity in girls with Turner's syndrome, although the effect diminished with time and excessive bone age advancement precluded improvement of predicted height.

   The efficacy of GH alone, or in combination with oxandrolone, in improving the height of girls with Turner's syndrome has been evaluated (Rosenfeld et al., 1986, 1992). Six-year data of this randomized trial reveal that 82% of girls with GH alone, and 92% of girls treated with GH and oxandrolone, have already exceeded their predicted adult heights. With 42 of the 62 subjects having completed growth, the mean height was 151.7 cm, or 5 feet, with the original projected height exceeded by 9 cm. Other trials have also demonstrated an increase in final height in individuals treated with GH (Takano et al., 1995). However, if consideration of GH treatment is entertained, it is best to refer the patient to an endocrinologist.

2. Secondary sexual characteristics in the female are achieved through the use of increasing doses of conjugated estrogens such as Premarin or with low doses of ethinyl estradiol at 100 ng/kg. Premarin therapy can be started at a dosage of 0.3 mg/day, increasing gradually, for 6 to 12 months, to 0.625–1.25 mg/day. At that time, to avoid unopposed estrogen stimulation of the endometrium, the clinician adds medroxyprogesterone acetate (Provera). The following schedule can then be used: Premarin, 0.625–1.25 mg/day for the first 25 days of each month, and Provera, 10 mg/day, added on days 17–25. Withdrawal flow will begin on about days 27–29. Treatment is restarted on day 1 of the next month. Transdermal administration of estradiol at doses of 50–100 µg/day is a potential alternative to orally administered conjugated estrogens. This approach can elicit the desired estrogenic effect without the pharmacological effect of orally administered estrogen on hepatic proteins.

3. Girls with a Y chromosome should have their gonads removed to prevent potential malignant neoplasias. Surgery should be followed by hormonal replacement during and after puberty.

Hypogonadotropic Hypogonadism

1. Females: Treat with hormonal therapy as already outlined here, until effective, easily administered gonadotropins become available.

2. Males: The preferred treatment is androgen therapy, in which testosterone enanthate in progressively higher doses ($25-100$ mg/m^2) can be given every 3 weeks. After 1 year, this dosage can be increased to $150-200$ mg/m^2. Some patients do better on lower doses given once every 2 weeks. Growth velocity should be followed in an attempt to maintain a normal pattern. Testosterone therapy will not induce spermatogenesis.

GnRH-related Hypogonadism   In males and females with hypogonadism caused by absent GnRH secretion, the pulsatile administration of GnRH can normalize gonadal function and induce fertility (Barbieri, 1992). This therapy is associated with high cost and the need for a high degree of compliance. It should be reserved for those individuals who desire fertility.

Gonadal Failure

1. Females: These patients are treated with hormonal therapy, as outlined in the previous section on Turner's syndrome.
2. Males: Males are treated with hormonal therapy, including testosterone in oil, as outlined previously.

Chronic Illness   Treatment of pubertal delay caused by chronic illness necessitates treating the underlying disorder. For example, enzyme replacement in cystic fibrosis, gluten-free diet in celiac disease, corrective surgery for congenital heart disease, and hyperalimentation in inflammatory bowel disease usually result in catch-up growth and maturity. Medications such as steroids or antimetabolites can inhibit growth. Catch-up growth can be observed after discontinuation of treatment with these drugs. In some cases the disease process is irreversible, such as in sickle cell anemia. The pubertal delay in sickle cell anemia is thought to be hypogonadism, possibly caused by a zinc deficiency. Zinc has been used with some early experimental success in alleviating this problem. In patients with chronic renal failure, there may be some growth after improved nutrition and hemodialysis or transplantation. However, many patients with chronic renal failure remain short. Recent studies suggest that GH can be administered to subjects with chronic renal failure before transplantation to improve height, and without causing deterioration of underlying renal function (Fine et al., 1994). Children with HIV infection who grow poorly and have body wasting may benefit from the anabolic effects of short-term GH administration; however, long-term use of such agents remains under investigation (Mulligan et al., 1993).

SHORT STATURE

Definition

Adult height is genetically determined; therefore any evaluation of short stature must be assessed with family members' height as a guide. Generally, the 3rd percentile is used as the lower limit of normal. Adolescents who fall below the 3rd percentile should be carefully evaluated for short stature.

Guidelines

An adolescent should be considered for an evaluation of short stature if:

1. A linear growth rate of less than $4.0-5.0$ cm/yr exists in the years before the normal age for peak linear growth velocity.
2. No evidence exists of a peak linear-growth-velocity year by age 16 in the male or age 14 in the female.

3. Distinct deceleration below the individual's established growth velocity occurs.
4. The adolescent's height is more than 2 SD from mid-parental height.
5. The adolescent's height is more than 3 SD below the mean. Adolescents whose height is between 2 and 3 SD below the mean deserve a careful history and physical examination, screening laboratory tests, and observation of growth for 6 months.

Differential Diagnosis

The differential diagnosis can be divided between those processes associated with normal puberty and those associated with simultaneous delay of puberty.

Short Stature without Pubertal Delay

1. Familial short stature
2. Isolated GH deficiency
3. Hypothyroidism (can also be associated with pubertal delay)
4. Congenital syndromes such as Down's, Noonan's, and Hurler's
5. Intrauterine growth retardation
6. Skeletal disorders; chondrodysplasias
7. Chronic illness
8. HIV infection

Short Stature with Pubertal Delay

1. Constitutional delay of puberty
2. Panhypopituitarism: Congenital and acquired
3. Congenital syndrome:
   a. Turner's and mixed gonadal dysgenesis
   b. Syndromes associated with hypogonadotropic hypogonadism
      — Prader-Labhart-Willi: Obesity, short stature, small hands and feet, almond-shaped palpebral fissures, mental deficiency, and cryptorchidism, with 50% having a deletion of chromosome 15 at region q11-13
      — Laurence-Moon-Biedl: Obesity, short stature, polydactyly, retinitis pigmentosa, mental deficiency, and genital hypoplasia
      — Alström's: Retinitis pigmentosa, diabetes mellitus, neurogenic deafness
      — Börjeson-Forssman-Lehmann: Obesity, short stature, severe mental deficiency, epilepsy, microcephaly, variable radiographic skeletal anomalies, and small genitalia
4. Glucocorticoid excess
5. Chronic illness
6. HIV infection

Evaluation of Short Stature

The evaluation of short stature is similar to that of delayed puberty. A thorough history is essential and should include:

1. Maternal pregnancy history: Medical illnesses and medication use
2. Birth weight and length, and estimate of gestational age: Important because premature infants with appropriate small weight tend to have a normal growth potential, whereas infants with intrauterine growth retardation who are inappropriately small for gestational age may not have catch-up growth

3. Complete review of systems: Especially renal and gastrointestinal
4. Growth history: Close review of symptoms (see Figs. 8.1 through 8.7, growth charts for various disease states)
5. Family history: Adult height and growth and pubertal patterns of all first- and second-degree relatives
6. Dietary history

A complete physical examination is the next step in the evaluation and should include:

1. Height and weight
2. Arm span and ratio of upper segment to lower segment
3. Sexual maturity ratings
4. A general physical examination, with special attention to the thyroid gland, ophthalmological examination, neurological examination, and stigmata of congenital syndromes

The laboratory evaluation of short stature should include:

1. Complete blood cell count and sedimentation rate
2. Urinalysis
3. Adjusted T_4 and TSH (for thyroid) determinations
4. Chemistry profile, including serum creatinine and liver enzymes
5. Bone age: Essential part of evaluation of short stature (The relationships between bone age, height age, and chronological age were discussed earlier in the chapter [see also Table 8.1]. A bone age equivalent to the chronological age suggests decreased growth potential [primordial short stature, genetic short stature, or skeletal dysplasia]. A significant delay in bone age increases the likelihood of endocrine or systemic disease as the cause of disordered growth. The bone age also provides an index for potential future growth.)
6. Other tests: Ordered as indicated by the history and physical examination (outlined earlier in the chapter) and include skull films; measurement of gonadotropin, GH, IGF-I (somatomedin-C), and IGFBP-3 levels; and x-ray films of the gastrointestinal tract

Constitutional Delay of Puberty   Most short stature in adolescents is either the result of constitutional delay of puberty or familial short stature. Guidelines for diagnosis were outlined earlier in the chapter.

Genetic or Familial Short Stature   Genetic or familial short stature is suggested by:

1. Normal history and physical examination findings
2. Birth weight and length that are often below the 3rd percentile for gestational age
3. Family history of short stature
4. Growth curve that generally parallels the 3rd percentile
5. Bone age that is appropriate for chronological age

Chronic Illness   Chronic renal disease and Crohn's disease are frequent causes of short stature at tertiary care hospitals. These diseases are usually diagnosed by an abnormal history, physical examination findings, or results of tests including screening CBC, sedimentation rate, urinalysis, and chemistry studies. Renal tubular acidosis can easily be overlooked as a cause of short stature. This process may be suggested by family history, urine pH, or serum bicarbonate values.

Endocrine Causes   Endocrine causes of short stature, such as hypothyroidism, GH deficiency, and adrenocortical excess, are uncommon. Hypothyroidism and adrenocortical excess can usually be detected by the patient's history, physical examination, or screening laboratory test. Adolescents with isolated GH deficiency can be difficult to differentiate from adolescents with constitutional delay in puberty. This is especially difficult during the time of expected peak linear growth velocity, when the growth of an adolescent with constitutional delay of puberty may seem to differ from the normal growth curve as other adolescents accelerate their growth velocities. Individuals with isolated GH deficiency have normal body proportions and often a high-pitched voice, a tendency toward hypoglycemia, a microphallus in boys, a childlike face, soft and finely wrinkled skin, and a large, prominent forehead. Currently the question of which individuals will benefit from GH therapy is being evaluated. It may be that other groups besides those with classic GH deficiency on standard pharmacological testing will benefit from GH use. These groups include certain individuals with previously classified "constitutional delay of puberty," genetic short stature, or intrauterine growth retardation, as well as patients with nonendocrine diseases such as renal failure and those requiring long-term glucocorticoid administration. However, which groups will benefit and the risk-benefit ratio are yet to be defined. It is clear, as seen in the studies of patients with Turner's syndrome, that GH deficiency will not remain the only criterion for treatment (Frasier and Lippe, 1990). Human growth hormone (hGH) has been removed from the market because of the potential of transmission of Creutzfeldt-Jakob disease. Only bioengineered GH is currently available. The possible benefit of using GnRH analogs to delay puberty and allow for a prolonged prepubertal growth period, thus increasing adult height, has been investigated. Although there are conflicting reports in the literature (Municchi et al., 1993; Lindner et al., 1993), there does not appear to be much benefit to ultimate adult height in delaying puberty with such agents.

Chromosomal Abnormality   The most common chromosomal abnormality causing short stature is Turner's syndrome, which occurs in 1 of every 2000 females born. However, because short stature is a part of the syndrome in virtually all cases, the incidence is much higher among females with short stature. The syndrome becomes a distinct possibility in the very short girl who does not exhibit a marked delay in bone age. The diagnosis requires a karyotype analysis for an adequate evaluation for mosaic patterns. The characteristics of Turner's syndrome were discussed earlier in the chapter.

Intrauterine Growth Retardation   Another cause of short stature is a "grab bag" category called primordial dwarfism, or intrauterine growth retardation. The patients are usually characterized by:

1. Small size for gestational age at birth
2. Slow growth from early infancy
3. Normal or minimally retarded epiphyseal maturation and thus normal bone age
4. Normal or minimally retarded sexual development
5. Normal physical examination findings (occasionally dysmorphic features compatible with a variety of syndromes) and normal laboratory test results
6. Normal growth hormone levels
7. Possible lower intellect
8. Normal growth pattern in the family

A host of maternal factors are associated with this problem, as well as abnormalities of the intrauterine environment.

Skeletal Dysplasias   Reduced growth characterized by skeletal dysplasias is related to an abnormality of the osseous and cartilage tissues. These disorders are suggested by:

1. Family history of skeletal dysplasias
2. Abnormal body proportions (abnormal U/L segment ratio)
3. Extremely retarded bone age
4. Abnormal osseous structures on x-ray examination

A benefit from surgical leg-lengthening procedures has been appreciated in the skeletal dysplasias.

Treatment of Short Stature

The treatment of most causes of short stature was reviewed earlier in the discussion of delayed puberty. Generally, hormone deficiencies such as hypothyroidism, hypopituitarism, and hypogonadism are treated with hormone replacement. Short stature as a result of chronic illness is treated by dealing with the underlying disorder. Disorders associated with abnormal growth potential, such as genetic short stature, intrauterine growth retardation, and skeletal dysplasias, may respond poorly to therapy, or the risk/benefit ratio may not yet be understood. Hormonal therapy with androgens for constitutional delay of puberty should be reserved for those males with significant emotional problems resulting from their short stature.

It is essential to be aware of the tremendous impact that short stature may have on an adolescent. Body image not only has become an increasing concern in our society but gains in importance as an adolescent gets older. The concerns and fears of the adolescent and of his or her family regarding short stature should be explored.

EXCESSIVE GROWTH—TALL STATURE

Tall stature is rarely a problem in boys because tallness is acceptable and even desired in males in our society. Even though tallness is becoming more acceptable among girls, there are still adolescent females or their parents who complain to physicians about excessive tallness.

Differential Diagnosis

1. Constitutional tall stature
2. Excess GH
3. Anabolic steroid excess
   a. Adrenal tumor
   b. Congenital adrenal hyperplasia, classic or nonclassic
   c. Precocious puberty
   d. Premature adrenarche
   e. Gonadal tumors
4. Hyperthyroidism
5. Miscellaneous
   a. Marfan's syndrome
   b. Neurofibromatosis
   c. Hypogonadism in the male
   d. Testicular feminization
   e. Homocystinuria
   f. Hereditary abnormalities of the skeleton
   g. Sotos syndrome

Evaluation

The most important information in evaluating tall stature is the family history of tallness in parents and siblings. If there is a family history of tallness and the history and physical examination findings are normal, the diagnosis is almost certainly familial tallness. If a family history of tallness is not found, then a more thorough search is indicated. Generally a complete history, physical examination, routine screening laboratory tests, and a determination of bone age are adequate to evaluate the outlined causes of tall stature. The bone age and sexual maturity rating are also essential to the evaluation. The adolescent girl who entered puberty early and is thus taller than her peers will have a corresponding advanced bone age and sexual maturity rating. More detailed tests such as GH and somatomedin determinations can be ordered as indicated. Also included in the evaluation of tallness should be the adolescent's and family's attitudes about tallness and the problems that may have arisen because of tallness.

Treatment in Females

Familial Tall Stature   Estrogens have been documented to decrease growth potential; however, because of possible side effects, estrogen therapy should be reserved for selected adolescents. Associated medical problems such as hyperglycemia, hypertension, hyperlipidemia, and thrombophlebitis would be a contraindication to estrogen therapy.

What is excessive height? Some adolescents are overwhelmed at 5 feet 6 inches (168 cm), whereas others are completely happy at 5 feet 10 inches (178 cm) or more. However, in general, estrogen therapy should be reserved for the adolescent female with a predicted height of more than 5 feet 11 inches to 6 feet (180–183 cm) and with indications that she (not her mother or father) is having psychological difficulties in coping with her height.

Timing of Treatment   Though the earlier the therapy, the greater the degree of height reduction, estrogen intervention should be delayed until the adolescent female is at least 9–10 years of age; puberty has started; and a height of about 5 feet 6 inches (168 cm) has been attained. This allows for evidence of spontaneous maturation. In addition, mature adult heights are more accurately predicted after the age of 10 years. In general, therapy is now started later than was previously recommended. Therapy should be delayed if the adolescent is unsure about undergoing treatment.

Estrogen Effects on Growth

1. Suppression of somatomedin
2. Acceleration of epiphyseal fusion

Dosage   Either ethinyl estradiol or conjugated estrogens (Premarin) are recommended. In either case, a progestational agent should be used each month to guard against unopposed estrogen stimulation of the endometrium. Both continuous and cyclic regimens of estrogen have been used. Studies using continuous regimens (Crawford, 1978; Van der Werff ten Bosch and Bot, 1981) indicate a greater height reduction, and the time until complete epiphyseal fusion is probably decreased.

1. Continuous regimen
   a. Ethinyl estradiol, 0.1–0.5 mg daily, or conjugated estrogens (Premarin), 2.5–10 mg daily; plus
   b. Norethindrone, 5 mg on the first 5 days of each month

2. Cyclic regimen
   a. Ethinyl estradiol on days 1–24, with a progestin added on days 18–24
   b. No hormones used for the remainder of the month

Duration of Therapy   Therapy should be continued until epiphyseal fusion is documented on hand and wrist radiographs. If therapy is stopped sooner, rebound growth may occur.

Side Effects   Potential side effects are similar to those of oral contraceptives. Usually side effects are mild, such as occasional nausea or breakthrough bleeding, or rare, such as hypertension or thrombophlebitis. There is no evidence of future disturbances of hypothalamic-pituitary-ovarian function. Gonadotropins usually recover within 1 to 2 months of the cessation of the estrogen therapy. No evidence that cancer develops as a result of estrogen therapy for tall stature has been demonstrated.

Follow-up

1. Visits every 3 months to evaluate height, weight, pubertal development, potential complications, and to perform a physical examination, including blood pressure determination
2. Gynecological assessment, including pelvic and breast examination and Pap smear every year
3. Skeletal age evaluation every 6–12 months
4. Height recorded at 3, 6, and 12 months, after treatment has been stopped, to detect growth increases

Treatment in Males

The treatment of boys has been studied less extensively. Treatment in one study (Zachmann et al., 1976) consisted of administration of a long-acting intramuscular testosterone preparation (Triolandren) at a dosage of 500 mg/m^2 given every 3 weeks. Side effects include weight gain, acne, edema, and a decrease in testicular volume, which returns to normal after therapy is stopped.

PRECOCIOUS PUBERTY

Sexual precocity is the development of sexual characteristics before the normal age.

1. "Isosexual precocity" refers to advanced sexual development appropriate for the phenotype of the child.
2. "Heterosexual precocity" refers to advanced sexual development at variance with the phenotype of the child (i.e., males are feminized and females are virilized)
3. "Incomplete precocious puberty" refers to the appearance of a single clinical pubertal change, such as premature thelarche (breast), premature adrenarche (axillary hair), and premature pubarche (pubic hair).
4. "Complete precocious puberty" refers to the appearance of advanced pubertal changes accompanied by hormonal effects elsewhere—pubic hair, axillary hair, and breast or phallus development. Complete precocious puberty includes true and pseudo forms:
   a. True precocious puberty: Release of gonadotropins with resultant puberty and potential fertility
   b. Pseudoprecocious puberty: Elevated levels of sexual hormones but low gonadotropin levels, with resultant advanced pubertal changes but an infertile state

Guidelines

1. Male: Any male achieving genital stage 2 before $9^1/_2$ years of age
2. Female: Any female with breast development or pubic hair development before the age of 8 years

Differential Diagnosis

Isosexual Precocious Puberty

1. True (gonadotropin levels elevated) complete forms
   a. Constitutional: Idiopathic
   b. Organic brain disease: Congenital anomalies such as septo-optic dysplasia, encephalitis, pinealomas, hypothalamic hamartomas, brain tumors in suprasellar region, meningitis, and trauma
2. Pseudo complete forms
   a. Gonadotropin-secreting tumors: Teratoma, hepatoblastoma, chorioepithelioma
   b. Gonadal tumors
      — Ovarian: Granulosa, theca-cell
      — Testicular: Leydig cell, adrenal rest tumor
   c. Adrenal: Tumor, congenital adrenal hyperplasia
   d. Hypothyroidism
   e. Iatrogenic or factitious androgen or estrogen abuse or other exposure to estrogen-containing makeup, hair creams, or oils
   f. McCune-Albright syndrome
   g. Hemihypertrophy syndrome
   h. Gonadotropin-independent precocious puberty (Wierman et al., 1985)
3. Incomplete forms
   a. Premature thelarche
   b. Premature adrenarche

Heterosexual Precocious Puberty

1. Female
   a. Ovarian: Arrhenoblastoma
   b. Adrenal: Congenital adrenal hyperplasia, virilizing tumor
   c. Androgen-producing teratoma
   d. Iatrogenic
2. Male
   a. Adrenal feminizing tumor
   b. Estrogen-producing teratoma
   c. Neurofibromatosis
   d. Iatrogenic

Evaluation

History   A complete history is important, and should include:

1. Information on intercurrent disease
2. History of drug ingestion, especially sex steroids
3. Family history, especially presence of similar conditions in family members
4. Chronology of development of secondary sexual characteristics, including breast development, pubic hair, axillary hair, and menses

5. Evaluation of growth history and growth spurt
6. History of head trauma
7. History of behavioral or emotional changes

Physical Examination   A complete physical examination should be performed, including:

1. Measurement of height and weight and evaluation of growth chart to determine the onset of increased linear-growth velocity
2. Evaluation of sexual maturity ratings, including gonadal size
3. A neurological examination
4. An ophthalmological examination
5. Careful testicular examination for evidence of masses
6. Abdominal, rectal, or pelvic examination, where applicable, to determine uterine and ovarian size
7. Evaluation for signs of hypothyroidism
8. Evaluation for evidence of estrogen stimulation
9. Evaluation for evidence of facial sebaceous glands, café au lait markings, and neurofibromatous lesions

Laboratory Examination   The laboratory evaluation of precocious puberty should proceed in a stepwise, logical fashion. The accompanying flow sheet (Fig. 8.8) for evaluating isosexual precocious puberty also includes diagnostic clues for each diagnosis. Thus, by evaluating bone age and gonadotropin levels after stimulation with GnRH (in those with advanced bone age), one can narrow the diagnostic possibilities tremendously. The bone age is extremely valuable. Retarded bone age and short stature suggest hypothyroidism. A bone age consistent with chronological age usually is seen with patients with incomplete precocious puberty. These patients need continued observation at regular intervals to monitor whether complete precocious puberty or signs of other illnesses are developing. An advanced bone age suggests a peripheral estrogen or androgen effect. If gonadotropins levels are low and there is no gonadotropin response to GnRH, pseudoprecocious puberty is diagnosed and the extra CNS source of hCG or sex steroids must be sought. If the gonadotropin levels are in the pubertal range or if there is a pubertal response to GnRH, then a search for a CNS lesion must be made before the diagnosis of idiopathic precocious puberty is made.

Treatment

Incomplete Forms   Generally, these forms are self-limited and will not progress.

True Sexual Precocity

Idiopathic   The natural history is variable. Observation for 6–12 months is advisable to determine whether the status is unchanged or changing rapidly. If unchanged, continued observation is in order. If the degree of sexual maturation has progressed rapidly, one should attempt to slow the process. Potent analogs of GnRH are used successfully for central precocious puberty. There is a down-regulating effect of these agents on the pituitary GnRH receptors, which inhibits gonadotropin release and causes diminished gonadal steroid production. These agents can be administered by the subcutaneous route or intranasally daily or in the long-acting "depo" form every 28 days. The accelerated linear-growth velocity, advancement of the skeletal age, and secondary sex characteristics regress with therapy (Kaplan and Grumbach, 1990). Other agents are used for pseudopuberty to diminish gonadal production of sex steroids or to inhibit the peripheral effect of these

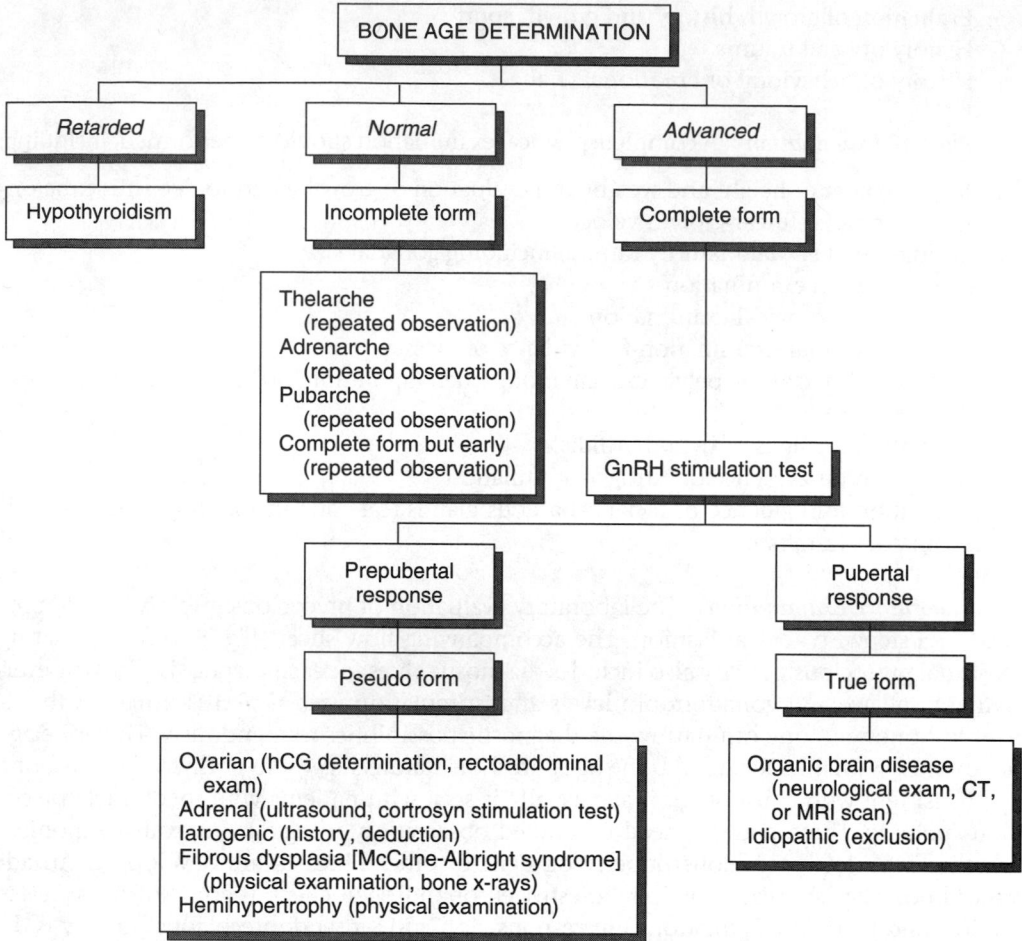

FIGURE 8.8.   Flow sheet for evaluation of isosexual precocious puberty. *MRI,* Magnetic resonance imaging. (Adapted from Brenner PE. Precocious puberty in the female. In: Mishell DR, Davajan VC, eds. Reproductive endocrinology, infertility, and contraception. © 1979 by FA Davis Co.)

hormones. These include testolactone, an inhibitor of aromatase activity, which has been used in girls with pseudoprecocious puberty caused by McCune-Albright syndrome. Medroxyprogesterone acetate can be used to inhibit ovarian and testicular steroidogenesis. Recently, an antifungal drug, ketoconazole, has been used to decrease testosterone production in males with gonadotropin-independent puberty. Spironolactone can be beneficial as an antiandrogen agent. Treatment should be continued until the child is able to handle the physical changes of puberty or until there has been normalization of the height prediction.

Organic Brain Disease   Treatment of the underlying disorder is provided.

Pseudosexual Precocity

1. Ectopic gonadotropin secretion: Tumor excision
2. Gonadal or adrenal tumors: Tumor removal
3. Congenital adrenal hyperplasia: Glucocorticoid treatment to suppress the adrenal gland

Psychosocial Management

Despite physical advancement, patients with precocious puberty rarely exhibit acceleration of intellectual or psychosocial development. Their social level is usually normal for their chronological age. Because of advanced physical development and increased strength, they may try to associate with older children. However, they are handicapped because of their lack of social skills. They may, moreover, become shy and inhibited because of their abnormal appearance as compared with their peers. Because of their potential fertility, it is important to consider sex education at an earlier age than usual.

BIBLIOGRAPHY

Adan L, Souberbielle JC, Brauner R. Management of the short stature due to pubertal delay in boys. J Clin Endocrinol Metab 1994;78:478.

Albanese A, Stanhope R. Investigation of delayed puberty. Clin Endocrinol 1995;43:105.

Allen D, Fost N. Growth hormone therapy for short stature: panacea or Pandora's box? J Pediatr 1990; 117:16.

Bailey JD, Park E, Cowell C. Estrogen treatment of girls with constitutional tall stature. Pediatr Clin North Am 1981;28:501.

Barnes HV. Recognizing normal and abnormal growth and development during puberty. In: Moss AV, ed. Pediatrics update: reviews for physicians. New York: Elsevier–North Holland Publishing, 1979:103.

Barnes N. Excessive growth. Arch Dis Child 1983;58:845.

Barbieri RL. Clinical applications of GnRH and its analogues. Trends Endocrinol Metab 1992;3:30.

Bercu BB, Shulman D, Root AW, et al. Growth hormone provocative testing frequently does not reflect endogenous GH secretion. J Clin Endocrinol Metab 1986;63:709.

Blum WF, Rainke MB. Use of insulin-like growth factor–binding protein 3 for the evaluation of growth disorders. Horm Res 1990;33(suppl):31.

Bramswig JH, Fasse M, Holthoff ML, et al. Adult height in boys and girls with untreated short stature and constitutional delay of growth and puberty: accuracy of five different methods of height prediction. J Pediatr 1990;117:886.

Brenner PE. Precocious puberty in the female. In: Mishell, DR, Davajan, VC, eds. Reproductive endocrinology, infertility, and contraception. Philadelphia: FA Davis, 1979.

Brown P, Gajdusek C, Gibbs CJ Jr, et al. Potential epidemic of Creutzfeldt-Jakob disease from human growth hormone therapy. N Engl J Med 1985;313: 728.

Buyse M, Feingold M. Growth abnormalities in genetic syndromes. Postgrad Med 1977;62:67.

Byard PJ. The adolescent growth spurt in children with cystic fibrosis. Ann Hum Biol 1994;21:229.

Cacciari E, Cicognani A, Pirazzoli P, et al. Differences in somatomedin-C between short-normal subjects and those of normal height. J Pediatr 1985;106:891.

Cameron N. Assessment of growth and maturation during adolescence. Hormone Res 1993;39:9.

Cara JF. Growth hormone in adolescence: normal and abnormal. Endocrinol Metab Clin North Am 1993; 22:533.

Conte FA, Grumbach MM. Estrogen use in children and adolescents: a study. Pediatrics 1978;62:1091.

Crawford, JD. Treatment of tall girls with estrogen. Pediatrics 1978;62:1189.

Dunkel L, Perheentupa J, Virtanen M, et al. Gonadotropin-releasing hormone test and human chorionic gonadotropin test in the diagnosis of gonadotropin deficiency in prepubertal boys. J Pediatr 1985a;107: 388.

Dunkel L, Perheentupa J, Virtanen M, et al. GnRH and HCG tests are both necessary in differential diagnosis of male delayed puberty. Am J Dis Child 1985b; 139:494.

Feuillan PP, Foster CM, Pescovitz OH. Treatment of precocious puberty in the McCune-Albright syndrome with the aromatase inhibitor testolactone. N Engl J Med 1986;315:1115.

Fine RN, Kohaut EC, Brown D, et al. Growth after recombinant human growth hormone treatment in children with chronic renal failure: report of a multicenter randomized double-blind placebo-controlled study. J Pediatr 1994;124:374.

Finkelstein JS, Neer RM, Biller BMK. Osteopenia in men with a history of delayed puberty. N Engl J Med 1992;326:600.

Frasier SD, Lippe BM. The rational use of growth hormone during childhood [Clinical Review 11]. J Clin Endocrinol Metab 1990;71:269.

Furlanetto RW. Insulin-like growth factor-1 measurements in the evaluation of growth hormone secretion. Horm Res 1990;33(suppl 4):25.

Harti-Henneberg C, Niirianeu AK, Rappaport P. Oxandrolone treatment of constitutional short stature in boys during adolescence. J Pediatr 1976;86:783.

Hill DE, Fisher RH. Chronic disease and short stature. Postgrad Med 1977;62:103.

Hoffman AR, Crowley WF Jr. Induction of puberty in men by long-term pulsatile administration of low-dose gonadotropin-releasing hormone. N Engl J Med 1982;307:1237.

Holland FJ, Fishman L, Bailey JD. Ketoconazole in the management of precocious puberty unresponsive to GNRH analogue therapy. N Engl J Med 1985;312: 1023.

Hopwood NJ, Kelch RP, Zipf NB, et al. The effect of synthetic androgens on the hypothalamic-pituitary-gonadal axis in boys with constitutionally delayed growth. J Pediatr 1979;94:657.

Kaplan SL, Grumbach MM. Pathophysiology and treatment of sexual precocity. J Clin Endocrinol Metab 1990;71:785.

Kletter GB, Kelch RP. Disorders of puberty in boys. Endocrinol Metab Clin North Am 1993;22:45.

Knudtzon J. Growth hormone therapy of short stature [Review]. Acta Paediatr Scand 1986;75:353.

Kritzler RK, Plotnick LP. The short child: a matter of time or cause for concern? Postgrad Med 1985;78:51.

LaFranchi S, Hanna CE, Mandel SH. Constitutional delay of growth: expected versus final adult height. Pediatrics 1991;87:82.

Lindner D, Job JC, Chaussain JL. Failure to improve height prediction in short-stature pubertal adolescents by inhibiting puberty with luteinizing hormone–releasing hormone analogue. Eur J Pediatr 1993;79:393.

Lipsky MS, Horner JM. The child with short stature. Am Fam Physician 1988;37:230.

Mahoney CP. Evaluating the child with short stature. Pediatr Clin North Am 1987;34:825.

Marin G, Domene HM, Barnes KM. The effects of estrogen priming and puberty on the growth hormone response to standardized treadmill exercise and arginine-insulin in normal girls and boys. J Clin Endocrinol Metab 1994;79:537.

Martha PM Jr, Gorman KM, Blizzard RM, et al. Endogenous growth hormone secretion and clearance rates in normal boys, as determined by deconvolution analysis: relationship to age, pubertal status, and body mass. J Clin Endocrinol Metab 1992;74:336.

Martinez A, Heinrich JJ, Domene H, et al. Growth in Turner's syndrome: long-term treatment with low-dose ethinyl estradiol. J Clin Endocrinol Metab 1987;65:253.

Mulligan K, Grunfeld C, Hellerstein MK, et al. Anabolic effects of recombinant human growth hormone in patients with wasting associated with human immunodeficiency virus infection. J Clin Endocrinol Metab 1993;77:956.

Municchi G, Rose SR, Pescovitz OH. Effect of deslorelin-induced pubertal delay on the growth of adolescents with short stature and normally timed puberty: preliminary results. J Clin Endocrinol Metab 1993; 77:1334.

Oberfield SE, Levine LS. The child with short stature. N Y State J Med 1986; January:15.

Oerter KE, Uriarte M, Rose SR, et al. Gonadotropin secretory dynamics during puberty in normal girls and boys. J Clin Endocrinol Metab 1990;71:1251.

Prader A. Pubertal growth. Acta Paediatr Jpn 1992;34: 222.

Rallison ML. Growth disorders in infants, children, and adolescents. New York: John Wiley & Sons, 1986.

Reynolds JM, Wood AJ, Eminson DM, et al. Short stature and chronic renal failure: what concerns children and parents? Arch Dis Child 1995;73:36.

Richman RA, Kirsch LR. Testosterone treatment in adolescent boys with constitutional delay in growth and development. N Engl J Med 1988;319:1563.

Rimoin DL, Borochowitz Z, Horton WA, et al. Short stature: physiology and pathology. West J Med 1986; 144:710.

Rivkees SA, Bode HH, Crawford JD. Long-term growth in juvenile acquired hypothyroidism: the failure to achieve normal adult stature. N Engl J Med 1988; 318:599.

Rogers DG. Puberty and insulin-dependent diabetes mellitus. Clin Pediatr 1992;31:168.

Root AW, Zamanillo J, Duckett G, et al. Gonadotropin-independent isosexual precocity in a boy with tuberous sclerosis: effect of ketoconazole. J Pediatr 1986; 109:1012.

Rosenfeld RG, Frane J, Attie KM, et al. Six-year results of a randomized, perspective trial of human growth hormone and oxandrolone in Turner syndrome. J Pediatr 1992;121:49.

Rosenfeld RG, Hintz RL, Johanson AJ, et al. Methionyl human growth hormone and oxandrolone in Turner syndrome: preliminary results of a prospective randomized trial. J Pediatr 1986;109:936.

Rosenfeld RG, Northcraft GB, Hintz RL. A prospective, randomized study of testosterone treatment of constitutional delay of growth and development in male adolescents. Pediatrics 1982;69:681.

Rosenfield RL. Low-dose testosterone effect on somatic growth. Pediatrics 1986;77:853.

Ross JL, Cassorla FG, Skerda MC, et al. A preliminary study of the effect of estrogen dose on growth in Turner's syndrome. N Engl J Med 1983;309:1104.

Schaefer F, Seidel C, Binding A, et al. Pubertal growth in chronic renal failure. Pediatr Res 1990;28:5.

Soliman AT, Khadir MM, Asfour M. Testosterone treatment in adolescent boys with constitutional delay of growth and development. Metabolism 1995;44: 1013.

Spagnoli A, Spadoni GL, Cianfarani S, et al. Prediction of the outcome of growth hormone therapy in children with idiopathic short stature. A multivariate discriminant analysis. J Pediatr 1995;126:905.

Speroff L, Glass RH, Kase NG. Abnormal puberty and growth problems. In: Clinical gynecologic endocrinology and infertility, 4th ed. Baltimore: Williams & Wilkins, 1989.

Stanhope R, Adams J, Brook CGD. Disturbances of puberty. Clin Obstet Gynecol 1985;12:557.

Takano K, Shizume K, Hibi I. Long-term effects of growth hormone treatment on height in Turner syndrome: results of a 6-year multicentre study in Japan. Committee for the Treatment of Turner Syndrome. Horm Res 1995;43:141.

Underwood LE. Report of the conference on uses and

possible abuses of biosynthetic human growth hormone. N Engl J Med 1984;311:606.

Underwood LE. Growth hormone therapy for short stature: yes or no? Hosp Pract. 1992;27:192.

Underwood LE, Van Wyk JJ. Normal and aberrant growth. In: Wilson JD, Foster DW, eds. Williams' textbook of endocrinology, 8th ed. Philadelphia: WB Saunders, 1992:1079.

Van der Werff ten Bosch JJ, Bot, A. Growth of tall girls without and during oestrogen treatment. Neth J Med 1981;24:52.

Vance ML, Thorner MO. Growth-hormone–releasing hormone: a clinical update. Ann Intern Med 1986; 105:447.

Weaver DS, Own GM. Nutrition and short stature. Postgrad Med 1977;62:93.

Wierman ME, Beardsworth DE, Mansfield MJ, et al. Puberty without gonadotropins: a unique mechanism of sexual development. N Engl J Med 1985;312:65.

Wilson DM, Kei J, Hintz RL, et al. Effects of testosterone therapy for pubertal delay. Am J Dis Child 1988; 142:96.

Wilson DM, Rosenfeld RG. Treatment of short stature and delayed adolescence. Pediatr Clin North Am 1987;34:865.

Wilson JD, Foster DW, eds. Williams' textbook of endocrinology, 7th ed. WB Saunders, 1985.

Wu FCW, Brown DC, Butler GE, et al. Early-morning plasma testosterone is an accurate predictor of imminent pubertal development in prepubertal boys. J Clin Endocrinol Metab 1993;76:26.

Zachmann M, Ferrandez A, Muurse G, et al. Testosterone treatment of excessively tall boys. J Pediatr 1976;88:116.

Zachmann M, Prader A. Anabolic and androgenic effect of testosterone in sexually immature boys and its dependency on growth hormone. J Clin Endocrinol Metab 1970;30:85.

CHAPTER 9
Thyroid Disease in Adolescents

Lawrence S. Neinstein and Francine Ratner Kaufman

Thyroid dysfunction increases in prevalence during the teen years. The onset can be of insidious or sudden onset. The most common presentation is of an asymptomatic goiter. However, hyperfunction or hypofunction does occur, sometimes manifested as menstrual irregularities, school dysfunction, or a change in behavior. These changes may be mistakenly ignored in the adolescent and credited as being normal adolescent reactions.

Changes in Thyroid Gland During Adolescence

1. Size: Doubles in size during puberty, reaching an average weight of 14 ± 5.2 g.
2. Hormonal changes
   a. Relative decreases occur in basal metabolic rate, total thyroxine (T_4), total T_3, thyroid-binding globulin, and thyroid-stimulating hormone (TSH).
   b. Relative increases occur in reverse T_3, thyroid-binding prealbumin, serum half-life of T_4, and volume of distribution of T_4.
   c. There are no changes in free T_4 or free T_3.

Thyroid Dysfunction Considerations in the Adolescent

Common Disorders

In order of frequency of clinical problems:

1. Goiter caused by chronic lymphocytic thyroiditis (Hashimoto's thyroiditis)
2. Simple nontoxic goiter
3. Graves' disease

Other Disorders

Other disorders, such as multimodular goiters, thyroid nodules, neoplasias, and other forms of acute suppurative thyroiditis, are rare in adolescents. Rallison et al. (1991) studied the incidence and natural history of thyroid diseases in adolescents. A total of 4819 school-age children, aged 11 to 18 years, were studied in 1965–1968 and restudied in 1985–1986. Initially 3.7% had an abnormal finding, including:

Problem	Rate per 1000 (1965–1968)
Diffuse hypertrophy	19.3
Chronic lymphocytic thyroiditis	12.7
Thyroid nodules (two with papillary carcinomas)	4.6
Hyperthyroidism or hypothyroidism	1.9

During the follow-up examination 20 years later, 1985–1986, the findings showed 298 (10.7%) with abnormalities, including:

Problem	Rate per 1000
Chronic thyroiditis	51.3
Simple goiters	28.7
Nodules (including 10 carcinomas)	23.2
Hypothyroidism	15.9
Hyperthyroidism	3.9

Of the 92 adolescents with "diffuse hypertrophy," 60% were healthy 20 years later, 20% were unchanged, and thyroiditis or colloid goiters had developed in a few.

Adolescent Goiter

There is no such condition as an "adolescent" goiter. Enlarged thyroid glands are indicative of dysfunction and require evaluation of the underlying disorder and appropriate therapy.

CLINICAL EVALUATION FOR THYROID DISEASE

1. History
   a. Family history of goiter, thyroiditis, other thyroid problems, or other autoimmune disease
   b. Drug history: Use of goitrogens, including lithium or iodine excess
   c. Menstrual history
   d. Change in weight
   e. Growth problems
   f. Change in behavior, sleep pattern, activity level, or function in school
   g. Change in bowel habits
2. Physical examination
   a. Height, weight
   b. Pulse, blood pressure
   c. Skin texture or lesions
   d. Adenopathy
   e. Presence of tremor
   f. Eye examination: Presence of exophthalmos or lid lag
   g. Deep-tendon reflexes: Slow or fast return phase
   h. Thyroid gland
      — Size
      — Shape
      — Nodularity
      — Consistency
      — Tenderness
      — Auscultation for bruits
3. Thyroid tests: Many are available, but only several are typically necessary for appropriate diagnosis. Common thyroid tests include:
   a. Serum total T_4 concentration: Total T_4 concentration is generally measured by either competitive protein-binding assay or radioimmunoassay (RIA). Most thyroid hormone is bound and inactive. Total T_4 is proportional to free T_4 if the level of thyroid-binding globulin (TBG) is normal.

b. T_3 resin uptake: This test is never useful when used alone. Rather, the test should be done only as an indirect measurement of TBG and to calculate the adjusted T_4 or T_4 index.

c. Adjusted T_4: A calculation using total T_4 and T_3 resin uptake with adjustment for changes in TBG levels. Adjusted T_4 is generally high in patients with hyperthyroidism. A few of these patients have only T_3 elevations (T_3 thyrotoxicosis). Conditions that alter TBG and thus total T_4 concentrations but yield a normal adjusted T_4 level include:
   — Factors increasing TBG: Oral contraceptives, pregnancy, heredity, acute hepatitis
   — Factors decreasing TBG: Androgens, cirrhosis, nephrosis, acromegaly, genetic, high-dose steroids
   — Drugs decreasing binding of T_4 and T_3: Salicylates, phenytoin (Dilantin), penicillin, heparin, barbital

d. Free T_4: Measures the percentage of free T_4 and is used to calculate the amount of free T_4. Because of the fluctuation between results obtained in different laboratories and the excellent accuracy of total T_4 and total T_3 levels, this test is rarely necessary.

e. Total T_3: Measures the total amount of T_3 in serum by radioimmunoassay. Useful in early or mild hyperthyroidism because the T_3 level rises earlier and more markedly than T_4. Not useful in evaluating hypothyroidism.

f. Free T_3: Measured in a manner similar to that of free T_4. An unreliable test at present. For quantitative aspects of total and free T_3 and T_4, see Table 9.1.

g. TSH: Serum TSH is measured by RIA. It is the most sensitive test for diagnosing primary hypothyroidism and separating thyroidal hypothyroidism (increased TSH level) from hypothalamic-pituitary hypothyroidism (low TSH level). Serum TSH concentration is markedly elevated in primary hypothyroidism. Sensitive TSH assays can distinguish normal TSH levels from suppressed levels (<0.7 µU/m). This is useful in diagnosing suppression of TSH caused by excessive thyroid supplementation or hyperthyroidism.

h. Thyroidal radioiodine uptake (RAIU): A measurement of thyroidal uptake of iodine 131 or 123. The chief value of this test is in the differential diagnosis of hyperthyroidism. RAIU is high or high-normal in hyperthyroid Graves' disease, in nodular goiter, or in Hashimoto's thyrotoxicosis. RAIU is low in factitious hyperthyroidism, in subacute thyroiditis, in abnormal location of the thyroid gland, or in patients with Graves' disease who have ingested iodine. [123]I is preferred because of the lower radiation dose.

i. Thyroid scan: A thyroid scan mainly evaluates morphologic features and functional status of the gland. It is useful in the differential diagnosis of the solitary nodule or in locating extrathyroidal tissue. [123]I or technetium (Tc) pertechnetate scans are preferred. Addition of a perchlorate discharge to the ^{123}I scan can be used to help differentiate Hashimoto's thyroiditis and inborn errors of thyroid hormone synthesis.

j. Thyroid antibodies: Levels of thyroid, thyroglobulin, and microsomal antibodies are elevated in most patients with Graves' disease and Hashimoto's thyroiditis. Antimicrosomal antibodies appear more sensitive (99% sensitivity) than antithyroglobulin antibodies (36% sensitivity) (Nordyke et al., 1993). Titers are lower in adolescents than adults. The presence of the specific thyroid-stimulating immunoglobulin (TSI)

TABLE 9.1.   Quantitative Aspects of Total and Free T_3 and T_4

Hormone	Mean Total (µg)	% Free	Mean Free Level (ng)
T_4	7.0	0.03	2.1
T_3	0.14	0.3	0.5

is seen in Graves' disease. This can be assayed at the time of diagnosis of Graves' disease and monitored as an indication of the resolution of the autoimmune process.

k. Thyrotropin-releasing hormone (TRH) test: This test is usually reserved for questionable cases of hyperthyroidism and for the differentiation of hypothalamic from pituitary hypothyroidism. Healthy patients have a positive response of increased TSH to a bolus (7 µg/kg, or 500 µg maximum) of intravenously administered TRH. The peak value exceeds 5 µU/mL and is usually less than 35 µU in normal persons. In hypothalamic hypothyroidism there is a late rise in the TSH concentration, and in pituitary hypothyroidism there is no response. In patients with hyperthyroidism, there is usually no elevation of the TSH level after a TRH injection. TRH also causes the release of prolactin, and abnormally elevated levels are seen in hypothalamic hypothyroidism and primary hypothyroidism.

l. Reverse T_3: An inactive isomer of T_3, produced from inner-ring deiodination of T_4. In nonthyroidal illness, such as starvation and anorexia nervosa, T_3 concentrations are low and reverse T_3 concentrations are elevated. In hypothyroidism, levels of both T_3 and reverse T_3 are low.

m. TBG by RIA: Direct measurement of TBG is done by RIA.

n. Thyroglobulin level: Thyroglobulin is leaked into the serum when there is destruction of thyroid parenchyma. The concentration is elevated in thyroid carcinoma.

EUTHYROID GOITER

The most common presentation of thyroid disease during adolescence is an asymptomatic goiter discovered by the teenager or his or her physician during a routine physical examination. The incidence is about 9/1000 per year, with the majority of affected teens being female.

CAUSES OF NONTOXIC ENLARGED THYROID GLANDS IN ADOLESCENCE

1. Common causes
    a. Hashimoto's thyroiditis
    b. Simple goiter
2. Uncommon causes
    a. Acute suppurative thyroiditis
    b. Subacute thyroiditis
    c. Primary thyroid neoplasms
    d. Goitrogen-inducted goiter

DIFFERENTIATION AND EVALUATION OF SIMPLE GOITER VERSUS HASHIMOTO'S THYROIDITIS

Table 9.2 compares typical symptoms in simple goiter versus Hashimoto's thyroiditis. If the adolescent is euthyroid, if results of thyroid function tests are normal, if no nodules are pal-

TABLE **9.2.**   Typical Characteristics of Simple Goiter versus Hashimoto's Thyroiditis

Characteristic	Simple Goiter	Hashimoto's Thyroiditis
Thyroid gland size	Variable	Variable
Thyroid gland consistency	Usually firm or pebbly	Usually irregular and firm
Family history	Positive in about 50% of cases	Positive in about 60% of cases
Thyroid function test results (thyroid index)	Normal	Usually normal; can have early hyperthyroidism and late hypothyroidism
Thyroid antibodies	Not detectable	Usually present

pable, and if there is no adenopathy or adherence of the gland to the neck structure, then no further diagnostic study is necessary. Thyroid antibodies are helpful in differentiating simple goiter from chronic lymphocytic thyroiditis (Hashimoto's thyroiditis). An uptake test and a thyroid scan are of some value in evaluating a nontoxic goiter, particularly if antithyroid antibodies are not present in high titers. If the uptake is decreased and patchy, and if there is a positive perchlorate discharge, these findings would be consistent with Hashimoto's (chronic lymphocytic) thyroiditis. Adolescents with chronic lymphocytic thyroiditis are at increased risk of having other immune disease, including diabetes mellitus, rheumatoid arthritis, systemic lupus erythematosus, adrenal insufficiency, hypoparathyroidism, vitiligo, pernicious anemia, and alopecia totalis.

A less-common presentation of euthyroid goiter in the adolescent is subacute thyroiditis. Characteristics of this disease include:

1. A self-limited illness, often following an acute viral illness
2. A thyroid gland that is usually tender, with mild enlargement
3. Usually no thyroid dysfunction
4. Absence of thyroid antibodies
5. An elevated erythrocyte sedimentation rate

TREATMENT OF SIMPLE GOITER

1. Indications for treatment
   a. Moderate-to-large goiter
   b. Cosmetic concerns of an enlarged goiter
   c. Pressure symptoms
   d. Progressively enlarging gland
2. Type of therapy
   a. Thyroid hormone: If indicated, best continued for life. Synthetic thyroxine is the best preparation, giving stable levels of T_4 and T_3 after about 3 weeks of treatment
   b. Dose: The replacement dose is about 0.1–0.15 mg/day. If there is only minimal thyroid enlargement and normal T_4 and TSH levels, gland size and thyroid hormone levels (T_4, TSH) should be evaluated every 6–12 months during adolescence

HYPOTHYROIDISM

Causes

Most hypothyroidism in adolescence is caused by chronic lymphocytic thyroiditis. Secondary pituitary and tertiary hypothalamic causes are rare.

Clinical Manifestations

1. Growth retardation and pubertal delay: Most common endocrine cause of delayed growth
2. Delayed bone maturation
3. Precocious puberty and galactorrhea
4. Menstrual disorders
5. Weight gain
6. Cutaneous manifestations
   a. Cold skin
   b. Decreased sweating
   c. Dry skin

    d. Edema of face and eyelids
    e. Erythema of cheeks
    f. Localized hyperkeratosis
    g. Pallor
    h. Thin epidermis
    i. Dry, brittle hair
    j. Patchy alopecia
    k. Sparse eyebrows
    l. Fine, downy hair
    m. Thickened, brittle nails
7. Usual signs of adult hypothyroidism: Lethargy, weakness, eyelid edema, cold intolerance, skin pallor, decreased memory, constipation, hoarseness, precordial pain, and anemia

Evaluation

Adjusted T_4 and TSH: TSH is the most sensitive indicator of primary hypothyroidism and can be used alone as a screen for hypothyroidism.

1. Low T_4 and high TSH concentrations indicate primary hypothyroidism.
2. Low T_4 and normal or low TSH concentrations indicate secondary hypothyroidism.

A TRH stimulation test can be performed. No TSH response indicates pituitary disease. A late rise in TSH concentration and failure to return to baseline at the completion of the test, coupled with elevated prolactin levels, indicate hypothalamic disease. An endocrine evaluation for cause and extent of hypothalamic or pituitary disease is also indicated. Low T_4 and normal TSH concentrations can also be seen in nonthyroidal illness, referred to as "sick" euthyroid. This also includes a low T_3 level and a normal or elevated reverse T_3 level. Low T_4 and normal TSH concentrations are also found in patients with TBG deficiency. Obtaining a TBG level by RIA confirms this diagnosis.

Therapy

Synthetic thyroxine is given in doses of 75–150 µg/day (1.6 µg/kg): 75–100 µg/day to most females and 100–150 µg/day to most males. The goals are T_4 levels in the normal range, normal and not oversuppressed levels of TSH, and resumption of growth. Hennessey et al. (1986) evaluated thyroid replacement therapy. A downward trend has occurred in the past 14 years because of an increased potency or bioavailability of thyroxine. The formulation was changed in 1982. Average replacement doses decreased from 169 to 112 µg during this period. Current average replacement doses equal about 127 ± 39 µg. Overtreatment with thyroxine should be avoided because it could lead to osteoporosis.

Initiation of Therapy   Usually, in adolescents, therapy can be started with a full dose of thyroxine. In older patients or those with heart disease, it should be started at 25 or 50 µg a day and increased by 25–50 µg/day each month. Chronically ill adolescents may need about 25–50 µg less than healthy teens. The serum thyroxine concentration returns toward normal within a few weeks of the start of therapy. Usually the teen will begin to improve clinically within 2 weeks and will become free of symptoms and signs by 3–6 months. The sensitive TSH measurements may decline slowly and remain elevated for up to 6–12 months. The higher the initial level, the longer it may take to return to normal. It is reasonable to check a TSH level 2 months after initiating therapy. However, the practitioner needs to be careful in altering doses at this point, because this can lead to overtreatment as a result of the slow decline in sensitive TSH levels. If the TSH level is not normal by 4 months and the free T_4 concentration has increased, it is reasonable to increase the dose by 25 µg/day. Repeated tests can be done 6–8 weeks after a change in dose. Once a teen is euthyroid and stable, he or she can be monitored at 6 months and then every year unless the condition again becomes symptomatic.

Subclinical Hypothyroidism   Patients with subclinical hypothyroidism are asymptomatic, and T_4 levels are usually normal but TSH levels are elevated. The individuals at highest risk for the development of clinical hypothyroidism are those who have both an elevated TSH concentration greater than 10 mU/L and an elevated concentration of thyroid antibodies. It is reasonable to treat individuals in the following categories:

1. TSH value greater than 10 mU/L
2. TSH value greater than 5 mU/L with a goiter or thyroid autoantibodies

HYPERTHYROIDISM

Hyperthyroidism is less common than euthyroid goiter in children and younger adolescents. Only 5% of patients with Graves' disease are less than 15 years of age. Hyperthyroidism becomes more common with age, particularly in women, affecting approximately 2% of women. The prevalence in females increases dramatically during late adolescence and young adult ages, with a peak at about age 25.

Causes of Hyperthyroidism in Adolescents

1. Common: Graves' disease (For practical purposes, almost all hyperthyroidism in adolescents is caused by Graves' disease.)
2. Uncommon
   a. Toxic nodular goiter: Single adenoma or multiple nodules
   b. Thyroiditis: Subacute, silent, or postpartum
   c. Iatrogenic illness: Exogenous intake of thyroxine
3. Rare
   a. Ectopic thyroid tissue (e.g., struma ovarii [ovarian teratoma containing thyroid tissue])
   b. Inappropriate TSH secretion: Pituitary tumor
   c. Exogenous iodide intake
   d. Thyroid cancer

Clinical Manifestations

1. Goiter
2. Change in school performance: Inability to complete tasks; untidy work
3. Emotional lability, nervousness, sleep disturbance
4. Weight loss and increased appetite
5. Muscle weakness and tremor
6. Eye changes (exophthalmos, ptosis, lid lag) less severe than in adults with hyperthyroidism
7. Menstrual changes: Amenorrhea, oligomenorrhea, or dysfunctional uterine bleeding
8. Cutaneous manifestations
   a. Eczema
   b. Erythema, or flushing
   c. Excoriations
   d. Fine, velvety or smooth skin

  e. Hyperpigmentation
  f. Moist skin and increased sweating
  g. Pretibial myxedema
  h. Pruritus
  i. Warm skin
  j. Thin, straight hair
  k. Brittle nails
  l. Alopecia
9. Other signs and symptoms similar to hyperthyroidism in adults: Nervousness, sweating, palpitations, heat intolerance, fatigue, diarrhea, tachycardia, wide pulse pressure, and tremor

Evaluation

The combination of TSH and T_4 index should confirm most cases of hyperthyroidism. If the TSH concentration is low but the T_4 concentration is normal, a T_3 level should be measured to evaluate for T_3 toxicosis.

1. TSH concentration
  a. Should be low in all forms of hyperthyroidism, except in TSH-secreting adenomas and ectopic TSH production.
  b. Normal TSH concentration nearly always excludes a diagnosis of hyperthyroidism, except in the rare individual with excessive TSH secretion.
  c. Sensitive TSH test alone may be recommended by some as a screen for hyperthyroidism.
2. Adjusted T_4 value
  a. If elevated, hyperthyroidism is confirmed. Pregnant women, those taking estrogens, or persons having an inherited increase in TBG production may have an elevated total T_4 concentration. However, their T_4 index or free T_4 and TSH values should all be normal.
  b. If normal and the TSH level is low, or if hyperthyroidism is suspected on examination, measure the total T_3 concentration. If the T_3 level is elevated, then hyperthyroidism (T_3 thyrotoxicosis) is indicated. If results are normal or borderline, a TRH stimulation test should be performed. If results of the TRH stimulation test show a normal TSH response, a euthyroid state is indicated. If a TSH response is absent, a probable hyperthyroid state is indicated.
3. Thyroid antibodies: Present, especially the specific TSI, in Graves' disease and in Hashimoto's thyrotoxicosis
4. Thyroid scan and uptake: Probably not indicated in an adolescent with hyperthyroidism, unless a nodule is present, factitious thyroid ingestion is suspected, or the patient lives in an area such as the Great Lakes area or Japan, where lymphocytic thyroiditis with spontaneously resolving hyperthyroidism (silent thyroiditis) is common
  a. Elevated uptake: Found in Graves' disease, toxic adenoma, toxic multinodular goiter, Hashimoto's thyrotoxicosis, and ectopic TSH production
  b. Decreased uptake: Found in thyroiditis, factitious thyroid ingestion, ectopic thyroid tissue, and metastatic functioning carcinoma

Therapy

Therapy for hyperthyroidism (Graves' disease) includes medical therapy, ablation with ^{131}I, and surgery.

Medical Therapy   Medical therapy should be started in all patients with hyperthyroidism. It is usually the primary modality in most adolescent patients. Medical therapy includes:

1. Symptomatic end-organ therapy with propranolol or another β-blocker. This measure is needed only if symptoms are moderate or severe and is discontinued as the euthyroid state is reached.
2. Antithyroid medication: Methimazole, carbimazole, or propylthiouracil (PTU). Methimazole is the active metabolite of carbimazole, and the conversion is almost 100%, so their effects and equivalent doses are comparable.
   a. Action
      — Inhibits iodine incorporation into tyrosine residues in thyroglobulin.
      — Reduces serum concentrations of thyrotropin-receptor antibodies.
      — Increases suppressor T-cell activity.
      — Propylthiouracil also inhibits peripheral conversion of T_4 to T_3.
   b. Metabolism: Peak blood levels are reached in 1 to 2 hours. PTU has a half-life of about 1–2 hours, whereas methimazole (Tapazole) has a half-life of about 3–5 hours.
   c. Indications: Major indications are for children, adolescents, young adults, and pregnant women with hyperthyroidism caused by Graves' disease. The choice of which antithyroid medication to use is based mainly on the practitioner's personal experience and preference. However, in many cases, methimazole is preferred because of compliance (in maintenance doses it can be used as a once-a-day drug) and a greater effect on decreasing the local thyroid immune response. In pregnant women, PTU is preferred because there is less placental transfer of the medication, a greater decrease in T_4-to-T_3 conversion, and some indication of possible congenital defects with methimazole. In most adolescents, an antithyroid medication should be tried in the hope of achieving a temporary or permanent remission.
   d. Doses
      — Methimazole: Started in a dose of about 10 mg twice a day. The dose may need to be reduced in 4–6 weeks as clinical and biochemical improvement takes place. The dose can be adjusted every 4–6 weeks until a maintenance dose is reached at about 5–10 mg/day.
      — PTU: Started in doses of 75–100 mg three times a day. This may be lowered, with time, to a maintenance dose of about 50–100 mg/day in divided doses.
   e. Follow-up: During the initial follow-up visits, the serum TSH concentration may remain low and thus is not a good indicator alone for adjusting dose levels. However, an elevated TSH concentration indicates that the medication dosage should be reduced. Virtually all patients with adequate compliance can reach the euthyroid state on these medications. A period of 2–4 months is usually required to attain this state, with the duration of treatment somewhat dependent on the size of the gland and the severity of the hyperthyroidism. When the euthyroid state is attained, TSI levels can be measured. If they have decreased or are no longer measurable, then the dose of medication may be reduced by 50% to 75%, so long as the teen remains euthyroid, which is assessed by monitoring with thyroid function tests. The majority of individuals receiving methimazole can be maintained on a single daily dose. In some individuals, antithyroid medication is reduced to a lesser degree and a small dose of thyroxine is added to maintain a euthyroid state. These measures can be taken to avoid a recurrence of a hyperthyroid state, which can occur in some individuals as they are weaned from antithyroid medication. However, because the antithyroid drugs have serious side effects, it is usually preferable to use as low a dosage as possible. Hashizume et al. (1991) found that treating individuals with methimazole, 30 mg/day

alone for 6 months and then 10 mg/day for 1 year, with thyroxine, 100 µg for 1 year, followed by thyroxine alone, reduced the recurrence rate to 1.7% as compared to a group treated without thyroxine (34.7% recurrence rate). Once a maintenance level is reached, the follow-up visits can be extended to 3 months.

f. Efficacy: Almost all individuals who take their medication will become euthyroid during treatment. The reported likelihood of a long-term remission ranges from 10–75%. Possible indicators of long-term remission include a small goiter and recent onset of disease. Many tests have been suggested to predict which patients will respond to medical therapy, but none has been consistently reliable. However, the presence of high titers of TSIs suggests that ongoing stimulation would still occur. Another factor in long-term remission is duration of therapy. Two years of treatment appears much more likely to induce a remission than 6–12 months of therapy. Thus most authorities recommend at least 12–24 months of suppression. After the initial treatment period, the drug dosage should be gradually discontinued while the adolescent is monitored for signs and symptoms of relapse. A relapse often occurs in the first few months after therapy has been discontinued, but individuals must be followed for life because many will have a relapse or hypothyroidism in future years. If a relapse occurs, the choices include another course of medical therapy, surgical intervention, or, depending on age, ^{131}I ablative therapy.

g. Minor side effects
    — Common: Pruritus, fever, rash, urticaria
    — Uncommon: Gastrointestinal distress, change in taste sensation, and production of insulin autoantibodies, causing hypoglycemia

h. Serious side effects (about 3/1000)
    — Rare: Agranulocytosis (<500 granulocytes/mm^3) occurs in about 0.5% of users. This is an idiosyncratic reaction but is probably less common in individuals receiving less than 30 mg of methimazole per day. It usually starts in the first 3 months of therapy and is manifested by an abrupt onset of fever, systemic toxic effects, and, often, mouth sores and pharyngitis. The abrupt onset makes routine monitoring of white blood cell counts useless in detecting this problem. Patients should be warned to stop using the medication at the first signs of fever, pharyngitis, or mouth sores. This is an absolute contraindication to further use of antithyroid medications. Transient leukopenia (<4000 leukocytes) occurs in up to 25% of children and 12% of adults and is not a reason to stop the medication.
    — Uncommon: Hepatitis (especially with PTU therapy), cholestatic jaundice (especially with methimazole), thrombocytopenia, aplastic anemia and lupuslike syndrome, nephrotic syndrome (with methimazole), and loss of taste (with methimazole).

^{131}I *Ablative Therapy*   Ablative therapy is highly successful in adults and has been increasingly used as a first line of therapy, although resulting hypothyroidism is common. However, the natural course of Graves' disease is toward hypothyroidism anyway. Although some institutions use ^{131}I in children and adolescents, its use is controversial because of concern over unknown long-term effects of radiation in the areas of cancer and fertility. There has been no evidence of an increased risk of thyroid cancer, leukemia, and most solid tumors; the risk of gastric cancer rises 10 years after treatment, and the risk of breast cancer rises (not significantly) after 30 years. Pregnancy is an absolute contraindication to radioiodine therapy. There is no evidence of an elevated risk of congenital abnormalities in the offspring of women previously treated with radioiodine.

There is significant controversy regarding the appropriate dose schedule, which varies from calculated doses to a fixed dose of 5 or 10 mCi. Radioiodine cures hyperthyroidism and decreases gland size in almost all individuals given multiple doses or a single large dose. Treated individuals need close monitoring for the development of hypothyroidism. There is concern that radioiodine may worsen Graves' ophthalmopathy (Franklyn, 1994) and should probably be avoided in individuals with active or progressive ophthalmopathy.

Surgery   Subtotal thyroidectomy has been advocated for patients who fail to benefit from or refuse medical therapy and for those with large goiters, especially with symptoms of compression or with cosmetic concerns. If the surgeon is experienced, the morbidity and mortality rates are low. Complications include hypothyroidism, hypoparathyroidism, and paralysis of the recurrent laryngeal nerve. Ideally, before surgery, individuals are treated with antithyroid medications until a euthyroid state is attained. Alternative short-term therapy includes β-blockers and potassium iodine to help reduce the risk of a postoperative thyrotoxic crisis (Franklyn, 1994). Relapse after surgery occurs in about 10% of individuals, usually within 5 years.

Dunn (1984) surveyed endocrinologists for preferences in treating Graves' disease. For a 19-year-old male or female, 67% preferred antithyroid medication for 1 year, 24% preferred radioactive iodine, and 9% preferred surgical intervention. If hyperthyroidism remained after medical therapy, there was a 50-50 split between surgery and radioactive iodine.

Pregnancy   Pregnant teens with hyperthyroidism should be treated with an antithyroid drug. The dose should be maintained at the lowest dose possible to keep the mother's T_4 level in the upper limit of the normal range. PTU is the preferred drug because less of it crosses the placenta or appears in breast milk.

Toxic Adenoma   Because of the permanent nature of a toxic thyroid adenoma or toxic multinodular goiter, this tumor should be treated with radioiodine.

THYROIDITIS

Although thyroiditis or a painful thyroid per se in an uncommon presentation in the adolescent, the thyroid enlargement associated with various types of thyroiditis is common. Table 9.3 outlines the differences between Hashimoto's and subacute thyroiditis. Among the

TABLE 9.3.   Hashimoto's versus Subacute Granulomatous Thyroiditis

Characteristic	Hashimoto's Thyroiditis (Chronic Lymphocytic)	Subacute Granulomatous Thyroiditis (de Quervain's)
Sex	F>>M	F>M
Family history	Positive	Negative
Associated with Graves' disease	Yes	No
Goiter	Moderate to large	Mild enlargement
Hyperthyroidism	Occasionally	No
Hypothyroidism	Occasionally	No
Painful thyroid gland	No	Yes
Vital prodrome	No	Yes
Uptake of ^{131}I	Increased in hyperthyroid; normal if euthyroid; decreased if hypothyroid	Decreased during acute phase
Thyroid antibodies	+ 80%	Not detectable
Erythrocyte sedimentation rate	Normal	Elevated
Biopsy specimen	Lymphocytic infiltration	Granulomatous thyroiditis
Prognosis	Overlaps with Graves' disease; frequent hypothyroidism	Benign course

forms of thyroiditis, Hashimoto's is the most common, with subacute granulomatous thyroiditis being about one-fortieth as common. Silent thyroiditis is very uncommon in adolescents, as is acute suppurative thyroiditis.

Acute Suppurative Thyroiditis

Acute suppurative thyroiditis is a rare form of thyroiditis caused by a bacterial, fungal, or parasitic infection and usually preceded by an infection elsewhere, such as an upper respiratory tract infection. Signs and symptoms include neck pain, fever, and dysphagia. The white blood cell count is usually elevated, and thyroid antibodies are not detected. Treatment is with analgesics, antibiotics, and surgical drainage if necessary. A fistula between the piriform sinus and the thyroid gland can contribute to the pathogenesis of acute suppurative thyroiditis and should be sought in such individuals (Szabo and Allen, 1989).

Subacute Granulomatous Thyroiditis

Subacute granulomatous thyroiditis (see Table 9.3) is a spontaneously remitting thyroid infection thought to be have a viral cause.

1. Clinical manifestations
   a. Abrupt onset
   b. Neck pain: Mild to severe
   c. Systemic symptoms common: Malaise, fever, fatigue, myalgias
   d. Thyroid slightly enlarged
   e. Mild to moderate signs of hyperthyroidism
   f. Tender thyroid gland
   g. Duration of 2–5 months
2. Laboratory findings
   a. Erythrocyte sedimentation rate often greater than 100 mm/hr
   b. White blood cell count often normal
   c. Initially: Iodine uptake low (often 0), elevated T_4 and T_3, followed by a period of normal uptake and subnormal results on thyroid function tests, followed by normal test results
3. Treatment: Salicylates; if severe, steroids

Subacute Lymphocytic Thyroiditis

Subacute lymphocytic thyroiditis is lymphocytic thyroiditis with spontaneously resolving hyperthyroidism, or silent thyroiditis. This form of thyroiditis has been thought to include as many as 14–23% of adult cases of hyperthyroidism, although recent studies outside the Great Lakes area suggest the prevalence to be in the 5% range. This is not a common cause of hyperthyroidism in adolescents; most cases occur in individuals more than 30 years of age. The cause is not known, and there is no evidence of a viral cause.

1. Clinical manifestations
   a. Mild to moderate hyperthyroid symptoms
   b. No signs of Graves' disease, such as exophthalmos or myxedema
   c. Enlarged, painless thyroid gland
   d. Abrupt onset of symptoms
   e. Firm, painless goiter

   f.   Often four phases: Hyperthyroid period (1–4 months), short euthyroid period, hypo-thyroid period (4–10 weeks), recovery
   g.   Recurrences in 10–50% of individuals
2. Laboratory findings
   a.   Low iodine uptake, in distinction from Graves' disease or Hashimoto's thyrotoxico-sis; complete suppression of TSH to TRH stimulation
   b.   Elevated antithyroglobulin antibodies in 25% and antimicrosomal antibodies in 60% of individuals
   c.   Erythrocyte sedimentation rate mildly elevated
   d.   Lymphocytic infiltration similar to Hashimoto's thyroiditis, as shown by biopsy (if done)
3. Treatment: Usually symptomatic, with β-blockers if necessary

Chronic Lymphocytic Thyroiditis

Chronic lymphocytic thyroiditis (Hashimoto's thyroiditis; see Table 9.3) is characterized by an autoimmune cause, a genetic predisposition, a strong female predilection, and a lympho-cytic infiltration of the thyroid gland. In almost all cases, thyroid antibodies are abundantly present. Although individuals may be in a hyperthyroid or a euthyroid state, the diagnosis is usually made because of a goiter and a hypothyroid state.

Diagnostic criteria include:

1. Firm goiter
2. Presence of antibodies
3. Elevated TSH level
4. Thyroid scan with "patchy uptake" (test not commonly needed)
5. Positive result on perchlorate discharge test (test not commonly needed)

Usually two or more of these findings are highly suggestive of Hashimoto's thyroiditis.

Treatment for the hypothyroidism is thyroid hormone replacement.

THYROID NODULES

Solitary thyroid nodules and thyroid cancer are uncommon during adolescence. Single nod-ules are four times more common in females than males. The differential diagnosis of soli-tary nonfunctional thyroid nodules includes:

1. Adenomas
2. Carcinomas
3. Cysts
4. Nodule of an unrecognized multinodular goiter
5. Other rare solitary lesions such as thyroiditis or developmental abnormalities

Evaluation

Evaluation of a thyroid nodule should include adjusted T_4, TSH, thyroid antibody, and thy-roglobulin levels. The initial major diagnostic step has become the fine-needle aspiration biopsy. In most centers the fine-needle aspiration biopsy is a safe and inexpensive test and leads to a better selection of which individuals require surgery. Results of the cytologic spec-imens are either benign, malignant, or indeterminate. The accuracy to cytologic diagnosis ranges from 70% to 97%. Individuals with benign results can be followed up safely.

Radionuclide scanning has been used in individuals with solitary nodules but cannot reliably distinguish between benign and malignant lesions. The scan is useful in those individual with thyrotoxicosis and a nodule. The scan can also be useful in individuals with an indeterminate biopsy result because a hyperfunctioning nodule is almost always benign. An ultrasound cannot distinguish benign nodules from malignant nodules.

High-risk factors include:

1. Male adolescent
2. Cold nodule on scan
3. Recent growth
4. Firm nodule
5. Cervical adenopathy
6. Solid lesion on ultrasound
7. Recurrent laryngeal, tracheal, or esophageal involvement
8. Multiple mucosal neuromas, suggestive of multiple endocrine neoplasia syndromes

Factors favoring benign lesion include:

1. Cystic lesion
2. Hyperfunctioning on scan
3. Elevated antibody levels
4. Family history of goiter

Management

1. Nodules with benign cytological features: These lesions can be either observed or treated with thyroxine. Thyroxine therapy is often instituted to try to reduce the size of the nodule or suppress further growth. There is little evidence that thyroxine suppression is of benefit in the treatment of benign hypofunctioning solitary nodules. In addition, there appears to be a risk of decreasing bone density in adults with thyroid suppressive therapy, although the risk to adolescents remains unknown.
2. Malignant lesions: Individuals with malignant lesions should undergo surgery with either a lobectomy or thyroidectomy, depending on the lesion. More extensive surgery is needed if lymph nodes are involved.
3. Nodules with indeterminate cytological results: Many experts recommend surgical excision for all individuals with a cytological result demonstrating indeterminate features. Radionuclide scanning is useful in these individuals because a "hot" scan indicates the ability to follow the teen's condition.
4. Cystic lesions: A cystic lesion should be aspirated. If the lesion is larger than 4 cm in diameter, it should be excised. If the cyst is less than 4 cm and there is either no fluid, cloudy fluid, serosanguineous fluid, or suspicious cytological features, it should be excised.

BIBLIOGRAPHY

Abbassi V, Shearin RB. Thyroid disease in the adolescent. J Curr Adolesc Med 1980;2:25.

Bahn RS, Heufelder AE. Pathogenesis of Graves' ophthalmopathy. N Engl J Med 1993;329:1468.

Barnes HV. Diffuse goiter in the euthyroid adolescent. J Curr Adolesc Med 1979;1:49.

Bayer MF. Effective laboratory evaluation of thyroid status. Med Clin North Am. 1991;75:1.

Bethune JE. Interpretation of thyroid function tests. Dis Mon 1989;35:541.

Boigon M, Moyer D. Solitary thyroid nodules. Separating benign from malignant conditions. Postgrad Med 1995;98:73.

Brody MB, Reichard RA. Thyroid screening: how to interpret and apply the results. Postgrad Med 1995; 98:54.

Brown J, Solomon DH, Beall GN, et al. Autoimmune thyroid disease, Graves', and Hashimoto's. Ann Intern Med 1978;88:379.

Celani MF, Mariani M, Mariani G. On the usefulness of levothyroxine suppressive therapy in the medical treatment of benign solitary, solid or predominantly solid, thyroid nodules. Acta Endocrinol (Copenh) 1990;123:603.

Clark OH, Duh QY. Thyroid cancer. Med Clin North Am 1991;75:211.

Collen RJ, Landaw EM, Kaplan SA, et al. Remission rates of children and adolescents with thyrotoxicosis treated with antithyroid drugs. Pediatrics 1980;65:550.

Cooper DS, Halpern R, Wood LC, et al. L-Thyroxine therapy in subclinical hypothyroidism: a double-blind, placebo-controlled trial. Ann Intern Med 1984;101:18.

Cooper DS, Korytkowski M. The treatment of hyperthyroidism. Mod Med 1988;56:94.

DeJong SA, Demeter JG, Jarosz H, et al. Thyroid carcinoma and hyperparathyroidism after radiation therapy for adolescent acne vulgaris. Surgery 1991;110:691.

De los Santos ET, Mazzaferri EL. Thyroid function tests: guidelines for interpretation in common clinical disorders. Postgrad Med 1989;85:333.

Dunn JT. Choice of therapy in young adults with hyperthyroidism of Graves' disease: a brief, case-directed poll of fifty-four thyroidologists. Ann Intern Med 1984;100:891.

Ehrmann DA, Sarne DH. Serum thyrotropin and the assessment of thyroid status. Ann Intern Med 1989;110:179.

Franklyn JA. The management of hyperthyroidism. N Engl J Med 1994;330:1731.

Gavin LA. Thyroid crises. Med Clin North Am 1991;75:179.

Gharib H. A strategy for the solitary thyroid nodule. Hosp Pract 1992;27:53.

Gharib H, James M, Charboneau W, et al. Suppressive therapy with levothyroxine for solitary thyroid nodules: a double-blind controlled clinical study. N Engl J Med 1987;317:70.

Graham GD, Burman KD. Radioiodine treatment of Graves' disease: an assessment of its potential risks. Ann Intern Med 1986;105:900.

Hamburger JI. The various presentations of thyroiditis: diagnostic considerations. Ann Intern Med 1986;104:219.

Hashizume K, Ichikawa K, Sakurai A, et al. Administration of thyroxine in treated Graves' disease: effects on the level of antibodies to thyroid-stimulating hormone receptors and on the risk of recurrence of hyperthyroidism. N Engl J Med 1991;324:947.

Hay ID. Thyroiditis: a clinical update. Mayo Clin Proc 1985;60:836.

Helfand M, Crapo LM. Screening for thyroid disease. Ann Intern Med 1990a;112:840.

Helfand M, Crapo LM. Monitoring therapy in patients taking levothyroxine. Ann Intern Med 1990b;113:450.

Hennessey JV, Burman KD, Wartofsky, L. The equivalency of two L-Thyroxine preparations. Ann Intern Med 1985;102:770.

Hennessey JV, Evaul JE, Tseng Y, et al. L-Thyroxine dosage: a reevaluation of therapy with contemporary preparations. Ann Intern Med 1986;105:11.

Herle AJV Rich P, Ljung BE, et al. The thyroid nodule. Ann Intern Med 1982;96:221.

Houston M, Hay ID. Practical management of hyperthyroidism. Am Fam Physician 1990;41:909.

Klein I, Levey GS. Silent thyrotoxic thyroiditis. Ann Intern Med 1982;96:242.

Klein I, Trzepacz PT, Roberts M, et al. Symptom rating scale for assessing hyperthyroidism. Arch Intern Med 1988;148:387.

Kuhel WI, Ward RF. Thyroid cancer in children. Lancet 1995;346:719.

Kung AW, Pun KK. Bone mineral density in premenopausal women receiving long-term physiological doses of levothyroxine. JAMA 1991;265:2688.

Lavin A, Nauss AH. Hypothyroidism in otherwise healthy hypercholesterolemic children. Pediatrics 1991;88:332.

Liaw YF, Huan MJ, Fan KD, et al. Hepatic injury during propylthiouracil therapy in patients with hyperthyroidism. Ann Intern Med 1993;118:424.

McConahey WM, Hay ID, Woolner LB, et al. Papillary thyroid cancer treated at the Mayo Clinic, 1946 through 1970: initial manifestations, pathologic findings, therapy, and outcome. Mayo Clin Proc 1986;61:978.

McFarland KF, Saleeby G. Graves' disease: manifestations and therapeutic options. Postgrad Med 1988;83:275.

Mazzaferri EL. Management of a solitary thyroid nodule. N Engl J Med 1993;328:553.

Mendel SJ, Brent GA, Larsen PR. Levothyroxine therapy in patients with thyroid disease. Ann Intern Med 1993;119:492.

Momotani N, Nog J, Oyanagi H, et al. Antithyroid drug therapy for Graves' disease during pregnancy: optimal regimen for fetal thyroid status. N Engl J Med 1986;315:24.

Mullin GE, Eastern JS. Cutaneous signs of thyroid disease. Am Fam Physician 1986;34:93.

Nikolai TF, Coombs GJ, McKenzie AK. Lymphocytic thyroiditis with spontaneously resolving hyperthyroidism and subacute thyroiditis: long-term follow-up. Arch Intern Med 1981;141:1455.

Nikolai TF, Coombs GJ, McKenzie AK, et al. Treatment of lymphocytic thyroiditis with spontaneously resolving hyperthyroidism (silent thyroiditis). Arch Intern Med 1982;142:2281.

Nordyke RA, Gilbert FI Jr, Miyamoto LA, et al. The superiority of antimicrosomal over antithyroglobulin antibodies for detecting Hashimoto's thyroiditis. Arch Intern Med 1993;153:862.

Prummel MF, Mourits MP, Berghout A, et al. Prednisone and cyclosporine in the treatment of severe Graves' ophthalmopathy. N Engl J Med 1989;321:1353.

Raab SS, Silverman JF, Elsheikh TM, et al. Pediatric thyroid nodules: disease demographics and clinical management as determined by fine-needle aspiration biopsy. Pediatrics 1995;95:46.

Rallison ML, Dobyns BM, Meikle AW, et al. Natural history of thyroid abnormalities: prevalence, incidence, and regression of thyroid diseases in adolescents and young adults. Am J Med 1991;91:363.

Ridgway EC. Clinician's evaluation of a solitary thyroid nodule [Clinical Review 30]. J Clin Endocrinol Metab 1992;74:231.

Rifat SF, Ruffin MT IV. Management of thyroid nodules. Am Fam Physician 1994;50:785.

Roberts JW, McKenney JF Jr. Answers to questions on thyroid nodules. Hosp Med 1986;22(July):25.

Rogers DG. Thyroid disease in children. Am Fam Physician 1994;50:344.

Ross DS. New sensitive immunoradiometric assays for thyrotropin. Ann Intern Med 1986;104:718.

Sawin CT, Surks MI, London M, et al. Oral thyroxine: variation in biologic action and tablet content. Ann Intern Med 1984;100:641.

Singer PA, Cooper DS, Levy EG, et al. Treatment guidelines for patients with hyperthyroidism and hypothyroidism. Standards of Care Committee, American Thyroid Association. JAMA 1995;273:808.

Surks MI, Chopra IJ, Mariash CN, et al. American Thyroid Association guidelines for use of laboratory tests in thyroid disorders. JAMA 1990;263:1529.

Szabo SM, Allen DB. Thyroiditis: differentiation of acute suppurative and subacute—case report and review of the literature. Clin Pediatr 1989;28:171.

Toft A. Thyroxine replacement therapy. Clin Endocrinol (Oxf) 1991;34:103.

CHAPTER 10
Gynecomastia

DEFINITION

Gynecomastia refers to a benign increase in glandular and stromal tissue associated with puberty. Gynecomastia must be differentiated from a lipoma and from fatty tissue of obese patients.

EPIDEMIOLOGY

1. Gynecomastia occurs in 19.6% of $10^1/_2$-year-old males, with a peak prevalence of 64% at 14 years and falling prevalence thereafter. Mean age at onset is 13 years 2 months. Approximately 4% of adolescents will have severe gynecomastia (>4.0 cm in diameter or about equal to mid-pubescent female breast) that persists into adulthood. Gynecomastia is also common during the neonatal period (60–90% of newborn infants) and between 50 and 80 years of age.
2. Relationship with puberty: Best correlated with biological events of puberty. Genital stage at onset of gynecomastia is as follows:

Genital stage 1	20%
Genital stage 2	50%
Genital stage 3	20%
Genital stage 4	10%

ETIOLOGY

Breast tissue of males and females is similar at birth and responds similarly to estrogens during childhood. At puberty, the breast tissue of boys demonstrates both ductal and periductal mesenchymal tissue proliferation. This tissue involutes and atrophies as testicular androgens increase to adult levels. In pubertal females, under the influence of both increasing estrogen and progesterone, breast tissue continues to undergo ductal enlargement, branching, and acini development. The hormonal levels determine the extent of breast tissue development. Because estrogens stimulate breast tissue development and androgens antagonize this effect, an increase in estrogen relative to testosterone can lead to gynecomastia.

Gynecomastia has been considered to result from an imbalance between circulating estrogens and androgens. Alterations in the ratio of estrogens to androgens have been demonstrated in individuals with gynecomastia related to Klinefelter's syndrome, thyrotoxicosis, cirrhosis, medications, adrenal and testicular neoplasm, primary hypogonadism, and malnutrition.

Mechanisms to account for an increase in estrogens or a decrease in androgens include:

1. Increase in serum estrogen concentrations
   a. Increase in estradiol secretion from testes (e.g., Leydig cell tumors)

210

    b. Excessive extraglandular conversion of androgens to estrogens by aromatase
- Overproduction of adrenal precursors; increased androstenedione converted by aromatase into estrone
- Overproduction of testicular precursors; increased conversion of testosterone to estradiol
- Enhancement of extraglandular aromatase activity
    - (1) Disease states (hyperthyroidism, liver disease)
    - (2) Increased body fat (obesity, ageing)
    - (3) Drugs (e.g., spironolactone)
    - (4) Idiopathic change (caused by persistence of a fetal form of aromatase)

    c. Increase in bioavailability of estrogens: Decrease in estrogens bound to sex-hormone–binding globulin (e.g., use of spironolactone and ketoconazole)

    d. Exogenous intake of estrogens: Oral intake of estrogens or topical use of estrogen creams

2. Decrease in serum androgen concentrations
    a. Impairment of testicular production in Leydig cells
- Primary hypogonadism
- Secondary hypogonadism through disorders of hypothalamus or pituitary
- Congenital enzyme defects
- Drug-induced inhibition of enzymes needed in testosterone synthesis (e.g., spironolactone, ketoconazole)
- Chronic stimulation of Leydig cells by high human chorionic gonadotropin (hCG) levels (e.g., hCG-secreting tumors); can lead to a reduction in testosterone biosynthesis
- Hyperestrogenic states leading to suppression of luteinizing hormone (LH) and testosterone secretion

    b. Increased hepatic clearance of androgens

    c. Increase in sex-hormone–binding globulin, leading to decrease in free testosterone (e.g., liver disease, hyperestrogenic states)

3. Alterations of estrogen and androgen receptors
    a. Androgen-receptor deficiency states (e.g., androgen insensitivity syndromes)

    b. Drug interference with androgen receptors (e.g., spironolactone, flutamide, cimetidine)

    c. Drugs that can mimic estrogens and stimulate estrogen receptor sites (e.g., digoxin; phytoestrogens in some marijuana preparations)

CLINICAL MANIFESTATIONS

1. Forms:
    a. Type I—One or more subareolar nodules, freely movable
    b. Type II—Breast nodules beneath areola but also extending beyond areolar perimeter
    c. Type III—Resembles breast development of sexual maturity rating 3 in the female

2. Bilaterality: Occurs in 77–95% of cases, with concurrent or sequential involvement of both breasts

3. Physical examination
    a. Types I and II gynecomastia—associated with a firm, rubbery consistency of the breasts (whereas type III is associated with a consistency similar to that of female breasts)
    b. Types I and II—usually associated with tenderness on palpation or when clothing touches the breast

DIFFERENTIAL DIAGNOSIS (adapted from Braunstein, 1993a)

1. Physiological: Pubertal gynecomastia
2. Drug exposure (Asterisk indicates that a strong relationship has been established; other drugs have been implicated through epidemiological studies, individual cases, or small groups of patients.)
   a. Hormones: Estrogens,* Testosterone,* Anabolic steroids*
   b. Psychoactive agents: Phenothiazines, diazepam, haloperidol, tricyclic antidepressants
   c. Cardiovascular drugs: Digoxin,* verapamil, captopril, methyldopa, nifedipine, enalapril, reserpine, minoxidil
   d. Antiandrogens or inhibitors of androgen synthesis: Cyproterone,* spironolactone,* flutamide*
   e. Antibiotics: Isoniazid, metronidazole, ketoconazole*
   f. Antiulcer medications: Cimetidine,* ranitidine, omeprazole
   g. Cancer chemotherapeutics, especially alkylating agents*
   h. Drugs of abuse: Marijuana, alcohol, amphetamines, heroin
   i. Other: Phenytoin, penicillamine
3. Pathological
   a. Renal failure and dialysis
   b. Recovery from malnutrition
   c. Primary gonadal failure: Including Klinefelter's syndrome and Reifenstein's syndrome
   d. Secondary hypogonadism
   e. Hyperthyroidism
   f. Liver disease, including cirrhosis and hepatoma
   g. Neoplasms
      — Testicular: Germ cell, Leydig cell, or Sertoli cell
      — Adrenal adenomas and carcinoma
      — Ectopic hCG production (especially lung, liver, and kidney cancer)
   h. Enzyme defects in testosterone biosynthesis
   i. Androgen insensitivity syndromes
   j. Excessive extraglandular aromatase activity
4. Pseudogynecomastia: Caused by adipose tissue in obese males or prominence of muscular adolescent males
5. Breast mass because of cancer, dermoid cyst, lipoma, hematoma, or neurofibroma

DIAGNOSIS

1. History: Careful history necessary to rule out drugs and systemic illness
2. Physical examination
   a. Findings suggestive of hypogonadism, hyperthyroidism, or hypothyroidism
   b. Testicular mass or atrophy
   c. Findings suggestive of liver disease
   d. Vertical and horizontal diameters of breast tissue (breast units = vertical diameter of breast × horizontal diameter)
   e. Differentiation of gynecomastia from pseudogynecomastia caused by excessive adipose tissue
      — Place teen in supine position, with the teen's hands behind his head. Examiner then places the thumb and forefinger at opposing margins of the breast
      — In gynecomastia, as the fingers are brought together, rubbery or firm breast tissue can be felt as a freely movable, and occasionally tender, disk of tissue concentric to the areola

— In pseudogynecomastia, no discrete mass is felt
— In other conditions, such as a lipoma or dermoid cyst, the mass is usually eccentric to the areola

In healthy pubertal males with a unilateral or bilateral, rubbery or firm mass, symmetrically subareolar, with no history of use of drugs associated with gynecomastia and with no renal, liver, or thyroid disease, the diagnosis is probable pubertal gynecomastia. No further tests are necessary in these teens. If associated drugs have been used, they should be discontinued and the teen reexamined in 1 month. At that time, breast tenderness, if present, should decrease and breast size may decrease.

If pubertal gynecomastia and drug, hepatic, and renal causes are ruled out, then a further endocrine diagnostic study is appropriate. The practitioner should order measurements of hCG, LH, serum testosterone, and estradiol. These tests will help in differentiating the cause of nonpubertal gynecomastia.

FINDINGS AND IMPLICATIONS OF SERUM hCG, LH, TESTOSTERONE, AND ESTRADIOL

1. Elevated hCG concentration: Perform testicular ultrasonography
   a. Mass found: Testicular germ cell tumor
   b. Normal sonogram: Extragonadal germ cell tumor or hCG-secreting neoplasm likely; chest film and abdominal computed tomography (CT) indicated
2. Decreased testosterone concentration
   a. Elevated LH concentration: Primary hypogonadism, including Klinefelter's syndrome, and testicular atrophy caused by mumps orchitis
   b. Normal or low LH concentration: Measure prolactin; magnetic resonance imaging (MRI) of hypothalamic pituitary area
      — Elevated prolactin level: Probably prolactin-secreting pituitary tumor
      — Normal prolactin level: Secondary hypogonadism
3. Elevated testosterone and elevated LH concentrations: Measure thyroxine (T_4) and thyroid-stimulating hormone (TSH)
   a. Elevated T_4 and low TSH concentrations: Hyperthyroidism (elevated testosterone is from the increase of sex-hormone–binding globulin, leading to an increase in total testosterone; the increase in LH with hyperthyroidism is less clear)
   b. Normal T_4 and TSH concentrations: Androgen resistance
4. Elevated estradiol and low or normal LH concentrations: Perform testicular ultrasonography
   a. Mass on sonogram: Leydig cell or Sertoli cell tumor
   b. Normal: Perform adrenal CT or MRI
      — Mass found: Adrenal neoplasm
      — No mass: Increased extraglandular aromatase activity
5. Normal concentrations of hCG, LH, testosterone, and estradiol: Idiopathic gynecomastia

THERAPY

1. Rule out other causes aside from pubertal gynecomastia. If other causes are diagnosed, they should be treated. If drugs are implicated, they should be discontinued, if possible.
2. Pubertal gynecomastia: In most individuals with pubertal gynecomastia, particularly with mild to moderate degrees, only reassurance and explanation of the process are needed. In most cases the condition will improve or resolve within 6–12 months.

3. Medical intervention
   a. Several drugs have been tried to reduce gynecomastia, including danazol, tamoxifen, clomiphene, dihydrotestosterone, and testolactone. None of these is approved by the U.S. Food and Drug Administration in the treatment of gynecomastia, and studies of the use of these medications in adolescent patients are minimal. Dihydrotestosterone can lead to a reduction in breast volume in 75% of individuals, with 25% having a complete response (Kuhn et al., 1983). However, this medication is not readily available. Danazol has some limited effectiveness but is associated with significant side effects and would not be recommended in the treatment of adolescents. Tamoxifen has been studied in two randomized, double-blind studies involving 16 patients. At a dosage of 10 mg twice a day, the drug has led to a statistically significant reduction in breast size and pain without side effects. Testolactone, an aromatase inhibitor, has also been found in an uncontrolled study to decrease pubertal gynecomastia without side effects.
   b. At present, medical therapy should be reserved for those individuals who have more than mild to moderate gynecomastia and who are significantly concerned about the condition. Tamoxifen could be used at an oral dose of 10 mg twice a day for a 3-month course. This should lead to a decrease in tenderness and pain, followed by reduction in size of breast tissue.
4. Surgical intervention: In adolescents with moderate to severe gynecomastia associated with psychological sequelae, surgical excision is recommended.

PROGNOSIS

Pubertal gynecomastia usually resolves in 12–18 months. In 27% of affected adolescents, the condition lasts for more than 1 year and in 7.7% more than 2 years. A small percentage of cases may persist into adulthood. There has been no proven relationship between gynecomastia and the development of breast cancer in males.

BIBLIOGRAPHY

Ardick KR. Holiday gynecomastia related to marijuana? Ann Intern Med 1993:119;253.

Biro FM, Lucky AW, Huster GA, Morrison JA. Hormonal studies and physical maturation in adolescent gynecomastia. J Pediatr 1990;116:450.

Bower R, Bell M, Ternberg J. Management of breast lesions in children and adolescents. J Pediatr Surg 1976; 3:337.

Braunstein GD. Gynecomastia. N Engl J Med 1993a;328: 490.

Braunstein GD. Diagnosis and treatment of gynecomastia. Hosp Pract 1993b;28:37.

Brenner P, Berger A, Schneider W, Axmann HD. Male reduction mammoplasty in serious gynecomastias. Aesthetic Plast Surg 1992;16:325.

Carlson HE. Current concepts: gynecomastia. N Engl J Med 1980;303:795.

Eberle AJ, Sparrow JT, Keenan BS. Treatment of persistent pubertal gynecomastia with dihydrotestosterone heptanoate. J Pediatr 1986;109:144.

Fagan TC, Johnson DG, Grosso DS. Metronidazole-induced gynecomastia. JAMA 1985;254:3217.

Kuhn JM, Roca R, Laudat MH, et al. Studies on the treatment of idiopathic gynaecomastia with percutaneous dihydrotestosterone. Clin Endocrinol 1983;19:513.

Large DM, Anderson DC. Twenty-four-hour profiles of circulating androgens and oestrogens in male puberty with and without gynecomastia. Clin Endocrinol 1979;11:505.

Lee PA. Pubertal gynecomastia. Br Med J 1976;1:1238.

Marynick SP, Nisula BC, Pita JC Jr, et al. Persistent pubertal macromastia. J Clin Endocrinol Metab 1980; 50:128.

Moore DC, Schlaepfer LV, Paunier L, et al. Hormonal changes during puberty. V. Transient pubertal gynecomastia: abnormal androgen-estrogen ratio. J Clin Endocrinol Metab 1984;58:492.

Nydick M, Bustos J, Dale JH, et al. Gynecomastia in adolescent boys. JAMA 1961;178:449.

Parker LN, Gray DR, Lai MK, et al. Treatment of gynecomastia with tamoxifen: a double-blind crossover study. Metabolism 1986;35:705.

Plourde PV, Kulin HE, Santner SJ. Clomiphene in the treatment of adolescent gynecomastia. Am J Dis Child 1983;137:1080.

Thompson DF, Carter JR. Drug-induced gynecomastia. Pharmacotherapy 1993;13:37.

Zachmann M, Eiholzer U, Muritano M, et al. Treatment of pubertal gynaecomastia with testolactone. Acta Endocrinol Suppl (Copenh) 1986;279:218.

Cardiovascular Problems

CHAPTER 11

Cardiac Risk Factors and Hyperlipidemia

Marc S. Jacobsen, Michael R. Kohn, and Lawrence S. Neinstein

One of the goals of adolescent health care is early intervention to prevent diseases that occur during adulthood. The pathogenesis of atherosclerosis begins in childhood and results from the interaction of environmental factors with the genetic endowment. Although not all the issues of identifying risk for cardiovascular disease are resolved, much has been learned. The effectiveness of interventions thus far described in reducing risk factors for children and adolescents has been demonstrated. Whether there is also a reduction in subsequent cardiac disease remains to be determined. However, it is now advisable to screen for risk factors and to provide appropriate management for those risk factors which are intervenable.

CARDIAC RISK FACTORS

Nonintervenable

1. Age
2. Sex (male)
3. Family history: Parent or grandparent, at 55 years of age or younger, with atherosclerosis or its sequelae
4. Parent with elevated cholesterol concentration (>240 mg/dL)

Intervenable

1. Smoking regularly
2. Hypertension: Systolic or diastolic blood pressure greater than the 95th percentile
3. Diet high in saturated fats, cholesterol, and total fats more than 30% of daily caloric intake
4. Dyslipidemia (modified from recommendations of the Expert Panel on Blood Cholesterol Levels in Children and Adolescents, 1992)
   a. Total cholesterol: More than 170 mg/dL
   b. Low-density lipoprotein (LDL) cholesterol: More than 130 mg/dL
   c. High-density lipoprotein (HDL) cholesterol: Less than 35 mg/dL
   d. Triglycerides: More than 150 mg/dL
5. Obesity: More than 30% above expected weight, or body mass index (BMI) above the 95th percentile for age

Section III CARDIOVASCULAR PROBLEMS

RISK FACTOR INTERVENTION

Practitioners must temper aggressive interventions with the knowledge that the efficacy of interventions in decreasing the rate of coronary artery disease (CAD) has been evaluated only in adults. Thus, the effect of such interventions in childhood and adolescents is more speculative. However, because early atherosclerotic lesions have already begun in the majority of adolescents and are worse in those with risk factors, it seems prudent to recommend a heart-healthy lifestyle to reduce atherosclerosis and CAD. This approach includes:

1. Promoting regular physical activity
2. Counseling on the importance of maintaining an ideal body weight
3. Advocating smoking prevention or cessation
4. Monitoring blood pressure and treating when persistently elevated
5. Recommending a heart-healthy diet—less than 30% of the total calories as fat, and low in saturated fat—for all individuals

Hypertension

The distribution of blood pressure in children and adolescents was described by the Second Task Force on Blood Pressure Control, and hypertension was classified, by age, as being "significant" or "severe" (Table 11.1). For adolescents with "significant" hypertension (i.e., diastolic blood pressure >86 mm Hg at 13–15 years of age or >92 mm Hg at 16–18 years) and no other risk factors, interventions should include a low-salt diet, weight reduction, and relaxation or other biofeedback techniques. Intervention for hypertension is covered in more detail in Chapter 12.

Cigarette Smoking

Cigarette smoke is an atherogenic risk factor due to alterations in lipids and fibrinogen. Smoking is associated with more cardiovascular deaths than cancer deaths. Most cigarette smoking begins early in adolescence, suggesting that this is an important period for prevention. Effective education programs must be developed and implemented at the national level, at the local school level, and in the practitioner's office. Every preteen and teen should be questioned regarding his or her smoking habits, and specific interventions should be targeted to prevent or extinguish smoking behavior.

Dyslipidemia

The primary therapy for hyperlipidemia during adolescence is modification of the diet, including a diet that is low in fat, saturated fats, and cholesterol. Regular physical activity is also indicated. Medications should be reserved for those teenagers with markedly high concen-

TABLE 11.1. Classification of Hypertension by Age Group

Age Group	Significant Hypertension (mm Hg)	Severe Hypertension (mm Hg)
Children (10–12 yr)	Systolic BP[a] >126	Systolic BP >134
	Diastolic BP >82	Diastolic BP >90
Adolescents (13–15 yr)	Systolic BP >136	Systolic BP >144
	Diastolic BP >86	Diastolic BP >92
Adolescents (16–18 yr)	Systolic BP >142	Systolic BP >150
	Diastolic BP >92	Diastolic BP >98

Adapted from Report of the Second Task Force on Blood Pressure Control in Children—1987. Pediatrics 1987;79:1–25.
[a]BP, blood pressure.

trations of lipids unresponsive to dietary therapy and with an extensive family history (see following section on hyperlipidemia).

Obesity

The best therapy for obesity is to prevent it. This requires curbing obesity early and particularly during the adolescent growth spurt. Without intervention, 8 out of 10 obese 12-year-old children will become obese adults. Exercise and other physical activity combined with dietary modifications are the best preventive measures, and some studies are showing positive results.

LIPID PHYSIOLOGY

Cholesterol and triglycerides are the major blood lipids. Cholesterol is a key constituent of cell membranes and a precursor of bile acids and steroid hormones. Cholesterol circulates in the bloodstream in spherical particles called lipoproteins containing both lipids and proteins called apoproteins. These particles consist of a core of triglycerides, cholesterol, and cholesterol esters, in varying amounts, surrounded by an outer shell of cholesterol and phospholipids. The apoproteins are embedded in the outer lipid layers (Fig. 11.1).

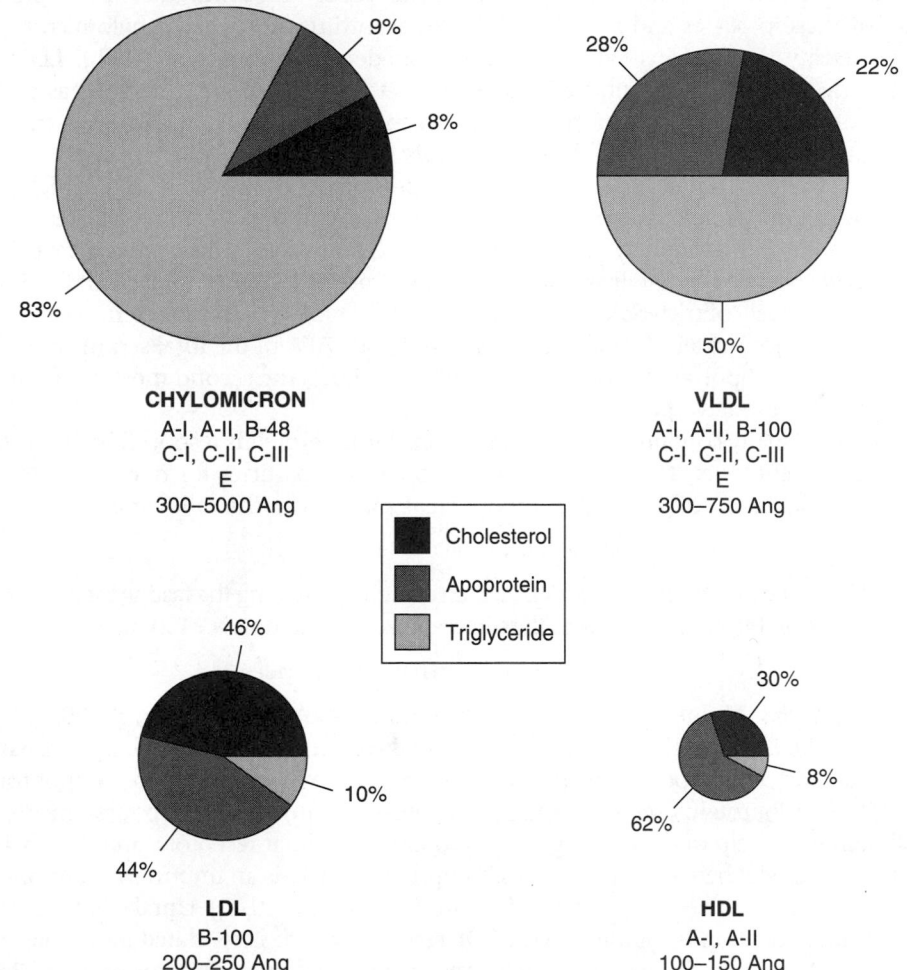

FIGURE 11.1.   Characteristics of lipoproteins. Apoproteins and volume are detailed below each lipoprotein. (Adapted from Hardoff D, Jacobson MS. Hyperlipidemia. Adolesc Med State Arts Rev 1992;3:475.)

TABLE 11.2.   Characteristics and Functions of Plasma Lipoproteins[a]

Ultracentrifugation	Electrophoresis	Density (g/mL)	Size (Å)	T (%)	C (%)	PH (%)	PR (%)
Chylomicron	Chylomicron	0.95	750–10,000	80–90	9	7	2
VLDL	Prebeta	0.95–1.006	300–800	50–70	20	18	7
LDL	Beta	1.019–1.063	200–230	9	47	23	21
HDL	Alpha	1.063–1.2	75–100	8	19	26	46

Adapted from Fleischmajer, R. A review of hypolipedemic drug therapy. Med Times 1981;December; and Lavie, C.J., et al. Management of lipids in primary and secondary prevention of cardiovascular diseases. Mayo Clin Prac 1988;63:605.
[a]T, triglycerides; C, cholesterol; PH, phospholipids; PR, protein.

1. Classification of lipoproteins: Five major classes of lipoproteins act as transport systems for cholesterol and triglycerides. They differ in physical and chemical characteristics and function, as well as in amounts of cholesterol, triglyceride, phospholipid, and protein. The lipoproteins can be separated by ultracentrifugation or electrophoresis, on the basis of differences in densities and surface properties. Table 11.2 summarizes the characteristics of these particles and their function. Ultracentrifugation yields chylomicrons, very low density lipoproteins (VLDL), intermediate-density lipoproteins (IDL), LDLs, and HDLs. Motility on electrophoresis yields the patterns commonly described as alpha-1, beta, prebeta, and broad beta (motility between beta and prebeta). However, this older designation, based on electrophoretic mobility, is no longer frequently used.
   a. *Chylomicrons:* Largest and least dense of the lipoproteins; composed mainly of triglycerides with a lipid/protein ratio of 99:1. Chylomicrons carry dietary fat as triglycerides from the intestine to the periphery of the body to be used for energy or deposition in fat cells.
   b. *VLDL:* Secreted by the liver and is the second major carrier of triglycerides. It is composed largely of triglycerides and contains less than 10% of the total serum cholesterol.
   c. *LDL:* Major carrier of cholesterol, containing 60–70% of the total serum cholesterol, and is an important factor in atherogenesis. (HDL is the second most important carrier of cholesterol.)
   d. *HDL:* Usually contains 20–30% of the total cholesterol. It is responsible for the transport of cholesterol back to triglyceride-containing particles for removal in the bile. The calculation of the proportion of LDL is made from the following formula:

   $$\text{Total cholesterol} = \text{LDL} + \text{HDL} + \text{VLDL}$$

   HDL is measured directly, and VLDL is estimated by dividing the fasting triglyceride concentration by 5 (true so long as the triglyceride concentration is <400 mg/dL). Therefore,

   $$\text{LDL} = \text{total cholesterol} - \text{HDL} - \text{triglycerides}/5$$

   e. *Apoproteins:* Numerous apoproteins, including A-I, A-II, A-IV, B-48, B-100, C-I, C-II, C-III, D, E-2, E-4, F, G, and H, are associated with lipoproteins. Each lipoprotein has a characteristic apoprotein profile. Lipoproteins may contain several apoproteins. These apoproteins serve as cofactors for enzymes involved in lipoprotein metabolism, they help in the binding of lipoproteins to cellular receptors, and they facilitate lipid transfer between lipoproteins. Apoprotein B-100 is an important component of VLDL and is the only apoprotein in LDL-cholesterol (LDL-C). Uptake of LDL by cells is dependent on its binding to the LDL receptor, which is regulated by apoprotein B-100. Abnormalities in both quality and quantity of these proteins, even in the absence of an elevated cholesterol concentration, may contribute to atherosclerosis.

TABLE 11.2.   *continued*

Origin	Destination	Function	Major Apoprotein
Intestine	Triglyceride storage and metabolizing cells, liver	Transport of dietary triglycerides	Apo A-I, A-4, B, C
Liver	Triglyceride storage and metabolizing cells	Transport of endogenously synthesized triglycerides and some cholesterol	Apo B, C-I, C-II, C-III, E
Metabolism of VLDL	Peripheral cells, liver	Transport of cholesteryl esters of intravascular and hepatic origin	Apo B
Intestine, liver	Liver, steroidogenic tissues	Reverse transport of cholesterol of peripheral origin	Apo A-I, A-II, D, E, C-1, C-2, C-3

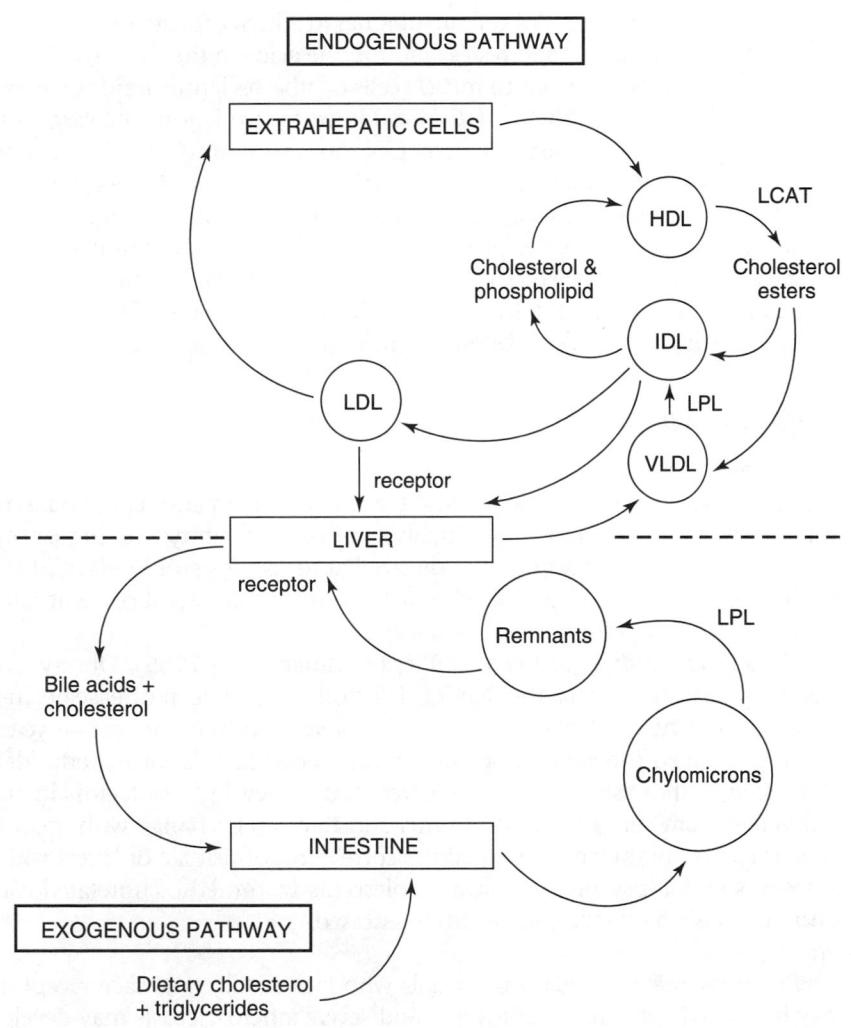

FIGURE 11.2.   Pathways of lipoprotein metabolism. *LCAT,* lecithin cholesterol acyltransferase; *LPL,* lipoprotein lipase. (From Weis S, Lacko AG. Pract Cardiol 1988;May:12–18.)

2. Lipoprotein circulation and sources (Fig. 11.2)
   a. Exogenous: Chylomicrons are formed in the gut wall after absorption of dietary fat. They are secreted into the lymph and enter the bloodstream, where the fatty acids are stored in adipose tissue, or are used in skeletal muscle and myocardium. Eventually they release almost all of their diet-derived triglyceride. This reaction is catalyzed by lipoprotein lipase. The chylomicron remnants are rapidly absorbed by the liver by specific receptors for these particles. In liver cells the remnants are degraded to free cholesterol, which is excreted into bile.
   b. Endogenous: The endogenous transport system includes VLDL, IDL, LDL, and HDL. Excess calories from carbohydrates and fatty acids are metabolized in the liver into triglycerides. The lipoproteins carrying these triglycerides are primarily VLDL, which moves to adipose tissue, where triglycerides are extracted; the result is the formation of IDL and LDL. The IDL particles are rapidly removed from circulation by LDL receptors in the liver.
      — LDL transports cholesterol to peripheral tissues. Besides the lipid component, LDL particles contain a single apoprotein B-100 molecule, the protein that binds to LDL receptors. After binding to LDL cell surface receptors, the LDL particles deliver cholesterol for synthesis of cell membranes in all cells; for steroid hormones in the adrenal glands, ovary, and testes; and for bile acids in the liver. The LDL-C found in macrophages and smooth muscle cells of atherosclerotic lesions enters by additional mechanisms. This LDL-C is modified by oxidation intravascularly and is taken up in lesions by oxy-LDL receptors and scavenger receptors. This process may provide alternative pathways for therapeutic intervention in the future.
      — HDL lipoproteins are secreted from the liver or intestine in a lipid-poor form or are made de novo in the plasma. As it matures, HDL accumulates cholesterol from tissues, including blood vessel walls, and thus has a major role in removing excess cholesterol and delivering it to the liver by means of the triglyceride-rich lipoproteins and cholesterol ester transfer protein.

LIPID PATHOPHYSIOLOGY

1. Epidemiological evidence
   a. In populations throughout the world there is a direct correlation between serum cholesterol levels and CAD rates. Individuals moving to a country with higher mean cholesterol levels gradually acquire the dietary habits, cholesterol levels, and CAD rates of their new country. In societies in which the total cholesterol concentration is less than 150 mg/dL, CAD is rare.
   b. Bogalusa Heart Study (Croft et al., 1986; Freedman et al., 1985): Observations from this study clearly show that the major risk factors of adult heart disease begin in childhood. Documented atherosclerotic changes were seen to occur by 5–8 years of age. This group noted the significance of environmental factors for hyperlipidemia, hypertension, and obesity. They also showed that the level of risk factors in childhood is different from that in the adult years and that levels change with growth phase. Most importantly they documented the correlation of risk factor levels with severity of lesions in autopsy material from adolescents who died of unrelated causes and who previously had been prospectively assessed.
2. Genetic evidence
   a. *Familial hypercholesterolemia:* Individuals who lack LDL cell surface receptor activity may have very high cholesterol levels, and severe atherosclerosis may develop in the first two decades of life. These individuals are referred to as having familial hypercholesterolemia. Those heterozygous for the LDL receptor defect account for 15% of premature CAD. Clinical manifestations such as xanthomas and other signs of cuta-

neous lipid deposition are generally seen in the fourth decade of life in heterozygotes and in adolescence in homozygotes.

b. *Familial combined hyperlipidemia (FCHL):* Autosomal dominant syndrome that affects approximately 1–2% of the population. Most, if not all, patients with this condition have elevated levels of LDL–apoprotein B (apoB). Abnormal metabolism of VLDL and partial lipoprotein lipase deficiency have also been described in association with this syndrome. Individuals with familial hypercholesterolemia (FH) account for a significant proportion of early CAD.

c. *Apoprotein E:* Three common alleles of apoprotein E (apoE), at a single-gene locus on chromosome 19, code for three isoforms of apoE: designated as apoE-2, apoE-3, and apoE-4. These are distinguished in the laboratory by isoelectric focusing. Both homozygous and heterozygous genotypes have been found. Increased cardiovascular risk is associated with apoE-2 and apoE-4, in comparison with the more common apoE-3.

3. Animal models: Atherosclerosis develops in animals fed diets elevating their serum cholesterol levels. In other animal experiments, a change of diet and the use of lipid-lowering drugs reduced elevated cholesterol levels and caused regression in atherosclerotic plaques.

4. Interventional trials: More than a dozen randomized clinical trials in adults have examined the effects of lowering cholesterol on CAD. These trials support the conclusion that lowering total and LDL-C levels reduces the incidence of CAD events. The degree of benefits is greatest in individuals who have other associated risk factors, such as cigarette smoking and hypertension. Examples of the most significant studies include:

a. *Coronary Primary Prevention Trial (CPPT):* A longitudinal double-blind study of asymptomatic men with hypercholesterolemia. This study demonstrated a decreased CAD risk of 2% for every 1% lowering of the serum cholesterol levels in adults with levels initially in the 250–300 mg/dL range.

b. *Helsinki Heart Study:* In this study the use of gemfibrozil lowered LDL-C by 8% and increased HDL-cholesterol (HDL-C) by 10%. This led to a 34% decrease in the incidence of CAD.

c. *Multiple Risk Factor Intervention Trial (MRFIT):* This study demonstrated that there is no threshold level of cholesterol for the development of atherosclerotic lesions. The study reported a relative risk of 0.7 with a level of 150 mg/dL, 1.0 with a level of 200 mg/dL, 2.0 with a level of 250 mg/dL, and 4.0 with a level of 300 mg/dL.

d. *Pathobiological Determinants of Atherosclerosis in Youth (PDAY):* This research group described the relationship of atherosclerosis in young men to serum lipoprotein cholesterol concentrations and smoking. A preliminary report demonstrated an association between commonly accepted risk factors (elevated LDL-C and low HDL-C concentrations and smoking) and the severity of atherosclerotic plaques in adolescents.

5. Relationship of particular lipoproteins

a. *LDL-C:* Studies show a positive relationship between the level of cholesterol, particularly LDL, and the frequency of CAD. There appear to be several outcomes for LDL. Any LDL that is not cleared by LDL receptors is metabolized by nonreceptor mechanisms, which may play a role in atherosclerosis. LDL molecules deposit their excess cholesterol at various tissue sites, including the intima of blood vessels.

b. *HDL-C:* Population studies suggest an inverse relationship between HDL-C and CAD. An HDL-C level less than 30 mg/dL carries a significantly increased risk of CAD. A level greater than 50 mg/dL yields a low risk, whereas octogenarians average more than 75 mg/dL. HDL has two components, HDL-2 and HDL-3. The former is considered a better indicator of negative CAD risk than is total HDL. Exercise raises the level of cardioprotective HDL-2, whereas ethanol raises HDL-3.

c. *Apoproteins:* Preliminary evidence suggests that apoproteins A-I, A-II, and B may be better than LDL, HDL, and total cholesterol in predicting the risk of CAD. Elevated levels of A-I and A-II are associated with a lower risk, and elevated apoB concentration is associated with a higher risk of CAD. Isoforms of apoE have also been implicated in cardiovascular risk, as noted previously.

d. *Ratios:* Correlation of CAD with the LDL/HDL ratio has also been examined in adults. The risk increases sharply with ratios that exceed 3.0. A ratio greater than 5.0 carries a very high risk of CAD. Individuals with CAD average a ratio greater than 5:1, whereas newborn infants have an average ratio of 2:1. Another ratio is that of total cholesterol to HDL-C. A ratio of less than 4.5 denotes below-average risk. However, the clinical use of ratios is problematic because LDL and HDL represent independent risk factors and respond differently to different interventions.

6. Other experimental work: Lipoprotein a (LP[a]) is a very large lipoprotein composed of apoB-100 and cholesterol, similar to LDL. In addition, this lipoprotein has a large glycoprotein, homologous to plasminogen, attached through a disulfide bond. It has no known physiologic function. Plasma levels appear to be genetically determined and associated with risk of cardiovascular disease. As yet there are no specific effective interventions, but LP(a) is under active investigation.

CLASSIFICATION OF HYPERLIPIDEMIAS

Historically, patients with hyperlipidemia have been classified into five major groups according to plasma lipoprotein patterns (lipoprotein phenotyping). More recent classifications of hyperlipidemia either are extensions of the earlier models based on more specific data obtained from newer laboratory techniques (Table 11.3) or are based on recently de-

TABLE 11.3.   Phenotypic Classification

1. Hypercholesterolemia with normal triglycerides
   a. Elevated LDL-C, type IIa
      — Primary: Familial hypercholesterolemia
                    Familial combined hypercholesterolemia
                    Mixed genetic-environmental hypercholesterolemia
      — Secondary: Anorexia nervosa
                    Acute intermittent porphyria
                    Biliary obstruction (lipoprotein X)
   b. Elevated HDL-C
                    Familial hyperalphalipoproteinemia
                    Idiopathic
2. Hypercholesterolemia and hypertriglyceridemia
   a. Elevated LDL-C and VLDL-C, type IIB
      — Primary: Familial hypercholesterolemia
                    Familial combined hypercholesterolemia
                    Familial LCAT[a] deficiency
      — Secondary: Hypothyroidism
                    Nephrotic syndrome
                    Cushing's syndrome/glucocorticoid therapy
   b. Dysbetalipoproteinemia, type III
3. Hypertriglyceridemia with normal cholesterol
   a. Elevated VLDL only, type IV
      — Primary: Familial hypertriglyceridemia
                    Familial combined hyperlipidemia

   — Secondary: Diabetes mellitus
                 Systemic lupus erythematosus
                 Alcohol
                 Nephrotic syndrome
                 Pancreatitis
                 Pregnancy
                 Hypothyroidism
                 Idiopathic hypercalcemia
                 Medications: Estrogens
   b. Elevated chylomicrons, type I
      — Primary: Lipoprotein lipase deficiency
                    Familial deficiency of apoprotein C-II
      — Secondary: Autoimmune hyperchylomicronemia: SLE
                    Diabetes mellitus
                    Alcohol
   c. Elevated VLDL and chylomicrons, type V
      — Primary: Familial hypertriglyceridemia
                    Familial combined hyperlipidemia
                    Apoprotein E (apoE-4 and apoE-2)
      — Secondary: Diabetes mellitus
                    Alcohol
                    Estrogen
4. Increased risk with normal or elevated cholesterol
   a. Hyperbetalipoproteinemia
   b. Lp(a) hyperlipoproteinemia

Adapted from Arden MR. Primary hyperlipidemias. In: Jacobson MS, ed. Atherosclerosis prevention: identification and treatment of the child with high cholesterol. London: Harwood Academic Publishers, 1991:30.
[a]LCAT, lecithin cholesterol acyltransferase.

TABLE 11.4.   Metabolic Classification of Dyslipoproteinemia in Children and Adolescents[a]

1. Disorders of LDL metabolism/disorders with increased LDL
   a. Decreased LDL removal
      — Familial hypercholesterolemia
      — Defective apoB-100
   b. Increased LDL production
      — Familial combined hypercholesterolemia
      — Hyperapobetalipoproteinemia
   c. Other
      — Polygenic hypercholesterolemia
2. Disorders of triglyceride rich lipoproteins
   a. Decreased removal (type 1 dyslipoproteinemia)
      — Lipoprotein lipase deficiency
      — ApoC-II deficiency (cofactor for LPL)
   b. Production of abnormal VLDL
      — Familial hypertriglyceridemia (AD)
   c. Decreased removal/increased production
      — Type V dyslipoproteinemia (AD)
      — Dysbetalipoproteinemia
3. Deficiency in HDL
   a. Increased HDL removal
   b. Decreased HDL production

From Kwiterovich PO Jr. Diagnosis and management of familial dyslipoproteinemia in children and adolescents. Pediatr Clin North Am 1990;37:1489.
[a]AD, autosomal dominant; LPL, lipoprotein lipase.

scribed genetic and metabolic disorders (Table 11.4). The nomenclature remains cumbersome and there is still much overlap, especially when attempts are made to reconcile these two systems. Previously well described syndromes, such as familial hypercholesterolemia, have been shown to have a specific genotype and yet may vary in phenotype. (ie., types IIa and IIb). Moreover, type IIa and IIb patterns of hyperlipidemia are associated with another syndrome, familial combined hyperlipoproteinemia. Finally, the lipoprotein phenotyping system fails to account for children and adolescents at risk of atherosclerosis as a result of hyperapobetalipoproteinemia or hypoalphalipoproteinemia, which have been described in the metabolic classification. Each of the two classification systems has clinical utility at present. It is hoped that as the field of molecular genetics advances, the two systems will be fused into one system on the basis of pathophysiology and the degree of risk (Breslow, 1991).

Familial forms of hyperlipidemia, identifiable in the standard clinical laboratory assessment, account for only 2% of cases, though they are responsible for more than 20% of premature CAD. The majority of cases of hyperlipidemia occur as a result of diet and lifestyle factors, in association with genetic polymorphism in apoE, lecithin cholesterol acyltransferase, lipoprotein lipase, and other lipid enzymes and cofactors. Hyperlipidemia also occurs as a result of medical conditions or the use of medications such as estrogens, isotretenoin, and β-adrenergic blockers.

1. Familial hypercholesterolemia (Table 11.5)
   a. Monogenic: An autosomal codominant disorder resulting from insufficient activity of the cell surface receptors for LDL. A number of different mutations in the LDL receptor gene occur in families, all of which result in the same phenotypic disease. Homozygous familial hypercholesterolemia is a rare disease, occurring in about one in a million individuals. Typically, individuals homozygous for this condition have coronary atherosclerosis in the 2nd or 3rd decade. Clinically, this condition may manifest in childhood and adolescence by the deposition of cholesterol esters in tendons (xanthomas), as well as in soft tissues of the eyelids (xanthelasma) and in the

TABLE 11.5.   Characteristics of Familial Hyperlipoproteinemias

Hyperlipoproteinemia	Phenotype	Cholesterol	Triglyceride	Xanthomas	Frequency (%)	Risk of CAD
Familial lipoprotein lipase deficiency	I	Nl	↑	Eruptive	Very rare	0
Familial hypercholesterolemia	IIa IIb	↑	↑	Tendon Tuberous xanthelasma	0.1–0.5	4+
Polygenic hypercholesterolemia	II	↑	Nl	Tuberous	5	2+
Familial dysbetalipoproteinemia	III	↑	↑	Palmar Planar Tuberous Tendon	Rare	4+
Familial combined hyperlipoproteinemia	IIa IIb IV Rarely V	↑	↑	Any type	1–2	3+
Familial hypertriglyceridemia	IV Rarely V	Nl	↑	Eruptive	1	1+

Adapted from Arky RA, Perlman AJ. Hyperlipoproteinemia. In: Rubenstein E, Federman DD, eds. Scientific American Medicine. New York: Scientific American, 1988.

cornea (arcus cornea). The mean cholesterol concentration in the heterozygous condition ranges from 250 to 500 mg/dL and in the homozygote from 500 to 1000 mg/dL. Homozygous individuals may respond poorly to drugs and require referral to specialists for consideration of more radical therapies. The heterozygous form has been estimated to occur in 1 in 200–500 individuals. A similar clinical presentation is observed in individuals with a heterozygous abnormality; however, the signs and symptoms tend to be milder and to develop later, about the 4th or 5th decade of life.

b. Polygenic: A common cause of type IIa hyperlipidemia, probably associated with a combination of multiple genetic abnormalities and environmental factors. Individuals with this condition lack typical features of familial hypercholesterolemia such as xanthelasma, arcus cornea, and tendinous xanthomas.

2. Familial defective apoB-100: A mutation in the apoB gene results in decreased affinity of LDL to the LDL receptor. The phenotypic expression of this condition in children has not been described. Homozygous and heterozygous genotypes are known. This condition may occur in as many as 1 in 500 people, but the defect appears to account for only a small percentage (<2%) of premature CAD.

3. Lipoprotein lipase deficiency: A rare condition associated with very high levels of triglycerides and normal cholesterol levels. Eruptive xanthomas may be present. Although the risk of atherosclerosis is not elevated, the individual is at risk of having pancreatitis, particularly when the triglyceride exceeds 500 mg/dL.

4. Familial dysbetalipoproteinemia: A very uncommon condition, occurring in about 1 in 5000 persons in the United States; it is seen only rarely in adolescence. In this condition the catabolism of VLDL remnants and of chylomicrons is delayed because an abnormal apoE alters the normal binding of VLDL remnants to LDL receptors. This problem should be suspected when triglyceride levels are somewhat higher than cholesterol levels in the presence of a significant cholesterol elevation. These individuals have an elevated risk of premature CAD and of peripheral vascular disease. They often are obese and have glucose intolerance, hyperuricemia, and tuboeruptive and palmar xanthomas. Caloric restriction is usually effective.

5. Familial hypertriglyceridemia: Autosomal dominant trait. Dietary factors, obesity, and a sedentary lifestyle are additional elements involved in the degree of expression.
6. Familial combined hyperlipidemia (FCHL): Affected individuals have high levels of LDL-C or triglycerides or both. This condition is usually not associated with tendinous xanthomas but is associated with premature CAD. Multiple lipoprotein phenotypes can occur in a single affected family. Affected individuals may have increases in VLDL alone, LDL alone, or VLDL plus LDL or chylomicrons. The diagnosis is made by a finding of multiple lipoprotein phenotypes in a single family when first-degree relatives are tested or when a typical pattern of modest elevation in concentrations of cholesterol and triglycerides is seen, together with a low HDL-C level. FCHL occurs in about 15% of patients with CAD before 60 years of age. The metabolic defect appears to be an overproduction of lipoproteins by the liver, as well as decreased catabolism in the periphery. Dietary therapy, along with physical exercise, plays an important role in treatment.

LIPID SCREENING AND MANAGEMENT

The process of screening and management differs for adolescents ($\leq$ age 20 years) and young adults (20–35 years), according to the National Cholesterol Education Program (NCEP). In addition to classification of lipid parameters, screening involves the identification of cardiovascular risk factors by history and physical examination.

History

1. Family history of premature cardiovascular diseases (<55 years of age) such as myocardial infarcts or other sequelae of atherosclerosis
2. Family history of dyslipidemia or hypertension
3. History of smoking
4. Dietary history: May use 24-hour recall history

Physical Examination

1. Signs of peripheral lipid deposition (xanthoma, xanthelasma, corneal arcus)
2. Weight, height, blood pressure, and sexual maturity rating
3. Body composition indexes: Adjunctively it may be useful to obtain an indication of body composition by measurement of mid upper arm circumference and standard skinfolds.

Screening in Adolescents

Normal values for adolescents and young adults are given in Table 11.6. The NCEP Expert Panel on Blood Cholesterol Levels in Children and Adolescents classifies risk on the basis of total cholesterol levels as follows:

Low risk	<170 mg/dL
Borderline risk	170–196 mg/dL
High risk	>200 mg/dL (95th percentile)

Giving dietary treatment to adolescents and young adults with the top 25% of cholesterol values is probably desirable but this has not been proven. Establishing such proof would be extremely difficult, requiring lengthy (30–40 years) longitudinal studies. Recommending drug treatment to the top 10% would be even more controversial and unproved until more is known about the risk/benefit ratio for such drugs in a younger population.

TABLE 11.6.   Lipid Values by Age and Sex

	Percentile							
	Cholesterol		Triglycerides		LDL-C		HDL-C	
Age (yr)	75th	90th	75th	90th	75th	90th	10th	25th
Males								
5–9	168	183	58	70	103	117	42	49
10–14	173	188	74	94	109	122	40	46
15–19	168	183	88	125	109	123	34	39
20–24	179	197	107	146	118	138	32	38
25–29	199	223	120	171	138	157	32	37
Females								
5–9	177	190	74	103	115	125	38	47
10–14	171	191	85	104	110	126	40	45
15–19	173	195	84	108	110	127	38	43
20–24	176	202	81	100	113	136	37	43
25–29	192	213	86	108	122	141	40	47

Adapted from The Lipid Research Clinics Population Studies data book. I. The prevalence study. Publication No. 80–1527. Bethesda, Maryland: National Institutes of Health, 1980.

At present, it seems reasonable to recommend that individuals in the borderline-risk group receive hygienic measures, including exercise instruction, nutritional advice such as the NCEP Step-1 prudent diet, and nonsmoking advice. Those in the high-risk group should receive all these measures plus dietary counseling by a dietitian and more frequent follow-up. Although the LDL-C level is more closely correlated with CAD risk, total cholesterol can be measured for follow-up to save on laboratory costs.

1. *Who:* If possible, all adolescents should be screened once during this age period. If not possible, then the following adolescents should be screened:
   a. Teens whose parents or relatives have had premature CAD or stroke, or clinical evidence of atherosclerosis before the age of 55 in male members and before age 60 in female members.
   b. Teens whose parents have elevated concentrations of lipoproteins
   c. Teens with hypertension or other significant cardiac risk factors
2. *How:* Serum lipids are best measured after a 12- to 14-hour fast; however, the total cholesterol level can be determined in a nonfasting sample because chylomicrons from dietary fat contribute essentially no cholesterol. If a nonfasting cholesterol level is borderline or above, a fasting sample should be obtained and analyzed for triglyceride, total cholesterol, and HDL-C with a calculation of LDL-C. Risk on the basis of LDL-C is as follows:

Acceptable	<110 mg/dL
Borderline	110–129 mg/dL
High risk	>130 mg/dL

Screening in Young Adults

The NCEP Expert Panel (1992) has made renewed recommendations for detection, evaluation, and treatment of high cholesterol concentrations in adults. The blood lipid levels that determine level of risk are higher for this age group because of the observed increase in total cholesterol and LDL-C with age.

1. Several changes in these most recent recommendations are important. For young adults, the following are most salient:

a. More attention is now paid to HDL-C. It is advised that HDL-C be measured as part of the first screening blood tests and that the level of HDL-C be considered a negative CAD risk factor.

b. There is now an increased emphasis on the role of physical activity and body weight as components of atherosclerosis prevention.

c. The presence of two or more other risk factors modifies the lipid level at which intervention is needed.

d. Secondary prevention for those with CAD is more aggressive and beyond the scope of this chapter (see summary NCEP report [Adult Treatment Panel II], JAMA 1993).

2. Recommendations for young adults between 20 and 35 years of age are as follows:

a. Serum cholesterol levels should be determined in every young adult regardless of family history at least once every 5 years. The concentration of HDL-C should be determined where accurate laboratories are available. In those without CAD, which will be the vast majority of 20- to 35-year-old adults, the following risk levels apply:

	Total Cholesterol	*HDL-C*	*LDL-C*
Desirable	<200 mg/dL	>35 mg/dL	<130 mg/dL
Borderline	200–239 mg/dL		130–159 mg/dL
High Risk	>240 mg/dL	<35 mg/dL	>160 mg/dL

The concentration of LDL-C is determined when either total cholesterol or HDL-C level is high or when two or more other risk factors are present along with a borderline total cholesterol level.

Management is based on the LDL-C level (Fig. 11.3). Yearly evaluation is indicated for anyone not in the desirable or borderline category without other risk factors. Borderline individuals with two or more risk factors or high-risk individuals receive more intensive dietary and exercise intervention.

b. Drug therapy should be considered in this age group (20–35 years) only when the LDL-C level is greater than 220 mg/dL, or when the LDL-C level is between 160 and 220 mg/dL in association with several other risk factors.

Hypertriglyceridemia

Moderate hypertriglyceridemia is not independently correlated with CAD. Severe hypertriglyceridemia (≥1000 mg/dL) is associated with an increased incidence of acute life-threatening pancreatitis and must be aggressively treated with diet, weight loss, and pharmacotherapy. The Framingham study has found that a triglyceride concentration greater than 150 mg/dL, in combination with an HDL level less than 35 mg/dL, is as good a predictor of CAD as is LDL elevation. Thus, in the presence of an elevated total cholesterol or a low HDL concentration, treatment with a diet low in fat and simple carbohydrates and an exercise program is recommended.

THERAPY FOR HYPERLIPIDEMIA

General Principles

1. Diagnose and treat secondary causes.
2. Reduce risk factors. Intervene with those risk factors that can be altered, including smoking and hypertension.
3. Start a heart-healthy diet. The principal treatment of hyperlipidemia in adolescents and adults is a diet with modified amounts of fat, saturated fat, and cholesterol. The goals of dietary therapy are to lower total cholesterol and LDL-C below the 90th percentile—

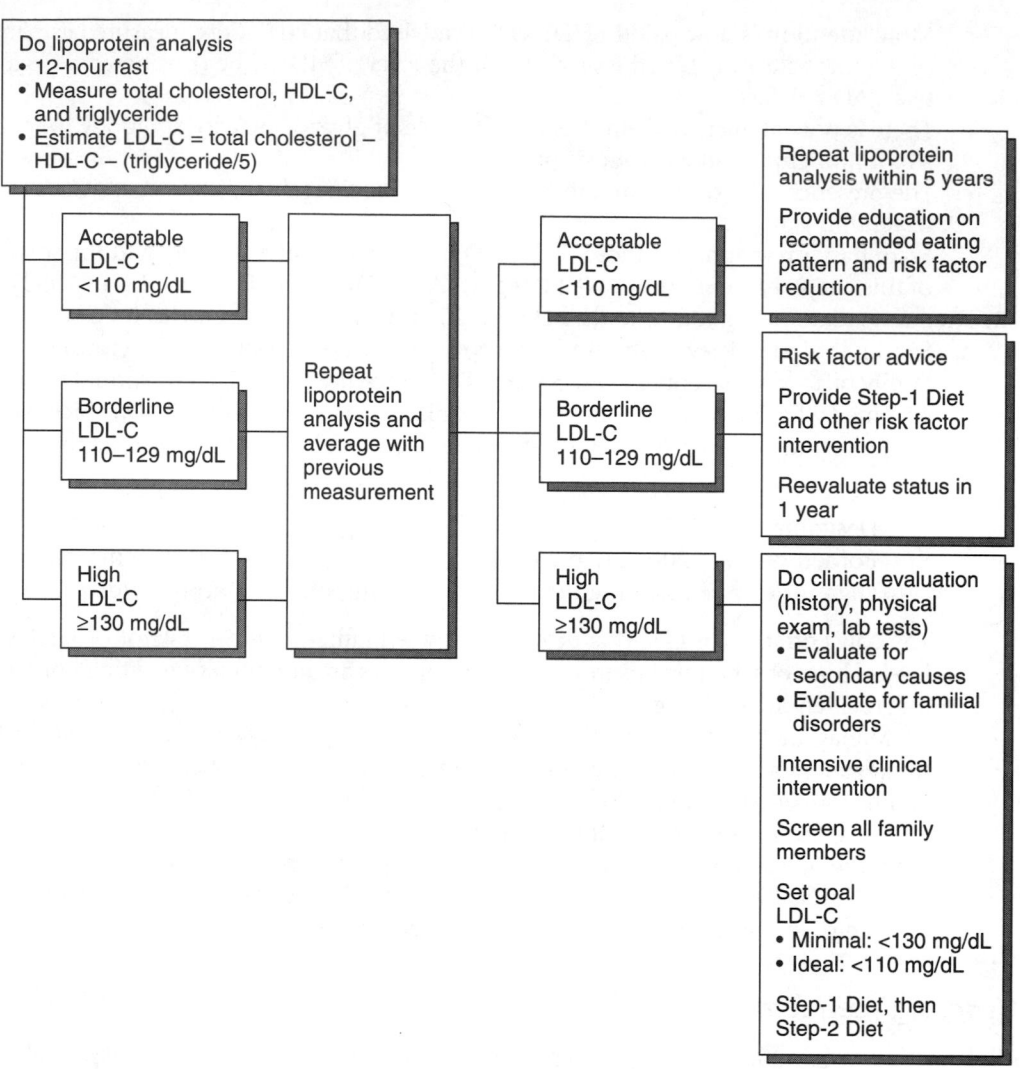

FIGURE 11.3.   Classification, education, and follow-up based on LDL-C in adolescents (<20 years). (From the National Cholesterol Education Programs Report of the Expert Panel on Blood Cholesterol Levels in Children and Adolescents. Pediatrics 1992;89(suppl):498.

preferably below the 75th percentile. Nutritional management is described in two steps as recommended by the NCEP Expert Panel on Blood Cholesterol Levels in Children and Adolescents, as shown in Table 11.7. If adherence to the NCEP Step-1 diet fails to achieve the minimal goals of therapy, the Step-2 diet should be prescribed.

The pediatric recommendations differ from those for adults in that careful consideration and monitoring of energy and micronutrient consumption are needed for support of normal growth and development. This is especially important during the adolescent growth years, when energy, protein, mineral, and vitamin requirements are increased. Nutritional counseling focusing on meeting fat and cholesterol recommendations while ensuring adequate macronutrient and micronutrient intake is needed.

4. Set dietary goals.
   a.   Reduced dietary fats

TABLE 11.7.   Dietary Therapy for High Blood Cholesterol Levels: Characteristics of Step-1 and Step-2 Diets for Lowering Blood Cholesterol Levels

Nutrient	Recommended Intake	
	Step-1 Diet	Step-2 Diet
Total fat	Average of no more than 30% of total calories	Same
Saturated fatty acids	<10% of total calories	<7% of total calories
Polyunsaturated fatty acids	≤10% of total calories	Same
Monounsaturated fatty acids	Remaining total fat calories	Same
Cholesterol	<300 mg/day	<200 mg/day
Carbohydrates	≈55% of total calories	Same
Protein	≈15–20% of total calories	Same
Calories	To promote normal growth and development and to reach or maintain desirable body weight	Same

  b. Reduced saturated fat and improved fatty acid balance
  c. Reduced dietary cholesterol
  d. Increased complex carbohydrates
      Achieving these dietary goals can be difficult for the teen, so help from a physician, a dietitian, and the family is crucial. Helpful suggestions include:

- Snacks: Most candies should be limited. Replace with graham crackers, Rye Krisp, melba toast, soda crackers, bagels, English muffins, and fruits and vegetables. Popcorn should be air popped.
- Desserts: Try fruits, low-fat yogurt, fruit ices, and jello.
- Cooking methods: Choose methods that use little or no fat, such as steaming, baking, or broiling.
- Eating away from home: Order entrees, potatoes, and vegetables without sauces or butter.
- Ask for salad dressings to be served on the side. Limit high-fat toppings such as bacon, crumbled eggs, cheese, and sunflower seeds.
- A regular exercise program is an important adjunct to a change in eating habits.
- Initiate diets that closely correspond to the adolescent's normal eating habits.
- Implement specific goals in a graduated fashion, rather than all at once.
- Family should participate in the dietary management and the exercise program.
- Stress the maintenance of ideal body weight, an exercise program, and the prevention of nicotine and alcohol use.

Dietary Therapy (Table 11.8)

1. Reduce dietary fats. Currently the typical fat intake of children in the United States is 36% of total energy consumption. To meet the goal of 30%, the teen must make several modifications in the use of "visible" and "invisible" fats. "Visible" fats include butter, margarine, oils, salad dressing, mayonnaise, cream, and gravies. They are often added to foods or used in preparation (e.g., fried chicken, French fries). "Invisible" sources of fat include oils and other fats incorporated into baked goods, processed foods (e.g., cold cuts, frozen meats, franks), whole milk, other dairy products, and snack foods (e.g., chips, doughnuts). Sources of fats should be identified in the adolescent's diet. The amount and frequency of consumption of high-fat food should be reduced and lower-fat alternatives given.
2. Reduce saturated fats and improve fatty acid balance. Saturated fatty acids with chain lengths of 12 carbons (lauric), 14 carbons (myristic), and 16 carbons (palmitic) have the

TABLE 11.8.   Recommended Diet Modifications to Lower Blood Cholesterol

	Step-1 Diet	
	Choose	Decrease
Fish, chicken, turkey, and lean meats	Fish, poultry without skin, lean cuts of beef, lamb, pork or veal, shellfish	Fatty cuts of beef, lamb, pork; spare ribs, organ meats, regular cold cuts, sausage, hot dogs, bacon, sardines, roe
Skim and low-fat milk, cheese, yogurt, and dairy substitutes	Skim or 1% fat milk (liquid, powdered, evaporated), buttermilk	Whole milk (4% fat): regular, evaporated, condensed; cream, half and half, 2% milk, imitation milk products, most nondairy creamers, whipped toppings
	Nonfat (0% fat) or low-fat yogurt	Whole-milk yogurt
	Low-fat cottage cheese (1% or 2% fat)	Whole-milk cottage cheese (4% fat)
	Low-fat cheeses, farmer or pot cheeses (all of these should be labeled no more than 2–6 g of fat per ounce)	All natural cheeses (e.g., blue, roquefort, camembert, cheddar, Swiss), low-fat or "light" cream cheese, low-fat or "light" sour cream, cream cheeses, sour cream
	Sherbet, sorbet	Ice cream
Eggs	Egg whites (2 whites equal 1 whole egg in recipes), cholesterol-free egg substitutes	Egg yolks
Fruits and vegetables	Fresh, frozen, canned, or dried fruits and vegetables	Vegetables prepared in butter, cream, or other sauces
Breads and cereals	Homemade baked goods using unsaturated oils sparingly, angel food cake, low-fat crackers, low-fat cookies	Commercial baked goods: pies, cakes, doughnuts, croissants, pastries, muffins, biscuits, high-fat crackers, high-fat cookies
	Rice, pasta	Egg noodles
	Whole-grain breads and cereals (oatmeal, whole wheat, rye, bran, multi-grain, etc.)	Breads in which eggs are a major ingredient
Fats and oils	Baking cocoa	Chocolate
	Unsaturated vegetable oils: corn, olive, rapeseed (canola oil), safflower, sesame, soybean, sunflower	Butter, coconut oil, palm oil, palm kernel oil, lard, bacon fat
	Margarine or shortenings made from one of the unsaturated oils listed above, diet margarine	
	Mayonnaise, salad dressings made with unsaturated oils listed above, low-fat dressings	Dressings made with egg yolk
	Seeds and nuts	Coconut

Reproduced, by permission, from The Expert Panel. Report of The National Cholesterol Education Program. Arch Intern Med 1988;148:49.

most hypercholesterolemic effect in humans. Stearic acid, an 18-carbon saturated fatty acid has been found to be less atherogenic than 12- to 16-carbon fatty acids. These 12- to 16-carbon fatty acids are found in certain vegetable oils (e.g., palm, coconut), animal fats, and whole-milk dairy products. The 18-carbon stearic acid is found in chocolate and beef.

Data from the 1988 Continuing Survey of Food Intakes by Individuals (CSFI) show that 14% of total calories is contributed to the diet from saturated fatty acids, a percentage that is above the recommended 10% limit. Therefore, when saturated fats are reduced to less than 10% of total calories, the balance of monosaturated and polyunsaturated fatty acids must be considered. Major sources of monosaturated fatty acids include peanuts, hazelnuts, avocado, lean beef, and poultry. Substituting these for fatty acids in the context of a low-fat diet can lead to a reduction in LDL-C, no elevation in triglycerides, and preservation of HDL-C.

The major categories of polyunsaturated fatty acids are omega-6 or omega-3 fatty acids, terms referring to the position of their double bond. Linoleic acid, the major omega-6 fatty acid in the diet, is found in vegetable oils such as safflower, sunflower seed, soybean, and corn oils. Omega-6 fatty acids, when used in the context of all dietary recommendations, lower total cholesterol and LDL-C concentrations without decreasing HDL-C. Taken in amounts greater than 10% of total calories, these fatty acids may cause subsequent lowering of HDL-C levels. The long-term safety of a diet high in polyunsaturated fats, in relation to the incidence of cancers, has not been established.

Omega-3 fatty acids are primarily found in cold-water fish (as eicosapentaenoic acid [EPA] and docosahexaenoic acid [DHA] and in soybean and walnut oils as linolenic acid. Omega-3 fatty acids given as fish oil supplements have been shown to lower elevated triglyceride levels in adult patients with hypertriglyceridemia and to improve the dyslipidemia in pediatric patients with systemic lupus erythematosus. Fish oil supplementation should be monitored medically for side effects such as decreased clotting time. In general, increasing the number of meals with cold-water fish (i.e., salmon, mackerel, bluefish, trout, and sablefish) to a minimum of twice weekly while decreasing fatty beef and poultry dishes would be beneficial.

3. Reduce dietary cholesterol. Dietary cholesterol will elevate both plasma concentrations of total cholesterol and LDL-C. The current consumption of cholesterol by children is less than 300 mg/day, which is almost within reach of the current recommendations. The following three suggestions are given to guide the patient with hyperlipidemia and his or her family:

   a. Eliminate visible egg yolks such as fried eggs and egg yolks used in home recipes and replace with egg whites or egg substitutes.
   b. Limit portions of cooked meat, chicken, and fish to 7–8 ounces daily; if lean cuts of beef and pork and controlled amounts of shellfish (six medium shrimp) are used, they can be incorporated into the diet and can provide a significant source of minerals and vitamins.
   c. Use skim milk or the lowest-fat dairy products available.

4. Increase complex carbohydrates. When fat is removed from an adolescent's diet, an energy deficit may occur. In the overweight or obese teenager this may aid in cessation of weight gain, but in the normal to underweight individual it may result in undesirable weight loss. Therefore, it is important to replace the fat energy with complex carbohydrate sources. Complex carbohydrates are found in fruits, vegetables, and starches such as pretzels, popcorn, bagels, unsweetened cereals, pasta, breads, corn, rice, and crackers.

   Fat-free baked products offer a wide variety of snacks for adolescents and encourage adherence to the diet regimen. It is important to note that these products are isocaloric with counterparts and contain a significant amount of simple sugar; therefore, they need to be limited for the patient with elevated triglyceride concentrations or weight or both.

Drug Therapy

The risk/benefit ratio for any drug therapy is unknown in adolescents. However, pharmacotherapy is considered when:

1. Supervised diet modification fails to lower LDL-C to acceptable levels or by at least 15% of baseline.
2. A parent has died or had severe atherosclerotic sequelae in his or her forties or younger.
3. The adolescent's LDL-C concentration is more than 190 mg/dL in the absence of other risk factors or more than 160 in the presence of any of the following: smoking, hypertension, xanthoma, diabetes, clinical signs of atherosclerosis.

TABLE 11.9.   Drug Therapy for High Blood Cholesterol Levels

Type of Drug	Mechanism of Action	Major Effects	Generic Name	Dose	Side Effects
Bile acid sequestrant	Binds bile intestine, LDL receptors in liver	Lowers total LDL-C	Cholestyramine Colestipol	1–2 packs	Constipation, abdominal discomfort
Nicotinic acid	Decreases production of VLDL in liver	Lowers total cholesterol and LDL-C and triglycerides; raises HDL-C	Niacin	500 mg	Flushing, itching, abdominal discomfort
HMG-CoA reductase inhibitor	Inhibits cholesterol synthesis; induces LDL receptor in liver	Lowers total cholesterol and LDL-C; may lower triglycerides and increase HDL-C	Lovastatin Pravastatin Simvastatin	20 mg with main meal	Headache, rash, muscle ache
Fibric acid	Increases activity of lipoprotein lipase; decreases triglyceride production in liver	Lowers triglycerides; raises HDL-C; modestly lowers total cholesterol and LDL-C	Gemfibrozil	600 mg t.i.d.	Abdominal discomfort, diarrhea, muscle ache, increased appetite
Butylphenol	Increases removal of LDL-C from blood; prevents LDL oxidations	Lowers total cholesterol and LDL-C; also lowers HDL-C	Probucol	500 mg	Electrocardiographic abnormalities, diarrhea, headache, rash, insomnia

Adapted from Hardoff D, Jacobson MS. Hyperlipidemia. Adolesc Med State Arts Rev 1992;3(1):473.

4. In the adult male less than age 35 who has no other risk factors, the NCEP recommends that drug therapy be delayed unless the LDL-C concentration is more than 220 mg/dL.

Table 11.9 summarizes mechanisms of action and major effects and lists recommended doses and side effects of the drugs used for hyperlipidemic conditions. These drugs are further detailed below.

Available Drugs

1. Bile acid sequestrants
   a. Cholestyramine (Questran), a hydrophilic, insoluble anion exchange resin powder
   Action: Interrupts the enterohepatic circulation of bile acids and binds bile acids in the intestine to form an insoluble complex, which is excreted in feces and thereby increases hepatic synthesis of bile acids from cholesterol. Depletion of the hepatic pool of cholesterol results in an increase in LDL receptor activity in the liver. This, in turn, stimulates removal of LDL from plasma and lowers the concentration of LDL-C. There may be an increase in hepatic VLDL production and thus an increase in triglycerides. The advantage of this drug in the treatment of adolescents is that there is no systemic absorption or toxic effects. However, the gastrointestinal side effects are frequent, leading to problems in compliance.
   Effects: Lowering of both total cholesterol and LDL-C levels by 15% to 30% at 16–24 g/day.
   Side effects:
   — Gastrointestinal effects include nausea, bloating, and constipation.

— Drug is difficult to take because it must be suspended in a liquid vehicle. If water is unsatisfactory, an unsweetened juice may improve palatability. Rapid ingestion may cause air swallowing.

— Bleeding tendencies, osteoporosis, or iron deficiency may result from poor absorption of vitamin K, calcium, or iron, but these complications are rare.

Dose: Powder, 16–24 g. Should be started at one pack (4 g of cholestyramine; 5 g orange-flavored filler) twice a day and gradually increased for a month to the full dose. The average dose is two or three packs (8–12 g) taken orally twice daily with meals.

b. Colestipol (Colestid)

Action, effects, and side effects: Similar to those of cholestyramine.

Dose: The average dose is one-and-a-half packs (7.5 g) taken orally twice daily with meals. The maximum adult dose is 30 g/day.

2. Nicotinic acid (niacin)

Action: Reduces VLDL production by inhibiting lipoprotein synthesis in the liver. Niacin is an effective drug but requires considerable physician and patient education because of side effects. However, at least in adults, the drug has proven efficacy and safety. It is also the least costly of the drugs.

Effects: Primarily reduces triglyceride levels but also lowers LDL-C levels and causes a slight rise in HDL. A dose of 3–4 g/day can result in a 40% decrease in triglyceride and VLDL levels, a 20% decrease in LDL levels, and a 30% increase in HDL levels. Nicotinic acid is particularly valuable in combination therapy with a bile acid sequestrant because of the complementary modes of action: niacin inhibiting LDL and VLDL production and the bile acid sequestrant increasing LDL excretion.

Side effects: The drug is poorly tolerated in the dosage needed for lipid lowering.

— Gastritis, peptic ulcer disease, vomiting, and diarrhea can occur.

— Liver function abnormalities can occur.

— Vasodilation with flushing is also a troublesome side effect.

Dose: The side effects can be reduced by starting with a small dose such as 50–100 mg with meals and gradually increasing for 1 month to 6 weeks. The average daily dose is 2–3 g, with a maximum dose of 6–9 g. The possibility of flushing as a side effect should be discussed. Since the flushing is due to prostaglandin effects, it can be ameliorated by taking one aspirin 30 minutes before each dose. Timed-release capsules may also decrease the side effects. Individuals taking niacin should have regular monitoring of aminotransferase, glucose, alkaline phosphatase, and uric acid values.

3. Inhibitors of 3-hydroxy-3-methylglutaryl–coenzyme A (HMG-CoA) reductase

a. Lovastatin (Mevacor)

Action: Competitively inhibits the rate-limiting enzyme in cholesterol biosynthesis. LDL receptor activity is also increased, leading to an increase in the rate of removal of LDL. However, long-term safety information is not available.

Effects: Causes an average reduction in the LDL-C concentration of 25–45%.

Side effects: Usually well tolerated. Side effects include changes in bowel function, headaches, nausea, fatigue, insomnia, skin rashes, and myositis. There is also an increase in aminotransferase levels in 1.9% of patients. Careful monitoring of liver function is essential. Myalgias occur in about 2.4% of individuals. Transient mild elevations in creatine kinase are commonly seen; in the few patients in whom markedly elevated levels and myositis develop, the drug should be discontinued. Preliminary results from the lovastatin adolescent trial on 65 adolescent males with familial hypercholesterolemia show efficacy similar to that seen in adults, with normal growth and development. Hence lovastatin may well become more commonly used in the future.

Dose: Usually the starting dose is 20 mg once daily with the evening meal, with increases to 40 mg and then 80 mg as a single evening dose or in divided doses. Liver function should be checked at the start of therapy, and tested every 4 to 6 weeks during the first 15 months of therapy, and then tested periodically.

    b. Pravastatin
Action, effects, and side effects: Similar to those of lovastatin.
Dosage: 10–40mg
    c. Simvastatin
Action, effects, and side effects: Similar to those of lovastatin.
Dosage: 5–40mg

4. Probucol (Lorelco)
Action: Increases rate of LDL catabolism; decreases LDL oxidation.
Effects: Lowers LDL-C by about 8–15% but with an associated reduction in HDL-C of up to 25%. The HDL/LDL ratio remains constant or is lowered. No extensive long-term studies are available for assessing the drug's safety or its effect on CAD risk.
Side effects: Minimal, with mostly minor gastrointestinal effects. Can cause a prolongation of the QT interval. Diarrhea, rash, and insomnia have been described.
Dose: 500 mg twice a day.

5. Fibric acid, or gemfibrozil (Lopid)
Action: Increases lipoprotein lipase (LPL) activity and decreases hepatic triglyceride production.
Effects: Reduces both VLDL and triglyceride levels. In some individuals, cholesterol levels may fall and HDL levels may rise. The drug is primarily used for lowering high levels of triglycerides.
Side effects: Biliary tract disease, and contraindicated in liver or kidney disease. Abdominal discomfort, diarrhea, muscle ache, and increased appetite can occur.
Dose: 1200 mg daily in two doses.

    Generally the bile acid sequestrants used together with nicotinic acid have been considered first-line agents. Probucol and gemfibrozil have been used as second steps. However, they are less effective in lowering LDL-C. Inhibitors of HMG-CoA reductase are perhaps the most effective agents, but the long-term side effects are unknown; they may well become first-line agents. Lovastatin is even more effective when used in conjunction with a bile acid sequestrant. Another issue for consideration is cost. The following are approximate costs based on the average wholesale price in 1994.

Cholestyramine (Questran)	$76/60
Nicotinic acid	$5.00/100
Gemfibrozil (Lopid)	$58/60
HMG-CoA reductase inhibitor (Mevacor), 20 mg	$120/60
Probucol (Lorelco)	$112/60

A summary of the major effects of drug therapy on lipids is listed in Table 11.10.

TABLE 11.10.   Major Effects of Drug Therapy on Lipids

Drug	Cholesterol	Triglycerides	HDL-C
Cholestyramine or colestipol	↓	No change or ↑	No change or ↑
Nicotinic acid	↓	↓	↑
Gemfibrozil or clofibrate	↓	↓	↑
Probucol	↓	No change	↓
Lovastatin	↓	No change or ↓	No change or ↑

6. Antioxidants

   Research by Steinberg and Witzum (1990) on the effects of oxidized LDL has suggested a therapeutic role for antioxidants in the treatment of elevated levels of LDL-C. These drugs have not been widely accepted in the treatment of adolescents and should be considered investigational.

Adherence to Drug Therapy

1. The teen must be well informed about the goals of drug treatment and the side effects.
2. It is important to start with small doses of drugs, especially if sequestrants and nicotinic acid are used.
3. The frequency of use of the medication and the impact on lifestyle must be discussed.
4. It is important to maintain regularly scheduled follow-ups with the teen.

SUDDEN DEATH

Most sudden deaths in adolescents outside of the three big causes of death in this age group (accidents, suicides, homicides) are related to the cardiovascular system. In a study of sudden and unexpected natural deaths in childhood and adolescence, Neuspiel and Kuller (1985) found that cardiovascular causes accounted for the largest group in adolescents. The other major contributors included infections, epilepsy, intracranial hemorrhage, and asthma.

1. Cardiovascular causes of sudden death in previously well adolescents include:
   a. Idiopathic hypertrophic subaortic stenosis or hypertrophic cardiomyopathy: the most common cause of sudden death, suggested by a triad of syncope, chest pain with dizziness, and a murmur at the left lower sternal border
   b. Anomalous origin of the left coronary artery
   c. Myocarditis
   d. Congestive cardiomyopathy
   e. Mitral valve prolapse: Unusual complication of mitral valve prolapse
   f. Aortic rupture, usually associated with Marfan's syndrome
   g. Idiopathic concentric left ventricular hypertrophy
   h. Prolonged QT syndrome
   i. Wolff-Parkinson-White syndrome and other preexcitation syndromes with tachyarrhythmias
   j. Coronary artery disease
   k. High-degree heart block
   l. Abnormality of the conduction system, such as sinoatrial node lesions or atrioventricular node lesions
2. Causes of sudden death in adolescents with prior cardiovascular disease include:
   a. Congenital aortic stenosis
   b. Congenital heart condition such as uncorrected tetralogy of Fallot (should be considered especially in adolescents with Down syndrome)
   c. Cyanotic heart disease with pulmonary stenosis
   d. Idiopathic hypertrophic subaortic stenosis or hypertrophic cardiomyopathy

If an adolescent is discovered to have one of the preceding syndromes, it is important to determine the pathophysiological severity and to consider the types of exercise that may present significant risks.

Evaluation

History   Of particular importance are symptoms of syncope, significant exercise intolerance, and exertional chest discomfort, and a family history of premature CAD, sudden death, syncope, or hypertension.

Physical Examination   Important findings include hypertension, abnormal cardiac rhythm, heart murmur, or Marfan's syndrome habitus.

Laboratory Tests   Exercise electrocardiography is useful in an adolescent with symptoms of exertional chest discomfort, syncope or exercise intolerance, or frequent ventricular arrhythmias. Routine screening with echocardiography or chest x-ray study is of little value. For further recommendations on limitations of these conditions for athletics, see Chapter 18.

SUPPORT MATERIALS

The following publications to assist in hypercholesterolemia therapy are available from the American Heart Association (7320 Greenville Ave., Dallas, TX 75231):

> *The AHA Diet* (publication No. 51-018-B): moderate, fat-controlled low-cholesterol meal plan
> *Cholesterol and Your Heart* (publication No. 50-069-A): explanation of what cholesterol is and why it is a risk factor
> *Recipes for Fat-Controlled, Low-Cholesterol Meals* (publication No. 50-020-B): recipes for healthy meals
> *AHA Cookbook* (publication No. 53-001-A): 250 recipes and a fat and cholesterol calorie chart
> In addition, the following is available from the National Cholesterol Education Program, National Heart, Lung, and Blood Institute (Box C-200, Bethesda, MD 20892): *Physician's Kit on High Blood Cholesterol*

BIBLIOGRAPHY

Anderson KM, Castelli WP, Levy D. Cholesterol and morality: 30 years of follow-up from the Framingham study. JAMA 1987;257:2176.

Arky RA, Perlman AJ. Cholesterol and mortality: 30 years of follow-up from the Framingham study. JAMA 1987;257:2176.

Baker AL, Roberts C, Gothing C. Dyslipidemias in childhood. An overview. Nurs Clin North Am 1995;30:243.

Becque MD, Katch VL, Rocchini AP, et al. Coronary risk incidence of obese adolescents: reduction by exercise plus diet intervention. Pediatrics 1988;81:605.

Berenson GS, ed. Causation of cardiovascular risk factors in children. New York: Raven Press, 1986.

Bharati S, Lev M. Sudden death in teenagers. Primary Cardiol 1985; January:73.

Blackett PR, Kittredge D. Hyperlipidemia in children. South Med J 1993;86:1083.

Breslow JL. Lipoprotein transport gene abnormalities underlying coronary heart disease susceptibility. Ann Rev Med 1991;42:357.

Castelli WP, Garrison RJ, Wilson PWF, et al. Incidence of coronary heart disease and lipoprotein cholesterol levels: the Framingham study. JAMA 1986;256:2835.

Castelli WP, Griffin GC. How to help patients cut down on saturated fat. Postgrad Med 1988;84:44.

Christensen B, Glueck C, Kwiterovich PO Jr, et al. Plasma cholesterol and triglyceride distributions in 13,665 children and adolescents: the prevalence study of the Lipid Research Clinics program. Pediatr Res 1980;14:194.

Clarke WR, Schrott HG, Leaverton PE, et al. Tracking of blood lipids and blood pressures in school-age children: the Muscatine study. Circulation 1978;58:626.

Consensus Conference. Lowering blood cholesterol to prevent heart disease. JAMA 1985;253:2080.

Cooper R, Allen A, Goldberg R, et al. Seventh-Day Adventist adolescents: life-style patterns and cardiovascular risk factors. West J Med 1984;140:471.

Cortner JA, Coates PM, Liacouras CA, et al. Familial combined hyperlipidemia in children: clinical expression, metabolic defects, and management. J Pediatr 1993;123:177.

Croft JB, Foster TA, Parker FC, et al. Transitions of cardiovascular risk from adolescence to young adulthood—the Bogalusa Heart Study. I. Effects of alterations in lifestyle. J Chronic Dis 1986;39:81.

Deedwania PC. Clinical perspectives on primary and secondary prevention of coronary atherosclerosis. Med Clin North Am 1995;79:973.

Dipalma JR. Lovastatin: cholesterol-lowering agent. Am Fam Physician 1987;36:189.

Donahue RP, Orchard TJ, Kuller LH, et al. Lipids and lipoproteins in a young adult population: the Beaver County Lipid Study. Am J Epidemiol 1985;122:458.

Dujovne CA, Harris WS. Approach to diagnosis and treatment of subjects at risk for dyslipidemia-induced, atherosclerotic cardiovascular disease. Pract Cardiol 1988;May:24.

Epstein LH, Valoski A, Wing RR, et al. 10-year follow-up of behavioral family- based treatment for obese 10-year-olds JAMA 1990;264:2519–2523.

Expert Panel. Report of the National Cholesterol Education Program Expert Panel on detection, evaluation, and treatment of high blood cholesterol in adults. Arch Intern Med 1988;48:36.

Freedman DS, Cresanta SR, Srinivasan SR, et al. Longitudinal serum lipoprotein changes in white males during adolescence: the Bogalusa Heart Study. Metabolism 1985;34:396.

Fripp RR, Hodgson JL, Kwiterovich PO, et al. Aerobic capacity, obesity, and atherosclerotic risk factors in male adolescents. Pediatrics 1985;75:813.

Gagliano NJ, Emans SJ, Woods ER. Cholesterol screening in the adolescent. J Adolesc Health 1993;14:104.

Gillman MW, Couples LA, Moore LL, et al. Impact of within person variability on identifying children with hypercholesterolemia: Framingham Children's Study. J Pediatr 1992;121:342.

Gosland IF, Crook D, Simpson R, et al. The effects of different formulations of oral contraceptive agents on lipid and carbohydrate metabolism. N Engl J Med 1990;323:1375.

Gotto AM Jr. Overview of current issues in management of dyslipidemia. Am J Cardiol 1993;71:3B.

Grundy SM. Cholesterol and coronary heart disease: a new era—state of the art review. JAMA 1986;256:2849.

Hardoff D, Jacobson MS. Hyperlipidemia. Adolesc Med State Arts Rev 1992;3(1):473–486.

Havel RJ, Hunninghake DB, Illingworth R, et al. Lovastatin (Mevinolin) in the treatment of heterozygous familial hypercholesterolemia: a multicenter study. Ann Intern Med 1987;107:609.

Havel RJ, Rapaport E. Management of primary hyperlipidemia. N Engl J Med 1995;332:1491.

Hunninghake DB, Stein EA, Mellies MJ. Effects of one year treatment with Pravastatin, an HMG-CoA reductase inhibitor, on lipoprotein a. J Clin Pharmacol 1993;33:574.

Huston TP, Puffer JC, Rodney WM. The athletic heart syndrome. N Engl J Med 1985;313:24.

Jacobson MS, ed. Atherosclerosis prevention: identification and treatment of the child with high cholesterol. London: Harwood Academic Publishers, 1991.

Jacobson MS, Copperman N, Haas T, et al. Adolescent obesity and cardiovascular risk: a rational approach to management. Ann N Y Acad Sci 1993;699:220.

Jones PH. A clinical overview of dyslipidemias: treatment strategies. Am J Med 1992;93:187.

Kahn JK. Reversing coronary atherosclerosis: how to put findings of recent trials to practical use. Postgrad Med 1993;94:50.

Kannel WB, Wilson PW. Efficacy of lipid profiles in prediction of coronary disease. Am Heart J 1992;124:768.

Kannel WB, Wilson PW. An update on coronary risk factors. Med Clin North Am 1995;79:951.

Kashyap ML. Hyperlipidemia: current recommendations and methods for making an accurate diagnosis. Mod Med 1987;55:56.

Kottke BA, Zinsmeister AR, Holmes DR Jr, et al. Apolipoproteins and coronary artery disease. Mayo Clin Proc 1986;61:313.

Kuritzky L. Dyslipidemia: drugs, diet, and common sense. Hosp Pract 1994;29:40.

Kwiterovich PO Jr. Diagnosis and management of familial dyslipoproteinemia in children and adolescents. Pediatr Clin North Am 1990;37:1489.

Larsen ML, Illingworth DR. Drug treatment of dyslipoproteinemia. Med Clin North Am 1994;78:225.

Laskarzewski P, Morrison JA, deGroot I, et al. Lipid and lipoprotein tracking in 108 children over a four-year period. Pediatrics 1979;64:584.

Lauer R, Shekelle RB. Childhood prevention of atherosclerosis and hypertension. New York: Raven Press, 1980.

Lauer RM, Clarke WR. Use of cholesterol measurements in childhood for the prediction of adult hypercholesterolemia: the Muscatine study. JAMA 1990;264:3034.

Lavie CJ, Gau GT, Squires RW, et al. Management of lipids in primary and secondary prevention of cardiovascular diseases. Mayo Clin Proc 1988;63:605.

Lipid Research Clinics Program. The Lipid Research Clinics Coronary Primary Prevention Trial results I and FII. JAMA 1984;251:351.

Lovastatin Study Group II. Therapeutic response to lovastatin (Mevinolin) in nonfamilial hypercholesterolemia: a multicenter study. JAMA 1986;256:2829.

Lovastatin Study Group III. A multicenter comparison of lovastatin and cholestyramine therapy for severe primary hypercholesterolemia. JAMA 1988;260:359.

Luckstead EF. Sudden death in sports. Pediatr Clin North Am 1982;29:1355.

Lueg MC, Anding RH. Hypercholesterolemia: new values, new strategies. Hosp Pract 1986;21:112.

Malloy MJ, Kane JP, Kunitake ST, et al. Complementarity of colestipol, niacin, and lovastatin in treatment of severe familial hypercholesterolemia. Ann Intern Med 1987;107:616.

Manninen V, Elo O, Frick H. Lipid alterations and decline in the incidence of coronary heart disease in the Helsinki Heart Study. JAMA 1988;260:641.

Maron BJ, Roberts WC, McAllister HA. Sudden death in young athletes. Circulation 1980;62:218.

McKenna WJ, Deanfiel JE. Hypertrophic cardiomyopathy: an important cause of sudden death. Arch Dis Child 1984;59:971.

Morrison JA, deGroot I, Edwards BK, et al. Lipids and lipoproteins in 927 schoolchildren, ages 6 to 17 years. Pediatrics 1978;62:990.

Morrison JA, Glueck CJ. Pediatric risk factors for adult coronary heart disease: primary atherosclerosis prevention. Cardiovasc Rev Rep 1981;2:1269.

Moss AJ, Schwarty PJ, Crampton RS. The long QT syndrome: a prospective international study. Circulation 1985;71:17.

National Cholesterol Education Program. Report of the Expert Panel on Blood Cholesterol Levels in Children and Adolescents. Pediatrics 1992;89(suppl): 495–500.

National Cholesterol Education Program, Adult Treatment Panel II. Summary of the second report of the National Cholesterol Education Program (NCEP) Expert Panel on Detection Evaluation and Treatment of High Cholesterol in Adults (Adult Treatment Panel II). JAMA 1993;269:3015.

Neuspiel DR, Kuller LH. Sudden and unexpected natural death in childhood and adolescence. JAMA 1985;254:1321.

Newman WP, Freedman DS, Voors AW, et al. Relation of serum lipoprotein levels and systolic blood pressure to early atherosclerosis: the Bogalusa Heart Study. N Engl J Med 1986;314:138.

Orchard TJ, Rodgers M, Hedley A, et al. Changes in blood lipids and blood pressure during adolescence. Br Med J 1980;280:1563.

Partinen M, Phil S, Strandberg T, et al. Comparison of effects on sleep of lovastatin and pravastatin in hypercholesterolemia. Am J Cardiol 1994;73:876.

Pathobiological Dermininants of Atherosclerosis in Youth. Relationship of atherosclerosis in young men to serum lipoprotein cholesterol concentrations and smoking: a preliminary report from the Pathobiological Determinants of Atherosclerosis Research Group. JAMA 1990;264:3018.

Pravastatin, simvastatin and lovastatin for lowering serum cholesterol concentrations. Med Lett Drugs Ther 1992;34:57.

Schwartz CJ, Valente AJ, Sprague EA. A modern view of atherogenesis. Am J Cardiol 1993;71:9B.

Stein EA, Glueck CJ, Morrison JA. Coronary risk factors in the young. Annu Rev Med 1981;32:601.

Steinberg D, Witzum JL. Lipoproteins and atherogenesis. JAMA 1990;264:3047.

Steiner NJ, Neinstein LS, Pennbridge J. Hypercholesterolemia in adolescents: effectiveness of screening strategies based on selected risk factors. Pediatrics 1991;88:269.

Stone NJ. Secondary causes of hyperlipidemia. Med Clin North Am 1994;78:117.

Truswell AS. Food carbohydrates and plasma lipids—an update. Am J Clin Nutr 1994;59:710S.

Walden CC, Hegele RA. Apolipoprotein E in hyperlipidemia. Ann Intern Med 1994;120:1026.

Weis S, Lacko AG. Role of lipoproteins in hypercholesterolemia. Pract Cardiol 1988;May:12–18.

Yeshurun D, Gotto AM Jr. Hyperlipidemia: perspectives in diagnosis and treatment. South Med J 1995;88: 379.

CHAPTER 12

Hypertension

Arno R. Hohn and Lawrence S. Neinstein

More than 30 million Americans, or about 15% of the population, have hypertension. Evidence suggests that only 1% or 2% of young people have persistent hypertension (Hohn, 1994). Most adults and teenagers with hypertension have idiopathic or primary hypertension—that is, no cause can be found for their blood pressure elevation.

Despite the low incidence of adolescent hypertension, it is imperative that blood pressures be measured when a teen is examined. The detection of elevated blood pressure and the evaluation for hypertension risk factors in the adolescent years may prevent later cardiovascular diseases, with their catastrophic consequences. In addition, the prevalence of secondary hypertension is somewhat higher in adolescents than in adults, so existing secondary causes should be identified and treated in the afflicted young person.

DEFINITION OF HYPERTENSION IN ADOLESCENCE

Mean systolic and diastolic blood pressures increase with age during the adolescent years. Figures 12.1 and 12.2 show blood pressures derived from the Second Task Force on Blood Pressure Control in Children (1987), appointed by the National Heart, Lung, and Blood Institute to provide guidelines for physicians. More recently, Rosner et al. (1993) presented information refining task force norms by adding considerations of height. However the task force's definitions of hypertension still hold and include:

1. Normal blood pressure: Systolic and diastolic blood pressures at less than the 90th percentile for age and sex
2. High normal BP: Average systolic and/or diastolic blood pressure consistently between 90th and 95th percentiles for age and sex
3. Significant hypertension: Systolic and/or diastolic blood pressures at greater than or equal to the 95th percentile for age and sex, with measurements obtained on at least three occasions
4. Serious hypertension: Systolic and/or diastolic blood pressures at greater than or equal to the 99th percentile for age and sex, with measurements obtained on at least three occasions

The Task Force on Blood Pressure Control in Children hypertension groups with "significant" hypertension and those with "severe" hypertension are compared in Table 12.1. In considering the levels for hypertension outlined in the table, the practitioner should take into account that larger adolescents (heavier and taller) have higher average blood pressures. As can be seen in Table 12.2, this is of particular importance in the tall adolescent, who may be mislabeled as hypertensive.

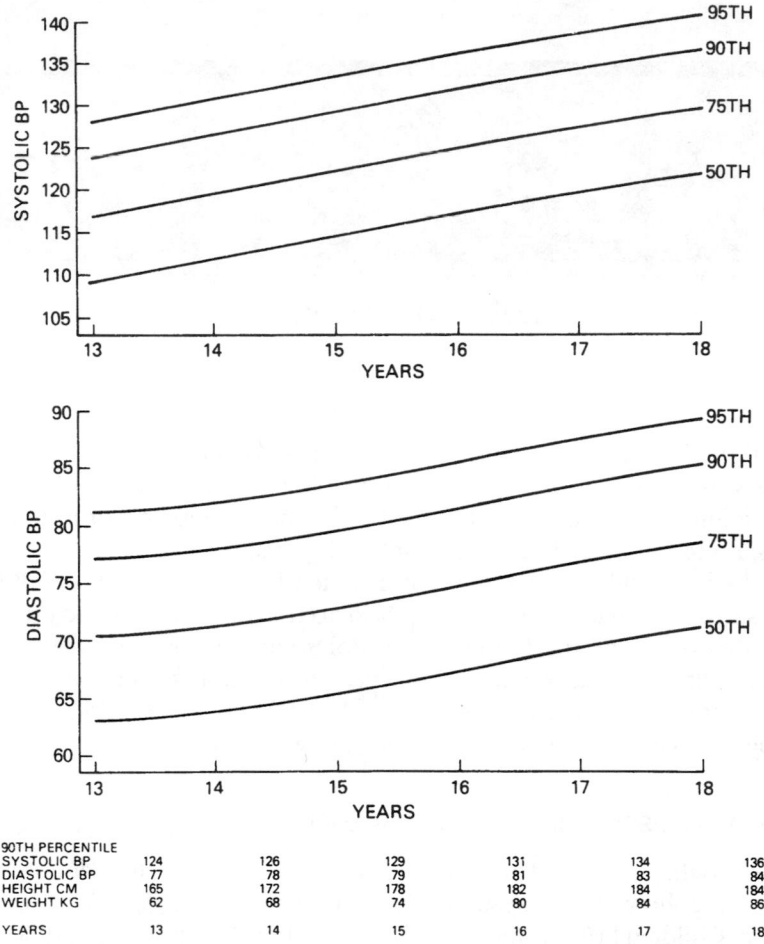

90TH PERCENTILE						
SYSTOLIC BP	124	126	129	131	134	136
DIASTOLIC BP	77	78	79	81	83	84
HEIGHT CM	165	172	178	182	184	184
WEIGHT KG	62	68	74	80	84	86
YEARS	13	14	15	16	17	18

FIGURE 12.1.   Age-specific percentiles of blood pressure (*BP*) measurements in boys, 13 to 18 years of age; Korotkoff phase V used for diastolic BP. (From National Heart, Lung, and Blood Institute's Task Force on Blood Pressure Control in Children. Washington, D.C.: U.S. Department of Health and Human Services, Public Health Services, National Institutes of Health, Jan 1987.)

TABLE 12.1.   Definitions of Significant versus Severe Hypertension in Adolescence

Age Group (yr)	"Significant" Hypertension (>95th percentile)	"Severe" Hypertension (>99th percentile)
10–12	Systolic BP ≥126[a]	Systolic BP ≥134
	Diastolic BP ≥82	Diastolic BP ≥90
13–15	Systolic BP ≥136	Systolic BP ≥144
	Diastolic BP ≥86	Diastolic BP ≥92
16–18	Systolic BP ≥142	Systolic BP ≥150
	Diastolic BP ≥92	Diastolic BP ≥98

[a]BP, blood pressure: measured in millimeters of mercury.

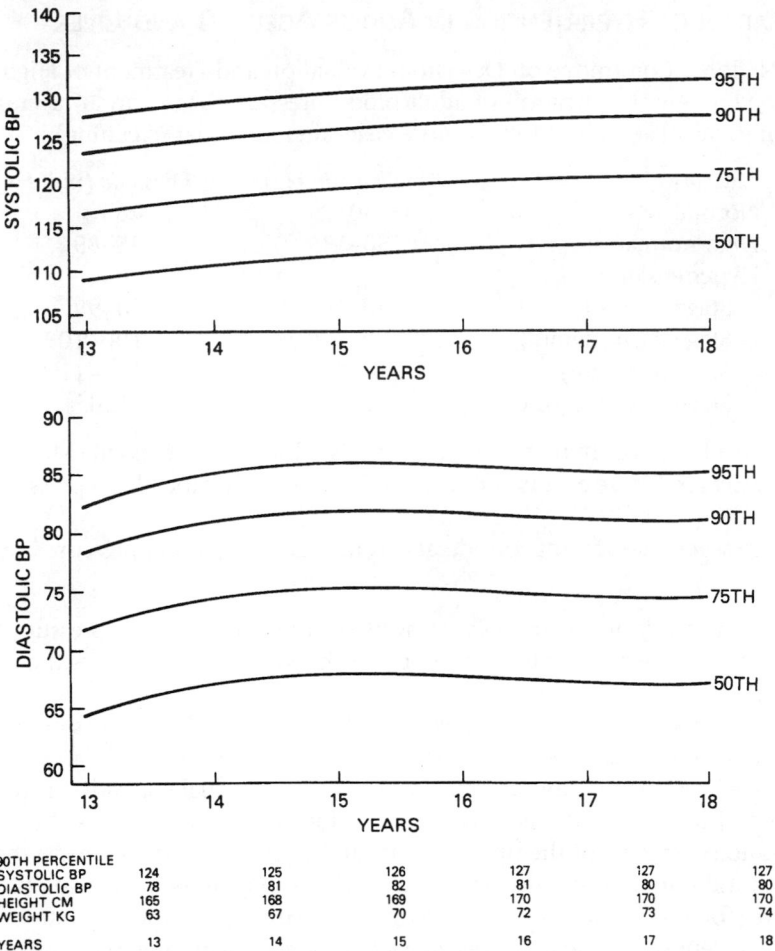

FIGURE 12.2.   Age-specific percentiles of blood pressure (*BP*) measurements in girls, 13 to 18 years of age; Korotkoff phase V used for diastolic BP. (From National Heart, Lung, and Blood Institute's Task Force on Blood Pressure Control in Children. Washington, D.C.: U.S. Department of Health and Human Services, Public Health Services, National Institutes of Health, Jan 1987.)

TABLE 12.2.   Significant Hypertension in Tall Adolescents

Age Group (yr)	Sex	Blood Pressure (mm Hg)	
		Systolic	Diastolic
10–12	Males	127	87
	Females	126	85
13–15	Males	136	89
	Females	131	88
16–18	Males	141	93
	Females	133	89

Adapted from Rosner B, Prineas RJ, Loggie JMH, et al. Blood pressure nomograms for children and adolescents, by height, sex and age, in the United States. J Pediatr 1993;123:871.

CLASSIFICATION OF HYPERTENSION IN ADULTS AGED 18 AND OVER

The Joint National Committee on Detection, Evaluation and Treatment of High Blood Pressure provided a new classification of adult blood pressure (based on an average of two or more readings taken at each of two or more visits after an initial screening):

Category	Systolic (mm Hg)	Diastolic (mm Hg)
Normal	<130	<85
High normal	130–139	85–89
Hypertension		
Stage 1 (mild)	140–159	90–99
Stage 2 (moderate)	160–179	100–109
Stage 3 (severe)	180–209	110–119
Stage 4 (very severe)	≥210	≥120

Although all stages of hypertension are associated with an increased risk of nonfatal and fatal cardiovascular disease events and renal disease, the higher the blood pressure, the greater the risk.

There are several important considerations in evaluating blood pressure in children and adolescents:

1. Although a variety of instruments are available to measure blood pressure, the mercury sphygmomanometer is generally accepted as the most accurate and is the instrument of choice.
2. Hypertension should not be diagnosed on the basis of a single measurement. Repeated measurements (at least three) on separate occasions are essential to diagnose hypertension. Using one isolated measurement may mislabel an individual with adverse consequences.
3. Proper cuff size is critical. The cuff should be long enough to encircle the arm and wide enough to cover 75% of the upper arm from the top of the shoulders to the olecranon. For practical purposes, use the largest cuff that fits the arm while leaving the antecubital fossa free for auscultation. It is better to choose a cuff slightly too big than one too small.
4. The adolescent should be in a quiet area and have sufficient time to relax—at least 5 minutes of rest. Measurements should be done with the adolescent in the sitting position, with the manometer at heart level. The arm (preferably the right) used for the measurement should be recorded in the chart. The adolescent should not have smoked or ingested caffeine within 30 minutes before measurement.
5. The cuff pressure should be released at a rate of 2–3 mm Hg per second. For diastolic blood pressure the fifth (disappearance) Korotkoff sound is usually accepted as more accurate in adolescents and adults.
6. A single blood pressure recorded at each visit is all that is usually necessary. Multiple pressures do not increase predictive value. Again, three pressures equal to or greater than the 95th percentile on three separate occasions are necessary for a diagnosis of hypertension.
7. Ambulatory monitoring, in which blood pressure measurements are obtained on an outpatient basis with recording devices, is not commonly needed in adolescents and young adults. However, for difficult diagnostic situations in which the blood pressures are repeatedly elevated in the office setting but normal out of the office, this type of monitoring can be helpful.

ETIOLOGY

The causes of hypertension vary among different age groups. In adolescents the prevalence of primary hypertension increases in comparison with younger children. This is particularly true

TABLE 12.3. Estimated Causes of Hypertension in Young People

Condition	Age Group	
	Adolescent (%)	Young Adult (%)
Congenital (including coarctation)	<1.0	<0.1
Renovascular (including thrombosis)	1.0	<0.4
Renal parenchymal disease	6.0	<4.0
Primary hypertension	91.0	95
Other	2.0	1
TOTAL	100	100

Adapted from Hohn AR. Guidebook for pediatric hypertension. Mount Kisco, New York: Futura Publishing, 1994.

for adolescents with mild hypertension. Renal parenchymal diseases are the most common secondary cause in the adolescent age group.

The medical literature has conflicting information concerning the causes of hypertension in young people. Studies finding a high incidence of secondary hypertension were, for the most part, small studies of patients seen in hypertension clinics. Information from large population studies show that primary hypertension is by far the most common cause of hypertension in the adolescent. Table 12.3 shows an estimation of the causes of hypertension in adolescents from data gathered from a number of population studies. Primary hypertension is thought to be the main cause of hypertension in young people.

EPIDEMIOLOGY

Prevalence

Extrapolating data from the medical literature on adolescent blood pressures coupled with the author's own experience using task force definitions of hypertension, places the prevalence of the disorder between 0.5% and 2% in young people. The importance of repeated measurements is demonstrated in a study of 3537 adolescents in New York (Kilcoyne et al., 1974). In that study, 5.4% of adolescents had systolic hypertension and 7.8% had diastolic blood pressures greater than 140/90 mm Hg on the first screening. The prevalence dropped to 1.2% and 2.4%, respectively, after rescreening. Likewise, Fixler et al. (1979) found in his survey of schoolchildren that 1.6% of 10,641 were hypertensive after three screenings. In Muscatine, Iowa, fewer than 1% of nearly 4000 adolescents were hypertensive after four screenings. Table 12.4 lists various prevalence studies of hypertension in adolescents.

Weight

Weight has long been held to have a positive relationship with blood pressure. More than half of hypertensive young people are obese. Higgins et al. (1984) suggested that if weight could be reduced in young people to below obesity levels (weight 20% above that given for height), the prevalence of hypertension would decrease by one-third.

Age

Blood pressure increases with age in a nonlinear fashion through adolescence. Pressure should remain constant once adult status is reached, as described by Oliver et al. (1977) in a primitive society. Unfortunately, in cultured societies that is not the case, and about one in six will manifest hypertension in adult life.

TABLE 12.4.   Results of Prevalence Studies of Hypertension in Young People

Author, Year Published	Number of Patients	Age (yr)	Position in which BP Taken	Definition of Hypertension[a] (mm Hg)	Race	Prevalence of Hypertension
Boynton and Todd, 1947 (U.S.)	72,210	16–30	Sitting	SBP 140 DBP 90	Not stated	7.36% male 1.12% female 5.87% male 2.18% female
Masland et al., 1956 (U.S.)	1,795	12–21	Not stated	BP 140/90	Not stated	1.4%
Boe et al., 1957 (Norway)	3,833	15–19	Sitting	SBP 150–160 DBP 90–95	White	1.04% female 3.01% male
Heyden et al., 1969 (U.S.)	435	15–25	Sitting	Average of 3 readings SBP 140 DBP 90	186 African-American 249 White	11.0%
Londe, 1966 (U.S.)	1,805	4–15	Supine	BP at 90th percentile, one reading Persistent BP at 95th percentile	92 African-American 1,713 White	12.4% male 11.6% female[b]
Wilber et al., 1972 (U.S.)	799	15–25	Sitting	SBP 160 DBP 95	All 79% African-American	1.0% 1.5%
Kilcoyne et al., 1974 (U.S.)	3,537[c]	14–19	Sitting	SBP 140 DBP 90	2,193 African-American 124 White 1,220 Hispanic	5.4% SBP 7.8% DBP
	(215/277)[d]					1.2% SBP 2.4% DBP
Lauer et al., 1974 (U.S.)	1,301	14–18	Sitting	SBP 140 DBP 90	96.4% African-American	8.9% SBP 12.2% DBP
Miller and Shekelle, 1976	13,231	15–16	Supine, 5–10 min	SBP 150 DBP 90	<1% African-American	4.6%[c] 2.3%[d]
Fixler et al., 1979	10,641	14 ± 0.03	Sitting, 4 min	Percentiles per 1977 Task Force	46% African-American 40 White 14 Latin	8.9%[c] 1.6%[d]

Adapted from Loggie JMH, Rauh LW. Persistent systemic hypertension in the adolescent. Med Clin North Am 1975;59:1371.
[a]SBP, systolic blood pressure; DBP, diastolic blood pressure; BP, blood pressure.
[b]Labile; 1.9% persistent.
[c]First screening test.
[d]Second screening test.

Salt and Other Nutrient Intake

Controversy prevails over the numerous studies concerning the relationship of sodium intake to blood pressure. For most individuals, little correlation exists. However, in certain salt-sensitive individuals, sodium restriction appears beneficial. For example, it has been suggested (Hohn et al., 1983) that African-American children from hypertensive families may be salt sensitive.

Other studies have found a link between potassium intake and both elevated and low blood pressure. However, efforts to correlate calcium and other divalent cations with blood pressure have been equivocal. Similarly correlations between blood pressure and vitamins A, C, and E, although suggestive, remain to be proven.

Dietary Fat and Fiber

Reduction in dietary intake of dietary fat and fiber together has been noted to reduce blood pressure. Triglyceride levels are also correlated with pressure levels.

Stress

Both physical stress and mental stress evoke changes in blood pressure. Indeed, the degree of change has been thought by some to be useful in predicting later life hypertension. This remains to be proven. However, exercise has been useful in the treatment of hypertension, and reduction of anxiety may also be beneficial.

Race

Although a significant determinant in adult blood pressure, race is not a factor in teens. As a rule, African-American adolescents have blood pressure levels similar to those of white adolescents. However, Voors et al. (1979) and Hohn et al. (1983) suggested that certain subgroups of African-American youths have higher pressures than their white counterparts. Rabinowitz et al. (1993) found a higher prevalence of hypertension among African-American females than among non-Hispanic females.

Genetics

Both familial-aggregation blood pressure studies, such as those of Zinner et al. (1971), and twin studies, such as those of Schieken (1993), indicate a strong positive correlation between hereditary influences and blood pressure measurements. The scheme for the natural history of hypertension presented in Figure 12.3 indicates the impact of the "gene pool."

Tracking (Maintenance of Rank Order with Time)

It has been said that the best predictor of future blood pressure is an individual's current pressure. However, evidence that adult hypertension is predictable by childhood blood pressures is controversial and correlation coefficients are generally low.

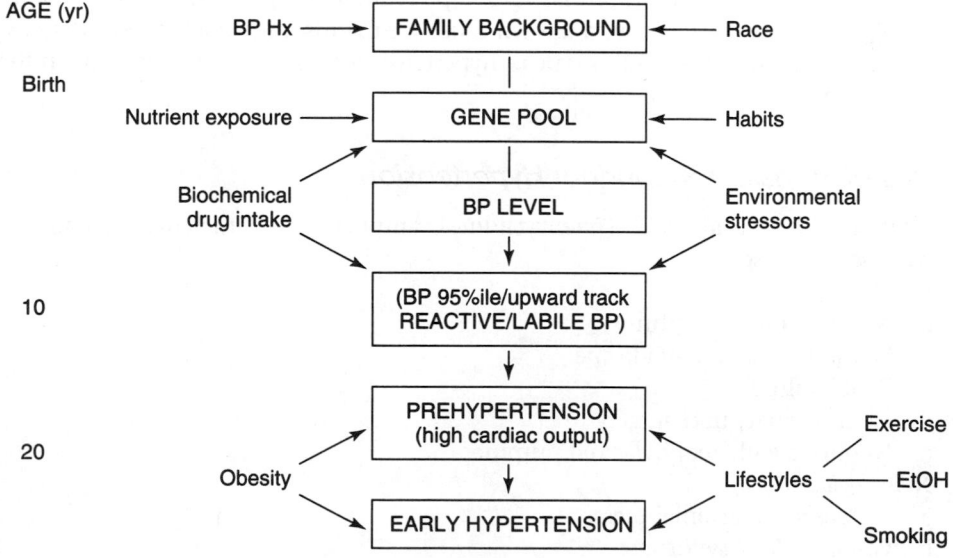

FIGURE 12.3. Natural history (*Hx*) scheme for hypertension. The impact of the "gene pool," although present at birth, does not manifest itself until later in life. *BP,* blood pressure; *EtOH,* alcohol. (Adapted from Hohn AR. Guidebook for pediatric hypertension. Mount Kisco, New York: Futura Publishing, 1994.)

Risk Factors for Later Life Primary Hypertension

About 1–2% of adolescents will be found to be hypertensive, and most of those will have primary hypertension. Yet, in at least 15%, hypertension will develop later in life. Early identification of those who ultimately will find themselves hypertensive might permit preventive programs to delay or avoid the disorder. Accordingly, those young people with risk factors for adult hypertension deserve special consideration. Lauer and Clarke (1989) monitored blood pressures in a large group of young people in Muscatine, Iowa, as they grew into adulthood. Risk factors that they and others found are listed below. Combinations of risk factors—for example, being young, African-American, obese, and from a hypertension-riddled family—may place a person at exceptional risk.

Hypertension Risk Factors

1. *Systolic blood pressure* greater than the 90th percentile: Doubles risk
2. *Family history* of two or more members with hypertension: Increases risk two to four times
3. *Weight* more than 20% above the norm for height: Two-thirds found to be hypertensive
4. *Race:* A greater than 10% higher incidence of hypertension in adulthood in African-Americans than in other racial groups (i.e., 25% will be found to be hypertensive later in life)
5. *Dietary cations:* Especially increased dietary sodium in salt-sensitive individuals and decreased potassium intake (may lead to higher blood pressures)
6. *Other risk factors:* Hyperlipidemia (or family history), stress, smoking, alcohol, drug intake, preeclampsia and eclampsia, and diabetes mellitus

Causes for Secondary Hypertension in Adolescence

More than 90% of hypertensive adolescents have no known cause for their disorder and are labeled as having primary or essential hypertension. Blood pressures are usually in the 95th–99th percentile range in essential hypertension. A small number of youths will be found to have serious hypertension (i.e., blood pressure >99th percentile). Such people will in all likelihood be found to have a known cause for the disorder labeled secondary hypertension. A number of causes of this type of hypertension are listed below, roughly in the order of frequency of occurrence.

Causes of Transient Secondary Hypertension

1. *Drug related:* Steroids, PCP (phencyclidine), amphetamines, mercury poisoning, oral contraceptive use
2. *Renal*
   a. Acute glomerulonephritis
   b. Hemolytic-uremic syndrome
   c. Renal failure
   d. Genitourinary tract surgery
   e. Nephritis with anaphylactoid purpura
3. *Neurological*
   a. Increased intracranial pressure
   b. Guillain-Barré syndrome
   c. Cervical and leg traction
4. *Vascular:* Painful sickle-cell crisis

5. *Metabolic*
   a. Hypercalcemia
   b. Hypernatremia
   c. Congenital adrenal hyperplasia
   d. Acute intermittent porphyria
6. *Miscellaneous*
   a. Burns
   b. Stevens-Johnson syndrome
   c. Postoperative status

Causes of Sustained Hypertension

1. *Renal*
   a. Bilateral obstructive uropathy
   b. Chronic glomerulonephritis
   c. Renal parenchymal disease (pyelonephritis, infarction, radiation, trauma)
   d. Renal artery lesions (stenosis, thrombosis, aneurysm)
      — Intrinsic: Fibromuscular hyperplasia, arteritis, thrombosis
      — Extrinsic: Compression
   e. Congenital defects (hypoplastic, polycystic kidney)
   f. Tumors
   g. Postrenal transplantation
   h. Familial nephritis
   i. Renal vein thrombosis
2. *Vascular*
   a. Coarctation of the aorta
   b. Aortitis; systemic disorders
3. *Endocrine*
   a. Pheochromocytoma
   b. Cushing's syndrome
   c. Primary aldosteronism
   d. Hyperparathyroidism
   e. Ovarian or adrenal tumors
   f. Congenital adrenal hyperplasia
   g. Neuroblastoma
4. *Metabolic*
   a. Diabetes mellitus with renal involvement
   b. Gouty nephropathy

DIAGNOSIS

Algorithm for Diagnosis

Schemes have been developed to assist in the diagnosis and management of various levels of hypertension. Figure 12.4 is a flow diagram for the identification and evaluation of hypertension in adolescents. Important aspects of this flowchart include:

1. Measuring blood pressure repeatedly during several visits.
2. Taking height into account. A blood pressure between the 90th and 95th blood pressure percentiles can be completely normal in an adolescent taller than the 90th growth per-

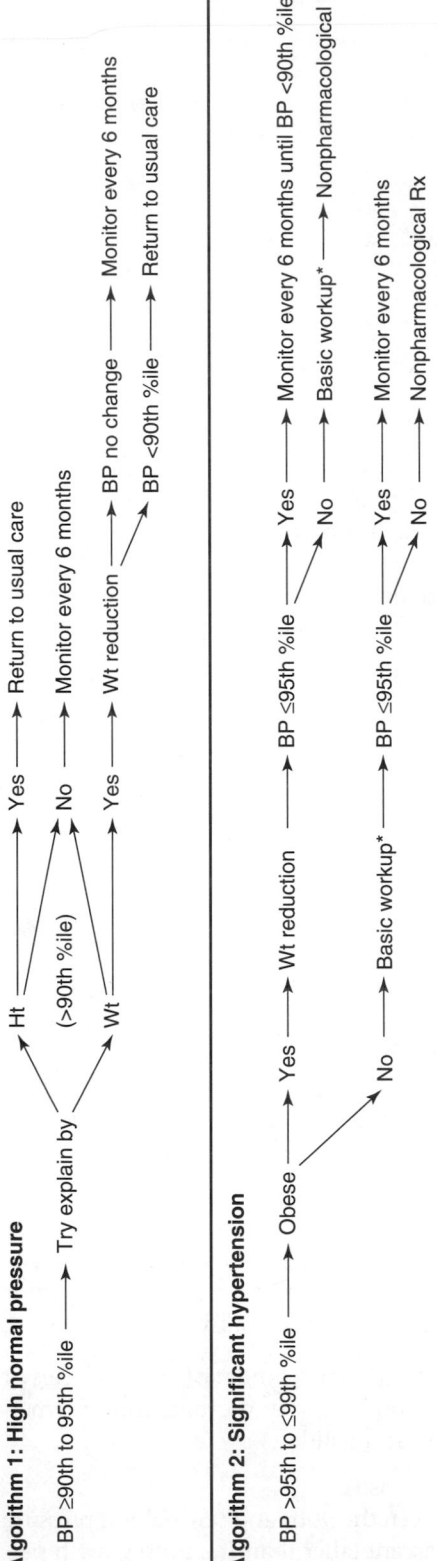
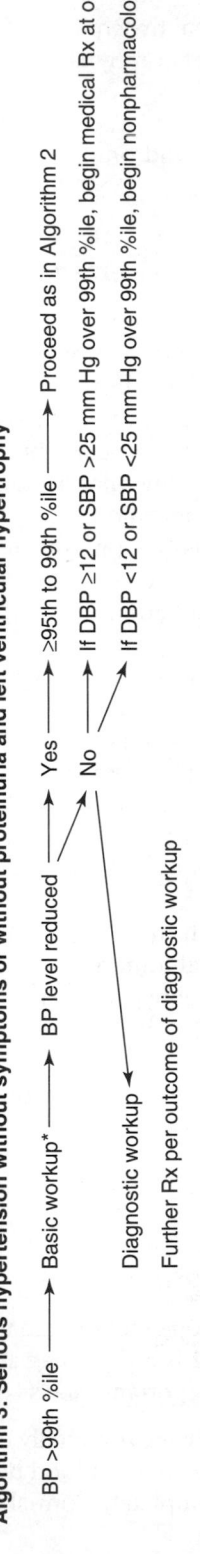

FIGURE 12.4. Algorithms for diagnostic study and treatment of persistent blood pressure (*BP*) ≥90th percentile (average of two measures repeated on next two visits). *Ht*, height; *wt*, weight; *DBP*, diastolic BP; *SBP*, systolic BP; *Rx*, treatment. (Adapted from Hohn AR. Guidebook for pediatric hypertension. Mount Kisco, New York: Futura Publishing, 1994.)

*Basic diagnostic workup = urinalysis, erythrocyte sedimentation rate, hemoglobin and hematocrit determinations, blood chemistry studies with electrolyte values.

centile for height. The 90th percentiles for heights are also shown on Figures 12.1 and 12.2.

3. Instituting and monitoring a weight reduction program for obese adolescents in the 90th–95th percentile.

4. Providing a diagnostic evaluation and giving nonpharmacological treatment—and possibly drug therapy if the blood pressure remains above the 95th percentile.

Avoidance of Mislabeling

Adolescents make fewer visits per year to health-care practitioners than do other age groups. However, each visit presents an opportunity to record blood pressure. About 10% of these young people will have a high initial blood pressure (≥95th percentile). They should be so labeled, not given a diagnosis of hypertension. Before a diagnosis of hypertension can be made, two subsequent blood pressure determinations on different days must also show a high systolic and diastolic pressure, or both. Only 1–2% of adolescents will fulfill this criteria and, by definition, have hypertension.

Type of Hypertension

Most young people with hypertension will have only a mild or moderate elevation of blood pressure—that is, their pressures will be at less than the 99th percentile. These people are generally symptom free and unaware of their pressure elevation. Mild to moderate hypertension in adolescents is more likely essential than secondary.

Another group, perhaps 1 in 1000 adolescents, will repeatedly have pressures at greater than the 99th percentile. They are more likely to have symptoms. Their moderately severe or severe hypertension is often a result of a renal, vascular, or endocrine problem. Secondary causes should be of higher concern in white females. A search must be made for one of the underlying causes of the disorder listed above.

Initial Diagnostic Study

The diagnostic evaluation needs to be tailored to the individual, taking into account the age, sex, race, family history, and level of hypertension. For example, a 12-year-old white female with no family history of hypertension and a diastolic blood pressure of 115 in all limbs would be a candidate for an aggressive evaluation for secondary causes and, in particular, renal parenchymal disease or renal artery stenosis. In contrast, a 17-year-old white male with a family history of hypertension and a diastolic blood pressure of 92 is not a good candidate for invasive studies to look for a secondary cause.

1. History: To perform a diagnostic study of a young person for hypertension requires that a detailed history be elicited. The history should aim at determining secondary causes, target-organ damage, and other cardiovascular risk factors. Look for evidence of urinary tract infections or renal disease, or for a patient or family history of hypertension, as well as at dietary, activity, and other habits. Be sure to ask specific questions regarding each of the following (a self-history form has been devised to aid in this process [Hohn, 1994]):
   a. Headache
   b. Chest pain or dyspnea
   c. History of muscle weakness
   d. Edema
   e. Pallor, flushing attacks, or palpitation

    f. Polydipsia, polyuria, or weight loss

    g. Change in hair, body habitus, or menses

    h. History of renal, thyroid, or heart disease

    i. Drug use

    j. Smoking history

    k. Dietary assessment, including sodium intake, alcohol use, and intake of cholesterol and saturated fats

    l. Family history of hypertension, myocardial infarction, diabetes, or strokes, with age at diagnosis

2. Physical examination: A thorough examination is also an essential part of the diagnostic study. The adolescent in question will often be found to be obese. The examination should include an exploration for evidence of a secondary cause or end-organ damage and an evaluation of:

    a. Blood pressure levels in both arms: Sitting and supine positions

    b. Pulses in all extremities

    c. Height and weight

    d. Neck: Carotid bruits or an enlarged thyroid gland

    e. Fundi: Arteriolar narrowing, arteriovenous nicking, hemorrhages, exudates

    f. Abdomen: Bruits, enlarged kidneys, masses, abnormal aortic pulsation

    g. Heart: Increased rate, size, precordial heave, clicks, murmurs, arrhythmias, third and fourth heart sounds

    h. Extremities: Diminished or absent arterial pulsations, bruits, edema

    i. Nervous system

    j. Body habitus: Pattern of obesity (e.g., "buffalo hump")

    k. Skin: Striae, café au lait spots, neurofibromas

3. Clinical signs of secondary causes of hypertension (Table 12.5) and the following considerations:

    a. Acute onset of hypertension in adolescents suggests acute renal disease.

    b. Severe hypertension suggests renal disease.

    c. Endocrine causes in adolescents are rare, and are unusual without clinical signs or symptoms.

    d. Bilaterally enlarged kidneys suggest polycystic disease.

4. Laboratory testing

    a. Reserved for those in whom secondary hypertension is suspected or in those whose blood pressure remains significantly elevated (95th–99th percentile) despite non-pharmacological measures (see below) for more than 6 months

    b. Unrevealing history and examination findings in most adolescents with persistent or severe hypertension or both, except for family history and obesity. Without positive historical or examination findings, only a basic set of laboratory tests should be done (limited testing will save time and health-care dollars):

        — Sedimentation rate

        — Hematocrit

        — Hemoglobin concentration

        — Urinalysis (with culture for females)

        — Blood chemistry panel (including blood urea nitrogen, creatinine, glucose) and electrolytes

    c. Additional laboratory tests: If secondary hypertension is suspected or if blood pressure remains elevated for longer than 6 months

        — Echocardiogram: Possible increase in left ventricular wall thickness (Thickness is thought to correlate roughly with time spent (hours, days) hypertensive. It is not seen in transient, or "white coat," hypertension.)

TABLE 12.5.   Clinical Clues to Secondary Causes of Hypertension[a]

Cause	History	Physical Examination	Laboratory
Coarctation of the aorta	Often asymptomatic fatigue of legs	Blood pressure in legs lower than in arms Femoral pulses decreased or delayed Systolic murmur Intercostal pulsations	Rib notching on chest x-ray Left ventricular hypertrophy
Unilateral renal parenchymal disease	Symptoms of urinary tract infection Fever History of trauma to flank Malignant hypertension	Rapidly progressive retinopathy Palpable hydronephrotic kidney CVA tenderness	Proteinuria Discrepancy in size or function of two kidneys Elevated creatinine
Renovascular disease	Trauma to abdomen or flank Hematuria	Bruit in abdomen or flank Café au lait spots or signs of neurofibromatosis	Discrepancy of size or function on pyelogram Increased plasma renin activity Arteriographic evidence of unilateral obstructive renal arterial lesions
Cushing's syndrome	Weight gain Weakness Change in habitus Easy bruising Amenorrhea	Truncal obesity Buffalo hump Moon facies Purple striae Hirsutism	Polycythemia Hyperglycemia Osteoporosis Elevated cortisols or abnormal suppression with dexamethasone
Primary aldosteronism	Periodic muscle weakness Paresthesias Polyuria Polydipsia Tetany	Chvostek's and Trousseau's signs present Tetany Muscle weakness	Alkaline pH Hypokalemia Elevated serum bicarbonate Elevated aldosterone secretion unresponsive to increased sodium intake Low plasma renin activity, unresponsive to low sodium
Pheochromocytoma	Episodes of flushing, sweating, palpitations Nervousness Weight loss Personality change Abdominal pain Family history of pheochromocytoma Paroxysmal hypertension Pallor, nausea, tremor	Paroxysmal hypertension Orthostatic hypotension Café au lait spots	Glucose intolerance Elevated urinary catecholamines, VMA, or metanephrine Elevated serum catecholamines Positive glucagon test result

[a]CVA, cerebrovascular accident; VMA, vanillylmandelic acid.

— Chest x-ray: Possible cardiomegaly
— Cholesterol and fasting triglyceride levels
— Urine culture if not previously done
— Uric acid concentration: If elevated, a marker for hypertension in young people

Further Diagnostic Tests for Specific Causes of Hypertension

In adolescents with severe hypertension or with signs or symptoms suggestive of a specific secondary cause, further diagnostic tests are indicated. The particular test needed depends on the suspected cause and the experience of the radiologists and laboratory that the practitioner is using. Consultation with someone knowledgeable about hypertension in young people would be helpful to pursue the most cost-effective and safest diagnostic evaluation. Many diagnostic studies have now become available to explore renal and endocrine causes. There is still controversy regarding which tests should be ordered and under what circumstances. Some of the tests include:

1. Renal studies
   a. Radiologic and radioisotope studies
      — Rapid-sequence intravenous pyelography
      — Renal ultrasonography
      — Renal radionuclide studies
   b. Renal angiography with measurement of renal vein renins (Timing of angiography depends on age of patient [earlier if younger], sex [earlier if female], and severity of hypertension [earlier if severe].)
   c. Digital subtraction angiography
   d. Computed tomography of the kidneys or adrenal glands
2. Hormonal studies
   a. Quantitation of urine catecholamines and metabolites
   b. Plasma catecholamines
   c. Peripheral plasma renin activity, serum and urinary aldosterone concentrations, and electrolyte determinations with and without salt loading
   d. Measurement of other hormones, such as free cortisol, in urine and plasma
   e. Measurement of aldosterone and cortisol in adrenal venous effluent
   f. Newer diagnostic tests (such as those utilizing converting enzyme inhibitors): Best left to the consultant in hypertension

THERAPY

Prevention

Optimally, measures to prevent or minimize the effects of hypertension should be applied to those adolescents prone to have the disorder later in life. The difficulty lies in finding those at risk and deciding what measures to apply. Data from young people for this purpose is lacking, and long-term follow-up information is unavailable. Nevertheless, a starting point for such a strategy is to consider those with the findings listed below as being at risk. They should be counseled about nonpharmacological treatments to maintain lower blood pressure and periodically monitored.

Normotensive adolescents who may benefit from nonpharmacological antihypertension measures include:

1. Those with consistently high-normal blood pressure (>90th percentile)
2. Those with a trend of upward-tracking pressures (>75th percentile) or pressures occasionally above the 95th percentile
3. Those who are obese, especially if parents are obese
4. Those with hyperlipidemia or a family history of the disorder, especially together with coronary artery disease or stroke
5. Those with diabetes mellitus
6. Those with two or more family members with treated hypertension, especially African-Americans

Criteria for Treatment

Most patients with definite hypertension at presentation will have some regression of blood pressure toward normal if monitored closely. Accordingly, it is wise to institute nonpharmacological measures while a basic diagnostic study is being done.

1. All patients with sustained severe hypertension (systolic or diastolic pressure >99th percentile; e.g., 150/98 mm Hg in 16- to 18-year-olds) require full diagnostic evaluation and either drug therapy or treatment of secondary causes.
2. Patients with continued mild hypertension (systolic or diastolic blood pressure between 95th and 99th percentiles; e.g., 142/92 mm Hg in 16- to 18-year-olds) should receive periodic blood pressure determination and nonpharmacological measures first.
3. The question of when to institute drug therapy for significant hypertension in adolescents is still controversial. Indications could include those with persistent significant hypertension (mild or moderate, 95th–99th percentile) unresponsive to nonpharmacological measures and with:
   a. African-American heritage, strong family history of hypertension, or both
   b. Other cardiovascular risk factors (see risk index for adolescents, Figs. 11.1 and 11.2)
   c. Evidence of target organ damage
4. Care must be exercised in labeling an adolescent as hypertensive because if the diagnosis is misapplied, it may lead to exclusion from activities or to future insurance problems.

Nonpharmacological Interventions

1. Weight reduction: Excess body weight is correlated closely with increased blood pressure. Weight reduction reduces blood pressure in a large proportion of hypertensive individuals who are more than 10% above ideal weight.
2. Avoidance of excess salt: Moderate sodium restriction in hypertensive individuals has been shown, on average, to reduce systolic blood pressure by 4.9 mm Hg and diastolic blood pressure by 2.6 mm Hg. Foods with high salt content are listed below.

Sauces	*Snack Foods*	*Excessive Soft Drinks*	*Meats and Seafood*	*Miscellaneous*
A-1 sauce	Corn chips	Coke (50 mg Na/12 oz)	Sausage	Bouillion
Relish	Pickles	Mountain Dew	Frankfurters	Olives
Soy sauce	Potato chips	(70 mg Na/12 oz)	Ham	Pizza
Worcestershire	Pretzels		Frozen	Sauerkraut
sauce	Salted popcorn		oysters	
	Salted peanuts			
	Chocolate			

Although there has been some evidence to suggest that potassium, calcium, or magnesium supplementation might theoretically be of benefit, at present none can be recommended. However, eating low-sodium, high-potassium foods could be recommended, as well as avoiding high-sodium, low-potassium foods. The adolescent should also still eat adequate daily amounts of calcium if on a salt-restricted diet. An increase in dietary fiber and a decrease in saturated fats could also be recommended for overall general health. Kaplan (1988) and others have reviewed the efficacy of other nonpharmacological measures.

3. Regular physical exercise. Regular aerobic physical activity, adequate to achieve at least a moderate level of physical fitness, may be beneficial for both prevention and treatment of hypertension. Regular aerobic physical activity can reduce systolic blood pressure in hypertensive patients by approximately 10 mm Hg.
4. Discontinuance of smoking and avoidance of alcohol excess, medications (except as directed by health-care providers), and drugs (e.g., cocaine, amphetamines). Although cigarette smoking is unrelated to hypertension, it is a major risk factor for cardiovascular disease and thus should be avoided by hypertensive individuals. Excessive alcohol intake can raise blood pressure and cause resistance to antihypertensive therapy.

5. Examination of other cardiovascular risk factors.
6. Use of methods such as behavior modification, biofeedback, and hypnosis.

Pharmacological Treatment

1. Antihypertensive medications are definitely indicated for those who have:
   a. Symptoms
   b. Dangerously high pressures (i.e., >12 mm Hg above the 99th percentile diastolic or >25 mm Hg above the 99th percentile systolic)
   c. Evidence of end-organ damage
2. If in doubt and the young person is free of symptoms, proteinuria, cardiomegaly, or echocardiographic evidence of left ventricular hypertrophy, it may be best to postpone drug treatment.
3. Adherence to drug therapy should be simple so that compliance will be increased in what may be a lifelong but asymptomatic problem.
4. Explicit education should be given regarding hypertension and the reasons for therapy.
5. The adolescent should be responsible for taking his or her own medication.
6. Antihypertensive agents should be chosen to obtain the maximum benefit with the fewest and least severe side effects. The ideal hypertensive agent would:
   a. Lower blood pressure in almost all hypertensive individuals
   b. Reverse specific pathogenic mechanisms
   c. Improve hemodynamics
   d. Be associated with few biochemical changes
   e. Be associated with few or no adverse reactions
   f. Have convenient once- or twice-a-day dosing
   g. Have a low cost
7. Unfortunately, the ideal antihypertensive agent does not exist. Initial therapeutic regimens have been debated. Many experts have recommended an individualized step-care approach, as suggested by the Joint National Committee (National High Blood Pressure Education Program) (1993) and shown in Figure 12.5. In this approach, a monotherapy drug regimen is superimposed on nonpharmacological therapy as initial treatment. Either a calcium entry blocker (CEB), angiotensin-converting enzyme (ACE) inhibitor, diuretic, or β-blocker may be used. Advocates of this approach recommend the following:
   a. Begin with a low dose of the chosen initial drug. CEBs and ACE inhibitors are preferred by many experts. However, only diuretics and β-blockers have been studied sufficiently to demonstrate a reduction in morbidity and mortality rates in association with antihypertensive therapy. ACE inhibitors are becoming more popular and more cost-effective. They may be especially helpful in the treatment of teens with high renin levels caused by renal disease. Preparations with once- or twice-daily dosing are available and can improve compliance. CEBs are also effective, offer convenient dosing schedules, and are generally well tolerated. Titrate the initial medication to a higher dose if necessary. If blood pressure control is still not achieved, proceed as follows:
   b. Add or substitute a small dose of either an ACE inhibitor or a thiazide diuretic or adrenergic inhibiting agent, whichever was not used in step a. Proceed to a full dose if necessary. If blood pressure control is still not achieved, proceed as follows:
   c. Add a third antihypertensive drug, usually a vasodilator or renin angiotensin inhibitor, or, preferably, obtain consultation from an expert in hypertension in young people.
   d. β-Blockers and diuretics have associated problems, including:
      — Diuretics: Hypokalemia, hypercholesterolemia, and hyperglycemia
      — β-Blockers: Elevated triglyceride levels and lowered high-density lipoprotein cholesterol levels

Step 1: Give Nonpharmacological Treatment

1. Weight control
2. Sodium restriction
3. Adequate dietary potassium and calcium
4. Low-fat, high-fiber diet
5. Exercise and relaxation response
6. Avoidance of alcohol, medications, other drugs

(If pressure not controlled, progress in steps but continue nonpharmacological treatment in all steps.)

Step 2: Start Initial Drug Treatment (Single Drug)

(Step 1 for DBP >99th percentile)
(+ Sx with nonpharmacological Rx)

1. Calcium entry blocker (CEB) *or*
2. ACE inhibitor *or*
3. β-Blocker *or*   } Use low dose
4. Diuretic

(If pressure remains uncontrolled)

Step 3: Add Second Drug of Different Class* or Substitute Another Drug of Same Class

*Diuretic *or* α_1-Blocker *or*
  β-Blocker *or*   Vasodilator *or*
  Calcium antagonist *or*   Central-acting α_2-agonist
  ACE inhibitor *or*

(If pressure still not controlled)

Step 4: Add Third Drug of Different Class or Substitute Second Drug

(Failure of pressure control)

Step 5: Provide Further Evaluation or Referral, or Add Third or Fourth Drug

Step-Down Program: Trial after prolonged pressure control

FIGURE 12.5.   Individualized step-care approach to hypertension therapy. *DBP,* diastolic blood pressure; *Sx,* symptoms; *Rx,* treatment. (From Hohn AR. Guidebook for pediatric hypertension. Mount Kisco, New York: Futura Publishing, 1994.)

e. ACE inhibitors and calcium blockers have the potential to control hypertension without the effects caused by β-blockers and diuretics. Though the long-term side effects and efficacy of these drugs are not yet known, midterm information is promising. Once-a-day dosing is the preferred initial therapy in most adolescents, and long-acting or sustained-release medications are available. ACE inhibitors and CEBs are popular as possible first choices for treating hypertension in adults and are seeing increasing use in pediatric circles.

8. Step-down therapy, or drug withdrawal, should not be forgotten. After an extended course of drug therapy and blood pressure control, a gradual reduction or withdrawal of medication can be attempted. This requires close observation and continuation of non-pharmacological therapy.

9. Classes of antihypertensive medications and specific drugs in each class are listed below. (Asterisk [*] indicates recommended or most used in class.) For doses, specific actions, and differences, as well as side effects, a reference such as the Pediatric Dosing Handbook and Formulary (Division of Pharmacy, Childrens Hospital of Los Angeles, 1994) must be consulted.

a. Diuretics
   — Loop-acting diuretics: Furosemide (Lasix)
   — Potassium-sparing agents: Spironolactone (Aldactone)
   — Thiazide diuretics: Hydrochlorothiazide (Hydrodiuril)*
b. Adrenergic inhibitors
   — β-Adrenergic antagonists: Atenolol (Tenormin)*; esmolol (Brevibloc); labetalol (Normodyne; Trandate); metoprololtartrate (Lopressor); nadolol (Corgard); pindolol (Visken); propranolol (Inderal); and timolol (Blocadren)
   — Central adrenergic inhibitors: Clonidine (Catapres); guanabenz (Wytensin); methyldopa (Aldomet)
   — α-Adrenergic receptor antagonists: Prazosin (Minipress)*
c. Vasodilators
   — Vascular smooth muscle relaxing agents: Diazoxide (Hyperstat); hydralazine (Apresoline)*; minoxidil (Loniten); nitroprusside (Nipride)
   — Slow-channel CEBs: Diltiazem HCl (Cardizem); nifedipine (Procardia)*; verapamil HCl (Calan; Isoptin)
d. ACE inhibitors
   — Captopril (Capoten)
   — Enalapril maleate (Vasotec)*
   — Enalapril maleate plus hydrochlorothiazide

SPECIAL POPULATIONS

1. African-Americans. The frequency of hypertension in African-Americans is among the highest in the world. Hypertension develops at an earlier age and is more severe in African-Americans than in whites. In African-Americans, diuretics have been proven to reduce hypertensive morbidity and mortality rates, and thus diuretics should be seriously considered for use in the absence of other conditions that prohibit their use. β-Blockers or ACE inhibitors are less effective in African-Americans; however, calcium antagonists and α_1-receptor blockers are as effective in African-Americans as in whites.
2. Females who take oral contraceptives. Most females who take oral contraceptives have a small increase in systolic and diastolic blood pressure but usually within normal range. Hormonal contraceptives, mainly those which contain estrogen, can increase angiotensinogen, leading to an increase in angiotensin II and an increase in blood pressure in some individuals. The risk of having overt hypertension appears to increase with age, duration of use, and body mass. Many of the studies of blood pressure and oral contraceptive agents involved higher doses of both estrogen and progesterone than are used currently.
3. Teens with asthma. In teens with asthma and hypertension, β-blocking drugs can worsen bronchoconstriction and therefore are relatively contraindicated. Methylxanthine and corticosteroids used to treat asthma can worsen hypertension.

HYPERTENSIVE EMERGENCIES

Rarely an adolescent will have signs of encephalopathy or heart failure at presentation and be found to have extraordinarily high blood pressure—that is, pressure 1.3 to 1.5 times the 95th percentile. This constitutes a true emergency and may have disastrous consequences unless efforts to lower the blood pressure are begun at once. The patient should be hospitalized and an intravenous line placed. If the patient is obtunded, intravenous sodium nitroprusside therapy should be started at a dose of 0.5 μg/kg and titrated as needed to slowly reduce the blood pressure toward the 99th percentile. When the patient becomes responsive, a change to oral medications is advocated. If the patient needing help is conscious when first seen, sublingual administration of nifedipine, 0.25 to 0.5 mg/kg every 30 minutes, is recommended until a decrease in blood pressure is seen or a maximum dose of 1 mg/kg is reached. At that point, maintenance therapy can be started or other drugs employed. The therapeutic goal in emergency cases is avoidance of hypotension or an excessively rapid lowering of the pressure. When adequate pressure control has been achieved, a vigorous search for the cause of the hypertension, if not known, must be made.

SUMMARY

As adolescents mature toward full adulthood, an increasing number will be found to have hypertension. Perhaps this progression can be delayed or avoided through the applications of the principles outlined in this chapter. At the very least, blood pressures should be taken when adolescents are seen for health care, regardless of the complaint.

When pressures are found to be repeatedly elevated, nonpharmacological antihypertensive measures (Fig. 12.5) should be started. They are good general health rules. Initially, in the absence of severe hypertension, a basic diagnostic study is all that is needed. Depending on the results, other tests may or may not be necessary. In most cases the blood pressure will regress toward normal levels during the study.

For the few adolescents with persistent serious hypertension, drug therapy is indicated. The individualized stepped-care approach, also displayed in Figure 12.5, is recommend. Very rarely, hypertension will be resistant to initial drug therapies. Such cases generally require consultation with an expert in the hypertension of young people.

BIBLIOGRAPHY

Boe J, Homerfelt S, Wedervang F. The blood pressure in a population: blood pressure readings and height and weight determinations in the adult population of the city of Berger. Acta Med Scand 1957;321(suppl):1.

Bottini PB, Carr AA, Rhoades RB, et al. Variability of indirect methods used to determine blood pressure: office vs mean 24-hour automated blood pressures. Arch Intern Med 1992;152:139.

Boynton RE, Todd RL. Blood pressure readings of 75,258 university students. Arch Intern Med 1947;80:454.

Brouhard BH. Hypertension in children and adolescents. Cleve Clin J Med 1995;62:21.

Cummings DM, Amadio P, Nelson L, et al. The role of calcium channel blockers in the treatment of essential hypertension. Arch Intern Med 1991;151:250.

Division of Pharmacy, Childrens Hospital of Los Angeles, Taketomo C, ed. Pediatric dosing handbook and formulary. Hudson, Ohio: Lexi-Comp, 1994.

Falkner B. Management of hypertension in children and adolescents. Am Fam Physician 1986;34:101.

Fifth Report of the Joint National Committee on Detection, Evaluation and Treatment of High Blood Pressure (JNC V). Arch Intern Med 1993;153:154.

Fixler DE, Laird WP, Fitzgerald V, et al. Hypertension screening in schools: results of the Dallas study. Pediatrics 1979;63:32.

Frohlich ED. Hypertension: 1986 evaluation and treatment—why and how. Post Grad Med 1986;80:28.

Goldring D, Hernandez A, Choi S, et al. Blood pressure in a high school population. II. Clinical profile of the juvenile hypertensive. J Pediatr 1979;95:298.

Goldring D, Londe S, Sivakoff M, et al. Blood pressure in a high school population. J Pediatr 1977;91:884.

Harris RD, Phillips RL, Williams PM, et al. The child-adolescent blood study. I. Distribution of blood pressure levels in Seventh Day Adventists (SDA). Am J Public Health 1981;71:1342.

Hediga ML, Schall JI, Katz SH, et al. Resting blood pressure and pulse rate distributions in black adolescents: the Philadelphia blood pressure project. Pediatrics 1984;74:1016.

Heyden S, Bartel AG, Hames CG, et al. Elevated blood pressure levels in adolescents, Evans County, Georgia. JAMA 1969;209:1683.

Higgins MW, Hinton PC, Keller JB. Weight and obesity as a predictor of blood pressure and hypertension. In: Loggie JMH, Horan MJ, Gruskin AB, et al, eds. National Heart, Lung, and Blood Institute workshop on juvenile hypertension. Proceedings of a symposium. New York: Biomedical Information, 1984:125.

Hohn AR. Guidebook for pediatric hypertension. Mount Kisco, New York: Futura Publishing, 1994.

Hohn AR, Riopel DA, Keil JE, et al. Childhood familial and racial differences in physiologic and biochemical factors related to hypertension. Hypertension 1983; 5:56.

Houston MC. Sodium and hypertension: a review. Arch Intern Med 1986;146:179.

Hunt JC, Frohlich ED, Moser M, et al. Devices used for self-measurements of blood pressure—revised statement of the National High Blood Pressure Education Program. Arch Intern Med 1985;145:2231.

Hypertension Prevention Collaborative Research Group. The effects of nonpharmacologic interventions on blood pressure of persons with high normal levels. JAMA 1992;267:1213.

Joint National Committee (National High Blood Pressure Education Program). The fifth report of the Joint National Committee on detection, evaluation and treatment of high blood pressure. Arch Intern Med 1993;153:154.

Kaplan NM. Maximally reducing cardiovascular risk in the treatment of hypertension. Ann Intern Med 1988;109:36.

Kaplan NM, Meese RB. The calcium deficiency hypothesis of hypertension: a critique. Ann Intern Med 1986;105:947.

Kilcoyne MM. Adolescent hypertension. Am J Med 1975;58:735.

Kilcoyne MM, Richter RW, Alsup PA. Adolescent hypertension. I. Detection and prevalence. Circulation 1974;50:1014.

Kim KE. Comparative clinical pharmacology of calcium channel blockers. Am Fam Physician 1991;43:583.

Kotchen TA, Havlick RJ. High blood pressure in the young. Ann Intern Med 1980;92:254.

Lauer RM, Clarke WR. Childhood risk factors for high adult blood pressure: the Muscatine study. Pediatrics 1989;84:633.

Lauer RM, Conner WE, Leaverton PE, et al. Coronary heart disease risk factors in school children: the Muscatine study. J Pediatr 1975;86:697.

Lieberman E. Pediatric hypertension, clinical perspective. Mayo Clin Proc 1994;69:1098.

Loggie JMH. Identification and management of juvenile hypertension. Postgrad Med 1979a;65:103.

Loggie JMH. Juvenile hypertension. In: Moss, AV, ed. Pediatrics update: reviews for physicians. New York: Elsevier-North Holland, 1979b;237–250.

Londe S. Blood pressure in children as determined under office conditions. Clin Pediatr 1966;5:71.

Masland RP, Heald FP, Goodale WT, et al. Hypertensive vascular disease in adolescents. N Engl J Med 1956; 255:894.

Materson BJ, Reda DJ, Cushman WC, et al. Single drug therapy for hypertension in men. N Engl J Med 1993;328:914.

Mehta SK. Pediatric hypertension: a challenge for pediatricians. Am J Dis Child 1987;141:893.

Moser M, Hebert P, Hennekens CH. An overview of the meta-analyses of the hypertension treatment trials. Arch Intern Med 1991;151:1277.

Moss AJ. Blood pressure in infants, children, and adolescents. West J Med 1981;134:296.

National Heart, Lung, and Blood Institute's Task Force on Blood Pressure Control in Children. Report of the Second Task Force on Blood Pressure Control in Children—1987. Washington, DC: U.S. Department of Health and Human Services, Public Health Service, National Institutes of Health, January 1987.

Neaton JD, Grimm Jr RH, Prineas RJ, et al. Treatment of mild hypertension study: final results. JAMA 1993; 270:713.

Oliver WJ, Cohen EL, Neel JV. Blood pressure, sodium intake and sodium-related hormones in the Yanomamo indians: a "no salt" culture. Circulation 1977; 52:146.

Rabinowitz A, Kushner H, Falkner B. Racial differences in blood pressure among urban adolescents. J Adolesc Health 1993;14:314.

Ram VS. Secondary hypertension: workup and correction. Hosp Pract 1994;29:137.

Rames LK, Clarke WR, Connor WE, et al. Normal blood pressure elevation in childhood: the Muscatine Study. Pediatrics 1978;61:245.

Reed WL. Racial differences in blood pressure levels of adolescents. Am J Public Health 1981;71:1165.

Rocchini AP. Adolescent obesity and hypertension. Pediatr Clin North Am 1993;40:81.

Rosner B, Prineas RJ, Loggie JMH, et al. Blood pressure nomograms for children and adolescents, by height, sex and age, in the United States. J Pediatr 1993;123: 871.

Schieken RM. Genetic factors that predispose the child to develop hypertension. Pediatr Clin North Am 1993;40:1.

Schieken RM. Hypertension and atherosclerosis in children. Curr Opin Cardiol 1994;9:130.

Second Task Force on Blood Pressure Control in Children. Report of the Second Task Force on Blood Pressure Control in Children—1987. Pediatrics 1987; 79:1.

Sinaiko AR, Gomez-Marin O, Prineas RJ. Effect of low sodium diet or potassium supplementation on adolescent blood pressure. Hypertension 1993;21: 989.

Vartiainen E, Tvomilehto J, Nissinen A. Blood pressure in puberty. Acta Pediatr Scand 1986;75:626.

Voors AWS, Berenson GS, Dalferes R, et al. Racial differences in blood pressure control. Science 1979; 204:1091.

Wilber JA, Millward D, Baldwin A, et al. Atlanta Community Blood Pressure Program: methods of community hypertension screening. Circ Res 1972;31 (suppl II):101.

Zinner SH, Levy PS, Kass EH. Familial aggregation of blood pressure in children. N Engl J Med 1971; 284:401.

CHAPTER 13

Heart Murmurs

Robert E. Stanton and Lawrence S. Neinstein

Cardiac murmurs may occur in approximately 50% of all children and often persist into adolescence. The vast majority of these murmurs have no underlying anatomic abnormality and are considered to be innocent or functional in origin. However, these terms are imprecise in that the term "functional" has been applied to physiological causes of murmurs, as in anemia, fever, hyperthyroidism, or pregnancy. Thus, the term *normal murmur* has been advocated to clearly indicate their benign nature. Yet approximately 1% of children are born with congenital heart disease and have murmurs related to a congenital defect that must be differentiated from the normal murmur. Failure to identify a murmur as normal may lead to anxiety or unnecessary restrictions. Failure to recognize murmurs of organic disease may have serious consequences because these lesions may serve as a focus for endocarditis. It is the task of the primary care physician to make the differentiation between the normal murmur and the organic murmur. The diagnosis begins with a thorough history and physical examination. If a diagnosis of congenital heart disease is already known, the algorithm is made simple.

History

1. Time of onset: Murmurs present at birth or in the first weeks of life suggest an organic basis, whereas murmurs first heard in early childhood or adolescence are more likely to be normal murmurs.
2. Cardiac symptoms: The symptomatic patient with decreased exercise tolerance, and excessive dyspnea and tachypnea on exertion may have an organic basis for the murmur.

Physical Examination

1. Appearance
   a. Presence of genetic abnormalities: Frequently associated with congenital heart disease, as in Down syndrome, Turner syndrome, or Marfan syndrome
   b. Cyanosis and clubbing: Strongly suggestive of congenital heart disease, as is the presence of a prominent or visibly hyperdynamic precordium
   c. Pectus excavatum deformity: Narrow anteroposterior diameter of the chest often associated with a normal murmur
2. Pulse in upper and lower extremities: Important component of the examination; observe for any discrepancies in intensity or timing
3. Blood pressures in arm and leg: Helpful component of evaluation for coarctation of the aorta; systolic gradient of 20 mm Hg between arm and leg consistent with coarctation of the aorta

4. Palpation: Presence of thrill, heave, or thrust over precordium an indication of pathological changes
5. Auscultation
   a. Second heart sound: The quality of the second heart sound (S_2) is of great diagnostic importance. The first component (aortic closure) and the second component (pulmonic closure) of S_2 should be equal. An accentuated pulmonary closure sound suggests pathological changes, as does a single S_2. There should be respiratory variation or splitting of the S_2 with widening of the separation on inspiration. Fixed splitting suggests an abnormality such as an atrial septal defect.
   b. Third heart sound (S_3): Ventricular filling heard at the lower left border is always abnormal after early infancy, as is a loud S_3 at the apex.
   c. Clicks: The presence of clicks is also an important clue to the diagnosis of organic disease. Ejection clicks heard in early systole are of either pulmonary or aortic origin. Pulmonary ejection clicks are best heard at the upper left sternal border and may be associated with valvar pulmonary stenosis, atrial septal defects, or pulmonary hypertension. Aortic ejection clicks are best heard at the lower left sternal border to the apex and may be associated with valvar aortic stenosis. Nonejection clicks are usually mid systolic and are present at the apex in association with mitral valve prolapse.
   d. Murmurs: The presence of a systolic or diastolic murmur requires careful analysis of its characteristics, including timing, intensity, duration, quality, and location. For practical purposes, all diastolic murmurs should be considered to be pathological.

DIAGNOSTIC CLUES OF INNOCENT MURMURS

1. History: Asymptomatic; onset in early childhood
2. Timing of murmur: Early systolic; almost never diastolic
3. Duration: Nonpansystolic
4. Intensity: Grade 3/6 or less
5. Radiation: Not extensive
6. Quality: Vibratory; no clicks
7. Location: Not maximal in aortic area
8. Change with position: Decrease while sitting
9. S_2: Normal splitting
10. Laboratory findings: Normal electrocardiogram (ECG) and chest x-ray film, although tests are generally unnecessary

DIAGNOSTIC CLUES TO PATHOLOGICAL MURMURS

1. History: Growth failure, decreased exercise tolerance, fainting, dizziness, chest pain
2. Signs: Clubbing, cyanosis, decreased or delayed femoral pulses, delayed or rapid carotid upstroke, apical heave
3. Murmur: Diastolic, pansystolic, continuous, loud, extensive radiation, including the back, increases with Valsalva maneuver

TYPES OF NORMAL MURMURS

A number of normal types of murmurs have been described. They have identifiable characteristics that allow them to be recognized by physical examination alone.

Still's Murmur

Still's murmur is the most common innocent precordial murmur.

1. Cause: Turbulence of flow in the left ventricular outflow tract
2. Quality
   a. Medium-pitched murmur with vibratory or buzzing quality
   b. Nonpansystolic
3. Location: Left lower sternal border and apex
4. Maneuvers: Murmur decreased on sitting or standing
5. Differential diagnosis
   a. Ventricular septal defect
   b. Mitral insufficiency
   c. Mitral valve prolapse
   d. Aortic stenosis
   e. Hypertrophic cardiomyopathy

Pulmonary Ejection Systolic Murmur

1. Cause: Turbulence of flow in the right ventricular outflow tract
2. Quality: Short mid-systolic murmur, grade 3/6 or less with normal splitting of S_2
3. Location: Left upper sternal area
4. Maneuvers: Murmur decreased by inspiration and sitting
5. Differential diagnosis
   a. Pulmonary stenosis
   b. Atrial septal defect
   c. Physiological flow murmur

Cervical Venous Hum

1. Cause: Turbulence of venous flow at the sharp angle made between the right subclavian vein and the superior vena cava
2. Quality: Continuous murmur with diastolic accentuation
3. Location: Heard best above the sternal end of clavicle; may be bilateral or unilateral; can be heard as low as third intercostal space
4. Maneuvers
   a. Murmur is increased by rotating the head away from the side being examined.
   b. Murmur is decreased or obliterated by jugular venous compression.
   c. Murmur is decreased with supine position.
5. Differential diagnosis: Murmur referred to base of heart can be confused with aortic or pulmonary stenosis

Supraclavicular Bruit

1. Cause: Turbulence at the site of branching of the brachiocephalic arteries
2. Quality: Short, early systolic murmur
3. Location: Maximal above the clavicles and lower portion of the sternocleidomastoid muscle; more common on right side
4. Maneuvers
   a. In 80% of patients the murmur is eliminated by compression of the subclavian artery against the first rib.

    b. Murmur is decreased by hyperextending the shoulders.

    c. Murmur is heard best in the sitting position with the bell of the stethoscope.

  5. Differential diagnosis: Murmur referred to base of heart can be confused with aortic or pulmonary stenosis

ORGANIC MURMURS

It is unusual for major congenital cardiac lesions to be diagnosed initially in adolescence. Yet, in the differential diagnosis of normal murmurs, a number of acyanotic lesions must be considered. A review of these lesions is included in Table 13.1.

Atrial Septal Defect

1. Hyperdynamic precordium with right ventricular lift; no thrill
2. Widely split and fixed S_2
3. Grade 3 or less systolic ejection murmur at upper left sternal border
4. Mid-diastolic rumble at lower left sternal border

TABLE 13.1.   Clues to Specific Organic Cardiac Lesions[a]

Diagnosis	Auscultation	Other Findings	Chest X-Ray	ECG
Patent ductus arteriosus	Continuous murmur with peak intensity at S_2; maximum left 2nd intercostal space	Wide pulse pressure	Prominent pulmonary artery	May be normal
Atrial septal defect	Wide fixed split S_2; mid-diastolic rumble at LLSB	RV lift	Prominent RV outflow	Incomplete RBBB
Pulmonary stenosis	Ejection click; wide split S_2; P_2 delayed and soft	RV lift	Prominent RV outflow; poststenotic dilation	RVH RAE
Aortic stenosis	Early systolic murmur, transmitted to neck; ejection click	LV lift; slow-rising pulse; paradoxical split S_2	LVE	LVH
Mitral regurgitation	Holosystolic murmur with radiation to axilla; soft S_1	LV lift	Big LA and LV	Left axis deviation; bifed P waves
Mitral valve prolapse	Mid-systolic click; mid- or late-systolic murmur			Abnormal T waves; arrhythmias
Idiopathic hypertrophic subaortic stenosis	Mid-systolic; loudest LLSB, increased with Valsalva maneuver and sitting	Rapid carotid upstroke, bisferious pulse	May have left ventricular and left atrial enlargement	LVH, may have Q waves
Ventricular septal defect	High-pitched, harsh holosystolic at LLSB	Thrill at LLSB	Normal	Normal if small VSD, LVH
Coarctation of aorta	Continuous or systolic precordial murmur	BP lower in legs than arms; diminished or delayed femoral pulses	Rib-notching LVH	

[a]BP, blood pressure; LA, left atrium; LLSB, left lower sternal border; LV, left ventricular; LVE, left ventricular enlargement; LVH, left ventricular hypertrophy; RAE, right atrial enlargement; RBBB, right bundle-branch block; RV, right ventricular; RVH, right ventricular hypertrophy; VSD, ventricular septal defect.

5. Laboratory findings
   a. ECG: rSr′ ECG pattern or right ventricular hypertrophy
   b. Chest x-ray: Cardiomegaly with increased pulmonary vascularity
   c. Echocardiogram: Diagnostic with visualization of defect

Ventricular Septal Defect

Shunt volume determines findings.

1. Hyperdynamic precordium with thrill; normal precordium with small shunt volume
2. Normal to accentuated S_2, depending on defect size
3. Grade 2–6 systolic murmur at lower left sternal border (Smaller defects may not be holo-systolic and have a high-frequency blowing quality.)
4. Mid-diastolic rumble of the apex with large shunt volume defects
5. Laboratory findings
   a. ECG: Normal in small defects; right ventricular hypertrophy, left ventricular hyper-trophy, or combined ventricular hypertrophy, depending on hemodynamics
   b. Chest x-ray: Normal in small defects; cardiomegaly with increased vascularity in the larger defects
   c. Echocardiogram: Visualization of larger defects; may be normal in very small defects

Patent Ductus Arteriosus

Shunt volume determines findings.

1. Hyperdynamic precordium with thrill; normal chest with small lesions
2. Grade 2–4 continuous murmur at upper left sternal border
3. Wide pulse pressure and bounding pulses, or normal with small lesions
4. Laboratory findings
   a. ECG: Normal, left ventricular hypertrophy, or combined ventricular hypertrophy, de-pending on hemodynamics
   b. Chest x-ray: Normal to cardiomegaly with increased vascularity
   c. Echocardiogram: Visualization of defect or shunt

Valvar Pulmonary Stenosis

Degree of obstruction determines the findings.

1. Right ventricular lift with thrill in more severe forms
2. Systolic ejection click at upper left sternal border
3. Normal to soft-wide split S_2, depending on severity
4. Grade 2–4 harsh systolic ejection murmur at upper left sternal border; may be heard in the back
5. Laboratory findings
   a. ECG: Normal to severe right ventricular hypertrophy
   b. Chest x-ray: Prominent pulmonary artery segment with normal vascularity
   c. Echocardiogram: Reasonable accuracy of the estimate of pressure gradient across pul-monary valve

Aortic Stenosis

Degree of obstruction determines findings.

1. Left ventricular thrust in more severe forms
2. Systolic thrill in suprasternal notch in more severe forms
3. Systolic ejection click at lower left sternal border to apex; not present in supravalvar or subvalvar types
4. Grade 2–4 long systolic ejection murmur at upper right sternal border; subvalvar murmur may be heard best at mid left sternal border.
5. High-frequency early diastolic decrescendo murmur of insufficiency, possibly in association with bicuspid aortic valve
6. Laboratory findings
   a. ECG: Normal to left ventricular hypertrophy, depending on severity
   b. Chest x-ray: Normal heart size with prominent ascending aorta; normal vascularity
   c. Echocardiogram: Reasonably reflects pressure gradient; localizes level of obstruction

Mitral Valve Prolapse

1. History of palpitations or chest pain
2. Normal heart sounds with nonejection mid-systolic click at the apex
3. Grade 1–3 apical systolic murmur with variable quality, from a harsh, honking, whooping murmur to a very soft murmur that may be absent in the supine position
4. Laboratory findings
   a. ECG: Abnormal T waves
   b. Chest x-ray: Normal
   c. Echocardiogram: Prolapse of mitral posterior leaflet

Mitral Valve Regurgitation

Findings depend on degree of regurgitation.

1. Normal to hyperdynamic precordium
2. Grade 2–4 high-frequency holosystolic apical murmur
3. Low-frequency apical mid-diastolic rumble with severe regurgitation
4. Laboratory findings
   a. ECG: May be normal with mild regurgitation; bifid P wave of left atrial enlargement
   b. Chest x-ray: Normal to cardiomegaly with large left atrium and left ventricle
   c. Echocardiogram: Mitral regurgitation

MANAGEMENT OF HEART MURMURS

On completion of a careful history and physical examination, it should be possible to differentiate normal murmurs from those with an organic basis. Electrocardiograms and chest x-rays do not add to the accuracy of a diagnosis of normal murmurs. In those situations in which there is uncertainty and a consideration of congenital heart disease, the electrocardiogram and chest x-ray may be helpful. However, in mild lesions with minimal cardiovascular stress, these also may be normal. An echocardiogram is a powerful but expensive diagnostic tool for consideration at this point. Yet, it has been shown that it is more cost-effective to refer these types of patients to a pediatric cardiologist than to obtain an echocardiogram before the referral.

Thus, management optimally requires a careful and systematic cardiovascular examination; judicial use of laboratory studies; referral, in selected cases, to a pediatric cardiologist; and, in the case of normal murmurs, confident reassurance.

BIBLIOGRAPHY

Castellotti DS, Makssoudian A, Mendes MC, et al. Heart murmur in pediatrics: innocent or pathologic? Rev Paul Med 1992;110:29.

Danford DA, Nasir A, Gumbiner C. Cost assessment of the evaluation of heart murmurs in children. Pediatrics 1993;91:365.

Liebman J. Diagnosis and management of heart murmur in children. Pediatr Rev 1982;3:321.

Luisada AA, Haring OM, Aravani C, et al. Murmurs in children: a clinical and graphic study of 500 children of school age. Ann Intern Med 1958;48:597.

Moss AJ. Clues in diagnosing congenital heart disease. West J Med 1992;156:392.

Rosenthal A. How to distinguish between innocent and pathologic murmurs in childhood. Pediatr Clin North Am 1984;31:1229.

Smith RT, Hohn AR. Normal heart murmurs in children. In: Conn RB, ed. Current diagnosis. Philadelphia: WB Saunders, 1985:464–468.

Smythe JF, Teixeira OHP, Demers PP, et al. Initial evaluation of heart murmurs: are laboratory tests necessary? Pediatrics 1990;86:497.

CHAPTER 14

Mitral Valve Prolapse

Mitral valve prolapse is one of the most commonly observed cardiac abnormalities in the adolescent age group. It is found in up to 12–17% of women of childbearing age. The finding is so prevalent that some authorities have suggested that mitral valve prolapse may not be a disease at all. Mitral valve prolapse is benign in most patients, but it can lead to serious complications in others, including chest pain, mitral regurgitation, infectious endocarditis, cerebral embolism, severe arrhythmia, and sudden death. A major difficulty with mitral valve prolapse is the relative inability to identify those adolescents who are at risk of having complications. Other names for this syndrome have included billowing mitral leaflet syndrome, Barlow's syndrome, posterior mitral leaflet syndrome, floppy valve syndrome, and mid-systolic click–late-systolic murmur syndrome.

ETIOLOGY

Genetics

Mitral valve prolapse is a genetically transmissible problem found in 30–50% of first-degree relatives of individuals with mitral valve prolapse. Transmission is suspected to be autosomal dominant, with a decrease in male expressivity. No chromosomal abnormalities are present.

Structural Abnormalities

1. Grossly: Abnormality of the anterior or posterior mitral valve leaflets, with redundancy and thickening of the leaflets
2. Histologically: Myxomatous degeneration of the mitral valve leaflets, with replacement of dense collagenous supporting tissue by loose, amorphous, acellular, hyalinized deposits. There is thickening of the leaflets with an increase in acid mucopolysaccharides in the spongiosa layer.
3. Functionally: Mitral valve prolapse can occur either because the mitral valve is too big (too much valve apparatus, as in Marfan syndrome) or because the left ventricular cavity is too small (as in hypertrophic cardiomyopathy, anorexia nervosa, straight back syndrome, pectus excavatum, atrial septal defect, or athlete's heart). Changes in left ventricular end-diastolic cavity size occur with changes in body position and can alter the quality and presence of the murmur.

Developmental Abnormality

A developmental abnormality was suggested in a study by Schutte et al. (1981) that demonstrated a narrower anteroposterior chest diameter and longer arm spans in patients without Marfan syndrome but with mitral valve prolapse. Further evidence is the report of pectus excavatum, straight back syndrome, or severe scoliosis in 75% of individuals with mitral valve prolapse.

Autonomic and Neuroendocrine Disturbance

Patients with mitral valve prolapse demonstrate an abnormal catecholamine excretion in response to stimuli, which suggests a hyperadrenergic state as the cause of a portion of the symptom complex.

EPIDEMIOLOGY

Prevalence

The prevalence of mitral valve prolapse in the literature has ranged from 1% to 17% (DeLeon, 1980), depending on the criteria for diagnosis. Recent reports have centered on 5–10% prevalence rates, with the prevalence in the pediatric age group (<18 years of age) reported to be 5%.

Sex

Females have higher prevalence rates by approximately 2–3:1, although they may be closer to 1:1 in children, with the ratio in adolescents probably falling in between.

Age

Mitral valve prolapse has been diagnosed in patients 2–84 years old. Symptomatic patients tend to be in their later-adolescent or young-adult years.

CLASSIFICATION

Mitral valve prolapse can be divided into three types:

1. Primary, or classic, prolapse: Idiopathic autosomal dominant disorder affecting the structure of the mitral valve. The valve leaflets will be thickened and elongated in association with myxomatous infiltration.
2. Secondary prolapse from myxomatous degeneration of mitral leaflets in individuals with connective tissue diseases such as Marfan or Ehlers-Danlos syndrome.
3. Prolapse of a normal mitral valve leaflet in individuals with papillary muscle dysfunction from ischemia or cardiomyopathy.

CLINICAL MANIFESTATIONS

Symptoms

It should be noted that all prevalence rates of symptoms are based on referral centers, where rates will be higher.

1. Palpitations: Approximately 40–50% prevalence rate. The palpitations may be unrelated to the occurrence of arrhythmias.
2. Chest pain: Approximately 40% prevalence rate. The pain tends to be precordial, is usually unrelated to effort, and is of longer duration than anginal pain. The cause is unknown, but suggested mechanisms have included mechanical stress on papillary muscle, coronary artery spasm, left ventricular dysfunction, and extracardiac conditions. Chest pain with mitral valve prolapse may not be related to the mitral valve prolapse. In one study of 17 pread-

olescents and adolescents with mitral valve prolapse and chest pain, 14 had abnormal findings on either esophageal manometry, the Bernstein test, an esophageal pH probe test, or esophagogastroscopy (Woolf et al., 1991). Ten of the patients had esophagitis or gastritis.

3. Dyspnea on exertion: Approximately 20–40% prevalence rate.
4. Fatigue: Approximately 12% prevalence rate.
5. Light-headedness: Approximately 12% prevalence rate.
6. Syncope: Approximately 2–4% prevalence rate. Moderate to severe orthostatic hypotension has been found in some patients with mitral valve prolapse and may account for the syncope (Santos et al., 1981).
7. Neuropsychiatric symptoms: A high prevalence of anxiety, panic attacks, and other psychiatric complaints (Vitiello et al., 1990). Although the rate of co-occurrence is high, there is no convincing evidence of a cause-and-effect relationship between the two disorders. Still, the relationship is clinically significant. If an individual with chest pain and mitral valve prolapse fails to respond to treatment, consider a panic disorder.
8. Asymptomatic: Approximately 25% prevalence rate.

Again, the true prevalence of these symptoms in the general population is unknown because these rates are based on referral or hospital-based patients.

Physical Findings

1. Click murmur auscultatory findings
   a. Systolic click and late systolic murmur, 31%
   b. Systolic click but no murmur present, 22%
   c. No systolic click but murmur present, 26%
   d. No click or murmur but positive findings on an echocardiogram, 21%
2. Murmur qualities: The murmur of mitral valve prolapse tends to be late systolic, high pitched, and best heard at the apex of the heart. The murmur and click have marked variability from beat to beat and from one examination to another. Maneuvers that decrease left ventricular volume (standing, Valsalva, and inspiration) move the click and maneuver closer to the first heart sound. Maneuvers that increase left ventricular end-diastolic volume (squatting, handgrip) delay the click and may diminish the murmur.
3. Associated physical abnormalities
   a. Increased association with Marfan syndrome
   b. Increased prevalence of scoliosis
   c. Increased prevalence of pectus excavatum
   d. Increase in anteroposterior diameter of the chest and length of the arm span
   e. Increased prevalence of orthostatic hypotension (Santos et al., 1981)
   f. Increased prevalence in individuals with anorexia nervosa: 9 of 28 patients versus 2 of 28 control subjects (Meyers et al., 1986)
   g. Increased prevalence in individuals with chronic lymphocytic thyroiditis: 41% versus 8% of control subjects (Marks et al., 1985)
   h. Increased prevalence in individuals with migraine headaches: 15% versus 7% of control subjects (Spence et al., 1984)

Laboratory Findings

1. Chest x-ray: Generally normal.
2. Electrocardiogram: Normal in more than 50% of patients. Abnormalities are nonspecific and include premature ventricular contractions, supraventricular tachyarrhythmias, bradyarrhythmias, and ST-T wave changes.

3. Echocardiogram: M-mode and two-dimensional echocardiography can visualize the mitral valve and confirm the presence of mitral valve prolapse. The degree of prolapse, amount of mitral regurgitation, severity of the deformity, thickness of the valve leaflets, and left ventricular function can also be evaluated. Certain echocardiographic features have been associated with a poor prognosis including thickened and redundant mitral valve leaflets.
4. Angiogram: An angiogram can confirm mitral valve prolapse but is an unnecessary diagnostic test unless other cardiac lesions are suspected.

DIAGNOSIS

The diagnosis of mitral valve prolapse should be suspected in adolescents with complaints of chest pain, palpitations, dizziness, syncope, dyspnea on exertion, or fatigue. If a systolic click or late systolic murmur is heard, an echocardiogram will confirm the diagnosis. An electrocardiogram (ECG) is indicated to check for arrhythmias. Teens with physical findings suggestive of mitral valve prolapse and significant symptoms should undergo chest x-ray, electrocardiography, echocardiography, Holter monitoring, and exercise testing. Teens with a murmur consistent with mitral regurgitation should undergo electrocardiography, chest x-ray, and echocardiography. If only a mitral valve prolapse murmur is found, then an ECG is indicated to check for arrhythmias. If an abnormal rhythm is present, a Holter monitor and exercise testing should be considered. Guidelines for the diagnosis of mitral valve prolapse (suggested by Perloff et al., 1986) follow.

Major Criteria

One or more major criteria establish a high probability of pathological mitral valve prolapse beyond a reasonable doubt.

1. Auscultation: Mid to late systolic clicks and late systolic murmur, or whoop alone or in combination at the cardiac apex.
2. Two-dimensional echocardiogram: Marked superior systolic displacement of mitral leaflets with coaptation point at or superior to annular plane, or mild to moderate superior systolic displacement of mitral leaflets with:
   a. Chordal rupture, *or*
   b. Doppler mitral regurgitation, *or*
   c. Annular dilation
3. Echocardiogram plus auscultation: Mild to moderate superior systolic displacement of mitral leaflets with:
   a. Prominent mid to late systolic clicks at the cardiac apex, *or*
   b. Apical late systolic or holosystolic murmur in young persons, *or*
   c. Late systolic whoop

Minor Criteria

One or more minor criteria suggest a need for periodic evaluation but are nondiagnostic for mitral valve prolapse.

1. Auscultation: Loud first heart sound with an apical holosystolic murmur
2. Two-dimensional echocardiogram
   a. Isolated mild to moderate superior systolic displacement of the posterior mitral leaflet
   b. Moderate superior systolic displacement of both mitral leaflets

3. Echocardiogram plus history: Mild-to-moderate superior systolic displacement of mitral leaflets with:
   a. Focal neurologic attacks or amaurosis fugax in a young person
   b. First-degree relatives with major criteria

COMPLICATIONS

Individuals with benign clicks and those who have mitral regurgitation should probably not be grouped under one diagnostic category, because the clinical significance can vary tremendously. The teen with a mid-systolic click and no mitral regurgitation will probably have an excellent clinical outcome. Most patients with mitral valve prolapse have no problems. In fact, by actuarial tables, their mortality rates are similar to rates in individuals without mitral valve prolapse. Complications include:

1. Arrhythmias: The most frequent complication. Arrhythmias occur in up to 40% of patients with mitral valve prolapse. They include premature ventricular contractions, supraventricular tachyarrhythmias, and bradyarrhythmias.
2. Infectious endocarditis: The risk of infective endocarditis for patients with mitral valve prolapse varies from 0.0175% to 0.052% per year, depending on the presence or absence of a regurgitant murmur (MacMahon et al., 1987). In the study of risk factors by Nishimura et al. (1985), all patients with endocarditis and mitral valve prolapse had redundant mitral valve leaflets.
3. Progressive mitral regurgitation: This complication is rare. In the Nishimura study (1985), progression to mitral valve replacement was best correlated with the left ventricular diastolic dimensions at initial presentation.
4. Sudden death: Estimates of this rare occurrence are as high as 1 in 53 persons with significant mitral regurgitation to 1 in 5400 persons with little or no mitral regurgitation (Kligfield et al., 1987). Nishimura et al. (1985) reported that the only association with sudden death was the presence of redundant mitral valve leaflets.
5. Stroke: There is a higher prevalence of mitral valve prolapse in young patients with stroke than in control subjects (Barnett et al., 1980). However, the true risk of stroke in individuals with mitral valve prolapse is unknown. One study estimated the risk of stroke in young patients with mitral valve prolapse to be about 0.02% per year (Wolf and Sila, 1987). The most likely cause is an embolism of a noninfective thrombus near or on the valve.

TREATMENT

1. Reassurance: The vast majority of adolescents and young adults with mitral valve prolapse are asymptomatic and have no complications. They should not be restricted in their activities, and serious sequelae need not be discussed.
2. Antibiotic prophylaxis: There is still some controversy regarding which individual with mitral valve prolapse should receive antibiotic prophylaxis. The American Heart Association suggests antibiotic prophylaxis for only those individuals with mitral valve prolapse complicated by mitral insufficiency, while acknowledging that complete information to guide therapy in this area is limited. Some experts also recommend prophylaxis whenever a thickened mitral valve leaflet is found on an echocardiogram. If prophylaxis is used, it is indicated for dental, gynecological, urological, and gastrointestinal procedures and surgery. Uncomplicated vaginal delivery and cesarean section rarely, if ever, precipitate endocarditis. It is recommended that prophylaxis be provided for those patients with mitral valve prolapse who have mitral insufficiency at the time of delivery and for those without mitral insufficiency if the delivery is complicated. See Table 14.1 for specific recommendations for prophylaxis.

TABLE 14.1. Antibiotic Prophylaxis[a]

Dental procedures
  1 Hr before procedure: Amoxicillin, 3 g PO, PLUS:
  6 Hr after initial dose: Amoxicillin, 1.5 g PO

  If penicillin allergic
    1 Hr before procedure: Erythromycin ethylsuccinate, 800 mg PO, or erythromycin stearate, 1 g PO, PLUS:
    6 Hr after procedure: Half of initial dose, OR

    1 Hr before procedure: Clindamycin, 300 mg PO, PLUS:
    6 Hr after initial dose: Clindamycin, 150 mg PO

Genitourinary and gastrointestinal procedures
  Standard regimen
    30 min before procedure: Ampicillin, 2 g IV or IM, plus gentamicin, 1.5 mg/kg IV or IM (maximum dose, 80 mg), AND
    6 Hr after initial dose: Amoxicillin, 1.5 g PO, OR
    8 Hr after initial dose: Repeat of parenteral regimen

  If penicillin allergic
    1 Hr before procedure: Vancomycin, 1 g IV for 1 hr, plus gentamicin, 1.5 mg/kg IV or IM (maximum dose, 80 mg), PLUS
    8 Hr after initial dose: Repeat of parenteral regimen

Adapted from Dajani AS, Bisno AL, Chung KJ, et al. Prevention of bacterial endocarditis: Recommendations by the American Heart Association. JAMA 1990;264:2919–2922.
[a]IM, intramuscularly; IV, intravenously; PO, per os (by mouth).

3. β-Blocking agents: β-Blocking agents are indicated for patients with mitral valve prolapse who have significant symptoms or significant arrhythmias.

4. Contraception: Controversy regarding the use of combination oral contraceptives by women with mitral valve prolapse is ongoing. Concern has been expressed that the abnormal hemodynamics of the mitral valve might promote thrombus formation with associated cerebrovascular accident. In one report, there was a 13.3 times increased risk of thromboembolic cerebrovascular insufficiency in oral contraceptive users with mitral valve prolapse compared with nonuser control subjects (Elam et al., 1986). However, all but one of the eight women with mitral valve prolapse who took oral contraceptives and who had a cerebrovascular accident either was a smoker or had a documented history of migraine headaches. Combination oral contraceptives could be used in women without a history of other cardiovascular risk factors, prior thrombotic complications, migraine headaches, symptomatic mitral valve prolapse, or overt mitral regurgitation. No studies have examined the use of progesterone-only contraceptive pills in these conditions, but the presumed negligible risk of altering coagulation parameters and causing embolic disease would make them a worthwhile alternative. Insertion of an intrauterine device should be preceded with antibiotic prophylaxis and should be avoided in women with overt mitral regurgitation.

5. Pregnancy: If there is no significant mitral regurgitation or other cardiac abnormality, there is no additional risk to the adolescent or her child during pregnancy and delivery.

BIBLIOGRAPHY

Alpert MA, Mukerji V, Sabeti M, et al. Mitral valve prolapse, panic disorder, and chest pain. Med Clin North Am 1991;75:1119–1133.

Barnett HJ, Boughner DR, Taylor W, et al. Further evidence relating mitral valve prolapse to cerebral ischemic events. N Engl J Med 1980;302:139.

Bergh PA, Hollander D, Gregori CA, et al. Mitral valve prolapse and thromboembolic disease in pregnancy: a case report. Int J Gynaecol Obstet 1988;27:133–137.

Beton DC, Brear SG, Edwards JD, et al. Mitral valve prolapse: an assessment of clinical features, associated conditions, and prognosis. Q J Med 1983;52:150.

Cheitlin MD. Mitral valve prolapse: an update. JAMA 1985;254:793.

Cheng TO. Mitral valve prolapse: when is it serious? Postgrad Med 1990;88:93–100.

Cheng TO. Office cardiology: controversies in the management of mitral valve prolapse. Mod Med 1991; 59:48–56.

Cowles T, Gotnik B. Mitral valve prolapse in pregnancy. Semin Perinatol 1990;14:34–41.

Davies AO, Mares A, Pool JL, et al. Mitral valve prolapse with symptoms of beta-adrenergic hypersensitivity. Am J Med 1987;82:193.

Degani S, Abinader EG, Scharf M. Mitral valve prolapse and pregnancy: a review. Obstet Gynecol Surv 1989; 44:642–649.

DeLeon AC. Mitral valve prolapse—etiology, diagnosis and management. Postgrad Med 1980;67:66.

Devereux RB. Recent developments in the diagnosis and management of mitral valve prolapse. Curr Opin Card 1995;10:107.

Elam MP, Viar MJ, Ratts TE, et al. Mitral valve prolapse in women with oral contraceptive–related cerebrovascular insufficiency. Arch Intern Med 1986; 146:73.

Fukuda N, Oki T, Iuchi A, et al. Predisposing factors for severe mitral regurgitation in idiopathic mitral valve prolapse. Am J Cardiol 1995;76:503.

Greenwood RD. Mitral valve prolapse in children. Postgrad Med 1986;80:257.

Kligfield P, Levy D, Devereux RB. Arrhythmias and sudden death in mitral valve prolapse. Am Heart J 1987; 113:1298–1307.

MacMahon SW, Roberts JK, Kramer-Fox R. Mitral valve prolapse and infective endocarditis. Am Heart J 1987;113:1291–1298.

Marks AD, Channick BJ, Adlin V, et al. Chronic thyroiditis and mitral valve prolapse. Ann Intern Med 1985;102:479.

Meyers DG, Starke H, Pearson PH, et al. Mitral valve prolapse in anorexia nervosa. Ann Intern Med 1986; 105:384.

Mitral valve prolapse and athletic participation in children and adolescents. American Academy of Pediatrics Committee on Sports Medicine and Fitness. Pediatrics 1995;95:789.

Moreau D, Weissman MM. Panic disorder in children and adolescents: a review. Am J Psychiatry 1992;149: 1306–1314.

Neinstein LS. Issues in reproductive management. New York: Thieme Publishing, 1994.

Nishimura RA, McGoon MD, Shub C, et al. Echocardiographically documented mitral valve prolapse: long-term follow-up of 237 patients. N Engl J Med 1985;313:1305.

Orencia AF, Petty GW, Khandheria BK, et al. Risk of stroke with mitral valve prolapse in population-based cohort study. Stroke 1995;26:7.

Pape L. Mitral valve prolapse: identifying and managing patients at risk for complications. Mod Med 1990;58:73–80.

Perloff JK, Child JS, Edwards JE. New guidelines for the clinical diagnosis of mitral valve prolapse. Am J Cardiol 1986;57:1124.

Procacci PM, Sauran SV, Schreiter SL, et al. Prevalence of clinical mitral valve prolapse in 1169 young women. N Engl J Med 1976;294:1086.

Rayburn WF, Fontana ME. Mitral valve prolapse and pregnancy. Am J Obstet Gynecol 1981;141:9–11.

Santos AD, Mathew PK, Hilal A, et al. Orthostatic hypotension: a commonly unrecognized cause of symptoms in mitral valve prolapse. Am J Med 1981;71:746.

Schutte JE, Gaffney FA, Blend L, et al. Distinctive anthropometric characteristics of women with mitral valve prolapse. Am J Med 1981;71:533.

Spence JD, Wong DG, Melendez LJ, et al. Increased prevalence of mitral valve prolapse in patients with migraine. Can Med Assoc J 1984;131:1457.

Sorrentino MJ. Mitral valve prolapse: avoiding complications of a progressive disease. Postgrad Med 1993; 93:63–66, 69–70, 79.

Vitiello B, Behar D, Wolfson S, et al. Diagnosis of panic disorder in prepubertal children. J Am Acad Child Adolesc Psychiatry 1990;29:782–784.

Wolf PA, Sila CA. Cerebral ischemia with mitral valve prolapse. Am Heart J 1987;113:1308–1315.

Woolf PK, Gewitz MH, Berezin S, et al. Noncardiac chest pain in adolescents and children with mitral valve prolapse. J Adolesc Health 1991;12:247.

Zua MS, Dziegielewski SF. Epidemiology of symptomatic mitral valve prolapse in black patients. J Nat Med Assoc 1995;87:273.

Zuppiroli A, Rinaldi M, Kramer-Fox R, et al. Natural history of mitral valve prolapse. Am J Cardiol 1995; 75:1028.

Orthopaedic Problems and Sports Medicine

SECTION V

Orthopedic Problems
and Sports Medicine

CHAPTER 15
Scoliosis and Kyphosis

Dale J. Townsend and Lawrence S. Neinstein

Many structural abnormalities of the spine such as meningomyelocele are discovered at birth or in early childhood. Some spinal conditions are discovered or worsen during adolescence, such as scoliosis and kyphosis. These latter problems are the topic of this chapter.

SCOLIOSIS

Scoliosis is a spinal condition in school-age children and adolescents involving a lateral curvature of the spine with a rotational component. While scoliosis can become a devastatingly crippling and deforming disease, it can be detected easily in adolescents, and therapy is available to prevent and correct major deformities. It is thus essential to examine adolescents for scoliosis and to refer them to a specialist when necessary.

Prevalence

The prevalence of scoliosis is dependent on the criteria used for the diagnosis. If 5- to 10-degree curves are included, the prevalence is 4–14% of children and adolescents. If only curves greater than 10 degrees are included, the prevalence falls to 2%. The prevalence of curves greater than 20 degrees is only 0.2–0.3%.

Classifications

Scoliosis has been classified in many ways: As structural versus nonstructural, by location, by age, and by origin. *Nonstructural scoliosis* may be identified by a spinal curve that corrects when the individual bends sideways toward the convex side of the curve. *Structural scoliosis* refers to a curve that fails to correct on side bending.

1. Idiopathic scoliosis: About 70–85% of all cases of scoliosis
2. Congenital scoliosis
   a. Vertebral: Myelomeningocele, hemivertebrae, vertebral bars, wedge vertebrae
   b. Extravertebral: Congenital rib fusions
3. Neuromuscular
   a. Neuropathic forms
      — Lower motor neuron disease (e.g., poliomyelitis, myelomeningocele, trauma)
      — Upper motor neuron disease (e.g., cerebral palsy, trauma, spinal tumors, syringomyelia)
   b. Myopathic forms
      — Progressive (e.g., muscular dystrophy)
      — Static (e.g., arthrogryposis)

4. Miscellaneous
   a. Mesenchymal disorders
      — Marfan syndrome, Ehlers-Danlos syndrome
   b. Metabolic disorders
      — Osteogenesis imperfecta
      — Rickets
   c. Neurofibromatosis
   d. Osteochondrodystrophies
      — Achondroplastic dwarfism
      — Diastrophic dwarfism
      — Mucopolysaccharidoses
      — Spondyloepiphyseal dysplasia
5. Acquired
   a. Postural scoliosis: A slight curve that disappears on lying down
   b. Compensatory scoliosis: Usually a result of a leg-length discrepancy; the pelvis dips down on the short side.
   c. Sciatic scoliosis: An irritative form secondary to pressure on a nerve root
   d. Hysterical scoliosis: A rare form secondary to a psychiatric condition
   e. Inflammatory scoliosis: Seen with a perinephric abscess or similar infection
   f. Traumatic: Secondary to spine fracture or dislocation
   g. Thoracogenic: Seen after thoracoplasty or thoracotomy
   h. Postradiation

Idiopathic Scoliosis

Adolescent idiopathic scoliosis is by far the most common form of scoliosis. It is defined by the Scoliosis Research Society as a lateral deviation of the spine of 11 or more degrees seen in the anteroposterior x-ray, and having no identifiable cause or associated syndrome. It is probably a genetic disease transmitted as an autosomal dominant trait with incomplete penetrance and variable expressivity. Approximately 7% of first-degree relatives and 12% of first-degree female relatives of affected girls have scoliosis. An earlier age of menarche (mean = 0.39 years early) but normal growth has been found in adolescent females with idiopathic scoliosis (Goldberg et al., 1993).

Sex Distribution   The female-to-male ratio increases with more significant curves. The ratio is 2:1 for curves 10–20 degrees and 10:1 for curves greater than 30 degrees.

Types

1. Infantile: Onset occurs between birth and 3 years of age, with males generally affected during their first year of life. The condition usually resolves spontaneously.
2. Juvenile: Onset occurs between 3 and 10 years of age; male and female distribution are about equal.
3. Adolescent: Onset occurs at age 10 until skeletal maturity. Seventy percent of affected individuals are female. This form has a tendency to progress with the growth spurt.

Symptoms   Scoliosis is usually asymptomatic and diagnosed from the complaint of a deformity or by routine physical examination. The incidence of back pain is not increased with idiopathic scoliosis even in adulthood. Painful scoliosis requires careful workup for an identifiable cause. Cardiorespiratory compromise is not clinically apparent until a thoracic curve is greater than 60 degrees, and not usually clinically significant until the curve is greater than 90 degrees.

Patterns of Curves   Four main curve patterns occur in idiopathic scoliosis:

1. Right thoracic curve: Upper end T4–T6, lower end T11–L1. This curve can result in a significant deformity and cardiopulmonary complications.
2. Thoracolumbar curve: Upper end T4–T6, lower end L2–L4. This curve is less cosmetically deforming than a thoracic curve but can cause a severe rib distortion.
3. Double major curves: Two curves of great prominence occur in this pattern. Double curves may be right thoracic, left lumbar; right thoracic, left thoracolumbar; left thoracic, right lumbar; and right thoracic, left thoracic.
4. Lumbar curves: Usually from T11–L5. In 65% of individuals the lumbar curve is left sided.

Most major curves are thoracic with the convexity to the right. Left thoracic dominant curves are associated with a higher incidence of intraspinal pathology.

Clinical Evaluation

History   History evaluation should include:

1. Age of onset
2. History of progression
3. Prior illness or trauma
4. Family history
5. Menstrual history of females

Physical Examination   The general examination should evaluate closely for:

1. Café au lait spots
2. Neuromuscular abnormalities
3. Cardiopulmonary abnormalities

The back examination should include:

1. Shoulder level: Check for unequal shoulder height.
2. Tips of scapula: Check for symmetry of elevation and distance from midline.
3. Lateral triangle symmetry: Check for symmetry of triangles formed by the arm hanging at the side, the lateral chest wall, and the hip prominence.
4. Trunk and head alignment: Drop a tape measure from the occiput down; it should center over the gluteal cleft.
5. Posterior chest wall asymmetry on forward bending: A rib hump may be unmasked with this technique.
6. Leg length: Check for equality of the distance of each leg between the anterior superior iliac spine and the medial malleolus.
7. Check side bending to evaluate flexibility and rigidity of curve.

The best screening test for scoliosis is the forward-bending test, in which an adolescent bends forward at the waist, with trunk parallel to the floor, legs straight, and arms dangling with fingers and palms together. This test increases the prominence of any rib humps. Postural scoliosis tends to improve with this maneuver or with side bending. Bunnell (1984), in an effort to decrease x-ray exposure, designed the inclinometer (scoliometer). This is a simple device that compares the horizon of the back with the horizontal plane, with the adolescent in the forward-flexed position. A tilt of less than 5 degrees correlates with an angle measured by x-ray of less than 20 degrees in more than 99% of individuals tested. The test is sensitive and fairly specific. Goldberg et al. (1995) found a sensitivity of the forward bend test in detecting or predicting 40 degrees scoliosis of 0.83 with a specificity of 0.99.

Although school screening has been widely advocated, there is some controversy over these mass screening programs (Goldberg et al., 1995). The disadvantage includes overdiagnosis leading to excessive radiographs and family concern.

Radiological Evaluation   If significant scoliosis is suspected, a radiograph should be obtained—an erect anteroposterior view of the spine from the occiput to the sacrum. An evaluation of bone age is also helpful to determine potential growth, as this may influence therapy. The amount of curvature is usually measured by the Cobb method (Fig. 15.1). In this technique a horizontal line is drawn at the inferior border of the inferiorly involved vertebra of the curve (*1*); another horizontal line is drawn at the superior border of the superiorly involved vertebra (*3*); perpendicular lines are drawn from each of the horizontal lines (*2* and *4*); and the intersecting angle is then measured (*5*).

Treatment

Congenital and neuromuscular scolioses require early orthopaedic intervention, as many require operative intervention, often before adolescence. The best treatment for adolescent idiopathic scoliosis is early detection, before the curve has progressed significantly. Most curves can be treated nonsurgically if treated early.

1. Exercises: Exercises by themselves accomplish nothing in structural scoliosis and are to be condemned as a sole treatment. They are helpful only in conjunction with braces or casts.
2. Electrical stimulation: Electrical stimulation via implantable or surface electrodes on the paraspinal muscles has been used for preventing progression of scoliosis. Numerous studies have shown this to be ineffective, and there is currently no role for its use in treating scoliosis.
3. Braces: Various braces, including the Milwaukee brace, Boston brace, and New York Orthopedic Hospital low-profile brace are available. Braces, in conjunction with exercises, can halt the progression of scoliosis. However, some data suggest that on long-term follow-up, many patients will lose some of the improvement they received from the brace. Braces are useful mainly in patients who have not reached skeletal maturity. It is important to consider that braces must be worn 23 hours a day for several years (until skeletal maturity), which often places a strain on the adolescent's developing identity and body image. Upadhyay et al. (1995) demonstrated that those patients who showed an increase in vertebral rotation or in Cobb angle after brace application were shown to have a greater risk of progression. These individuals had progression of curves leading to brace failure in 93% of patients and 79% of these required surgery. The patients with no change in both vertebral rotation and Cobb angle after bracing also often experienced frequent brace failure (69%). Reduction in both Cobb angle and vertebral rotation after bracing was predictive of a good outcome in 97% of cases with no patients in this group requiring surgery. Most of the patients with lumbar scoliosis (91%) showed such reductions.
4. Surgery: Surgery generally involves placement of spinal metal rods, as well as spinal fusion, to partially correct and stabilize the curve.
5. Patient management (Table 15.1): Adolescents with curves of less than 10–20 degrees can be observed with serial x-rays every 6–12 months, depending on the degree of curve and age of the adolescent. Younger patients with greater curves need closer follow-up and can be referred to specialists or clinics dealing with scoliosis. Adolescents with curves greater than 15–20 degrees definitely need referral for evaluation and close follow-up. Growing children and adolescents with curves in the 30- to 40-degree range or 20- to 30-degree range with a documented increase of 5–10 degrees will usually require a brace and an exercise program. Mature adolescents with curves greater than 50–60 degrees or younger adolescents with curves greater than 40 degrees generally require surgery.

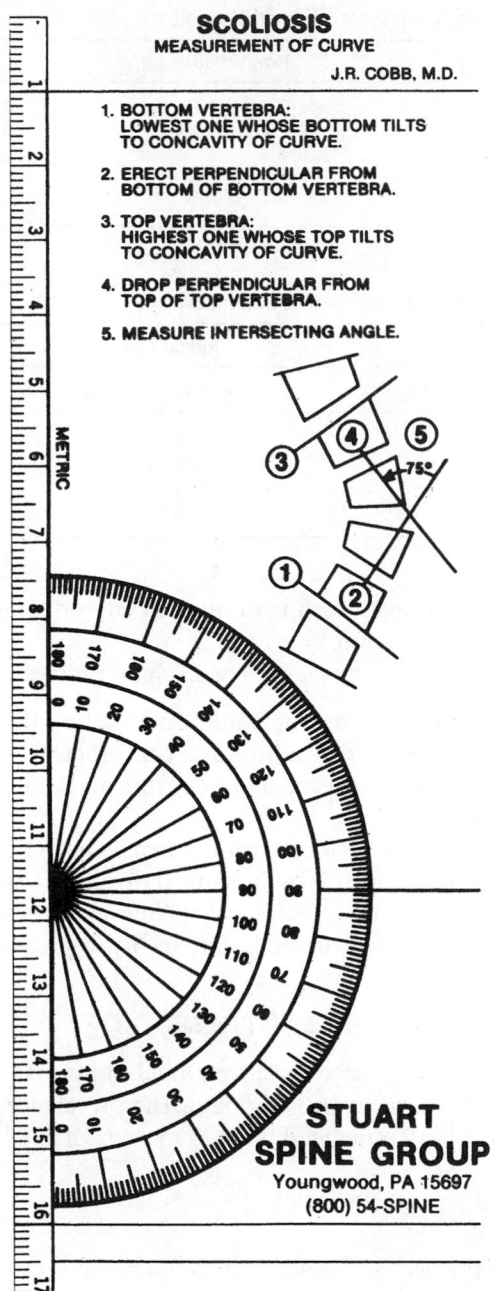

FIGURE 15.1.   Diagram shows the Cobb method of measuring the spinal curve caused by scoliosis. (Reproduced with permission from Stuart Spine Group, Youngwood, Pennsylvania.)

6. Prognosis: Curves of 5–10 degrees are of questionable significance. Over 90% never progress and are not associated with any cosmetic or physiological consequences. Even most curves between 10 and 15 degrees in growing individuals do not significantly increase. Factors indicating an increased risk of progression during adolescence include:
   a. Sex: Females have a tenfold increased risk of progression over males.
   b. Size of curvature when first seen: A larger curve carries an increased risk of progression.

TABLE 15.1.   Management of Adolescent Idiopathic Scoliosis

Curve Size (Degrees)	Progression	Therapy
0–25		Serial observation
25–30	5–10 degrees	Brace
30–40		Brace
>40		Surgery if immature
>50		Surgery (adult)

TABLE 15.2.   Risk of Progression of Idiopathic Scoliosis

| Initial curve | Age at Presentation | | | |
	Girls, 10–12 yr	Girls, 13–15 yr	Girls, >15 yr	Boys
<19	25%	1%	<1%	3%
20–29	60%	40%	10%	6%
30–59	90%	70%	30%	
>60	100%	90%		

   c. Age at presentation: Curves starting during puberty or before menarche have an increased chance of progression.
   d. Location of curve: Lumbar curves are less likely to progress than thoracic curves.

Curves of less than 50 degrees during adulthood are usually not associated with significant increases. Larger curves during adulthood can progress $1/2$–1 degree per year. The progression of curves during pregnancy is unpredictable and can be associated in some individuals with large increases.

A curve of 20–29 degrees in a 10- to 12-year-old female has a 60% chance of progression, but only a 10% risk in a girl over age 15. In the same individuals a curve of 30–59 degrees has a risk of progression of 90% and 30%, respectively (Table 15.2). Peterson et al. (1995) found several radiological findings and chronological age to be highly predictive of a progressive curve.

SCHEUERMANN'S DISEASE (JUVENILE KYPHOSIS)

Scheuermann's disease is defined as an relatively rigid abnormal increase in the posterior convexity of the thoracic spine of unknown origin. The prevalence is about 1% in the adolescent population, with a peak onset at about 12–15 years of age.

Pathogenesis

Although the cause of kyphosis is unknown, the pathogenesis is more clear. There is a change in the matrix of the vertebral plate due to changes in the collagen-proteoglycans ratio. This leads to alterations in the ossification process.

Clinical Manifestations

1. Back deformity: Round deformity may be the initial complaint, or it may be an incidental finding. The adolescent may present with:
   a. Thoracic kyphosis: 75% of cases occur in the midthoracic spine, 25% in the thoracolumbar spine, and rarely in the lumbar spine alone
   b. Forward displacement of the shoulders

   c. Winging of the scapula

   d. A head and neck carried forward from their center of gravity

   e. Protuberant abdomen

2. Back pain: Over one-half of patients present with persistent back pain localized in an involved area. The prevalence of pain is related to age, occurring in about 22% of adolescents at the onset of the process and about 60% of individuals by the time of skeletal maturation. The pain is usually aggravated with activity and is most intense at the apex of the kyphotic curve. Flexion and extension of the spine may aggravate the pain.

3. Forward bending may increase the kyphotic curve. Spine hyperextension fails to correct the curve. This distinguishes Scheuermann's disease from "adolescent postural roundback."

4. Tenderness to palpation may be present in up to 70% of individuals on palpation of the kyphotic dorsal vertebrae.

Diagnosis

Diagnosis includes evaluation of:

1. Clinical appearance: The relatively rigid kyphosis that does not correct with hyperextension of the spine

2. X-ray: Radiological examination is necessary for diagnosis. Lateral x-ray findings include:

   a. Anterior vertebral wedging in the area of excessive kyphosis

   b. Irregularities of the vertebral endplates and narrowing of the disc spaces in the affected spine segments

   c. Schmorl's nodules: Occasional abnormal protrusions of intervertebral disc material into the vertebral bodies causing radiolucent pockets bulging from the disc spaces

Normal thoracic kyphosis ranges from 20–40 degrees (using the Cobb method on the lateral x-ray as described for treatment of scoliosis in Fig. 15.1). Scheuermann's disease typically presents with kyphosis greater than 40 degrees with the associated vertebral abnormalities described above.

Treatment

Treatment is controversial, and not all patients require intervention. The indications for therapy, the natural history, the relationship between pain and treatment, and the effect of treatment on the condition are all unclear. Treatment modalities include braces, exercises, and surgery. Postural exercises seem to have little value but have been recommended in mild cases. Bracing can improve the back pain symptoms and decrease the kyphosis in lesser curves. Operative correction (spinal fusion) is rarely indicated—only in skeletally mature patients with chronic pain and large curves (generally over 70 degrees).

BIBLIOGRAPHY

Ascani E, Bartolozzi P, Logroscino CL, et al. Natural history of untreated idiopathic scoliosis after skeletal maturity. Spine 1986;11:784.

Ascani E, Montanaro A. Scheuermann's disease. In: Bradford DS, Hensinger R, eds. Pediatric spine. New York: Thieme Publishers, 1985:307–324.

Bertrand S, Drvaric D, Lange N, et al. Electrical stimulation for idiopathic scoliosis. Clin Orthop 1992;276:176.

Bunnell WP. An objective criterion for scoliosis screening. J Bone Joint Surg [Am] 1984;62:31.

Connolly PJ, Von Schroeder HP, Johnson GE, et al. Adolescent idiopathic scoliosis. Long-term effect of instrumentation extending to the lumbar spine. J Bone Joint Surg Am 1995;77:1210.

Goldberg CJ, Dowling FE, Fogarty EE. Adolescent idiopathic scoliosis—early menarche, normal growth. Spine 1993;18:529.

Goldberg CJ, Dowling FE, Fogarty EE, et al. School scoliosis screening and the United States Preventive Services Task Force. An examination of long-term results. Spine 1995;20:1368.

Green NE. Adolescent idiopathic scoliosis. Spine State Art Rev 1990;4(1):211.

Hungerford DS. Spinal deformity in adolescence. Early detection and non-operative management. In: Barnes HV, ed. Symposium on adolescent medicine. Med Clin North Am 1975;59:1517.

Karol L. Male adolescent idiopathic scoliosis. West J Med 1993;159:482.

Keim HA. Back deformities. In: Symposium on common orthopedic problems. Pediatr Clin South Am 1977;24:871.

Keim HA. Scoliosis. Clin Symp (CIBA Pharmaceutical Co.) 1978;30(1):1.

Lonstein JE, Carlson JM. The prediction of curve progression in untreated idiopathic scoliosis during growth. J Bone Joint Surg 1984;66A(7):1061.

Murrell GA, Coonrad RW, Moorman CT, et al. An assessment of the reliability of the Scoliometer. Spine 1993;18:709.

Nachemson AL, Peterson LE. Effectiveness of treatment with a brace in girls who have adolescent idiopathic scoliosis. A prospective, controlled study based on data from the Brace Study of the Scoliosis Research Society. J Bone Joint Surg Am 1995;77:815.

Peterson LE, Nachemson AL. Prediction of progression of the curve in girls who have adolescent idiopathic scoliosis of moderate severity. Logistic regression analysis based on data from the Brace Study of the Scoliosis Research Society. J Bone Joint Surg Am 1995; 77:823.

Pinto WC, Avanzi O, Dezen E. Common sense in the management of adolescent idiopathic scoliosis. Orthop Clin North Am 1994;25:215.

Pizzutillo PD. Idiopathic scoliosis and kyphosis. In: Schafer M, ed. Instructional course lectures. Park Ridge, Illinois: American Academy of Orthopaedic Surgeons, 1994:185–191.

Rinsky LA. Advances in management of idiopathic scoliosis. Hosp Pract 1992;27:49.

Rinsky LA, Gamble JG. Adolescent idiopathic scoliosis. West J Med 1988;148:182.

Shaughnessy WJ. Management of adolescent idiopathic scoliosis. Curr Opin Rheumatol 1993;5:301.

Song K, Herring JA. Early recognition and assessment of idiopathic scoliosis. J Musculoskel Med 1993;10(4): 63.

Song K, Herring JA. Management options for idiopathic scoliosis. J Musculoskel Med 1993;10(11):40.

Tachdjian MO. The spine. In: Wickland Jr EH, ed. Pediatric orthopedics. Philadelphia: WB Saunders, 1990: 2183–2404.

Thompson GH. Back pain in children. In: Schafer M, ed. Instructional course lectures. Park Ridge, Illinois: American Academy of Orthopaedic Surgeons, 1994: 221–230.

Tolo V. Spinal deformity. In: Pine J, ed. Pediatric orthopaedics in primary care. Baltimore: William & Wilkins, 1993:83–102.

Upadhyay SS, Nelson IW, Ho EK, et al. New prognostic factors to predict the final outcome of brace treatment in adolescent idiopathic scoliosis. Spine 1995; 20:537.

US Preventive Services Task Force. Screening for adolescent idiopathic scoliosis. JAMA 1993;269(20): 2664.

Weinstein SL, Ponseti I. Curve progression in idiopathic scoliosis. J Bone Joint Surg 1983;65A(4):447.

Weinstein SL, Zavala DC, Ponseti I. Idiopathic scoliosis: long-term follow-up and prognosis in untreated patients. J Bone Joint Surg 1981;63A(5):702.

Winter RB. Spinal problems in pediatric orthopaedics. In: Morrissy RT, ed. Lovell and Winter's Pediatric orthopaedics. 3rd ed. Philadelphia: JB Lippincott, 1990: 625–702.

CHAPTER 16

Common Orthopaedic Problems

Lawrence S. Neinstein and Dale J. Townsend

This chapter discusses several orthopaedic problems encountered frequently in adolescents, including Osgood-Schlatter disease, patellofemoral syndrome (chondromalacia patellae), subluxation and dislocation of the patella, osteochondritis dissecans, slipped capital femoral epiphysis, spondylolysis and spondylolisthesis, and "growing pains."

OSGOOD-SCHLATTER DISEASE

Osgood-Schlatter disease is a painful enlargement of the tibial tubercle at the insertion of the patellar tendon. It is a common problem, especially among active adolescent males.

Etiology

During development of the anterior tibial tubercle, a small ossification center develops in the largely cartilaginous tubercle. With developing muscle mass during puberty, this small area comes under great traction stress from the patellar tendon, and small fragments of cartilage or of the ossification center can be avulsed. The problem is often aggravated by activities that involve quadriceps femoris contraction, such as running and jumping, with resultant additional stress on the tubercle.

Epidemiology

1. Males have a greater prevalence than females.
2. Mean age of onset: Onset usually coincides with the period of rapid linear growth.
   a. Females: 10 years, 7 months
   b. Males: 12 years, 7 months
   In a study by Yashar et al. (1995), the average chronological age in adolescents with Osgood-Schlatter disease was the same as the average bone age. This is in contrast to slipped capital femoral epiphysis in which physeal abnormalities and skeletal maturation anomalies do occur.

Clinical Manifestations

1. Pain and soft tissue swelling over the tibial tubercle
2. Tenderness and warmth over the tibial tubercle
3. Normal knee joint with full range of motion
4. Unilateral involvement more common than bilateral involvement
5. Duration usually several months but can last longer

Diagnosis

1. History: Pain at the tibial tubercle, aggravated by activity and relieved by rest
2. Physical examination: Tenderness and swelling of the tibial tubercle
3. X-ray: Not essential for diagnosis but taken only to eliminate the possibility of other processes. The x-ray may reveal:
   a. Soft tissue swelling anterior to tibial tubercle
   b. A radiopaque fragment in the tendon anterior to the tibial tubercle

Therapy

1. Explanation: Careful explanation of the condition to the adolescent and to his or her parents is essential to alleviate fears and misconceptions.
2. Restriction of activity: Curtailment of activity for 2–4 weeks is usually sufficient for improvement, allowing return to sports thereafter. Some individuals recommend adolescents to curtail activities that cause pain for a period of 2 months. However, it may be difficult to convince the athletic adolescent to rest, especially without parental or coach support.
3. Immobilization: If symptoms are severe or fail to respond to restriction of activity, immobilization with a knee immobilizer or cylinder cast for a few weeks is effective.
4. Steroids: Corticosteroid injections are contraindicated, as they may weaken the tendon.
5. Nonsteroidal anti-inflammatory drugs, ice: These may provide symptomatic pain relief only.
6. Knee pads: Knee pads should be used for activities where kneeling or direct knee contact may occur.

Prognosis

The prognosis is excellent, but adolescents should be informed that the process may recur if excessive activity is performed. Usually when growth is completed, the problem stops, leaving only a prominent tubercle.

PATELLOFEMORAL SYNDROME (CHONDROMALACIA PATELLAE)

Patellofemoral syndrome, patellar malalignment syndrome, or chondromalacia patellae is a frequent cause of knee pain among adolescents, accounting for as much as 70–80% of knee pain problems in females and 30% in males. It is also the leading cause of knee problems of athletes. The term *patellar malalignment syndrome* is commonly used today, as it is a better descriptive term for part of the pathophysiology of the condition. The condition has traditionally been known as chondromalacia patellae. However, this term implies actual softening and damage of the patellar articular cartilage, and in fact, many individuals have no changes in their articular surface.

Etiology

Patellar malalignment syndrome often is a result of abnormal biomechanical forces that occur across the patella. Even in an individual with normal anatomy, the force that occurs in this area, especially when the body is supported with one leg and the knee is partially flexed, is tremendous. Abnormal forces can result because of:

1. Quadriceps femoris muscle imbalance or weakness or abnormality in the attachment of the vastus medialis
2. Altered patellar anatomy, such as a small or high-riding patella

3. Increased femoral neck anteversion, with associated knee valgus and external tibial torsion, which increases lateral stress on the patella
4. Increased Q angle: The angle found between a line drawn from the anterosuperior iliac spine through the center of the patella and a line from the center of the patella to the tibial tubercle (normal: <15 degrees)
5. Variations in the patellar facet anatomy

Chondromalacia patellae implies actual degeneration of the patellar cartilage, similar to the process of cartilage degeneration that can occur elsewhere in the body. This is characterized microscopically by cartilage softening and swelling, then fissuring and fibrillation. The cause of this cartilage degeneration is multifactorial, involving one or more of the following:

1. Direct trauma: Especially common with injuries to the anterior aspect of the patella from a fall on the flexed knee
2. Indirect trauma: Frequent repetitive activity involving knee flexion and extension such as hiking, jogging, and calisthenics
3. Abnormal anatomic variations: Accompanied by resultant abnormal biomechanical forces affecting the patellofemoral joint as previously described
4. Disease affecting cartilage systemically: Rheumatoid arthritis, sepsis, and recurrent hemarthrosis

Epidemiology

1. Common in both male and female athletes
2. Higher prevalence among females in the general population, but a higher prevalence among males in athletic populations

Clinical Manifestations

1. The pain of chondromalacia patellae or patellofemoral syndrome is characterized by:
   a. Peripatellar or retropatellar location
   b. Relation to activity: The pain usually increases with activity such as running, squatting, or jumping, and decreases with rest. Often the pain is most acute immediately on getting up to start an activity after a period of sitting.
   c. Insidious onset
2. Positive movie or theater sign: Prolonged sitting with flexed knee is uncomfortable.
3. Pain is often severe on ascending or descending stairs.
4. Knees may buckle or give out, especially when going up or down stairs.
5. Crepitus or a grating sensation may be felt, especially with climbing stairs.
6. History of injury to the patella area may be present.
7. Symptoms are bilateral in one-third of adolescents.
8. Two-thirds of patients have at least a 6-month history of pain.
9. Physical examination
   a. Inspection of the adolescent with chondromalacia patellae or patellofemoral syndrome may reveal several anatomic abnormalities:
      — Patellar malalignment or squinting patella: With the adolescent's feet together, the two patellae may be displaced anteromedially. This is often found associated with a Q angle of greater than 15 degrees. The Q angle is a measurement of the extensor mechanism alignment and was described previously.
      — External tibial torsion
      — Genu varum
      — Prominent knee fat pads

b. Tenderness of the articular surface of the patella is elicited by knee extension and by displacing the patella medially and laterally while palpating the under surface. When asked to point to the area of pain, most adolescents will rub one or two fingers up and down the medial side of the patella; some adolescents will rub the lateral side. Usually the pain cannot be further localized to an exact spot.

c. Retropatellar crepitation may be determined by palpating for crepitus with one hand over the knee during flexion and extension. Crepitation is only significant if associated with pain.

d. Dynamic patellar compression test, or "grind sign," may be performed by compressing the superior aspect of the patella between thumb and index finger as adolescent actively tightens the quadriceps in 10 degrees of flexion. Pain is elicited if chondromalacia patellae is present. Direct compression of the patella against the femur with the knee flexed will also elicit pain.

e. Knee range of motion is usually normal.

f. Joint effusion usually does not occur but can be present in severe cases.

g. Decreased bulk of the area around the vastus medialis on the affected side may be present. Thigh circumference should be checked comparing normal to involved side.

Diagnosis

The diagnosis is usually made by compatible history and physical examination. X-rays are usually of little help but are important in evaluating for other conditions. The x-rays should include anteroposterior, lateral, tunnel, and tangential views. Arthroscopy is useful in difficult diagnostic cases. Other conditions causing knee pain in the adolescent include meniscal lesions, Osgood-Schlatter disease, tendonitis of the patellar tendon, recurrent dislocation of the patella, infrapatellar fat pad lesions, and osteochondritis dissecans. Always remember that many hip disorders present as vague knee or thigh pain.

Treatment

Treatment consists of four major components.

1. Control of symptoms
   a. Rest and avoidance of activities such as running, jumping, climbing, and squatting that produce patellofemoral compression forces: Walking and swimming are good exercises to continue. If the condition is severe, then immobilization with a cylinder cast or knee immobilizer may be necessary.
   b. Nonsteroidal anti-inflammatory agents or aspirin for 6–12 weeks
   c. Warm soaks
2. Muscle strengthening: As soon as tolerated, muscle-strengthening exercises should be performed once a day. Initially, these should be isometric quadriceps exercises. Strengthening of the vastus medialis is particularly important. The exercises should be done with a weighted boot or on an exercise machine with the knee in full extension. The weight should be held for 5 seconds and repeated in three sets of 10 repetitions. When the affected leg can tolerate 50% of the weight of the normal leg, the exercises can be done in increasing degrees of flexion until, finally, isotonic exercises can be performed.
3. Graduated running: After symptoms are controlled and 30 pounds of weight are held, a graduated running program can be instituted. Ice may be helpful just following exercise.
4. Maintenance: When the condition is under control, a maintenance program of quadriceps and hamstring exercises should be done two to three times a week. Most adolescents respond to medical management. Some severe cases will require corrective surgery.

SUBLUXATION AND DISLOCATION OF THE PATELLA

Subluxation and lateral dislocation of the patella are prevalent in the 2nd and 3rd decades of life, with a slightly higher prevalence in females. Instability of the patellofemoral joint may permit the patella to dislocate partially out of the intercondylar groove. The patella then snaps back into place, in contrast to a complete dislocation in which the patella continues to complete lateral dislocation. These episodes usually occur while the quadriceps is contracting with the knee in flexion and the foot fixed to the ground. Symptoms include pain, giving way of the knee, a popping or grinding sensation, and swelling. Physical findings may be similar to chondromalacia patellae, which is frequently associated with recurrent subluxation or dislocation. Subluxation of the patella can mimic the clinical picture of a torn meniscus. Complete dislocation is usually a dramatic event and is easy to diagnose, with the patella visible on the lateral side of the joint. With incomplete healing, there may be recurrent dislocation of the patella, which can lead to eventual osteoarthritis.

Treatment

1. Subluxation of the patella
   a. Advise regarding the use of quadriceps-strengthening exercises.
   b. Temporarily restrict or modify activity.
   c. Use elastic support to stabilize lateral side of patella.
   d. Perform surgery only if all other therapy fails.
2. Dislocation of the patella
   a. Reduction often occurs spontaneously.
   b. Gentle straightening of the knee by lifting the foot may allow the patella to slide into place.
   c. X-rays should be taken, since the dislocation and reduction may generate sufficient force to fracture bone in up to 10% of cases.
   d. Immobilize the knee in a cylinder cast or knee immobilizer for 3 weeks, followed by range of motion and quadriceps-strengthening exercises.
3. Recurrent dislocation: This problem generally requires surgical treatment to realign the pull of the quadriceps mechanism.

OSTEOCHONDRITIS DISSECANS

Osteochondritis dissecans is a condition of focal avascular necrosis in which bone and overlying articular cartilage separate from the medial femoral condyle or, less commonly, the lateral femoral condyle. The peak incidence is in the adolescent age group. The clinical course and treatment vary according to the age of onset, with children and young adolescents having a better prognosis than older adolescents and adults.

Etiology

The exact cause is unknown. Postulated factors include:

1. Trauma: Approximately 40% of patients have a history of knee trauma. A history of definite and severe injury is most common in older patients. Impingement of the tibial spine on the medial femoral condyle may play a role.
2. Ischemia: The evidence for obstruction of blood supply as a cause has been postulated, but evidence is lacking.

3. Epiphyseal development: In younger patients with osteochondritis, an accessory nucleus in the epiphyseal area may make the femoral condyle more vulnerable to trauma. Some adolescents have variants of normal growth that may simulate osteochondritis dissecans on x-ray, causing the condition to be overdiagnosed in younger adolescents.
4. Heredity: Heredity plays a minor role in some patients.

Clinical Manifestations

1. Onset in childhood and early adolescence
   a. History
       — An intermittent nonspecific knee pain usually related to activity is a common symptom.
       — Extension movements of the knee may cause swelling and soreness.
       — Symptoms often present for months to years prior to consultation.
   b. Examination
       — The adolescent may walk with the tibia in external rotation on affected side.
       — Localized tenderness over the site of the lesion is best detected with the knee in 90 degrees of flexion and palpation of the femoral condyles.
       — A small, firm, movable mass may be palpable in the joint, indicating the presence of loose bodies.
       — Quadriceps atrophy may be present.
       — Effusion is present on rare occasions.
       — Check for a positive Wilson's sign. Flex knee to 90 degrees; internally rotate the tibia on the femur and extend the knee slowly with tibia in internal rotation. If the sign is positive, pain will occur as the knee reaches 30 degrees of flexion. This pain is often relieved by external rotation of the tibia.
       — Thirty percent of individuals may have bilateral signs.
2. Onset in late adolescence and young adulthood
   a. History
       — Either insidious onset or history of specific injury with immediate onset of pain and swelling may be present.
       — Locking or acute swelling may occur if a bone fragment becomes loose.
       — Usually unilateral involvement is seen.
       — Synovial effusion is more common in younger patients than in older ones.
   b. Examination: The findings are similar to those found in younger patients, except young adults have a higher prevalence of swelling and unilateral involvement.
3. Radiological picture: Anteroposterior, lateral, and tunnel views should be taken. X-ray examination often reveals a well-circumscribed area of subchondral bone separated from the remaining femoral condyle by a crescent-shaped radiolucent line. The separate bone may appear sclerotic or fragmented. The lesion may not be seen on a standard anteroposterior view; the lesion may best be appreciated on the tunnel view. The medial femoral condyle is involved in 75–85% of cases, while approximately 15% of cases involve the lateral femoral condyle. In addition to the femoral condyle, the patella, femoral head, and talus may be involved.
4. Juvenile versus adult osteochondritis: See Table 16.1.

Treatment

1. Childhood and early adolescence
   a. Restrict symptom-producing activities.

TABLE 16.1.   Juvenile versus Adult Osteochondritis

Characteristics	Juvenile	Adult
Age	5–15	15–30
Epiphyses	Open	Closed
Bilateral	30% of cases	10% of cases
Onset	Insidious	Acute
Injury	Minor factor	Major factor
Prognosis	Excellent	Fair
Complications	Seldom	Occasionally

   b. Immobilize with cast or knee immobilizer if symptoms are severe.

   c. Advise regarding use of isometric quadriceps-strengthening exercises.

   d. Aspirin and nonsteroidal anti-inflammatory agents are not routinely used but are useful if pain or effusion is present.

   e. Healing usually occurs within 6–12 months.

   f. If there is a detached fragment, therapy usually requires surgical intervention.

2. Older adolescents and adults: Orthopaedic consultation is necessary for possible arthroscopy or surgery for either removal or internal fixation of the fragment. Surgery is particularly important in teenagers with progressive fragment formation, increasing bony sclerosis, or articular changes.

SLIPPED CAPITAL FEMORAL EPIPHYSIS

Slipped capital femoral epiphysis is a disease in which the anatomical relationship between the femoral head and neck is altered secondary to a disruption of the epiphyseal plate.

Etiology

The femoral head slips posteriorly, inferiorly, and medially on the femoral metaphysis. This occurs through the cartilaginous hypertrophied cell layer of the epiphysis. The condition tends to occur in adolescents because of:

1. The increased weight burden at adolescence
2. A decreased resistance to the added weight burden secondary to a shift in the femoral epiphysis from a horizontal to an oblique position
3. Increased stress to an area that has not reached bony maturity

A chronic gradual slip accounts for 80% or more of cases of slipped capital epiphysis during adolescence and is usually related to the combination of obesity and slow maturation. Acute slips occur secondary to severe trauma, such as a fall or an automobile accident, and are more common in younger children than adolescents. Most cases of slipped capital epiphysis are unrelated to an endocrine disorder, although the disease has been associated with hypopituitarism, hypogonadism, and hypothyroidism. Endocrine abnormalities are often associated with bilateral slips, and occur more often in the extremes of the adolescent age group (before age 9 or after age 16).

Epidemiology

1. Sex: Males have a greater prevalence than females by between 2:1 to 4:1.
2. Incidence: A sample study (Kelsey, 1971) found the incidence per 100,000 individuals in Connecticut in the under-25-year-old population to be:

African-American males	7.79
African-American females	6.68
White males	4.74
White females	1.64

3. Season: Onset of symptoms occurs more frequently in spring and summer.
4. Average age of onset: Usually symptoms occur shortly before or during period of accelerated growth. In females the range is 10–13 years of age; in males 12–15 years of age.
5. Hip involved: Left hips are affected more frequently in males. No difference is noted in females. Unilateral cases occur three times more frequently than bilateral.
6. Weight of affected patients: Approximately 88% of patients are obese, with 50% of cases at or above the 95th percentile of weight for age and the 97th percentile of weight for height.
7. Bone age: Seventy percent of affected patients have skeletal maturation that is 6 months or more retarded.

Clinical Manifestations

1. Symptoms
   a. Pain: Pain is localized to hip or groin in 80% of patients. Thigh or knee pain may be present secondary to obturator nerve referral. This can occur without hip pain.
   b. Click in the hip occurs.
2. Signs
   a. Internal rotation is diminished and adduction of hip is decreased.
   b. Decreased flexion of the hip is present.
   c. Affected leg often is held in slight external rotation and adduction.
   d. With passive hip flexion, the femur abducts and externally rotates.
   e. Limp: A limp is present in 50% of patients. The adolescent with acute slippage may not be able to bear weight on the affected extremity.

Diagnosis

1. History and physical examination: Consistent signs and symptoms are present. The condition should be considered in any adolescent with hip or knee pain or a limp.
2. X-ray changes: Anteroposterior and frog-leg lateral roentgenograms of the pelvis should be taken.
   a. Earlier and more subtle slips are seen on the frog-leg lateral views better than on the anteroposterior views. More advanced slips show the obvious slippage inferiorly and posteriorly of the femoral head epiphysis on both anteroposterior and frog-lateral films.
   b. Early changes include epiphyseal widening and rarefaction.
3. Bone scan: A bone scan may show increased uptake at the involved epiphyseal plate.

Treatment

Orthopaedic referral is required, as surgery is the only reliable treatment. Further slippage can be prevented with the introduction of threaded screws across the epiphyseal plate in situ (reduction of the slip is seldom, if ever, indicated). Treatment should be performed as early as possible, since greater slippage leads to a worse prognosis. Avascular necrosis can occur with acute, large slips. Premature degenerative joint disease is a frequent late development in many severe, chronic slips, even with fixation. For moderate and severe cases, corrective osteomies can be performed to improve gait and range of motion.

SPONDYLOLYSIS AND SPONDYLOLISTHESIS

Spondylolysis represents a defect in one or both vertebral pars interarticularis. If forward displacement of a vertebra occurs, the condition is called spondylolisthesis. The condition is rare below the age of 5 and increases in prevalence between the ages of 5–8 to about 5%, which is the prevalence found in adult populations. The condition is probably a result of a stress fracture in the pars interarticularis, resulting in permanent nonunion. The condition is twice as common in males than in females and in the white population than in nonwhite populations. Repeated stress and genetic predisposition may increase the incidence of the problem.

The problem is most common in the lumbar spine, particularly in the L5. Usually spondylolysis is asymptomatic and is found unexpectedly on x-rays taken for other reasons. Spondylosis may become symptomatic, particularly in individuals involved in repetitive hyperextension of the back, such as in dance and gymnastics; the prevalence in female gymnasts is 11%, and the condition is found in 15–20% of dancers complaining of back pain. The pain may be precipitated by trauma. The area of the defect in the pars interarticularis may develop a pseudarthrosis, with the formation of bony or cartilaginous deformities at the defect. With movement these can cause nerve root irritation and pain. Treatment usually consists of abdominal strengthening exercises and hamstring flexibility exercises, if the individual is active.

Spondylolisthesis occurs when the spondylolytic vertebra is displaced anteriorly to the vertebrae below it. This occurs most commonly between L5 and S1. Symptoms usually involve pain near the involved vertebra and can cause sensory and motor changes if a spinal nerve root is compressed. On examination, the involved area will be tender and the spinous process of the slipped vertebra may be prominent. The pain can often be increased by hyperextension of the leg. Further sensory findings may be present if spinal nerve root compression is present. Because of the L5 location of most of the cases, sensory findings are most common on the dorsomedial aspect of the foot and the hallux. The condition is best demonstrated on oblique films, although anteroposterior and lateral films should also be obtained. Recognition of structures on the oblique film is facilitated by the structures' similarity to the appearance of a Scotty dog, as follows: pedicle, the eye; superior articular process, the ear; inferior articular process, the forelimb; transverse process, the nose; and arch, the body. Slippage is usually graded by the percentage of the underlying vertebral body that has slipped over. Grade I equals a slippage of 0–25% of the anteroposterior diameter of the vertebral body below; grade II equals 26–50% slippage; grade III, 51–75%; and grade IV, 76–100%. Generally, a slippage of less than 50% does not cause major problems and does not curtail most activities. A slippage of greater than 50% would probably preclude the individual from strenuous activities. The chance of progressive slippage is most marked in individuals between the ages of 9 and 15. Further progression is rare after age 18.

In individuals with an acute presentation, a bone scan may be helpful. With an abnormal bone scan at the pars interarticularis, rest for several months may be indicated. There is a chance in these individuals for healing of a presumed acute fracture. In individuals with a normal bone scan, the prognosis for healing of the lesion is negligible.

Consultation with an orthopaedist is usually necessary if either pain or slippage is present. Spondylolysis and mild spondylolisthesis can usually be managed with mild back exercises and braces. Cases that do not respond to therapy, especially those with severe slippage, may require removal of any bony defect and spinal fusion.

"GROWING PAINS"

Pain in the lower limbs is not uncommon among children and younger adolescents. Many causes are possible and include:

1. Trauma: Fractures, dislocation, contusion
2. Infection: Osteomyelitis, septic arthritis, abscess, cellulitis
3. Vascular: Hemophilia, sickle cell anemia, hemangioma
4. Congenital: Tarsal coalition, dislocation of hip
5. Slipped femoral capital epiphysis
6. Osgood-Schlatter disease
7. Osteochondritis dissecans
8. Chondromalacia patellae
9. Rheumatic: juvenile rheumatoid arthritis, polymyositis
10. Leukemia

Most of these causes are well delineated by history, physical examination, and appropriate laboratory tests. However, "growing pains" may be difficult to define and diagnose and are a diagnosis of exclusion. Some practitioners question the existence of "growing pains."

Etiology

The cause is unknown, but implicated factors include rapid growth, puberty, fibrositis, weather, and psychological factors.

Epidemiology

1. Prevalence: The prevalence of growing pains is reported at between 4% and 50% of children and adolescents. A study of 2200 school children revealed a prevalence of 12.5% in males and 18.4% in females (Oster, 1972).
2. Age: The prevalence of growing pains increases after age 5 and peaks at age 13 in males and age 11 in females.

Clinical Manifestations

1. Pain
   a. Intermittent pain or ache usually localized to the muscles of the legs and thighs: The most common sites are the front of the thighs and calves and behind the knees. Less commonly involved sites include the back, shoulder, arm, and groin.
   b. Bilateral pain is usually present.
   c. Pain usually occurs late in the day, in the evening, or at night.
2. No loss of mobility
3. No tenderness, erythema, or swelling
4. No fever or symptoms of systemic disease
5. Normal laboratory study and x-rays.

Diagnosis

There is no simple approach to a definite diagnosis. A thorough evaluation should include:

1. A consistent history of no symptoms of systemic disease
2. Normal findings from physical examination
3. Normal laboratory findings including normal complete blood count level, sedimentation rate, and x-rays (other tests such as rheumatoid factor and an antinuclear antibody as clinically indicated)

Treatment

Conservative therapy involving reassurance, heat, massage, and nonsteroidal anti-inflammatory medications or aspirin is usually sufficient.

BIBLIOGRAPHY

Aronson DD, Loder RT. Slipped capital femoral epiphysis in black children. J Pediatr Orthop 1992;12:74.

Atar D, Lehman WB, Grant AD. Growing pains. Orthop Rev 1991;20(2):133.

Binazzi R, Felli L, Vaccari V, et al. Surgical treatment of unresolved Osgood-Schlatter lesion. Clin Orthop 1993;289:202.

Bradley J, Dandy DJ. Osteochondritis dissecans and other lesions of the femoral condyle. J Bone Joint Surg 1989;71B:518.

Browne JE. Runners and their afflictions. Hosp Med 1986;(suppl):13.

Busch MT, Morrissy RT. Slipped capital femoral epiphysis. Orthop Clin North Am 1987;18:637.

Carney BT, Weinstein SL, Noble J. Long-term follow-up of slipped capital femoral epiphysis. J Bone Joint Surg 1988;70B:174.

Causey AL, Smith ER, Donaldson JJ, et al. Missed slipped capital femoral epiphysis: illustrative cases and a review. J Emerg Med 1995;13:175.

Davidson K. Patellofemoral pain syndrome. Am Fam Physician 1993;48:1254–1262.

DeHaven KE, Dolan WA, Mayer PJ. Chondromalacia patellae and the painful knee. Am Fam Physician 1980;21:117.

Deluca SA, Rhea JT. Slipped femoral epiphysis. Am Fam Physician 1984;29:159.

DiStefano VJ. How I manage osteochondritis dissecans. Physician Sportsmed 1986;14:135.

Edmonson AS. Spondylolisthesis. In: Crenshaw AH, ed. Campbell's operative orthopaedics, vol 4. St. Louis: CV Mosby, 1987.

Eilert RE. Adolescent anterior knee pain. In: Heckman JD, ed. Instructional course lectures. Park Ridge, Illinois: American Academy of Orthopaedic Surgeons, 1993;497–516.

Fredrickson BE, Baker D, McHolick WJ, et al. The natural history of spondylolysis and spondylolisthesis. J Bone Joint Surg 1984;66A:699.

Fulkerson JP, Kalenak A, Rosenberg TD, et al. Patellofemoral pain. In: Eilert RE, ed. Instructional course lectures. Park Ridge, Illinois: American Academy of Orthopaedic Surgeons, 1992;57–71.

Henry JH. The patellofemoral joint. In: Nicholas JA, Hershman EB, eds. The lower extremity and spine in sports medicine. St. Louis: CV Mosby, 1986.

Hensinger RN. Current concepts review: spondylolysis and spondylolisthesis in children and adolescents. J Bone Joint Surg 1989;71A:1098.

Horn BD, Moseley CF. Current concepts in the management of pediatric hip disease. Curr Opin Rheumatol. 1992;4:184.

Insall J. Current concepts review: patellar pain. J Bone Joint Surg 1982;64A:147.

Johnson AC. How spondylolysis can be repaired. Patient Care 1983;17:73.

Kelsey JL. Incidence and distribution of slipped capital femoral epiphysis in Connecticut. J Chronic Dis 1971;23:567.

Kujala UM, Kvist M, Heinonen O. Osgood-Schlatter's disease in adolescent athletes: retrospective study of incidence and duration. Am J Sports Med 1985;13:236.

LaBrier K, Oneill DB. Patellofemoral stress syndrome: current concepts. Sports Med 1993;16:449.

Loder RT, Wittenberg B, DeSilva G. Slipped capital femoral epiphysis associated with endocrine disorders. J Pediatr Orthop 1995;15:349.

Morita T, Ikata T, Katoh S, et al. Lumbar spondylolysis in children and adolescents. J Bone Joint Surg Br 1995; 77:620.

Morrissy RT. Slipped capital femoral epiphysis. In: Morrissy RT, ed. Lovell and Winter's Pediatric orthopaedics. 3rd ed. Philadelphia: JB Lippincott, 1990: 885–904.

Oster J. Recurrent abdominal pain, headache, and limb pain in children and adolescents. Pediatrics 1972; 50:429.

Oster J, and Nielsen, A. Growing pains. Acta Paediatr Scand (suppl) 1972;61:329.

Pizzutillo PD, Hummer CD. Non-operative treatment for painful adolescent spondylolysis or spondylolisthesis. J Pediatr Orthop 1989;9:538.

Rosenberg ZS, Kawelblum M, Cheung YY, et al. Osgood-Schlatter lesion: fracture or tendinitis? Scintigraphic, CT, and MR imaging features. Radiology 1992;185:853.

Ruffin IV MT, Kiningham RB. Anterior knee pain: the challenge of patellofemoral syndrome. Am Fam Physician 1993;47:185.

Sandow MJ, Goodfellow JW. The natural history of anterior knee pain in adolescents. J Bone Joint Surg 1985;67:36.

Staheli LT. The lower limb. In: Morrissy RT, ed. Lovell and Winter's Pediatric orthopaedics. 3rd ed. Philadelphia: JB Lippincott, 1990:741–766.

Stanitski CL. Anterior knee pain syndromes in the adolescent. J Bone Joint Surg 1993;75:1407.

Stanitski CL. Knee overuse disorders in the pediatric and adolescent athlete. In: Heckman JD, ed. Instructional course lectures. Park Ridge, Illinois: American Academy of Orthopaedic Surgeons, 1993:483–495.

Tachdjian MO. Joints. In: Wickland Jr EH, ed. Pediatric orthopedics. Philadelphia: WB Saunders, 1990:1410–1599.

Tachdjian MO. The spine. In: Wickland Jr EH, ed. Pediatric orthopedics. Philadelphia: WB Saunders, 1990: 2183–2404.

Taylor PM. Osteochondritis dissecans as a cause of posterior heel pain. Physician Sportsmed 1982;10:53.

Teitz CC. Sports medicine concerns in dance and gymnastics. Pediatr Clin North Am 1982;29:1399.

Thompson GH. Back pain in children. In: Schafer M, ed. Instructional course lectures. Park Ridge, Illinois: American Academy of Orthopaedic Surgeons, 1994: 221–230.

Tolo V. Back pain. In: Pine J, ed. Pediatric orthopaedics in primary care. Baltimore: Williams & Wilkins, 1993: 103–122.

Tolo V. Hip and thigh. In: Pine J, ed. Pediatric orthopaedics in primary care. Baltimore: Williams & Wilkins, 1993:135–168.

Tolo V. Knee. In: Pine J, ed. Pediatric orthopaedics in primary care. Baltimore: Williams & Wilkins, 1993: 169–192.

Weiker GG. The dancer's spine. Emergency Med 1982; 14:28.

Wells D, King JD, Roe TF, et al. Review of slipped capital femoral epiphysis associated with endocrine disease. J Pediatr Orthop 1993;13:610.

Winter RB. Spinal problems in pediatric orthopaedics. In: Morissy RT, ed. Lovell and Winter's Pediatric orthopaedics, 3rd ed. Philadelphia: JB Lippincott, 1990: 625–702.

Wood JB, Klassen RA, Peterson HA. Osteochondritis dissecans of the femoral head in children and adolescents: a report of 17 cases. J Pediatr Orthop 1995;15:313.

Yashar A, Loder RT, Hensinger RN. Determination of skeletal age in children with Osgood-Schlatter disease by using radiographs of the knee. J Pediatr Orthop 1995;15:298.

CHAPTER 17

Back Pain

Back pain (in particular, lower back pain) is one of the most common complaints among adult patients and the most common cause of disability in individuals younger than 45. While back pain is very unusual in prepubertal and young adolescent patients, middle and older adolescents not infrequently complain of back pain.

PREVALENCE

The prevalence of backaches increases with age, with the lowest prevalence in children and adolescents. However, back pain, particularly lower back pain, can be relatively common in older adolescents.

Studies of lower back pain in adolescents:

1. Turner et al., (1989): Less than 2% of the clients in an orthopaedic practice of children younger than 15 complained of back pain.
2. Grantham (1977): Back pain was experienced by 11.5% of adolescent male students in an English school.
3. Balague et al. (1988): Back pain affected 27% of Swiss school students.
4. Fairbanks et al. (1984): Back pain affected 26% of English school students.
5. Olsen et al. (1992): Back pain was experienced by 30.4% of 1242 American adolescents aged 11–17. Of those with back pain, one-third had a history of needing to restrict their activity, and 7.3% sought medical attention for back pain.

ETIOLOGY

The etiology of back pain varies with age. The younger the individual, the more likely that back pain is not related to musculoskeletal strain. The major causes of back pain in the adolescent are listed below in their general order of prevalence.

1. Ligamentous strain
2. Traumatic lower back derangement
3. Spondylolysis and spondylolisthesis: These problems may be particularly common in acute low back pain in adolescent athletes. Micheli et al. (1995) compared the etiology of back pain in adolescent athletes to that in adults. Sixty-two percent of the adolescents had an abnormality of their posterior elements associated with the onset of back pain. Forty-seven percent of the 100 adolescents were ultimately shown to have a spondylolysis stress fracture of the pars interarticularis. Only 5% of adult subjects had spondylolysis associated with low back pain. Discogenic back pain was the final diagnosis in 48% of the adults but was the final diagnosis in only 11% of the adolescent athletes. Muscle-tendon strain was also more common in the adults than in adolescent athletes (27% versus 6%).
4. Functional back pain secondary to somatization disorder or conversion reaction

5. Scheuermann's disease (juvenile kyphosis)
6. Inflammatory process
   a. Disc space infection
   b. Osteomyelitis
   c. Rheumatoid variant such as Reiter's syndrome or ankylosing spondylitis
   d. Bacterial endocarditis
7. Gastrointestinal diseases (cholecystitis, pancreatitis, and penetrating ulcers) and renal diseases (pyelonephritis, nephrolithiasis, and perinephric abscess)
8. Referred pain: Intrapelvic pathology such as endometritis
9. Osteoid osteoma: A benign tumor of bone that can involve the posterior elements of the vertebrae and lead to back pain; sclerosis of one of the posterior elements of the vertebrae usually revealed by radiological examination
10. Congenital anomalies of the spine
11. Spinal cord tumor or leukemia
12. Scoliosis: Causes backache when severe
13. Metabolic or endocrine diseases
    a. Cushing's disease
    b. Osteoporosis
    c. Acromegaly
    d. Hyperparathyroidism
    e. Osteomalacia
14. Herniated lumbar disc: Uncommon in adolescents

EVALUATION

In most individuals with acute back pain, the cause is never known, but the course is almost always benign and self-limited. However, to eliminate the possibility of a more serious condition, a thorough history and physical examination are basic requisites.

1. History
   a. The history should include:
      — Characteristics of the pain including, severity, type, onset and duration, prior treatment and limitations, exacerbating and alleviating maneuvers
      — History of trauma and athletic and work history
      — Systemic symptoms: Fever, iritis, urethritis, arthritis
      — Family history of spondylitis
      — Neurologic symptoms, including bladder or bowel changes
   b. Specific conditions
      — Tumors: Back pain occurring at rest, especially at night, is a common feature of vertebral involvement with a neoplastic process. Constant back pain, associated neurological deficits, and rigidity of the spine on attempted movement may be associated with tumors. Other suggestive historical information includes prior history of a malignant tumor and unexplained weight loss.
      — Spondylolysis and spondylolisthesis: Back pain may radiate to buttocks or thighs. There may be a history of hyperextension activities of the spine such as gymnastics or ballet.
      — Infection: Discitis and osteomyelitis of a vertebrae can lead to significant back pain. Discitis is most common in younger children and usually affects the lumbar region and is associated with *Staphlococcus aureus.* The pain may radiate to the hip, leg, or abdomen and may lead to a gait disturbance. A history of another site of infection such as urinary tract infection, skin infection, or intravenous drug use may be suggestive of an infectious spinal process.

- Spondyloarthropathy: The back pain associated with spondyloarthropathies is associated with insidious onset, worsening of symptoms in the morning and with rest, a decrease in symptoms with activity, an onset before 30 years of age, and pain that persists over 3 months.
- Scoliosis: Back pain is not usually a feature of scoliosis and should suggest the possible presence of another disorder.

Severe back pain in an adolescent is more likely associated with a pathologic condition than a muscular strain and should be more carefully evaluated. Writhing pain suggests a possible intra-abdominal condition. Unrelenting pain suggests cancer or an infectious process.

2. Physical examination: This should include examination in the standing, sitting, and supine positions.

a. Standing position
   - Asymmetry: Check for pelvic or leg length discrepancies.
   - Curvatures: Check for kyphosis or scoliosis and perform forward-bending examination.
   - Percuss spine for local tenderness.
   - Check gait, including heel and toe walking.
   - Range of motion: Most adolescents should be able to bend to within 15 cm of their toes regardless of the problem. Individuals with paraspinal muscle spasm will tend to arch their lumbar area while bending their spine at the hips.
   - Midline defects: Midline defects including dimpling, hypertrichosis, hemangiomatosis, cutaneous nevi, and soft tissue masses may be a clue to an underlying spinal abnormality such as spina bifida.

b. Sitting position
   - Test knee, ankle, and Babinski's sign.
   - Test muscle strength of lower extremities.
   - Perform distraction leg-raising test: Ask individual to straighten his or her leg while seated. Patients with a disc problem arch backward in tripod position to take pressure off sciatic nerve. Results of this test should correlate with results of straight leg–raising in supine position.

c. Supine position
   - Measure leg length from anterosuperior iliac spine to medial malleolus. A difference greater than 2.5 cm should be evaluated.
   - Check for muscle atrophy by measuring girth of each leg a fixed measured distance above and below the patella.
   - Perform sensory examination.
   - Perform straight leg–raising test: Teen should be on back with one leg flexed at the hip and knee and sole of that foot on the table as you test the other leg. Pain radiating down the back of the second leg when this leg is lifted and the knee extended is a positive test. An unequivocal test is indicated when pain occurs when the angle between the back of the thigh and the table is less than 60 degrees. Pain when this angle is greater than 60 degrees may be caused by muscular irritability. The examiner can also lift the leg to the point of pain and then lower the leg 5 degrees and dorsiflex the foot. This will stretch the sciatic nerve and is another sign of nerve impingement. If pain occurs in the opposite leg while lifting one leg, a positive crossed straight leg–raising sign is present. This has been highly correlated with a herniated disc.
   - Femoral stretch test: With the teen facing down and the knees straight, lift one leg backward, extending the hip but keeping the knee straight. This test stretches the femoral nerve, and pain radiating into the anterior thigh indicates L-2, L-3, and L-4 nerve root irritation.

With chronic back pain a rectal examination is indicated to look for decreased sphincter tone, suggesting pressure on nerve roots from a tumor or herniated disc. In addition, the circumferences of the upper and lower legs should be measured to look for muscle atrophy.

3. Specific conditions
   a. Tumors: Neurological deficits may be present, including weakness and bowel and bladder dysfunction.
   b. Spondylolysis and spondylolisthesis: The teen may have hyperlordosis. Stiffness and limited straight leg raising from hamstring spasm or tautness may be present. Localized tenderness may occur at L-5 to S-1. Neurologic deficits may be present if significant slippage has occurred.
   c. Infections: Tenderness may be well localized over affected vertebrae.
   d. Herniated disc: Pain commonly radiates down the leg. In more advanced cases a herniated disk is associated with muscle weakness, atrophy, and decrease in sensation and reflexes.
   e. Functional pain: Tests for nonorganic etiology
      — Press on head with gentle downward pressure. If patient collapses or complains of severe pain, the problem may be functional.
      — Gently palpate paraspinous muscles. Complaints of severe pain or falling to the floor may be indicative of a nonorganic problem.
      — Holding teen's wrists next to his or her hips, turn teen's body side to side. Since this does not cause stress on the muscles or nerve roots, it should not cause any significant pain.
      — Perform Burn's test. Have teen kneel on regular chair and touch the floor with his or her fingertips. If teen cannot reach within 15 cm of floor, the test is considered positive and possibly indicative of a nonorganic cause.

Diagnosis

Radiological examination should be done in adolescents with chronic back pain (more than 3 months). Other indications for radiologic examination include a history of serious trauma; known cancer; pain at rest; unexplained weight loss; drug or alcohol abuse; point tenderness; treatment with corticosteroids; or temperature above 38°C; or when clinical manifestations are consistent with the diagnosis of scoliosis, kyphosis, spondylolisthesis, or ankylosing spondylitis or demonstrate a neuromotor deficit. In the absence of history or physical findings suggestive of serious disease, spine films have a low diagnostic yield. Lumbar spine radiographs are estimated to be the largest source of gonadal irradiation in the United States.

With chronic back pain a complete blood count, sedimentation rate, and urinalysis should be obtained.

1. Tumors: History and physical examination consistent with possible tumor should lead to routine radiological examination and then magnetic resonance imaging (MRI) as needed.
2. Spondylolysis and spondylolisthesis: Plain radiographs including anteroposterior, lateral, and oblique views can confirm the diagnosis.
3. Infections: With discitis, plain radiographs show disc space narrowing and irregularities or erosions of the endplate. This finding may not be present for the first 2–3 weeks. A bone scan may show positive results much earlier. With osteomyelitis, there is usually erosion and collapse of the vertebral bodies on plain films. A disc aspiration or biopsy for culture is needed to identify the organism involved.

4. Herniated disc: Plain radiographs usually show no abnormal findings, and the diagnosis may require an MRI scan.
5. Functional back pain: Diagnosis can be made based on negative results from evaluation and radiographs and positive results from psychosocial assessment.

TREATMENT

Most acute back pain will resolve in a relatively short period of time; 70% in 1 week, 80% by 2 weeks, and 90% by 2 months. For many of the causes of back pain the treatment is directed at the specific cause:

1. Tumors: Appropriate surgical treatments, radiation therapy, or chemotherapy.
2. Spondylolysis and spondylolisthesis: For adolescents with symptomatic nonprogressive spondylolisthesis, decreased activities and anti-inflammatory medications can be tried. In some individuals immobilization in a cast or orthotic device may be necessary. In adolescents with significant progression of their slippage (more than 50% slip), refractory pain, neurological deficit, or gait disturbance, surgical stabilization with spinal fusion of the vertebra that has slipped is probably necessary. Acute or symptomatic spondylolysis can be treated with a supportive brace or body cast to promote healing of fracture and prevent anterior displacement.
3. Infections: Discitis can be treated with rest and anti-inflammatory medication. The use of antibiotics is controversial and is probably best used if there is a suspicion of infection based on presence of fever, high sedimentation rate, positive results from blood culture or disc space aspirate, or failure of response to conservative therapy. An osteomyelitis requires aspiration or needle biopsy of the involved area with appropriate antibiotics, depending on culture results.
4. Herniated disc: Treatment includes trial of bed rest and anti-inflammatory medications for several weeks. An individual with significant neurological findings that fail to respond to conservative management may need surgical intervention.
5. Functional back pain: Treatment includes appropriate individual and family counseling for identified problem.

For back pain secondary to muscular or ligamentous strain the treatment includes back exercise, weight reduction, anti-inflammatory medications and sometimes a change in activities. For acute strain, cryotherapy using ice in a towel or a wet towel that has been kept in the freezer is helpful. It can be applied for 15–20 minutes, four times a day for at least the first 3 days. After this time, cold can be replaced with heat using a heating pad or moist hot towel.

Sample recommendations and back exercises for individuals with chronic or recurrent musculoskeletal back pain are discussed below.

General Recommendations: Acute Back Strain

1. Never bend from the waist only; bend at the hips and knees.
2. When standing for a prolonged time, place one foot on a step to reduce back strain.
3. Never lift a heavy object higher than the waist.
4. Never sleep on the abdomen; it is best to sleep on one side with hips and knees bent. Use a firm mattress or put a $^3/_4$-inch plywood board under a soft mattress.
5. When sitting, place the spine up against the back of a chair, and be sure one or both knees are higher than the hips.
6. Shoes should have low heels.

Back Exercises

Back exercises should be begun slowly and increased slowly over time.

1. Knee hug
   a. Lie on back with pillow under head; inhale.
   b. Slowly raise knees to chest.
   c. Clasp knees with hands and hold for count of 10.
   d. Repeat three times and build slowly to 20 per day.
2. Cat backs
   a. Get on all fours on the floor.
   b. Arch back up like a cat and then down as far as possible.
   c. Repeat three times and build slowly to 20 per day.
3. Leg lifts
   a. Lie on stomach with arms at sides.
   b. Raise each leg in turn, to a height of 1 foot off the floor.
   c. Start with three lifts of each leg and build slowly to 20 per day.
4. Back flattener
   a. Lie on back, knees raised, with feet on floor and hands over head.
   b. Tighten stomach and buttock muscles at same time to flatten back against floor.
   c. Hold for count of 10. Repeat three times and build slowly to 20 per day.
5. Shoulder lifts
   a. Lie flat on stomach with arms at side.
   b. Lift both shoulders 6 inches off the floor.
   c. Start with three and build slowly to 20 per day.
6. Posture check
   a. Stand with back to wall. Press heels, rump, shoulders, and head against wall.
   b. Move feet forward and bend knees so back slides down a few inches.
   c. Tighten abdominal and buttock muscles so lower back is flat against wall.
   d. Hold this position and walk feet back so back slides up the wall.
   e. Standing straight, walk away from wall and around the room.
7. Sit-ups (should be started several weeks after exercises have begun)
   a. Lie flat on back with knees bent.
   b. Sit up to an upright position while grasping knees.
   c. Return to starting position.
   d. Start with three and build slowly to 20 per day.

BIBLIOGRAPHY

Balague F, Dutoit G, Waldburger M. Low back pain in schoolchildren. Scand J Rehabil Med 1988;20:175.

Carey TS, Garrett J, Jackman A, et al. The outcomes and costs of care for acute low back pain among patients seen by primary care practitioners, chiropractors, and orthopedic surgeons. The North Carolina Back Pain Project. N Engl J Med 1995;333:913.

Deyo RA, Diehl AK. Lumbar spine films in primary care: current use and effects of selective ordering criteria. J Gen Intern Med 1986;1:20.

Deyo RA, Diehl AK, Rosenthal M. Reducing work absenteeism due to backache: a random clinical trial. N Engl J Med 1986;315:1064.

Deyo RA, Mayer TG, Pedinoff S, et al. An attack on low back pain. Patient Care 1987;21:106.

Deyo RA, Rainville J, Kent DL. What can the history and physical examination tell us about low back pain? JAMA 1992;268:760.

Dyment PG. Low back pain in adolescents. Pediatr Ann 1991;20:170.

Fairbanks J, Pynsent PB, Poortvliet JA, et al. Influence of anthropometric factors and joint laxity in the incidence of adolescent back pain. Spine 1984;9:461.

Frazier LM, Carey TS, Lyles MF, et al. Selective criteria may increase lumbosacral spine roentgenogram use in acute low-back pain. Arch Intern Med 1989; 149:47.

Frymoyer JW. Back pain and sciatic. N Engl J Med 1988; 318:291.

Grantham VA. Backache in boys—a new problem. Practitioner 1977;218:226.

Hall H. A simple approach to back-pain management. Patient Care 1992;26:77.

Hastings DE. Back pain: a multifaceted syndrome. Postgrad Med 1977;62:159.

Hockberger R. Low back pain. Emerg Med 1986;16:123.

Jenner JR, Barry M. ABC of rheumatology. Low back pain. Br Med J 1995;310:929.

King HA. Evaluating the child with back pain. Pediatr Clin North Am 1986;33:1489.

Micheli LJ, Wood R. Back pain in young athletes. Significant differences from adults in causes and patterns. Arch Pediatr Adolesc Med 1995;149:15.

Olsen TL, Anderson RL, Dearwater SR, et al. The epidemiology of low back pain in an adolescent population. Am J Pub Health 1992;82:606.

Pedinoff S, Pinals RS, Schwartz SA, et al. A rational workup for low-back pain. Patient Care 1991;25:43.

Shekelle PG, Adams AH, Chassin MR, et al. Spinal manipulation for low-back pain. Ann Intern Med 1992; 117:590.

Staheli LT. Pain of musculoskeletal origin in children. Curr Opin Rheumatol 1992;4:748.

Turner PG, Green JH, Galasko CSB. Back pain in childhood. Spine 1989;14:812.

Wipf JE, Deyo RA. Low back pain. Med Clin North Am 1995;79:231.

Guidelines in Sports Medicine

Albert Hergenroeder and Lawrence S. Neinstein

More than 20 million children and adolescents participate in organized sports in the United States. While some health-care professionals caring for adolescents do not treat injuries on the playing field, almost all will do preparticipation examinations and treat acute and chronic injuries in their practice. This chapter addresses several areas: the preparticipation sports examination, the classification of sports, conditioning, rehabilitation, exclusion from sports for special conditions, diagnosis and treatment of common injuries (including head and neck injuries), drug use in young athletes, and game site equipment.

PREPARTICIPATION SPORTS EXAMINATION

The American Medical Association's (AMA's) Guidelines for Adolescent Preventive Services (GAPS) recommends that an annual preventive service visit be conducted each year during the adolescent period, with a complete physical examination at least once during early adolescence, middle adolescence, and late adolescence. *In addition*, the American Academy of Pediatrics recommends that adolescents involved in strenuous activity should have a sports-specific examination on entry into junior and senior high school and that such an examination be updated by an annual questionnaire emphasizing recent injuries or any health condition affecting sports participation. The student must have annual physician clearance to continue participating, which requires the physician review an updated health history and perform the directed physical examination discussed below.

The preseason examination is not a comprehensive health maintenance visit that addresses topics such as drug use, sexual activity, violence, mental health, organic disease complaints, screening tests, and immunizations. Unfortunately, the preparticipation sports examination is used as a poor substitute for the annual comprehensive health evaluation for many teens. Establishing mechanisms wherein teens receive annual comprehensive health maintenance visits *and* have directed preparticipation sports examinations should be a priority. This discussion of the preseason examination assumes that the athlete is receiving regular maintenance care, and the preparticipation sports examination is in addition to their routine care.

Objectives

The major objective of the preparticipation sports examination is to identify those musculoskeletal and other medical conditions that could be worsened by sports participation. Specifically, the examination should be designed to:

1. Identify conditions that preclude participation in specific sports.
2. Diagnose treatable conditions and undetected disease.
3. Develop treatment and rehabilitation plans for problems.
4. Prevent further injuries by identifying and treating musculoskeletal abnormalities, especially unrehabilitated injuries.

5. Advise the athlete which sports he or she can participate in, if a condition exists that precludes participation in specific sports.
6. Fulfill legal and insurance requirements.

The preparticipation sports examination has been shown to be helpful in identifying adolescents at risk for orthopaedic injury, but its usefulness for identifying adolescents at risk for sudden cardiac death or for other undiagnosed chronic medical disorders is not substantiated (AMA, 1994). The true-positive rate for identifying athletes who should be disqualified from participation varies from 1.6 per 1000 to 12.8 per 1000 with the false-positive rate varying from 11.8 per 1000 to 79.5 per 1000.

Examination Design

Ideally, the preseason examination should occur 3–4 weeks before preseason practice to allow time for evaluation and treatment of problems. Figure 18.1 is a sample preparticipation health examination record developed by Hulse and Strong.

Medical History   The most productive portion of the preparticipation examination is the medical history. About 70% of orthopaedic and other medical problems causing dis-

---

PREPARTICIPATION HEALTH EXAMINATION RECORD

School_____ ☐☐

| Last Name | First Name | Middle Initial | Grade _____ ☐☐ |

Age ☐☐   Race: ☐ Black ☐ White ☐ Other   Sex: ☐ Male ☐ Female

This application to compete in interscholastic athletics is entirely voluntary on my part and is made with the understanding that I have not violated any of the eligibility rules and regulations of the State Association.

_____   _____
Date   Signature of Student

Parent's or Guardian's Permission & Release
"I hereby give my consent for the above-named student to represent his or her school in the athletic activities except those indicated on this form by the examining physician, provided that such athletic activities are approved by the State Association. I also give my consent for the student to accompany the school team on any of its local or out-of-town trips."

The Richmond County Board of Education has no responsibility to provide first aid at any of the games, and the parents understand that the risk of injury is assumed by the student and parents when they are executing this form. However, in the event physicians, physical therapists, physician's assistants, nurses, or other persons trained in the rendering of first aid are available, as volunteers or otherwise, and render aid to any student injured during the course of any such activities or travel, then the parents do hereby release and forever discharge such persons and the Richmond County Board of Education from any liability arising out of any first aid or immediate treatment of injuries.

_____   _____
Typed or Printed Name of Parent or Guardian   Signature of Parent or Guardian

_____   _____   _____
Address   Phone   Date

FIGURE 18.1. Sample preparticipation health examination record. (Reproduced by permission from Hulse E, Strong WB. Participation evaluation for athletics. Pediatrics in Review 1987;9:176–177.)

Figure continued through page 308.

HEALTH HISTORY

(To be completed by Student and Parents **prior to examination**)

Yes	No	Has this student had any:
1. ☐	☐	Chronic or recurrent illness?
2. ☐	☐	Illness lasting over one week?
3. ☐	☐	Hospitalizations?
4. ☐	☐	Surgery other than tonsillec-tomy?
5. ☐	☐	Missing organs (eye, kidney, testicle)?
6. ☐	☐	Allergy to any medication?
7. ☐	☐	Problems with heart or blood pressure?
8. ☐	☐	Chest pain with exercise?
9. ☐	☐	Dizziness or fainting with exercise?
10. ☐	☐	Dizziness, fainting, frequent headaches, or convulsions?
11. ☐	☐	Concussion or unconscious-ness?
12. ☐	☐	Heat exhaustion, heat stroke, or other problems with heat?

Yes	No	Does this student:
13. ☐	☐	Wear eyeglasses or contact lens?
14. ☐	☐	Wear dental bridges, braces, plates?
15. ☐	☐	Take any medication?
		Is there any history of:
16. ☐	☐	Injuries or recurring medical treatment?
17. ☐	☐	Neck injury?
18. ☐	☐	Knee injury?
19. ☐	☐	Knee surgery?
20. ☐	☐	Ankle injury?
21. ☐	☐	Other serious joint injury?
22. ☐	☐	Broken bones (fractures)?
23. ☐	☐	Is there any reason why this student should not participate in sports?
24. ☐	☐	Has any family member died suddenly at less than 40 years of age of causes other than an accident?
25. ☐	☐	Has any family member had a heart attack at less than 55 years of age?

Date of last known tetanus (lock jaw) shot:_____

Use this space to **explain** any of the **above numbered YES answers** or to provide any additional information.

_____

_____

_____

_____

FIGURE 18.1.   *continued*

qualification are detected by the medical history alone. The medical history may be completed by the athlete or parents and reviewed by the physician prior to the examination. The history should be sports specific, relatively brief, and should assess for:

1. Past injuries causing the athlete to miss a game or practice: The practitioner may need to ask, for example, "Have you ever had a muscle pull? A pinched nerve? A back injury? The practitioner may have to ask the same question in different ways: Have you ever fractured a bone? Have you ever broken a bone?" (Some athletes are very concrete and think a break and a fracture, for instance, are two different things. Other athletes may not volunteer information if they think it will result in exclusion from sports participation.)
2. A loss of consciousness or memory following a head injury
3. Previous exclusion from sports for any reason
4. Past or present conditions or illnesses requiring ongoing physician care
5. Prior surgery and sequelae

PHYSICAL EXAMINATION

Date _____

Height ⬜⬜   Vision: Right ⬜⬜⬜ / ⬜⬜⬜   Normal 1 ⬜ without glasses (Check one)

Weight ⬜⬜⬜   Left ⬜⬜⬜ / ⬜⬜⬜   2 ⬜ with glasses

Pulse rate ⬜⬜⬜   Abnormal 3 ⬜ without glasses

Blood pressure ⬜⬜⬜ / ⬜⬜⬜   4 ⬜ with glasses

	Normal	Abnormal	Not Examined	Comments	Examiner	Problem Code	
1. Eyes							
2. Ears, nose, throat							
3. Mouth and teeth							
4. Neck (soft tissue)							
5. Cardiovascular							
6. Chest and lungs							
7. Abdomen							
8. Genitalia-hernia							
9. Sexual maturity							
10. Skin and lymphatics							
11. Neck							
12. Spine							
13. Shoulders							
14. Arms and hands							
15. Hips							
16. Thighs							
17. Knees							
18. Ankles							
19. Feet							
20. Neurological							

Based on this history and physical examination, the following abnormalities were found and may need treatment.

1. _____

2. _____

3. _____

FIGURE 18.1.   *continued*

PARTICIPATION RECOMMENDATIONS

1. ☐ There were no history or physical findings on this examination that would prohibit this student from participating in competitive athletics.
2. ☐ This student should have the following health problems evaluated or treated prior to participating in competitive athletics:

   _____

3. ☐ This student has health problems that would prohibit him or her from participating in competitive athletics.

   _____
   Physician

FIGURE 18.1. *continued*

6. Allergies, asthma, or exercise-induced bronchospasm
7. Medications
8. Tetanus immunization
9. A history of a cardiac murmur, extra beats, dizziness, irregular heartbeat, chest pain, or presyncope or syncope with exercise
10. A family history of cardiovascular disease, especially sudden cardiac death, at an early age
11. The menstrual history in females
12. A history of relatively rapid increase or decrease in body weight and the athlete's perception of their current body weight

Physical Examination   The examination should be a directed examination emphasizing the identification of medical problems that could worsen the athlete's performance or conditions that might be worsened by athletic participation. The preparticipation examination should de-emphasize those aspects of the physical examination that would not influence whether an athlete can compete in a particular sport. This preparticipation examination philosophy is based on two principles:

1. Most athletes in the adolescent age group are healthy.
2. Most athletes have had previous medical evaluations. (This assumption was discussed above.)

Many conditions that preclude participation in sports are picked up in the preadolescent age group and are not subtle. For example, congenital heart disease and hemophilia typically will be detected before adolescence. Subtle presentations of congenital defects or acquired diseases, however, may be undetected. The most commonly detected abnormalities on preseason examinations are previously undetected and unrehabilitated musculoskeletal injuries. The annual preparticipation examination, especially for teenagers, should serve as quality control for the diagnosis and rehabilitation of injuries. With this in mind the physical examination should include an assessment of:

1. Height and weight used to estimate ideal body weight: Obesity is not a reason for exclusion but would require mention to the athlete, parent, and coach of the increased risk of heat illness and how that risk might be reduced.
2. Blood pressure and pulse: Blood pressure should be taken in the right arm with the athlete sitting. Athletes with hypertension should be evaluated further but not excluded from participation unless the hypertension is severe. Participation in sports for teens with hypertension is discussed later. Pulse can be as low as 25 bpm in highly trained aerobic athletes. Pulse in the 40–50 bpm range is routine and does not need evaluation if the athlete is asymptomatic.

3. Visual acuity and pupil equality: Teens with visual acuity less than 20/40 in one or both eyes should be referred for further evaluation but are not excluded from participation. Athletes who are legally blind (<20/200) need to wear protective eyewear during sports but are not excluded from any sport if protective eyewear is worn. Anisocoria is important to note prior to a closed head injury.

4. Skin: Particularly evaluating for infections that are highly contagious (i.e., varicella or impetigo). Players with these infections must be noninfectious before returning to sports in which skin-to-skin contact is possible.

5. Teeth and mouth: Teeth and mouth must be examined only if the history suggests an acute problem.

6. Cardiac examination: Document the presence of murmurs, clicks, and rubs. Normal or physiological murmurs are characteristically less than IV or VI systolic murmurs that decrease from supine to standing, with no diastolic component, with a normal physiological split S_2. The murmur of hypertrophic cardiomyopathy, if one is present, may sound like a normal murmur, except that it may increase in intensity from supine to standing.

7. Abdomen: Organomegaly is a disqualifying condition for contact sports. A single kidney is a contraindication for participation in contact sports.

8. Genitalia in males: An undescended testicle is not a contraindication to contact sports, but the player should wear a protective cup. An evaluation for the unidentified testis is necessary. If one testis is undescended, the player can play all sports if he wears a protective cup. Genitalia in females do not need examination unless there is a specific complaint.

9. Sexual maturation stage: Tanner stage assessment for sexual maturity is appropriate for males; however, it has no role in deciding whether a teen should play a given sport. Tanner stage assessment is not indicated in the preseason examination in females, unless the athlete has a specific complaint.

10. Orthopaedic screening: Orthopaedic screening should include muscle strength, range of motion, and joint stability testing and evaluation for structural abnormalities of major joints such as the ankle, knee, shoulder, elbow, and back. A screening examination has been outlined by many organizations. The screening examination includes (listed in parentheses are diagnoses to consider if the examination is abnormal):

    a. Body symmetry (Fig. 18.2): Observe the adolescent standing with arms at their sides dressed in shorts and a shirt that allows inspection of the distal quadriceps muscles and acromioclavicular joints, respectively. Look for:
    — Head tilted or turned to side (consider primary cervical spine injury, primary or secondary trapezius or cervical muscle spasm)
    — Asymmetry of shoulder heights (trapezius spasm, shoulder injury, scoliosis)
    — Enlarged acromioclavicular joint (previous acromioclavicular joint sprain, shoulder separation)
    — Asymmetrical iliac crest heights (scoliosis or leg length difference, back spasm)
    — Swollen knee, prominent tibial tuberosity (any knee injury, Osgood-Schlatter disease): Ask the athlete to contract ("tighten") the quadriceps muscles; look for atrophy of the vastus medialis obliquus, a characteristic of any knee or lower extremity injury in which the athlete avoids normal use of that leg.
    — Swollen ankle (unrehabilitated ankle sprain)

    b. Neck examination (Fig. 18.3): The neck examination is especially important in players with a previous history of neck injury and brachial plexopathy (referred to as "stingers" or "burners"). Have the athlete do the following maneuvers:
    — Look at floor (cervical flexion)
    — Look at ceiling (cervical extension)
    — Look over left shoulder; right shoulder (left and right rotation, respectively)

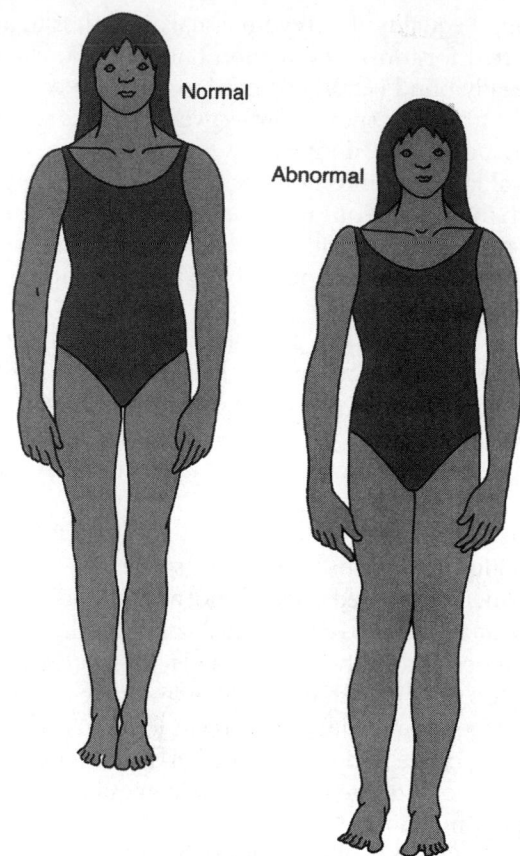

Normal

Abnormal

FIGURE 18.2.   Body symmetry. (Used with permission of Ross Products Division, Abbott Laboratories, Columbus, OH 43216, from For the practitioner, © 1981 Ross Products Division, Abbott Laboratories.)

— Put right ear on right shoulder; left ear on left shoulder (right and left lateral flexion)
— Look for limited or asymmetrical motion (neck injury or congenital cervical abnormalities). *Any athlete with limitation of range of motion, weakness, or pain with neck examination is excluded from contact sports until further evaluation.*

c. Shoulder examination

— Have the athlete raise arms from the side and touch hands above head keeping elbows extended (full abduction). Look for:
  (1) Asymmetrical elevation of shoulder before arms reach 90 degrees (shoulder weakness, shoulder instability, impingement syndrome)
  (2) Inability to raise arms to full abduction position (shoulder weakness, impingement syndrome, or apprehension from subluxation or dislocation)
— Athlete holds arms in front of body (forward flexion) and to the side (90 degrees abduction, Fig. 18.4). Examiner attempts to push hands down. Look for:
  (1) Asymmetric atrophy or fasciculations of anterior and middle deltoid muscles and pain or weakness (may be indicative of a variety of shoulder problems)
— Athlete puts hands behind head (maximal external rotation or abduction). Look for:
  (1) Inability to get hand behind head (i.e., lack of external rotation of shoulder) or apprehension (shoulder subluxation or dislocation); an athlete with limitation of motion should be evaluated further before he or she is cleared for further participation

Normal

Abnormal

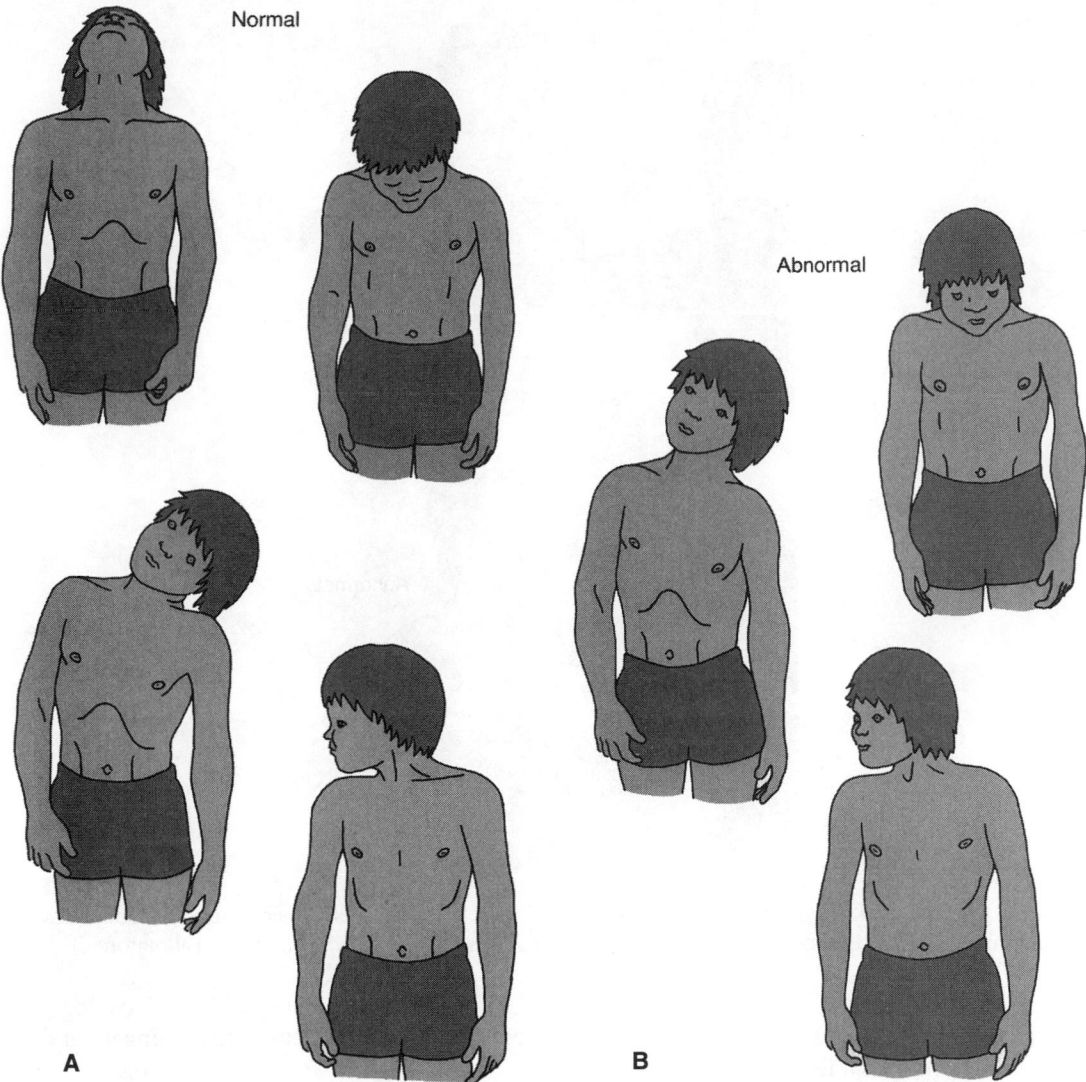

A   B

FIGURE 18.3.   Neck symmetry. (Used with permission of Ross Products Division, Abbott Laboratories, Columbus, OH 43216, from For the practitioner, © 1981 Ross Products Division, Abbott Laboratories.)

   d. Elbow
      — Athlete extends and flexes elbows with arms to the side (90 degrees abduction, Fig. 18.5). Look for:
      — Asymmetrical elbow extension or flexion (prior dislocation or fracture, osteochondritis dissecans)
      — With arms at sides and elbows flexed 90 degrees, athlete pronates and supinates forearms (Fig. 18.6). Look for:
      (1) Asymmetrical loss of motion (residual of forearm fractures, Little Leaguer's elbow, osteochondritis dissecans of elbow, radial head or navicular fracture)
      The etiology of a limitation of range of motion of the elbows should be established before a young athlete is cleared for participation, especially in throwing sports.

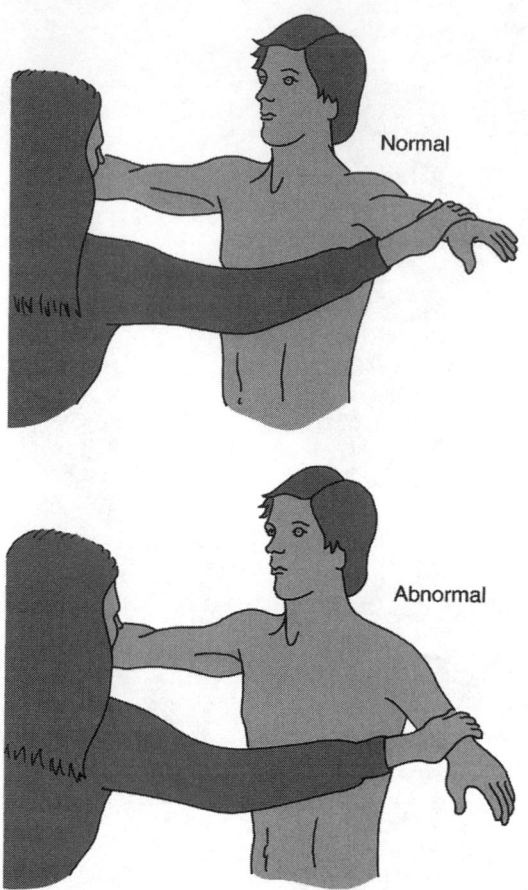

FIGURE 18.4.   Shoulder symmetry. (Used with permission of Ross Products Division, Abbott Laboratories, Columbus, OH 43216, from For the practitioner, © 1981 Ross Products Division, Abbott Laboratories.)

— With arms at sides and elbows flexed 90 degrees, athlete spreads fingers and makes a fist (Fig 18.7). Look for:

(1) Lack of finger flexion, swollen joints, finger deformities (residuals of sprains, fractures)

Hand injuries should be evaluated and recommendations for sports participation based on the severity of the injury and the specific sport the athlete desires to play. Typically, the athlete is not excluded from participation.

e. Back and leg observation

— Athlete stands facing away from examiner (Fig. 18.8). Look for:

(1) Asymmetry of waist (scoliosis or leg length difference)
(2) Elevated shoulder (scoliosis or trapezius spasm from shoulder or neck injury)
(3) Depressed shoulder (scoliosis or muscle weakness)
(4) Prominent rib cage (scoliosis)
(5) Increased lordosis (spondylolysis, tight hip flexors, weak hamstrings)

Idiopathic scoliosis is not a contraindication for sports participation in almost all cases, unless the angle is severe. If pain is present, the diagnosis is not idiopathic scoliosis, and the definitive diagnosis should be established.

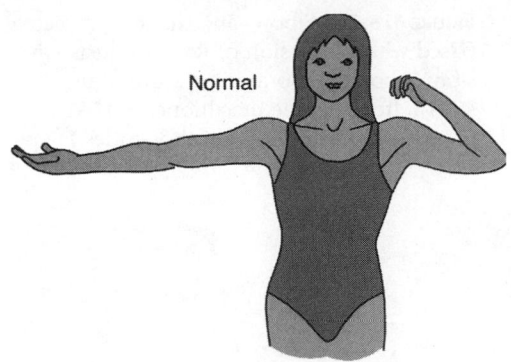

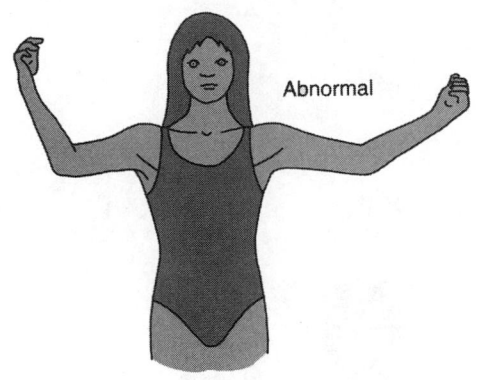

FIGURE 18.5.   Elbow and hand symmetry. (Used with permission of Ross Products Division, Abbott Laboratories, Columbus, OH 43216, from For the practitioner, © 1981 Ross Products Division, Abbott Laboratories.)

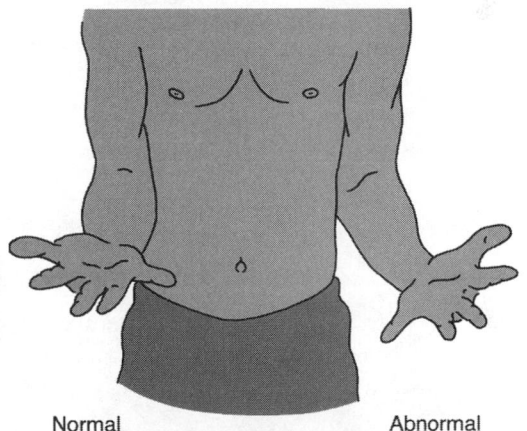

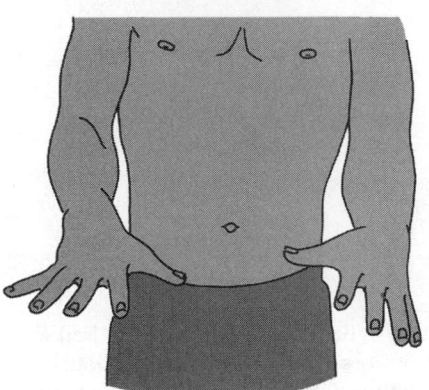

FIGURE 18.6.   Elbow and hand symmetry. (Used with permission of Ross Products Division, Abbott Laboratories, Columbus, OH 43216, from For the practitioner, © 1981 Ross Products Division, Abbott Laboratories.)

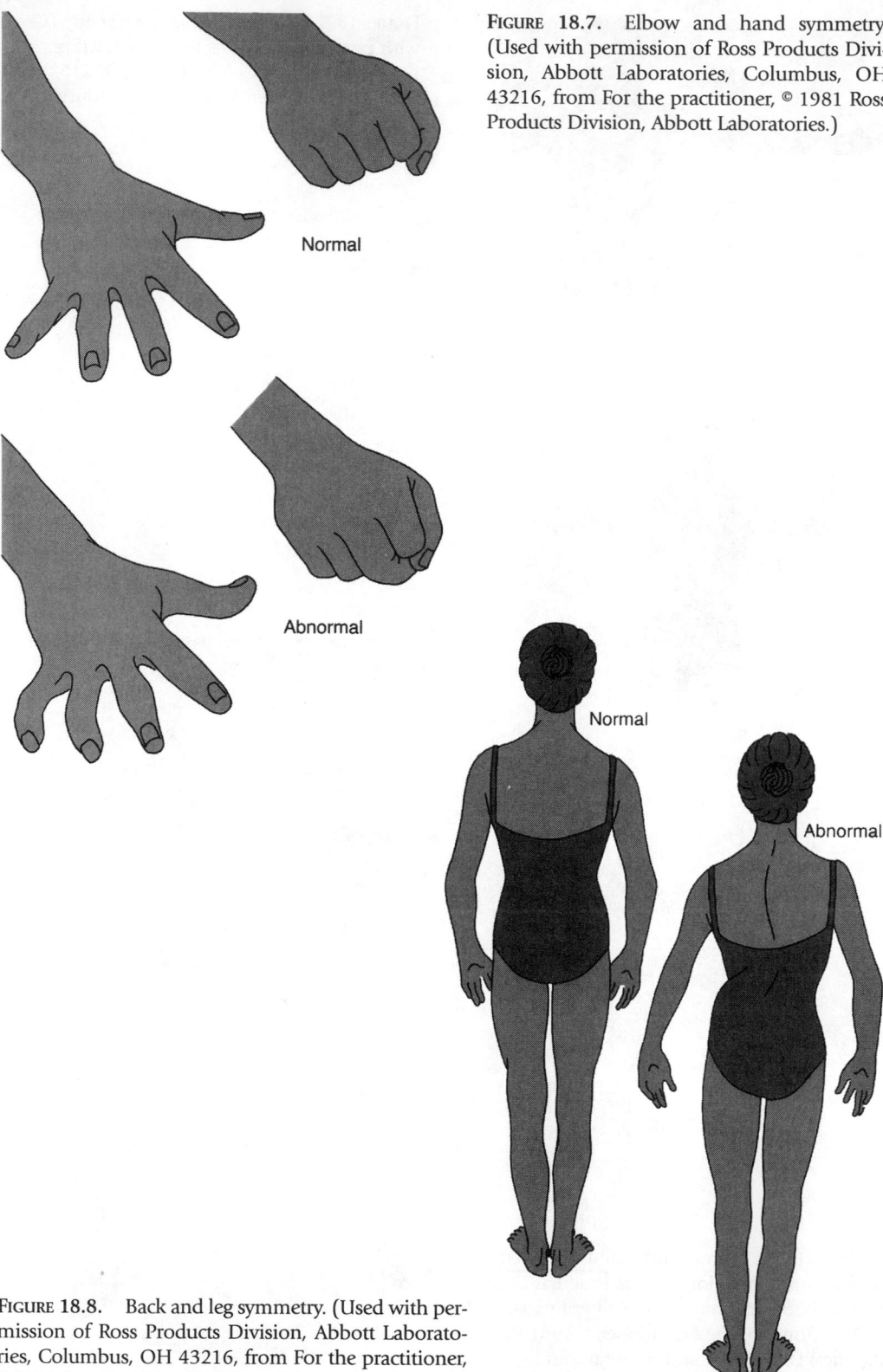

FIGURE 18.7. Elbow and hand symmetry. (Used with permission of Ross Products Division, Abbott Laboratories, Columbus, OH 43216, from For the practitioner, © 1981 Ross Products Division, Abbott Laboratories.)

Normal

Abnormal

Normal

Abnormal

FIGURE 18.8. Back and leg symmetry. (Used with permission of Ross Products Division, Abbott Laboratories, Columbus, OH 43216, from For the practitioner, © 1981 Ross Products Division, Abbott Laboratories.)

— Athlete bends forward at waist and hips (lumbar flexion) to touch toes (Fig. 18.9). Look for:
  (1) Twisting or deviating of side (paraspinous muscle spasm)
  (2) Asymmetrical prominence or rib cage (scoliosis)
  (3) Inability to obliterate lumbar lordosis (spondylolysis, paraspinous muscle spasm)
— Standing straight, athlete rises onto toes (Fig. 18.10). Look for:
  (1) Asymmetry of heel elevation (calf weakness or restricted ankle motion from sprain or fracture)
  (2) Asymmetry of gastrocnemius muscle (atrophy from incompletely rehabilitated ankle or leg injury)
— Athlete rises onto heels. Look for:
  (1) Asymmetry of forefoot and toe elevation (weakness of ankle dorsiflexors or limitation of ankle motion from ankle fracture or sprain)
  If asymmetry on toe or heel raising is detected, further evaluation and treatment is indicated before clearing the athlete for full sports participation.
f. Hip and knee screening
— Have the athlete slowly assume a painless squatting position (buttocks on heels) (Fig. 18.11). If the athlete cannot do this, then further evaluation is indicated. Ask him or her to take four steps forward in this squatting position ("duck walk"), turn 180 degrees in this squatting position and take four more steps. Look for:

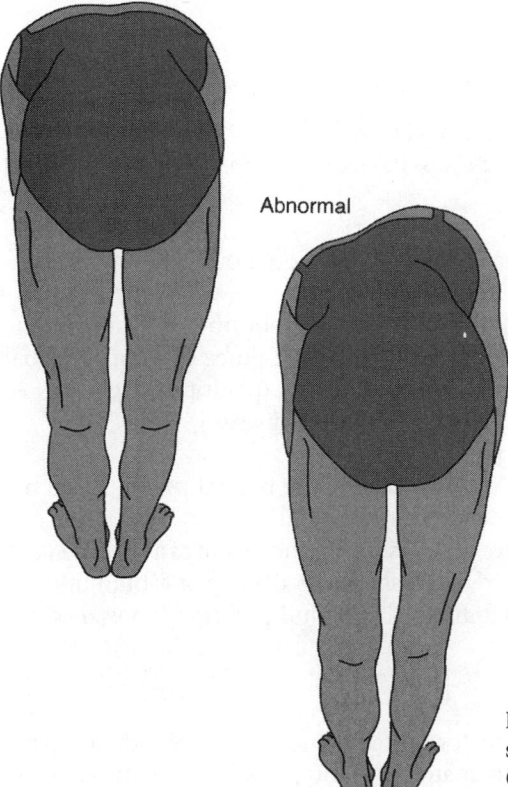

Normal

Abnormal

FIGURE 18.9.   Back symmetry. (Used with permission of Ross Products Division, Abbott Laboratories, Columbus, OH 43216, from For the practitioner, © 1981 Ross Products Division, Abbott Laboratories.)

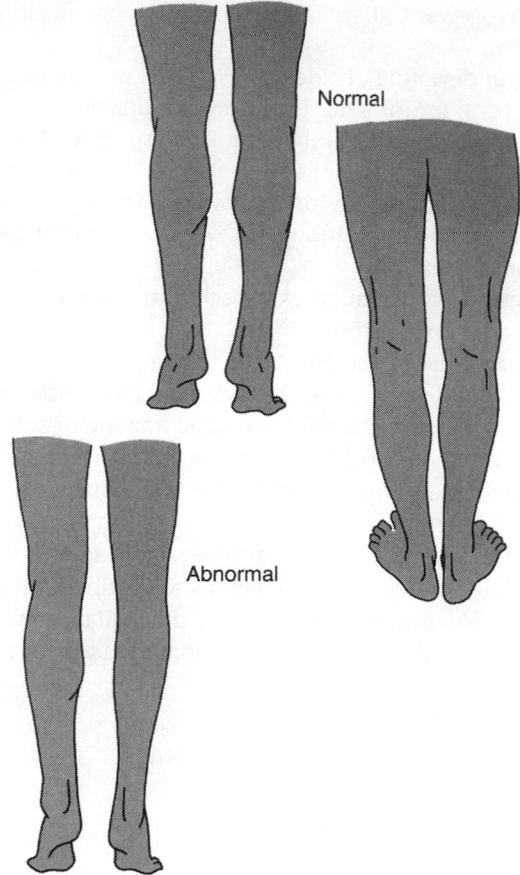

FIGURE 18.10.   Leg symmetry. (Used with permission of Ross Products Division, Abbott Laboratories, Columbus, OH 43216, from For the practitioner, © 1981 Ross Products Division, Abbott Laboratories.)

(1) Asymmetry of heel height off ground (limited ankle motion or Achilles tendon tightness from tendinitis or injury)

(2) Asymmetrical knee flexion (i.e., difference in heel to buttock height from the rear view or inability to get down as far on one side [knee effusion, residual limitation of motion from sprain, torn meniscus, quadriceps tightness or weakness, patellofemoral pain, Osgood-Schlatter's disease])

(3) Pain at any point in the range of knee flexion

The etiology of the pain should be established and the patient rehabilitated before allowing return to participation without restrictions.

g. Ankle screening: Have the athlete hop five times as high as he or she can on each foot. Inability to do so suggests an undiagnosed or unrehabilitated ankle or foot injury. The ankle should be evaluated and fully rehabilitated before full participation is allowed.

Laboratory Tests

Blood for hemoglobin and a dipstick of the urine for protein, glucose, and blood have been recommended as screening tests for athletic participation. Although the hemoglobin may be indicated in teenagers who do not have ongoing general medical care, it is not recommended

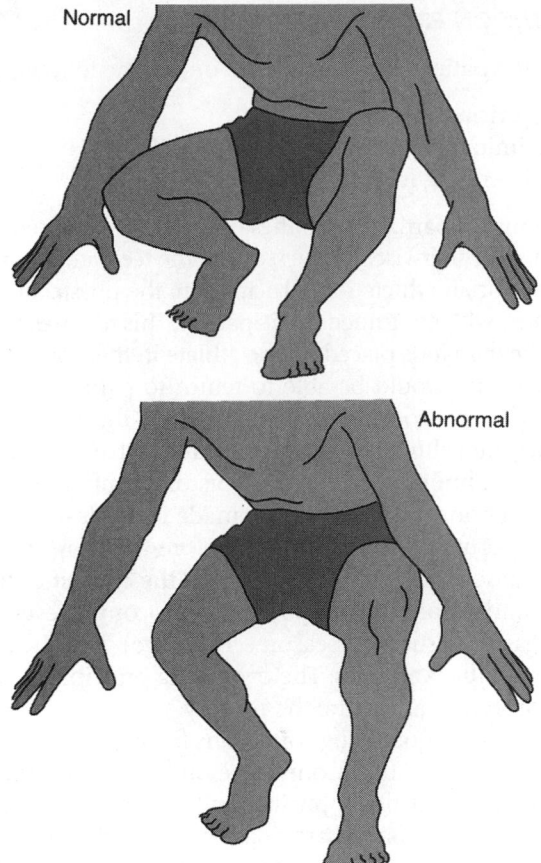

Normal

Abnormal

FIGURE 18.11.   Leg symmetry. (Used with permission of Ross Products Division, Abbott Laboratories, Columbus, OH 43216, from For the practitioner, © 1981 Ross Products Division, Abbott Laboratories.)

for teens who are receiving care regularly and are asymptomatic. There is a particular problem diagnosing anemia in highly trained aerobic athletes who have a reduced hematocrit due to intravascular volume expansion, but their oxygen-carrying capacity is normal. The urine dipstick is not indicated in the absence of symptoms that suggest genitourinary tract dysfunction (Vehaskari and Rapola, 1982). Screening for iron deficiency in menstruating female athletes, especially if they run long-distance events, by measuring serum ferritin is advocated by some experts. However, empiric iron therapy may be the most cost-effective approach to preventing iron deficiency in healthy female athletes (Elliot, 1991).

Some centers use isokinetic or isotonic equipment to screen for muscle weakness, especially quadriceps and hamstring weakness or imbalance. This testing may be reasonable if the equipment is available to the athletes at no extra cost and if used to evaluate athletes with previous injuries where there is question about their recovery. However, the utility for screening all athletes has not been established. Weakness can be screened for using the history and physical examination.

Estimating body composition using anthropometric measurements (i.e., skinfold) is indicated in wrestling as prediction equations for minimum wrestling weight have been established. Using skinfold measurements as screening tests is not indicated for all athletes but can be used for individual patients who need to gain or lose weight.

CLEARANCE OR EXCLUSION FROM SPORT

After the examination, the patient should be given one of the following recommendations:

1. Full clearance for participation
2. Participation with limitations (give exact restrictions)
3. Clearance withheld pending further evaluation

If there are restrictions on participation, these should be discussed with the athlete and a parent, coach, or guardian. Otherwise, the message to the teen athlete may be misinterpreted. If a physician does not clear an athlete for participation, the physician should be prepared to discuss the risks associated with continued participation. This requires an understanding of the medical problem and the demands placed on the athlete in that sport. For instance, a football lineman with an ankle sprain would be able to return to participation earlier than a ballet dancer. The physician must also consider how important is this sport versus another activity? Some young athletes may be willing to switch to another activity with a lower risk of reinjury.

In any athlete with an abnormality noted on history or physical examination, the diagnosis accounting for the abnormality should be made and, ideally, successful treatment or rehabilitation of the abnormality accomplished before allowing full sports participation. However, each case must be evaluated individually in the context of the age of the patient, the severity of the injury, the sport, how important the upcoming event is to the athlete (i.e., a state championship game versus a preseason scrimmage), and the sequelae if the athlete is injured further, among other variables. The overriding principle, however, should be that the health of the athlete should always be the priority.

Tables 18.1 and 18.2 list disqualifying conditions for sports participation recommended by the American Academy of Pediatrics Committee on Sports Medicine and Fitness (1994). These are guidelines only and may not apply in specific cases. The usefulness of Table 18.2 is limited because the recommendation to participate is qualified in the majority of conditions. Athletes may choose to participate in a sport against medical advice, under the domain of the Americans with Disabilities Act, preventing discrimination based on physical limitations. This does not mean the physician should approve the athlete against his or her best judgment, but the athlete may choose to participate even against the physician's advice or attempt to obtain permission to play from another physician.

A strenuous sport can place dynamic (volume) or static (pressure) demands on the cardiovascular system. A classification system taking into account these considerations is available in Table 18.3. The practical value of this classification is still unknown as the current knowledge regarding the relative risks of these two types of exercise for different cardiovascular conditions is limited.

Regarding exercise physiology and sports participation in children and youth with chronic illnesses the reader is referred to the bibliography (Bar-Or, 1983).

Management of Cardiac Conditions

Cardiac Conditions Any athlete complaining of true angina, syncope, presyncope, or palpitations while exercising, independent of the physical examination, should be excluded from participation until evaluated further. Full evaluation should include an electrocardiogram, a continuous ambulatory (Holter) monitor, a maximal stress test, and an echocardiogram with Doppler flow studies. The majority of young athletes who die a sudden cardiac death during sports are asymptomatic prior to the event, and when they have had symptoms, seldom has the correct diagnosis been made. The best reference for giving guidance to athletes with cardiac conditions is the 26th Bethesda Conference (1994).

TABLE 18.1.   Classification of Sports by Contact

Contact or Collision	Limited Contact	Noncontact
Basketball	Baseball	Archery
Boxing[a]	Bicycling	Badminton
Diving	Cheerleading	Body building
Field hockey	Canoeing or kayaking (white water)	Bowling
Football	Fencing	Canoeing or kayaking (flat water)
Flag	Field	Crew or rowing
Tackle	High jump	Curling
Ice hockey	Pole vault	Dancing
Lacrosse	Floor hockey	Field
Martial arts	Gymnastics	Discus
Rodeo	Handball	Javelin
Rugby	Horseback riding	Shot put
Ski jumping	Racquetball	Golf
Soccer	Skating	Orienteering
Team handball	Ice	Power lifting
Water polo	Inline	Race walking
Wrestling	Roller	Riflery
	Skiing	Rope jumping
	Cross-country	Running
	Downhill	Sailing
	Water	Scuba diving
	Softball	Strength training
	Squash	Swimming
	Ultimate Frisbee	Table tennis
	Volleyball	Tennis
	Windsurfing or surfing	Track
		Weight lifting

Reproduced by permission from Committee on Sports Medicine and Fitness. Medical conditions affecting sports participation. Pediatrics 1994;94:757–760. Copyright 1994.
[a]Participation not recommended.

Specific Cardiac Conditions

1. Mitral valve prolapse (see Chapter 14)
   a. The estimated prevalence in the general populations is 5% (Jeresaty, 1979).
   b. Mitral valve prolapse is generally a benign, asymptomatic condition. Patients can have palpitations, dizziness, supraventricular and ventricular arrhythmias, and chest pain in which case they should be excluded from sports until fully evaluated. Sudden cardiac death in patients with mitral valve prolapse who die while exercising is rare. There are 12 case reports to date. A midsystolic click, with or without a late systolic murmur, is the auscultatory hallmark of this condition. Mitral valve prolapse is a clinical diagnosis not requiring echocardiography unless a murmur is present, in which case an echocardiogram is indicated to assess for mitral insufficiency.
   c. Patients with mitral valve prolapse can participate in all competitive sports unless the following exist:
      — A history of syncope documented to be arrhythmogenic in origin
      — A family history of sudden death associated with mitral valve prolapse
      — Repetitive forms of supraventricular and ventricular arrhythmias particularly if exaggerated by exercise
      — Moderate to marked mitral regurgitation
      — Prior embolic event
   d. Athletes with mitral valve prolapse *and* any of the above symptoms can only participate in low-intensity sports (Table 18.3).

Table 18.2.   Medical Conditions and Sports Participation[a]

Condition	May Participate?
Atlantoaxial instability (instability of the joint between cervical vertebrae 1 and 2)	Qualified yes
Explanation: Athlete needs evaluation to assess risk of spinal cord injury during sports participation.	
Bleeding disorder	Qualified yes
Explanation: Athlete needs evaluation.	
Cardiovascular diseases	
Carditis (inflammation of the heart)	No
Explanation: Carditis may result in sudden death with exertion.	
Hypertension (high blood pressure)	Qualified yes
Explanation: Those with significant essential (unexplained) hypertension should avoid weight and power lifting, body building, and strength training. Those with secondary hypertension (hypertension caused by a previously identified disease), or severe essential hypertension, need evaluation.	
Congenital heart disease (structural heart defects present at birth)	Qualified yes
Explanation: Those with mild forms may participate fully; those with moderate or severe forms, or who have undergone surgery, need evaluation.	
Dysrhythmia (irregular heart rhythm)	Qualified yes
Explanation: Athlete needs evaluation because some types require therapy or make certain sports dangerous, or both.	
Mitral valve prolapse (abnormal heart valve)	Qualified yes
Explanation: Those with symptoms (chest pain, symptoms of possible dysrhythmia) or evidence of mitral regurgitation (leaking) on physical examination need evaluation. All others may participate fully.	
Heart murmur	Qualified yes
Explanation: If the murmur is innocent (does not indicate heart disease), full participation is permitted. Otherwise the athlete needs evaluation (see congenital heart disease and mitral valve prolapse above).	
Cerebral palsy	Qualified yes
Explanation: Athlete needs evaluation.	
Diabetes mellitus	Yes
Explanation: All sports can be played with proper attention to diet, hydration, and insulin therapy. Particular attention is needed for activities that last 30 minutes or more.	
Diarrhea	Qualified no
Explanation: Unless disease is mild, no participation is permitted, because diarrhea may increase the risk of dehydration and heat illness. See "Fever" below.	
Eating disorders	Qualified yes
Anorexia nervosa	
Bulimia nervosa	
Explanation: These patients need both medical and psychiatric assessment before participation.	

Reproduced by permission from Committee on Sports Medicine and Fitness. Medical conditions affecting sports participation. Pediatrics 1994;94:757–760. Copyright 1994.

[a]This table is designed to be understood by medical and nonmedical personnel. In the "Explanation" section, "needs evaluation" means that a physician with appropriate knowledge and experience should assess the safety of a given sport for an athlete with the listed medical condition. Unless otherwise noted, this is because of the variability of the severity of the disease or of the risk of injury among the specific sports in Table 18.1, or both.

2. Asymmetric septal hypertrophy or hypertrophic cardiomyopathy (HCM)
   a. HCM is a primary abnormality of the myocardium manifested by an asymmetrically hypertrophied, nondilated left ventricle in the absence of a cardiac or systemic disease that could cause left ventricular (LV) hypertrophy.
   b. Mechanism of sudden death is not established but a common factor seems to be arrhythmia.
   c. If symptoms are present, which in many cases they are not before the sudden death, they include exertional dyspnea, angina pectoris, fatigue, or syncope.
   d. Increased intensity of murmur from supine to standing may be present.

TABLE 18.2.   *continued*

Condition	May Participate?
Eyes	
Functionally one-eyed athlete	Qualified yes
Loss of an eye	
Detached retina	
Previous eye surgery or serious eye injury	
Explanation: A functionally one-eyed athlete has a best corrected visual acuity of <20/40 in the worse eye. These athletes would suffer significant disability if the better eye was seriously injured as would those with loss of an eye. Some athletes who have previously undergone eye surgery or had a serious eye injury may have an increased risk of injury because of weakened eye tissue. Availability of eye guards approved by the American Society for Testing Materials (ASTM) and other protective equipment may allow participation in most sports, but this must be judged on an individual basis.	
Fever	No
Explanation: Fever can increase cardiopulmonary effort, reduce maximum exercise capacity, make heat illness more likely, and increase orthostatic hypotension during exercise. Fever may rarely accompany myocarditis or other infections that may make exercise dangerous.	
Heat illness, history of	Qualified yes
Explanation: Because of the increased likelihood of recurrence, the athlete needs individual assessment to determine the presence of predisposing conditions and to arrange a prevention strategy.	
HIV infection	Yes
Explanation: Because of the apparent minimal risk to others, all sports may be played that the state of health allows. In all athletes, skin lesions should be properly covered, and athletic personnel should use universal precautions when handling blood or body fluids with visible blood.	
Kidney: absence of one	Qualified yes
Explanation: Athlete needs individual assessment for contact or collision and limited contact sports.	
Liver: enlarged	Qualified yes
Explanation: If the liver is acutely enlarged, participation should be avoided because of risk of rupture. If the liver is chronically enlarged, individual assessment is needed before collision/contact or limited contact sports are played.	
Malignancy	Qualified yes
Explanation: Athlete needs individual assessment.	
Musculoskeletal disorders	Qualified yes
Explanation: Athlete needs individual assessment.	
Neurologic	
History of serious head or spine trauma, severe or repeated concussions, or craniotomy.	Qualified yes
Explanation: Athlete needs individual assessment for collision or contact or limited contacted sports, and also for noncontact sports if there are deficits in judgment or cognition. Recent research supports a conservative approach to management of concussion.	
Convulsive disorder, well controlled	Yes
Explanation: Risk of convulsion during participation is minimal.	
Convulsive disorder, poorly controlled	Qualified yes
Explanation: Athlete needs individual assessment for collision or contact or limited contact sports. Avoid the following noncontact sports: archery, riflery, swimming, weight or power lifting, strength training, or sports involving heights. In these sports, occurrence of a convulsion may be a risk to self or others.	

Table continued on following page.

- e. The athlete may have a family history of early sudden death, particularly related to exercise.
- f. Diagnosis is made by demonstrating LV wall thickness of more than 15 mm, although some highly trained athletes can have LV thickness to 16 mm and some patients with HCM, especially young, growing adolescents, can have LV thickness of less than 15 mm.
- g. Athletes with HCM must be evaluated by a cardiologist before participation.

Table 18.2.   *continued*

Condition	May Participate?
Obesity	Qualified yes
Explanation: Because of the risk of heat illness, obese persons need careful acclimatization and hydration.	
Organ transplant recipient	Qualified yes
Explanation: Athlete needs individual assessment.	
Ovary: absence of one	Yes
Explanation: Risk of severe injury to the remaining ovary is minimal.	
Respiratory	
Pulmonary compromise including cystic fibrosis	Qualified yes
Explanation: Athlete needs individual assessment, but generally all sports may be played if oxygenation remains satisfactory during a graded exercise test. Patients with cystic fibrosis need acclimatization and good hydration to reduce the risk of heat illness.	
Asthma	Yes
Explanation: With proper medication and education, only athletes with the most severe asthma will have to modify their participation.	
Acute upper respiratory infection	Qualified yes
Explanation: Upper respiratory obstruction may affect pulmonary function. Athlete needs individual assessment for all but mild disease. See "Fever" above.	
Sickle cell disease	Qualified yes
Explanation: Athlete needs individual assessment. In general, if status of the illness permits, all but high exertion, collision or contact sports may be played. Overheating, dehydration, and chilling must be avoided.	
Sickle cell trait	Yes
Explanation: It is unlikely that individuals with sickle cell trait (AS) have an increased risk of sudden death or other medical problems during athletic participation except under the most extreme conditions of heat, humidity, and possibly increased altitude. These individuals, like all athletes, should be carefully conditioned, acclimatized, and hydrated to reduce any possible risk.	
Skin: boils, herpes simplex, impetigo, scabies, molluscum contagiosum	Qualified yes
Explanation: While the patient is contagious, participation in gymnastics with mats, martial arts, wrestling, or other collision or contact or limited contact sports is not allowed. Herpes simplex virus probably is not transmitted via mats.	
Spleen, enlarged	Qualified yes
Explanation: Patients with acutely enlarged spleens should avoid all sports because of risk of rupture. Those with chronically enlarged spleens need individual assessment before playing collision or contact or limited contact sports.	
Testicle: absent or undescended	Yes
Explanation: Certain sports may require a protective cup.	

   h. Recommendations for participation in sports are:
      — Athletes with the unequivocal diagnosis of HCM should not participate in most competitive sports with the possible exception of those of low intensity (Table 18.3). This applies to athletes with and without evidence of LV outflow obstruction.
      — It may be that the recommendations for sports participation may be more liberal for athletes older than 30, as the risk for sudden cardiac death may be reduced.
 3. Coronary artery anomalies
   a. Rare overall: Anomalies should be suspected if evaluation of syncope or chest pain during exercise is normal.
   b. May lead to sudden death: Identification before death is difficult as many patients are asymptomatic prior to the sudden death.
   c. Physical examination is typically normal.
   d. Cardiac consultation prior to participation is mandatory if this condition is suspected.
   e. If identified, the athlete should be excluded from all sports participation.
 4. Myocarditis
   a. The incidence in young athletes is controversial due to the imprecise criteria for diagnosis.

TABLE 18.3.   Classification of Sports by Strenuousness

High to Moderate Intensity			
High to Moderate Dynamic and Static Demands	High to Moderate Dynamic and Low Static Demands	High to Moderate Static and Low Dynamic Demands	Low Intensity (Low Dynamic and Low Static Demands)
Boxing[a]	Badminton	Archery	Bowling
Crew or rowing	Baseball	Auto racing	Cricket
Cross-country skiing	Basketball	Diving	Curling
Cycling	Field hockey	Equestrian	Golf
Downhill skiing	Lacrosse	Field events (jumping)	Riflery
Fencing	Orienteering	Field events (throwing)	
Football	Ping-pong	Gymnastics	
Ice hockey	Race walking	Karate or judo	
Rugby	Racquetball	Motorcycling	
Running (sprint)	Soccer	Rodeoing	
Speed skating	Squash	Sailing	
Water polo	Swimming	Ski jumping	
Wrestling	Tennis	Water skiing	
	Volleyball	Weight lifting	

Reproduced with permission from Committee on Sports Medicine and Fitness. Medical conditions affecting sports participation. Pediatrics 1994;94:757–760. Copyright 1994.
[a]Participation not recommended.

b. The process is characterized by an inflammatory infiltrate of the myocardium with necrosis or degeneration of myocytes. The disease progresses through active, healing, and healed phases and arrhythmias may occur at any time.

c. Recommendations regarding sports participation
— Athletes in whom a presumptive diagnosis has been made should be excluded from all competitive sports for 6 months and then ventricular function evaluated at rest and with exercise before allowing return to sports.
— Athletes can return to sports when ventricular function and dimensions are normal and clinically relevant arrhythmias are absent on ambulatory monitoring.
— There is no strong evidence for endomyocardial biopsy as a precondition for returning to sports participation.

d. Regarding the athlete with an acute febrile illness characterized by fever and myalgia, it seems prudent to withhold that athlete from competition; however, there are no data to support that this protects from sudden death. In athletes diagnosed with sudden death related to myocarditis, there seems to be no temporal pattern related to a recent febrile illness and the sudden death.

5. Systemic hypertension
a. Although hypertension is associated with an increased risk for sudden death and complex ventricular arrhythmias, to date it has not been incriminated as cause of sudden cardiac death in young, competitive athletes.
b. Table 18.4 lists severe hypertension by age group. Athletes with less than severe hypertension in the absence of end organ damage and heart disease have no restrictions. Those with severe hypertension should be held out of sports, especially high static sports (Table 18.3) until their blood pressure is better controlled.

Maturational Issues

There is controversy regarding the role of avoidance of contact sports in adolescents before full puberty and in the role of segregating youth based on sexual maturity ratings. New York State has adopted a voluntary Selection Classification Age Maturity Program. The program

TABLE 18.4. Classification of Severe Hypertension in Adolescents[a]

	Severe Hypertension Stage 3	Very Severe Hypertension Stage 4
Child 10–12 yr[b]		
Systolic	135–144	≥145
Diastolic	90–94	≥95
Adolescent 13–15 yr[b]		
Systolic	150–159	≥160
Diastolic	95–99	≥100
Adolescent 16–18 yr[b]		
Systolic	160–179	≥180
Diastolic	100–109	≥110
Adult >18 yr[c]		
Systolic	180–209	≥210
Diastolic	110–119	≥120

Adapted from 26th Bethesda Conference. Recommendations for determining eligibility for competition in athletes with cardiovascular abnormalities. Med Sci Sports Exerc 1994;26:S223–S283.
[a]Blood pressure values are based on the average of three or more readings taken at each of two or more visits after the initial screening. These definitions apply to individuals who are not taking antihypertensive drugs and are not acutely ill.
[b]To be consistent with the classification in adults these levels are adapted from the recommendations in the Report of the Second Task Force on Blood Pressure Control in Children. Pediatrics 1987;79:1–25.
[c]These levels are adapted from the Fifth Report of the Joint National Committee on Detection, Evaluation, and Treatment of High Blood Pressure (JNC V). Arch Intern Med 1993;153:154.

uses five criteria to match students with other peers based on similar physical and athletic ability. These criteria include the type of sport; the level of competition; the degree of agility, endurance, strength, and speed; proficiency in the sport; and a physical examination, including sexual maturity. There are no data based on a well-designed study to support the hypothesis that matching athletes by maturity level reduces injuries. It has been demonstrated that injury rates increase with increased pubertal maturation.

Conditioning and Physical Fitness

An expert panel has recommended that adolescents meet the following two physical activity guidelines (Physical activity guidelines, 1994):

1. All adolescents should be physically active daily, or nearly every day, as part of play, games, sports, work, transportation, recreation, physical education, or planned exercise in the context of family, school, and community activities.
2. Adolescents should engage in three or more sessions per week of activities that last 20 minutes or more at a time and that require moderate to vigorous levels of exercise exertion.

The majority (over 80%) of adolescents meet guideline 1 and are physically active on a daily basis with physical activity defined as any bodily movement produced by skeletal muscles that results in energy expenditure (Pate, 1994). There is a great deal of interindividual variability, and girls and older adolescents are less likely to satisfy guideline 1. Approximately one-half of adolescents appear to be meeting guideline 2 with exercise defined as planned, structured, and repetitive bodily movement done to improve or maintain one or more components of physical fitness. Compared to adults, adolescents are physically active, but engage in little structured exercise and are at risk of becoming sedentary adults.

Fitness has four principal components:

1. Body composition
2. Cardiovascular fitness (maximum oxygen consumption [Vo_2] max being the gold standard)
3. Strength
4. Flexibility

Although a common notion is that the fitness of today's youth is poor, the only component of fitness that has been documented to have declined in the past three decades is body composition: obesity has increased both in teens and young adults (Gortmaker et al.,1987; Indexes, 1994).

With respect to reducing obesity, adolescents need both reduced caloric intake and increased energy expenditure (Hergenroeder and Phillips, 1994).

Regarding improving cardiovascular fitness, a recommended training program would include aerobic exercise (continuous large muscle contractions that involve maintenance of 60–90% of the maximum heart rate), for 20–25 minutes, three to four times per week. Training should be tailored to the adolescent's current level of fitness, desired level of fitness, motivation, and discipline to adhere to a training regimen. Examples of aerobic activity are listed in Table 18.3 as high dynamic exercise.

Regarding strength training, it is established that just as in adults, prepubescent and pubescent subjects can increase strength safely by resistance training. The training program should include close adult supervision, a preparticipation examination, and the use of well-maintained equipment (including sturdy shoes). Guidelines for resistance training in teens have been reviewed (Blimpke, 1993). Resistance training is associated with strength gains and neuromuscular adaptation in *preadolescents* but is not associated with muscle hypertrophy. Short-term resistance training has no effect on somatic growth or body composition, and is not associated with increased injury rate or recovery, or improved sports performance. Muscle hypertrophy will occur in pubertal subjects. One standard resistance training program includes:

1. Establishing a 10 repetition maximum (the maximum weight that can be lifted 10 times), called 10 rep max
2. One set of 10 repetitions at 50–75% of the 10 rep max
3. A second set at 75% of the 10 rep max
4. A third set at 100% of the 10 rep max, doing as many repetitions as possible

Ideally, over 4–6 weeks, the exercises should then progress to three to four sets of 10 to 20 repetitions, with addition of more weight when 20 repetitions are easily performed. *One repetition maximum weight lifting should be avoided as it is a mechanism of injury.* The weight should be lifted through the entire range of motion of the joint to avoid loss of flexibility. Warm-up and cool-down periods, which could include stretching exercises, should accompany each session. Three sessions per week, on alternate days, allowing for a day of rest in between weight training sessions, is adequate. Gains in strength are more resistant to detraining compared to gains in aerobic fitness, with up to 50% of the strength capacity retained for a year or more in a person who is no longer training.

Regarding flexibility, there is no study demonstrating that stretching in healthy, previously uninjured subjects, prevents injuries. However, asymmetry or loss of flexibility must be recognized and treated, as improving flexibility and strength in previously injured athletes will decrease the likelihood of subsequent injuries. A flexibility program for injured joints should include pain-free stretches. If a healthy teen desires a stretching program, the following may be offered:

1. The program should consist of stretching before and after each practice or competition.
2. Each stretch should be held statically for 20 seconds, for 5–10 repetitions, and with a frequency of 3–5 days per week.

INJURIES

Injury Prediction

Factors that may predispose the athlete to injury include:

1. Weakness or inflexibility related to a previous injury
2. Accelerated growth
3. Training errors, including too rapid increases in pace, distance, repetitions, weight, or resistance, are the most common factor in overuse injuries
4. Inappropriate equipment (improper shoes, equipment not sized appropriately)
5. Change in the environment such as running up hills or on a banked track compared to a flat surface

Injury Prevention

There are several established ways of preventing injuries:

1. Recognize and fully rehabilitate old injuries. This may be the most important function of the preseason examination (Keller et al., 1989).
2. Minimize environmental hazards to injury. Breakaway bases (bases in baseball and softball that are not anchored to the ground) have been associated with fewer and less significant ankle and lower leg injuries from sliding. The incidence of serious neck injuries decreased after the trampoline was removed from gymnastics competition (Conference on Sports, 1992).
3. Enforce rules to eliminate high risk for injury behavior. Serious neck injuries in football dropped significantly after spear tackling was made illegal in football (Mueller and Cantu, 1991).

As mechanisms of injury are elucidated, preventive measures can be planned. This underscores the need for continued research in the etiology of sports injuries. Recommendations about injury prevention that are not based on data are not useful. For instance, textbooks and sports medicine experts commonly speak of preseason strengthening and improved flexibility as methods of injury prevention. This has not been demonstrated in athletes without pre-existing injuries that require specific rehabilitation.

An excellent review of the approach to the epidemiology of youth sports has been published (Conference on Sports, 1992).

Event Coverage and Sideline Decisions

In general, athletes should not be allowed to return to participate in sports until the following criteria have been satisfied:

1. The injury has been diagnosed.
2. The examiner is reasonably certain that the injury will not worsen with continued play.
3. The examiner is reasonably certain that continued participation (with the injury) will not result in a secondary injury.
4. The athlete has achieved full range of motion and strength in the injured joint.

The following are examples of injuries or conditions that preclude returning to sports until the previous criteria are fulfilled.

1. Unconsciousness, however brief
2. Inappropriate responses after head trauma
3. Any neurological abnormalities
4. Obvious swelling
5. Limited range of motion
6. Pain within the normal range of motion
7. Bleeding
8. An injury the examiner does not know how to handle
9. Obvious loss of normal function
10. Any time the athlete feels injured and does not desire to return to play

The above criteria and the examples given must be put into context. The author has sent players back into football games with ankle sprains and upper extremity injuries who did not strictly meet these criteria, but the situation was assessed on the sideline with the athlete and a decision made that the athlete could return to play. Strict adherence to these guidelines is unrealistic, as a proportion of athletes would miss a significant part of the season if their injury had to be back to 100% of baseline.

The physician caring for the athlete should be familiar with common injuries and their therapy. A few are discussed in the following section. For further information on specific injuries, see the bibliography of this chapter.

Concussion

Definition   Concussion is a traumatically induced alteration in mental status, not necessarily associated with loss of consciousness. The following lists a grading scale for concussion (Kelly et al., 1991):

1. Grade 1 concussion: Characterized by having confusion without posttraumatic amnesia and *without* loss of consciousness
2. Grade 2 concussion: No loss of consciousness but posttraumatic amnesia
3. Grade 3 concussion: Loss of consciousness or altered mental status at 24 hours

Note: These definitions are more conservative than those before 1990 listed below.

1. Grade 1 concussion: Confusion or amnesia for less than 30 minutes
2. Grade 2 concussion: Plus or minus loss of consciousness but never more than 5 minutes; if there is no loss of consciousness, posttraumatic amnesia lasts for more than 30 minutes but less than 24 hours.
3. Grade 3 concussion: Loss of consciousness for more than 5 minutes or altered mental status for more than 24 hours
4. Evaluation: Complete neurological examination including a mental status examination

Return to Contact Sports   The following guidelines are designed to prevent brain edema secondary to cerebrovascular congestion. This phenomenon is most common in the pediatric age group, but it has been described in adolescents and young adults (Kelly et al., 1991). Repeated blows to the head can predispose the brain to vascular congestion from autoregulatory dysfunction. Thus, an asymptomatic period is recommended before return to contact sports, depending on the severity of the injury.

1. Grade 1 concussion
   a. First concussion: They may return if asymptomatic in 20 minutes (no headaches, no dizziness, oriented, memory is intact at rest, and after sprinting and doing a few push-ups). If there are symptoms after the injury, they are out for the game. They need to

be asymptomatic for 1 week before they are allowed to have contact again. In the meantime, they can do cardiovascular fitness training.

   b. Second concussion: If it is the second concussion of the season (grade 1), they can return in 2 weeks if they are asymptomatic for 1 week.

   c. Third concussion: If it is their third grade 1 concussion of the season, they are out for the season, and they may return next season if they are asymptomatic.

  2. Grade 2 concussion

   a. First concussion: They are out of the game and back after 1 week of being asymptomatic. If they have symptoms, then consider admission to the hospital, although this is not typical. If there are no symptoms, they can be followed at home. If they continue to be symptomatic at 7 days, a computed tomography (CT) scan is indicated.

   b. Second concussion: With a second concussion in a season, they are out for a minimum of 1 month and may return if they are asymptomatic after 1 week.

   c. Third concussion: With a third grade 2 concussion, they are out for the season. They may return next season if they are asymptomatic at least 3–4 months.

  3. Grade 3 concussion: All should be sent to the hospital and CT scan should be considered.

   a. First concussion: With the first grade 3 concussion, they can return to play after they are asymptomatic for 2 weeks with rest and exertion.

   b. Second concussion: With the a second grade 3 concussion in a season, they are terminated for the season and can only play a noncontact sport the next continuous season. For instance, if they are injured in football in the fall, they cannot play hockey in the winter, but they could play a contact sport in the spring.

   c. Third concussion: After three grade 3 concussions, advise noncontact sports.

These guidelines address concussions in a season; however, there clearly are sequelae of repeated concussions over years as discussed below.

Sequelae of Chronic Head Trauma

Large Forces Over Time: Boxing   The average age of the heavyweight boxing champion at the time they won their first title is approximately 26 years of age. Most likely there is neuromuscular deterioration secondary to chronic injury in boxing which has various manifestations. Dementia pugilistica was the description given to the punchy boxer in 1928 and also occurs in other sports characterized by repeated head trauma. This syndrome includes:

1. Injury in and around the third ventricle leading to memory deficits, emotion lability, and euphoria
2. Injury to the inferior cerebellar tonsils, manifest as slurred speech and abnormal balance
3. Degeneration of the basal ganglia leading to Parkinson's disease
4. Diffuse neuronal loss leading to a picture that is similar to Alzheimer's disease

Neuropsychiatric abnormalities can persist for up to 6 months after a concussion (not only in sports). This has led to the definition of the postconcussion disorder described below (Diagnostic and Statistical Manual, 1994):

1. History of head trauma including loss of consciousness, posttraumatic amnesia
2. Evidence of difficulty of attention (concentrating, shifting focus of attention, performing simultaneous cognitive tasks) or memory
3. Three or more of the following occur shortly after the injury and last 3 months or more:
   a. Easily fatigued
   b. Disordered sleep
   c. Headache

    d. Dizziness

    e. Irritability or aggression with little provocation

    f. Anxiety or depression

    g. Change in personality (social or sexual inappropriateness)

    h. Apathy or lack of spontaneity

Note: Dementia (decreased cognition, memory, or any of the above) due to a single head injury is usually not progressive. If the dementia or behavior is progressively worse, consider another diagnosis, such as hydrocephalus or major depressive disorder.

Cervical Spinal Injuries

General Management

1. When a player's head or neck is injured, initially, a spinal cord injury must be assumed to be present and the patient not moved until a diagnosis is established that allows movement. If the chance of a cervical spine injury exists, the patient is immobilized and transported to an emergency room.

2. If the patient is unconscious, has neck pain or radiating pain to an extremity, has paresis or paresthesia, presence of a cervical spine injury should be assumed. The athlete should be immobilized on a board and transported to an emergency room.

3. If there is no motor or sensory abnormality on examination of the extremities, the patient is conscious, and there is no neck pain, the patient can be allowed to walk off the field for further evaluation. If at any time the patient complains of radiating pain, paresthesia, or neck pain, the physician should consider that a cervical spine fracture is present and initiate appropriate procedures. The first priority is to determine if the patient's cardiopulmonary status is stable. The second priority is to do no harm, which in the case of a potential unstable cervical spine fracture or dislocation means allowing no one to move the athlete, including taking off the helmet or rolling the patient over, until the appropriate emergency personnel are present—at which time the cervical spine should be stabilized and the patient transported. Physicians who cover football games especially, or any athletic event potentially, should be comfortable stabilizing and preparing for transport an athlete with a potential cervical spine fracture. This can only be learned by hands-on training.

    Cervical Muscle Strain   Cervical muscle strains are common and painful. The mechanisms of injury include rapid acceleration of a muscle(s) due to a collision or a quick movement causing the muscle to tear or repetitive contractions causing muscle fatigue and eventually muscle tearing. There should be no motor or sensory deficits on examination. The athlete will complain of pain typically in the trapezius area. There will be tenderness over the muscle body, limitation of range of motion, and pain with resistance. Midline pain and tenderness are consistent with a cervical fracture and should be treated as such in the acute setting. Any player without full range of motion and strength is excluded from further contact. Ice, nonsteroidal anti-inflammatory drugs (NSAIDs), and physical therapy should be initiated immediately. There is almost never an indication for a soft cervical collar. The player should receive physical therapy and start exercises at home. Clearance for return to contact occurs when the athlete has normal range of cervical motion and strength.

    "Stingers" or "Burners"   A "stinger" is a common neck injury in contact sports, resulting from direct brachial plexus trauma, often occurring when a player hits another opponent with his head. The player describes a burning pain in the distribution of a branch of the brachial plexus. The athlete can return to full participation when motor and sensory examination of the extremity is normal. Full recovery may occur in seconds or minutes or, in severe cases, months.

Lumbar Spine and Lower Back Injuries

The common causes of lower back pain in adolescents include:

1. Muscle strains: The diagnosis is typically made on the history of an acute pain while lifting in the lumbar-flexed position (bent forward). Muscle contusions occur with direct trauma to the area.

2. Spondylolysis: Lumbar spondylolysis is a stress fracture of the pars interarticularis. The fracture may follow a single traumatic event but more likely occurs following multiple microtraumas to the pars interarticularis while the athlete is in the lumbar-extended position. This occurs in many sports, especially ballet, gymnastics, and weight lifting. The athlete may have had pain for years before the diagnosis is made. On examination, *the hallmark of spondylolysis is reproduction of pain when the patient assumes a lumbar-extended position while standing.* The diagnosis is made by x-ray, oblique view of the lumbar spine, or with a bone scan. Treatment consists of relative rest, exercises to improve lumbar flexibility, and abdominal and lumbar strengthening. The patient may miss a few months to 12 months of sports. If not treated, the spondylolysis can progress to spondylolisthesis characterized by slippage of the vertebral body anterior to the next most distal vertebral body. The risk of slippage may be greatest during the most rapid stages of bony growth; therefore, aggressive, conservative management in adolescents is critical.

3. Disc herniation: Although uncommon in teens, disc herniation occurs often enough that physicians must recognize it. The presentation may include the classic sciatica, but it may be manifest as acute or chronic lower back, hip, or leg pain. Straight leg test should be positive, but this is not 100% sensitive. A magnetic resonance imaging (MRI) scan is not necessary unless the patient does not respond to conservative management or there is question about the diagnosis. Routine x-rays may show disc space narrowing. Management is with anti-inflammatory medication, relative rest, and physical therapy. The player can return to play when the examination is normal.

4. Sacroiliitis: This pain is typically chronic in nature. On examination the patient may have positive results from a Patrick test. The Patrick test involves having the teen, while lying supine, place the lateral malleolus of the tested leg on the opposite knee. Then the examiner presses the teen's flexed knee toward the examining table. Hip pain indicates a positive result. An x-ray of the sacroiliac joints should be obtained and consideration given to evaluating the patient further for rheumatological disease. Treatment is with relative rest, NSAIDs, and physical therapy.

5. Other causes of lower back pain include infection and neoplasia. These should be considered in patients with fever, or other constitutional signs or in patients who do not respond to initial therapy.

   See Chapter 17 for further discussion of back pain.

General Indications for Referral to an Orthopaedic Surgeon for Patients with Acute Trauma of an Extremity

Evaluation, treatment, and criteria for referral for specific injuries are discussed below. There are general criteria, however, for immediate consultation regardless of the injury site. They include:

1. Obvious deformity
2. Acute locking: The joint cannot be moved actively or passively past a certain point.

3. Penetrating wound of major joint, muscle, or tendon
4. Neurological deficit
5. Joint instability perceived by athlete or elicited by physician
6. Bony crepitus

If the primary physician evaluating the patient has training in the evaluation and functional rehabilitation of musculoskeletal injuries, the physician will have a higher threshold for referral.

Treatment and Rehabilitation of Injuries

General Concepts   The prevention of long-term sequelae of injury depends on complete rehabilitation, manifest as full, pain-free range of motion and normal strength. The general principles of the initial phase of rehabilitation, regardless of the specific injury, includes:

1. *Rest*
2. *Ice*
3. Compression
4. Elevation

This protocol will be discussed below for specific injuries.

The next phase of rehabilitation has the goals of establishing full range of motion and strength. As range of motion is improving the athlete should simultaneously work on strengthening. When range of motion is normal and strength is 80–90% of the uninvolved side, the athlete can start back into functional activities that approximate the sports-specific activity, in a graduated activity.

Knee Injury

History of the Injury   Based on the description of the mechanism of injury and the history of pain, the physician should be able to suggest the likely structures injured.

1. Knee pain that occurs while running straight, no trauma or fall
   a. Chronic pain: Likely to be patellofemoral dysfunction (PFD).
   b. Acute pain: Consider osteochondritis dissecans and pathologic fracture. *Any teen with knee pain without a history of trauma and with an equivocal examination that does not pinpoint the diagnosis should have an x-ray examination of the knee. In addition, if the hip examination is abnormal, x-rays of the hip are needed to rule out slipped capital femoral epiphysis.* Osgood-Schlatter disease and PFD do not necessarily need x-rays to establish a diagnosis.
2. Knee injury that occurs with weight bearing, cutting while running, or with an unplanned fall: Consider internal derangement including ligamentous and meniscal tears and fracture. A player who injures the knee while cutting, without being hit or having direct trauma, has a torn anterior cruciate ligament tear until proven otherwise.
3. A valgus injury to the knee (a force delivered to the outside of the knee, directed toward midline) is likely to tear the medial collateral ligament, possibly the anterior cruciate ligament, and either the medial or lateral meniscus.
4. Chronic anterior knee pain that worsens with going up stairs, after sitting for prolonged periods, or after squatting or running is likely to be PFD. *In general,* if the patient does not give a history of the knee giving out, locking, sharp pain, effusion, the sensation of something loose in the knee, or the sensation that something tore with the initial injury, the injury is probably not significant. If there is hemarthrosis within 24 hours after the injury, internal derangement is present and a diagnosis must be sought. At the game site

or if evaluating the patient within an hour or so after the injury, the best indicator of severity of injury of the lower extremity is the ability to bear weight and walk pain free. If the athlete can do this, he or she probably has not suffered a major injury and does not require immediate referral.

Physical Examination

- Observation of gait: Weight bearing? limping?
- Inspection for swelling, discoloration
- Vastus medialis obliquus (VMO) contraction looking for reduced bulk and tone
- Peripatellar palpation (Tenderness over the tibial tuberosity is diagnostic of Osgood-Schlatter disease; peripatellar pain is characteristic of PFD.)
- Quadriceps and hamstring flexibility
- Evidence of meniscal tears (McMurray and modified McMurray tests)
- Evidence of ligamentous instability including valgus, varus testing (for medial collateral and lateral collateral ligaments, respectively)
- Lachman and pivot shift tests (anterior cruciate ligament) and sag sign and posterior drawer (posterior cruciate ligament)

Indications for Plain Knee X-Rays

- Pain with motion and weight bearing
- Rapidly expanding effusion
- A history of a "loose body or "something floating"
- Uncertain diagnosis

Anteroposterior, lateral, and oblique views are standard. The sunrise view details the patellofemoral joint and should be ordered as needed.

MRI in the acutely injured knee is not necessary in many cases. In experienced hands, the MRI adds little to the diagnosis and should be reserved for diagnostic dilemmas and patients who do not respond to conservative management.

Management of Acute Knee Injuries

- Establish a working diagnosis.
- Perform x-ray examination on all patients.
- Relative rest: Prescribe crutches if the patient cannot bear weight without pain. A soft knee immobilizer or a hinged brace applied by a physical therapist is indicated in the first few days after the injury.
- Apply ice for 20 minutes three to four times per day.
- Start isometric quadriceps contractions on the first day if possible. If the patient cannot contract the quadriceps, order a stimulation unit to contract the quadriceps until the patient is able to do so.
- Elevate the leg as much as possible.
- Use compression wrap.
- Prescribe NSAID regimen.
- Refer to physical therapy.

Management of Chronic Knee Pain due to Patellofemoral Dysfunction

- The diagnosis is based on a history of knee pain, with peripatellar pain on examination as discussed above.
- Refer to physical therapy.

- Some patients benefit from orthotics if they are pronators and do not respond to conventional, first-line therapy. Likewise, some patients respond to neoprene knee sleeves.
- A 10-day course of NSAIDs may be useful if there is pain with activities of daily living.
- Return to sports can be gradual and progressive.

Ankle Injuries   Ankle injuries are the single most common acute injury in adolescent athletes. The diagnosis and treatment of ankle injuries in adolescents is the same as in adults, with the exception that teens may have open growth plates, which may be the primary injury site compared to an adult, where the primary injury is likely to be torn ligaments.

Acute Ankle Injury

1. Mechanism of injury
   a. Inversion (turning the ankle under or in): Constitutes 85% of acute ankle injuries
   b. Eversion: Generally more serious because of higher risk of syndesmosis injury and fracture
2. Physical Examination
   a. Acute injury: The best time to examine the patient is immediately after injury when the examination can be informative. Unfortunately, the patient commonly presents with diffuse swelling, tenderness, and decreased range of motion hours to days after the injury. The physical examination will be limited in diagnosing specific lesions at this point. At a minimum the examination should include:
      — Inspection for gross abnormalities, asymmetry, vascular integrity
      — Palpation for bony tenderness
      — Testing for weight bearing
   b. The physical examination may be more informative 3–4 days after the injury when the patient has appropriately used rest, ice, compression, and elevation.
      — Inspect for swelling and ecchymosis.
      — Assess active range of motion in six directions.
         (1) Plantar flexion; plantar flexion and inversion; plantar flexion and eversion
         (2) Dorsiflexion; dorsiflexion and inversion; dorsiflexion and eversion.
      — Assess resisted range of motion in the same six directions.
      — Palpate for potential fracture at a minimum of five sites: Proximal fibula, distal fibula, distal tibia, base of fifth metatarsal, and along the entire ankle joint line.
      — Attempt passive range of motion: Plantar flexion and dorsiflexion, talar tilt, anterior drawer.
      — Assess for pain-free weight bearing with normal gait and then heel and toe walking.
3. Associated injuries: Complications associated with ankle sprains
   a. Up to 15% of all complete ligament tears have an associated fracture, the most common sites being the talus, the fifth metatarsal, fibula, and tibia. If there is bony tenderness in patients with open epiphyses, assume a fracture is present even if the x-ray results are negative. Immobilize without weight bearing for 1 week; if tenderness persists, cast for 2 weeks. If a fragment is present, it does not always require casting or surgery. If the fragment is small and does not appear to be in the joint space, then treat conservatively and monitor.
   b. Tibiofibular syndesmosis injury occurs in approximately 5% of ankle sprains. These are more serious injuries than the typical lateral ligament sprain. On examination there is tenderness proximal to the joint line along the syndesmosis. Pressing the midshaft together and then releasing the pressure may worsen the pain.

    c. Talar fractures occurs in approximately 7% of ankle sprains in patients who are treated in an emergency room. The patient will complain of delayed healing, catching, locking, or persistent pain. Initial x-ray examination results may be negative. Subsequent x-rays or CT scan may be required.

    d. Peroneal subluxation is seen in approximately 0.5% of ankle sprains. Tenderness occurs along the tendon sheath, posterior and superior to the lateral malleolus.

4. X-ray examination: Patients who present with inability to bear weight, point tenderness, or diffuse edema that precludes a thorough physical examination should have an x-ray examination. Anterosposterior, lateral, and mortise views are standard. Stress films are not indicated.

5. Treatment: Acute phase

    a. The goal is to limit disability. Successful treatment is not defined only by the absence of pain, but also with return to full range of motion, strength, and proprioception.

    b. Rest: Advise the athlete to do nothing that hurts.

    c. Ice: Never heat in first 72 hours. Apply ice for 20 minutes at a time, three to four times per day.

    d. Compression: If using an elastic wrap, always wrap distal to proximal from the base of the toes to midcalf.

    e. Compression and stability can be provided by an air stirrup, which should be used for all acute sprains not complicated by fracture.

    f. Elevation: During the first 2–3 days, elevate the ankle as much as possible.

    g. If discussing the injury by phone, advise patients to seek treatment immediately.

    h. NSAIDs: Prescribe NSAIDs or acetaminophen for pain relief and theoretically to control inflammation, but NSAIDs do not affect the outcome per se.

    i. Casting is recommended for most fractures but not indicated otherwise. Casting should not be routine for ankle sprains, as it actually delays recovery. The air stirrup provides stability to inversion and eversion but it also allows for active dorsiflexion and plantar flexion, which is key in early rehabilitation.

6. Rehabilitation must start as soon as possible.

    a. Relative rest: Progress off crutches as soon as possible; do pain-free exercise.

    b. Stretching: Primary soleus, gastrocnemius, by doing calf stretches.

    c. Strengthening: Band exercises, toe to heel walking, pain free, and progressive. This can be done with the air stirrup on.

    d. Proprioceptive retraining: Raising on toes with little support (1 or 2 fingers on a chair) and eyes closed for 5 minutes a day.

    e. Functional progression of exercise, for instance: toe walking → walking at a fast pace → jogging → jogging and sprinting → sprinting and jogging on curves → figure of eight running → back to playing.

    f. The air stirrup can be worn in competition, most comfortably with low-cut or three-quarters height shoes, and provides excellent stability.

Chronic Ankle Instability   The leading causes of chronic ankle instability and pain are:

1. Strength deficits
2. Loss of flexibility
3. Loss of proprioception
4. Intra-articular pathology

In the evaluation all causes must be considered and rehabilitated specifically. A sports medicine–trained physical therapist is invaluable in this regard.

Large Muscle Contusions   The prototype injury in this category is the quadriceps contusion. This injury occurs from a direct blow to the thigh. It occurs in all sports and is very common in football, even though the players wear thigh pads. The athlete's presentation can range from feeling a mild discomfort or "charley horse" after the game to being unable to bear weight immediately after the trauma. The pathophysiology of the injury is bleeding in and around the quadriceps muscle as a result of the contusion. The quadriceps immediately goes into spasm, resulting in pain and disability. If the bleeding is not arrested immediately, the bleeding can be substantial.

On examination the physician needs to consider a femoral fracture, which would be characterized by severe pain and the inability to bear weight. The examination of a quadriceps contusion is characterized by more diffuse tenderness over the body of the quadriceps muscle and typically they can bear weight but may not be able to extend the knee actively. With passive flexion of the knee while the athlete is in the prone position, the patient will experience pain as the quadriceps, which is in spasm, is stretched. The injury can be graded as the degrees of passive flexion that the patient will permit:

1. More than 90 degrees—mild injury: If treated appropriately, player will probably return to competition within 3–5 days.
2. Between 60 and 90 degrees—moderate injury: Player will probably return to play in 2–4 weeks if treated appropriately.
3. Less than 60 degrees—severe injury: Player may be out for the season.

Treatment   The key is to stop further bleeding by applying ice for 20 minutes. When not icing, apply a tight compression wrap around the thigh and have the patient elevate the leg. The player should keep the knee in full flexion as much as possible during the first 24 hours after the injury. NSAIDs should not be given, as they may promote decreased clotting. Therefore, acetaminophen is the drug of choice.

The patient should start isometric quadriceps contractions as soon as possible. In moderate to severe injuries treatment by a sports-trained physical therapist is essential. In experienced hands the use of ultrasound can promote rapid recovery from this injury. Therapy that is too timid or too aggressive can retard recovery. If the bleeding is extensive and the athlete is reinjured before the hematoma has resolved, the athlete risks developing myositis ossificans, which can be career threatening and require surgical excision if functional ability is compromised.

Shin Splints and Stress Fractures of the Lower Leg   Patients with shin splints or stress fractures of the lower leg experience lower extremity pain that initially appears toward the end of exercise. If untreated and the athlete continues in the exercise that caused the injury, the pain will occur earlier in the exercise period and persist longer after the exercise is over. It can occur in any weight-bearing athlete but is most common in runners. A common presentation is medial shin pain. The principal two diagnoses to consider are medial tibial stress syndrome (shin splints) and medial tibial stress fracture, which will be discussed here. Other diagnostic possibilities include compartmental syndromes and vascular abnormalities, which will not be discussed.

On examination the pain of shin splints should be more diffuse and tenderness closer to the muscle, rather than bone, at the muscle-bone interface along the medial tibia. In stress fractures of the medial tibia the pain should be more pinpoint and over bone and not muscle. There is an injury spectrum from shin splints to stress reaction to stress fracture, which can be difficult to distinguish clinically. Further diagnostic studies may be indicated. Fractures can occur in any bone and are most common in the tibia and fibula.

Plain x-rays of patients with shin splints will appear normal, but unfortunately, most of the plain x-rays of patients with tibial stress fractures will also appear normal, at least in the first few weeks of the injury. The most sensitive test to diagnose stress fractures has been the bone scan. This is being challenged, but not yet replaced, by the use of magnetic resonance imaging. If the bone scan is normal then the physician can be more confident that the diagnosis is shin splints due to medial tibial stress syndrome.

A single best treatment protocol for shin splints and stress fractures of the medial tibia has not been established. One treatment protocol includes:

1. Relative rest: This means doing nothing that hurts within 24 hours of the activity. Alternative activities such as swimming, cycling, and pool running (running in the deep end of a pool supported by a buoyant vest or jacket) can be used to maintain the patient's fitness level while the leg injury is recovering. After 7–10 days the patient can start on a walking program and progress to a jogging program over 10–14 days, as long as they remain pain free. At any point in this functional rehabilitation progression if pain reappears, the athlete should have 2–3 pain-free days before resuming the walk-jog program. After jogging for 7–10 days, they can progress to sprinting and then jumping as long as they remain pain free.
2. Ice each day for 20 minutes directly to the site.
3. Provide pronation control if appropriate.
4. Increase shock absorption of the patient's shoes.
5. Stretch and strengthen the dorsiflexors (anterior tibialis), plantar flexors (posterior tibialis, gastrocnemius, soleus), everters (peroneal muscles).
6. NSAIDs can be used in shin splints for 7–10 days but should not be used long-term, as they may mask the pain and allow the athlete to return to activity too rapidly. NSAIDs should probably not be used for stress fractures, as the number of pain-free days is part of the index for return to the next level of activity in the functional rehabilitation progression.

It is difficult to predict when athletes will recover sufficiently from stress fractures and shin splints to return to exercise or competition. As long as they follow a functional rehabilitation program as outlined above under relative rest they at least will be involved in some rehabilitation activity toward full activity. Avoid projecting a day that the athlete will return to competition, as the athlete is likely to be disappointed when that prediction is wrong.

The Female Athlete

The number of female adolescents participating in sports has increased dramatically. In general, female athletes have injury rates that are similar to males in the same sport with the exception of the anterior cruciate ligament injury rate in female basketball players, which appears to be higher. Females and males also get similar injuries; therefore all that has been discussed to this point applies to males and females alike.

Breast Injuries

Although breast injuries are uncommon, 72% of female athletes experience sore or tender breasts after exercise. Specific brands of supporting bras for sports are listed below.

Champion: Full line of athletic bras. Designed for sports that produce high motion and medium motion. Prices: about $20–35.
Sportjock Supplex Action Bra and Super S'Port Bra. Price: about $20.
Gilda Marx, Danskin, and Reebok make a full line of athletic bras with various colors, designs, patterns. Designed more for dance, aerobics, and walking. Very fashionable bras; often worn as tops. Price: $15–25.

Insport: Full line of athletic bras. Price: $20–23.

Moving Comfort: Designed for medium-busted women, for medium support. Price: $25–30.

Osteopenia

A special area of concern for female athletes is osteopenia associated with amenorrhea or oligomenorrhea with or without the presence of eating disorders. Runners with amenorrhea have higher rates of stress fractures than do eumenorrheic runners. The long-term consequences of amenorrhea and osteopenia during the second decade may be increased risk of osteoporosis in the postmenopausal period. Bone mineral density measurements are indicated in women with amenorrhea of more than 6 months. Treatment of osteopenia should include:

1. Alterations in training to maintain a high level of fitness but also allowing for weight gain to a weight closer to expected for age and height: This assumes the coach will be understanding, which is often times not the case.
2. Hormonal supplementation with estrogen or progestin in the form of oral contraceptive pills (OCPs): It has not been established that OCPs increase bone density, but there is one preliminary report that suggests they do work in improving lumbar spine and total body bone density in women with hypothalamic amenorrhea (Hergenroeder, 1995). Conjugated estrogens (0.625 mg/day for 21 days per month) with medroxyprogesterone have not been effective in improving bone density in women with hypothalamic amenorrhea or ovarian failure (Emans et al., 1990; Warren et al., 1994). One report demonstrated an improvement of bone density with use of medroxyprogesterone 10 mg/day, 10 days per month in adult women but that has not been replicated and is not an accepted treatment protocol for adolescents (Prior, 1994).
3. Psychological counseling for athletes with eating disorders
4. Daily elemental calcium intake of 1500 mg/day

DRUG USE IN ATHLETES (Wadler and Hainline, 1989; Anderson and McKeag, 1989)

1. Epidemiology: The use of drugs to enhance performance has always been and will remain a part of athletic competition. The use of ergogenic aids has increased, or at least our recognition of the use of these drugs has increased in athletes over the past 20 years. Drug use by intercollegiate athletes has been found in the following frequencies (Puffer, 1988):

Drug	Percentage of Athletes
Alcohol	88
Amphetamines	8
Anabolic steroids	6.5
Anti-inflammatory medication	31
Caffeine	68
Cocaine	17
Marijuana	36

In general, the use of all recreational drugs appears to be no higher in athletes than nonathletes. Some drugs appear to be used less (smoking cigarettes), and some (anabolic steroids) are used more by athletes. Drugs are available starting in junior high school. The major categories of drugs used to improve performance by athletes include stimulants, pain relievers, and anabolic steroids (Wadler and Hainline, 1989).

2. Therapeutic drugs: Over-the-counter analgesics, decongestants, antihistamines, laxatives, antidiarrheal agents, and weight loss medications are commonly used by athletes. Athletes should be asked specifically about these medications during office or training room visits, as they may not perceive them as important as prescription drugs and not report their use. In addition, these medications have important side effects that can affect performance, and some of these preparations are banned by sports governing bodies (National Collegiate Athletic Association and United States Olympic Committee). Physicians are encouraged to use the Athletic Drug Reference published annually when advising athletes, especially college and elite athletes, about medication and prescription drug use.
3. Performance enhancing drugs
   a. Stimulants: Stimulants have been used extensively to combat psychological and muscular fatigue. These substances are banned by the International Olympic Committee (IOC) and can be detected by urine tests.
      — Amphetamines: Fine motor coordination and performance on tasks requiring prolonged attention have been shown to improve with amphetamine use. Side effects include anxiety, restlessness, tremors, tachycardia, irritability, confusion, and poor judgment, and these occur at higher doses.
      — Cocaine: Regarding the potential ergogenic effects of cocaine, no literature is available. Effects include increased heart rate, reflexes, and blood pressure, with accompanying euphoria. In the inexperienced user, reflexes are often more rapid, but desynchronous, leading to a decrement in athletic performance. Lethal toxicity can occur unexpectedly, particularly with intravenous use, as the dosages of cocaine on the street vary widely. Symptoms of acute overdose are difficult to treat and include arrhythmias, seizures, hyperthermia, and death. Metabolites can be found in the urine within 24–36 hours and up to 4 days after acute ingestion.
      — Caffeine: Caffeine is probably the most commonly used stimulant. Several studies have documented increased muscle work output for endurance activities. Significant side effects mimic those for other stimulants. In addition, caffeine has a direct diuretic effect, making it contraindicated in prolonged exertion. Caffeine is banned by the IOC in amounts greater than 12 µg/mL (approximately 4–8 cups of coffee or 8–16 cups of cola).
   b. Anabolic steroids: Anabolic steroid use is associated with increased muscle size and strength, especially in athletes who are weight training when the steroid use is initiated and who are consuming a high-calorie diet. The increase in strength is due in part to the increased aggressiveness of training associated with steroid use. There is no evidence that steroid use enhances aerobic power. These drugs may be injected or taken orally and are often freely available from peers and coaches. Buckley et al. (1988) report that 6.6% of 12th grade male students have used anabolic steroids. About 21% indicated their primary source was a health professional. Serious side effects include:
      — Risk of hepatic damage manifest as elevated liver-specific enzymes: The risk of hepatic neoplasms is unknown, as the reports to date are anecdotal.
      — Decreased high-density and increased low-density lipoprotein cholesterol levels
      — Oligospermia and azoospermia with decreased testicular size
      — Premature epiphyseal closure in pubertal athletes
      — Acne
      — Masculinization in women manifested as deepening of the voice, acne, and hair loss
      — Feminization in men manifested as gynecomastia and a high voice
      — Adverse psychological effects including increased aggressiveness and rage in some athletes
      — Increased use of other illicit drugs

Injected steroids are detectable in the urine for 6 months or longer. Orally administered anabolic steroids disappear from the urine after days to weeks.

   c. Narcotic analgesics: Narcotic analgesics are not perceived as "ergogenic aids" per se in that although they may allow an athlete to perform who is in pain from an injury, they do not enhance athletic performance. In standard doses there also does not appear to be a detriment. However, they may be abused as analgesics in an attempt to return to play in spite of pain. The effects of psychomotor retardation include sedation, dysphoria, and nausea and vomiting.

4. Recreational drugs
   a. Smokeless tobacco: The use of smokeless tobacco among preprofessional and professional baseball players is estimated to be 30–40% (Ernster et al., 1990), compared to 4–11% for the same age group in the general population. Cigarette smoking is less common in the baseball players. Complications of smokeless tobacco include oral cancer, periodontal disease, oral leukoplakia, and mouth and gum irritation. Smokeless tobacco may have a performance-enhancing effect on cognitive tasks. There does not appear to be a demonstrable effect on reaction time, and there is not a demonstrable ergogenic effect. The perception of benefit and cultural support for smokeless tobacco use in sports, such as baseball, football, and rodeo, sustain its use.
   b. Alcohol: Alcohol is the leading drug of abuse among high school and college students, regardless of whether they are involved in sports. Alcohol has become entwined in the fabric of sport in America through sponsorship use of athletic events. Beer producers spend large percentages of their advertising budgets on sports. This financial relationship between alcohol and sports appears unlikely to change, and to the extent that advertising alcohol influences drinking behaviors, alcohol abuse will remain a problem for adolescents and young adults. Alcohol use acutely and chronically impairs athletic performance by impairing cognition and visual-motor coordination. However, athletes who significantly abuse alcohol may not have impaired performance until the problem is chronic. Physicians and trainers should attempt to diagnose and refer for treatment at the early and middle stages of alcohol abuse and not wait until performance deteriorates.

5. Testing for performance-enhancing drugs
   a. The readers are encouraged to contact the National Collegiate Athletic Association (913-339-1906) or the United States Olympic Committee (1-800-233-0393, Drug Control Hotline). The following five components should be included in a drug testing program at an institution:
     — A written policy regarding the purpose of the drug prevention program, the methods of collection, and consequences: In developing this plan, representatives from coaches, parents, athletes, medical staff, and physicians should be involved.
     — An educational component must be prepared and used.
     — Testing: Actual testing must take place, preferably at random.
     — Discipline for those who test positive: The mechanism of feedback to the player and coaches must be established. The physician should not be in the role of administering any disciplinary action, rather should work with the athlete to identify a problem if it exists and facilitate appropriate care.
     — A process for evaluation of treatment for drug users must be implemented.

EMERGENCY PROCEDURES AND EQUIPMENT

Emergency procedures and equipment should be planned prior to the sports season. The coach, trainer, and other health personnel should have a clear idea of their role in an emergency. Although it is often not arranged that a physician be available for games, a physician's presence is highly desirable. Important aspects of emergency procedures, as well as equipment, are listed below.

1. Emergency procedures
    a. Ensure that first-aid equipment and well-trained personnel are available.
    b. Have a telephone in close proximity for summoning emergency medical assistance. A cellular phone is ideal.
    c. Know which emergency room facilities are available.
    d. Call for adequately equipped and staffed emergency transport vehicles.
    e. Communicate with the receiving emergency facility to ensure the availability of necessary personnel and equipment and that the receiving emergency room staff receive a first-hand account of the injury and treatment at the injury site before transfer.
    f. During and after the physician administers care to the athlete at the injury site, the physician should document all pertinent historical, physical examination, and treatment data.
2. Medical equipment: The medical equipment necessary for event coverage depends on the event and the environment in which it is played. For instance, blankets are not necessary for indoor events and events in warm weather. Below is an all-inclusive list of supplies. These supplies should be procured in advance of the season. Most trainers will have this equipment on site.
    a. Equipment: An asterisk indicates supplies that are necessary independent of the event and the environment.
        — Applicators (swabs)*
        — Adhesive bandages*
        — Bandage scissors*
        — Povidone-iodine (Betadine) ointment and solution*
        — Blankets
        — Blood pressure apparatus*
        — Clipper or razors for shaving areas to be taped*
        — Crutches*
        — Cups for drinking*
        — Elastic tape (1 inch, 3 inch)
        — Eye patches*
        — Felt pads*
        — Finger splints*
        — Fire extinguisher (provided by school)
        — Flashlight or penlight*
        — Fluor-I-Strip*
        — Foam bandage (3 inch)
        — Forceps*
        — Gauze rolls (2 inch)
        — Gauze pads (4 inch × 4 inch)*
        — Gloves, sterile and nonsterile*
        — Heel cups for bruised heels*
        — Ice, coolers, and plastic bags that seal*
        — Nail cutters*
        — Ophthalmoscope, otoscope*
        — Protective pads (elbows, knees, etc., provided by school)
        — Record system
        — Scalpel

 — Scissors*
 — Skin adherent for taping*
 — Slings (triangular bandages)*
 — Soap
 — Spine board*
 — Splints (regular, inflatable)*
 — Stockinettes
 — Suction cups for contact lens removal*
 — Sterile suture set*
 — Steri-strips, assorted*
 — Stethoscope*
 — Swiss army knife or knife and Phillips screwdriver*
 — Tape, adhesive
 — Tape cutters (shark or bandage scissors)*
 — Thermometer*
 — Tongue depressors
 — Tongue forceps
 — Tracheotomy tube*
 — Tufskin*
 — Turkey baster (to suction vomitus from the mouth of an unconscious patient)
 — Wrist watch*
 — Wraps (elastic, nonelastic)

b. Medications: The asterisks indicate medication that should be at the game site. The other medications can be stored in the training room or the student health service observation unit.
 — Acetaminophen*
 — Aerosolized albuterol with a metered dose inhaler*
 — Antacids*
 — Antifungal ointment, powder
 — Dexamethasone or methylprednisolone (provided by the ambulance crew for spinal cord injury)*
 — Diazepam, injectable (ambulance crew)*
 — Diphenhydramine, oral and injectable*
 — Ear drops (Auralgan Otic Drops and Cortisporin Otic Drops)
 — Electrolyte solution, oral*
 — Electrolyte solution, injectable with intravenous setup*
 — Epinephrine (Adrenalin) 1:1000*
 — Lidocaine hydrochloride 2% with and without epinephrine nose drops*
 — Loperamide, 2 mg tablets*
 — Ophthalmological irrigation solution and eye cup*
 — Prednisone tablets
 — Prochlorperazine (Compazine) injectable and suppository
 — Sunscreen
 — Tetanus toxoid
 — Topical anesthetic (lidocaine or tetracaine-adrenaline-cocaine solution)
 — Topical steroid
 — Zinc oxide

c. Resuscitation equipment
 — Oral airways, all sizes
 — Ambu bag with face mask and adapter for endotracheal tubes

— Endotracheal tubes, cuffed, all sizes
— Laryngoscope kit
— Cricothyroidotomy kit
— Syringe (large) and large suction catheter
d. Resuscitation medications
— Epinephrine 1:10,000
— Lidocaine
— Sodium bicarbonate 50 mEq
— Lactated Ringer's solution
— Morphine
— Meperidine (Demerol) 100 mg
— Intravenous tubing and needles

BIBLIOGRAPHY

General

Allen JG, Overbaugh KA. The adolescent athlete. Part III: the role of nutrition and hydration. J Pediatr Health Care 1994;8:250.

American Academy of Pediatrics. Sports medicine: health care for young athletes. Evanston, Illinois: American Academy of Pediatrics, 1991.

American Academy of Pediatrics, Committee on Sports Medicine and Fitness. Pediatrics 1994;94:757–760.

American Medical Association. AMA guidelines for adolescent preventive services (GAPS) recommendations and rationale. Baltimore: Williams & Wilkins, 1994.

American Medical Association Board of Trustees. Athletic preparticipation examinations for adolescents. Arch Pediatr Adolesc Med 1994;148:93.

Anderson J. Stretching. Bolinas, California: Shelter Publications, 1980.

Anderson W, McKeag D. Replication of the national study of substance use and abuse habits of college student athletes. In: Mission KS, ed. Technical report. Overland Park, Kansas: National Collegiate Athletic Association, 1989.

Bar-Or O. Pediatric sports medicine for the practitioner: from physiologic principles to clinical applications. New York: Springer-Verlag, 1983.

Bering JR, Steen SN. Sports nutrition for the 90's. Gaithersburg, Maryland: Aspen Publishers, 1991.

26th Bethesda Conference. Recommendations for determining eligibility for competition in athletes with cardiovascular abnormalities. Med Sci Sports Exerc 1994;26:S223–S283.

Blimpke, CJ. Resistance training during preadolescence. Sports Med 1993;15:389.

Bouchard C, Shepard RJ, Stephens T, eds. Physical activity, fitness and health. International proceedings and consensus statement. Champaign, Illinois: Human Kinetics Publishers, 1994.

Buckley WE, Yesalis CE, Friedl KE. Estimated prevalence of anabolic steroid use among male high school seniors. JAMA 1988;260:3441.

Buckman MT. Gastrointestinal bleeding in long-distance runners. Ann Intern Med 1984;101:127.

Caldwell GL Jr, Safran MR. Elbow problems in the athlete. Orthop Clin North Am 1995;26:465.

Conference on sports injuries in youth: surveillance strategies. Proceedings. [NIH publication 93–3444]. Washington, DC: National Institutes of Health, Department of Health and Human Services, Public Health Services, 1992.

Council on Scientific Affairs, American Medical Association. Ensuring the health of the adolescent athlete. Arch Fam Med 1993;2:446.

Diagnostic and statistical manual of mental disorders. 4th ed. Washington DC: American Psychiatric Association, 1994.

Durant RH, Pendergrast RA, Seymore C, et al. Findings from the preparticipation athletic examination and athletic injuries. Am J Dis Child 1992;146:85.

Durant RH, Seymore C, Linder CW, et al. The preparticipation examination of athletes: comparison of single and multiple examiners. Am J Dis Child 1985; 139:657.

Elliot DL, Goldberg L, Loprinzi M. Management of suspected iron deficiency: a cost-effectiveness model. Med Sci Sports Exerc 1991;23:1332.

Ernster VL, Grady DG, Greene JC, et al. Smokeless tobacco use and health effects among baseball players. JAMA 1990;264:218.

Forman ES, Dekker AH, Javors JR, et al. High-risk behaviors in teenage male athletes. Clin J Sport Med 1995;5:36.

Futterman LG, Lemberg L. Sudden death in athletes. Am J Crit Care 1995;4:239.

Garrick JG. Orthopedic preparticipation screening examination. Ped Clin North Am 1990;37:1047.

Garrick JG, Requa R. Injuries in high school sports. Pediatrics 1978;61:465.

Garrick JG, Webb DR. Sports injuries: diagnosis and management. Philadelphia: WB Saunders, 1990.

Goldberg B, Saraniti A, Whitman P, et al. Pre-participation sports assessments: an objective evaluation. Pediatrics 1979;66:736.

Gortmaker SL, Dietz WH, Sobol AN, et al. Increasing pediatric obesity in the US. Am J Dis Child 1987;14:535.

Hackett P, Rennie D. The incidence, importance, and prophylaxis of acute mountain sickness. Lancet 1976;2:1149.

Hergenroeder AC. Diagnosis and treatment of ankle injuries. A review. Am J Dis Child 1990;144:809.

Hergenroeder AC, Garrick JG, eds. Sports medicine. Pediatr Clin North Am 1990;37.

Hergenroeder AC, Phillips S. Advising teenagers and young adults about weight gain and loss through exercise and diet: practical advice for the physician. In: Shenker IR, ed. Monographs in clinical pediatrics: adolescent medicine. London: Harwood Academic Publications, 1994:113–116.

Indexes of obesity and comparisons with the previous national survey data in 9- and 10-year-old black and white girls: The National Heart, Lung, and Blood Institute Growth and Health Study. J Pediatr 1994;124:675.

Irrgang JJ, Delitto A, Hagen B, et al. Rehabilitation of the injured athlete. Orthop Clin North Am 1995;26:561.

Johnson MD. Tailoring the preparticipation exam to female athletes. Physician Sportsmed 1992;20:61.

Johnson MD, Kibler WB, Smith D. Keys to successful preparticipation exams. Physician Sportsmed 1993; 21:109.

Johnson TS, Rock PB. Current concepts: acute mountain sickness. N Engl J Med 1988;319:841.

Keene JS, Lange RH. Diagnostic dilemmas in foot and ankle injuries. JAMA 1986;256:247.

Keller CS, Noyes FR, Buncher R. The medical aspects of soccer injury epidemiology. Am J Sports Med 1989; 15:230.

Kelly JP, Nichols JS, Filley CM, et al. Concussion in sports: guidelines for the prevention of catastrophic outcome. JAMA 1991;266:2867.

Kreipe RE, Gewanter HL. Physical maturity screening for participation in sports. Pediatrics 1985;75:1076.

Landers DM, Crews DJ, Boutcher SH, et al. The effects of smokeless tobacco on performance and psychophysiological response. Med Sci Sports Exerc 1992; 24:895.

Maron BJ, Roberts WC, McAllister HA, et al. Sudden death in young athletes. Circulation 1980;62:218.

Mast EE, Goodman RA, Bond WW, et al. Transmission of blood-borne pathogens during sports: risk and prevention. Ann Intern Med 1995;122:283.

Mayne BR. A team physician's bag. Physician Sportsmed 1981;9:85.

McClain LG, Reynolds S. Sports injuries in a high school. Pediatrics 1989;84:446.

Micheli LJ, Wood R. Back pain in young athletes. Significant differences from adults in causes and patterns. Arch Pediatr Adolesc Med 1995;149:15.

Mitchell JH, Haskell WL, Raven PB. Classification of sports. Med Sci Sports Exerc 1994;26:S242.

Mueller FD, Cantu RC. National Center for Catastrophic Sports Injury Research: eighth annual report (1982–1990). Chapel Hill, North Carolina: University of North Carolina, 1991.

Nelson MA. Medical exclusion from participation in sports. Pediatr Ann 1992;21:149.

Nickerson HJ, Holubets MC, Weiler BR, et al. Causes of iron deficiency in adolescent athletes. J Pediatr 1989; 114:657.

Overbaugh KA, Allen JG. The adolescent athlete. Part II: injury patterns and prevention. J Pediatr Health Care 1994;8:203.

Pate RR, Long BJ, Heath G. Descriptive epidemiology of physical activity in adolescents. Pediatr Exerc Sci 1994; 6:434.

Physical activity guidelines for adolescents. Pediatr Exerc Sci 1994;6:299–463.

Purcell JS, Hergenroeder AC. Physical conditioning in adolescents. Curr Opin Pediatr 1994;6:373.

Reid DC. Sports injury assessment and rehabilitation. New York: Churchill Livingston, 1992.

Reider B, ed. Sports medicine: the school-age athlete. Philadelphia: WB Saunders, 1991.

Rifat SF, Ruffin MT 4th, Gorenflo DW. Disqualifying criteria in a preparticipation sports evaluation. J Fam Prac 1995;41:42.

Ross Laboratories. For the practitioner: orthopedic screening examination for participation in sports. Columbus, Ohio: Ross Laboratories, 1978.

Safran MR. Elbow injuries in athletes. A review. Clin Orthop 1995;310:257.

Speca JM, Cowell HR. Minibike and motorcycle accidents in adolescents: a new epidemic. JAMA 1976; 232:55.

Stewart JG, Ahlquist DA, McGill DB, et al. Gastrointestinal blood loss and anemia in runners. Ann Intern Med 1984;100:843.

Van Camp SP, Bloor CM, Mueller FO, et al. Nontraumatic sports death in high school and college athletes. Med Sci Sports Exerc 1995;27:641.

Vehaskari V, Rapola J. Isolated proteinuria: analysis of a school-age population. J Pediatr 1982;101:661.

Vinger PF, Tolpin DW. Racket sports: an ocular hazard. JAMA 1978;239:2575.

Wadler GI, Hainline B. Drugs and the athlete. In: Ryan AJ, ed. Contemporary exercise and sports medicine series. Philadelphia: FA Davis, 1989.

Wight JN Jr, Salem D. Sudden cardiac death and the "athlete's heart." Arch Intern Med 1995;155: 1473.

Female Athletes

Barnett NP, Wright P. Psychological considerations for women in sports. Clin Sports Med 1994;13:297.

Cann CE, Martin MC, Genant HK, et al. Decreased spinal mineral content in amenorrheic women. JAMA 1984;251:626.

Constantini NW, Warren MP. Physical activity, fitness, and reproductive health in women: clinical observations. In: Bouchard C, Shepard RJ, Stephens T, eds. Physical activity, fitness and health. Champaign, Illinois: Human Kinetics Publishers, 1994.

Constantini NW, Warren MP. Special problems of the female athlete. Bailleres Clin Rheumatol 1994;8:199.

Constantini NW, Warren MP. Menstrual dysfunction in swimmers: a distinct entity. J Clin Endocrinol Metab 1995;80:2740.

Drinkwater BL, Bruemner B, Chesnut III CH. Menstrual history as a determinant of current bone density in young athletes. JAMA 1990;263:545.

Drinkwater BL, Nilson K, Ott S, et al. Bone mineral density after resumption of menses in amenorrheic athletes. JAMA 1986;256:380.

Emans SJ, Grace E, Hoffer FA, et al. Estrogen deficiency in adolescents and young adults: impact on bone mineral content and effects of estrogen replacement therapy. Obstet Gynecol 1990;76:585.

Heinonen A, Oja P, Kannus P, et al. Bone mineral density of female athletes in different sports. Bone Miner 1993;23:1.

Hergenroeder AC, Klish WJ, Smith EO, et al. A randomized clinical trial of bone mineral density changes in young women with hypothalamic amenorrhea treated with oral contraceptive pills. J Invest Med 1995;43(suppl 1):23A.

Hergenroeder AC, Klish WJ, Smith EO, et al. A randomized clinical trial of the effect of taking oral contraceptive pills over 12 months on bone mineral density in young women with hypothalamic amenorrhea [Abstract]. Pediatr Res 1995;37:6A.

Lebrun CM. Effect of the different phases of the menstrual cycle and oral contraceptives on athletic performance. Sports Med 1993;16:400.

Loucks AB. Physical activity, fitness, and female reproductive morbidity. In: Bouchard C, Shepard RJ, Stephens T, eds. Physical activity, fitness and health. Champaign, Illinois: Human Kinetics Publishers, 1994.

Marcus R, Cann C, Madvig P, et al. Menstrual function and bone mass in elite women distance runners: endocrine and metabolic features. Ann Intern Med 1985;102:158.

Nattiv A, Agostini R, Drinkwater B, et al. The female athlete triad. The inter-relatedness of disordered eating, amenorrhea, and osteoporosis. Clin Sports Med 1994;13:405.

Neinstein LS. Menstrual dysfunction in pathophysiologic states. West J Med 1985;143:476.

Shangold MM. How I manage exercise-related menstrual disturbances. Physician Sportsmed 1986;14:113.

Tanner SM. Preparticipation examination targeted for the female athlete. Clin Sports Med 1994;13:337.

Warren MP, Fox RP, De Rogatis AJ, et al. Osteopenia in hypothalamic amenorrhea: a 3-year study [Abstract]. Endocrine Society Annual Meeting, Anaheim, California, 1994.

Wilson JH, Wolman RL. Osteoporosis and fracture complications in an amenorrhoeic athlete. Br J Rheumatol 1994;33:480.

Yeager KK, Agostini R, Nattiv A, et al. The female athlete triad: disordered eating, amenorrhea, osteoporosis. Med Science Sports Exerc 1993;25:775.

Drug Use and Athletes

Buckley WE, Yesalis III CE, Friedl KE, et al. Estimated prevalence of anabolic steroid use among male high school seniors. JAMA 1988;260:3441.

Cowart VS. Erythropoietin: a dangerous new form of blood doping. Physician Sportsmed 1989;17:115.

DuRant RH, Rickert VI, Ashworth CS, et al. Use of multiple drugs among adolescents who use anabolic steroids. N Engl J Med 1993;328:922.

Ghaphery NA. Performance-enhancing drugs. Orthop Clin North Am 1995;26:433.

Hallagan JB, Hallagan LF, Snyder MB. Anabolic-androgenic steroid use by athletes. N Engl J Med 1989; 321:1042.

Johnson MD. Anabolic steroid use in adolescent athletes. Pediatr Clin North Am 1990;37:1111.

Puffer JC. Drugs and doping in athletes. In: Mellion MB, ed. Office management of sports injuries and athletic problems. Philadelphia: Handley & Belfus, 1988.

Strauss R, ed. Drugs and performance in sports. Philadelphia: WB Saunders, 1987.

Wadler GI, Hainline B. Drugs and the athlete. In: Ryan A, ed. Contemporary exercise and sports medicine series. Philadelphia: FA Davis, 1989.

Yeasalis CE, Bahrke MS. Anabolic-androgenic steroids. Current issues. Sports Med 1995;19:326.

Ankle

Bahr R, Karlsen R, Lian O, et al. Incidence and mechanisms of acute ankle inversion injuries in volleyball. A retrospective cohort study. Am J Sports Med 1994; 22:595.

Barrett JR, Tanji JL, Drake C, et al. High- versus low-top shoes for the prevention of ankle sprains in basketball players. A prospective randomized study. Am J Sports Med 1993;21:582.

Gooch JL, Geiringer SR, Akau CK. Sports medicine. 3. Lower extremity injuries. Arch Phys Med Rehabil 1993;74:S438.

Griffin LY. Common sports injuries of the foot and ankle seen in children and adolescents. Orthop Clin North Am 1994;25:83.

Hergenroeder AC. Diagnosis and treatment of ankle injuries. A review. Am J Dis Child 1990;144:809.

Karlsson J, Lansinger O. Chronic lateral instability of the ankle in athletes. Sports Med 1993;16:355.

Keene JS, Lange RH. Diagnostic dilemmas in foot and ankle injuries. JAMA 1986;256:247.

Kvist M. Achilles tendon injuries in athletes. Sports Med 1994;18:173.

Liu SH, Jason WJ. Lateral ankle sprains and instability problems. Clin Sport Med 1994;13:793.

Mascaro TB, Swanson LE. Rehabilitation of the foot and ankle. Orthop Clin North Am 1994;25:147.

Seto JL, Brewster CE. Treatment approaches following foot and ankle injury. Clin Sports Med 1994;13: 695.

Smith RW, Reischl SF. Treatment of ankle sprains in young athletes. Am J Sports Med 1986;14:465.

Stiell IG, Greenberg GH, McKnight D, et al. Decision rules for the use of radiography in acute ankle injuries. JAMA 1993;269:1127.

Yeung MS, Chan KM, So CH, et al. An epidemiological survey on ankle sprain. Br J Sport Med 1994;28:112.

Knee and Thigh

Albright JP, Powell JW, Smith W, et al. Medial collateral ligament knee sprains in college football. Effectiveness of preventive braces. Am J Sports Med 1994;22:12.

Buhari SA, Singh S, Wong HP, et al. Tibial tuberosity fractures in adolescents. Singapore Med J 1993;34:421.

Caborn DN, Johnson BM. The natural history of the anterior cruciate ligament-deficient knee. A review. Clin Sports Med 1993;12:625.

Davidson K. Patellofemoral pain syndrome. Am Fam Physician 1993;48:1253.

Gooch JL, Geiringer SR, Akau CK. Sports medicine. 3. Lower extremity injuries. Arch Phys Med Rehabil 1993;74:S438.

Hutchinson MR, Ireland ML. Knee injuries in female athletes. Sports Med 1995;19:288.

Kujala UM, Kvist M, Heinonen O. Osgood-Schlatter's disease in adolescent athletes. Am J Sports Med 1985;13:236.

LaBrier K, Oneill DB. Patellofemoral stress syndrome. Current concepts. Sports Med 1993;16:449.

Maffulli N, Binfield PM, King JB, et al. Acute haemarthrosis of the knee in athletes. A prospective study of 106 cases. J Bone Joint Surg 1993;75:945.

Main WK, Hershman EB. Chronic knee pain in active adolescents. Physician Sportsmed 1992;20:139.

Shelbourne KD, Rowdon GA. Anterior cruciate ligament injury. The competitive athlete. Sports Med 1994;17:132.

Wickiewicz TL, Edwards JC. Sports-related injuries to the shoulder and knee. Surg Annu 1993;25:193.

Young JL, Laskowski ER, Rock MG. Thigh injuries in athletes. Mayo Clin Proc 1993;68:1099.

Zarins B, Adams M. Knee injuries in sports. N Engl J Med 1988;318:950.

Shoulder

Boublik M, Hawkins RJ. Clinical examination of the shoulder complex. J Orthop Sports Phys Therapy 1993;18:379.

Bowyer BL, Gooch JL, Geiringer SR. Sports medicine. 2. Upper extremity injuries. Arch Phys Med Rehabil 1993;74:S433.

Copeland S. Throwing injuries of the shoulder. Br J Sports Med 1993;27:221.

Jobe FW, Pink M. Classification and treatment of shoulder dysfunction in the overhead athlete. J Orthop Sport Phys Therapy 1993;18:427.

Jobe FW, Pink M. The athlete's shoulder. J Hand Ther 1994;7:107.

Markey KL, Di-Benedetto M, Curl WW. Upper trunk brachial plexopathy. The stinger syndrome. Am J Sports Med 1993;21:650.

Meister K, Andrews JR. Classification and treatment of rotator cuff injuries in the overhand athlete. J Orthop Sports Phys Therapy 1993;18:413.

Silliman JF, Dean MT. Neurovascular injuries to the shoulder complex. J Orthop Sports Phys Therapy 1993;18:442.

Wickiewicz TL, Edwards, JC. Sports-related injuries to the shoulder and knee. Surg Annu 1993;25:193.

Baseball

American Academy of Pediatrics Committee on Sports Medicine. Risk of injury from baseball and softball in children 5 to 14 years of age. Pediatrics 1994;93:690.

Centers for Disease Control and Prevention. Sliding-associated injuries in college and professional baseball—1990–1991. JAMA 1993;269:1925.

Dorsey JK, Benton R. Saving young arms and batters' heads [Letter]. Pediatrics 1993;91:679.

Basketball

Sickles RT, Lombardo JA. The adolescent basketball player. Clin Sports Med 1993;12:207.

Dance

Bauman PA, Singson R, Hamilton WG. Femoral neck anteversion in ballerinas. Clin Orthop Related Res 1994;May:57.

Khan K, Brown J, Way S, et al. Overuse injuries in classical ballet. Sports Med 1995;19:341.

Fehlandt AF Jr, Micheli LJ. Lumbar facet stress fracture in a ballet dancer. Spine 1993;18:2537.

Garrick JG, Requa RK. Ballet injuries. An analysis of epidemiology and financial outcome. Am J Sports Med 1993;21:586.

Greer JM, Panush RS. Musculoskeletal problems of performing artists. Baillieres Clin Rheumatol 1994;8:103.

Hardaker JWT Jr, Vander Woude LM. Dance medicine. An orthopaedist's view. N C Med J 1993;54:67.

Harrington JT, Crichton KJ, Anderson IF. Overuse ballet injury of the base of the second metatarsal. A diagnostic problem. Am J Sports Med 1993;21:591.

Jeresaty RM. Mitral valve prolapse. New York: Raven Press, 1979.

Karlsson MK, Johnell O, Obrant KJ. Bone mineral density in professional ballet dancers. Bone Miner 1993;21:163.

Milan KR. Injury in ballet: a review of relevant topics for the physical therapist. J Orthop Sports Phys Therapy 1994;19:121.

Petrucci GL. Prevention and management of dance injuries. Orthop Nurs 1993;12:52.

Quirk R. Common foot and ankle injuries in dance. Orthop Clin North Am 1994;25:123.

Schon LC. Foot and ankle problems in dancers. Md Med J 1993;42:267.

Schon LC, Biddinger KR, Greenwood P. Dance screen programs and development of dance clinics. Clin Sports Med 1994;13:865.

Van de Meulebroucke B, Dereymaeker G. Stress lesions of the forefoot in ballet dancers. Acta Orthop Belg 1994;60:S47.

Warren MP, Brooks-Gunn J, Hamilton LH, et al. Scoliosis and fractures in young ballet dancers. N Engl J Med 1986;314:1348.

Young N, Formica C, Szmukler G, et al. Bone density at weight-bearing and nonweight-bearing sites in ballet dancers: the effects of exercise, hypogonadism, and body weight. J Clin Endocrinol Metab 1994;78:449.

Golfing

Batt ME. Golfing injuries. An overview. Sports Med 1993;16:64.

Gymnastics

Wadley GH, Albright JP. Women's intercollegiate gymnastics. Injury patterns and "permanent" medical disability. Am J Sports Med 1993;21:314.

High-Altitude Problems

Grissom CK, Roach RC, Sarnquist FH, et al. Acetazolamide in the treatment of acute mountain sickness: clinical efficacy and effect on gas exchange. Ann Intern Med 1992;116:461.

Hsia CC. Southwestern Internal Medicine Conference: pulmonary complications of high-altitude exposure. Am J Med Sci 1994;307:448.

Jacobson ND. Acute high-altitude illness. Am Fam Physician 1988;38:135.

Johnson TS, Rock PB. Current concepts: acute mountain sickness. N Engl J Med 1988;319:841.

Krasney JA. A neurogenic basis for acute altitude illness. Med Sci Sports Exerc 1994;26:195.

Leon Velarde F, Arregui A, Vargas M, et al. Chronic mountain sickness and chronic lower respiratory tract disorders. Chest 1994;106:151.

Selland MA, Stelzner TJ, Stevens T, et al. Pulmonary function and hypoxic ventilatory response in subjects susceptible to high-altitude pulmonary edema. Chest 1993;103:111.

Tso EL, Wagner TJ Jr. What's up in the management of high-altitude pulmonary edema? Md Med J 1993; 42:641.

Hockey

Bjorkenheim JM, Syvahuoko I, Rosenberg PH. Injuries in competitive junior ice-hockey. 1437 players followed for one season. Acta Orthp Scand 1993;64:459.

Boyle PM, Mahoney CA, Wallace WF. The competitive demands of elite male field hockey. J Sports Med Phys Fitness 1994;34:235.

Pattersson M, Lorentzon R. Ice hockey injuries: a 4-year prospective study of a Swedish elite ice hockey team. Br J Sports Med 1993;27:251.

Pelletier RL, Montelpare WJ, Stark RM. Intercollegiate ice hockey injuries. A case for uniform definitions and reports. Am J Sports Med 1993;21:78.

Reynen PD, Clancy WG Jr. Cervical spine injury, hockey helmets, and face masks. Am J Sports Med 1994; 22:167.

Stuart MJ, Smith AM, Nieva JJ, et al. Injuries in youth ice hockey: a pilot surveillance strategy. Mayo Clin Proc 1995;70:350.

Running

Janisse DJ. Indications and prescriptions for orthoses in sports. Orthop Clin North Am 1994;25:95.

Jones BH, Cowan DN, Knapik JJ. Exercise, training and injuries. Sports Med 1994;18:202.

Paty JG Jr. Running injuries. Curr Opin Rheumatol 1994;6:203.

Shorten MR. The energetics of running and running shoes. J Biomech 1993;26:41S.

van Mechelen W, Hlobil H, Kemper HC, et al. Prevention of running injuries by warm-up, cool-down, and stretching exercises. Am J Sports Med 1993;21: 711.

Skating

Calle SC. In-line skating injuries, 1987 through 1992 [Letter]. Am J Public Health 1994;84:675.

Calle SC, Eaton RG. Wheels-in-line roller skating injuries. J Trauma 1993;35:946.

Schieber RA, Branche-Dorsey CM, Ryan GW. Comparison of in-line skating injuries with rollerskating and skateboarding injuries. JAMA 1994;271:1856.

Young CC, Mark DH. In-line skating. An observational study of protective equipment used by skaters. Arch Fam Med 1995;4:19.

Skiing

Bladin C, Giddings P, Robinson M. Australian snowboard injury data base study. A four-year prospective study. Am J Sport Med 1993;21:701.

Colbeck SC. A review of the friction of snow skis. J Sports Sci 1994;12:285.

Ekeland A, Holtmoen A, Lystad H. Lower extremity equipment-related injuries in alpine recreational skiers. Am J Sports Med 1993;21:201.

Ekeland A, Nordsletten L. Equipment related injuries in skiing: recommendations. Sports Med 1994;17: 283.

Nicholas R, Hadley J, Paul C, et al. Snowboarder's fracture: fracture of the lateral process of the talus. J Am Board Fam Pract 1994;7:130.

Paletta GA, Warren RF. Knee injuries and alpine skiing. Treatment and rehabilitation. Sports Med 1994;17:411.

Tough SC, Butt JC. A review of fatal injuries associated with downhill skiing. Am J Forensic Pathol 1993;14:12.

Tough SC, Butt JC. A review of 19 fatal injuries associated with backcountry skiing. Am J Forensic Med Pathol 1993;14:17.

Volleyball

Schafle MD. Common injuries in volleyball. Treatment, prevention and rehabilitation. Sports Med 1993;16:126.

Underwater Sports

Edge CJ. Medical aspects of scuba diving. Standards for diabetic divers are workable [Letter]. Br Med J 1994; 309:340.

Kinsinger JW, Brian JE Jr. Medical qualification of sport scuba divers. J Ark Med Soc 1993;89:552.

Neuman TS, Bove AA, O'Connor R, et al. Asthma and diving. Ann Allergy 1994;73:344.

Obafunwa JO, Busuttil A, Purdue B. Deaths of amateur scuba divers. Med Sci Law 1994;34:123.

Dermatological Disorders

CHAPTER 19

Acne

Anita S. Pakula and Lawrence S. Neinstein

Acne is the most common skin disease evaluated by health-care practitioners and is most prevalent in adolescents. Although 85% of adolescents have acne to some degree, the importance of this disease cannot be measured in numbers alone but must take into account the psychosocial consequences. The impact on self-esteem and body image of the developing teenager can affect social interactions, school performance, and eventual employment.

ETIOLOGY

The pilosebaceous units (well-developed sebaceous glands with miniature hairs) located in highest concentration on the face, upper chest, and upper back are the sites for the development of acne. The key pathogenic factors of acne vulgaris are (*a*) androgen-induced increased sebum production, (*b*) abnormal keratinization of sebaceous and follicular epithelium; (*c*) proliferation of *Propionibacterium acnes,* and (*d*) inflammation.

1. Androgenic hormones (gonadal and adrenal) stimulate both enlargement and increased activity of sebaceous glands on the face, neck, and upper trunk. The sebaceous glands are androgen-sensitive appendages of hair follicles whose function is the secretion of lipids to lubricate the skin and hair. Serum dehydroepiandrosterone sulfate (DHEA-S) appears to be the earliest marker for the development of acne (Lucky et al., 1991; Stewart et al., 1992). Although testosterone levels are normal in most acne patients, local conversion to the end-organ effector dihydrotestosterone may be increased in acne-bearing skin. Furthermore, androgens may decrease the linoleic acid concentration in the sebum of acne patients, contributing to abnormal keratinization and obstruction of the pilosebaceous ducts (Morello et al., 1976).
2. Abnormal keratinization of the sebaceous and follicular ducts results in retention hyperkeratosis and microcomedo formation (comedogenesis).
3. The excessive sebum and the anaerobic environment created by the plugged follicle results in the colonization and proliferation of the anaerobic diphtheroid, *P. acnes.*
4. This bacteria triggers immune and nonimmune inflammatory reactions by the following mechanisms:
   a. Lipases are produced that are capable of hydrolizing the triglycerides of sebum into irritating and comedogenic free fatty acids.
   b. Chemotactic factors are released that attract leukocytes. Hydrolytic enzymes released by these neutrophils can produce breaks in the walls of the follicle, leading to the disruption of follicular contents, leakage into the dermis, and resultant inflammation.
   c. Complement pathways and host response are activated.

CLINICAL DISEASE

Types of lesions include comedones, inflammatory papules, pustules, nodules, true cysts, and scars. Each is discussed next.

Comedones

Comedones are the earliest sign of acne often appearing 1–2 years before puberty.

1. Microcomedo: Microcomedos are impactions of keratin, lipids, bacteria, and rudimentary hair within the sebaceous follicle. These are small and subclinical and are seen only on magnification or biopsy specimens from acne patients. They are the precursor to all acne lesions.
2. Open comedo (blackhead)
   a. The epithelium-lined sac is filled with keratin and lipids and has a dilated orifice.
   b. The black coloration comes from melanin pigment.
   c. Usually the keratinous material is sloughed, and no inflammation occurs unless traumatized.
3. Closed comedo (whitehead)
   a. Minimally palpable lesion is 1–3 mm in size with microscopic opening preventing the escape of contents.
   b. Active lesions may resolve spontaneously; if the follicular wall ruptures superficially, the lesion becomes an inflamed pustule, and deeper inflammation results in a papule or nodule.

Papules

Papules are inflammatory lesions measuring less than 5 mm in diameter.

1. Superficial papules resolve in 5–10 days, with little scarring except postinflammatory hyperpigmentation (especially in adolescents with dark complexions).
2. Deep papules usually have more intense inflammation. These can take weeks to resolve and may result in scarring.

Pustules

Pustules are lesions with a visible central core of purulent material.

Nodules

Nodules are inflammatory lesions measuring 5 mm or greater and can result as pustules rupture and form abscesses. Nodules commonly occur around the earlobes, neck, and jawline.

True Cysts

True cysts are lined by epithelium and are the rare residual lesions of healed pustules or nodules.

Scars

Types of scarring include:

1. Ice pick or depressed scars
2. Perifollicular fibrosis, characterized by a yellow ring around follicle remnants

3. Hypertrophic scars and keloids, which tend to form on the chest, back, jawline, and ears and are more common in dark complected individuals

Location

1. The face is the area most prominently affected.
2. The back, chest, buttocks, upper arms, and thighs are also commonly affected areas.
3. Acne typically spares the axilla, hands, forearms, calves, and feet.

Grading

A widely accepted and standardized system for grading acne does not exist, but any classification scheme should take into consideration morphology, distribution, complications, response to therapy, and impact of disease on the individual. At present, it is recommended that acne be classified by the predominant type of lesion, such as comedonal, papulopustular, or nodular, and is then graded as mild, moderate, or severe.

Timing

1. Acne may appear as early as 5–8 years of age and seems to correlate with pubertal maturation. The prevalence and severity increases with advancing pubertal development. The prevalence of acne peaks between the ages of 14 and 17 in females and 16 and 19 in males.
2. Acne varies from a short, mild course to a severe disease lasting 10–15 years.
3. Many adolescents do not have resolution of their acne by 20 years of age.
4. Males tend to have more severe acne for a shorter time.
5. Females tend to have a milder disease for a longer time.

DIFFERENTIAL DIAGNOSIS

Nonacne Lesions

1. Adenoma sebaceum: The most common cutaneous manifestation of tuberous sclerosis, presenting as pink to red facial papules that develop in childhood or puberty. The lesions represent angiofibromas.
2. Flat warts: Skin-colored papules that may spread (Koebner phenomenon) with trauma.
3 Perioral dermatitis: Small, 1- to 3-mm erythematous papules or papulopustules of the chin, nasolabial folds, or periorbital areas that may be accompanied by scaling. A granulomatous variant exists. Topical corticosteroids can induce or aggravate this condition. Related to acne rosacea. Treated with topical or oral antibiotics. Topical metronidazole is very effective.
4. Hidradenitis suppurativa: Disease of apocrine follicles of axilla, groin, buttocks, and periareolar areas manifested by multiheaded comedos; deep, tender nodules; and scarring.

Subtypes of Acne

1. Neonatal acne
   a. Stimulation of sebaceous glands by maternal and neonatal androgens derived from the hyperactive neonatal adrenal gland. The lesions are usually closed comedos on the nose, forehead, and cheeks. Spontaneous resolution occurs in 1–3 months.

b. Infantile acne usually presents between the third and sixth months, and it may be associated with an increased risk of developing acne vulgaris during adolescence (Chew, et al., 1990). Males are more commonly affected.

c. Inflammatory acne lesions may occur.

2. Gram-negative folliculitis

a. Usually caused by a secondary colonization with *Escherichia coli, Klebsiella, Pseudomonas, Enterobacter,* or *Proteus* spp. during broad-spectrum antibiotic use.

b. Can produce multiple pustules and nodules with a predilection for the perinasal area.

c. Suspected in an adolescent patient with acne who is doing poorly or flaring on antibiotics.

d. Use culture results for guiding diagnosis and therapy. Isotretinoin (Accutane) is effective.

3. Cosmetic acne

a. Less common since the advent of noncomedogenic cosmetics, but occlusive moisturizing creams, cocoa butter, vitamin E oil, and pomades may create comedonal acne.

4. Occupational acne

a. Certain products can cause obstruction to sebaceous follicles, including mineral oil, crude petroleum, coal tar, and pitch.

b. Halogenated aromatic hydrocarbons can also cause an acneform eruption.

5. Drug-induced acne

a. Drugs involved include androgens, adrenocorticotropic hormone (ACTH), steroids (oral and topical), barbiturates, phenytoin, isoniazid, rifampin, lithium, bromides, and iodines.

b. These drugs can also exacerbate pre-existing acne.

c. Steroid acne is typically a monomorphous eruption of papules or papulopustules that resolves without scarring. It does not produce comedones, nodules, and scars. It may involve areas, such as extremities, that are not normally affected in acne vulgaris (Hurwitz, 1989).

6. Acne conglobata

a. Acne conglobata is a severe, suppurative, often chronic form of nodular acne most often occurring in white males.

b. The back is often severely affected, along with the thighs, buttocks, and upper arms.

7. Acne fulminans

a. This rare form of noduloulcerative acne has an abrupt onset often accompanied by fever, leukocytosis, anemia, polyarthritis, and, rarely, osteolytic bone lesions (Karvonen, 1993).

b. Abrupt onset is associated with the following: Large necrotic nodules and ulcerations.

8. Acne mechanica: This form occurs at sites of physical trauma such as the chin from helmet straps and shoulders and upper back from shoulder pads.

9. Acne Excoriee des Jeunes Filles: Most frequently seen in adolescent girls who excoriate or manipulate the acne lesions; severe scarring and even mutilation may result. It is usually associated with emotional stress.

THERAPY

General

Several considerations are important in treating adolescents with acne:

1. Practitioners must appreciate the significance of this problem to adolescents. The short- and long-term consequences of acne to the adolescent's emotional well-being should not be underestimated.
2. Most adolescents treat themselves and will often heed peer suggestions more readily than those of a physician. Thus, practitioners must emphasize the role and necessity of compliance.
3. Practitioners must understand the route, timing, and dose of the drugs administered. Use only a few drugs and know them well.
4. Make sure the adolescent understands how to use the medications.
5. Do not promise instant success. Point out that:
   a. Therapy with topical agents often causes acne to look worse in the first 3–4 weeks.
   b. Improvement may take months.
6. Explain side effects of all medications used.
7. Perform a thorough history and physical examination. The female patient should also be examined for the presence of hirsutism, alopecia, and obesity. She should be asked about her menstrual cycle and use of oral contraceptives.
8. Treat according to severity, as follows:
   a. Mild comedonal acne may respond to over-the-counter or prescription acne preparations such as salicylic acid or benzoyl peroxide. Table 19.1 lists common over-the-counter preparations.

TABLE 19.1. Over-the-Counter Products

Product	Preparation	Manufacturer	Active Ingredient[a]	Concentration (%)
Acne-Aid	Cream	Stiefel	BPO	10
Benoxyl	Lotion	Stiefel	BPO	5, 10
Clear by Design	Gel	SmithKline Beecham	BPO	2.5
Clearasil	Cream, lotion	Richardson-Vicks	BPO	10
	Cleanser		SA	0.5
	Clearstick		SA	1.25, 2.0
	Pads		SA	1.25, 2.0
Fostex	Bar, cream	Bristol-Myers	Sulfur, SA	2.0
	10% Bar		BPO	10
	Super strength wash, cream, gel		BPO	10
Loroxide	Lotion	Dermik	BPO	5.5
Neutrogena	On-the-Spot lotion	Neutrogena	BPO	2.5
	Acne wash		SA	2.0
	Acne mask		BPO	5.0
Noxzema	Clear Ups lotion	Noxell	BPO	10
	On-the-Spot lotion		BPO	10
	Clear Ups gel and pads		SA	0.5
Oxy	Cleanser	SmithKline Beecham	SA	0.5
	Lotion		BPO	5, 10
	10 wash		BPO	10
	Clean pads		SA	0.5,[b] 2.0
	Night Watch lotion		SA	1.0, 2.0
Panoxyl	Bar	Stiefel	BPO	5, 10
Rezamid	Lotion	Summers	Sulfur	5
			Resorcinal	2.0
SAStid	Soap	Stiefel	Precipitated sulfur	10
Sebasorb	Lotion	Summers	SA	2.0
Stri-Dex	Pads	Sterling Health	SA	0.5,[b] 2.0

[a]BPO, benzoyl peroxide; SA, salicylic acid.
[b]Sensitive skin formulas use lower concentration of alcohol.

   b. Moderate-to-severe comedonal acne may respond to the addition of tretinoin (Retin-A) at bedtime.

   c. Mild inflammatory acne may respond to the addition of a topical antibiotic or 5% benzoyl peroxide with 3% erythromycin (Benzamycin) gel.

   d. Unresponsive or moderate-to-severe inflammatory acne requires the addition of a systemic antibiotic.

   e. Nodular or nodulocystic acne that does not respond to oral antibiotics should be treated with isotretinoin (Accutane) by an experienced practitioner.

Topical Agents

A list of topical agents available is provided in Table 19.2.

1. Benzoyl peroxide
   a. Actions
      — Bacteriocidal effect on *P. acnes* with low potential for resistance
      — Mild comedolytic action, decreases free fatty acids
   b. Dose
      — Benzoyl peroxide is available in 2.5%, 4%, 5%, and 10% concentrations.
      — The aqueous gels are better tolerated than compounds prepared in an alcohol and acetone vehicle. Benzoyl peroxide in the gel form also appears to have better penetration and higher effectiveness than benzoyl peroxide in soaps, washes, and lotions.
      — Gradually increase concentration as tolerated.
   c. Adverse side effects
      — Peeling and irritation
      — Contact dermatitis (about 1–2%)
2. Tretinoin or retinoic acid (Retin-A)
   a. Action: Decreases follicular plugging, making it very useful in comedonal acne
   b. Dose and usage
      — Close supervision and instruction are required.
      — The following concentrations are available: 0.025%, 0.05%, and 0.1% cream; 0.01% and 0.025% gel; and 0.05% liquid.
      — The cream is the least irritating, followed by the gel and the liquid.
      — Start with the 0.025% cream or 0.01% gel every other night 30 minutes after washing face and gradually increase to a daily regimen. If not effective, increase the concentration as tolerated.

TABLE 19.2.   Topical Therapy for Acne

Benzoyl peroxide
5% Benzoyl peroxide with 3% erythromycin
Benzoyl peroxide-sulfur
Tretinoin
Salicylic acid
α-Hydroxy acids
Resorcinol
Resorcinol-sulfur
Sulfacetamide-sulfur
Topical antibiotics
Clindamycin
Erythromycin
Metronidazole
Tetracycline

— Using benzoyl peroxide in the morning and tretinoin in the evening is often the most effective. Caution should be used with concomitant topical medication, as skin irritation can become excessive.

— After 1 or 2 weeks of therapy, some irritation will occur. If severe, therapy can be stopped for a short time. After 3–4 weeks, a pustular eruption can occur, indicating the dislodging of microcomedos; treatment should continue.

— Avoid sun exposure because of the photosensitizing properties of tretinoin. If used during summer months, SPF 15 or higher sunscreen should be used.

— Use with caution on black and Asian patients, since tretinoin can cause hyperpigmentation or hypopigmentation.

c. Adverse side effects
   — Peeling and irritation
   — Hyperpigmentation or hypopigmentation
   — Sun sensitivity

3. Other peeling agents
   a. Washes and lotions
      — Usually contain either salicylic acid, resorcinol, sulfur, or α-hydroxyacids
      — Are not as effective as benzoyl peroxide and tretinoin
   b. Abrasive scrubs and vigorous washing: Should be avoided, as they irritate the skin and may result in inflammation
   c. Cryotherapy with carbon dioxide acetone slush or liquid nitrogen: May increase peeling, but usually not necessary
   d. Sunlight or ultraviolet light
      — Does not appear to affect acne significantly, and potential risks of photoaging and carcinogenesis outweigh any benefits.

4. Topical antibiotics include tetracycline, erythromycin, clindamycin, and metronidazole. Topical antibiotics allow direct application and have negligible systemic side effects. Although they can be effective for mild-to-moderate inflammatory acne, topical antibiotics cannot replace systemic antibiotics in more severe cases. Preparations include:
   a. Tetracycline (Topicycline): The agent is applied twice a day, but it is not recommended because it may cause black-light fluorescence.
   b. Erythromycin (e.g., A/T/S solution, T-Stat solution, Erygel, Akne-mycin): Available in solutions, gels, pads, and ointment; applied twice daily.
   c. Clindamycin (Cleocin T solution, C/T/S): Available in a solution, lotion, gel, and pledget; applied twice daily. Pseudomembranous colitis has rarely been reported to occur with topical use (Parry and Rha, 1986).

Systemic Therapy

1. Antibiotics
   a. Actions
      — Decrease population of *P. acnes*
      — Reduce amount of free fatty acids
      — May depress inflammatory response in the pilosebaceous follicle
   b. Usage (summarized in Table 19.3)
      — Drugs used include tetracycline, doxycycline, minocycline, erythromycin, clindamycin, trimethoprim-sulfamethoxazole, and dapsone.
      — None are indicated for noninflammatory comedonal acne.
      — Dapsone and clindamycin, because of serious side effects, should be reserved for severe or recalcitrant acne.

TABLE 19.3.   Systemic Antibiotic Therapy

Drug	Dose	Advantages	Disadvantages
Tetracycline	250 mg–1500 mg/day	Inexpensive	Poor compliance, gastrointestinal upset
Doxycycline	50–200 mg/day	Inexpensive, improved compliance	Photosensitivity, esophageal ulceration
Minocycline	50–200 mg/day	Low resistance, low photosensitivity	Expensive, vertigo-like symptoms, Löffler-like syndrome, lupus-like reaction, rare tooth and skin discoloration
Erythromycin	500–1000 mg/day	Inexpensive	Gastrointestinal upset, frequent resistance
Trimethoprim-sulfamethoxazole	1–2 double strength tablets per day	Effective in Gram-negative folliculitis, lipophilic	Bone marrow suppression, drug eruptions
Clindamycin	300–450 mg/day	Effective	Limited to short-term use, pseudomembranous colitis

— Oral antibiotics can be used in combination with topical therapy.

— The initial dose of tetracycline or erythromycin should be 500–1000 mg in two divided doses daily. This dose may be decreased after about 4 weeks, depending on response. Tetracycline binds with calcium, so milk products should be avoided within 2 hours of a dose. Some patients may require up to 2 g of tetracycline daily, but consider switching to another preparation if these doses are required for a prolonged period of time.

— Minocycline is extremely effective and well tolerated. Doses from 50–200 mg daily are used. Dizziness, tinnitus, and nausea may be experienced at higher doses. Tooth discoloration and skin pigmentation have rarely been reported.

  c. Side effects
— Tetracycline: Associated with gastrointestinal upset and candida vaginitis and rarely a drug eruption, anemia, neutropenia or phototoxicity. Tetracycline should not be used in children less than 8 years of age or adolescent females who are pregnant.

— Doxycycline: Frequently causes photosensitivity.

— Erythromycin: Nausea; vomiting; diarrhea; candida vaginitis; occasional drug eruptions.

— Routine laboratory monitoring is generally not necessary in healthy adolescents receiving long-term oral antibiotic therapy. However, if a patient has a pre-existing condition or develops symptoms, appropriate laboratory tests should be performed.

2. 13-cis-Retinoic acid or isotretinoin (Accutane): 13-cis-retinoic acid has dramatically reversed the course of acne in many individuals with severe nodulocystic or recalcitrant acne. Because of significant toxicity, the drug is still reserved for treatment of severe nodular or recalcitrant acne. The use of the drug should be reserved for practitioners experienced with its use. Careful laboratory monitoring is also required.

  a. Actions: The drug is a synthetic vitamin A derivative that affects keratinization by suppressing sebum production and diminishing the growth of *P. acnes*.

  b. Usage: Isotretinoin is usually given in a daily dose of 1 mg/kg divided into two doses. The range can be up to 2 mg/kg/day with these higher doses reserved for back and chest lesions or for patients who failed an initial course of isotretinoin. The length of therapy is 15–20 weeks, with clinical improvement often continuing after discontinuation of the medication. Relapse is less likely to occur if a dose of 1 mg/kg/day is used or a total cumulative dose of 120 mg/kg of body weight is reached; however, there appears to be no additional benefit of cumulative doses of greater than 150 mg/kg of body weight. Because of the teratogenic effects of the drug, it should only be prescribed to female adolescents who are on effective contraception for at least 1 month prior to beginning therapy, during therapy, and for 1 month after completing therapy. The potential effects on the fetus should be communicated in both oral and written forms.

   c. Laboratory monitoring should include:
- Baseline: Complete blood count (CBC), liver function tests, cholesterol, triglycerides, and urinalysis. In females, a serum or urinary pregnancy test with a sensitivity of at least 50 mIU/mL should be obtained within 1 week of starting therapy. Female patients should be instructed to start therapy on the second or third day of their next normal menstrual period.
- Two weeks after beginning therapy: Repeat cholesterol and triglycerides.
- At 4 weeks and monthly thereafter: Repeat baseline tests, including serum or urine pregnancy test, but urinalysis is optional.
- End of therapy: Repeat CBC, liver function tests, cholesterol, triglycerides, and pregnancy test.

   d. Side effects:
- Mucocutaneous
  - (1) Cheilitis, 90%
  - (2) Xerosis, 78%
  - (3) Dry mouth, 70%
  - (4) Epistaxis, 46%
  - (5) Conjunctivitis, 40%
  - (6) Desquamation, 16%
  - (7) Hair loss (thinning, not balding), 9%
  - (8) Other: vaginal dryness, urethritis
- Musculoskeletal
  - (1) Arthralgias and myalgias, 16%
- Hyperostosis: Mainly a problem when drug is used for prolonged periods of time in other dermatologic conditions
- Decreased night vision
- Headaches, 5%
- Pseudotumor cerebri, rare
- Depression
- Photosensitivity, 5–10%
- Elevated cholesterol (7%) and triglyceride (25%) levels
- Elevated liver function tests, 15%
- Renal: Proteinuria and hematuria
- Hematologic: Elevated erythrocyte sedimentation rate (40%), leukopenia, elevated platelets (10–20%)
- Skin rash: Occasional pyogenic granuloma-like lesions (hypergranulation tissue); *Staphylococcus aureus* skin colonization and infections
- Cheilitis and hypertriglyceridemia: Tend to be dose related

3. Hormonal: The major role for hormonal intervention is in individuals with an endocrine problem such as polycystic ovary syndrome or congenital adrenal hyperplasia. Hormonal therapy includes:
   a. Estrogens: Estrogen in a dose of 50 µg or more of ethinyl estradiol is effective in suppressing sebaceous gland activity, but the potential side effects preclude its use in most female patients. However, newer oral contraceptives that contain less androgenic progestins such as desogestrel (Desogen, Ortho-Cept) or norgestimate

(Ortho-Cyclen, Ortho Tri-Cyclen) may lessen acne. For side effects, see Chapter 43, section on oral contraceptives. Estrogens cannot be used in males because of the feminizing side effects.

  b. Corticosteroids: The use of high doses of corticosteroids should be reserved for the treatment of acne conglobata, acne fulminans, and the acute flare of acne precipitated by initiating isotretinoin therapy. Prednisone 5.0–7.5 mg or dexamethasone 0.25–0.5 mg are effective in reducing adrenal androgen production.

  c. Antiandrogens: The agents available are not approved for use in the treatment of acne, and the side effects usually result in poor compliance. However, spironolactone, cyproterone acetate, and flutamide have been used with some success, particularly in female patients with other signs of androgen excess.

Acne Surgery

1. Comedone extraction: Open comedones can be easily removed with a comedo extractor. Closed comedones require puncture with a needle or lancet first. One should avoid extensive surgical treatment, since manipulation can lead to scarring.
2. Incision and drainage: Do not incise acne pustules and nodules, because of possible resultant scarring.
3. Intralesional corticosteroids: Injection of 0.05–0.1 mL of 1.0–2.5 mg/mL triamcinolone acetonide into each papulonodular or cystic lesion is recommended.
4. Rehabilitation: After acne lesions have become quiescent, young adults may explore surgical options for scars. At present, alternatives include collagen implants for isolated shallow depressions, punch excision and grafting, chemical peels, dermabrasion, and laser resurfacing.

General Measures

1. Diet: No evidence exists that foods such as cola, chocolate, nuts, or french fries increase acne severity. Unless a patient notices dramatic differences with certain foods, dietary restrictions are unnecessary.
2. Hygiene: Overemphasis on compulsive scrubbing is unnecessary and may itself cause a dermatitis. Mild soaps or cleansers should be used to wash the face three times a day.
3. Stress: Stress has a reciprocal effect on acne. Stress seems to make acne worse, and reciprocally, acne increases adolescents' anxiety levels and decreases their self-image. Continued support must be given to the affected adolescent.

BIBLIOGRAPHY

Bergfeld WF. The evaluation and management of acne: economic considerations. J Am Acad Dermatol 1995; 32:S52.

Bershad S, Rubinstein A, Paterniti JR Jr, et al. Changes in plasma lipids and lipoproteins during isotretinoin therapy for acne. N Engl J Med 1985;313:981.

Berson DS, Shalita AR. The treatment of acne: the role of combination therapies. J Am Acad Dermatol 1995; 32:S31.

Chew EW, Bingham A, Burrows D. Incidence of acne vulgaris in patients with infantile acne. Clin Exp Dermatol 1990;15:376.

Cunliffe WJ. Unemployment and acne. Br J Dermatol 1986;115:379.

Eady EA, Farmery MR, Ross JI, et al. Effects of benzoyl peroxide and erythromycin alone and in combination against antibiotic-sensitive and -resistant skin bacteria from acne patients. Br J Dermatol 1994;131: 331.

Guidelines of care for acne vulgaris. J Am Acad Dermatol 1990;22:676.

Healy E, Simpson N. Acne vulgaris. Br Med J 1994;308: 831.

Hurwitz RM. Steroid acne. J Am Acad Dermatol 1989; 21:1179.

Hurwitz S. Disorders of the sebaceous and sweat glands. In: Hurwitz S, ed. Clinical pediatric dermatology. 2nd ed. Philadelphia: WB Saunders, 1993;136–163.

Hurwitz S. Acne vulgaris: pathogenesis and management. Pediatr Rev 1994;15:47.

Kaidbey KH, Kligman AM. Pigmentation in comedones. Arch Dermatol 1974;109:60.

Kaminer MS, Gilchrest BA. The many faces of acne. J Am Acad Dermatol 1995;32:S6.

Karvonen SKL. Acne fulminans: report of clinical findings and treatment of twenty-four patients. J Am Acad Dermatol 1993;28:572.

Krowchuk DP, Stancin T, Keskinen R, et al. The psychosocial effects of acne on adolescents. Pediatr Dermatol 1991;83:332.

Layton AM, Henderson CA, Cunliffe WJ. A clinical evaluation of acne scarring and its incidence. Clin Exp Dermatol 1994;19:303.

Layton AM, Knaggs H, Taylor J, et al. Isotretinoin for acne vulgaris—10 years later: a safe and successful treatment. Br J Dermatol 1993;129:292.

Lehucher-Ceyrac D, Weber-Buisset MJ: Isotretinoin and acne in practice: a prospective analysis of 188 cases over nine years. Dermatology 1993;186:123.

Leyden JJ. New understandings of the pathogenesis of acne. J Am Acad Dermatol 1995;32:S15.

Leyden JJ, James WD. Staphylococcal aureus infections as a complication of isotretinoin therapy. Arch Dermatol 1987;123:606.

Lucky AW. Endocrine aspects of acne. Pediatr Clin North Am 1983;30:495.

Lucky AW. Update on acne vulgaris. Pediatr Ann 1987; 16:29.

Lucky AW. Hormonal correlates of acne and hirsutism. Am J Med 1995;98:89S.

Lucky AW, Biro FM, Huster GA, et al. Acne vulgaris in early adolescent boys: correlations with pubertal maturation and age. Arch Dermatol 1991;127:210.

Lucky AW, Biro FM, Huster GA, et al. Acne vulgaris in premenarchal girls. Arch Dermatol 1994;130:308.

Morello AM, Downing DT, Strauss JS. Octadecadienoic acids in the skin surface lipids of acne patients and normal subjects. J Invest Dermatol 1976;66:319.

Nguyen QH, Kim YA, Schwartz RA. Management of acne vulgaris. Am Fam Physician 1994;50:89.

Parry MF, Rha CK. Pseudomembranous colitis associated with the topical administration of clindamycin phosphate. Arch Dermatol 1986;122:583.

Pochi PE, Ceilley RI, Coskey RJ, et al. Guidelines for prescribing isotretinoin (Accutane) in the treatment of female acne patients of childbearing potential. J Am Acad Dermatol 1988;19:920.

Poliak SC, DiGiovanna JJ, Gross EG, et al. Minocycline-associated tooth discoloration in young adults. JAMA 1985;254:2930.

Report of the Consensus Conference on Acne Classification. J Am Acad Dermatol 1991;24:495.

Stainforth JM, Layton AM, Taylor JP, et al. Isotretinoin for the treatment of acne vulgaris: which factors may predict the need for more than one course? Br J Dermatol 1993;129:297.

Stewart ME, Downing DT, Cook JS, et al. Sebaceous gland activity and serum dehydroepiandrosterone sulfate levels in boys and girls. Arch Dermatol 1992; 128:1345.

Sykes NL Jr, Webster GF: Acne: a review of optimum treatment. Drugs 1994;48:59.

Winston, MH, Shalita AR. Acne vulgaris: pathogenesis and management. Pediatr Clin North Am 1991;38: 889.

Yankosky DM, Pochi PE. Acne vulgaris in childhood: pathogenesis and management. Dermatol Clin 1986;4:127.

CHAPTER 20

Miscellaneous Dermatological Disorders

Lawrence S. Neinstein and Anita S. Pakula

While acne is the most prevalent skin disorder during adolescence, other diseases such as seborrhea, eczematous dermatitis, fungal infections, warts, and several other conditions are common at this time. Most of these disorders are mild, but to the adolescent concerned about body image and popularity, a skin problem may assume the importance of a serious illness. Effective therapy and understanding of the adolescent's feelings may lead to a strong alliance between patient and physician. Acne was discussed in Chapter 19. This chapter describes other skin problems commonly encountered during adolescence.

ECZEMATOUS DERMATITIS

Eczematous dermatitis is a superficial inflammatory response to multiple exogenous and endogenous agents of the skin that includes a poorly defined group of problems whose etiology is often either multifactorial or unknown. The two major groups of dermatitis affecting adolescents are contact dermatitis and atopic dermatitis.

Contact Dermatitis

Clinical Manifestations

1. Distribution: Areas that have been exposed to the inciting agent, often including the hands, eyelids, genitalia, and legs.
2. Lesions: Tendency for confluency, sharp borders, or straight lines. The lesions tend to have vesicles or bullae, oozing, and fissuring.

Types

1. Irritant dermatitis: A nonimmunologically mediated dermatitis that occurs in all individuals exposed to the agent in potent enough doses. Prior exposure is not required. Irritants include:
   a. Alkalis: Soaps, detergents, bleaches, cleansers
   b. Acids: Hydrochloric acid, nitric acid, oxalic acid, carbolic acid, acetic acid, and salicylic acid
   c. Insecticides
   d. Hydrocarbons: Oils and tars
   e. Fiberglass

360

2. Allergic contact dermatitis: A cell-mediated reaction that occurs in patients specifically sensitive to the offending agent. Prior exposure is required for a reaction. Agents commonly include:
   a. Rhus (poison ivy, oak, or sumac) dermatitis typically has a linear pattern.
   b. Nickel and other metals, particularly mercury and chromium
   c. Rubber compounds
   d. Dichromates: A common cause of shoe dermatitis; also found in metals, paint, cement, and photographic chemicals
   e. Clothing dyes or chemical finishes (i.e., formaldehyde resin)
   f. Adhesive tape: The rubber component or the glue
   g. Cosmetics: Hair dyes, hair sprays, artificial nails, nail hardeners, lipsticks, eye makeup, preservatives, sunscreens, perfumes, and mouthwashes

Diagnosis

1. Typical vesicular, erythematous lesions in a well-defined patch or an arrangement corresponding to the distribution of contact
2. History of exposure to an offending agent
3. Patch testing helpful in allergic contact dermatitis

Treatment

1. Find offending agent and eliminate exposure.
2. In acute reactions, apply cool Burow's compresses for 30 minutes several times daily.
3. Apply topical corticosteroid creams.
4. Antihistamines may help decrease the associated pruritus.
5. For widespread, severe, contact dermatitis, a course of systemic corticosteroids tapered over 2–3 weeks is indicated. The initial dose can be approximately 40–60 mg/day with decreases of 5 mg/day.

Atopic Dermatitis

Atopic dermatitis is a common, chronic, pruritic dermatitis also known as atopic eczema and allergic eczema, which typically has its onset in childhood and may improve or continue in adolescence.

Clinical Manifestations

1. Hereditary predisposition: A positive family history of atopy (asthma, allergic rhinitis, atopic dermatitis) is present in two-thirds of individuals.
2. Association with other atopic conditions: Fifty percent of individuals concurrently have either asthma or allergic rhinitis.
3. Course is chronic and fluctuating.
4. Pruritus: Itching is often severe.
5. Typical morphology and distribution: In adolescence the morphology resembles the adult pattern of flexural lichenification and involvement of the face, neck, and hands.
6. Skin lesions: The essential lesions are dry, slightly elevated, flat-topped papules that tend to coalesce to form lichenified, scaly plaques. The plaques may become excoriated, exudative, or crusted.
7. Dry skin is a common association.
8. Seasonal variation in disease activity is common.

9. Elevated IgE often occurs.
10. Keratosis pilaris: Follicular hyperkeratosis on the lateral upper arms and thighs is commonly associated with atopic dermatitis.
11. Pityriasis alba: Scaly, hypopigmented patches (typically on the face, neck, trunk and extremities of children and adolescents between the ages of 3 and 16 years) represent a nonspecific dermatitis that may be a variant of atopic dermatitis. The teen is usually asymptomatic, but pruritus may occur.

Complications

1. Infections: Increased susceptibility to herpes simplex virus, *Staphylococcus aureus, Trichophyton rubrum*, warts, and molluscum contagiosum
2. Eye: Increased prevalence of cataracts, keratoconus, recurrent conjunctivitis, periorbital darkening, and retinal detachment
3. Exfoliative dermatitis

Differential Diagnosis

1. Seborrheic dermatitis: Greasy, scaly scalp; distribution more likely to include scalp, eyebrows, and ears
2. Contact dermatitis: History of contact with an offending agent; scaling and fissuring of lesions
3. Tinea corporis or pedis: Sharp margins; confirmed by positive findings from potassium hydroxide examination
4. Scabies: Distribution usually includes web spaces of hands, groin, buttocks, axilla; positive skin scraping for mites or eggs
5. Psoriasis: Well-demarcated erythematous plaques with silvery scale; predilection for extensor surfaces; nail pitting common, but not specific

Treatment

1. Avoid hot water; decrease number of baths and showers.
2. Avoid soaps, detergents, and overheated rooms.
3. Acute weeping lesions: Use tepid, wet dressings with Burow's solution (aluminum acetate).
4. Dry skin lesions: Use an emollient such as Aquaphor, Eucerin, Shepard's, or Lubriderm.
5. Apply topical corticosteroid cream or ointment (see Table 20.1 for classification of topical corticosteroids by potency).
6. Use oral antihistaminic agent.
7. Use oral antistaphylococcal antibiotics if a secondary infection is present.

Other Types of Eczematous Dermatitis

1. Lichen simplex chronicus: One or more lichenified plaques probably secondary to repeated local trauma such as rubbing or scratching
2. Dyshidrotic eczema (pompholyx): Recurrent crops of vesicles on palms and soles and sides of fingers and toes; exacerbated by stress and frequent exposure to water
3. Seborrheic dermatitis: Greasy scaling patches on scalp, eyebrows, nasolabial area, intertriginous areas, and chest
4. Nummular dermatitis: Minute vesicles and papules that enlarge to form discrete, erythematous, coin-shaped patches

TABLE 20.1.   Classification of Commonly Used Topical Corticosteroids According to Potency[a]

Drug	Generic Name
I. Superpotency[b]	
Diprolene gel or ointment, 0.05%	Betamethasone dipropionate
Psorcon ointment, 0.05%	Diflorasone diacetate
Temovate cream or ointment, 0.05%	Clobetasol propionate
Ultravate cream or ointment, 0.05%	Halobetasol propionate
II. High Potency	
Cyclocort ointment, 0.1%	Amcinonide
Diprolene AF cream, 0.05%	Betamethasone dipropionate
Diprosone ointment, 0.05%	Betamethasone dipropionate
Elocon ointment, 0.1%	Mometasone furoate
Florone ointment, 0.05%	Diflorasone diacetate
Halog cream, 0.1%	Halcinonide
Lidex cream or gel or ointment, 0.05%	Fluocinonide
Maxiflor ointment, 0.05%	Diflorasone diacetate
Maxivate ointment, 0.05%	Betamethasone dipropionate
Topicort cream or ointment, 0.25%	Desoximetasone
III. Potent	
Aristocort A ointment, 0.1%	Triamcinolone acetonide
Cyclocort cream or ointment, 0.1%	Amcinonide
Diprosone cream, 0.05%	Betamethasone dipropionate
Elocon cream, 0.1%	Mometasone furoate
Florone cream, 0.05%	Diflorasone diacetate
Halog ointment or emollient cream or solution, 0.1%	Halcinonide
Lidex-E cream, 0.05%	Fluocinonide
Maxiflor cream, 0.05%	Diflorasone diacetate
Maxivate cream, 0.05%	Betamethasone dipropionate
Valisone ointment, 0.1%	Betamethasone valerate
IV–V. Medium potency	
Cordran cream or ointment, 0.05%	Flurandrenolide
Cutivate cream or ointment, 0.05%	Fluticasone propionate
Diprosone lotion, 0.05%	Betamethasone dipropionate
Kenalog lotion or cream or ointment, 0.1%	Triamcinolone acetonide
Locoid cream, 0.1%	Hydrocortisone butyrate
Synalar cream or ointment, 0.025%	Fluocinolone acetonide
Westcort cream or ointment, 0.2%	Hydrocortisone valerate
VI. Low potency	
Aclovate cream or ointment, 0.05%	Alclometasone dipropionate
DesOwen cream or ointment or lotion, 0.05%	Desonide
Synalar cream or solution, 0.01%	Fluocinolone acetonide
Tridesilon cream, 0.05%	Desonide
Valisone lotion, 0.05%	Betamethasone valerate
VII. Lowest potency	
Topicals with hydrocortisone, dexamethasone, flumethalone, prednisolone, and methylprednisolone.	

Adapted from Stoughton RB, Cornell RC. Review of superpotent steroids. Semin Dermatol 1987;6:72–76.
[a]Compounds are listed alphabetically, not by strength, within each classification. Potency varies according to the corticosteroid, its concentration, and its vehicle, with ointments generally being more potent than creams.
[b]Use of superpotent steroids should be limited to 2 weeks or less.

Pyoderma

Types

1. Acne: See Chapter 19 for discussion.
2. Folliculitis: Infection of a hair follicle is common and usually involves *S. aureus* or streptococci. The infection is usually superficial and is characterized by tiny pustules near affected hair follicles, surrounded by an area of erythema. Common locations include the scalp, extremities, buttocks, and perioral and perinasal areas. Treatment involves local

hygiene with antibacterial soaps or cleansers and a topical antibiotic ointment. Systemic antibiotics are unnecessary in uncomplicated cases.

   Pseudofolliculitis barbae is a noninfectious, inflammatory condition occurring in men with curly hair, caused by reentry of curved hairs after shaving. Treatment consists of either growing a beard or shaving with either a sharp razor or electric razor. Tretinoin (Retin-A), α-hydroxyacids, and mild topical corticosteroids have been used with limited success.

3. Impetigo: Although most common in children, impetigo does occur in adolescents. It is characterized by discrete and coalescent lesions that begin as vesicles, quickly become pustular, and then rupture, leaving a thick yellowish crust. The lesions are usually related to group A β-hemolytic streptococci or *S. aureus*. Localized infection can be treated with topical mupirocin (Bactroban), but more extensive or recurrent disease requires treatment with systemic antibiotics. Resistance to erythromycin and penicillin is being seen with increasing frequency.
4. Pseudomonas folliculitis or hot tub dermatitis: Pruritic papulopustular eruptions typically appear 1–2 days after exposure to a whirlpool, hot tub, or swimming pool, with a predilection for areas covered by a swimsuit, axillae, and upper arms. Usually resolves in 7–14 days, rarely associated with constitutional symptoms or systemic infection.
5. Furuncles: Staphylococcal abscesses develop around hair follicles. Multiple lesions may coalesce to form a carbuncle. Treatment includes warm compresses, antistaphylococcal antibiotics, and incision and drainage of fluctuant lesions. Recurrent or chronic furunculosis requires eradication of the staphylococcal carrier state.

PAPULOSQUAMOUS ERUPTIONS

Eruptions consisting of scaly patches and plaques that occur with some frequency during adolescence include psoriasis, pityriasis rosea, seborrheic dermatitis, fungal infections, drug eruptions, and secondary syphilis (for a discussion, see Chapter 63).

Psoriasis

Psoriasis affects between 1–3% of the population with the onset being between the ages of 10 and 20 years in nearly 25%.

Etiology   Although the cause of psoriasis is unknown, the role of heredity is becoming more apparent as genetic linkage is being identified.

Precipitating Factors

1. Streptococcal pharyngitis
2. Trauma
3. Stress

Clinical Manifestations

1. Appearance: Round, circumscribed, erythematous plaques with a silvery "micaceous" scale. Small or guttate lesions are often associated with streptococcal pharyngitis.
2. Distribution: Scalp, trunk, elbows and knees are common sites. Nails may show pitting, onycholysis, and oil spots. Inverse psoriasis is limited to the umbilicus and intertriginous areas.
3. Symptoms
   a. Pruritus is variable.

b. Psoriatic arthritis, which is a seronegative polyarthritis, is uncommon in adolescence.
c. Emotional stress and depression may be present.

Diagnosis   Diagnosis of psoriasis is based on typical appearance, location of lesions, or rarely skin biopsy results.

Treatment   Psoriasis may remit spontaneously or as a result of therapy, but recurrences are almost certain. Treatment depends on the severity, duration, and site of disease and on the emotional state and treatment preference of the adolescent.

1. Evaluation and avoidance of precipitating factors
2. Topical therapy should be tried first and can include:
   a. Topical corticosteroids
   b. Tar: Preparations such as Estar gel or Balnetar solution may be more cosmetically pleasing to the adolescent.
   c. Anthralin
   d. Calcipotriene (Dovonex) ointment: A synthetic vitamin D_3 analog useful in treating limited psoriasis
   e. Intralesional corticosteroids: Useful for localized psoriatic plaques; potential side effects—atrophy and hypopigmentation.
   f. Phototherapy with ultraviolet B (UVB) alone or in combination with topical tar preparations; UVA combined with oral or topical psoralens reserved for severe, recalcitrant psoriasis
3. Systemic therapy is rarely indicated in adolescents because of the potential long-term side effects.

Pityriasis Rosea

Pityriasis rosea is a self-limited disorder of unknown cause frequently occurring during adolescence.

Clinical Manifestations

1. Lesions: Oval, salmon-colored papular and macular, 1- to 2-cm scaly lesions, whose long axes follow the body's lines of cleavage in "Christmas tree" distribution. The lesions typically have a fine cigarette-paper-like scale peripherally.
2. Herald patch: The rash is usually preceded by a large, 2- to 6-cm single lesion known as the "herald patch." The interval between the herald patch and other lesions is usually between 2 and 21 days.
3. Distribution: Symmetrical, occurring mainly on the trunk, upper arms, and lower neck, with occasional involvement of face, scalp, hands, and feet.
4. Pruritus: Ranges from very mild to severe.
5. Other systemic symptoms: Constitutional symptoms are rare.

Differential Diagnosis

1. Tinea corporis
2. Secondary syphilis
3. Seborrheic dermatitis

Treatment

1. Reassurance: Condition spontaneously resolves within 6–8 weeks.
2. Antihistamines or topical corticosteroids: Use if pruritus is significant.

Seborrheic Dermatitis

Seborrheic dermatitis is a chronic inflammatory disease of the skin, limited to areas of excessive sebaceous gland activity.

Clinical Manifestations

1. Distribution: Usually involves the scalp, eyebrows, forehead, lips, ears, nasolabial creases, axilla, chest, inframammary folds, umbilicus, and groin
2. Appearance: Dry, moist, or greasy scales often crusted with yellow patches of various sizes
3. Pruritus: May or may not be present
4. Course marked by many remissions and exacerbations

Differential Diagnosis

1. Psoriasis
2. Tinea corporis
3. Pityriasis rosea
4. Atopic and contact dermatitis

Treatment

1. Scalp should be shampooed two to three times weekly with either a tar (Ionil T Plus, Pentrax, Zetar), selenium sulfide (Selsun), sulfur (Sebulex), zinc (Zincon, DHS Zinc), or ketoconazole 2% (Nizoral) shampoo.
2. Hydrocortisone 1–2.5% or, if necessary, low-potency nonfluorinated topical corticosteroids may be used sparingly for short periods of time on the face. Many topical corticosteroid preparations are available in a solution for the scalp.

Fungal Infections

The dermatophytoses are the most common fungal disease of the skin. The three principal genera responsible are *Trichophyton, Microsporum,* and *Epidermophyton.* These are responsible for tinea capitis, tinea corporis, tinea pedis, tinea barbae, tinea cruris, and tinea unguium (onychomycosis). Other common superficial fungal infections in adolescents include tinea or pityriasis versicolor caused by *Pityrosporum orbiculare* and *Candida albicans,* which is the causative agent in many cases of intertrigo, paronychia, vaginitis, and pruritus ani.

Dermatophytoses

1. Tinea capitis: Tinea capitis is a dermatophyte infection of the scalp and hair follicles, most commonly caused by *Trichophyton tonsurans.* It most commonly presents as an enlarging scaly patch of alopecia often consisting of broken hairs (black dots). A granulomatous mass, a kerion, can develop in response to the infection. Some of these fungi are spread by contact with objects such as combs, brushes, and hats, and others from cats and dogs. The diagnosis can be made by either fluorescence of the infected hairs with a Wood's lamp, examination of the hairs with potassium hydroxide, or culture of infected hairs. Some studies show that only one-third of individuals will have positive results from examination of a potassium hydroxide specimen, so one cannot necessarily rely on the potassium hydroxide examination alone. If the diagnosis is in question, a culture can be taken. Treatment is with systemic griseofulvin microsize 250–500 mg/day or ultramicrosize 330–375 mg/day. Treatment is continued for 6–8 weeks, or at least 2 weeks after

a negative culture. Itraconazole 100 mg/day has been used in resistant cases or in patients who cannot tolerate griseofulvin. In addition, topical selenium sulfide 2.5% or keto-conazole 2% shampoo should be used twice weekly to reduce the shedding of spores.

2. Tinea barbae: A dermatophyte infection of the bearded area. This disease is more common in adolescents living in rural areas who work with farm animals. The involvement is mostly one-sided on the neck or face and results in either deep nodular suppurative lesions or superficial, crusted, partially bald patches. Treatment is with griseofulvin 500 mg daily for 4–6 weeks.

3. Tinea corporis: This dermatophyte infection may involve any area of the body except for the scalp, beard, face, hands, feet, and groin. It is characterized by a gradually expanding, circular, red ring with a raised margin containing scales and minute vesicles. Pruritus is common. There is a tendency for central healing. The diagnosis is confirmed by a potassium hydroxide examination of a skin scraping or a culture of the fungus. The differential diagnosis includes the other papulosquamous eruptions. If the lesions are localized, topical therapy can be chosen from a variety of agents (Table 20.2). If the lesions are widespread or resist local therapy, griseofulvin 500 mg daily for approximately 4 weeks is effective. Treat sources of infection such as pets, infected family members or other close contacts, including those that occur during sports such as wrestling.

4. Tinea cruris: Commonly called "jock itch" or "crotch rot," this is a common dermatophyte infection of the groin in adolescent males. The lesions are usually found on the upper and inner surfaces of the thighs, especially during summer months. Typical lesions are bilateral or unilateral, crescent shaped, reddish, and scaly, with sharply defined, raised borders. The scrotum is usually unaffected. The diagnosis is generally made on the basis of clinical appearance, negative findings from Wood's lamp examination, and the presence of branching hyphae on potassium hydroxide wet mount. Cultures of the scales can be performed, if necessary, for diagnosis. Differential diagnosis of common groin eruptions includes:

TABLE 20.2. Topical Antifungal Drugs and Coverage

Drug	Coverage		
	Candida	Dermatophyte	Tinea Versicolor
Imidazole compounds			
Clotrimazole (Lotrimin, Mycelex)	+	+	+
Econazole nitrate (Spectazole)	+	+	+
Ketoconazole (Nizoral)	+	+	+
Miconazole nitrate (Monistat-Derm, Micatin Zeasorb-AF powder)	+	+	+
Oxiconazole nitrate (Oxistat)		+	
Sulconazole nitrate (Exelderm)		+	+
Iodinated trichlorophenol			
Haloprogin (Halotex)		+	+
Pyridone-ethanolamine salt			
Ciclopirox olamine (Loprox)	+	+	+
Allylamine compounds			
Naftifine HCL (Naftin)		+	
Terbinafine HCL (Lamisil)		+	
Polyenes			
Amphotericin B (Fungizone)	+		
Nystatin(Mycostatin)	+		
Undecylenic acid			
Desenex, Pedi-Dri, Pedi-Pro, Cruex		+	
Tolnaftate			
Tinactin, Aftate, Tritin, Ting		+	?

Adapted from Cohn M. Superficial fungal infections. Postgrad Med 1992;91:249.

    a. Tinea cruris

    b. Candidiasis
- Eruptions are more inflammatory.
- The margins are less discrete, with individual satellite papules or pustules outside the confluent area.
- The scrotum is commonly affected.
- A potassium hydroxide preparation reveals budding yeast and pseudohyphae.

    c. Erythrasma
- The rash appears as a well-defined pinkish or brownish patch.
- The rash fluoresces a coral red under a Wood's lamp.
- Potassium hydroxide preparation may show negative results, but Gram's stain may show Gram-positive filamentous rods (*Corynebacterium minutissimum*).

    d. Psoriasis
- Often accompanied by psoriatic lesions elsewhere
- Negative findings from potassium hydroxide preparation and Wood's lamp examination
- Biopsy helpful

    e. Intertrigo
- Red, macerated, foul-smelling skin in inguinal creases
- Obesity a predisposing factor

    f. Seborrheic dermatitis
- Erythematous eruption with a well-demarcated, nonraised border
- Typical lesions elsewhere
- Negative findings from potassium hydroxide wet mount and Wood's lamp examination

    g. Neurodermatitis
- Leathery, lichenified, mottled eruption with ill-defined borders
- Negative findings from potassium hydroxide preparation and Wood's lamp examination

    h. Irritant dermatitis
- History of use of sprays, soaps, detergents, or medication

    i. Other pruritic groin rashes include scabies, pediculosis pubis, miliaria. Treatment of some of these other common groin eruptions includes:
- Candidiasis: Topical nystatin, ketoconazole, or miconazole cream two to three times a day
- Erythrasma: Topical erythromycin two times a day or systemic erythromycin 250 mg four times a day
- Psoriasis: Low-potency topical corticosteroids
- Intertrigo: Keep affected area dry and use drying powders
- Seborrheic dermatitis: Low-potency (class VI–VII) topical corticosteroids
- Neurodermatitis: Low-potency topical corticosteroids

5. Tinea pedis: A dermatophyte infection involving the soles of the feet and the toe webs. Early signs are scaling, maceration, and fissuring of the toe webs. This can extend to scaling, redness, and vesicular eruptions on the soles. Tight-fitting occlusive footwear and warm, humid weather predispose the adolescent to infection. The infection is often transmitted through shared bath and shower facilities. Potassium hydroxide examination will reveal branching hyphae. Tinea pedis can be confused with intertrigo, erythrasma, candidiasis, dyshidrosis, psoriasis, and contact dermatitis. Treatment for tinea pedis consists of:

    a. Employ a regimen of soaks or wet compresses with Burow's or Domboro's solution for 15–30 minutes two to four times daily.

b. Secondary bacterial infection should be treated with topical or oral antibiotics depending on severity.

c. A topical antifungal agent can be helpful; but if infection is severe or unresponsive, a course of griseofulvin microsize 500 mg/day or ultramicrosize 660–750 mg/day for 4–8 weeks may be helpful.

d. If there is a severe inflammatory response or an "id" reaction (see item 7), a short, 1-week course of topical or systemic steroids is helpful.

e. Keep feet dry and well aerated; sandals should be worn if possible or white cotton socks with shoes.

f. Use a prophylactic program of drying the feet thoroughly after baths, and then use a medicated powder such as Tinactin or Zeasorb-AF, once the infection is over.

6. Tinea unguium: Tinea unguium is a dermatophyte infection of the nail plate. Onychomycosis includes all infections of the nail caused by any fungus, including dermatophytes and yeast. The infection begins with a white or yellow discoloration of the distal part of the nail. The nail subsequently becomes thickened, brittle, elevated, and deformed. Identification of the causative organism is essential for therapy. It is important to sample the nail layer near the nail bed for culture. Various nail dystrophies, including psoriasis, may be confused with onychomycosis. Griseofulvin is the most effective cure, but therapy may require more than a year of treatment; thus, griseofulvin should be reserved for motivated adolescents. The alternative to systemic therapy is removal of the nail plus topical therapy. Sporanox 100 mg twice daily for 3 months has recently been approved.

7. Dermatophytid: An "id" reaction is a cutaneous or systemic reaction to the fungal antigen borne through the bloodstream from the primary fungal focus to sensitized areas of the skin. The condition is often associated with dermatophytoses of the scalp and feet, and rarely causes systemic problems including fever, anorexia, adenopathy, and leukocytosis. The reaction may consist of a widespread follicular, scaly eruption or may be limited to a vesiculobullous or scaly eruption of the hands. The former is more commonly associated with tinea capitis and the latter with tinea pedis.

Tinea (Pityriasis) Versicolor

1. Clinical manifestations: Scaly hypopigmented or hyperpigmented macules or patches typically located over the upper trunk and arms, and occasionally the face and neck caused by *Pityrosporum orbiculare*. The lesions are usually asymptomatic.

2. Predisposing factors: Humidity, hyperhidrosis, heredity, diabetes, systemic corticosteroids.

3. Diagnosis: Made by observation of hyphae and spores (spaghetti and meatballs) on potassium hydroxide wet mount. Wood's light examination is helpful in showing yellowish or brownish fluorescence.

4. Differential diagnosis: Pityriasis alba, vitiligo, pityriasis rosea, seborrheic dermatitis, and syphilis.

5. Treatment

a. Topicals: Selenium sulfide 2.5% shampoo, zinc pyrithione shampoo or soap, sulfur-salicylic acid, Tinver lotion (25% sodium thiosulfate, 1% salicylic acid, and 10% alcohol). Usually these agents are used in the shower or overnight as tolerated daily for 2 weeks, then several times a month for maintenance. Topical antifungals of the imidazole class are effective but expensive for large areas of involvement.

b. Systemic ketoconazole (Nizoral) 400 mg as a single dose or taken on 2 consecutive days has been shown to be effective, as has 200–400 mg daily for 5–10 days. Hepatitis, however, has been reported with short courses of ketoconazole.

Drug Eruptions

A skin rash is one of the most common side effects of drug administration. Many drugs can cause skin reactions of various types. The most commonly implicated drugs are sulfamethoxazole, ampicillin, penicillin, gentamicin, cephalosporins, barbiturates, and isoniazid. Other drugs used by adolescents that cause skin eruptions less often are diphenhydramine, aspirin, aminophylline, codeine, and tetracycline. The following are various skin eruptions and implicated agents.

1. Maculopapular or morbilliform rash

   Ampicillin or amoxicillin: Reaction
      rate is nearly 90% in patients
      with infectious mononucleosis.
   Barbiturates
   Carbamazepine
   Diazepam and related compounds
   Erythromycin
   Furosemide

   Gold
   Isoniazid
   Penicillin
   Phenytoin
   Salicylates
   Sulfonamides
   Tetracycline
   Thiazides

2. Urticaria

   Nonimmunologic
   Aspirin
   Contrast media
   Opiates
   Nonsteroidal anti-inflammatory drugs

   Immunologic
   Barbiturates
   Penicillin
   Sulfonamides
   Tetracyclines

3. Erythema multiforme: Generalized erythematous macules or bullae with targetoid lesions. Mucosae may be involved and fever may accompany more severe reactions.

   Allopurinol
   Barbiturates
   Bromides
   Chloramphenicol
   Gold salts
   Griseofulvin

   Hydralazine
   Penicillin
   Phenothiazines
   Phenylbutazone
   Phenytoin
   Salicylates

   Sulfonamides
   Tetanus antitoxin
   Tetracycline
   Thiazide diuretics
   Vaccines (measles, polio, diphtheria)

4. Erythema nodosum

   Bromides
   Codeine

   Oral contraceptives
   Penicillin

   Salicylates
   Sulfonamides

5. Exfoliative dermatitis

   Allopurinol
   Barbiturates
   Codeine
   Gold
   Isoniazid

   Penicillin
   Phenyl
   Phenothiazines
   Phenytoin

   Quinacrine
   Sulfonamides
   Tetracycline
   Vitamin A

6. Acneform eruptions

   Adrenocorticotropic hormone (ACTH)
   Androgenic hormones
   Bromides

   Corticosteroids
   Hydantoins
   Iodides

Isoniazid	Phenobarbital
Lithium	Vitamin B_{12}
Oral contraceptives	

7. Photosensitive eruptions

Coal tar	Griseofulvin	Sulfonamides
Disinfectants	Phenothiazines	Tetracyclines
Dyes	Psoralens	Thiazide diuretics
Essential oils		

8. Fixed drug eruptions: One or few erythematous or hyperpigmented ovoid lesions sometimes containing bullae. They occur in same location with repeated exposure to the inciting drug.

Barbiturates	Penicillin	Quinacrine
Erythromycin	Phenolphthalein	Sulfonamides
Gold	Pseudoephedrine	Tetracycline
Metronidazole	hydrochloride	Trimethoprim

Secondary Syphilis

For a discussion, see Chapter 63.

SKIN GROWTHS

Warts: Verrucae

1. Etiology: *Papillomavirus* (DNA virus of papovavirus family). Many different human papilloma virus (HPV) types have been identified. Although there is some association between HPV type and the clinical type of wart, this is not a 100% correlation. HPV types 2 and 4 are associated with common warts.
2. Epidemiology
   a. Age: Peak prevalence is between ages 10 and 19; thereafter, the prevalence decreases.
   b. Prevalence: Seven percent to 10% of general population.
   c. Transmission: Inoculation occurs by direct or indirect contact from one person to another; autoinoculation is common. Local trauma promotes inoculation.
   d. Incubation: 1–6 months.
3. Clinical manifestations: The clinical classification and appearance of a wart is dependent on the wart's location on the skin.
   a. Verruca vulgaris
      — Single or multiple in occurrence
      — Most frequently occur on hands, fingers and periungually, but can occur anywhere
      — Usually sharply circumscribed, firm hyperkeratotic papules 1–5 mm in diameter when located on hands
      — Filiform warts, projecting as threadlike structures often when located on neck and face
   b. Verruca plana (flat warts)
      — Flat skin-colored or pink lesions, 1–3 mm, smooth and slightly raised
      — Commonly occur on face, dorsa of hands, wrists, and knees
      — Often numerous and may occur in a linear pattern from spreading of the virus as a result of scratching or trauma such as shaving

    c. Verruca plantaris (plantar warts)
- Occur on the plantar surface of feet, usually at points of pressure
- Do not extend above the skin surface; covered by hyperkeratotic material
- May occur as an isolated lesion or in groups (mosaic warts)
- May appear as multiple small black points, which represent thrombosed blood vessels

    d. Condylomata acuminata (venereal warts): Moist, polypoid warts located in genital area and may be transmitted venereally. These are discussed in Chapter 66.

4. Treatment: Warts vary in natural history. Some warts disappear spontaneously after several months or years, while others remain unchanged or spread. Recurrence rate is high regardless of choice of therapy.

    a. Cryotherapy: Application of liquid nitrogen is an effective method of treating most warts and usually causes less skin scarring than electrodesiccation. Flat warts tend to be resistant to therapy and should be treated minimally to avoid scarring. Light freezing with liquid nitrogen is of value. Topical tretinoin can also be used to treat flat warts. The procedure for freezing warts is as follows:
- Dip cotton applicator in liquid nitrogen.
- Apply only long enough to turn wart white.
- Avoid freezing surrounding tissue, especially near digital vessels and nerves at the sides of fingers.
- Over 1–2 weeks, a blister forms, becomes hemorrhagic, and peels off with part or all of wart.
- The procedure may need to be repeated.

    b. Electrodesiccation and curettage: This treatment requires expert skill to avoid unnecessary destruction and scarring.

    c. Acid: Trichloroacetic acid and bichloroacetic acid are especially useful in plantar warts. The treatment is as follows:
- Pare the wart.
- Paint the wart with acid and work into wart with needle or toothpick by carefully sticking wart several times.
- Can dress with salicylic acid pads. May repeat in 1 week.

    d. Podophyllin: Condylomata acuminatum can effectively be treated with 20–25% podophyllin in benzoin, or trichloroacetic acid (80–90%).

    e. Carbon dioxide laser surgery, bleomycin, tretinoin, 5-fluorouracil, and immunotherapy have been used to treat recalcitrant warts.

Molluscum Contagiosum

Molluscum contagiosum is a common, viral-caused growth. For more information, see Chapter 66.

Parasitic Skin Infections

1. Pediculosis: See Chapter 67.
2. Scabies: See Chapter 67.

MISCELLANEOUS SKIN CONDITIONS

Vitiligo

Vitiligo is an acquired, disfiguring disease characterized by the loss of melanin, resulting in depigmented areas of the skin. It is associated with ocular abnormalities, autoantibodies, thyroid disease, diabetes mellitus, and leukotrichia (depigmentations of the hair).

Epidemiology

1. Age of onset: Fifty percent of cases begin in the second and third decade of life.
2. Prevalence: Vitiligo occurs in approximately 1–2% of the population. Prevalence increases to 8–20% if hyperthyroidism, thyroiditis, pernicious anemia, juvenile diabetes mellitus, or uveitis is present.

Etiology   The cause is unknown, but autoimmune mechanisms are speculated.

Clinical Manifestations

1. Depigmented, well-circumscribed, cutaneous white macules, several millimeters to several centimeters, appear on the skin, usually noticed first during the summer months.
2. Any area can be affected, but the face and extremities are most common.
3. Usually the distribution is bilateral and symmetrical.
4. Wood's light examination is helpful in identifying early lesions.

Differential Diagnosis   Morphea (localized scleroderma), pityriasis alba, and tinea versicolor may be confused with vitiligo.

Treatment   Although treatment is difficult, it is improving.

1. Use of sunscreens for photoprotection and avoidance of sun
2. Use of a cover-up cosmetic such as Dermablend or Covermark
3. A 2- to 3-month trial of a low- to mid-potency topical corticosteroid
4. Topical or oral psoralens followed by long wavelength ultraviolet radiation (UVA) radiation: Must be used with great caution and administered by a practitioner experienced in their use
5. Autologous skin grafts
6. Spontaneous repigmentation rarely occurs

Sunburn

Teenagers often spend long days at the beach or are involved in athletic activities without attempting to protect their skin from the sun. Sunburn can be a frequent summer problem. Recommendations to adolescents include:

1. Midday exposure: Avoid exposure from 10 AM to 3 PM, when the sun's short ultraviolet rays are at their peak. Adjust 1 hour for daylight savings time.
2. Acclimating: Gradually increase exposure time to sun.
3. Clothing: Wear protective clothing and a hat when possible.
4. Sunscreens: Sunscreens do not prevent a tan but they do lessen burning. A sunprotective factor (SPF) of 15 or greater with a broad spectrum of coverage should be used regularly (Table 20.3).
5. Temperature: The cooling effect of water and wind at the beach decreases the ability to detect sunburn; therefore, the adolescent must be educated to the sun's strong effects.
6. Medications: Certain medications can increase photosensitivity. These include griseofulvin, oral contraceptives, diphenhydramine, phenothiazines, psoralen, sulfonamides, tetracyclines, and tranquilizers.

Photoallergic reactions are uncommon, immunologically mediated responses to small amounts of the offending agent. Phototoxic reactions appear as an exaggerated sunburn and occur in nearly all individuals with sufficient exposure to the offending drug.

TABLE 20.3.   Sunscreens and Protective Spectrum[a]

	Spectrum
Chemical	
PABA	UVB
Cinnamates	UVB
Benzophenones	UVB (some UVA)
Parsol 1789 (butylmethoxydibenzoyl-methane)	UVA
Physical	
Zinc oxide	UVA/UVB
Titanium dioxide	UVA/UVB

[a]PABA, *p*-aminobenzoic acid; UVA, ultraviolet A; UVB, ultraviolet B.

Urticaria

Urticaria, or hives, is an extremely common problem occurring in 15–20% of adolescents.

Appearance   Appearance is that of transient, discrete, erythematous wheals, which may coalesce and form large edematous patches with raised borders. Simple urticaria involves only the superficial layers of the skin, while angioedema is a deeper reaction involving both skin and the mucous membranes. Severe pruritus or stinging sensations can occur.

Classifications

1. Acute urticaria: Onset of less than 6 weeks.
2. Chronic urticaria: Duration of greater than 6 weeks.
3. Drug induced: Penicillin and sulfonamides are the most common drugs involved.
4. Food: Urticaria after eating most commonly involves ingestion of nuts, fish, eggs, fresh berries, shellfish, or food additives. Some of these reactions are immunologically related, while others are caused by direct release of histamine.
5. Inhalants: Many airborne particles such as pollen, animal dander, and mold spores can induce urticaria.
6. Insect and arthropod bites and stings.
7. Infections: Various bacterial, virus, and parasitic infections have been suggested as possible causes of urticaria.
8. Neoplasias: Hodgkin's disease has been associated with urticaria.
9. Thyroid disease
10. Physical urticarias
11. Cholinergic urticaria: This reaction can be triggered by heat, exercise, or stress. Cholinergic urticaria is produced by the reaction of acetylcholine on the mast cell. It is characterized by highly pruritic, punctate wheals 1–3 mm in diameter. These wheals are surrounded by large areas of erythema. The palms and soles are always spared. Aquagenic urticaria may be a form of cholinergic urticaria that produces a similar reaction on contact with water. The diagnosis can be confirmed by either soaking a foot in hot water, exercising the adolescent, or using a methacholine (Mecholyl) skin test. These will all reproduce the lesions.
12. Heat urticaria
13. Cold urticaria: Localized or generalized hives develop with exposure to cold air or water, rarely accompanied by syncope, hypotension, and drowning. Hereditary and acquired variants exist. The diagnosis may be confirmed in most cases with an ice cube test. Cyproheptadine (Periactin) is helpful, but desensitization may be necessary.
14. Pressure urticaria: Urticaria in response to slight pressure, such as sitting or clapping.
15. Solar urticaria

16. Vibratory urticaria
17. Dermatographism: Characterized by the development of localized wheals and erythema, following stroking of the skin with a blunt instrument.
18. Contact urticaria: Caused by direct contact with certain chemicals, plants, and arthropods (caterpillars).

Treatment

1. Avoid the inciting factor, if known. Use of elimination diets may be helpful in determining a specific food involved.
2. Antihistamines are effective, but primarily in acute urticaria. Hydroxyzine (Atarax) 25 mg three times a day is the drug of choice in cholinergic urticaria and dermatographism.
3. Epinephrine is useful if the urticaria is associated with angioedema.
4. Systemic steroids are beneficial in severe acute reactions, especially with associated angioedema.
5. Cold baths or showers may be helpful in relieving some of the itching.

Hereditary Angioedema

Hereditary angioedema is an autosomal dominant disease resulting in sudden attacks of edema of the soft tissue or mucous membranes of the pharynx and larynx. Gastrointestinal edema can occur, causing nausea, vomiting, and severe abdominal pain. Laryngeal edema can cause death. Often, hereditary angioedema first appears during adolescence and can occur as frequently as every 2 weeks. Attacks can be precipitated by stress or trauma or can occur spontaneously. A low level of C1 esterase inhibitor is found in 85% of patients, while in the other 15% the inhibitor is nonfunctional. The decrease or nonfunctional C1 esterase inhibitor allows for increased activity of the complement system.

Diagnosis The serum C4 level is used as a screening test, as it is reduced even when the patient is asymptomatic. The C2 level is reduced during attacks. If these levels are reduced and the C1 inhibitor protein level is normal, a functional assay should be performed.

Treatment Treatment of acute episodes involves administration of epinephrine, ethacrynic acid, or metalluride and, if necessary, tracheostomy. Antihistamines and corticosteroids are generally not effective. Prophylactic treatment involves the use of ε-aminocaproic acid, danazol, or stanozolol.

Hair Loss

Hair loss can be extremely frightening and traumatic to an adolescent. Evaluating an adolescent with a complaint of hair loss involves a thorough history and physical examination and an understanding of hair physiology.

Hair Physiology Scalp hair grows at the rate of 0.35 mm/day. The rate is faster in females and in summer months. The average daily loss is 25–100 hairs from a total of about 100,000. Eighty percent to 90% of hair is in the growing, or anagen, phase. Anagen hairs have a heavy external root sheath that looks like a gelatinous capsule around the lower third of the hair. Ten percent to 15% of hair is in the resting, or telogen, phase. These hairs have a smooth shaft ending in a short bulbous root. Approximately 5% or less of hairs are in a transitional or catagen phase.

Hair Conditions

1. Male pattern baldness: This is produced in genetically susceptible individuals, resulting in a loss of hair secondary to the effects of androgenic hormones. Usually only scalp hair

is involved. Baldness usually does not occur until the late twenties or thirties, but premature alopecia can occur in the teens or early twenties.

2. Telogen effluvium: Acute illness, surgery, or other severe stress can stop hair growth and cause hairs to go into the telogen phase. When hair resumes growth 6–10 weeks later, resting hair is shed. This condition presents as acute general hair loss 2–4 months after a stressful event. Illness, surgery, "crash dieting," parturition, discontinuation of oral contraceptives, anticoagulants, and hypervitaminosis A have been known to trigger an episode of telogen effluvium.

3. Anagen effluvium: Anagen effluvium is hair loss occurring during the growing phase. Common causes include antimitotic drugs used for chemotherapy, immunosuppressive drugs, warfarin (Coumadin), heparin, arsenic, and gentamicin. In anagen effluvium, the hair develops a focal weakness above the bulb so that the anagen bulb is usually not shed with the hair.

4. Alopecia areata: Alopecia areata is characterized by rapid and complete hair loss in patches, usually involving the scalp, bearded area, eyebrows, or eyelashes. If the hair loss involves the entire scalp, the condition is referred to as alopecia totalis, and if the loss includes the whole body, alopecia universalis. Alopecia areata may be associated with pitting of the nails. The tendency is for spontaneous recovery, but the prognosis is worse with decreasing age and increasing involvement. In 25% of cases, the condition is permanent.
   a. Etiology: Autoimmunity, atopy, hereditary factors, and stress are all implicated; however, the cause is still unknown.
   b. Diagnosis: Clinical presentation of sharply circumscribed patches of alopecia with exclamation point hairs at the periphery of the bald patch.
   c. Differential diagnosis: Tinea capitis, early lupus erythematosus, and trichotillomania.
   d. Treatment: Reported successes have included intralesional corticosteroids, topical corticosteroids alone or in combination with topical minoxidil (Rogaine), anthralin, dinitrochlorobenzene (DNCB), squaric acid dibutyl ester, diphencyprone, and photochemotherapy (PUVA).

5. Hair loss secondary to physical factors
   a. Traction alopecia: Hair loss at the margin of scalp, occurring primarily in African-American females and in women who wear hair tightly braided.
   b. Hot comb alopecia
   c. Trichotillomania: Irregular patches of hair loss secondary to breaking or removal of hairs on the scalp, eyebrows, or eyelashes by plucking, twirling, or rubbing. It is associated with emotional stress, or less commonly a psychiatric disorder.

6. Scalp disease: Hair loss can occur secondary to various scalp diseases, including psoriasis, fungal disease, seborrhea, or eczema.

7. Metabolic disorders: Hair loss can be found with iron deficiency, hypothyroidism, hyperthyroidism, diabetes mellitus, or hypopituitarism.

8. Systemic diseases: Hair loss can be seen with lupus erythematosus.

9. Scarring alopecia: This form of irreversible hair loss is the end result of a variety of inflammatory processes or trauma. Some dermatologic conditions that may result in scarring include discoid lupus erythematosus, scleroderma, lichen planus, acne keloidalis, folliculitis decalvans, and dissecting cellulitis of the scalp.

10. Hair-shaft structural defects: Various defects in hair structure can result in hair loss. These defects are often associated with abnormalities of the skin, teeth, breast, nails, and bones. Metabolic disorders and mental retardation can also occur. These conditions include pili torti, monilethrix, trichorrhexis, pili annulati, and Menkes' kinky-hair syndrome. A discussion of these conditions can be found in Hurwitz (1993).

Evaluation

1. History: An extensive history is indicated, including the onset and duration of hair loss, drug use, skin or scalp disease, and recent stress, surgery, illness, or dietary changes.
2. Physical examination: Check especially for evidence of seborrhea, scalp disease, or an endocrine disorder.
3. Pull test: Lightly grasp about 20 hairs and pull gently. Normally 1 or 2 telogen hairs will come out. In an adolescent with hair-shaft damage, telogen effluvium, alopecia areata, or anagen effluvium, hair pulls out in great quantities. If many hairs pull out, microscopic examination of the hairs will determine if anagen or telogen hair loss is present.
4. Examine scalp closely and perform a potassium hydroxide test if indicated. A fungal culture of the hair and scalp may also be productive.
5. A complete blood count, urinalysis, liver function tests, thyroid studies, serum ferritin, and a fasting blood glucose are ordered as indicated.
6. Referral to a dermatologist may be necessary for further evaluation and scalp biopsy if diagnosis is in question.

Tattoos

Tattoos may be a problem among adolescents. The tattoo may have been applied as a result of a dare, peer pressure, or gang participation. Numerous reactions can occur:

1. Hypersensitivity to the dye
2. Unsanitary methods have resulted in hepatitis, tuberculosis, and syphilis. Concern about transmission of human immunodeficiency virus (HIV) infection exists.
3. Keloids can form.

Treatment is not entirely satisfactory; but with the advent of new lasers, treatment has resulted in less scarring than older methods such as excision, dermabrasion, or carbon dioxide laser surgery.

Primary Syphilis and Herpes Simplex

For a discussion of primary syphilis and herpes simplex, see Chapters 64 and 65.

Hyperhidrosis

Hyperhidrosis is excessive sweating in response to heat or emotional stimuli. Treatment with topical aluminum chloride preparations such as Certain-Dri, Xerac AC, or Drysol is often beneficial. Systemic anticholinergic agents, glutaraldehyde, and iontophoresis have been also been used with varying degrees of success.

Bromhidrosis

Bromhidrosis is malodorous sweating that may be apocrine or eccrine in origin and is caused by bacteria. Good hygiene includes the use of antibacterial soaps, topical antibiotics, antiperspirants, Burow's or potassium permanganate soaks, and absorbent powders.

Pink Pearly Penile Papules

Pink pearly penile papules are a normal occurrence in about 15% of postpubertal males. The lesions appear as elongated papillae, about 1–3 mm in diameter, located on the coronal margin of the penis, especially the anterior border. They often appear in one to five rows and are usually of uniform size and shape. The color tends to be pearly white. Microscopically, they have a normal epidermal appearance except for absent pigment in the basal layer. In contrast, condylomata acuminata tend to be of less uniform size and shape, change over time, and are not neatly arranged around the corona of the penis. No treatment is necessary except reassurance.

Acanthosis Nigricans

Acanthosis nigricans appears as a gray-brown thickening of the skin. It is manifested as symmetrical, velvety, papulomatous plaques, with increased skinfold markings. The lesions are commonly located on the base of the neck axilla, groin, and antecubital fossa. The lesions may also occur on the dorsum of the hand, elbow, periumbilical skin, and mucous membranes. It is commonly found during a routine physical examination in an otherwise healthy obese adolescent. Occasionally, a parent is concerned as to why the teen does not wash themselves.

Acanthosis can be classified into benign and malignant. The vast majority of acanthosis nigricans lesions in adolescents are not associated with a malignancy. The common associations in teens are obesity, diabetes mellitus, and HAIRAN syndrome (hyperandrogenism, insulin resistance, and acanthosis nigricans) and other endocrinopathies.

The condition is difficult to treat. Benzoyl peroxide, and tretinoin (Retin-A) have been tried but without any controlled studies demonstrating efficacy.

BIBLIOGRAPHY

Cobb MW. Human papillomavirus infection. J Am Acad Dermatol 1990;22:547.

Cohn MS. Superficial fungal infections: topical and oral treatment of common types. Postgrad Med 1992;91:239.

Dunagin WG, Millikan LE. Drug eruptions. Med Clin North Am 1980;64:983.

Dunn JF Jr. Vitiligo. Am Fam Physician 1986;33:137.

Dunn JF Jr. Pseudofolliculitis. Am Fam Physician 1988;38:169.

Elder JT, Nair RP, Sun-Wei G, et al. The genetics of psoriasis. Arch Dermatol 1994;130:216.

Farber EM, Nall L. Guttate psoriasis. Cutis 1993;51:157.

Fenske NA, Johnson SA. Major causes of alopecia, with suggestions for history taking, work up, and therapy. Postgrad Med 1976;60:79.

Fisher AA. Contact dermatitis. Philadelphia: Lea & Febiger, 1986.

Fragola LA Jr, Watson PE. Common groin eruptions: diagnosis and treatment. Postgrad Med 1981;69:159.

Greaves MW. Chronic urticaria. N Engl J Med 1995;332:1767.

Greaves MW, Weinstein GD. Treatment of psoriasis. N Engl J Med 1994;332:581.

Grimes PE. Vitiligo: an overview of therapeutic approaches. Dermatol Clin 1993;11(20):325.

Guercio-Hauer C, Macfarlane DF, Deleo VA. Photodamage, photoaging and photoprotection of the skin. Am Fam Physician 1994;50:327.

Headington JT. Telogen effluvium: new concepts and review. Arch Dermatol 1993;129:356.

Helm TN. Evaluation of alopecia. JAMA 1995;273:897.

Howard R, Frieden IJ. Tinea capitis: new perspectives on an old disease. Semin Dermatol 1995;14:2.

Hurwitz S. Clinical pediatric dermatology. Philadelphia: WB Saunders, 1993.

Jacobs PH. Ketoconazole use in tinea versicolor. West J Med 1987;147:547.

Laude TA. Approach to dermatologic disorders in black children. Semin Dermatol 1995;14:15.

Levy ML. Disorders of the hair and scalp in children. Pediatr Clin North Am 1991;38(4):905.

Mahmood T. Urticaria. Am Fam Physician 1995;51:811.

Mallory SB, Watts JC. Sunburn, sun reactions, and sun protection. Pediatr Ann 1987;16:77.

McBurnery EI. Vitiligo: Clinical picture and pathogenesis. Arch Intern Med 1979;139:1295.

Nielson TA, Reichel M. Alopecia: diagnosis and management. Am Fam Physician 1995;51:1513.

Obrien JM. Common skin problems of infancy, childhood, and adolescence. Prim Care 1995;22:99.

Odom R. Diagnosis and treatment of common fungal infections. Mod Med 1987a;55:34.

Odom R. A practical review of antifungals. Mod Med 1987b;55:59.

Parish LC, Witkowski JA. Cutaneous bacterial infections: how to manage primary, secondary and tertiary lesions. Postgrad Med 1992;91:119.

Perret CM, Steijlen PM, Happle R. Alopecia areata: pathogenesis and topical immunotherapy. Int J Dermatol 1990;29:83.

Przybilla B, Eberlein-Konig B, Rueff F. Practical management of atopic eczema. Lancet 1994;343:1342.

Sahn EE. Alopecia areata in childhood. Semin Dermatol 1995;14:9.

Seville RH. Stress and psoriasis: the importance of insight and empathy in prognosis. J Am Acad Dermatol 1989;20:97.

Sterling GB. Sunscreens: a review. Cutis 1992;50:221.

SECTION VI

Neurological Disorders

CHAPTER 21

Epilepsy

Wendy G. Mitchell and Lawrence S. Neinstein

Epilepsy is the most common chronic neurological condition in adolescents. It is defined as recurrent, usually transient, episodes of disturbed central nervous system (CNS) function (seizures), excluding extracerebral causes such as syncope, hypoglycemia, or episodic psychiatric syndromes. Epilepsy has been reported since Biblical times and has been seen differently by different cultures. Views have ranged from veneration of epileptics as mystics to imprisoning them or placing them in mental hospitals. As recently as 1965 two states prohibited marriage if a person had epilepsy, and until the early 1970s immigration into the United States was prohibited for people with epilepsy. The majority of adolescents with epilepsy have the potential for excellent control with medication and high likelihood of eventual remission of their epilepsy. Recent advances in basic science have contributed to the understanding of mechanisms of epilepsy and seizures. New medications and surgical techniques have improved the outcome of severe, intractable epilepsy. Despite this, fears, prejudices, and social stigma remain common. Epilepsy is thus somewhat more challenging to treat in teens than other chronic illnesses.

Epilepsy is a difficult condition for patients of all ages. However, for the adolescent concurrently undergoing the stresses of peer relationships, independence, and body image, epilepsy can be especially trying. The goals of management of epilepsy include proper diagnosis, evaluation, treatment of underlying etiologies, appropriate use of anticonvulsant drugs, and recognizing and dealing with the many associated psychosocial problems.

ETIOLOGY

Seizures are caused by an excessive discharge of a population of cortical neurons. The location and pattern of spread of activity determine the clinical expression. Seizures may be due to acute physiological or neurological disturbances or due to epilepsy. Recurrent *unprovoked* seizures are the hallmark of epilepsy. The diagnosis of epilepsy does not imply a specific etiologic factor in the individual. Epilepsy may be genetic, idiopathic, or secondary, due to remote insult to the nervous system. Acutely, seizures may also be provoked by infection, trauma, metabolic disturbances, drugs, drug withdrawal, or fever. Seizures that occur *only* in the setting of an acute provocation are not generally classified as epilepsy, although in some epileptics, specific stimuli or situations provoke seizures.

EPIDEMIOLOGY

1. Prevalence: One in 200 in the general population, with a higher prevalence in children.
2. Incidence: Annual incidence is 1:1000.

3. Onset: Peak periods for the onset of idiopathic and age-related primary epilepsies are during the early school years and during adolescence. The onset of secondary (remote symptomatic) seizures is highest during infancy and in the geriatric age group but may occur at any age.

4. Gender: Epilepsy occurs slightly more often in males than in females (relative risk for males 1.1–2.4 in various studies).

5. Socioeconomic, racial, and ethnic factors: In the United States and Western Europe, epilepsy is slightly more common among lower socioeconomic groups. Epilepsy is more common in Mexico and Central America, and in immigrants from these areas in the United States, at least partially due to the high incidence of cerebral cysticercosis. Epilepsy is more prevalent among African-Americans than whites in the United States.

6. Mental retardation and cerebral palsy are associated with higher rates of epilepsy, as well as lower rates of complete remission of childhood-onset epilepsy.

7. Epilepsy is associated with increased risk of death, including sudden unexplained death, but risk in adolescents with epilepsy is small.

CLINICAL MANIFESTATIONS

Classifications: Table 21.1 lists classifications of seizures, based on international classifications.

Seizure Components

The progression of a seizure is characterized by several temporal components, variably present:

1. Prodrome: Altered behavior or mood occurring hours to days prior to the actual seizure; infrequent.

TABLE 21.1. Classifications of Seizures

Generalized seizures: Bilaterally symmetrical, both in clinical and electroencephalographic manifestations, without focal features.
1. Tonic-clonic, generalized convulsive, grand mal
2. Tonic seizures
3. Clonic seizures
4. Absence seizures
   a. Simple (impaired consciousness only): Classic petit mal
   b. Atypical: Disturbed consciousness plus myoclonic component, automatisms, autonomic component, or abnormality of postural tone
5. Akinetic (atonic) seizures
6. Myoclonic seizures

Partial seizures: Clinical and electroencephalographic onset is localized to one part of the brain (focal).

Simple partial seizures: No impairment of consciousness
1. Motor symptoms
2. Sensory symptoms
3. Autonomic symptoms
4. Special sensory (visual, auditory, olfactory, gustatory)
5. Psychic symptoms (fear, déjà vu, jamais vu, euphoria)

Complex partial seizures: Partial seizure with impairment of consciousness, includes most seizures described as "psychomotor." Seizure may begin with impairment of consciousness or as a simple partial seizure and progress to impaired consciousness.

Partial with secondary generalization: Either partial simple or complex partial seizures may secondarily generalize, producing a tonic-clonic or clonic convulsion similar to a primary generalized convulsion. A partial simple seizure may progress via a complex partial seizure or directly to a secondarily generalized seizure.
1. Simple partial seizures progressing to generalized seizures
2. Complex partial seizures progressing to generalized seizures
3. Simple partial seizures progressing to complex partial seizures progressing to generalized seizures

---

2. Aura: Altered sensation or psychic symptom occurring just prior to other ictal manifestations. The aura is actually part of the seizure, representing a simple partial seizure, usually with sensory, special sensory, or psychic symptoms.
3. Ictus: The observed seizure event, usually with motor activity.
4. Postictal state: Altered neurological function ranging from coma to mild lethargy, hemiplegia to minimal focal motor dysfunction, lasting minutes to 24 hours.

Grand Mal Seizures (Generalized Tonic-Clonic Seizures)

1. Aura: May have brief, nondescript aura.
2. Ictus
   a. Tonic phase: Forceful, postural contractions in flexion or extension. Usually early phase, momentary to several minutes, occasionally longer, may include:
      — Deviation of head
      — A cry at the onset
      — Loss of consciousness at start of seizure
      — Fall to ground
      — Bites tongue or cheeks
   b. Clonic phase: Bilateral, generally symmetric, brisk jerking movements. Clonic movements have a discernible fast-slow component, as distinguished from other types of movement (writhing, sustained posturing, random bilateral nonsynchronous movements), which are less likely a part of a convulsion.
   c. After tonic-clonic phase, the patient usually becomes flaccid, with or without incontinence of urine or stool, as seizure stops.
3. Postictal state
   a. Early: Unconscious state, with decreased tone and reflexes. Patients may have fixed pupils.
   b. Recovery phase: Sleeplike state, but patient is responsive to arousal.
   c. Late phase: Confusion or headache.

Petit Mal and Other Absence Seizures

1. Prodrome: None, but often cluster on arising in morning.
2. Aura: None; abrupt onset of ictus.
3. Ictus: Brief period (few seconds to 30 seconds) of blank staring.
   a. Loss of consciousness, usually without fall.
   b. Typical absence: Minor automatisms; may have blinking of eyes, movement of fingers common.
   c. Complex absence: Associated with automatisms, myoclonic movements or loss of tone; may be longer than 30 seconds.
4. Postictal: No postictal confusion, but amnesia of seizure is usual.
5. One-third of absence seizures remit during adolescence (most likely in childhood-onset simple absence; less likely in adolescent-onset absence).
6. The electroencephalogram (EEG) is characteristic, showing 3-Hz spike and wave activity in typical petit mal. Other absence syndromes show generalized polyspike wave discharges, slow spike wave (Lennox-Gastaut syndrome), or 4- to 5-Hz spike wave (juvenile myoclonic epilepsy of Janz).
7. Specific epileptic syndromes with onset in adolescence combine absence with myoclonic seizures and occasional grand mal seizures, most prominent on arising in the morning. Early morning myoclonus may be viewed as "normal" by the patient and not reported without specific questioning (juvenile myoclonic epilepsy of Janz).

8. Patients with absence or absence plus myoclonic seizures are more likely to be photosensitive than those with other seizure types. "Videogame"-related seizures are generally limited to these patients.

Myoclonic Seizures

1. Myoclonic jerks are brisk, irregular, and may involve trunk or extremities, symmetrically or asymmetrically. Jerks may be of small amplitude or massive, causing the patient to fall.
2. Patient is generally aware of the jerks if they are isolated. They may be unaware if myoclonic jerks are part of absence seizures.
3. Differential diagnosis includes tics, nonepileptic myoclonus, and other movement disorders.
4. Etiologies
   a. Myoclonic seizures, usually on arising in the morning, with adolescent onset, are a characteristic part of juvenile myoclonic epilepsy. Absence or generalized tonic-clonic seizures often occur in these patients.
   b. Myoclonic seizures may be part of an epileptic encephalopathy such as Lennox-Gastaut syndrome, beginning in early childhood and continuing in adolescence.
   c. Photomyoclonus may occur with exposure to strobe or strobelike conditions in teens with photosensitive epilepsy. They may have other generalized seizures, or this may be their only symptom.
   d. A variety of degenerative conditions, including progressive myoclonic epilepsies, sialidosis, and subacute sclerosing panencephalitis (SSPE), may present in the teens and may be accompanied by myoclonic seizures.
5. There is no prodrome, aura, or postictal period.
6. EEG usually shows bursts of spike wave or polyspike and wave in a generalized distribution. Photosensitivity may be demonstrated on EEG using strobe.

Partial Simple Seizures

1. Benign focal epilepsy of childhood (also known as benign Rolandic epilepsy) is the most common cause of focal motor seizure in childhood and early adolescence.
   a. Seizures are partial simple seizures usually involving face or arm; seizures may secondarily generalize.
   b. Episodes occur during drowsiness or sleep onset, or on awakening.
   c. Seizures resolve by the midteens.
   d. There is no underlying structural lesion.
2. Partial simple seizures with onset in adolescence or adulthood are more commonly associated with structural pathology (tumor, arteriovenous malformation, head injury, malformation, stroke).
3. Sensory phenomena (aura) may be the only manifestation of a brief limited seizure.
4. Ictus: Most partial simple seizures are focal motor.
   a. Consciousness is retained. Speech arrest may occur with dominant hemisphere seizure origin (usually with seizure involving right face, left brain in right-handed person).
   b. Clonic activity may "march" up an extremity or spread from arm to face or arm to leg, and so on (or vice versa).
5. Postictal: Headache, postictal hemiparesis (Todd's paralysis).
6. EEG
   a. Benign focal epilepsy of childhood is associated with central-temporal spikes, which are more commonly seen in light sleep. EEG abnormality is commonly bilateral, even if all observed seizures were on same side.
   b. Other partial seizures may be associated with spikes or slowing in a unilateral distribution.

Partial Seizures with Complex Symptomatology

Partial seizures with complex symptomatology are seizures of focal onset with altered consciousness. Older terms include *psychomotor seizures* and *temporal lobe seizures,* although not all partial complex seizures originate in the temporal lobe and not all temporal lobe seizures are complex partial (may be simple partial).

1. May begin at any age.
2. Structural pathology is more common than in generalized epilepsies or benign focal epilepsy of childhood. Mesial temporal sclerosis may cause seizures of temporal lobe origin with onset in adolescence.
3. Prodrome: Patients may report that "they know a seizure is coming."
   a. May occur hours or days prior to a seizure.
   b. Includes mood change, headache, change in appetite.
4. Typical partial complex seizures consist of the following sequence. Any of the sequence may be omitted other than the altered state of consciousness.
   a. Aura: Initial sensory, autonomic, or psychic symptoms lasting seconds to minutes; common phenomena include fear, déjà vu, "rising feeling" in abdomen, tingling, and visual, auditory, olfactory, or gustatory hallucination. Flushing or pallor may be observed. Consciousness is generally retained, and patient remembers this part of the seizure.
   b. Blank stare with impairment of responsiveness and consciousness: The patient is motionless, does not remember events clearly during this phase, if at all.
   c. Automatisms: Hand wringing, picking, lip smacking, walking aimlessly, grunting, gagging, or swallowing. While destructive or injurious behavior may occur, directed deliberate violence does not. Consciousness is impaired or lost during this phase, and the patient does not remember it. Frontal lobe origin complex partial seizures may produce thrashing, agitated movements, bicycling leg movements, or pelvic thrusting, which are difficult to distinguish from hysterical behavior.
   d. Postictal state: Confusion, stupor, headache, and lethargy may last seconds to hours.
5. Precipitants: Sleep deprivation, alcohol, or drug ingestion.
6. EEG: Focal spikes in temporal, frontal, or parietal areas, usually unilateral. EEG findings may be normal. Special procedures such as sleep deprivation, special leads, and prolonged monitoring may be useful for diagnosis.

Features that help to differentiate various seizures reported as "little seizures" or "staring spells" (partial complex, petit mal, and atypical absence) are listed in Table 21.2.

DIFFERENTIAL DIAGNOSIS

Seizures

1. Symptomatic seizures (due to acute systemic disturbance or trauma)
   a. Acute metabolic disturbance (i.e., hypoglycemia, hyponatremia, hypocalcemia)
   b. Acute CNS infection (i.e., encephalitis, meningitis)
   c. Intoxication (cocaine, alcohol, phencyclidine [PCP], phenylpropanolamine, inhalants)
   d. Drug or alcohol withdrawal (barbiturates, sedatives, benzodiazepines after prolonged use)
   e. Acute head trauma (impact seizure, seizure in first few days after significant head trauma)

TABLE 21.2.   Features of Absence and Complex Partial Seizures

Type	Aura	Loss of Consciousness	Duration	Automatisms
Petit mal	None	Immediate	5–20 sec	Occasional simple automatisms
Absence atypical	None	Immediate	5–45 sec	Occasional automatisms
Complex partial	Often	Gradual or partial in some patients	5 sec–5 min	Frequent, more complicated

    f. Syncopal seizure: Brief tonic or clonic seizure occurring after primary syncope
    g. Acute stroke
  2. Acquired (symptomatic or secondary) epilepsies due to remote history of CNS insult
    a. Cerebral malformations: Macroscopic or microscopic (cortical dysgenesis)
    b. Intrauterine infections (cytomegalovirus [CMV], toxoplasmosis)
    c. Perinatal insults
    d. Postneonatal infections (meningitis, encephalitis, brain abscess)
    e. Posttraumatic epilepsy
    f. Tuberous sclerosis
    g. Brain tumors, other mass lesions
    h. Vascular malformations, infarctions
    i. Cysticercosis
    j. Genetic due to progressive or degenerative conditions
    k. Unknown, but presumed symptomatic: Epileptic encephalopathies such as Lennox-Gastaut syndrome and early myoclonic encephalopathy
  3. Idiopathic epilepsy (also called age-related epilepsies)
    a. Primary generalized epilepsies
    b. Benign focal epilepsy of childhood

Other Paroxysmal Events That May Suggest Seizure Activity

  1. Vasovagal syncope
  2. Migraine
  3. Cardiac disease
    a. Arrhythmias
    b. Low-output states
    c. Mitral valve prolapse
  4. Hyperventilation and anxiety states
  5. Orthostatic hypotension
  6. Sleep disturbances
    a. Narcolepsy: Catalepsy, sleep attacks, sleep paralysis, hypnagogic hallucinations
    b. Drowsiness or sleep attacks in patients with obstructive sleep apnea or sleep deprivation
    c. Sleepwalking and other parasomnias
    d. Night terrors
  7. Movement disorders
    a. Tics
    b. Paroxysmal kinesiogenic choreoathetosis
    c. Stiff-man syndrome and other syndromes of continuous muscle fiber activity

TABLE 21.2.   *continued*

Postictal State	Memory of Event	EEG	Associated Abnormalities
None	None	3-Hz spike wave	Twenty percent have grand mal as well; mentally normal
None	None	Slow spike wave or polyspike	Myoclonus, drop attacks, grand mal; mental retardation more common
Frequent	Partial in some patients	Focal spikes	May have secondary generalization; structural lesions may underlie disorder

    d. Dystonias (paroxysmal torticollis, activity-related dystonias, dystonia musculorum deformans, drug-related)
8. Pseudoseizures (hysterical symptoms)
9. Episodic "staring" and inattention
    a. Attention deficit disorder
    b. Disorders of arousal

DIAGNOSIS

History

Epilepsy is primarily a clinical diagnosis based on the history. An astute observer of the event is more important than any "test."

1. Review the following with the observers of the event:
    a. What was the teen doing before the episode began: Sleeping, quiet, watching TV, exercising, reading, anxious?
    b. Where did the event occur?
    c. What time of day?
    d. What was the first abnormality noted? Did the teen seem to be aware something was wrong?
    e. What happened during the seizure?
    f. Could teenager be aroused? Respond to commands? At what point did unresponsiveness start? How long did unconsciousness last?
    g. Was there incontinence of urine or stool?
    h. What happened after the seizure?
2. Review the following with the patient:
    a. What was the last event he or she remembers before the seizure?
    b. Could patient hear or understand people talking during the seizure? Could he or she respond?
    c. What happened after the seizure? What is the first thing recalled after the event?
    d. Precipitating events: Sensory stimulation, activity, drugs, meals, medications, sleep pattern, stress, menses
    e. Prior seizures or similar events
3. Family history of epilepsy, neurocutaneous syndromes, other neurological conditions
4. Perinatal history, particularly birth injury, prematurity, maternal infections
5. History of CNS infections or trauma
6. Drug history, including prescribed, over-the-counter, and "street" drugs and alcohol

Physical Examination

1. Perform general physical examination for evidence of systemic disease.
2. Skin: Look for café au lait spots, depigmented macules, adenoma sebaceum, Shagreen patch, and subungual fibromas.
3. Eyes: Perform fundiscopic examination for papilledema.
4. Neurological examination: Look for evidence of focal abnormalities. Observe gait, movements at rest and active for evidence of movement disorder as alternative explanation of symptoms.
5. Blood pressure: Assess pressure while teen is lying and standing.
6. Pulse: Check for irregularities, if arrhythmia is suspected.
7. Cardiac examination: Check for evidence of mitral valve prolapse, heart failure, or other abnormalities that might lead to arrhythmias.
8. Hyperventilation: Hyperventilate for 1–2 minutes to induce an episode if absence (petit mal) seizures are suspected or if symptoms are thought to be directly due to hyperventilation.

Laboratory Tests

1. Complete blood count and routine chemistry panel are indicated prior to initiating anticonvulsant therapy (as baseline). Platelet count should be included if valproic acid or carbamazepine are to be used.
2. In an apparently well teenager without underlying medical problems, electrolytes, calcium, phosphorus, or magnesium have a very low yield for finding a cause of seizures. Blood sugar measurements may be helpful if hypoglycemia is suspected *only* if drawn while the patient is symptomatic. These tests are not indicated on a routine basis in most teens with seizures.
3. EEG: Routine study should consist of waking EEG, hyperventilation, and photic stimulation. Hyperventilation is particularly useful if absence (petit mal) seizure is suspected. Photic stimulation is especially helpful if patient reports that seizures occur when exposed to videogames, TV, rapid flashing lights, or in the car. Sleep study (sleep deprived if possible) increases the yield in patients with complex partial seizures, benign focal epilepsy of childhood, and some generalized epilepsies.
4. Neuroimaging: Computed tomography (CT) scan or magnetic resonance imaging (MRI) are indicated for focal seizures (except clear-cut benign focal epilepsy of childhood), seizures associated with neurological abnormalities or papilledema, neurocutaneous stigmata, or suspected degenerative conditions.
5. Lumbar puncture is indicated if infection or hemorrhage is suspected.

Grand Mal Seizures versus Syncopal Episode

Table 21.3 compares grand mal seizures and syncopal episodes.

TABLE 21.3.   Grand Mal Seizures versus Syncopal Episodes

Component	Grand Mal	Syncope
Preictal	May have prodome; aura may occur at time of loss of consciousness	Variable—may experience faint or dizzy feeling
Ictus	Violent body spasms; often cries out; sweaty appearance; may have incontinence after tonic-clonic component; coma after seizure	No stereotype; no abrupt onset; slowly falls to floor; cold and clammy May have mild twitching
Postictal	Gradual return to consciousness; confusion	Rarely, confusion

TABLE 21.4.   Hysterical Seizures versus Epilepsy

Hysterical Seizures	Epileptic Seizures
Observed or observers nearby	Observed or unobserved
Bizarre motor activity, back arching, pelvic thrusting	Usually stereotypic for particular patient; automatisms of complex partial seizures may vary with activity and environment; generalized convulsions usually tonic, clonic
No incontinence	
During ictus: Active pupillary reflex, normal corneal reflex	
May occur in patients with epilepsy; may have abnormal EEG interictally, but no change during episode	May be incontinent of urine and stool
	May have dilated unreactive pupils and lose corneal reflex during event
	Rhythmic spikes, slowing or electrodecremental EEG during episode, but may be normal
	Twofold or threefold increase above baseline serum prolactin after convulsion or partial complex seizure is nearly invariable

Hysterical Episodes (Pseudoseizures) versus Epilepsy

Table 21.4 compares pseudoseizures and epilepsy.

THERAPY

After the diagnosis of epilepsy is made, two major components of therapy exist: Drug therapy to control the seizures and counseling regarding psychosocial issues.

Anticonvulsant Therapy

General Guidelines

1. Start with a single anticonvulsant medication.
2. Increase the medication slowly by time increments equal to five times the half-life of the drug until seizures are controlled or toxicity occurs, except when control is urgent (frequent seizures or status epilepticus).
3. Use serum levels only as guidelines: Clinical response is more important. Do not overuse levels. At least five half-lives are necessary for medication level to reach steady state after starting or altering dosage.
4. Give medication each day based on half-life: Give a drug more frequently only with refractory seizures or demonstrated rapid metabolism.
5. Teen should have close follow-up, including monitoring of seizure frequency, physical examination, and evaluation for drug toxicity. *Note:* Frequent follow-up also allows for early detection of nonmedical effects (social, academic, independence, vocational).
6. Substitute a second drug only when the first is pushed to tolerance without controlling the seizure, unless allergic or serious idiosyncratic effects are evident. When the second drug is at adequate serum levels, wean the first. Polytherapy is reserved for refractory patients unresponsive to trials of monotherapy with at least two to three different anticonvulsants at maximum tolerated levels.
7. Discontinuation criteria: Medications may be tapered and discontinued after patient is seizure free for 2–4 years. Estimated risk for recurrence on tapering is 30–40%, greatest during the period of taper or in the first 6 months after discontinuation of the medication. Risk factors for recurrence are somewhat controversial but include the following in at least some studies:
   a. Mental retardation or neurological abnormalities

   b. Long duration of seizures or large number of seizures before full control with medication

   c. Partial seizures (other than the benign focal epilepsies of childhood such as Rolandic epilepsy)

   d. Abnormal EEG findings despite seizure-free period (highest risk: combination of focal slowing and focal epileptiform spikes)

   e. Adolescent-onset seizures less likely to remit than seizures with onset in earlier childhood

Medication should be tapered one drug at a time (generally sedating drugs first), tapering each drug over 6 weeks to 3 months.

Drugs for Specific Seizure Types

1. Generalized tonic-clonic seizures (grand mal), either primarily or secondarily generalized:
   a. Phenobarbital: Least expensive, can be given once a day.
   b. Carbamazepine (Tegretol): Generics are usable if *same* generic is consistently available; avoid switching brands.
   c. Phenytoin (Dilantin): Brand name capsules can be used once a day. Generic capsules or chewable tablets must be divided b.i.d. or t.i.d.
   d. Valproic acid (Depakene or Depakote): Depakote is preferred.
   e. Primidone (Mysoline): Reserve for refractory patients.
   f. Lamotrigine (Lamictal): Recently released, but not yet approved for use in patients under 12 years.

   Many practitioners favor either phenobarbital or carbamazepine. Phenytoin is an effective medication but may cause unacceptable side effects (gum hypertrophy, hirsutism), particularly in children and early adolescents. In patients with *mixed* generalized seizures (i.e., generalized tonic-clonic, plus myoclonic or absence), carbamazepine or phenytoin occasionally may induce or exacerbate myoclonic or drop attacks (rare). Valproic acid, preferably in the long-acting capsules (Depakote), is the drug of choice in mixed generalized epilepsies (grand mal plus myoclonic or absence).

2. Petit mal epilepsy
   a. Ethosuximide (Zarontin): Standard therapy, usually well tolerated.
   b. Valproic acid (Depakote or Depakene): First choice if absence and generalized tonic-clonic seizures coexist.
   c. Clonazepam (Klonopin), other benzodiazepines: Occasionally effective as monotherapy.
   d. Felbamate (Felbatol): This relatively new drug is effective for several seizure types including generalized convulsive (tonic-clonic) and absence seizures. It is only approved for children with Lennox-Gastaut syndrome (mixed generalized epilepsy). A high incidence of aplastic anemia associated with felbamate has limited use of this medication to refractory patients able to give informed consent to its risks.
   e. Lamotrigine (Lamictal): Newly released for adults and teens.

3. Simple partial seizures (focal motor, focal sensory)
   a. Carbamazepine (Tegretol): See above regarding generic forms.
   b. Phenobarbital
   c. Phenytoin (Dilantin): See above regarding generic forms.
   d. Primidone (Mysoline): Reserve for refractory patients.
   e. Gabapentin (Neurontin): Adjunctive treatment of partial onset seizures has been approved for patients over age 14 years. Probably not suitable for monotherapy. This is the only available anticonvulsant that is not metabolized and does not change me-

tabolism of other medications. Consider in multisystem disease when alteration of drug metabolism of other agents is important.

    f. Lamotrigine (Lamictal): See above.

    g. Felbamate (Felbatol): See above. Not yet approved for partial seizures in children and risky due to adverse effects. Reserve for extremely refractory patients.

Note: The use of gabapentin, lamotrigine, and felbamate should only be undertaken in direct consultation with a neurologist with expertise in treatment of epilepsy.

  4. Complex partial seizures

    a. Medications used are generally the same as for simple partial seizures.

    b. Clorazepate (Tranxene) is occasionally useful as an adjunct drug.

    c. Gabapentin (Neurontin) is a new anticonvulsant that appears to be useful for partial seizures as an adjunctive agent.

Table 21.5 provides metabolism guidelines for first-line antiepileptic drugs. Following is an outline of drug side effects and other problems with anticonvulsant therapy.

Side Effects of Anticonvulsant Drugs

Adverse effects of anticonvulsants can be divided into two major groups: *Dose-related* and *idiosyncratic* reactions unrelated to drug level. Mild sedation is common with initiation of any anticonvulsant. This effect generally wanes after a few weeks. Sedation and ataxia with initiation of treatment is more significant with carbamazepine, so that treatment is generally started at low doses and raised over several weeks. Potential reproductive effects are also important to consider in teenage girls of childbearing potential.

Dose-Related Effects

1. Toxic CNS effects are shared among most anticonvulsants.

    a. Excessive levels (or deliberate overdoses) produce ataxia, nystagmus, and sedation progressing to coma, with respiratory and cardiac depression at extremely high doses.

    b. Movement disorders (chorea) may be seen at toxic drug levels, primarily with phenytoin or carbamazepine.

2. Non-CNS dose-related effects are common.

    a. Alterations in vitamin D metabolism produce "chemical rickets," generally without clinical abnormalities. Clinical rickets is occasionally seen in multihandicapped patients receiving anticonvulsants but having limited sun exposure and lacking vitamin D supplementation.

    b. Folate metabolism is altered, producing megaloblastic changes, usually without anemia.

    c. Thyroid function tests are commonly altered without clinical evidence of hypothyroidism.

    d. Gastrointestinal: Gastric distress is common with valproic acid and ethosuximide. Avoidance of side effects from both drugs improves if dose is divided or given with food.

3. Drug interactions are also common.

    a. Virtually all anticonvulsants induce hepatic microsomal enzymes, increasing clearance of themselves (autoinduction), each other, and a variety of other medications including steroids, estrogens, anticoagulants, and so forth. An exception is the recently introduced anticonvulsant, gabapentin (Neurontin), which is excreted unchanged in the urine and does not affect other drug metabolism.

    b. Conversely, several drugs significantly inhibit metabolism of carbamazepine and to a lesser extent phenytoin. The most commonly encountered is erythromycin (and the

TABLE 21.5.   Metabolism and Dosing Guidelines for First-Line Antiepileptic Drugs Used as Monotherapy[a]

Generic Name (Brand Name)	Serum Half-life	Time to Steady State	Therapeutic Levels
Phenytoin (Dilantin)	24 ± 12	5–10 days	10–20 µg
Phenobarbital (Luminal)	72 ± 16	14–21 days	15–40 µg/mL
Primidone (Mysoline)	12 ± 6 for primidone[b] 72 ± 16 for phenobarbital metabolite	14–21 days for metabolites	8–12 µg/mL primidone 15–40 µg/mL phenobarbital
Carbamazepine (Tegretol, Epitol)	12 ± 3 chronic; 36 ± 12 naive[c]	3–5 days	5–13 µg/mL
Ethosuximide (Zarontin)	30 ± 6	7–14 days	40–100 µg/mL
Valproic acid (Depakene, Depakote)	12 ± 6[d]	2–5 days	50–120 µg/mL
Clonazepam (Klonopin)	24 ± 12	5–10 days	Not helpful[e]

[a]Monotherapy pharmacokinetics differ for chronic-use versus antiepileptic drug–naive patient. Patients switched to monotherapy with phenytoin, barbiturates, or carbamazepine from another enzyme-inducing antiepileptic drug generally need higher doses.
[b]Primidone has several active metabolites including phenobarbital and PEMA. While primidone has a relatively short half-life, other metabolites have long half-lifes and a steady-state may take 14–21 days to achieve.
[c]Carbamazepine metabolism autoinduces in many patients (much more rapid elimination after first few weeks of treatment). Repeated dosage adjustments are often necessary in the first few months of use.
[d]Depakote is slow release with variable absorption and later peaks, but is metabolized to valproic acid with same elimination kinetics as Depakene and generics.
[e]Serum levels of benzodiazepines are not helpful in predicting therapeutic response. Alterations in receptors produce marked tolerance. Serum levels are occasionally useful in suspected ingestions or overdose, or to check compliance.

newer macrolides, clarithromycin, and azithromycin). These competitively inhibit carbamazepine metabolism to an extent that previously stable patients may develop significant toxicity less than 24 hours after addition of the antibiotic. A similar effect is seen with propoxyphene (Darvon). These drugs should be avoided in a patient taking carbamazepine.

c. Isoniazid (INH) inhibits both carbamazepine and phenytoin metabolism. Since it is generally used on a long-term basis, the anticonvulsant drug can be adjusted to account for the decreased clearance.

Idiosyncratic (Non-Dose Related)   The following side effects may occur with any anticonvulsant.

1. Allergic reactions: Skin rash, Stevens-Johnson syndrome, lupuslike syndromes, and even death can occur with any anticonvulsant, although most reported cases are associated with phenobarbital, phenytoin, or carbamazepine.
2. Bone marrow toxicity, usually reversible, has been reported with several anticonvulsants. Fatal aplastic anemia has been reported with carbamazepine, primarily in older adults.

TABLE 21.5. *continued*

Toxic Levels	Daily Dosage	Minimum Daily Dosage	Preparations
>20 µg/mL	3–8 mg/kg 250–400 mg/day	1 (Dilantin Capsules; 2–3 Dilantin Tablets, generic capsules, suspension)	Dilantin Capsules: 100 mg, 30 mg Dilantin Infatabs: 50 mg Liquid: 25 mg/5 mL; 125 mg/5 mL Generic capsules: 100 mg
>40 µg/mL (much higher may be tolerated if used chronically)	1–5 mg/kg 90–200 mg/day	1	Tablets: 15 mg, 30 mg, 60 mg 100 mg (essentially all generic) Liquid: 20 mg/5 mL
>15 µg/mL primidone	10–15 mg/kg 500–1000 mg/day	2	Tablets: 50 mg, 250 mg Liquid: 250 mg/5 mL
>15 µg/mL	20 mg/kg (start lower) 400–1800 mg/day	2	Tablets: 100 mg, 200 mg Liquid: 100 mg/mL
>150 µg/mL	10–40 mg/kg 500–1500 mg/day	2 (1 for low doses, if tolerated)	Capsules: 250 mg Liquid: 250 mg/5 mL
>120 µg/mL	15–60 mg/kg 750–3000 mg/day	2 (Depakote); 3 (Depakene)	Capsules: 125 mg, 250 mg, 500 mg Depakote: 250 mg Depakene or generic Sprinkle capsules: 125 mg Depakote Liquid: 250 mg/5 mL (Depakene, generic)
Not helpful	0.02–0.05 mg/kg 1–20 mg/day	2	Tablets: 0.5 mg, 1 mg, 2 mg

Shortly after its widespread release, an excess incidence of aplastic anemia was found with felbamate (Felbatol), severely limiting its current use.

3. Hepatic toxicity and metabolic abnormalities are seen in patients receiving valproic acid, primarily in infants, but rarely can occur with any anticonvulsant, at any age. These may include hyperammonemia, lactic acidosis, and Reye's-like syndrome.

4. Adenopathy, "mononucleosis syndrome," and pseudolymphoma are primarily associated with hydantoins.

5. Hair loss: Moderate hair thinning is relatively common with valproic acid. Frank alopecia does not occur. Other anticonvulsants may produce hair loss as part of allergic reactions.

6. Weight changes: Weight gain is most frequently problematic with valproic acid. Weight loss is common with felbamate, particularly at higher doses, and with valproic acid in young children.

Reproductive There is a moderately increased risk of abnormal pregnancy outcome in women with epilepsy, regardless of specific drug treatment.

1. Facial malformations, particularly cleft palate, microcephaly, congenital heart disease, and minor malformations such as hypoplastic nails have been related to phenytoin, trimethadione (Tridione), and possibly other anticonvulsants as well. Some authors feel that these nonspecific malformations are more frequent in offspring of epileptic mothers, regardless of treatment.

2. Open neural tube defects may be more frequent in fetuses exposed to valproic acid.

3. It is difficult to pick an anticonvulsant that is "completely safe." Risk of fetal damage must be balanced against risk of recurrent convulsions if medications are withdrawn.

4. There is no reason to withhold oral contraceptives from a woman receiving anticonvulsants, but higher estrogen doses may be needed due to more rapid metabolism of the component hormones.

Specific Adverse Effects

Phenytoin (Dilantin)

1. Dose related
   a. CNS: Nystagmus, ataxia, sedation, decreased motor speed, increased seizures at toxic levels
   b. Endocrine: Induction of vitamin D metabolism; clinical rickets only with poor intake and decreased sun exposure (i.e., institutionalized individuals not eating dairy products or taking supplements)
   c. Gingival hyperplasia: Particularly a problem with poor oral hygiene or orthodontic appliances
   d. Hypertrichosis
   e. Soft tissue thickening: Particularly orbital ridges, lips, nose
   f. Reproductive: Reports of malformations including microcephaly, nail hypoplasia, facial anomalies, cardiac defects, and mental retardation occurring in up to 10% (highest estimate) of fetuses exposed to phenytoin during gestation; risk probably substantially lower
2. Idiosyncratic
   a. Hematologic: Megaloblastic anemia (mild megaloblastic changes are common and dose related), pseudolymphoma (fever, adenopathy, rash, hepatosplenomegaly)
   b. Allergic or immunologic: Lupus syndrome, rash, Stevens-Johnson syndrome
   c. Hepatitis

Barbiturates (Phenobarbital, Primidone, Mephobarbital [Mebaral])

1. Dose related
   a. CNS: Sedation, irritability; overdoses produce coma and respiratory and cardiac depression; worsening symptoms in patients with coexisting attention deficit disorder
   b. Psychiatric: Increased incidence of depression, particularly in patients with family history of a major affective disorder
   c. Reproductive: Unknown risk of malformations; thought to be lower than with phenytoin or valproic acid
2. Idiosyncratic
   a. Allergic or immunologic: Lupus syndrome, rash, Stevens-Johnson syndrome
   b. Hepatitis
   c. Hematologic: Megaloblastic anemia

Carbamazepine (Tegretol, Epitol)

1. Dose related
   a. CNS: Dizziness, ataxia, drowsiness, diplopia, visual symptoms, particularly at beginning of treatment or with high doses
   b. Hematologic: mild depression of white blood count is common and reversible
   c. Gastrointestinal: Nausea, vomiting, anorexia (uncommon)
   d. Reproductive: Unknown risk of fetal malformations; thought to be less teratogenic than phenytoin, but evidence is poor
2. Idiosyncratic
   a. Hematologic: Irreversible aplastic anemia reported but extremely rare in children and young adults
   b. Allergic or immunologic: Rash, Stevens-Johnson syndrome

c. Hepatitis
d. Hyponatremia, usually asymptomatic

Ethosuximide (Zarontin), Methsuximide (Celontin)

1. Dose related
    a. CNS: Fatigue, lethargy, dizziness (at high levels)
    b. Gastrointestinal: Nausea, abdominal distress, vomiting (usually preventable by dividing dose or giving medication with food)
2. Idiosyncratic
    a. Hematologic: Granulocytopenia
    b. Allergic or immune: Skin rash, lupuslike syndrome

Valproic Acid (Depakene, Depakote)

1. Dose related
    a. CNS: Sedation, ataxia at very high doses or in combination with other anticonvulsants are common. Fine tremor may occur at high dose levels.
    b. Gastrointestinal: Nausea, vomiting, abdominal distress are common (much less common with Depakote; if using Depakene liquid, give with food).
    c. Hepatic: All patients taking valproic acid have mildly elevated liver enzymes (SGOT, SGPT, LDH, generally about two to three times baseline values). These are not clinically significant.
    d. Metabolic: Serum ammonia is elevated to about two to three times baseline values in patients taking valproic acid. Severe elevations may be associated with idiosyncratic reactions or very high doses. Lactic acidosis may occur at high doses, leading to growth failure. Serum carnitine may be reduced. Supplementation with oral carnitine has been advocated by some to prevent depletion.
    e. Changes in appetite: Approximately 10% of patients experience significant weight gain. Weight loss or failure to thrive occurs with high doses, usually associated with significant anorexia. Look for lactic acidosis, hyperammonemia, or depleted levels of free carnitine in patients with weight loss.
    f. Reproductive: There is an increased risk of open neural tube defects in fetuses exposed to valproate.
2. Idiosyncratic
    a. Hepatotoxicity: Fatal hepatotoxicity resembling Reye's Syndrome occurs primarily in children under 2 years of age receiving polytherapy. Adolescents on monotherapy have a very low incidence of severe toxicity. Monitoring of liver functions will not always prevent this syndrome, which may occur without warning.
    b. Hematologic: A rare but partially dose-related syndrome resembling idiopathic thrombocytopenic purpura (ITP) may cause profound thrombocytopenia and bleeding. It generally reverses promptly with discontinuation of valproic acid. Mild thrombocytopenia commonly occurs with intercurrent viral illness and may reverse spontaneously or with lowered doses.

Benzodiazepines: Clonazepam (Klonopin), Clorazepate (Tranxene), Diazepam (Valium)

1. Dose related
    a. CNS: Sedation, ataxia, and behavioral disturbances are most prominent on initiation of treatment or after dosage increases, waning with continued administration.

2. Idiosyncratic
   a. Systemic, allergic, or hematologic side effects are rare with benzodiazepines.
   b. Increased salivation may complicate management of the multihandicapped patient or one with severe respiratory disease.

Felbamate (Felbatol)

1. Dose related
   a. CNS: Sedation, ataxia, dizziness, insomnia, and headache are common.
   b. Non-CNS: Appetite decreases, dyspepsia, and nausea are prominent, particularly with high doses in the first few months of therapy. Weight loss can be substantial but is usually regained.
2. Idiosyncratic
   a. A significant incidence of severe aplastic anemia, leading to death in about one-third of known cases, has been attributed to this medication. Use should be restricted to patients refractory to all other medication, in the hands of experienced epileptologists, and with adequate informed consent.
   b. Death due to liver dysfunction has also been reported. See preceding cautions.
   c. Allergic: Itching, rash, and other allergic symptoms ranging from trivial through Stevens-Johnson syndrome have been reported.
   d. Psychiatric: Agitation, hallucinations, aggressive behavior, and frank psychosis have been reported.

Gabapentin (Neurontin)

1. Dose related
   a. CNS: Sedation, dizziness, ataxia, diplopia are common.
   b. Non-CNS: Anorexia, dyspepsia, weight gain are occasionally seen.
2. Idiosyncratic: To date, few if any allergic or organ-system toxicities have been reported.
3. Other important information: Unlike *all* other anticonvulsants, gabapentin is not metabolized but is excreted unchanged in the urine. Administration of gabapentin does not affect other drug levels. Dose adjustment is necessary for patients with renal impairment, depending on creatinine clearance.

Lamotrigine (Lamictal)

1. Dose related
   a. CNS: Sedation, dizziness, ataxia, diplopia
2. Idiosyncratic
   a. Rashes, including Stevens-Johnson syndrome
   b. Liver dysfunction, including hepatic necrosis (single case report)

Other Problems with Anticonvulsant Therapy

1. Since teenagers in whom epilepsy is well controlled often have no symptoms except for the drug side effects, it is tempting for them to take their medications only intermittently. These and other compliance problems are common (see suggestions for improving compliance at the end of this chapter).
2. Medications may increase preexisting behavior problems and occasionally cause depression.
3. Some drugs can increase seizure frequency as the dose is increased.

Other Important Treatment Issues

The care of the epileptic teen extends beyond drug therapy. Total care involves dispelling myths and educating, providing for community resources, and providing counseling for the teen's voiced or unvoiced concerns.

Dispelling Myths and Educating   Many myths about epilepsy can be eliminated by reassuring the teenager that:

1. Epilepsy is not contagious.
2. The seizures may disappear with age.
3. Most seizures can be prevented with medication.
4. Epilepsy does not lower the teenager's intelligence.
5. He or she can participate in almost all activities.
6. Epilepsy is not a "mental illness."

The parent should also be given the above reassurances, in addition to the following:

1. There is no need to feel guilty. It is unlikely that anything the parent did (or did not do) caused the epilepsy.
2. There is no need for special schooling solely due to epilepsy.
3. Neither epilepsy nor anticonvulsants cause learning disabilities or cognitive loss.

The teen and family should be educated regarding the following:

1. Diagnosis
2. Importance of careful observation and record keeping
3. Avoidance of precipitating factors, if any
4. Side effects of medication
5. Prognosis and follow-up
6. Precautions and restrictions, particularly regarding driving, swimming, bicycle and motorcycle riding, until seizure control is assured: State requirements regarding reports to Department of Motor Vehicles should be explained. Restrictions may need to be imposed regarding use of hazardous equipment such as power tools.
7. For women and adolescent girls of childbearing age, the need for adequate birth control while receiving most anticonvulsant drugs

Family members should be aware of first aid for seizure episodes:

1. Generalized convulsion (tonic, tonic-clonic, clonic)
   a. Help the person into a lying position if there is adequate warning.
   b. Do not try to restrain the person.
   c. Clear the area of dangerous objects.
   d. Remove glasses and loosen tight clothing.
   e. Turn the head to one side (or roll person onto their side) to allow saliva to drain out.
   f. *Do not* put anything into the person's mouth.
   g. Family members should be given specific criteria to call for paramedic help: If seizure lasts longer than 5–10 minutes, or if seizures cluster without recovery, call for emergency medical help. Specific advice should be individualized, based on the patient's seizure history.
   h. Report what you observe.
2. Partial seizures (simple and complex)
   a. Do not restrain person.
   b. Remove harmful objects from area.

3. Petit mal
   a. No first aid is necessary.
   b. Protect from harm if in dangerous situation until episode passes.

Community Resources   Teenagers and parents should be provided with references and should be informed of community resources about epilepsy. Many local epilepsy societies sponsor job search training; some have vocational training and placement programs. Some sponsor teen groups for peer support, camps, and family programs. The Epilepsy Foundation of America has a library of videotapes, pamphlets, and other educational materials for patients and families.

Epilepsy Foundation of America
4351 Garden City Drive
Landover, MD 20785

Local chapters can be located through the national offices or are often listed in telephone directories under "Social Service Organizations."

Miscellaneous Concerns

1. Sports and activity: No need for restriction of activities except for swimming alone, scuba diving, mountain climbing, or bicycling in areas with traffic. Contact sports are generally restricted until seizures are controlled.
2. Medical identification: The teen with epilepsy should wear a medical identification bracelet or necklace. This may avoid unnecessary trips to emergency facilities or unneeded testing if a seizure occurs away from home.
3. Driving: Health-care professionals should be aware of their state's driving laws regarding epilepsy. These should be explained to the teen, with the reasons for the laws. The wish to be seizure free to receive a license may enhance compliance. Laws regarding mandatory reporting to the state's Department of Motor Vehicles vary among the states.
4. School: The adolescent's school should be informed if seizures are a recurring problem. If the teenager has been seizure free for an extended time, there often is no need to inform the teachers of diagnosis, as this may cause unnecessary restrictions and lowered expectations.
5. Anticipate other concerns: Seizures, because of their unpredictable and abrupt onset, threat of injury, and embarrassment can have profound effects on the developing adolescent. Try to anticipate and be sensitive to these concerns. Early teens may be concerned about whether their body is normal. Middle teens will have concerns about their peers, driving, and sports restrictions. Older adolescents will be more concerned regarding vocational planning and perhaps future health insurance.
6. Compliance: As stated earlier, compliance can be a significant problem in dealing with an epileptic teenager. Suggestions for improving compliance include:
   a. Provide clear explanations of drugs used and their side effects.
   b. Give adolescent responsibility for taking medications.
   c. Discuss possible consequences of noncompliance with teen, such as recurrent seizures and inability to get or keep a driver's license.
   d. Referral to a teen group sponsored by a local chapter of the Epilepsy Foundation of America may be helpful.
   e. "Day of the week" pillboxes filled and checked weekly, with parental supervision, may enable a young teen to manage his or her own medications.

BIBLIOGRAPHY

Aicardi J. Epilepsy in children. New York: Raven Press, 1986.

Brent DA, Crumrine PK, Varma RR, et al. Phenobarbital treatment and major depressive disorder in children with epilepsy. Pediatrics 1987;80:909–917.

Bronen RA. Epilepsy: the role of MR imaging. Am J Roentgenol 1992;159:1165.

Camfield PR, Camfield CS. The prognosis of childhood epilepsy. Semin Pediatr Neurol 1994;1:102–110.

Camfield CS, Camfield PR, Gordon KE, et al. Predicting the outcome of childhood epilepsy—a population-based study yielding a simple scoring system. J Pediatr 1993;122:861–868.

Carranco E, Kareus J, Co S, et al. Carbamazepine toxicity induced by concurrent erythromycin therapy. Arch Neurol 1985;42:187–188.

Cascino GD. Epilepsy: contemporary perspectives on evaluation and treatment. Mayo Clin Proc 1994;69:1199.

Centers for Disease Control and Prevention. Prevalence of self-reported epilepsy—United States, 1986–1990. JAMA 1994;272:1893.

Chadwick D. Do anticonvulsants alter the natural course of epilepsy? Br Med J 1995;310:177.

Chigier E. Compliance in adolescents with epilepsy or diabetes. J Adolesc Health 1992;13:375.

Dodson WE, Pellock JM. Pediatric epilepsy: diagnosis and therapy. New York: Demos Publications, 1993.

Durner M, Greenberg DA, Delgado-Escueta AV. Is there a genetic relationship between epilepsy and birth defects? Neurology 1992;42:63.

Emerson R, O'Sourza BJ, Vining EP. Stopping medication in children with epilepsy. N Engl J Med 1981;304:1125.

French J. The long-term therapeutic management of epilepsy. Ann Intern Med 1994;120:411.

Graf WD, Chatrian GE, Glass ST, et al. Video game-related seizures: a report on 10 patients and a review of the literature. Pediatrics 1994;93:551.

Grunewald RA, Panayiotopoulos CP. Juvenile myoclonic epilepsy. A review. Arch Neurol 1993;50:594.

Harden CL. New antiepileptic drugs. Neurology 1994;44:787.

Hart RG, Easton JD. Carbamazepine and hematological monitoring. Ann Neurol 1982;11:309–312.

Hiilesmaa VK. Pregnancy and birth in women with epilepsy. Neurology 1992;42:8.

Holmes GL, Sackellares JC, McKiernan J, et al. Evaluation of childhood pseudoseizures using EEG telemetry and videotape monitoring. J Pediatr 1980;97:554–558.

Lamotrigine for epilepsy. Med Lett Drugs Ther 1995;37:21.

Laxer KD. Guidelines for treating epilepsy in the age of felbamate, vigabatrin, lamotrigine, and gabapentin. West J Med 1994;161:309.

Luther JS, McNamara JO, Carville S, et al. Pseudoepileptic seizures: methods and video analysis to aid diagnosis. Ann Neurol 1982:12:458–462.

Mattson RH. Current challenges in the treatment of epilepsy. Neurology 1994;44:S4.

Mattson RH, Cramer JA, Colline JF, et al. Comparison of carbamazepine, phenobarbital, phenytoin, and primidone in partial and secondary generalized tonic-clonic seizures. N Engl J Med 1985;313:145–151.

Mattson RH, Rebar RW. Contraceptive methods for women with neurologic disorders. Am J Obstet Gynecol 1993;168:2027.

Mitchell WG, Chavez JM. Carbamazepine versus phenobarbital for partial onset seizures in children. Epilepsia 1987:28:56–60.

Mitchell WG, Lee H, Chavez JM, et al. Academic underachievement in children with epilepsy. J Child Neurol 1991;6:65–72.

Mitchell WG, Zhou Y, Chavez JM, et al. Effects of antiepileptic drugs on reaction time, attention and impulsivity in children. Pediatrics, 1993;91:101–105.

Nash JL. Pseudoseizures: etiologic and psychotherapeutic considerations. South Med J 1993;86:1248.

Nelson KB, Ellenberg JH. Predictors of epilepsy in children who have experienced febrile seizures. N Engl J Med 1976;295:1029.

Parks BR Jr, Dostrow VG, Noble SL. Drug therapy for epilepsy. Am Fam Physician 1994;50:639.

Ramsay RE. Clinical efficacy and safety of gabapentin. Neurology 1994;44:S23.

Samoil D, Grubb BP, Kip K, et al. Head-upright tilt table testing in children with unexplained syncope. Pediatrics 1993;92:426.

So EL. Update on epilepsy. Med Clin North Am 1993;77:203.

Tennison M, Greenwood R, Lewis D, et al. Discontinuing antiepileptic drugs in children with epilepsy. New Engl J Med 1994;330:1407–1410.

Thurston JH, Thurston DL, Hixon BB. Prognosis in childhood epilepsy. N Engl J Med 1982;306:831.

Wilder BJ. The treatment of epilepsy: an overview of clinical practices. Neurology 1995;45(suppl 2):S7.

Wolfe DA, Grubb BP, Kimmel SR. Head-upright tilt test: a new method of evaluating syncope. Am Fam Physician 1993;47:149.

Wyler AR. Modern management of epilepsy. Recommended medical and surgical options. Postgrad Med 1993;94:97.

Yearby MS. Problems and management of the pregnant woman with epilepsy. Epilepsia 1987:28(suppl 3):S29–S36.

CHAPTER 22

Headaches

Wendy G. Mitchell and Lawrence S. Neinstein

Recurrent headaches are a frequent problem in adolescents and adults, accounting for numerous physician visits and lost days of work and school. Most recurrent headaches are not associated with severe organic pathology, but may be important signs of stress, anxiety, or depression. In contrast, the single severe acute headache, particularly in a patient without prior headache history, may be due to significant central nervous system (CNS) or systemic disease.

PAIN-SENSITIVE AREAS: WHAT HURTS IN THE HEAD?

In general, the brain parenchyma and dura are insensitive to pain. Pain-sensitive areas include:

1. Intracranial
   a. Cranial nerves (CN) V, IX, and X (Most intracranial structures are innervated by CN V.)
   b. Dural arteries
   c. Major venous sinuses
   d. Dura at base of skull
   e. Intracavernous and proximal intracranial portions of the carotid arteries
2. Extracranial
   a. Skin, fascia, muscles, and blood vessels of scalp
   b. Upper cervical nerve roots
   c. Muscles of the neck
   d. Sinuses, teeth
   e. Eyes, eye muscles

MECHANISMS OF PAIN

1. Vascular dilation: Distention of pain-sensitive cranial arteries causes headaches. This mechanism is involved in migraine headaches and in many headaches associated with fever, systemic infection, metabolic disturbances, and vasodilator drugs. Migraine headaches may be associated with vasoactive agents, including serotonin, bradykinin, norepinephrine, prostaglandins, and histamine. The role of these vasoactive substances may be casual or reactive. There is increasing evidence that migraine is neurally initiated, rather than a direct response of the vascular system, with vascular changes being a secondary phenomena. The "aura" of migraine headaches and the neurological manifestations of complicated migraine are due to vasoconstriction of intracranial arteries, leading to ischemia in affected areas of the brain.
2. Muscular contraction: Increased muscular contraction of the head and neck muscles can lead to a headache. This mechanism of headaches is involved in tension and psychogenic

headaches, but may be a secondary source of pain in migraine. Patients with migraine commonly have muscle contraction and tenderness as a result of the headache, rather than as a primary event.

3. Traction: Traction of pain-sensitive structures intracranially may cause headache. Examples include mass lesions such as brain tumor, brain abscess, subdural hematoma, and increased intracranial pressure. Brain tumors rarely cause pain directly unless pain-sensitive cranial nerves are involved, intracranial pressure is increased, or there is traction on meninges.

4. Inflammation of pain-sensitive areas: Examples include meningitis (either aseptic or bacterial), sinusitis, dental disease, orbital inflammation, and vasculitic syndromes involving intracranial or extracranial vessels.

EPIDEMIOLOGY

1. Prevalence
   a. Approximately 40% of children by age 7 have headaches, 66% by age 12, and 75% of adolescents by age 15. Most of these headaches are infrequent and nondisabling.
   b. Migraine headaches: Twenty-five percent of migraineurs first develop symptoms during childhood. There is about a 4% prevalence rate among individuals aged 7 through 15. However, migraine is commonly underdiagnosed if mild or infrequent, and prevalence may be higher.
2. Sex: Headaches occur in about equal prevalence among males and females until around age 12. At that time headaches become more common in females due to the increasing prevalence of migraine headaches in females.
3. Types: Most headaches in adolescents and adults are either vascular headache (migraine), muscular contraction headaches, or a combination of both. Secondary causes, such as a brain tumor, are uncommon. Cluster headaches usually start during late adolescence or later but can start as early as 8 years of age. Depressive headaches may present in preteens or teens, at times with denial of other depressive symptoms.

DIFFERENTIAL DIAGNOSIS AND CHARACTERISTICS (Table 22.1)

Acute, Nonrecurrent (First or Worst) Headaches

While this may be the first attack of episodic, recurrent headaches it is important to rule out serious, potentially life-threatening etiologies:

1. Febrile patient
   a. Meningitis: Bacterial, viral, tuberculosis (TB), other aseptic
   b. Brain abscess or other intracranial infection
   c. Encephalitis
   d. Sinusitis
   e. Nonspecific headache due to fever
   f. Associated with other infections: Headache is a common symptom in strep throat, influenza, mononucleosis, and rubeola.
2. Afebrile patient
   a. Subarachnoid hemorrhage (arteriovenous malformation [AVM], aneurysm with acute bleed)
   b. Intraparenchymal hemorrhage (AVM, venous angioma, trauma)
   c. Other (cysticercosis, acute obstructive hydrocephalus)
   d. Headache following a seizure (postictal)

Table 22.1. Headache Presentations

Type of Headache	Onset	Location	Pain Quality
Common migraine	Gradual	Unilateral or bilateral	Throbbing, pulsating
Classic migraine	Gradual	Unilateral	Throbbing, pulsating
Muscle contraction	Variable, usually afternoon	Occipital, bilateral, frontal, bandlike	Steady pressure, dull
Cluster	2 AM to 3 AM, abrupt	Unilateral, orbital, or temporal	Burning, boring, excruciating
Mass lesions	Gradual or sudden, but usually recent	Focal or general	Varied, often dull ache
Pseudotumor (benign increased intra-cranial pressure)	Variable	Vertex or diffuse	Dull
Depressive	Prolonged, constant	Generalized	Dull, unvarying

    e. Cerebral ischemia, particularly if other neurological findings or predisposing factors (i.e., sickle cell disease) are present
    f. Severe hypertension
    g. Acute dental disease
    h. Eye or orbit: Acute glaucoma, inflammatory disease of orbit

Recurrent Headaches (Episodic, Complete Recovery Between Episodes)

1. Muscle-tension type headaches (MTTH): There is now significant doubt in the neurological literature that muscle tension headaches exist, other than in situations of direct neck muscle trauma. Many headache experts consider "tension headaches" to be *mostly* misdiagnosed vascular headaches.
    a. Bandlike, bilateral, steady pain, occipital more than temporal
    b. *Lacking the following:* Throbbing, nausea, vomiting, photophobia, associated neurological symptoms
    c. Often gradual in onset, related to stress or fatigue
    d. May be caused by minor trauma to neck muscles, whiplash, muscle strain
    e. May be caused by tempomandibular joint dysfunction
2. Migraine (also known as vascular headache)
    a. Classic migraine 10–15%
      — "Aura" of sensory disturbances: Visual changes, numbness, tingling, dizziness, vertigo, syncope are common.
      — Throbbing, unilateral, usually frontal or temporal pain occur.
      — Anorexia, nausea, vomiting are often accompanying symptoms.
      — Phonophobia, photophobia are common.
      — Sleep often relieves migraine.

Table 22.1.   *continued*

Duration	Associated Symptoms	Prodomata	Precipitating Factors
Hours to days	Nausea, vomiting, chills, fever, photophobia, weakness, fatigue	Paresthesias, dizziness, mood disturbance, minutes to hours before pain	Alcohol, chocolate, cheese, red wine, glare
4–8 hours or longer	As in common migraine	Scotomata, sensory paresis, weakness, 10–20 minutes before pain	As in common migraine
Hours to day	Weakness, fatigue	None	Stress
Minutes to hours, usually 30–40 minutes	Unilateral, lacrimation, conjunctival infection, rhinorrhea, ptosis, sweating, miosis	None	Alcohol
Varied	Neurological signs	None	Cough, bending, exercise
Variable, may occur during sleep or early morning	Visual obscurations and papilledema	None	Vitamin A or D overdosage, steroid treatment or withdrawal, obesity, endocrine abnormalities, tetracyclines
Days to months	Depression may be masked; anorexia; sleep disturbances; anhedonia; school phobia	None	Factors causing depression; family history of affective disorders common

— Family history is often positive. Although parent may not describe his or her headaches as migraine, more careful history of family members' headache pattern often reveals vascular headaches.
— A childhood history of motion sickness or cyclic vomiting is common.
— Pattern of headaches varies over time. Exacerbations or onset may be precipitated by puberty, college, or other life stresses.
— In some subjects, episodes may be precipitated by certain foods, including chocolate, tyramine-containing cheeses, red wines, and foods containing monosodium glutamate (MSG) or nitrates or nitrites.
— History of relief with ergot compounds or specific serotonin agonists (sumatriptan, dihydroergotamine) is supportive of diagnosis.
   b. Common migraine 80–90%
      — As above, but lacking aura
      — May be bilateral, variable in pain distribution
   c. Variant migraine 5–10%
      — Hemiplegic migraine: Often familial, presents with hemiplegia, aphasia, or speech disturbances, followed by headache and associated symptoms as above. Headache is generally contralateral to hemiplegia. Headache may be less symptomatic than hemiplegia.
      — Confusional migraine: More common in younger children but may continue into teens. A period of confusion and disorientation is usually followed by vomiting, deep sleep, and waking feeling well. Headache may not be reported by child and generally is not prominent.
      — Abdominal migraine: Episodic abdominal pain with nausea or vomiting, followed by or accompanied by headache. However, headache may be minimal or absent. Aura may precede pain. Relief of episodes by sleep or antimigraine therapies supports diagnosis.

— Basilar migraine: Dizziness, vertigo, syncope, dysarthria common, preceding variable headache and vomiting. Headache may be minimal or even absent. Common in adolescent girls.
— Ophthalmoplegic migraine: Abnormal eye movements, sometimes with near-complete ophthalmoplegia and diplopia, are followed by more typical migraine symptoms.

3. Cluster headaches less than 5% in children, teens
   a. Male predominance
   b. Steady burning or pain, usually localized behind one eye, sudden onset, extremely severe but brief
   c. Rhinorrhea, lacrimation, conjunctival injection on same side common
   d. Horner's syndrome ipsilaterally during attack common
   e. During clusters, multiple daily episodes, often in early morning hours, awakening patient from sleep
   f. Differential diagnosis includes occult dental disease, acute glaucoma, tic douloureux.

Note: Several rare metabolic disorders may mimic migraine, including mitochondrial diseases; mitochondrial myopathy, encephalopathy, lactacidosis, and strokelike episodes (MELAS) syndrome; and several organic acidurias. If metabolic disease is suspected, blood for lactate, pyruvate, ammonia and urine for organic acids should be collected during the episodes.

Chronic Headaches (Variable But Essentially Continuous or Increasing Since Onset)

1. Intracranial mass lesions
   a. While many patients with brain tumors have headaches, very few patients with headaches have brain tumors.
   b. Headaches due to brain tumors commonly are accompanied by other neurological symptoms such as vomiting, diplopia, unsteadiness, weakness, neuroendocrine abnormalities or personality and behavioral changes.
   c. Findings from neurological examination and fundoscopic examination are often abnormal.
2. Hydrocephalus (with or without mass):
   a. May be relatively constant, often worse in morning.
   b. Aquaductal stenosis may present in teens, even if congenital.
   c. Head may be large, but this is not universal.
   d. Pain is usually dull, vertex, and not very severe.
   e. Pain may be increased by straining, bowel movements, coughing, or bending.
3. Post–lumbar puncture headaches
   a. Headache is positional, often abruptly relieved by recumbency.
   b. Headache, nausea, and vomiting may be severe if patient is upright.
   c. Primary treatment is 1–2 days of recumbency.
   d. If not relieved in several days and severe, epidural blood patch provides relief in about 90%, but may cause some lower back discomfort.
   e. Salt and fluid loading and abdominal binders are of limited efficacy.
   f. Occasionally, spontaneous or post–traumatic occult cerebrospinal fluid (CSF) leaks may present identically. Opening pressure on spinal tap is extremely low.
4. Pseudotumor cerebri (also called benign intracranial hypertension): Increased intracranial pressure without mass.

   a. Papilledema is common. Visual fields may be abnormal, including enlarged blind spot or constricted peripheral fields.
   b. Visual obscuration (transient dimming or loss of vision with straining or position change) may be present.
   c. Pain is usually dull, vertex.
   d. Pseudotumor cerebri is more common in females, obese patients.
   e. May be caused by excessive vitamin A or D intake.
   f. May be caused by tetracycline intake.
   g. There is a risk of permanent visual loss if untreated.
5. "Transformed migraine": Migraine attacks may go from episodic to chronic, essentially continuous pain.
   a. Excessive use of symptomatic medication (analgesics, ergots) may contribute.
   b. Other migrainous symptoms are usually present, but may only be present in retrospect.
6. Depressive headaches
   a. "All day, all the time, every day, no relief."
   b. Other overt depressive symptoms may be absent.
   c. Excessive disability (school absenteeism, social isolation) is common.
   d. Family history often positive for affective disorders.
   e. Often responsive to antidepressant medications and supportive psychotherapy.
7. Post-traumatic (head trauma)
   a. Headaches usually have mixed migrainous and "tension" quality.
   b. Diminish gradually over time.
   c. Minor trauma may precipitate episodic migraines.
8. Local extracranial disease
   a. Chronic sinusitis
   b. Dental disease, including temporomandibular joint (TMJ) dysfunction
   c. Glaucoma
   d. Other orbital inflammatory lesions
   e. Vasculitis involving extracranial vessels (rare in teens)
9. Human immunodeficiency virus (HIV) or acquired immunodeficiency syndrome (AIDS)
   a. Chronic or recurrent headaches are common.
   b. May be due to HIV, coexisting other infections (intracranial, sinus, ear), or treatment, including antiretroviral agents.
10. Pregnancy
   a. Early pregnancy may be associated with headache, nausea, and vomiting.
   b. Pregnancy may exacerbate migraines.
11. Chronic meningitis or other inflammatory conditions
   a. CNS sarcoidosis may present with meningeal or parenchymal involvement.
   b. TB, fungal, or other recurrent or chronic "aseptic" meningitis may present with sustained or recurrent headaches.
12. Headaches due to other medical conditions: Headache may be intermittent or continuous. Hypoxia, hypercarbia, significant hypertension, severe anemia, uremia, dialysis, and certain medications may cause nonspecific throbbing or dull headache. This is particularly important in treating adolescents with other chronic conditions such as cystic fibrosis, chronic pulmonary disease, renal failure, sickle cell anemia, cancer, organ transplants, or cyanotic congenital heart disease. Treatment is generally aimed at the underlying condition and symptomatic relief of pain. Treatment options may be severely limited by the underlying condition for patients with migraine coexisting with other chronic illnesses.

DIAGNOSIS

In the evaluation of the chronic or recurrent headache patient, the history is (nearly) everything! The rest is the examination!

1. Onset: Age at first episode, events or illnesses surrounding onset, temporal pattern of headaches (time of day, day of week, season), frequency.
2. Pattern and chronology of pain: Have the patient describe a typical headache episode in detail
   a. Prodrome
   b. Location
   c. Quality (pounding, dull, sharp, sticking)
   d. Change in quality or location as headache progresses
   e. Associated autonomic symptoms (sweating, pallor, flushing, palpitations)
   f. Nausea, vomiting, anorexia
   g. Duration
   h. Severity, limitation of activities
   i. Response to medications, sleep
3. Preceding and accompanying symptoms, particularly visual or other neurological symptoms
4. Precipitants of specific episodes, or at onset of headaches
   a. Stress: Family, school, peers
   b. Illnesses
   c. Foods: Nitrate- or nitrite-containing foods, MSG, chocolate, nuts, cheeses, other specific suspect foods
   d. Medications: Intake of over-the-counter medications (i.e., phenylpropanolamine in decongestants or diet pills)
   e. Exertion
   f. Caffeine intake or withdrawal
   g. Alcohol intake
   h. Toxic exposures, particularly lead, hydrocarbons
   i. Physical exposures: Bright or flashing lights, temperature changes, strong odors
5. Other associated illnesses or symptoms, including HIV risks. Changes in menstrual pattern or galactorrhea may suggest pituitary lesion or pregnancy.
6. Medications (prescribed, over-the-counter)
   a. Analgesics
   b. Birth control pills
   c. Other medications used for headaches (acute or prophylactic)
   d. Tetracycline
7. Vitamin consumption, particularly fat-soluble vitamins (A, D, E), unusual diets, supplements
8. Substance abuse
9. Depression or mood disorders
10. School phobia or school avoidance, other secondary gains
11. Behavior between attacks: Any recent personality change, change in school performance
12. Family history
    a. Migraine
    b. Epilepsy
    c. Other headaches
    d. Affective disorders

Physical Examination

The physical examination should include a good general physical examination plus a careful neurological examination. If possible, the patient should be examined both during a typical episode and when free of symptoms. Pertinent physical findings include:

1. Vital signs: Elevated blood pressure or temperature
2. Eyes, ears, nose, and throat: Sinus tenderness, acute or chronic otitis, poor dentition, refractive error
3. General physical examination: Café au lait spots, signs of systemic illness, galactorrhea
4. Neck: Nuchal rigidity, spasm or tenderness of cervical neck muscles, or "trigger points"
5. Funduscopic examination: Papilledema, narrowing of vessels, optic atrophy
6. Neurological examination: Mental status, cranial nerves, motor, sensory examination, gait, coordination

Laboratory Tests

In patients with recurrent headaches separated by periods of complete recovery, laboratory and radiological workup are seldom indicated in the presence of a normal physical examination. Laboratory and radiological workup should be guided by the history and physical examination; that is, sinus films may be indicated if facial tenderness or nasal discharge suggest sinusitis. Neuroimaging (computed tomography or magnetic resonance imaging) is indicated if an abnormal result from neurological examination or papilledema is present or if the head circumference is over the 95th percentile without other explanation. Neuroimaging is *not* generally needed for long-standing, recurrent headaches with complete clearing of symptoms between episodes in the face of normal neurological and funduscopic examinations.

In contrast, an acute severe headache in a patient with no prior headache history must be considered more closely, as underlying systemic or CNS pathology may be life threatening.

THERAPY

Rule 1: Not having headaches is better than getting rid of it once it occurs. Rule 1B: Not taking pills every day is better than taking pills. Look for precipitants, particularly avoidable ones.

Rule 2: Do not underestimate the role of reassurance. Teens and parents are often more concerned that the headache is caused by a brain tumor than by the discomfort of the headache itself. Once reassured, often treatment beyond simple analgesics is neither necessary nor desired by the patient.

1. Headache diary: The patient should be encouraged to understand causes and precipitants for their headaches. Keeping a headache diary can be therapeutic itself, even if no specific precipitants are ever identified. The diary is kept for a variable period, usually until at least three typical headache episodes have occurred, or up to 3 months if no attacks occur while keeping the diary. Patient (with help of parent) records a *detailed* diary of headaches, medication intake, and results as well as activities, foods, stresses, sleep pattern, and physical environment. The following items can be important in uncovering the precipitating factors in recurrent headaches:
   a. Foods: Chocolate, nuts, cola, caffeine-containing beverages, cheeses. (Best to record *all* food intake in diary.)
   b. Food additives: Monosodium glutamate (MSG), nitrates and nitrites. Nitrates and nitrites are present in nearly all cured meats such as hot dogs, bacon, sausage, ham,

lunch meats. MSG is not always clearly listed on food labels. Foods commonly high in MSG include dried soups and noodles, dried flavoring packets for taco or spaghetti sauces, and some snack foods.

   c. Physical stimulants: Bright light exposure, rapidly moving or strobe light (or strobe effect when driving). Temperature changes, exercise, sexual activity.

   d. *All medications*, including over-the-counter medications and birth control pills, for headache or any other condition.

   e. Alcohol or other substance intake.

   f. Obvious allergic symptoms (rashes, asthma, allergic rhinitis).

   g. Stresses: School, tests, emotional stressors.

   h. Sleep pattern: Deviations from usual pattern, particularly excessive sleep, may precipitate headaches.

2. Treatment of tension-type headaches

   a. A brief period of relaxation or a nap often brings relief.

   b. Simple physical measures: Massage or stretching exercises of neck muscles or warm or cold compresses may help, particularly with relaxation. Biofeedback is occasionally effective but is expensive and requires a very motivated patient and family.

   c. Simple analgesics (acetaminophen, nonsteroidal anti-inflammatory drugs [NSAIDs], aspirin), if not used excessively, are often effective.

   d. Combined analgesic-sedative drugs (butalbital [Fiorinal], other combinations) should be used sparingly, if at all.

   e. Mixed tension-vascular headaches, if very frequent and disabling, may be treated on a prophylactic basis with low-dose tricyclic antidepressants, usually amitriptyline.

3. Migraine headaches: Things to do on a *trial* basis for all migraine patients:

   a. Wear sunglasses, brimmed hat, or visor whenever in bright sun. In many communities a "doctor's note" is needed to allow hat or sunglasses during outdoor activities at school.

   b. Avoid strobes or strobelike conditions.

   c. Try diet eliminating MSG and nitrates or nitrites.

   d. Stabilize caffeine intake (same amount every day) or wean off completely.

   e. Trial eliminating all alcohol.

4. Medications for acute episodic migraine treatment (classic, common, or variant) in patient with relatively infrequent headaches.

   a. Simple analgesics, taken as soon as possible at onset of episode (acetaminophen, NSAIDs such as ibuprofen, naproxen) often abort migraine, without need for stronger medications. Caffeine (either as tablet NoDoz or beverage) may potentiate the effect of the analgesic.

   b. Antiemetic, either orally, rectally, or parenterally: Promethazine (Phenergan), chlorpromazine (Thorazine), or prochlorperazine (Compazine) combined with or followed by an analgesic is very helpful if nausea or vomiting are prominent. Use of a sedating antiemetic will often allow oral analgesic to be tolerated and promote sleep, as well as relieving nausea and vomiting.

   c. Sedative-analgesic combinations: Small doses of a short-acting sedative such as barbiturate with acetaminophen or aspirin are reasonable if headaches are infrequent and relieved by sleep. Multiple preparations and brands are available (butalbital [Fiorinal], meprobamate with aspirin [Equagesic]).

   d. Ergot derivatives work best for classic migraine but work for some common migraines. Ergotamine must be used immediately at onset of symptoms. Medication should be available to the teen at all times, including in school. Sublingual, oral, rectal, or inhaled preparations are available, with multiple brand names. Cafergot combines ergotamine and caffeine. Other preparations mostly contain only ergotamine, usually ergotamine tartrate, 1–2 mg per dose.

e. Sumatriptan, a specific serotonin agonist is administered by subcutaneous injection or orally. It is not yet labeled for use in children or adolescents. The "self-injection" syringes are only available in a 6-mg dose, which may be too high for a smaller teen. Fractional doses (2–3 mg) may be used from unit-dose vials using a regular syringe and needle. As subjective sensory phenomena may be very worrisome to the patient, the first dose should always be given under direct medical supervision. If successful and well tolerated, the teen or parents may be instructed in administration at home, particularly if episodes are infrequent but very severe. *Do not use for hemiplegic migraines.* Oral sumatriptan is available in the United States. The adult dose is 25 mg once or twice. Doses for teens are not yet established.

f. Dihydroergotamine (intravenous [IV] or intramuscular [IM] injection): DHE-45, given 10–15 minutes after a parenteral dose of antiemetic (commonly metoclopramide [Reglan] or chlorpromazine [Thorazine]), may provide rapid relief of migraine symptoms, even several hours after onset. Several small doses may be given under direct supervision in an emergency room or office. Occasionally, the patient or family may be taught to self-administer DHE at home for severe episodes. *Do not use for hemiplegic migraines.*

g. Inhaled high-flow oxygen may relieve cluster headaches rapidly. Cluster headache patients often carry a small tank of oxygen with them at all times and become psychologically dependent on the availability of this treatment modality if it is effective at relieving their severe attacks of pain.

h. Thorazine (chlorpromazine) 10 mg IV (single dose) has been reported to relieve migraine pain rapidly.

Warning: If headaches are frequent (i.e., more than twice a week), beware of analgesic or ergot overuse syndromes! This may convert intermittent migraine to chronic "transformed" migraine.

4. Prophylactic treatment: Adolescents with severe recurrent attacks causing significant school absenteeism or functional limitations should be considered for prophylactic treatment. Prophylactic treatment is generally indicated in migraines accompanied by significant neurological deficits (hemiplegic migraine, for example), even if the episodes are infrequent. Prophylactic treatment may be preferred even in patients responsive to ergotamine, due to inability to carry medications in school. Continue treatment until headache pattern has markedly improved for approximately 6 months, then consider a trial of a taper off medication.

a. β-blockers: Propranolol is effective in approximately 70% of adolescents with severe migraine, although there have been few well-controlled studies. The initial dose is 40–80 mg, divided b.i.d. or t.i.d. Higher dosages (up to 240 mg/day) may be used. The effect is not immediate. Usually, a gradual decrease in headache frequency is seen over several weeks to months. Side effects include fatigue, depression, decreased exercise tolerance, particularly at high doses. Severe asthma, insulin-dependent diabetes, or depression are contraindications. Other β-blockers (i.e., atenolol) may also be effective.

b. Tricyclic antidepressants (amitriptyline, imipramine, desipramine): Amitriptyline (Elavil) is useful for prophylaxis of migraine or mixed tension-vascular headaches. Initial daily dose is 10–25 mg at bedtime, increased gradually as needed to 75–100 mg/day. Side effects include sedation, dry mouth, arrhythmias, hypotension, and decreased tolerance of warm environments.

c. Low-dose aspirin or NSAIDs (ibuprofen, naproxen) used in chronic, low doses may effectively prevent migraine attacks. NSAIDs may be particularly effective in menstrual migraine if started a day or two prior to expected symptomatic periods.

d. Cyproheptadine (Periactin): The usual dosage is 2–4 mg t.i.d. A major side effect is sedation. Significant weight gain occasionally occurs.

e. Anticonvulsants: Valproic acid (Depakote), low-dose phenobarbital, and possibly phenytoin (Dilantin) have been reported to prevent migraine. The dose used often is lower than that necessary for seizure control.

f. Calcium channel blockers (verapamil, nimodipine), have been used with some success for migraine prophylaxis.

g. Clonidine (Catapres) has occasionally be reported to been useful.

h. Ergonovine maleate may be administered daily for migraine prophylaxis. Dosage is 0.2 mg b.i.d. or t.i.d. for 4–6 weeks.

i. Methysergide (Sansert): Significant risks make this a last choice in most circumstances. It should not be used continuously for more than 6 months, due to risk of retroperitoneal and pericardial fibrosis. Close follow-up is essential. However, this is a very effective modality for patients with refractory, frequent migraines.

5. "Transformed migraine," chronic migraine, if severe and disabling

a. IV dihydroergotamine (DHE-45), usually combined with Reglan or Thorazine, is given over 2–4 days on an adjusted every-8-hour schedule. This requires hospitalization, close supervision, and dosage titration over the first few doses.

b. Short courses of high-dose corticosteroids may end the episode. Usually, high-dose prednisone (2 mg/kg/day) or dexaminethasone (Decadron) are used for about 5 days.

c. Withdrawal of chronic (overused or daily use) non-narcotic and narcotic analgesics and ergots is essential. This may require hospitalization.

PROGNOSIS

Childhood onset migraines may remit during adolescence or young adulthood. Adolescent onset migraines often continue into adulthood. However, teen should be reassured that even people with a strong tendency to migraine do not have frequent attacks throughout life. Patterns of occurrence are highly variable.

BIBLIOGRAPHY

Barron TF, Ostrov BE, Zimmerman RA, et al. Isolated angiitis of CNS: treatment with pulse cyclophosphamide. Pediatr Neurol 1993;9(1):73–75.

Bateman DN. Sumatriptan. Lancet 1993;341:221.

Battistella PA, Ruffilli R, Cernetti R, et al. A placebo-controlled crossover trial using trazodone in pediatric migraine. Headache 1993;33(1):36–39.

Baumel B. Migraine: a pharmacologic review with newer options and delivery modalities. Neurology 1994;44:S13.

Caviness VS, Phil D, O'Brien P. Headache. N Engl J Med 1980;302:446.

Dexter SL. Rebreathing aborts migraine attacks. Br Med J 1982;284:312.

Diamond S, Freitag FG, Solomon GD, et al. Migraine headache: working for the best outcome. Postgrad Med 1987;81:174-183.

DuBose CD, Cutlip AC, Cutlip WD 2nd. Migraines and other headaches: an approach to diagnosis and classification. Am Fam Physician 1995;51:1498.

Ferrari MD. Sumatriptan in the treatment of migraine. Neurology 1993;43:S43.

Fleisher DR, Matar M. The cyclic vomiting syndrome: a report of 71 cases and literature review. J Ped Gastroenterol Nutr 1993;17(4):361–369.

Friedman AP. Current concepts in the diagnosis and treatment of chronic recurring headache. Med Clin North Am 1972;56:1257.

Garvey MJ, Tollefson GD, Schaffer CB. Migraine headaches and depression. Am J Psychiatry 1984;141: 986–988.

Gascon GG. Chronic and recurrent headaches in children and adolescents. Pediatr Clin North Am 1984; 31:1027–1051.

Henry P, Allens H. Subcutaneous sumatriptan in the acute treatment of migraine in patients using dihydroergotamine as prophylaxis. French Migraine Network Bordeaux-Lyon-Grenoble. Headache 1993; 33(8):432–435.

Hoffert MJ. Treatment of migraine: a new era. Am Fam Physician 1994;49:633.

Igarashi M, May WN, Golden GS. Pharmacologic treatment of childhood migraine. J Pediatr 1992;120 (4 Pt 1):653–657.

Johannes CB, Linet MS, Stewart WF, et al. Relationship of headache to phase of the menstrual cycle among young women: a daily diary study. Neurology 1995; 45:1076.

Kaiser RS. Depression in adolescent headache patients. Headache 1992;32:340.

Kumar KL, Cooney TG. Headaches. Med Clin North Am 1995;79:261.

Larson EB, Omenn GS, Lewis H. Diagnostic evaluation of headache: impact of computerized tomography and cost effectiveness. JAMA 1980;243:359.

Ling W, Oftedal G, Weinberg W. Depressive illness in childhood presenting as severe headache. Am J Dis Child 1970;120:122–124.

Lipton RB, Stewart WF. Migraine in the United States: a review of epidemiology and health care use. Neurology 1993;43:S6.

Lipton RB, Stewart WF, Celentano DD, et al. Undiagnosed migraine headaches. A comparison of symptom-based and reported physician diagnosis. Arch Intern Med 1992;152(6):1273–1278.

MacDonald JT. Childhood migraine: differential diagnosis and treatment. Postgrad Med 1986;80:301–306.

McGrath PJ, Humphreys P, Keene D, et al. The efficacy and efficiency of a self-administered treatment for adolescent migraine. Pain 1992;49(3):321–324.

Mathew NT, Dexter J, Couch J, et al. Dose ranging efficacy and safety of subcutaneous sumatriptan in the acute treatment of migraine. US Sumatriptan Research Group. Arch Neurol 1992;49:1271.

Neighbor ML. Sumatriptan—a new treatment of migraine. Western J Med 1993;159(5):597–598.

Prensky AL, Sommer D. Diagnosis and treatment of migraine in children. Neurology 1979;29:506.

Raskin NH. Acute and prophylactic treatment of migraine: practical approaches and pharmacologic rationale. Neurology 1993;43:S39.

Rapoport AM. Recurrent migraine: cost-effective care. Neurology 1994;44:S25.

Rothner AD. Headaches in children and adolescents. Postgrad Med 1987;81:223–230.

Rothner AD. Management of headaches in children and adolescents. J Pain Symptom Manage 1993;8:81.

Schulman EA, Silberstein SD. Symptomatic and prophylactic treatment of migraine and tension-type headache. Neurology 1992;42:16.

Sheftell FD. Chronic daily headache. Neurology 1992; 42:32.

Shinnar S, D'Souza BJ. The diagnosis and management of headaches in children. Pediatr Clin North Am 1981;29:79.

Solbach MP, Waymer RS. Treatment of menstruation-associated migraine headache with subcutaneous sumatriptan. Obstet Gynecol 1993;82:769.

Solomon GD, Steel JG, Spaccavento LJ. Verapamil prophylaxis of migraine. JAMA 1983;250:2500–2502.

Tfelt-Hansen P. Sumatriptan for the treatment of migraine attacks—a review of controlled clinical trials. Cephalalgia 1993;13(4):238–244.

Welch KM. Drug therapy of migraine. N Engl J Med 1993;329(20):1476–1483.

CHAPTER 23

Syncope and Vertigo

Wendy G. Mitchell and Lawrence S. Neinstein

Up to 30% of healthy teenagers experience some type of syncopal episode during their adolescence. Many terms are used by patients to describe their complaints. Symptoms may include light-headedness, floating feelings, faintness, spinning sensations, loss of consciousness, and seizure episodes. It is best to try to divide these complaints into either syncopal or near syncopal episodes, vertigo, nonspecific dizziness, or seizures. Each category has separate implications and therapy. Vague feelings of dizziness and faintness may fit into any of these categories.

SYNCOPE

Syncope implies a brief loss of consciousness, usually lasting several seconds to a minute or so, with loss of postural tone followed by spontaneous recovery without resuscitation. While the vast majority of episodes are neurocardiogenic (vasovagal), any condition that decreases cerebral perfusion, cardiac or noncardiac, as well as metabolic disturbances and psychiatric conditions, may cause syncope. Conversely and complicating the evaluation in some instances is the phenomena of syncopal convulsions, in which a primarily syncopal episode precipitates a brief generalized seizure.

In most studies of syncope, syncope of unknown origin (often termed simple syncope) and vasovagal syncope account for the majority of cases. A study of syncope in children and adolescents conducted at the Cleveland Clinic found the following causes (Gordon et al., 1987):

Unknown causes	27/73
Vasovagal reaction	17/73
Psychogenic causes	8/73
Hyperventilation	4/73
Febrile seizures	3/73
Adjustment disorder	2/73

1 each: Sick sinus syndrome, anxiety, trauma, carotid sinus hypersensitivity, diabetes mellitus, hysterical conversion, migraine, DeMorsier's syndrome, behavior disorder, myocardial disease, atrioventricular (AV) nodal reentry tachycardia, and muscular dystrophy.

A serious disorder was found in only 4%.

The following problems may also cause dizziness without syncope, or "near syncope."

Noncardiac Causes

Syncope Due to Decreased Cerebral Perfusion Pressure

1. Vasodepressor episode, vasovagal syncope, neurocardiogenic syncope, common faint

a. The most frequent cause of syncope among teenagers and adults, accounting for most syncopal episodes.

b. Duration: May last for a few seconds to a few minutes.

c. Onset: Gradual. Patient generally is aware that something is wrong.

d. Precipitating factors: Acute stress including fear, anxiety, pain, hunger, overcrowding, fatigue, injections, and the sight of blood. Alcohol and exposure to cold or heat can also precipitate an attack. Prolonged standing, particularly without movement, may contribute.

e. Attack description
   — Early phase: The early phase is characterized by an elevated pulse, elevated blood pressure, and increased cardiac output. Symptoms include feelings of apprehension and anxiety, light-headedness, feeling of warmth.
   — Middle phase: Pulse, heart rate, blood pressure, and cardiac output fall. Symptoms include pallor, nausea, sweating, belching, yawning, mydriasis, weakness, cold hands, and faintness.
   — Faint: If the blood pressure drops below 60–70 mm Hg, loss of consciousness will occur. There is gradual loss of muscle tone and a fall to the ground.
   — Syncopal seizures: In some individuals, a brief tonic or clonic seizure will be precipitated by syncope. It always *follows* the preceding syncopal symptoms. It is more likely if the patient faints while sitting or is kept from assuming the recumbent position on loss of consciousness.
   — Recovery: Consciousness generally returns in under 1 minute, often with a brief period of perceived inability to respond despite awareness of the environment. Patient may report fatigue, malaise, weakness, nausea, and headache for up to an hour after fainting.

f. Position: Episodes generally occur while the patient is in the sitting or standing position. Prolonged standing for hair combing or braiding is a common precipitant in adolescent and preadolescent girls. Assuming recumbent or head-down position may prevent progression of the episode to full loss of consciousness.

g. Pathophysiology: The exact pathophysiology is still not completely understood. However, the initial phase is characterized by an increase in catecholamine release. The second phase is characterized by a dilation of the vascular bed, with a shift in blood flow to the muscles and a drop in cardiac output. In many patients there is also an increase in vagal tone, leading to a marked decrease in heart rate.

2. Hyperventilation: Hyperventilation is a frequent cause of dizziness in the adolescent, although syncope less frequently follows. Symptoms of hyperventilation include:

a. Respiratory: Subjective shortness of breath secondary to increased thoracic respiratory efforts; chest pain either secondary to pressure on the diaphragm from gastric distention or related to thoracic muscle strain; increased thoracic breathing, sighing, and yawning.

b. Cardiovascular: Palpitations, tachycardia, and precordial pain.

c. Neurological: Paresthesias in extremities or periorally, light-headedness, dizziness, disorientation, impaired thinking, tetany, seizures, syncope, and headaches.

d. Gastrointestinal: Epigastric pain usually related to aerophagia; dry mouth; belching; bloating; and flatulence.

e. Musculoskeletal: Muscle pains and cramps, tremors, stiffness, and muscle spasm.

f. Psychiatric: Anxiety, depression, phobias, insomnia, sensations of unreality, and nightmares.

g. General: Fatigue, weakness, and exhaustion, particularly as attack subsides.

h. Pathophysiology: The alkalosis from hyperventilation leads to cerebral vasoconstriction and a decrease in perfusion in the brain. It is estimated that cerebral blood flow is decreased by 2% for each drop of 1 mm Hg in arterial partial pressure of carbon dioxide. Other physiological effects of hyperventilation and resulting alkalosis include a decrease in peripheral release of oxygen secondary to the Bohr effect on oxyhemoglobin, a decrease in ionized calcium level, hypophosphatemia, and possible coronary vasospasm. Attacks often occur during stressful situations, and the adolescent may be unaware of the hyperventilation.

3. Orthostatic hypotension: Orthostatic hypotension is uncommon in adolescents. It is considered to be a drop in systolic blood pressure of more than 20 mm Hg and a drop in diastolic pressure of more than 10 mm Hg or an increase in heart rate of more than 20 bpm on attaining an upright position. Good reviews of this problem are found in Kroenke (1985) and Schatz (1984b). Causes include:

   a. Inadequate homeostatic mechanisms: Prolonged bed rest, exhaustion after intense exercise, pregnancy, anorexia nervosa, heat exposure, fever, marijuana use.

   b. Reduced effective blood volume: Hemorrhage, dehydration, burns, diabetes insipidus, hemodialysis, adrenal insufficiency, and varicose veins.

   c. Medication and street drugs: Antihypertensives, phenothiazines, antidepressants, narcotics, sedatives, calcium channel blockers, alcohol.

   d. Autonomic neuropathies: Pure autonomic neuropathies may be autoimmune or familial (familial dysautonomia). Mixed motor and motor-sensory neuropathies may include autonomic neuropathy and may be genetic or acquired due to autoimmune phenomena (Guillain-Barré syndrome, chronic immune demyelinating polyneuropathy), diabetes, nutritional or uremic or metabolic causes, heavy metal poisoning, porphyria, pernicious anemia, vincristine toxicity, or chronic hydrocarbon toxicity (glue sniffing, gasoline sniffing).

   e. Spinal cord injury, transverse myelitis, spinal cord tumor, or syringomyelia may cause autonomic dysfunction. Orthostatic hypotension (and positional hypertension) are particularly common with acute paraplegia due to spinal injury from any cause.

   f. Hydrocephalus and posterior fossa tumors may occasionally cause orthostatic hypotension.

   g. Miscellaneous: Syndromes of neurotransmitter excess including carcinoid syndrome, systemic mastocytosis, and pheochromocytoma.

4. Subclavian steal syndrome: An uncommon cause of syncope related to occlusion in the proximal subclavian artery. This can lead to reversal of blood flow in the adjacent vertebral artery if vascular resistance in the arm decreases (during exercise), causing blood to flow away from the brain.

5. Micturition syncope: More commonly reported in adults, but has been reported in older adolescents and young adults. Usually not associated with any serious illnesses when it occurs in this age group. Condition most commonly occurs after rising at night for urination. Rapid emptying of the bladder leads to a reflex vasodilation and a resultant decrease in cerebral blood flow, with sudden loss of consciousness.

6. Cough syncope: Rare in the adolescent. This is caused by prolonged bout of severe coughing, bringing about a decrease in cardiac output from an increase in intrathoracic pressure. Most commonly reported in adolescents with severe chronic lung disease (cystic fibrosis, severe asthma).

7. Cerebro-occlusive disease: Extremely rare in the adolescent, unless some predisposing factor such as sickle cell anemia, vasculitis, or vascular anomaly exists.

8. Migraine: Adolescents with migraine headaches have syncopal episodes, vertigo, or dizziness preceding or accompanying migraine headaches. Migraines characterized by vertigo, dizziness, or ataxia are generally classified as basilar artery migraine. Vertigo, dizziness, or syncope may be presenting complaint and more prominent than the headache (see Chapter 22).

Syncope Due to Metabolic Causes

1. Hypoglycemia: Hypoglycemia is characterized by a gradual onset of anxiety, weakness, sweating, palpitations, and tremor. Recovery is prompt with carbohydrate intake, but no relief is obtained on recumbency. Symptomatic hypoglycemia other than in the context of insulin-dependent diabetes is very rare in adolescents and is commonly overdiagnosed by patients and families.
2. Hypoxia (high altitude): Hypoxia significant enough to produce syncope without other predisposing causes is extremely rare.

Syncope Due to Neuropsychological Factors Hysterical syncope is characterized by an unanxious patient who, in the presence of others, gracefully slumps to the floor without injury. There are generally no blood pressure or pulse changes or associated physiological changes.

Cardiac Causes

Cardiac syncope, although not common in the adolescent, occurs with enough frequency that this condition must be considered. Cardiac causes of syncope should be considered in the adolescent with a history of syncope of sudden onset, syncope during vigorous exercise, or syncope occurring in a recumbent position. Several conditions can cause cardiac syncope:

1. Mitral valve prolapse: This condition, discussed in Chapter 14, can lead to symptoms of dizziness and syncope. Underlying mechanisms include arrhythmias, a hyperadrenergic state, and orthostatic hypotension.
2. Cardiac arrhythmias and conduction disturbances: Heart block, sinus node dysfunction, paroxysmal atrial tachycardia (PAT), and drug-induced arrhythmias.
   a. PAT usually causes weakness or faintness but not syncope. The onset and end are very abrupt.
   b. Conduction disturbances may be due to primary cardiac condition or may accompany systemic conditions such as muscular dystrophies, myotonic dystrophy, Friedreich's ataxia, or mitochondrial cytopathies, particularly Kearns-Sayre syndrome.
   c. Syndrome of prolonged QT interval is familial and predisposes to a variety of arrhythmias, including the potential for sudden death.
3. Left ventricular dysfunction: Cardiomyopathy
4. Obstructive cardiovascular disease
   a. Left ventricular outflow obstruction: Aortic stenosis and idiopathic hypertrophic subaortic stenosis (IHSS).
   b. Pulmonary outflow obstruction: Pulmonary hypertension, pulmonary embolism, severe pulmonary stenosis due to congenital heart anomalies.
   c. Left ventricular inflow obstruction: Mitral stenosis, left atrial myxoma.
5. Pericardial tamponade

VERTIGO

Vertigo is a true movement sensation in which the world seems to revolve around the patient or the patient senses that he or she is spinning. Vertigo is much less common in the adolescent than nonspecific dizziness, light-headedness, or syncope. Causes of true vertigo may be either peripheral or central.

1. Peripheral
   a. Vestibular neuritis (acute labyrinthitis): Usually a result of an acute viral or bacterial infection or local trauma. This usually resolves over several days. Vertigo is generally intense, position sensitive, and accompanied by nausea and vomiting.

    b. Benign positional vertigo: Characterized by a spinning sensation after quick movements of the head or body. The attacks last seconds to minutes, occur abruptly, and are unassociated with nausea or vomiting. Cause is unknown in most patients.

    c. Ototoxic drugs: Aminoglycosides, diuretics (furosemide), aspirin, caffeine, phenytoin (Dilantin), and alcohol may cause transient or permanent vertigo.

    d. Acoustic neuromas: Vertigo with or without tinnitus and hearing loss in the affected ear. Bilateral acoustic neuromas are associated with neurofibromatosis type 2, often with onset in adolescence.

    e. Ménière's disease: Rare in adolescents. This is characterized by vertigo, tinnitus, and hearing loss secondary to an increase in endolymph. Symptoms are generally intermittent.

    f. Motion sickness

    g. Ear obstruction (i.e., cerumen compacted against tympanic membrane)

2. Central lesions of the brainstem or cerebellar tracts involving vestibular input or vestibulo-ocular pathways may cause vertigo. Central lesions causing true vertigo are often accompanied by ataxia or other motor signs due to involvement of adjacent structures. Cerebellar or brainstem lesions may be caused by:

    a. Tumors, including of brainstem, cerebellum

    b. Demyelinating diseases (i.e., multiple sclerosis)

    c. Vasculitis (lupus, isolated central nervous system [CNS] angiitis)

    d. Cerebral infarctions (stroke)

    e. Infections of the nervous system (encephalitis) or postinfectious inflammatory demyelination

    f. Migraine (although nonspecific dizziness is more common)

    g. Brain injury due to head trauma

3. Seizures: Occasionally, vertigo may be the primary or initial symptom of a complex partial seizure (see Chapter 21).

DIAGNOSIS

The history is the most crucial part of the evaluation in any of these conditions, as it allows differentiation of syncope from vertigo and seizures. The history is also helpful in identifying the specific etiology of the problem within each of these categories. It is unusual to find a cause for syncope as a result of conducting a multitude of tests if the diagnosis is not suggested by the history and physical examination. In most cases diagnosis is established by history (and negative physical and neurological examination) alone, and treatment is easily established. Batteries of tests (computed tomography [CT] scan, electroencephalogram [EEG], electrocardiogram [ECG], Holter monitor, blood chemistries) ordered nonselectively rarely determine cause.

History

1. Description of the episode and of any previous attacks helps define the nature of the attack. If the teen cannot describe the attack, it is helpful to get a description from another witness. Description of color changes (initial pallor versus initial cyanosis or flushing) may help distinguish syncope from seizure.

2. Circumstances preceding the attack, such as a stressful situation or environmental circumstances that might predispose to a common faint or hyperventilation.

3. Precipitating factors: Stress, recent infection (labyrinthitis), fasting (hypoglycemia), exercise, position, and environmental factors such as heat, crowding, stuffy room.

TABLE 23.1.   Common Faint versus Seizure

Characteristics	Common Faint	Seizure
Warning	Usually prodromal symptoms	Aura common
Duration	Brief	Prolonged
Position at onset	Usually erect	Any position
Color change	Pallor frequent	Flushing or cyanosis
Convulsions	Rare	Common
Urinary incontinence	Rare	Common
Postictal state	None	Disorientation, headaches

TABLE 23.2.   Peripheral versus Central Vertigo

Characteristics	Peripheral Vertigo	Central Vertigo
Onset	Usually paroxysmal	Seldom paroxysmal
Intensity	Severe	Seldom severe
Duration	Usually short	Longer
Influence of head position	Frequent	Seldom
Autonomic nervous system symptoms	Definite	Less intense or absent
Tinnitus	Frequent	Seldom present
Deafness	Frequently present	Seldom present
Disturbances of consciousness	Seldom present	More frequently present
Focal neurologic deficits	Infrequent	Frequent
Associated symptoms	Nausea, vomiting	Visual, headaches

4. Alleviating factors: Recumbency, food, sudden movements.
5. Suddenness of onset: A common faint is gradual, while cardiac syncope and seizures may be sudden in onset.
6. Position during attack: A common faint is always in the sitting or standing position, while cardiac syncope or seizures may occur in any position.
7. Duration of the attack is important.
8. Convulsive activity during the attack, urinary incontinence, or tongue biting suggesting epilepsy.
9. See Table 23.1 for distinguishing features of common faint versus seizure.
10. The history may also be helpful in differentiating peripheral from central vertigo (Table 23.2).

Physical Examination

1. General physical examination with special emphasis on:
   a. Blood pressure: Both arms (to check for subclavian steal syndrome) and changes with positional maneuvers (orthostatic hypotension)
   b. Skin and mucous membranes for evidence of anemia or dehydration
   c. Cardiac examination
      — Mitral valve prolapse: Midsystolic click and late systolic murmur
      — IHSS: Bisferious carotid pulse with brisk upstroke, double apical pulse, precordial thrill, paradoxic split S_2, and loud S_4
      — Increased intensity of systolic murmur during the strain phase of the Valsalva maneuver
      — Aortic stenosis: Basal systolic ejection murmur
      — Pulmonic stenosis: Loud basal systolic murmur heard best to the left of the sternum

— Left atrial myxoma: Rare, suspected in the presence of mitral diastolic murmurs or early diastolic sounds

2. Neurological examination, with emphasis on:
   a. Evidence of cranial nerve deficits, particularly 3, 4, 6, 7, and 8; funduscopic examination
   b. Focal motor deficits
   c. Tendon reflexes: Loss, asymmetry, hyperreflexia
   d. Cerebellar function: Truncal or appendicular ataxia
   e. Nystagmus with straight gaze: Horizontal suggests peripheral etiology, whereas vertical and diagonal nystagmus are more suggestive of central etiology.
   f. Sensory abnormalities: Peripheral sensory loss suggesting neuropathy

3. Special examination procedures
   a. Hyperventilation: Have the adolescent hyperventilate for 2–3 minutes. Ask the adolescent to describe the sensations to determine if they are similar to the presenting symptomatology. This should not be performed if teen has sickle cell anemia, epilepsy, or cardiac or renal disease.
   b. If vertigo is a symptom, then also have the adolescent perform:
      — Quick head turn
      — Valsalva maneuver
      — Sudden turn while walking
      — Nylen-Bárány test: Have adolescent sit at the edge of a table. Holding onto the adolescent's head, have the adolescent abruptly lie back as you place his or her head 45 degrees below the table and at a 45-degree angle to one side. Repeat the test with head at a 45-degree angle to the opposite side.

   These tests are often positive in benign positional vertigo.

4. Laboratory procedures
   The history and physical examination suffice to make the diagnosis in the majority of causes of dizziness and syncope. However, certain tests are beneficial in other circumstances.
   a. Tilt-table testing: Tilt-table testing is helpful to document that syncope and dizziness are vasovagal (neurocardiogenic) if history alone is not adequate. While tilt-table testing is somewhat time consuming and costly, it may avoid using multiple other tests nonselectively. In tilt-table testing the patient's pulse, blood pressure, and symptoms are monitored first in a supine position, then in a head-up 65-degree tilt for 15 minutes. If tilting does not reproduce the symptoms, graded infusions of isoproterenol are given, first in supine, then in head-up tilt position. Positive test results are defined as reproduction of syncopal or presyncopal symptoms and either a vasodepressor response (mean arterial blood pressure drop of 25 mm Hg or more) or cardioinhibitor response (heart rate decrease of 45 bpm or more) or both. Rechallenge after administration of metoprolol to determine if β-blockers will inhibit the response may be helpful in assessing whether treatment will prevent syncope.
   b. Cardiac syncope: If cardiac syncope is suspected, then an ECG is necessary. Depending on the underlying mechanism and disease suspected, an echocardiogram, Holter monitor, and treadmill test may be useful. In some instances the conduction disturbances are not delineated without intracardiac electrocardiography with and without atrial pacing.
   c. Vertigo: For prolonged vertigo unassociated with an acute infection or vertigo that seems positional in origin, referral to a neurologist or otolaryngologist is advisable for further evaluation and testing.
   d. Seizures: If a seizure disorder is suspected, then an EEG may be useful. If complex partial seizures are suspected, arrange to have the EEG done after overnight sleep deprivation, with recording of natural sleep, to increase yield.

e. Hypoglycemia: Hypoglycemia is commonly "diagnosed" by patients and family members without evidence. If hypoglycemia is suspected, temporary provision of a home blood sugar monitoring system for use while the patient is symptomatic may be substantially more useful than several blood sugars drawn when the patient is asymptomatic, or prolonged oral glucose tolerance testing. If blood sugar is found to be low on home testing, further evaluation is necessary. Referral to an endocrinologist should be considered if symptomatic hypoglycemia is documented and not due to an obvious cause such as skipping meals.

f. Metabolic: If a metabolic cause is suspected, serum sodium, potassium, magnesium, and creatinine tests should be ordered. More specialized testing, such as for adrenal insufficiency, may be indicated in rare situations.

THERAPY

Therapy is dependent on the specific condition diagnosed. For the vasodepressor syndrome (simple syncope), therapy is reassurance and making sure that the patient assumes a recumbent or head-down position when symptoms start. If patient is prone to fainting with prolonged standing, contracting the leg muscles also helps in increasing venous return and cardiac output. If episodes are very frequent and do not respond to simple measures, β-blockers may inhibit the cardiodepressor response.

The treatment for hyperventilation is reassurance, education about the physiology of hyperventilation, and teaching of a strategy to deal with hyperventilation and precipitating stressors. This can include having the patient breathe into a paper bag or teaching diaphragmatic breathing. The teenager should be instructed to place one hand on the abdomen and the other on the chest. The adolescent should then practice breathing so that the lower hand moves while the upper hand is held still.

Syncope, dizziness, and vertigo associated with migraine should be treated as migraine (see Chapter 22).

Treatment of vertigo is difficult. For the short-term treatment of vertigo and vomiting associated with acute labyrinthitis, antiemetics or mild sedatives may be useful, but all cause drowsiness.

Benign positional vertigo may respond to deconditioning maneuvers (i.e., repeatedly provoking the vertigo with position change to gradually suppress the response).

Vertigo associated with significant CNS disease is problematic, as long-term treatment with sedating medications is generally unacceptable, and nonsedating medications usually are ineffective. Central vertigo due to acute CNS lesions such as strokes generally decreases or abates entirely, but this process may take months or years.

Epileptic vertigo is rare, but generally responds to anticonvulsant drugs (see Chapter 21).

BIBLIOGRAPHY

DiMarco JP, Garan H, Harthorne WJ, et al. Intracardiac electrophysiologic techniques in recurrent syncope of unknown cause. Ann Intern Med 1981;95:542.

Gordon TA, Moodie DS, Passalacqua M, et al. A retrospective analysis of the cost-effective workup of syncope in children. Cleve Clin Q 1987;54:391.

Goroll AH, May LA, Mulley AG. Evaluation of dizziness. In: Goroll AH, May LA, Mulley AG, eds. Primary care medicine. Philadelphia: JB Lippincott, 1995.

Grubb BP, Temesy-Armos P, Moore J, et al. The use of head-upright tilt table testing in the evaluation and management of syncope in children and adolescents. Pacing Clin Electrophysiol 1992;15:742.

Hanna DE, Hodgens JB, Daniel WA Jr. Hyperventilation syndrome. Pediatr Ann 1986;15:708.

Hannon DW, Knilans TK. Syncope in children and adolescents. Curr Probl Pediatr 1993;23:358.

Kapoor WN. Evaluation and management of the patient with syncope. JAMA 1992;268:2552.

Kapoor WN. Workup and management of patients with syncope. Med Clin North Am 1995;79:1153.

Kapoor W, Karpf M, Levey GS. Issues in evaluating patients with syncope. Ann Intern Med 1984;100:755.

Kapoor WN, Karpf M, Wieand S, et al. A prospective evaluation and follow-up of patients with syncope. N Engl J Med 1983;309:197.

Kapoor WN, Peterson JR, Karpf M. Micturition syncope: a reappraisal. JAMA 1985;253:796.

Kroenke K. Orthostatic hypotension. West J Med 1985; 143:253.

Kroenke K, Lucas CA, Rosenberg ML. Causes of persistent dizziness. A prospective study of 100 patients in ambulatory care. Ann Intern Med 1992;117:898.

Lerman-Sagie T, Lerman P, Mukamel M. A prospective evaluation of pediatric patients with syncope. Clin Pediatr 1994;33:67.

Linzer M, Varia I, Pontinen M, et al. Medically unexplained syncope: relationship to psychiatric illness. Am J Med 1992;92:18S.

Magarian GJ, Middaugh DA, Linz DH. Hyperventilation syndrome: a diagnosis begging for recognition. West J Med 1983;138:733.

Maragos NE, Neel HB, McDonald TJ. Dissection of dizziness. Postgrad Med 1981;69:109.

McCowan R, Tone L, Thorpe C, et al. The use of head-up tilt table testing in the evaluation of unexplained syncope. W Va Med J 1992;88:233.

Missri JC, Alexander S. Hyperventilation syndrome: a brief review. JAMA 1978;240:2093.

Mott SH, Packer RJ, Soldin SJ. Neurologic manifestations of cocaine exposure in childhood. Pediatrics 1994;93:557.

Myer CM III. The dizziness of children. Emerg Med 1986;30:49.

Naccarelli GV. Evaluation of the patient with syncope. Med Clin North Am 1984;68:1211.

O'Marcaigh AS, MacLellan-Tobert SG, Porter CJ. Tilt-table testing and oral metoprolol therapy in young patients with unexplained syncope. Pediatrics 1994; 93:278.

Ormerod AD. Syncope. Br Med J 1984;288:1219.

Ozme S, Alehan D, Yalaz K, et al. Causes of syncope in children: a prospective study. Int J Cardiol 1993;40:111.

Radack KL. Syncope: cost-effective patient workup. Postgrad Med 1986;80:169.

Samoil JD, Grubb BP, Kip K, et al. Head-upright tilt table testing in children with unexplained syncope. Pediatrics 1993;92:426.

Schatz IJ. Orthostatic hypotension: diagnosis and treatment. Hosp Pract 1984a;19:59.

Schatz IJ. Orthostatic hypotension: functional and neurogenic causes. Arch Intern Med 1984b;144:773.

Smith CW Jr. Hyperventilation syndrome. Postgrad Med 1985;78:73.

Strieper MJ, Auld DO, Hulse JE, et al. Evaluation of recurrent pediatric syncope: role of tilt table testing. Pediatrics 1994;93:660–662.

CHAPTER 24

Sleep Disorders

Martin M. Anderson and Lawrence S. Neinstein

Sleep disturbances occur with less frequency in adolescents than in children or adults but are not uncommon as either a presenting symptom or positive item on a review of systems. Sleep disorders include insomnias, hypersomnias (narcolepsy and other causes of excessive daytime sleepiness), and parasomnias (nightmares, night terrors, sleepwalking, and nocturnal enuresis). Sleep disturbances in adolescents may represent a reaction to anxiety or depression, drug abuse (hallucinogens, alcohol, barbiturates), scheduling irregularities (naps, late hours), or a specific sleep disorder (narcolepsy, night terrors).

SLEEP PHYSIOLOGY

Sleep is divided into rapid eye movement (REM) sleep and nonrapid eye movement (NREM) sleep. Studies of sleep physiology are carried out using polysomnography, which usually includes electroencephalogram (EEG), electro-oculogram (EOG), electromyogram (EMG), and measures of respiratory function such as air flow and oxygen saturation.

Rapid Eye Movement Sleep

REM sleep, which occupies 15–30% of sleep time, is characterized by a high autonomic arousal state including increased cardiovascular and respiratory activity, very low voluntary musculature tone, and rapid synchronous nonpatterned eye movements. The EEG pattern shows a low-voltage variable frequency resembling the awake state. Most dreams occur during REM sleep.

Nonrapid Eye Movement Sleep

NREM sleep occupies 70–85% of sleep time and is divided into four stages:

1. Stage 1: Very light sleep, characterized on EEG by alpha waves similar to the quiet awake state.
2. Stage 2: Medium-deep sleep, characterized on EEG by sleep spindles of 12–16 cps.
3. Stages 3 and 4: Progressively deeper sleep, characterized on EEG by general slowing of frequency and increase in amplitude. Muscular and cardiovascular activity are decreased and little dreaming occurs.

SLEEP PATTERN

Normal sleep usually consists of a brief period of stage 1 and stage 2, followed by a lengthier interval of stages 3 and 4. After about 70–100 minutes of NREM sleep, a 10-minute to 25-

minute REM period occurs. This cycle is repeated four to six times about every 90 minutes throughout the night. The REM periods usually increase by 5–30 minutes each cycle.

Adolescents probably require a minimum of 9 hours of sleep per night to awake refreshed and rested. However, the amount of sleep they actually get is usually much less than what they need. On the average, on school nights, 10- to 11-year-olds sleep about $9\frac{1}{2}$ hours, 12- to 13-year-olds about 9 hours, 14- to 15-year-olds about $7\frac{3}{4}$ hours, 16- to 17-year-olds about $7\frac{1}{2}$ hours, and 18-year-old college freshmen about 7 hours. The adolescent often tries to make up for the sleep deficit accumulated during the week by sleeping much longer on weekends.

Sleep History

Any adolescent with a sleep disturbance should be questioned about:

1. Type of sleep disturbances
2. Frequency and duration of disturbances
3. Prior sleep problems
4. Daytime symptoms
5. Family history of sleep disorders
6. Age of onset
7. Bedtime habits: Amount of sleep, what time the adolescent goes to sleep, what time he or she awakens, and what is done before sleep
8. Treatment previously tried
9. Psychosocial history
10. Medications and drug history, including over-the-counter medications, alcohol, coffee, and other stimulants

Having an adolescent keep a 1-week sleep diary, listing bedtimes, nighttime symptoms, time on awakening, daytime fatigue or sleepiness, and daytime naps can be a very helpful tool in evaluating a sleep disturbance.

Specific Sleep Disorders

To treat a sleep problem, one must define the specific disorder. Disorders include:

1. Insomnias: Insomnias are the most frequent sleep disorders in adolescents. They involve either a problem falling asleep, staying asleep, or awakening too early.
   a. Delayed sleep phase syndrome: Inability to fall asleep at an appropriate time. This is accompanied by extreme difficulty in arising in the morning. If allowed to fall asleep naturally, the adolescent will fall asleep easily, albeit very late, and will awaken refreshed after 9–10 hours of sleep. If awakened, they will get up and attend school or work but may, once there, have difficulty staying awake. Delayed sleep phase syndromes can be associated with nighttime insomnia as well as day time sleepiness.
   b. Motivated sleep delay: Appears similar to delayed sleep phase syndrome, but in this case the adolescent has a conscious desire to stay up late at night and sleep late into the afternoon even if it means being late for school. However, if motivated by something he or she really wants to do, they can awaken early by themselves. This is probably a form of school refusal syndrome.
      Insomnia frequently occurs secondary to situational stress, anxiety, or poor sleeping habits. A history of stress and irregular activity is helpful in the diagnosis. Other less common causes of insomnia include any physical illness associated with pain or

discomfort and substance abuse or withdrawal (especially stimulants, alcohol, or sedatives).

2. Hypersomnias (excessive daytime sleepiness): The rigorous schedule required of adolescents by school, employment, and extracurricular activities often results in adolescents' receiving less than the 9–10 hours of sleep they require. This chronic sleep deprivation may cause complaints of fatigue or difficulty staying awake during school or work. It may adversely affect school or work performance and result in stimulant use to stay awake, moodiness, and even automobile accidents related to falling asleep at the wheel. Insufficient sleep is by far the most common cause of hypersomnia in adolescents. Specific sleep disorders are listed below.

3. Narcolepsy
   a. Onset commonly occurs between the ages of 10 and 25 years old.
   b. Characterized by
      — Sleep attacks: Intrusive and debilitating periods of sleep during the day which may last a few seconds to 30 minutes and are often precipitated by sedentary, monotonous activity; more frequent after meals and later in the day. No amount of sleep can restore the individual to full alertness.
      — Cataplexy: Brief (seconds to 2 minutes), sudden loss of muscle tone while conscious, often in response to emotional or sudden stimulation.
      — Sleep paralysis: Temporary loss of muscle tone occurring at the onset of sleep or just before awakening.
      — Hypnagogic and hypnopomic hallucinations: False visual or auditory perceptions that occur just before sleep (hypnagogic) or on awakening (hypnopomic).
      — May have automatic activity during periods of altered consciousness.
   c. Frequency of components
      — Sleep attacks: 100%
      — Sleep attacks and catalepsy: 70%
      — Sleep paralysis: 50%
      — Hallucinations: 25%
      — All four: 10%
   d. Evidence of genetic transmission: The exact genetic transmission of narcolepsy is unclear. However, it is strongly associated with human lymphocyte antigens (HLA) antigen haplotypes DR15,DQ6 (old nomenclature DR2,DQW).
   e. Narcolepsy is diagnosed using both overnight polysomnography and daytime multiple sleep latency test (MSLT). The overnight polysomnography will exclude other sleep disorders, such as sleep apnea. The MSLT is the most specific test for narcolepsy. It will show a shortened time to sleep onset (sleep latency) and early onset of REM sleep.

4. Parasomnias: Undesirable physical events that occur during sleep.
   Sleep starts: Jerking motions that occur during the transition between wakefulness and sleep. These are normal events in 60–80% of people.
   Partial arousals: Somnambulism (sleepwalking) and night terrors (sleep terrors, pavor nocturnus) are both disorders of impaired arousal.
   a. Both conditions occur early at night, about 60–90 minutes after sleep onset, during the rapid transition from deep NREM sleep to a light NREM sleep.
   b. Both usually begin in childhood or early adolescence and disappear by older adolescence.
   c. About 40% of 6- to 16-year-old children have at least one episode of sleep walking, and 1–3% experience night terrors.
   d. A positive family history can be found in one or both parents in over 60% of cases.
   e. Associated psychopathology is uncommon if the onset is in childhood, but is more common with an onset during adolescence or adulthood.

f. Characteristics
  — Sleepwalking
    (1) Usually lasts from 1–30 minutes.
    (2) The individual usually has a low level of awareness manifested by clumsiness.
    (3) The individual usually has a blank expression, with indifference to the environment.
    (4) There is usually no recall of the experience.
  — Night terrors (sleep terrors)
    (1) Intense anxiety, fear, and sensation of doom
    (2) Autonomic discharge (tachycardia, tachypnea, sweating)
    (3) Vocalizations in the form of screams, moans, or gasps
    (4) Little recall
g. Psychological disturbances are suggested as a more likely cause of the night terrors or sleepwalking if the onset is after age 12, the condition has persisted for several years, there is a negative family history, and there is maladaptive daytime behavior.
h. Hysterical phenomena such as fugue states are suggested by a more alert state, more purposeful movements, and longer duration.
5. Nightmares (dream anxiety attacks)
  a. Affect about 5% of the population.
  b. Onset usually before age 10; more suggestive of psychological cause if onset is after this age.
  c. Often associated with fear of attack, falling, or death.
  d. Drug withdrawal, especially from barbiturates or alcohol, can lead to nightmares.
  e. Table 24.1 differentiates nightmares from night terrors.
  f. Sleep paralysis, hypnagogic and hypnopomic hallucinations: although frequently seen in narcolepsy, they can occur in non-narcoleptics.
6. Nocturnal enuresis (see Chapter 26)
  a. Approximately 1–5% of adolescents are enuretic.
  b. Enuresis is independent of stage of sleep.
  c. Enuresis may be primary or secondary.
    — Primary: Without a several-month period of dryness since infancy. Primary enuresis may involve a maturational delay and is often associated with a positive family history. There are two prominent theories of its cause:
      (1) That it is a maturational delay in neuromuscular control of the bladder.
      (2) That it is related to a blunting of the diurnal antidiuretic hormone (ADH) secretion, resulting in an increased nocturnal urine production that exceeds the functional bladder capacity.
    — Secondary: Relapse of enuresis after at least a several-month dry period. Secondary enuresis should prompt further evaluation of an organic cause such as di-

TABLE 24.1.   Nightmares versus Night Terrors

Characteristic	Night Terrors	Nightmares
Vocalization	Intense	Limited
Autonomic activity	Marked increase	Slight increase
Arousal	Difficult	Easy
Motility	Marked	Limited
Recall	Minimal	Vivid
Sleep stage	NREM sleep	REM sleep

abetes or infection or a psychological cause such an acute stressor (death, divorce, new baby in family, natural disaster).

TREATMENT

Insomnia

1. Counseling regarding any existing situational stresses.
2. Regularize bedtime and awakening hours. Try to have the adolescent arise at a similar hour each day. Avoid excessive sleep on weekends. Avoid trying to force sleep when not tired.
3. Have adolescent schedule time other than bedtime to think about problems.
4. Teach relaxation techniques.
5. Daily exercise, but not close to bedtime.
6. Curtail alcohol, coffee, tea, cola, or other stimulant drugs.
7. Bedroom environment should be for sleep only (i.e., no television in bedroom).
8. Keep bedroom dark and as quiet as possible.
9. Avoid daytime naps.
10. Severe cases due to sleep phase delays may need chromotherapy (an adjustment of sleep waking schedule performed by an expert in sleep disorders). The motivated sleep delay syndrome is especially hard to treat and may need the involvement of a psychologist or psychiatrist.

Somnambulism

1. Protect patient by removing harmful objects and locking doors.
2. Reassurance, if onset is during childhood, that problem should resolve.

Night Terrors (Sleep Terrors)

1. Reassurance that problem should resolve by itself.
2. Psychological evaluation and treatment indicated where psychopathology is present.
3. Benzodiazepines, tricyclic antidepressants, relaxation techniques, or mental imagery may be used to suppress night terrors.
4. Avoid sleep deprivation. Try to regularize sleep and wake schedule.

Nightmares (Sleep Anxiety Attacks)

1. Evaluation and treatment of any underlying psychological stresses or fears.
2. Evaluation and treatment of any associated alcohol or other drug abuse problems.

Nocturnal Enuresis (see Chapter 26)

Treatment for nonorganic enuresis can include:

1. Drink less fluid in the 2 hours before bedtime.
2. Urinate before going to bed.
3. The adolescent should be responsible for laundering and changing linens. Consider placing a dry towel under the patient to decrease the need for linen changes.
4. Elimination of guilt or blame. Positive rewards and praise for dry nights.

5. Exercises to improve control of urinary stream and to increase bladder capacity.
6. Behavior techniques, especially the new, smaller alarm systems, are the most effective methods for treating enuresis and have the lowest relapse rate.
7. Medications are not as effective in the long term as are behavioral techniques, especially the alarm. However, they have more immediate effects and can be used in conjunction with behavioral techniques.
   a. Imipramine (Tofranil) is effective, but relapse is common after stopping the medication.
   b. Desmopressin (DDAVP) is also quite effective and has fewer potential side effects than imipramine. It also has a high relapse rate after its discontinuation and is currently quite expensive.

Narcolepsy

1. Drugs: Methylphenidate (Ritalin) is the drug of choice for sleep attacks.
   a. Administer at least 1 hour after meals to allow for absorption.
   b. Titrate to lowest effective dose.
   c. Avoid late afternoon or evening doses.
2. Imipramine is the drug of choice for catalepsy and sleep paralysis.
   a. Requires only 10–75 mg/day.
   b. Avoid evening dose.
3. Avoid dangerous activities such as driving an automobile or scuba diving.
4. Naps: Short scheduled naps during the day may prevent sleep attacks.

Other Hypersomnias

1. Treatment of any underlying disorder.
2. Treatment of delayed sleep phase syndrome by chromotherapy if severe (more than 3–4 hours out of phase).
3. Increase the amount of nighttime sleep with the understanding that teens need 9–10 hours of sleep but often get much less, thus are chronically sleep deprived, resulting in excessive daytime sleepiness.

SLEEP DISORDER CLINICS

For severe sleep disorders or diagnostic dilemmas, referral to a sleep disorder clinic can help. Appendix II to this book contains a partial listing of institutions specializing in the treatment of sleep disorders.

BIBLIOGRAPHY

Aldrich MS. Narcolepsy. Neurology 1992;42(suppl 6):34.

Allsopp MR, Zaiwalla Z. Narcolepsy. Arch Dis Child 1992;67:302.

Andrade MM, Benedito-Silva AA, Domenice S, et al. Sleep characteristics of adolescents: a longitudinal study. J Adol Health 1993;14(5):401.

Bloom DA. The American experience with desmopressin. Clin Pediatr 1993;Special ed:28.

Carskadon MA. Patterns of sleep and sleepiness in adolescents. Pediatrician 1990;17:17.

Carskadon MA, Vieira C, Acebo C. Association between puberty and delayed phase preference. Sleep 1993; 16(3):258.

Evans JHC, Meadow SR. Desmopressin for bed wetting: length of treatment, vasopressin secretion, and response. Arch Dis Child 1992;67:184.

Ferber R. Sleep schedule-dependent causes of insomnia and sleepiness in middle childhood and adolescence. Pediatrician 1990;17:13.

Friman PC, Warzak WJ. Nocturnal enuresis: a prevalent,

persistent, yet curable parasomnia. Pediatrician 1990; 17:38.

Hjalmas K, Bengtsson B. Efficacy, safety and dosing of desmopressin for nocturnal enuresis in Europe. Clin Pediatr 1993;Special ed:19.

Hogg RJ, Husmann D. The role of family history in predicting response to desmopressin in nocturnal enuresis. J Urol 1993;150:444.

Hublin C, Kaprio J, Partinen M, et al. The prevalence of narcolepsy: an epidemiological study of the Finnish twin cohort. Ann Neurol 1994;35(6):709.

Kales A, Kales JD. Sleep disorders. N Engl J Med 1974; 290:487.

Kales A, Soldatos CR, Kales JD. Sleep disorders: insomnia, sleepwalking, night terrors, nightmares, and enuresis. Ann Intern Med 1987;106:582.

Kales A, Vela-Bueno A, Kales JD. Sleep disorders: sleep apnea and narcolepsy. Ann Intern Med 1987;106: 434.

Kales JD, Kales A, Bixler ED, et al. Resource for managing sleep disorders. JAMA 1976;241:2413.

Knudsen UB, Rittig S, Norgaard JP, et al. Long-term treatment of nocturnal enuresis with desmopressin. Urol Res 1991;19:237.

Kupfer DJ, Reynolds CF. Sleep disorders. Hosp Pract 1983;100:101.

Mahowald MW, Rosen GM. Parasomnias in children. Pediatrician 1990;12:17.

Milter MM, Hajdukovic R, Erman MK. Treatment of narcolepsy with methamphetamine. Sleep 1993;16(4):306.

Norgaard JP, Djurhuus JC. The pathophysiology of enuresis in children and young adults. Clin Pediatr 1993;Special ed:5.

Rivinus TM, Ferber R. Practical approaches to sleep disorders in childhood. Med Times 1979;107:71.

Rushton HG. Evaluation of the enuretic child. Clin Pediatr 1993;Special ed:14.

Soldatos CR, Kales A, Kales JD. Management of insomnia. Annu Rev Med 1979;30:301.

Terho P. Desmopressin in nocturnal enuresis. J Urol 1991;145:818.

Zarcone V. Narcolepsy. N Engl J Med 1973;288:1156.

Genitourinary Disorders

CHAPTER 25

Genitourinary Tract Infections

Genitourinary tract infections, common in adolescents, include cystitis, pyelonephritis, asymptomatic bacteriuria, and urethritis.

CYSTITIS

Epidemiology

1. Cystitis is three to five times more common in females than males. The prevalence is shown below:

	Male	Female
Infants	1–2%	0.5%
Young children	0.1%	1.5%
College students	<0.01%	5.0%

2. Ten percent to 20% of females have at least one episode of acute cystitis during adolescence or young adulthood. Foxman (1990) found that 30% of young women had a least one recurrence within 6 months of the first infection.
3. Risk factors for infection
   a. Females: Females are at greater risk than males because of a short urethra, which has close proximity to vaginal and rectal microorganisms. Risk factors for a urinary tract infection include:
      — Poor perineal hygiene
      — Tight panty hose
      — Coitus: New sexual partner or start of sexual activity
      Strom et al. (1987) examined risk factors in females for symptomatic bacteriuria and found that intercourse in the previous 48 hours, diaphragm use in the previous 48 hours, not urinating after intercourse, and a history of urinary tract infection were correlated with an increased risk of urinary tract infection. There was no correlation in this study between infections and the use of oral contraceptives or tampons, nor with the direction of wiping after a bowel movement. Risk factors included:
      — Delayed postcoital micturition
      — Pregnancy
      — Diaphragm use
      — History of recent urinary infection
      — Insertion of foreign body
      — Anatomical abnormalities, including urethral stenosis, neurogenic bladder, nephrolithiasis, and vesicoureteral reflux.
      — Blood group B or AB nonsecretor
      — P_1 blood group phenotype (epithelial cell receptors facilitate bacterial attachment)

   b. Males
      — Risk factors and pathophysiology are less understood in males. In non-sexually-
        active adolescent males, bladder and renal infections may be a result of structural
        or functional abnormalities of the urinary tract. Risk factors include:
      (1) Blood group B or AB nonsecretor
      (2) P_1 blood group phenotype (epithelial cell receptors facilitate bacterial at-
          tachment)
      (3) Homosexuality in association with *Escherichia coli* exposure through anal
          intercourse
      (4) Sexual partner with vaginal colonization by uropathogens
      (5) Lack of circumcision, which is associated with greater colonization of glans
          by *E. coli*
      (6) CD4⁺ cell counts of less than 200/mL blood

Microbiology

Females   The most common organism in adolescent females with acute cystitis is *E. coli*
(75–90%). *Staphylococcus saprophyticus* is probably the second most common cause of urinary
tract infection in young women (>10%). Other gram-negative organisms cause most of the
remainder of the infections. In chronic or recurrent infections, *Klebsiella* sp., enterococci,
Pseudomonas aeruginosa, *Enterobacter* sp., *Proteus* sp., *Staphylococcus aureus*, *Streptococcus fae-
calis*, and *Serratia marcescens* play a more common role than in acute infections.

Males   About three-fourths of urinary tract infections in adolescent and young adult
males are due to gram-negative bacilli, but *E. coli* infections are not nearly so common as in
females. Gram-positive organisms, especially enterococci and coagulase-negative staphylococci, account for about one-fifth of infections. *Trichomonas vaginalis* is a rare cause of bacteriuria in males, usually involving an infection of the urethra or prostate. *Gardnerella vaginalis* can
also occasionally cause infections in males.

Symptoms

Females

1. Dysuria
2. Frequency, hesitancy, and urgency
3. Lower abdominal pain
4. Low-grade fever
5. Gross hematuria

Symptoms caused by infections in the genitourinary tract are difficult to localize. For example, dysuria and dyspareunia in the female can be related to infections in either the bladder, urethra, or vulva. However, the location of the dysuria is occasionally helpful. The dysuria
associated with cystitis or urethritis is often described as internal pain, whereas external pain
is more often associated with other conditions such as a vulvar inflammation or a herpes simplex infection.

Males   Aside from the preceding symptoms, males may also have symptoms associated
with genitourinary infections in the prostate, epididymis, seminal vesicles, and testes.

Differential Diagnosis of Acute Dysuria

The most common complaint arousing suspicion of cystitis is dysuria. The following are considerations in the differential diagnosis of cystitis and dysuria:

Females Table 25.1 lists the pathogens, incidence of pyuria and hematuria, urine culture findings, and signs and symptoms of acute dysuria in women.

1. Acute urethritis secondary to *Chlamydia trachomatis, Neisseria gonorrhoeae,* or herpes simplex virus.
2. Vulvovaginitis due to *Candida* or *Trichomonas.*
3. Local dermatitis: Includes irritations from chemicals and other agents such as soap, contraceptive agents and foams, and feminine hygiene products.
4. Subclinical pyelonephritis: Some females with only dysuria have an upper urinary tract infection. These infections may be more difficult to eradicate. There are no reliable and simple methods to distinguish them from lower urinary tract infections.
5. Acute urethral syndrome: The presence and frequency of dysuria in women with urine cultures showing between 10^2 colony-forming units (CFU) and 10^5 organisms per milliliter has in the past been termed the urethral syndrome or the dysuria-pyuria syndrome. However, studies in the past decade have shown that many women with symptomatic cystitis have fewer than 10^5 CFU/mL. Thus this lower figure of 10^2 CFU/mL may have good sensitivity and specificity in treating urinary tract infections. Kunin et al. (1993) reevaluated acute urinary symptoms and "low count" bacteriuria ($>10^2-10^4$ CFU/mL) in women. *E. coli* and *S. saprophyticus* were the only microorganisms statistically associated with urinary tract symptoms and pyuria. This revision of bacterial counts has lessened or eliminated the need for the category of urethral syndrome or dysuria-pyuria syndrome. The small group of symptomatic women with no growth on urine culture need close evaluation for infections with *C. trachomatis, Mycobacterium tuberculosis,* herpes simplex virus, *Candida,* or *T. vaginalis.* The practitioner is reminded that about 10% of symptom-free women have low bacterial counts and up to 20% of asymptomatic women have pyuria. Patients with dysuria and pyuria and no evidence of cystitis or vaginitis may have

TABLE 25.1. Differential Diagnosis of Acute Dysuria in Women

Condition	Pathogen	Pyuria	Hematuria	Urine Culture	Signs, Symptoms
Cystitis	*E. coli, S. saprophyticus, Proteus, Klebsiella* sp.	Usually	Sometimes	$10^2->10^5$	Acute onset, severe symptoms, dysuria, frequency, urgency, suprapubic or low back pain, suprapubic tenderness
Urethritis	*C. trachomatis, N. gonorrhoeae,* herpes simplex virus	Usually	Rarely	$<10^2$	Gradual onset, mild symptoms, vaginal discharge or bleeding, lower abdominal pain, new sexual partner, cervical or vaginal lesions on examination
Vaginitis	*Candida* sp., *T. vaginalis*	Rarely	Rarely	$<10^2$	Vaginal discharge or odor, pruritus, dyspareunia, external dysuria, no frequency or urgency, vulvovaginitis on examination

Adapted from Stamm WE, Hooton TM. Management of urinary tract infections in adults. N Engl J Med 1993;329:1329.

a favorable response to tetracycline or doxycycline. No benefit from antibiotic therapy has been found in patients who do not have pyuria.

6. Causes of dysuria: In a study of 53 adolescent females with a complaint of dysuria, Demetriou et al. (1982) found the following causes:

   a. 41% had a vaginitis caused by *Candida, T. vaginalis,* or *G. vaginalis.*
   b. 17% had a urinary tract infection.
   c. 17% had a vaginitis and a urinary tract infection.
   d. 10% had a sexually transmitted infection (caused by *N. gonorrhoeae, Chlamydia,* or herpesvirus).
   e. 15% had another cause (e.g., local infection, trauma, or acute urethral syndrome).

Males   In males the major diseases in the differential diagnosis of cystitis and dysuria include:

1. Gonococcal urethritis and nongonococcal urethritis
2. Prostatitis
3. Irritation from agents such as spermicidal foam.

Diagnosis

1. History
   a. Are there symptoms suggestive of vulvovaginitis, such as an abnormal vaginal discharge or vaginal itching? With a vaginal infection, symptoms of frequency and urgency are less common.
   b. Does the teen use any medications or irritants such as douches, feminine hygiene products, strong soaps, bubble bath, or contraceptive products that could cause a local dermatitis?
   c. Is the teen sexually active? If so, sexually transmitted diseases, including a cervicitis or urethritis caused by *C. trachomatis, N. gonorrhoeae,* or *T. vaginalis,* become a concern.
   d. Are there signs of upper genitourinary tract disease? Fever and flank pain suggest acute pyelonephritis.
   e. Are there factors suggestive of a subclinical pyelonephritis, such as underlying urinary tract disease, diabetes mellitus, urinary infections in childhood, three or more previous urinary tract infections, or acute pyelonephritis in the past?
2. Physical examination
   a. In both sexes an examination of the abdomen and flank for tenderness should be performed. In addition, the genital area should be examined for a local dermatitis.
   b. In females, a pelvic examination should be performed if the teen is sexually active or if there is history of a vaginal discharge.
   c. In males, the physical examination should include inspection and palpation of the genitals to check for urethral discharge, meatal erythema, inflammation of the glans penis, penile lesions, an enlarged or tender epididymis or testis, or inguinal lymphadenopathy.
3. Laboratory studies
   a. Microscopic examination of urine
      — The presence of one or more bacteria per oil immersion field of uncentrifuged urine has an 80–95% correlation with bacteriuria in which the bacteria count is 10^5/mL. This examination may also be performed on a gram-stained specimen of unspun urine.
      — A count of more than 10 organisms per oil immersion field on a centrifuged unstained sediment also correlates with positive culture results. Pyuria with five or

more leukocytes per high-power field of urine sediment on spun urine has a poorer correlation. Sources of error with the latter include variable volumes of urine, variable time and speed of centrifugation, and inconsistent resuspension volume. However, analysis of unspun urine for leukocytes in a counting chamber does give reproducible results and is significant if the count is greater than 10 leukocytes/mm^3. Urine should be examined within 2 hours of collection. Presence of pyuria is a good indicator that antibiotic therapy will be helpful. Individuals with no recognized pathogen rarely have pyuria and usually do not respond to treatment. A positive finding with a leukocyte esterase dipstick has a sensitivity of about 75–96% in detecting pyuria associated with an infection.

b. Urine culture
  — A bladder or renal infection usually correlates with a colony count of more than 100,000 CFU/mL. However, a colony count of more than 100 CFU/mL usually indicates an infection in the presence of symptoms and pyuria. A urine culture is not mandatory for adolescent females, particularly with a first episode. If therapy fails, or for males, a culture is recommended. Cultures are also indicated for females with pyuria without bacteriuria. Cultures are recommended for males because the organisms are less predictable. Independent predictors of a positive urine culture result include a history of a prior urinary tract infection, back pain, microscopic pyuria, hematuria, and bacteriuria (Wigton et al., 1985).
  — Posttreatment cultures also require reevaluation. The vast majority of recurrences are symptomatic. In most instances, follow-up cultures are indicated only for patients with acute pyelonephritis, a complicated infection, or during pregnancy.

c. Culture alternatives: Several rapid culture kits available for office use, including:
  — Dipslide: Best studied and most reliable kit culture technique. The test is inexpensive and yields high sensitivity and specificity rates (generally <1% false-positive and false-negative results).
  — Filter-paper techniques yield false-negative rates of 3–20% and false-positive rates of 2–23%.
  — Several other chemical tests use nitrate glucose oxidase or catalase to detect the presence of bacteriuria. These tests are neither highly sensitive nor specific.

4. Other tests
  a. Females: In females, three infections within 1–2 years is an indication for a full evaluation, which may include an ultrasonography and voiding cystourethrography. However, in postpubertal females with uncomplicated cystitis, evaluation after recurrent episodes is unlikely to find significant abnormalities that would change the therapy or prognosis. Table 25.2 outlines recommended use of urinalysis and urine culture in women with acute dysuria. Figure 25.1 is a flow diagram for evaluation of women with internal dysuria.
  b. Males: Although some authorities recommend a full investigation after the first infection, this is probably of greater importance in the young child or infant. In adolescent males, an investigation with more invasive tests is probably not indicated after the first infection, unless there is evidence in the history or physical examination of a possible renal abnormality or there is no response to therapy. This is particularly true for males who are sexually active. Krieger et al. (1993) evaluated acute urinary tract infection in healthy university men. The incidence was 5 of 10,000 males per year. Of this group of males, 92% responded to a single course of antibiotics. None of the men in this study had neurological or anatomical abnormalities, and all the radiographic findings were normal. The major risk factor was a history of sexual activity in the previous month.

Table 25.2.   Recommended Use of Urinalysis and Urine Culture in Women with Acute Dysuria

Suspected Cause and Clinical Findings	Diagnostic Tests and Expected Results
Acute pyelonephritis Fever, rigors, nausea, vomiting, flank pain, costovertebral angle tenderness	Urinalysis: Pyuria and bacteriuria Urine culture: >100,000 bacteria/mL Urine Gram stain: Gram-negative bacilli or gram-positive cocci

Subclinical pyelonephritis
  Underlying urinary tract disease
  Diabetes mellitus
  Immunocompromised state
  Urinary tract infection before age 12 years
  Symptoms for 7–10 days before seeking care
  Documented relapsing infection with same organism
  Three or more urinary infections in past year
  Acute pyelonephritis in past year
	Urinalysis: Pyuria and bacteriuria
	Urine culture: >100,000 bacteria/mL

Chlamydial urethritis
  Sexual partner with recent urethritis
  New sexual partner
  Gradual onset
  Absence of hematuria
  Mucopurulent cervical discharge
	Urinalysis: Pyuria without bacteriuria

Gonococcal urethritis
  Sexual partner with recent urethritis
  Recent history of documented gonorrhea
	Urinalysis: Pyuria without bacteriuria
	Gram stain of purulent discharge from urethral or cervical os: Gram-negative intracellular diplococci
	Gonorrhea culture on Thayer-Martin media: *Neisseria gonorrhoeae*

Vaginitis Symptoms of vaginal discharge, itch, or irritation	Vaginal examination: Abnormal discharge Microscopic examination of abnormal discharge: Budding yeast and pseudohyphae, trichomonads, "clue cells"
Lower urinary tract bacterial infection None of the above clinical indicators, but presence of pyuria; also associated with suprapubic tenderness, hematuria, urgency, frequency, and prior history of bacterial cystitis	Urinalysis: Pyuria and bacteriuria
No apparent infectious pathogen None of the above clinical indicators and absence of pyuria	Urinalysis: No pyuria, no bacteriuria

Adapted from Komaroff AL. Urinalysis and urine culture in women with dysuria. Ann Intern Med 1986;104:212.

Recurrent Infections in Female Adolescents

About 20% of young women will have recurrent infections. Most of these adolescents and young women do not have anatomical or functional abnormalities of the urinary tract. Recurrent cystitis should be documented at least once by culture. Those females with a relapse (recurrent infection with original pathogen within 2 weeks after completion of therapy) should have an evaluation for an occult source of infection or urologic abnormality.

PYELONEPHRITIS

Pyelonephritis is an infection of the renal pelvis and medulla. The clinical manifestations include:

1. Symptoms of acute cystitis
2. Fever
3. Costovertebral tenderness
4. Elevated leukocyte count and erythrocyte sedimentation rate

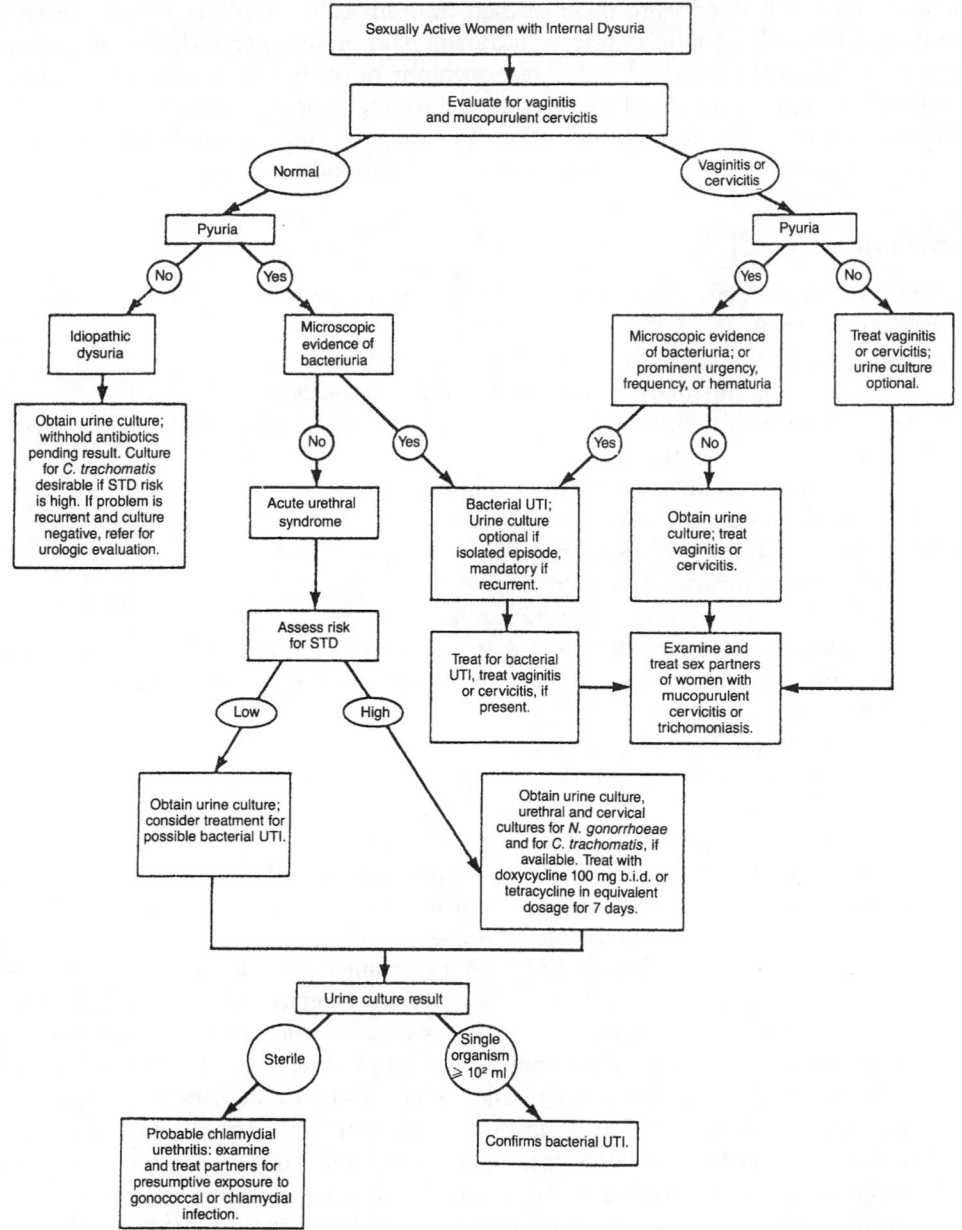

FIGURE 25.1. Flow diagram for evaluation of women with internal dysuria. (Reproduced, by permission, from Holmes KK. Lower genital tract infection in women: cystitis, urethritis, vulvovaginitis, and cervicitis. In: Holmes KK, Mardh PA, Sparling PF, Weisner PJ, eds. Sexually transmitted diseases. © 1990 by McGraw-Hill Book Co., New York.)

5. Urinalysis revealing leukocytes and bacterial casts
6. Positive urine culture result

The range of symptoms varies from cystitis with mild flank pain to those of septicemia. Most acute pyelonephritis in female adolescents and young women is caused by *E. coli* (>80%), and most of these organisms are in a uropathogenic subgroup. Pyuria and gram-negative bacteria are usually present on examination of the urine. Urine culture specimens should always be obtained from these women, and, in addition, blood culture specimens from those who are hospitalized. If fever and flank pain persist after 72 hours of treatment, then cultures should be repeated and ultrasonography or computed tomography should be considered to evaluate for an abscess. Routine imaging procedures for pyelonephritis in young women are not indicated. Indications for imaging studies include recurrent pyelonephritis, slow resolution, persistent hematuria, or childhood infection.

Treatment

1. Acute, uncomplicated infections in females (*E. coli, S. saprophyticus, Proteus mirabilis, Klebsiella pneumoniae*)
   a. No complicating problems: Use a 3-day oral regimen of either:
      — Trimethoprim-sulamethoxazole, 160 mg/800 mg every 12 hours, OR
      — Trimethoprim, 100 mg every 12 hours, OR in older adolescents a 3-day regimen of a quinolone, such as;
        (1) Norfloxacin, 400 mg every 12 hours
        (2) Ciprofloxacin, 250 mg every 12 hours
        (3) Ofloxacin, 200 mg every 12 hours
        (4) Lomefloxacin, 400 mg daily
        (5) Enoxacin, 400 mg every 12 hours
   b. Complicating problems such as diabetes, or a history of a recent urinary tract infection, or symptoms for more than 1 week: Consider the use of a 7-day regimen of a medication listed above.
   c. Pregnancy: Consider 7-day regimen of:
      — Amoxicillin, 250 mg given orally every 8 hours
      — Nitrofurantoin, 100 mg four times a day
      — Cefpodoxime proxetil, 100 mg every 12 hours
      — Trimethoprim-sulfamethoxazole, 160/800 mg every 12 hours
      Single-daily-dose short-term therapy: Numerous trials have been conducted with single-dose regimens of amoxicillin, trimethoprim-sulfamethoxazole, or single-dose quinolone therapy. These studies have studied both 1-day single-dose therapy and 3-day single-daily-dose therapy. However, the use of a single dose, and in particular 1-day therapy, remains controversial. In general, amoxicillin seems to be less effective given as a single dose than as a 7–10 day course. Studies using single-dose trimethoprim-sulfamethoxazole have yielded mixed results. Quinolones have also been studied in this regard. Norfloxacin is approved in Canada for 3-day treatment of cystitis. Saginur and Nicolle (1992) compared a single-dose of norfloxacin with the 3-day b.i.d. regimen. The 3-day regimen was more effective especially if *S. saprophyticus* was involved. Iravani (1993) conducted a large multicenter study comparing single-dose fleroxacin therapy with a 7-day course of fleroxacin or ciprofloxacin. Though all three regimens had similar clinical cure rates and relapse rates, the single-dose 1-day therapy had a slightly lower bacteriological eradication rate. Gaudreault et al. (1992) found that single daily doses of trimethroprim-sulfadiazine for 3 days had similar cure rates and relapse rates, as with longer-term therapy in children. This study included both males and females. Overall, a 3-day course of antibiotics appears to ensure greater success than the single-dose antibiotic regimens.
2. Acute, uncomplicated pyelonephritis in females (*E. coli, P. mirabilis, K. pneumoniae, S. saprophyticus*): Avoid amoxicillin and first-generation cephalosporins because 20–30% of organisms are resistant.
   a. Mild to moderate illness with no nausea or vomiting. Initial outpatient oral therapy is acceptable in adolescents with a community-acquired infection not associated with severe systemic symptoms or known complications. Oral therapy can include either:

— Trimethoprim-sulfamethoxazole, 160/800 mg every 12 hours for 10–14 days
— Quninolones for older adolescents and young adults:
  (1) Norfloxacin, 400 mg every 12 hours for 10–14 days
  (2) Ciprofloxacin, 500 mg every 12 hours for 10–14 days
  (3) Ofloxacin, 200–300 mg every 12 hours for 10–14 days
  (4) Lomefloxacin, 400 mg every day for 10–14 days
  (5) Enoxacin, 400 mg every 12 hours for 10–14 days
b. Severe illness requiring hospitalization: Parenterally administered antibiotics, including either:
— Trimethoprim-sulfamethoxazole, 160/800 mg every 12 hours
— Ceftriaxone, 1–2 g/day
— Ciprofloxacin, 200–400 mg every 12 hours
— Ofloxacin, 200–400 mg every 12 hours, *or*
— Gentamicin, 1 mg/kg every 12 hours (with or without ampicillin)
Use these until fever has resolved and then treat with oral antibiotics, using either:
— Trimethoprim-sulfamethoxazole, 160/800 mg every 12 hours for 10–14 days
— Norfloxacin, 400 mg every 12 hours for 14 days
— Ciprofloxacin, 500 mg every 12 hours for 14 days
— Ofloxacin, 200–300 mg every 12 hours for 14 days
— Lomefloxacin, 400 mg every day for 14 days, *or*
— Enoxacin, 400 mg every 12 hours for 14 days
c. Pregnancy: Hospitalization recommended, with parentally administered antibiotics, either:
— Ceftriaxone, 1 to 2 g/day
— Gentamicin, 1 mg/kg every 12 hours (with or without ampicillin)
— Trimethoprim-sulfamethoxazole, 160/800 mg every 12 hours
— Aztreonam, 1 g every 8 to 12 hours
Use these until fever has resolved and then treat with oral antibiotics, either:
— Amoxicillin, 500 mg given orally every 8 hours for 14 days
— Cefpodoxime proxetil, 200 mg every 12 hours for 14 days
— Trimethoprim-sulfamethoxazole, 160/800 mg every 12 hours for 14 days
3. Complicated urinary tract infections in females (*E. coli, Proteus, Klebsiella* sp., *Pseudomonas* sp., *serratia* sp., enterococci, staphylococci)
a. Mild to moderate illness with no nausea or vomiting: Administer either:
— Norfloxacin, 400 mg every 12 hours for 10–14 days
— Ciprofloxacin, 500 mg every 12 hours for 10–14 days
— Ofloxacin, 200–300 mg every 12 hours for 10–14 days
— Lomefloxacin, 400 mg every day for 10–14 days
— Enoxacin, 400 mg every 12 hours for 14 days
b. Severe illness requiring hospitalization: Administer parenteral antibiotics, either:
— Ampicillin, 1 g every 6 hours, and gentamicin, 1 mg/kg every 8 hours
— Ciprofloxacin, 200–400 mg every 12 hours
— Ofloxacin, 200–400 mg every 12 hours
— Ceftriaxone, 1–2 g every day
— Aztreonam, 1 g every 8–12 hours
— Ticarcillin-clavulanate, 3.2 g every 8 hours
— Imipenem-cilastatin, 250–500 mg every 6–8 hours
c. Use one of the regimens listed above until fever is gone, and then give oral therapy with either:
— Trimethoprim-sulfamethoxazole, 160/800 mg every 12 hours for 14–21 days
— Norfloxacin, 400 mg every 12 hours for 14–21 days

— Ciprofloxacin, 500 mg every 12 hours for 14–21 days
— Ofloxacin, 200–300 mg every 12 hours for 14–21 days
— Lomefloxacin, 400 mg every day for 14–21 days
— Enoxacin, 400 mg every 12 hours for 14–21 days

   d. Contraindications: Fluoroquinolones should not be used in pregnancy and are not approved for use in adolescents less than 16 years of age. Trimethoprim-sulfamethoxazole is not approved for use in pregnancy but has been widely used. Gentamicin should be used with caution during pregnancy because of the risk of toxic effects on fetal eighth-nerve development.

4. Recurrent infections: Recurrent cystitis in females should be managed by either continuous prophylaxis, postcoital prophylaxis, or therapy initiated by the patient.

   a. Continuous prophylaxis: Use either:
— Trimethoprim, 100 mg, daily, OR
— Trimethoprim-sulfamethoxazole, 40/200 mg daily, OR
— Nitrofurantoin, 50–100 mg daily, OR
— Norfloxacin, 200 mg daily, OR
— Cephalexin, 250 mg daily

   b. Postcoital prophylaxis: Use either:
— Trimethoprim-sulfamethoxazole, 40/200 mg, OR
— Nitrofurantoin, 50–100 mg, OR
— Cephalexin, 250 mg

   c. Patient-administered single-dose therapy: An alternative to prophylaxis in the compliant individual is self-medication initiated at the time that symptoms appear, with either a single-dose or a 3-day regimen. This was as efficacious and cost-effective as continuous prophylaxis in a study by Wong et al. (1985). Patient-initiated therapy is best for individuals with only one or two episodes per year.

   d. Nonantibiotic measures: Nonantibiotic prevention of recurrent urinary tract infections includes:
— Voiding after intercourse
— Discontinuing use of a diaphragm
— Emptying the bladder frequently
— Acidifying the urine

5. Treatment of urinary tract infections in males: Less information is known about short-term, single-dose therapy in males. Males should probably receive a 7- to 10-day course. However, in less compliant males a 3-day regimen of norfloxacin or trimethoprim-sulfamethoxazole could be used.

ASYMPTOMATIC BACTERIURIA

The prevalence of asymptomatic bacteriuria (reproducible growth of more than 10^5 CFU/mL) ranges from about 1% to 7%. There is a tendency toward spontaneous cure. Progressive renal impairment is rare, except in individuals whose infection begins in childhood. Asymptomatic bacteriuria during pregnancy is a risk factor for the development of acute pyelonephritis, for lower fetal birth weight, and for a higher incidence of prematurity. Treatment is mainly indicated for:

1. Pregnant females
2. Males
3. Females with either an underlying renal tract abnormality or immunocompromising disease

Treatment should be with appropriate antibiotics selected on the basis of culture sensitivities.

NONGONOCOCCAL URETHRITIS

Nongonococcal urethritis (NGU) is an inflammation of the urethra unassociated with gonococcal infection.

Etiology

1. *Chylamydia trachomatis:* There is clear evidence that certain genotypes cause about 40% of the cases of NGU.
2. *Ureaplasma urealyticum* (T-strain *Mycoplasma*): Reliable data implicate this organism as a cause of about 20–30% of additional cases of NGU.
3. In the remainder of cases, the cause is uncertain. Other possibilities include *Gardnerella vaginalis,* herpes simplex virus, *Staphylococcus saprophyticus, Escherichia coli,* and *Trichomonas vaginalis.*

Epidemiology

1. Incidence: Extremely common among sexually active men. In England, it is the most frequently recorded sexually transmitted disease. Approximately 2–3 million cases occur yearly in the United States.
2. Transmission: Sexual contact is the means of transmission.

Clinical Manifestations

1. Discharge: Scanty or moderate, watery discharge (Some patients have no discharge, whereas some have copious, purulent discharge, which usually starts 8–14 days after contact.)
2. Dysuria
3. Rarely, hematuria
4. Occasionally, history of cystitis in female sexual partners

Diagnosis

1. Clinical history
2. Positive finding with leukocyte esterase dipstick
3. Gram stain of urethral discharge
   a. More than five polymorphonuclear cells per oil immersion field indicates urethritis.
   b. The lack of intracellular gram-negative diplococci suggests nongonococcal urethritis.
4. Urine
   a. A leukocyte count of more than 10 cells per high-power dry field of the urine sediment from the first 10–15 mL of a urine stream indicates urethritis.
   b. The leukocyte esterase dipstick test can also be used.
   c. The urine sediment test, although often unnecessary if a discharge is present, is helpful in determining the presence or absence of urethritis.
5. Urethral culture if Gram stain of the discharge is negative: Culture or nonculture technique for gonorrhea and chlamydial infection

Therapy

1. Recommended regimen
   a. Doxycycline, 100 mg orally twice daily for 7 days, OR
   b. Azithromycin, 1 g orally in a single dose

2. Alternative regimens
   a. Erythromycin base, 500 mg given orally four times daily for 7 days, OR
   b. Erythromycin ethylsuccinate, 800 mg given orally, four times daily for 7 days
   c. For a patient who cannot tolerate high-dose erythromycin schedules: One of the following regimens:
      — Erythromycin base, 250 mg given orally four times a day for 14 days, OR
      — Erythromycin ethylsuccinate, 400 mg given orally four times a day for 14 days

Note: Patients with persistent or recurrent objective signs of urethritis after adequate treatment of themselves and their partners warrant further evaluation for less common causes of urethritis. In addition, in some individuals with persistent infections, a longer (14–21 days) course of antibiotics may be effective. Finally, sexual partners must be treated.

PROSTATITIS

Etiology

Prostatitis is an inflammatory reaction confined to the prostate gland. In adolescents, prostatitis is an unusual condition. Acute prostatitis in adolescents is often associated with infection. The organisms probably reach the prostate as a result of a urethral infection, by reflux of infected urine into the prostatic ducts, or by lymphogenous or hematogenic spread. Although it is often assumed that sexually transmitted diseases and, in particular, infection with *Neisseria gonorrhoeae* and *Chlamydia trachomatis,* cause a large percentage of the cases of acute prostatitis in adolescents and young adults, proof through adequate studies has not been achieved. Coliform bacteria, *Staphylococcus saprophyticus, Mycoplasma hominis, Ureaplasma urealyticum,* and *Trichomonas vaginalis* have also been implicated as causative agents. In one study of 409 patients with prostatitis—males aged 19 years and older—the most frequent organism isolated was *U. urealyticum* (de la Rosette et al., 1993). The cause or causes of noninfectious prostatitis and chronic prostatitis are even more unclear.

Diagnosis

1. In acute bacterial prostatitis, symptoms include:
   a. Pain: Penoscrotal, suprapubic, perineal, groin, or back, or pain that occurs during ejaculation
   b. Bladder symptoms: Frequency, dysuria, hesitation
   c. Systemic symptoms: Chills, fever, malaise
   d. Other symptoms: Hematospermia, hematuria
2. In nonacute prostatitis the symptoms are less dramatic and may include frequency, urgency, and dysuria.
3. The only method for documenting prostatitis is the segmental culture technique.
   a. Four specimens are collected, including:
      — First-voided 10 mL urine
      — Midstream urine
      — Prostatic secretions during prostatic massage
      — First-voided 10 mL after prostatic massage
   b. In individuals with bacterial prostatitis, the third and fourth specimens should grow more colonies than the first two. The presence of more leukocytes in the first specimen suggests urethritis, and growth primarily in the second specimen suggests cystitis. However, because the meaning and interpretation of this test are not standardized and the test is time-consuming, expensive, and uncomfortable, it should not be performed routinely in adolescents.

Treatment

In the acutely inflamed prostate gland, antibiotics have good penetration; however in males with recurrent prostatic infections, treatment is hampered by the lack of good antibiotic penetration. The best antibiotics for prostatic infections include trimethoprim, erythromycin, doxycycline, and tetracycline. The quinolones, including ofloxacin, also have good penetration into the prostate.

HEMATOSPERMIA

Bloody ejaculate is an unusual condition but can occur in adolescent males. The adolescent may notice a reddish discoloration of his semen either after masturbation or on removing a condom after intercourse. This condition may cause extreme anxiety or feelings of guilt. The teen may be concerned about a malignancy or fear that his behavior has caused the condition. In adolescents, the condition is usually either idiopathic and self-limited or related to an infectious disease such as a gonococcal or chlamydial urethritis. Aside from evaluation for a urinary tract infection, prostatitis, or sexually transmitted urethritis, an extensive examination should not be performed unless the initial findings are negative and the condition is persistent.

BIBLIOGRAPHY

Abrahamsson A, Hansson S, Jodal U, et al. *Staphylococcus saprophyticus* urinary tract infections in children. Eur J Pediatr 1993;152:69.

Adler J. Diagnosis of dysuria in adolescent girls. Postgrad Med 1984;76:206.

Ansbach RK, Dybus KR, Bergeson R. Uncomplicated *E. coli* urinary tract infection in college women: a retrospective study of *E. coli* sensitivities to commonly prescribed antibiotics. J Am Coll Health 1995;43:183.

Bergeron MG. Treatment of pyelonephritis in adults. Med Clin North Am 1995;79:619.

Bowie WR, Alexander R, Stimson JB, et al. Therapy for nongonococcal urethritis. Ann Intern Med 1981;95:306.

Brumfitt W, Hamilton-Miller JM. A comparative trial of low dose cefaclor and macrocrystalline nitrofurantoin in the prevention of recurrent urinary tract infection. Infection 1995;23:98.

Colleen S, Mardh PA. Prostatitis. In: Holmes KK, Mardh PA, Sparling PF, et al., eds. Sexually transmitted diseases. 2nd ed. New York: McGraw-Hill, 1990.

Davison JM, Sprott MS, Selkon JB. The effect of covert bacteriuria in schoolgirls on renal function at 18 years and during pregnancy. Lancet 1984;2:651.

de la Rosette JJMCH, Hubregtse MR, Meuleman EJH, et al. Diagnosis and treatment of 409 patients with prostatitis syndromes. Urology 1993;41:301.

Demetriou E, Emans SJ, Masland RP Jr. Dysuria in adolescent girls: urinary tract infection or vaginitis? Pediatrics 1982;70:299.

Durbin WA Jr, Peter G. Management of urinary tract infections in infants and children. Pediatr Infect Dis J 1984;3:564.

Fihn SD, Johnson C, Roberts PL, et al. Trimethoprim-sulfamethoxazole for acute dysuria in women: a single-dose or 10-day course: a double-blind, randomized trial. Ann Intern Med 1988;108:350.

Fine JS, Jacobson MS. Single-dose versus conventional therapy of urinary tract infections in female adolescents. Pediatrics 1985;75:916.

Fletcher MS, Herzberg Z, Pryor JP. The aetiology and investigation of haemospermia. Br J Urol 1981;53:669.

Forland M. Urinary tract infection: how has its management changed? Postgrad Med 1993;93:71.

Foxman B. Recurring urinary tract infection: incidence and risk factors. Am J Public Health 1990;80:331.

Gaudreault M, Beland M, Girodias JB, et al. Single daily doses of trimethoprim/sulphadiazine for three or 10 days in urinary tract infections. Acta Paediatr 1992;81:695.

Holmes KK. Lower genital tract infection in women: cystitis, urethritis, vulvovaginitis, and cervicitis. In: Holmes KK, Mardh PA, Sparling PF, et al., eds. Sexually transmitted diseases. 2nd ed. New York: McGraw-Hill, 1990.

Hooton TM. A simplified approach to urinary tract infection. Hosp Pract 1995;30:23.

Iravani A. Multicenter study of single-dose and multiple-dose fleroxacin versus ciprofloxacin in the treatment of uncomplicated urinary tract infections. Am J Med 1993;94:89S.

Johnson JR, Stamm WE. Urinary tract infection in women: diagnosis and treatment. Ann Intern Med 1989;111:906.

Johnson MAG. Urinary tract infection in women. Am Fam Physician 1990;41:565.

Komaroff AL. Urinalysis and urine culture in women with dysuria. Ann Intern Med 1986;104:212.

Krieger JN, Ross SO, Simonsen JM. Urinary tract infections in healthy university men. J Urol 1993;149:1046.

Kunin CM, White LV, Hua Hua T. A reassessment of the importance of "low count" bacteriuria in young women with acute urinary symptoms. Ann Intern Med 1993;119:454.

Latham RH, Running K, Stamm WE. Urinary tract infections in young adult women caused by *Staphylococcus saprophyticus*. JAMA 1983;250:3063.

Leigh DA. Prostatitis—an increasing clinical problem for diagnosis and management. J Antimicrob Chemother 1993;32(suppl A):1–9.

Lipsky BA. Urinary tract infections in men: epidemiology, pathophysiology, diagnosis, and treatment. Ann Intern Med 1989;110:138.

Marshall VG, Fuller NL. Hemospermia. J Urol 1982; 128:151.

Merrick MV, Notghi A, Chalmers N, et al. Long-term follow-up to determine the prognostic value of imaging after urinary tract infections. Part 1: reflux. Arch Dis Child 1995;72:388.

Merrick MV, Notghi A, Chalmers N, et al. Long-term follow-up to determine the prognostic value of imaging after urinary tract infections. Part 2: scarring. Arch Dis Child 1995;72:393.

Millar LK, Wing DA, Paul RH, et al. Outpatient treatment of pyelonephritis in pregnancy: a randomized controlled trial. Obstet Gynecol 1995;86:560.

Ohkawa M, Yamaguchi K, Tokunaga S, et al. *Ureaplasma urealyticum* in the urogenital tract of patients with chronic prostatitis or related symptomatology. Br J Urol 1993;72:918.

Papp GK, Hoznek A, Hegedus M, et al. Hematospermia. J Androl 1994;15:31S.

Rouse DJ, Andrews WW, Goldenberg RL, et al. Screening and treatment of asymptomatic bacteriuria of pregnancy to prevent pyelonephritis: a cost-effectiveness and cost-benefit analysis. Obstet Gynecol 1995; 86:119.

Saginur R, Nicolle LE. Single-dose compared with 3-day norfloxacin treatment of uncomplicated urinary tract infection in women. Arch Intern Med. 1992; 152:1233.

Sheinfeld J, Schaeffer AJ, Cordon-Cardo C, et al. Association of the Lewis blood-group phenotype with recurrent urinary tract infections in women. N Engl J Med 1989;320:773.

Silber TJ, Kastrinakas M. Hematospermia in adolescents and young adults. Pediatrics 1986;78:708.

Smellie JM, Rigden SP, Prescod NP. Urinary tract infection: a comparison of four methods of investigation. Arch Dis Child 1995;72:247.

Stamm WE, Hooton TM. Management of urinary tract infections in adults N Engl J Med 1993;329:1329.

Stamm WE, McKevitt M, Counts GW. Acute renal infection in women: treatment with trimethoprim-sulfamethoxazole or ampicillin for two or six weeks. Ann Intern Med 1987;106:341.

Stapleton A, Latham RH, Johnson C, et al. Postcoital antimicrobial prophylaxis for recurrent urinary tract infection: a randomized, double-blind, placebo-controlled trial. JAMA 1990;264:703.

Strom BL, Collins M, West SL, et al. Sexual activity, contraceptive use, and other risk factors for symptomatic and asymptomatic bacteriuria: a case-control study. Ann Intern Med 1987;107:816.

Wigton RS, Hoellerich VL, Ornato JP, et al. Use of clinical findings in the diagnosis of urinary tract infection in women. Arch Intern Med 1985;145:2222.

Wong ES, McKevitt M, Running K, et al. Management of recurrent urinary tract infections with patient-administered single-dose therapy. Ann Intern Med 1985;102:302.

Zhanel GG, Harding GKM, Guay DRP. Asymptomatic bacteriuria: which patients should be treated? Arch Intern Med 1990;150:1389.

CHAPTER 26

Enuresis

Lawrence S. Neinstein and Diane Tanaka

Enuresis is the involuntary passage of urine, usually during sleep, occurring more than once a month. Although often considered a childhood problem, enuresis is also found in adolescents, causing major emotional problems and family stress. Primary enuresis is defined as enuresis with no periods of prior consistent dryness. In secondary enuresis, patients have a history of 3–6 months of prior dryness.

ETIOLOGY

Most cases of enuresis are related to nonorganic causes. In these patients the causes may be multifactorial.

Organic Causes

1. Neurological lesions
   a. Myelomeningocele, the most common neurological cause of enuresis
   b. Mental retardation
   c. Spinal cord injury
2. Urological abnormalities
   a. Recurrent urinary tract infections can be a cause of enuresis.
   b. Obstructive lesions: Controversy exists over the role and prevalence of urological lesions in enuresis. The prevalence of urological abnormalities in patients with enuresis ranges in different studies from 2% to 97%.
   c. Detrusor instability: Khan et al. (1993) found that the mean threshold volume at which detrusor instability was demonstrated was 200 mL in enuretic patients. The mean bladder capacity of age-matched nonenuretic patients was 325 mL.
3. Renal concentrating defects (e.g., sickle cell anemia)
4. Diabetes mellitus and diabetes insipidus

Genetic Causes

1. A family history of enuresis is common. Prevalence in such cases follows:

Relatives with Enuresis	Prevalence of Enuresis in Offspring
Both parents	77%
One parent	44%
No parents	15%

2. Prevalence in an identical twin of an enuretic twin is 68%.

Sleep Disorder

Enuresis may be associated with incomplete sudden arousal from a deep sleep. In these cases, there is difficulty in arousing the patient. However, recent studies have demonstrated that most enuretic patients are normal sleepers and that enuresis can occur during any stage of sleep.

Developmental Delay

A developmental delay in adequate neuromuscular maturation of the bladder and an immaturity of central nervous system inhibition of the micturition reflex during sleep have been postulated. There are differing opinions among experts as to the role of these problems in the pathophysiology of enuresis.

Small Functional Bladder Capacity

Some patients with enuresis demonstrate small bladder capacity.

Psychological Factors

There is an increased prevalence of emotional difficulties in patients with enuresis. However, this may often be a result of the enuresis. The majority of enuretic patients are psychologically normal.

Vasopressin Levels

Some individuals with nocturnal enuresis may have an insufficient nocturnal rise in the concentration of antidiuretic hormone and a nocturnal urine production up to four times the volume of their functional bladder capacity. As children approach adolescence, a faulty circadian rhythm of arginine vasopressin (AVP) secretion may be the paramount pathogenetic factor.

EPIDEMIOLOGY

1. Prevalence: Decreasing prevalence occurs with increasing age.
   a. Age 4: 30%
   b. Age 5: 14–20%
   c. Age 6: 10%
   d. Age 10: 5–10%
   e. Age 12: 3%
   f. Age 15: 2–3%
   g. Age 18: 1–2%
   h. Army recruits: 0.1–2.5% (according to studies of this group)
2. Sex: Male/female ratio is 3:2.
3. Race: More African-American teens are affected than white teens.
4. Timing: Seventy-five percent to 90% of teens have nocturnal enuresis only, whereas 10–25% of teens have nocturnal and daytime enuresis.

DIAGNOSIS

There is disagreement regarding evaluation of enuresis in children and adolescents. One should remember that significant organic lesions are infrequent, and most are detectable by history, physical examination, and simple laboratory tests. The prevalence of organic lesions is higher in adolescents than in children. The prevalence of a psychological or organic cause is higher in secondary and daytime enuresis.

History

The history should include:

1. Severity of enuresis
   a. Nocturnal only or daytime
   b. Number of nights per week
2. Type of enuresis (primary or secondary)
3. History of urinary tract infections
4. Toilet-training history
5. Family history of enuresis
6. Prior therapeutic modalities
7. Adolescent's and family's adjustment to the problem
8. Member of the family responsible for changing sheets and laundry
9. History of any sleep disorders, such as night terrors or unusually deep sleep
10. General psychosocial review of family, peers, and school
11. Voiding history of straining to urinate or low-velocity stream

Physical Examination

1. Check blood pressure.
2. Abdomen: Check for masses.
3. Genitourinary tract: Check the urethral meatus for evidence of stenosis. Observe or have a nurse observe the urinary stream to see whether it is full and forceful versus narrow or dribbling.
4. Perform a neurological examination.
   a. Gait
   b. Lower extremity: Motor and sensory
   c. Deep-tendon reflexes
   d. Perineal sensation
   e. Rectal sphincter tone
   f. Bulbocavernosus reflex

Laboratory Tests

1. Urinalysis: Glucose, protein, white blood cells, specific gravity (should be >1.025 g after 14-hour fluid restriction)
2. Urine culture
3. Bladder capacity: Self-measurement of urine output after holding urine as long as possible (should be >350 mL)
4. Intravenous pyelogram and voiding cystourethrogram: Mainly if there is daytime wetting, abnormal findings on physical examination, or abnormal urinalysis findings

THERAPY

If a urological lesion is discovered, then referral to a urologist for appropriate management is recommended. As stated, no organic lesions are present in the majority of adolescents. In these teens, the cause of enuresis is generally multifactorial and includes genetic predisposition, small bladder capacity, a sleep disorder, developmental delay, or abnormal secretion of AVP. Therapy includes:

1. Motivational counseling: Regardless of any other modalities chosen, motivational counseling is helpful. Studies indicate that counseling alone leads to a 25–70% remission rate. Through motivational counseling, the teen learns to assume responsibility and become an active participant in the management program. In such a program the practitioner:
   a. Reassures the adolescent and family that this problem is common to many teens. The parents and the teen should not feel guilty about "causing" the problem.
   b. Gives the adolescent an active role by putting him or her in charge of changing the sheets and placing them in the laundry machines. The parents should be encouraged to take a backseat position in dealing with the problem.
   c. Reduces secondary friction caused by enuresis.
   d. Gives positive reinforcement for dryness.
   e. Provides close initial follow-up with the practitioner.
2. Alarm systems: The use of alarm systems is perhaps the best therapy for functional enuresis.
   a. Types: Older alarms required elaborate pad-and-bell systems. Newer alarms are lightweight, easy to use, and relatively inexpensive ($50–$60). The alarms consist of two clips attached to the teen's underwear and connected to a wrist alarm or pajama-collar alarm. The alarm buzzes if a small amount of wetness occurs on the underwear. Alarms are available from:

      Nytone ($48.50)   Wet-stop ($55)
      Medical Products, Inc.   Palco Laboratories
      2424 South 900 West   8030 Soquel Dr.
      Salt Lake City, UT 84119   Santa Cruz, CA 95062
      801 973-4090   800 346-4488

   b. Basis for using alarm: The alarm awakens the teen and usually leads to a contraction of the external bladder sphincter. If the teen can be conditioned to associate bladder distention with awakening and subsequent inhibition of further urination, he or she will become conditioned to awakening in response to bladder distention before urination. The alarm system can take weeks to several months to work. With time, the teen awakens earlier and earlier with less wetting of the bed. The alarm should be continued until 3 weeks after dryness has been achieved.
   c. Instructions: Instructions are included with each alarm but should be carefully reviewed with parent and teen. The teen should hook up the alarm himself or herself; have a flashlight or bedside lamp near the bed; and remind himself or herself to wake up and stop the urine flow at the moment the alarm is heard. When the alarm buzzes, the teen should:
      — Stop the alarm by disconnecting the electrodes.
      — Go to the bathroom and empty his or her bladder.
      — Put on dry pajamas and reconnect the alarm.
      — Put a towel over wet spot on the bed or change the sheets.
   d. Results: Long-term cure rates average 70%. Relapses average about 10% and respond to repeated use of the alarm.
3. Bladder exercises: Because some patients with enuresis have a small bladder capacity, exercises have been used to increase bladder tone and size. The technique involves having the patient hold his or her urine as long as possible when the urge to urinate occurs. The patient may also be encouraged to interrupt the urinary stream, which may help the patient to withstand uninhibited bladder contractions. Recording urine volumes helps to

measure progress. This technique has been primarily utilized in children and has a success rate of about 35%. However, because this method not only has lower success rates than newer methods (i.e., desmopressin acetate [DDAVP], alarm systems) but uses negative experiences and potentially intensifies the struggle between parent and teen, it cannot be highly recommended.

4. Medications: No drug exists that is adequately safe and effective for curing enuresis. The major drugs available include:

    a. DDAVP: Newest medication used for enuresis; drug of choice for many experts
        — Action: DDAVP is a synthetic analog of arginine vasopressin that counteracts a possible insufficient nocturnal rise in vasopressin levels in some individuals with nocturnal enuresis.
        — Dosage: The medication comes as a nasal spray that delivers 10 μg per spray or as a graduated intranasal tube (Rhinal Tube) that delivers doses of 5, 10, 15, and 20 μg per spray. The usual initial dose is 20 μg. However, the dose may need to be adjusted either upward or downward, to between 10 and 40 μg/mg per day; this amount can be given in one dose at night or twice a day. Some individuals may respond to a dose as low as 5 μg/day. The Rhinal Tube must be used if 5 μg doses are required. This medication can be used as an adjunct to motivational counseling and the use of an alarm system.
        — Results: DDAVP was approved for the treatment of nocturnal enuresis at the end of 1989. The response to desmopressin improves with increasing age in patients with nocturnal enuresis. Therefore, the best results are seen in patients more than 10 years of age. A family history of nocturnal enuresis at more than 10 years of age and a normal bladder capacity are also predictors of a positive response to desmopressin. Seventy percent of patients with nocturnal enuresis who receive desmopressin stop their bedwetting completely or reduce it significantly. A positive effect of the medication is seen within a few days and is maintained as long as the drug is administered. Most patients have a relapse after drug withdrawal, especially if the therapy drug is stopped abruptly. Therefore, the drug should be tapered off slowly. Long-term lasting treatment, at least 1 year, is becoming more routine. During long-term therapy, treatment-free windows of approximately 3-month intervals are essential to avoid treating a child who has become dry.
        — Side effects: Side effects include transient headache and nausea. Nasal congestion, rhinitis, nosebleeds, abdominal cramps, and sore throats have also been reported. These symptoms usually disappear with a reduction in dose. In Europe, from 1974 to June 1992, only 21 patients using desmopressin had water intoxication.
        — Oral desmopressin: Stenberg and Lackgren (1993) found that oral desmopressin is as effective as intranasal desmopressin and as safe, with similar adverse effects (e.g., headache and abdominal pain). However, at least a tenfold increase in the desmopressin dosage is required in comparison with intranasal dosage. The drug is currently in clinical trials, and approval is pending. Preliminary effective doses for oral desmopressin therapy have ranged from 200 to 400 μg.

    b. Imipramine (Tofranil)
        — Action: The exact pharmacological action is not well understood. Possible mechanisms include the drug's antidepressant action (unlikely, since the antienuritic effects are immediate), alterations in sleep and arousal mechanisms, and anticholinergic effects. Imipramine is also thought to increase excretion of antidiuretic hormone from the posterior portion of the pituitary gland. Studies have also shown that the drug acts as a weak peripheral anticholinergic and antispasmodic agent.
        — Dosage: 50–75 mg at bedtime. The clinical response to the drug correlates with plasma levels. The optimal dose, based on weight, is 0.9–1.5 mg/kg per day. Drug

efficacy may also be influenced by the timing of administration. For example, teens who wet the bed before 1 AM may benefit from late-afternoon administration of the drug. A new sustained-release form of imipramine, Tofranil-PM, may therefore work better.

— Results: Response rate is 25–40%; relapse rate is 40–60%. The relapse rate is higher when the drug is stopped abruptly or prematurely. The maximal effect of imipramine usually occurs in the first week of therapy. However, one should continue therapy for 1–2 weeks before deciding on efficacy and whether to adjust dosage. The current recommendation is to treat for 3–6 months and then taper the drug by decreasing the dose, frequency, or both for 3–4 weeks. If the patient has a relapse, one can repeat a course of therapy. The drug is most beneficial for occasional use when dryness is necessary (e.g., trips, vacations, parties).

— Side effects: Nervousness, gastrointestinal distress, syncope, and anxiety can occur; the drug is dangerous if there is an overdose.

c. Oxybutynin (Ditropan)

— Action: Antispasmodic action reduces uninhibited detrusor muscle contraction and increases bladder capacity. Therefore, it may be most beneficial for patients with small-capacity bladders who also have daytime frequency or enuresis associated with uninhibited bladder contractions.

— Dosage: A dosage of 5 mg three times a day is usually given.

— Results: A success rate of 90% was reported in one study of individuals with daytime enuresis, bladder instability, or both. The drug is rarely helpful in treating patients with only nocturnal enuresis.

— Side effects: Anticholinergic effects are present.

Monda et al. (1995) evaluated continence rates with observation, imipramine, desmopressin, or alarm therapy. The patients were weaned from therapy 6 months after inclusion in the study. Of the 50 patients under observation 6% were continent at 6 months and 16% were continent within 12 months. Of 44 patients treated with imipramine 36% were continent at 6 months on medication; however, only 16% were continent at 12 months, off medication. With desmopressin, 68% of 88 patients were continent at 6 months but only 10% were continent at 12 months. However, of the 79 patients treated with alarm therapy 63% were continent at 6 months and 56% were dry at 12 months. Thus although the three forms of therapy improved continence over observation alone, only the bed-wetting alarm system demonstrated persistent effectiveness.

5. Hypnosis: Noncontrolled studies of success with the treatment of enuresis using hypnosis have been reported (Johnson, 1981; Olness, 1979). The technique usually involves suggestions that the adolescent wake up when the urge to urinate occurs and go to the bathroom. Hypnosis may be successful in treating enuresis in patients who are highly motivated. Banerjee and Srivastav (1993) found that 72% of children whose enuresis was treated with hypnosis had a positive response, and at 9-month follow-up, 68% of patients in the hypnosis group had maintained a positive response.

PROGNOSIS

Reported spontaneous cure rates (Forsythe and Redmond, 1974) are as follows:

1. Ages 5–9: 14%/yr
2. Ages 10–14: 16%/yr
3. Ages 15–19: 16%/yr
4. After age 20: 3%/yr

BIBLIOGRAPHY

Ack M, Norman ME, Schmitt BD. A conservative approach to enuresis. Patient Care 1984;18:54.

Ack M, Norman ME, Schmitt BD. Enuresis: the role of alarms and drugs. Patient Care 1985;19:75.

Banerjee S, Srivastav A, Palan BM. Hypnosis and self-hypnosis in the management of nocturnal enuresis: a comparative study with imipramine therapy. Am J Clin Hypn 1993;36:113.

Bloom D. The American experience with desmopressin. Clin Pediatr 1993;July (Spec No):28–31.

Crawford JD. Treatment of nocturnal enuresis. J Pediatr 1989;114:687.

Forsythe WI, Redmond A. Enuresis and spontaneous cure rate. Arch Dis Child 1974;49:259.

Fritz GK, Rockney RM, Yeung AS. Plasma levels and efficacy of imipramine treatment for enuresis. J Am Acad Child Adolesc Psychiatry 1994;33:60.

Hjalm~os K, Bengtsson B. Efficacy, safety, and dosing of desmopressin for nocturnal enuresis in Europe. Clin Pediatr 1993;July (Spec No):19–24.

Hogg RJ, Husmann D. The role of family history in predicting response to desmopressin in nocturnal enuresis. J Urol 1993;150:444.

Johnson RL. Use of hypnosis with enuretic adolescents. J Curr Adolesc Med 1981;2:39.

Kales A, Soldatos CR, Kales JD. Sleep disorders: insomnia, sleepwalking, night terrors, nightmares, and enuresis. Ann Intern Med 1987;106:582.

Key DW, Bloom DA, Sanvordenker J. Low-dose DDAVP in nocturnal enuresis. Clin Pediatr 1992;31:299.

Khan Z, Starer P, Singh VK, et al. Role of detrusor instability in primary enuresis. Urology 1993;41:189.

Matthiesen TB, Rittig S, Djurhuus JC, et al. A dose titration and an open 6-week efficacy and safety study of desmopressin tablets in the management of nocturnal enuresis. J Urol 1994;151:460.

Miller K. Concomitant nonpharmacologic therapy in the treatment of primary nocturnal enuresis. Clin Pediatr 1993;July (Spec No):32.

Miller K, Atkin B. Drug therapy for nocturnal enuresis: current treatment recommendations. Drugs 1992;44:47.

Miller K, Goldberg S, Atkin B. Nocturnal enuresis: experience with long-term use of intranasally administered desmopressin. J Pediatr 1989;114:723.

Moffatt MEK, Kato C, Bless IB. Improvements in self-concept after treatment of nocturnal enuresis: randomized, controlled trial. J Pediatr 1987;110:647.

Monda JM, Husmann DA. Primary nocturnal enuresis: a comparison among observation, imipramine, desmopressin acetate and bed-wetting alarm systems. J Urol 1995;154:745.

Norgaard JP, Djurhuus JC. The pathophysiology of enuresis in children and young adults. Clin Pediatr 1993;July (Spec No):5.

Olness K. The use of self-hypnosis in the treatment of childhood nocturnal enuresis. Clin Pediatr 1979;14:273.

Patient Education Aid. Dealing with enuresis. Patient Care 1984;18:110.

Patient Education Aid. Using an alarm to stop bedwetting. Patient Care 1985;19:174.

Rushton HG. Older pharmacologic therapy for nocturnal enuresis. Clin Pediatr 1993;July (Spec No):10.

Rushton HG. Evaluation of the enuretic child. Clin Pediatr 1993;July (Spec No):14.

Schmitt BD. Nocturnal enuresis: an update on treatment. Pediatr Clin North Am 1982;29:21.

Schmitt BD. New enuresis alarms: safe, successful, and child-operable. Contemp Pediatr 1986;September:1.

Schmitt BD. Overcoming bed-wetting in the teen years. Contemp Pediatrs 1992;9:77.

Shu SG, Lili YP, Chi CS. The efficacy of intranasal DDAVP therapy in children with nocturnal enuresis. Chung-Hua I Hsueh Tsa Chih 1993;52:368.

Stenberg A, Lackgren G. Treatment with oral desmopressin in adolescents with primary nocturnal enuresis: efficacy and long-term effect. Clin Pediatr 1993;July (Spec No):25.

CHAPTER 27

Asymptomatic Proteinuria and Hematuria

Paul S. Kurtin and Lawrence S. Neinstein

ASYMPTOMATIC PROTEINURIA

Asymptomatic proteinuria, defined as proteinuria not associated with hematuria, hypertension, or renal insufficiency, is a common finding on a screening urinalysis in adolescent patients. For the majority of these teens, no significant renal disease is present and the long-term prognosis is excellent. However, even the presence of proteinuria unassociated with significant renal disease can be important for the adolescent and family by causing problems in acceptance for employment or the armed services and by causing concerns about long-term prognosis. The objective in evaluating these adolescents is to establish the significance of the proteinuria, search noninvasively for treatable underlying conditions, and select those few patients who need referral for more extensive evaluation, including renal biopsy.

Etiology

1. Increased glomerular permeability (e.g., primary or secondary glomerulopathies [minimal change disease, lupus erythematosus, membranous nephropathy])
2. Increased production of abnormal proteins (e.g., monoclonal gammopathies)
3. Decreased tubular reabsorption of proteins (e.g., tubular disease [Fanconi's syndrome, aminoglycoside nephrotoxicity], chronic interstitial nephritis)
4. Miscellaneous (e.g., functional proteinuria [fever, exercise, congestive heart failure], and orthostatic proteinuria)

Epidemiology

1. Prevalence: Two to five percent of healthy adolescents have protein in their urine on a dipstick test of a random urine sample. This prevalence falls with repeated testing, and a diagnosis of persistent proteinuria should be based on three separate urine tests.
2. Peak age: The prevalence peaks at about age 16.

Clinical Manifestations

Small amounts of protein in the urine are normal, and most individuals excrete 30–130 mg of protein per day. The maximum normal amount is 150 mg/day for adolescents and adults. "Isolated asymptomatic proteinuria" refers to excretion of more than 150 mg/day by a person without clinical signs or symptoms. The presence of hypertension, edema, hypoalbuminemia, or hyperlipidemia suggests more profound renal abnormalities. Orthostatic (postural) proteinuria, which is proteinuria while upright but not while recumbent, is common in teens. It is characterized by:

1. An asymptomatic state
2. Age at onset: 10–20 years
3. Dipstick urine findings
    a. PM: 1–3+
    b. AM: Negative finding
    c. Urine sediment: Negative finding
4. Quantitative protein excretion
    a. Supine: 10–75 mg in 12 hours
    b. Upright: 150–1200 mg in 12 hours
5. Renal function: Normal

Differential Diagnosis

1. Mild asymptomatic proteinuria (excretion of protein: <500 mg/m^2 in 24 hours)
    a. Benign persistent proteinuria
    b. Orthostatic or postural proteinuria (proved with split 24-hour urine collection)
    c. Pyelonephritis (usually with fever and pyuria)
    d. Renal tubular disorders
    e. Chronic interstitial nephritis
    f. Congenital dysplastic lesions
    g. Other: Exercise, trauma (with hematuria), fever, congestive heart failure (severe)
2. Moderate proteinuria (excretion of protein: 500–2000 mg/m^2 in 24 hours)
    a. Acute poststreptococcal glomerulonephritis
    b. Primary glomerulonephritis
    c. Hereditary chronic nephritis
    d. Systemic diseases: Systemic lupus erythematosus
3. Severe proteinuria (protein excretion: >2000 mg/m^2 in 24 hours; usually >3.5 g), typically associated with edema, hypoalbuminemia, and hypercholesterolemia
    a. Idiopathic glomerulonephritis: Minimal change disease, focal sclerosis, membranous or membranoproliferative glomerulonephritis
    b. Systemic disease: Systemic lupus erythematosus; amyloidosis (in setting of chronic inflammatory disease or familial Mediterranean fever)
    c. Less common
        — Infections: Bacterial endocarditis, hepatitis, malaria
        — Toxins: Mercury, heroin, gold, penicillamine
    d. Uncommon
        — Allergens: Bee stings
        — Mechanical: Pericarditis, renal vein thrombosis
        — Cancer: Hodgkin's disease, lymphoma
        — Pregnancy
        — Congenital: Fabry's and Alport's syndromes

Diagnosis

The qualitative dipstick test for protein will detect protein levels greater than 10–30 mg/dL. An initial positive test result should be confirmed on two more repeated tests because many

TABLE 27.1.   Causes of False-Positive Test Results for Proteinuria

Cause	Dipstick Method	Protein Precipitation Methods

Highly concentrated urine
    Because the dipstick provides only a qualitative reading, proteinuria
    (2+) in a highly concentrated urine with a specific gravity of 1.030
    may have different (less) significance than proteinuria (2+) in a
    dilute urine of specific gravity 1.010.
	+	+

Gross hematuria	+	+
Contamination with antiseptic (chlorhexidine or benzalkonium)	+	–
Highly alkaline urine	–	–
Radiographic contrast media (affects specific gravity more than proteinuria)	–	+
High levels of cephalosporin or penicillin analogs	–	+
Sulfonamide metabolites	–	+

Adapted from Abuelo JF. Proteinuria: diagnostic principles and procedures. Ann Intern Med 1983;98:186.

individuals will have transient proteinuria and then have negative findings on subsequent evaluation. False-positive test results should be considered (Table 27.1). If proteinuria is confirmed, then a more thorough history, physical examination, and laboratory evaluation are indicated to rule out significant disease. A useful screening test is a spot protein/creatinine ratio. A random urine sample is analyzed for protein and creatinine. When both are expressed in milligram amounts, a ratio of less than 0.1 is normal and a ratio greater than 10 signifies nephrotic-range proteinuria. This test is also useful for monitoring the course of proteinuria without performing more burdensome, timed urine collections.

History   Inquire about:

1. Recent upper respiratory tract infection or pyoderma
2. Edema
3. Skin rashes, arthralgias, or photosensitivity
4. Flank pain
5. Diabetes mellitus (10–14 years of diabetes usually required before clinical detection of proteinuria; detection of microalbuminuria possible at earlier stages of disease)
6. Intoxications, drug history, bee stings, and other allergic history
7. Family history of renal disease

Physical Examination   Check for:

1. Blood pressure; height and weight percentiles
2. Vision and hearing screening, especially if hereditary nephritis is a consideration
3. Edema
4. Rash
5. Abdominal mass
6. Joint examination
7. Cardiac examination
8. Signs of systemic diseases

Laboratory Tests   Include in evaluation:

1. Urinalysis
    a. Dipstick tests: Protein, glucose, and blood should be tested. If the dipstick test result is positive for protein, a repeated dipstick test at another time or times should be performed. If protein is still present, a 24-hour quantitative test should be performed.

    b. Microscopic examination for casts and cells: Examination of sediment is crucial because abnormal results suggest an underlying renal problem. Red blood cell (RBC) casts suggest glomerulonephritis; white blood cell casts suggest pyelonephritis or interstitial nephritis.

2. Twenty-four-hour urine specimen for protein: Because a dipstick test provides only a qualitative measurement of urinary protein, a quantitative test is required to determine whether the 24-hour amount is abnormal and to provide a baseline value for monitoring of the patient's condition and consideration of any potential interventions.

    a. The test should be performed in the following manner to test for orthostatic proteinuria at the same time:

       — At 7 AM, the teenager voids and discards first morning urine; subsequent urine is then collected in the first bottle (bottle A).

       — At 8 PM that evening, the teenager lies in bed for 2 hours and then voids into bottle A at 10 PM.

       — All urine during the night should go into the second bottle (bottle B).

       — At 7 AM the next day, the teenager voids into bottle B, and the collection period has ended.

    b. The sum of the amounts of protein in the urine in the two bottles equals the 24-hour protein content. With orthostatic proteinuria, the total will be greater than 150 mg and usually less than 1 g. The urinary protein collected during the recumbent period should be less than 75 mg. The ratio of protein in bottle A to protein in bottle B can also be used to diagnose orthostatic proteinuria; a ratio of 5:1 or greater is consistent with orthostatic proteinuria. Total urinary creatinine should also be measured during the 24-hour urine collection so that creatinine clearance can be estimated. The serum creatinine concentration is also required to calculate the creatinine clearance. If the 24-hour collection demonstrates postural proteinuria or a 24-hour total of less than 500 mg, then no further diagnostic study is indicated. Follow-up should be done every 6 to 12 months to monitor for increasing proteinuria, a rising serum creatinine concentration, or the development of hematuria or hypertension. Although unusual, significant glomerulopathies can begin with orthostatic proteinuria that later becomes persistent.

3. If the protein value is more than 500 mg with no postural proteinuria, then further evaluation is indicated. It should include serum urea nitrogen and creatinine concentrations; complete blood cell count; concentrations of albumin, antinuclear antibody, and cholesterol; hepatitis B screening tests; complement levels (CH_{50}, C3, C4); and an antistreptolysin O titer. Not all tests need be done at once. The clinical history and physical examination should direct the order and amount of testing. If signs or symptoms suggest:

    a. Hepatitis: Measure liver enzymes and hepatitis B surface antigen

    b. Recent streptococcal infection: Determine serum complement and antistreptococcal enzyme titers

    c. Systemic lupus erythematosus: Determine antinuclear antigen and complement levels

4. Renal ultrasonography: Order if abnormal renal function or nonpostural proteinuria is present. This test yields useful information, such as the number of kidneys present (1/1000 people are born with a single kidney, a finding that could influence subsequent evaluation and treatment), the size of the kidneys (small kidney size reflects chronic disease), and echogenicity. Although nonspecific, increased renal echogenicity reflects "medical renal disease" that may require further evaluation.

5. Renal biopsy: Because of the limited number of treatment options for many renal lesions, the frequent use of therapeutic trials, and the ability to diagnose common lesions on the basis of the history and laboratory findings, the indications for a renal biopsy are now more limited than in the past. A biopsy can help define the nature of the renal disease if

the history, physical examination, and laboratory tests are not revealing. A biopsy can also define the severity of the lesion and help in determining its prognosis. This information is very important for teens and their families confronted with a diagnosis of renal disease. Refer to a nephrologist for further evaluation and consideration for renal biopsy when:

a. A 24-hour protein concentration is greater than 1000 mg.
b. The diagnosis is unclear and significant disease is suspected because of the presence of proteinuria, hematuria, hypertension, or renal insufficiency.
c. The nephrotic syndrome is present and has not responded to a therapeutic trial of corticosteroids for minimal change disease.
d. Renal function is deteriorating.
e. The patient, family, or both express a need for prognostic information.

With a careful history, physical examination, urinalysis, and 24-hour urinary protein test, one should be able to identify those adolescents with significant proteinuria and thus determine which teenagers will need follow-up only, versus those who need referral for more expert monitoring or renal biopsy.

Prognosis and Follow-up

Isolated Proteinuria   In general, the prognosis for asymptomatic orthostatic or persistent proteinuria (excretion of <500 mg protein in 24 hours) is good. A study of the 1937 Yale University class revealed a prevalence of proteinuria of 13.8% (Baskin et al., 1972). On 30-year follow-up the group with proteinuria had mortality rates similar to those of the rest of the class. Another group of patients with orthostatic proteinuria was followed for 15 years (Robinson, 1971). At the end of that time, 50% still had proteinuria but no significant renal dysfunction. That group has now been followed up for nearly 35 years with few adverse effects of the proteinuria. Table 27.2 outlines the risk of chronic renal disease with recommended follow-up.

Nonisolated Proteinuria   Dependent on underlying cause of proteinuria:

Gross or Microscopic Hematuria   Usually indicative of glomerular disease when associated with significant proteinuria. Two more common diagnoses in adolescents (especially after an upper respiratory tract infection) include IgA nephropathy (Berger's disease) and poststreptococcal glomerulonephritis. In the absence of clinical manifestations of a chronic illness, with protein excretion of less than 1 g/day and with other normal findings on screening tests, follow-up with twice-yearly blood pressure checks, urinalysis, and determination

TABLE 27.2.   Risk of Chronic Renal Disease and Recommended Follow-up

Pattern of Protein Excretion	Risk of Chronic Renal Failure	Recommended Evaluation	Interval
Transient Intermittent	None		
(<150 mg/day)	None	None	
(>150 mg/day)	Very slight, if any	Blood pressure, urinalysis	1 yr
Constant	20% after 10 yr (depending on exact lesion)	Blood pressure, urinalysis, BUN,[a] serum creatinine	0.5–1 yr
Orthostatic	Very slight, if any	Blood pressure, urinalysis, monitor change in pattern or amount of proteinuria	1–2 yr

Adapted from Abuelo JE. Proteinuria: diagnostic principles and procedures. Ann Intern Med 1983;98:186.
[a]BUN, blood urea nitrogen.

of serum creatinine values is sufficient. IgA nephropathy can be distinguished from acute poststreptococcal glomerulonephritis (PSGN) by the absence of an incubation period separating the onset of an acute infection from the onset of hematuria. Acute PSGN should have an incubation period of 7–10 days. Patients with IgA nephropathy often are found to have persistent microscopic hematuria with intermittent episodes of gross hematuria associated with acute, intercurrent illnesses.

Associated with Systemic Disease

1. Acute illnesses such as Henoch-Schönlein purpura and PSGN usually carry a good prognosis.
2. Chronic illnesses such as lupus erythematosus or a vasculitis usually carry a more guarded prognosis that is dependent on the entire disease process and not just the renal involvement.
3. Azotemia or urinary protein excretion greater than 2 g is usually associated with significant underlying renal disease. Evaluation and therapy for proteinuria associated with a chronic systemic disease, for azotemia, or for proteinuria in the nephrotic range are beyond the scope of this manual and should be carried out in consultation with a subspecialist.

HEMATURIA

Hematuria is defined as the excretion of abnormal quantities of RBCs in the urine. Most authorities accept 2–4 erythrocytes per high-power field (HPF) on a resuspended centrifuged urine sediment specimen as normal. The orthotolidine-impregnated paper strips will give a positive result with a urine specimen that contains as few as 3–5 RBCs/HPF. Hematuria must be differentiated from pigmenturia from such causes as myoglobinuria, hemoglobinuria, porphyrinuria, and exogenous pigments.

Epidemiology

1. Fewer than 3% of healthy individuals excrete more than 3 RBCs/HPF.
2. Several studies have examined the prevalence of hematuria in school-aged children and young adults.
   a. Vehaskari et al. (1979) examined 8954 school-aged children and found a prevalence of 4.1% in at least 1 of 4 urine specimens for 2 days. One percent had 2 or more specimens indicative of hematuria.
   b. Dodge et al. (1976) studied 6070 school-aged children and found that 0.5% had hematuria on at least 2 of 3 specimens.
   c. Froom et al. (1984) examined 1000 symptom-free air force personnel aged 18–33 years and found that 5.2% had 2–4 RBCs/HPF at any one time for a period of 15 years. The cumulative incidence of 2–4 RBCs during the 15 years was 38.7% on at least 1 occasion, 16.1% on 2 or more occasions, and 7.9% on 3 or more occasions. The cumulative incidence was 25.7%, 10.7%, and 5.6% for at least 1 specimen, 2 specimens, and 3 specimens, respectively, with 3–5 RBCs/HPF. Only one patient had significant pathological changes. No others had significant renal disease.

Differential Diagnosis

Although the differential diagnosis of hematuria is extensive, the common conditions in adolescents are much fewer and are listed and discussed here separately. In addition, use of a systematic evaluation will narrow the diagnostic possibilities. The causes of hematuria can be divided into renal parenchymal, urinary tract, and systemic coagulation disturbances. False hematuria must also be considered.

Renal Parenchymal Diseases

1. Glomerular diseases
   a. Primary
      - IgA nephropathy (Berger's disease)
      - Membranous or membranoproliferative glomerulonephritis
      - Focal glomerulonephritis or glomerulosclerosis
   b. Secondary
      - Glomerulonephritis associated with connective tissue diseases, hemolytic uremic syndrome, or Henoch-Schönlein purpura
      - Glomerulonephritis associated with infections such as streptococcal infection, shunt infections, or infective endocarditis
   c. Hereditary: Alport's syndrome, polycystic kidney disease, medullary sponge kidney
   d. Benign familial hematuria: Primary renal hematuria with thin basement membrane
2. Nonglomerular diseases
   a. Vascular diseases
      - Malignant hypertension
      - Loin-pain hematuria syndrome
      - Arteriovenous malformation
      - Renal arterial emboli
   b. Papillary necrosis: Sickle cell disease, diabetes mellitus, alcoholism, analgesic abuse
   c. Trauma: Severe, as in injuries from motor vehicle accidents or contusions from contact sports
   d. Acute bacterial pyelonephritis
   e. Neoplasms

Urinary Tract Disease

1. Hypercalciuria or renal calculi
2. Inflammatory: Urethritis, cystitis, or prostatitis
3. Neoplasms or arteriovenous malformation within bladder

Coagulopathies   Rarely, hematuria is caused by coagulopathy without structural abnormalities in the genitourinary tract or without the use of instruments such as Foley catheters. Included are:

1. Thrombocytopenia
2. Congenital or acquired coagulation defect
3. Use of heparin or warfarin sodium (Coumadin)

False Hematuria   False hematuria can be caused by vaginal bleeding, factitious hematuria, and pigmenturia, including endogenous (porphyrinuria, hemoglobinuria, myoglobinuria) and exogenous (foods and drugs) forms of pigmenturia.

Etiology

The most common causes of microscopic hematuria in adolescents are hypercalciuria, acute infections, trauma, overexercise, renal stones, benign recurrent hematuria, and hereditary nephritis. The most common causes of gross hematuria are IgA nephropathy, trauma, hyper-calciuria, and infections.

Diagnosis

The health-care practitioner must first differentiate between true hematuria and false hematuria.

1. True hematuria: Positive dipstick finding, RBCs on spun urine, clear spun urine, and clear spun serum (unnecessary unless myoglobinuria or hemoglobinuria is suspected)
2. Hemoglobinuria: Positive dipstick finding, negative result of microscopic examination, red spun urine, and pink spun serum
3. Myoglobinuria: Positive dipstick finding, negative result of microscopic examination, orange-red or brown spun urine, clear spun serum
4. Porphyrins or exogenous pigments: Negative dipstick finding, negative result of microscopic examination, red spun urine, clear spun serum
5. Menstruation: Must be ruled out because menstrual blood can easily contaminate urine specimen

The history, physical examination, and screening laboratory tests are usually adequate to exclude significant pathological changes.

History

1. Pattern of hematuria: Microscopic versus macroscopic. Macroscopic, or gross, hematuria is more likely with severe trauma, severe cystitis, or IgA nephropathy. The relationship to intercurrent illnesses may indicate possible poststreptococcal glomerulonephritis or IgA nephropathy.
2. Family history of renal disease or hematuria: Suggestive of hereditary nephritis, benign familial hematuria, or polycystic kidneys. Family history of vision problems or hearing loss with renal disease may indicate hereditary nephritis.
3. Associated symptoms are as follows:
   a. Dysuria, frequency: Cystitis, urethritis, or (rarely) hypercalciuria
   b. Colic: Renal stones
   c. Weight gain: Nephrotic syndrome
   d. Fever: Cystitis, pyelonephritis, or a systemic illness
   e. Joint pain and rashes: Systemic lupus erythematosus or Henoch-Schönlein purpura
   f. Hearing loss: Hereditary nephropathy
   g. Bleeding tendency: Coagulopathy
   h. Previous heart murmurs or tooth extractions: Endocarditis
   i. Loin pain: Loin-pain hematuria syndrome
   j. Blood clots: Lower genitourinary tract disease
4. Drug history: Analgesic abuse, or use of warfarin (Coumadin), heparin, or oral contra-ceptives
5. Relation to exercise: Short-term hematuria after long-distance running or heavy exer-cise—suggestive of possible athletic hematuria

Physical Examination

1. Blood pressure: Elevated blood pressure associated with hematuria suggests renal abnormality.
2. Skin: Petechiae are suggestive of thrombocytopenia. Rashes may indicate connective tis-sue disease. Ecchymosis is suggestive of Henoch-Schönlein purpura.

3. Corneal and lens abnormalities and hearing loss suggest hereditary nephritis.
4. Abdomen: Check for masses and renal enlargement (polycystic disease).

Laboratory Tests   As with proteinuria, the incidence of hematuria falls with repeated examinations. Therefore, significant hematuria should be confirmed on repeated urinalyses before an extensive evaluation is undertaken. Urine should be examined to determine the presence or absence of RBC casts and proteinuria. RBC casts or dysmorphic RBCs, suggest a renal parenchymal origin, usually either glomerulonephritis or interstitial nephritis, and the need for further evaluation. Significant proteinuria would also suggest a glomerular cause and the need for further evaluation. Although blood in the urine can cause some proteinuria, even heavy bleeding usually results in less than 1 g/24 hr. If there are no RBC casts or a qualitative proteinuria (greater than 1+), the evaluation will depend on the history and the physical examination findings. Because idiopathic hypercalciuria is now recognized as an important cause of microscopic hematuria, it is useful to obtain a calcium/creatinine ratio on a spot, random urine sample. A ratio of less than 0.21 is normal. If the ratio is greater, hypercalciuria is overwhelmingly the cause of the hematuria and no further evaluation is required.

1. With signs or symptoms suggestive of infection, obtain a urine specimen for culture.
2. Basic laboratory tests should be ordered, as discussed above with proteinuria, and should include a complete blood cell count, platelet estimation, and determinations of creatinine and complement levels.
3. If coagulopathy is suspected, then order determinations of the prothrombin time, partial thromboplastin time, platelet count, and bleeding time, as indicated.
4. For African-American patients, order sickle cell screening or hemoglobin electrophoresis to evaluate for sickle cell trait.
5. In adolescents with signs and symptoms suggestive of connective tissue disease or proteinuria and RBC casts, order the following tests: Antinuclear antigen (ANA), anti-DNA antibody, third and fourth components of complement (C3 and C4), antistreptolysin O titer (ASO), audiography, serum albumin, cholesterol, quantitative urinary protein, and creatinine clearance.
6. Check urine of first-degree relatives for hematuria. The presence of hematuria in a parent, sibling, or child of an adolescent may indicate either benign familial hematuria (if family members are well) or hereditary nephritis (if family members have renal disease).

Additional Tests   If, after evaluation, the diagnosis is unclear and hematuria is persistent or recurrent, then one should obtain a renal sonogram to look for structural causes of hematuria such as cysts or hydronephrosis. If the diagnosis is still unclear, the next step, if the patient has lower tract symptoms of dysuria or urgency and the RBC morphologic features are normal, is cystoscopy. In the presence of RBC casts and significant proteinuria, a renal biopsy is indicated. In the absence of proteinuria or RBC casts, the indications for renal biopsy are less clear. Trachtman et al. (1984) studied 76 such children and adolescents and found that the most common diagnoses were hereditary nephritis, IgA nephropathy, thinning of the glomerular basement membrane, and C3 staining. The chances of finding a lesion of known significance (i.e., hereditary nephritis and IgA nephropathy) were most enhanced by selecting individuals with either a history of gross hematuria or a family history of renal disease or hematuria in a first-degree relative. The recommendation was for renal biopsy in individuals with microscopic hematuria persistent for more than 6 months, with either one episode of gross hematuria or a positive family history. As discussed above, because treatment of the renal causes of hematuria (other than hypercalciuria) is limited, and because most systemic diseases can be diagnosed without a biopsy, the indications for a biopsy are limited and include the additional presence of proteinuria, hypertension, or renal insufficiency. Without such a history, almost all individuals will have either normal biopsy findings or changes not indicative of significant pathological changes. If gross hematuria persists without an obvious cause, renal angiography can be considered in looking for vascular causes of the hematuria.

Specific Conditions

1. Marathon runner's hematuria: Gross or microscopic hematuria associated with many forms of exercise, including baseball, track, football, hockey, boxing, cross-country skiing, swimming, crew, lacrosse, rugby, and basic military training. The typical history is one of a normal urine before exercise, with hematuria on the first specimen voided after exercise, lasting up to 24–48 hours, possibly in association with dysuria and suprapubic discomfort. The cause is unclear, but the condition seems unrelated to the duration of sustained activity. It may be caused by either a decrease in renal plasma flow, local trauma to the bladder, or leakage of blood from spiral vessels in the adventitia of minor calyces. It is less of a problem in children than older adolescents and adults. The prognosis is excellent unless another renal problem is the underlying cause.

2. Loin-pain hematuria syndrome: A cause of hematuria found mainly in young females receiving oral contraceptives. The condition occurs with recurrent bouts of gross or microscopic hematuria with or without dysuria but almost always with unilateral or bilateral loin pain. The blood pressure and renal function are normal. Protein excretion is usually less than 1 g/day. The renal biopsy shows C3 deposits in arterioles by fluorescence microscopy. Treatment has not been satisfactory. The use of birth control pills should be discontinued.

3. IgA nephropathy (Berger's disease): A relatively common cause of gross hematuria in young adults. It is associated with IgA and IgG deposits in the mesangium. Eighty percent of patients are between 16 and 35 years of age. The male/female ratio is 6:1. Symptoms include recurrent bouts of hematuria (usually gross) after upper respiratory tract infections. The disease may be associated with dysuria and flank pain. The urinary protein concentration is usually more than 1 g/day. Renal function is usually normal, but a moderate percentage of individuals (40%) may progress to renal insufficiency. Poor prognostic signs include hypertension, renal insufficiency, and persistent proteinuria (protein excretion >1 g/day. Serum IgA levels are elevated in 50% of patients. The diagnosis is made by the characteristic history or renal biopsy. No treatment is available. Henoch-Schönlein purpura may cause similar renal lesions but is associated with nonthrombocytopenic vasculitic purpura, arthralgias, and abdominal pain. These two conditions may represent different parts of the spectrum of a similar pathogenic process.

4. Hereditary nephritis (Alport's syndrome) and polycystic kidney disease: The adult form of polycystic kidney disease, which usually manifests itself in the second or third decade of life with hematuria and hypertension. It is an autosomal dominant disease. Familial nephritis in males often has an early onset of renal insufficiency. The renal disease is often accompanied with abnormalities of the lens and retina and high-frequency hearing loss.

5. Benign familial hematuria: A condition characterized by glomerular hematuria (RBC casts), nonprogressive renal disease, and normal renal function in many affected family members. It is often associated with thinning of the glomerular basement membrane. The inheritance is autosomal dominant. The diagnosis is suggested by (*a*) the presence of hemoglobin or RBC casts in the urine of the adolescent, in addition to that of a parent or sibling, (*b*) absence of renal insufficiency in the patient, and (*c*) no history of renal failure or of auditory abnormalities in the affected family members. The disease is more common in females. Table 27.3 is helpful in differentiating benign familial hematuria from hereditary nephritis and IgA nephropathy.

TABLE 27.3.   Differentiation of Benign Familial Hematuria from Hereditary Nephritis and IgA Nephropathy

Clinical Feature	Familial Hematuria	Alport's Syndrome	IgA Nephropathy
Presentation	Microscopic hematuria	Proteinuria, hypertension, or renal failure	Gross or microscopic hematuria or proteinuria
Deafness	No	Yes	No
Familial end-stage renal disease	No	Yes	No
Sex ratio	2:1 F	5:1 M	2:1 M
Blood pressure	Normal	Elevated	Normal
Protein excretion	<0.5 g	>0.5 g	>0.5 g
Creatinine	Normal	Elevated	Normal
Family urine specimens	Abnormal	Abnormal	Normal

Adapted from Blumenthal SS, Fritsche C, Lemann J Jr. Establishing the diagnosis of benign familial hematuria. JAMA 1988; 259:2263.

BIBLIOGRAPHY

Proteinuria

Abitbol C, Zilleruelo G, Freundlich M, et al. Quantitation of proteinuria with urinary protein/creatinine ratios and random testing with dipsticks in nephrotic children. J Pediatr 1990;116:243.

Abuelo JF. Proteinuria: Diagnostic principles and procedures. Ann Intern Med 1983;98:186.

Baskin AM, Freedman LR, Davis JS, et al. Proteinuria in Yale students and 30- year mortality experience. J Urol 1972;108:617.

Chevalier RL. Proteinuria in children: does it warn of a renal disorder? Diagnosis 1986;8:113.

Dodge WF, West EF, Smith EH, et al. Proteinuria and hematuria in school children: epidemiology and natural history. J Pediatr 1976;88:327.

Fang LST. Evaluation of proteinuria. In: Goroll AH, May LA, Mulley AH, eds. Primary care medicine. Philadelphia: JB Lippincott, 1995.

Ginsberg JM, Chang BS, Matarese RA, et al. Use of single voided urine samples to estimate quantitative proteinuria. N Engl J Med 1983;309:1543.

Levey AS, Lau J, Pauker SG, et al. Idiopathic nephrotic syndrome: puncturing the biopsy myth. Ann Intern Med 1987;107:697.

Potter EV, Lipschultz SA, Abidh S, et al. Twelve- to seventeen-year follow-up of patients with poststreptococcal acute glomerulonephritis in Trinidad. N Engl J Med 1982;307:725.

Robinson RR. Orthostatic proteinuria: definition and prognosis. The Kidney 1971;4:1.

Springberg PD, Garrett LE, Thompson AL, et al. Fixed and reproducible orthostatic proteinuria: results of a 20-year follow-up study. Ann Intern Med 1982;97:516.

Stapleton FB: Morphology of urinary red blood cells: a simple guide in localizing the site of hematuria. Pediatr Clin North Am 1987;34:561.

Stapleton FB, Noe HN, Roy S, et al. Hypercalciuria in children with urolithiasis. Am J Dis Child 1982;136:675.

Stewart DW, Gordon JA, Schoolwerth AC. Evaluation of proteinuria. Am Fam Physician 1984;29:218.

Thompson AL, Durrett RR, Robinson RR. Fixed and reproducible orthostatic proteinuria: results of a 10-year follow-up evaluation. Ann Intern Med 1970;73:235.

West CD. Asymptomatic hematuria and proteinuria in children: causes and appropriate diagnostic studies. J Pediatr 1976;89:174.

Hematuria

Blau EB. Hematuria in children: is it a cause for alarm? Postgrad Med 1986;79:65.

Blumenthal SS, Fritsche C, Lemann J Jr. Establishing the diagnosis of benign familial hematuria. JAMA 1988; 259:2263.

Brewer ED, Benson GS. Hematuria: algorithms for diagnosis. I. Hematuria in the child. JAMA 1981;246:877.

Cilento BG Jr, Stock JA, Kaplan GW. Hematuria in children. A practical approach. Urol Clin North Am 1995;22:43.

Dodge WF, West EF, Smith EH. Proteinuria and hematuria in schoolchildren: epidemiology and early natural history. J Pediatr 1976;88:327.

Fairly KF, Birch DF. Hematuria: a simple method for identifying glomerular bleeding. Kidney Int 1982; 21:105.

Froom P, Ribak J, Benbassat J. Significance of microhaematuria in young adults. Br Med J 1984;288:20.

Glassock RJ. Hematuria and pigmenturia. In: Massry SG, Glassock RJ, eds. Textbook of nephrology. Baltimore: Williams & Wilkins, 1983:1.

Hoover DL, Cromie WJ. Theory and management of exercise-related hematuria. Physician Sportsmed 1981; 9:91.

Mohr DN, Offord KP, Owen RA, et al. Asymptomatic microhematuria and urologic disease: a population-based study. JAMA 1986;256:224.

Mokulis JA, Arndt WF, Downey JR, et al. Should renal ultrasound be performed in the patient with microscopic hematuria and a normal excretory urogram? J Urol 1995;154:1300.

Trachtman H, Weiss RA, Bennett B, et al. Isolated hematuria in children: indications for a renal biopsy. Kidney Int 1984;25:94.

Vehaskari VM, Rapola J, Koskimies O, et al. Microscopic hematuria in schoolchildren: epidemiology and clinicopathologic evaluation. J Pediatr 1979;95:676.

CHAPTER 28
Scrotal Disorders

Martin M. Anderson and Lawrence S. Neinstein

MALE GENITAL EXAMINATION

Examination of the male genitalia is a crucial part of the examination of the teenager. It is a relatively easy examination to learn because the male genitalia are readily accessible for palpation. Female examiners should note that in a study of male adolescents (Neinstein et al., 1989), males felt equally comfortable with either male or female examiners during this part of the examination. Before beginning the examination, the examiner should make sure that his or her hands are warm.

1. Inspect pubic area: Note sexual maturity rating, local pathological conditions such as scabies, crabs, warts, or molluscum contagiosum.
2. Inspect groin and inner aspect of thighs: Note swelling from lymphadenitis or herniation or the presence or absence of fungal infection.
3. Inspect penile meatus: Check for presence of discharge, erythema, warts, or hypospadius.
4. Inspect prepuce: Check for phimosis.
5. Inspect penile glans: Check for redness (*Candida* infection, balanitis, or contact dermatitis) and ulcerations (herpes, syphilis, trauma). It is important to replace the foreskin to the original position after examination to prevent the foreskin from constricting the penile shaft.
6. Inspect corona: Check for pink, pearly penile papules. These are normal small skin appendages located on the corona in as many as 15% of teenagers (Neinstein and Goldenring, 1984).
7. Inspect shaft: Check for ulcers and warts. Warts may be present in many more males than was originally suspected. Many of these cases will be detected only by close examination, by colposcopy, or with acetic acid staining. The role of colposcopy or acetic acid staining in the examination of these warts needs to be clarified further.
8. Inspect scrotum: Check for redness or other lesions.
9. Inspect testes: Check for gross enlargement (hydrocele, infection, tumor, or hernia) or for gross asymmetry suggesting possible atrophy or cryptorchidism on one side.
10. Palpate inguinal area: Check for lymphadenopathy or hernia mass.
11. Palpate testes: Check size, shape, and presence of tenderness or masses. The adult testes are about 4–5 cm long and 3 cm wide but vary from one person to another. Examine all parts of the testicle between the thumb and first two fingers.
12. Palpate epididymis: The epididymis lies on the posterior wall of the testes. It attaches at the upper part of the testicles and runs down the back of the testicles. The epididymis becomes the vas deferens and leaves the testicle as part of the spermatic cord. Tenderness and swelling in this area usually indicate epididymitis.

13. Palpate vas deferens: Check for varicocele. Occasionally a hydrocele of the cord may be present.
14. Check for hernia.

CRYPTORCHIDISM

Cryptorchidism refers to an undescended testis that cannot be drawn into the scrotum. The normal testicular descent occurs in the eighth month of fetal life. If a testis cannot be drawn into the scrotum by the third or fourth month of life, there is little evidence to suggest that it will spontaneously descend later.

Epidemiology

The prevalence of cryptorchidism in newborn infants is 3.4%, decreasing to 0.7% by 9 months of age. This prevalence stays the same throughout childhood and adolescence.

Diagnosis

When a testis is not palpable in the scrotum, gentle massage should be performed along the line of descent from the anterosuperior spine, medially, and downward to the pubic tubercle. If the testis is not truly undescended, it should become palpable in the scrotum. If cryptorchidism is present, the teen should be examined for stigmata of associated disorders (i.e., Noonan's, Klinefelter's, and Kallmann's syndromes and trisomy 13, 18, or 21).

Complications

1. Infertility: Data suggest that potential fertility in the cryptorchid testis may be significantly impaired compared to normal testicular fertility, regardless of patient age at the time of discovery of the undescended testis. The fertility index of the descended mates of unilateral undescended testes may also be somewhat impaired in certain age groups. Fertility is significantly hampered in patients with bilateral cryptorchid testes if the condition is not corrected by age 6 years.
2. Malignancy: Five to twelve percent of all malignant testicular tumors occur in people with a history of an undescended testis. The relative risk of tumors in such individuals is increased about 10–40 times. Moreover, the risk is increased even if the testis is brought down into the scrotum. In the United Kingdom Testicular Cancer Study (1994), a significant association of testicular cancer with undescended testis (odds ratio, 3.82; 95% confidence interval, 2.24–6.52) was found. In this study the excess risk associated with undescended testis was eliminated in men who had had an orchidopexy before the age of 10 years.

Therapy

Therapy for cryptorchidism in teenagers should be corrective surgery. These teens should be aware of the increased risk of testicular cancer and should be taught testicular self-examination.

SCROTAL SWELLING AND MASSES

Evaluation

This section discusses the general approach to the adolescent with a scrotal mass or a painful scrotum (Fig. 28.1).

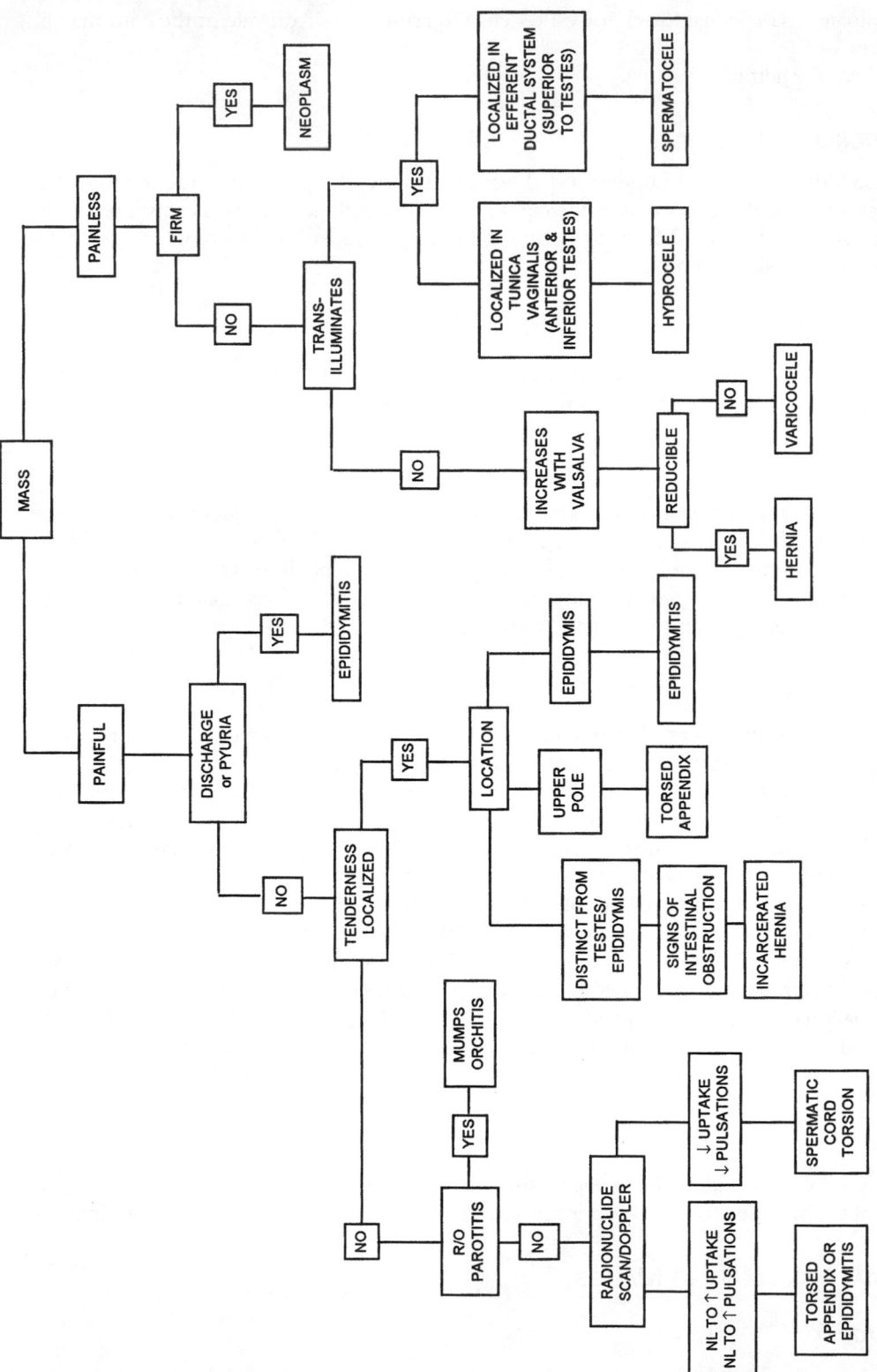

Figure 28.1.   Diagnostic approach to scrotal masses. (Adapted from Schlossberger N. Male reproductive health. I. Painful scrotal masses. Adolesc Health Update 1992;4[3]:1–8; and Klein BL, Ochsenschlager DW. Scrotal masses in children and adolescents: a review for the emergency physician. Pediatr Emerg Care 1993;9[6]:351.)

History

The adolescent should be questioned regarding:

1. Pain: Abrupt onset suggestive of torsion; lack of pain suggestive of a tumor or cystic mass
2. Trauma
3. Recent change in testicular size
4. Sexual activity: Epididymitis a rare occurrence without a history of sexual activity or genitourinary abnormalities
5. Prior history of pain: Torsion often preceded by episodes of mild pain

Examination

1. Inspect testes.
   a. In torsion the affected testis is often higher than the contralateral side. With infections the affected testis is often lower.
   b. In torsion the affected testis and often the contralateral testis lie horizontally instead of in the usual vertical position, secondary to the congenital defect involved.
2. Carefully palpate the testicular surfaces, the epididymis and cord (posterior structures), and the head of the epididymis (lateral structure).
   a. Isolated swelling and tenderness of the epididymis suggests epididymitis.
   b. A tender, pea-sized swelling at the upper pole of the testis suggests torsion of the appendix testis.
   c. Generalized swelling and tenderness of both the testis and the epididymis can be found in either testicular torsion or epididymitis with orchitis.
   d. Presence of a cremasteric reflex makes torsion less likely.
   e. Prehn's sign: Lack of pain relief with elevation of the testis is *not* a reliable test for torsion.
3. If a painless mass is present (Fig. 28.1):
   a. Palpate to assess location.
      — Mass associated with testis is more likely a tumor.
      — Mass unassociated with testis is less likely a tumor.
      — "Bag of worms" on left spermatic cord is probably a varicocele.
      — Mass located near the epididymis is likely a spermatocele or hydrocele.
      — Mass that is separate from testis/epididymis, that intensifies with straining (Valsalva), and that is reducible is likely a hernia.
   b. Transilluminate the mass with a light source: clear transillumination suggests a hydrocele or spermatocele. Absence of transillumination suggests a testicular tumor or, if mass is separate from the testis/epididymis, a hernia.

Laboratory Evaluation

1. Urinalysis: The presence of a positive leukocyte esterase on a urine dipstick or leukocytes on microscopy (especially if there are more than 20 white blood cells per high-power field) is suggestive of epididymitis rather than torsion.
2. Gram stain: In cases of a painful scrotum and a history of urethritis or dysuria, a urethral Gram stain is helpful. Gram-negative diplococci suggest a gonococcal epididymitis. A negative Gram stain suggests either a chlamydial epididymitis, an orchitis, or torsion.
3. Doppler and scans: In cases of a painful scrotum where torsion is suspected, a Doppler flow study, a nuclear scan, or both are crucial. If these are not readily available, then ex-

plorative surgery to examine for torsion is indicated. In cases of torsion, the scan and Doppler study will show a decreased flow to the affected side. Color Doppler ultrasonography may be the most reliable test for diagnosing testicular torsion.

It should be stressed that torsion is a surgical emergency. In cases of painful swelling of the testis, when the diagnosis of epididymitis is not clear and a scan or Doppler study is not immediately available, urological consultation and explorative surgery are indicated.

Differential Diagnosis

1. Painless scrotal mass or swelling
   a. Hydrocele
   b. Spermatocele
   c. Varicocele
   d. Hernia
   e. Testicular tumor
   f. Idiopathic scrotal edema
2. Painful scrotal mass or swelling
   a. Torsion of spermatic cord
   b. Torsion of appendix testis
   c. Epididymitis
   d. Orchitis
   e. Trauma resulting in hematoma
   f. Hernia
   g. Henoch-Schönlein syndrome

TORSION (Fig. 28.2A)

Etiology

Normally the testes are covered anteriorly with a mesothelial structure, the tunica vaginalis. The posterior surface lies bare. In some males the tunica vaginalis more completely surrounds the testes. This causes the testes to lie like "bell clappers" in the scrotal cavities. With this deformity, a testis can twist on the spermatic cord, compromising circulation. Aside from torsion at the spermatic cord, appendages of the testes and epididymis can occasionally undergo torsion.

Epidemiology

Peak age prevalence is 12–18 years. The additional weight of the testes at puberty leads to increased prevalence at that time. The prevalence is increased tenfold in teens with an undescended testis.

Clinical Manifestations

1. Onset is usually abrupt and occasionally starts at night.
2. Fifty percent of teenagers have had brief prior episodes of scrotal pain.
3. Pain may be isolated to the scrotum or radiate to the abdomen.
4. Physical examination shows:
   a. Testis is tender and swollen.

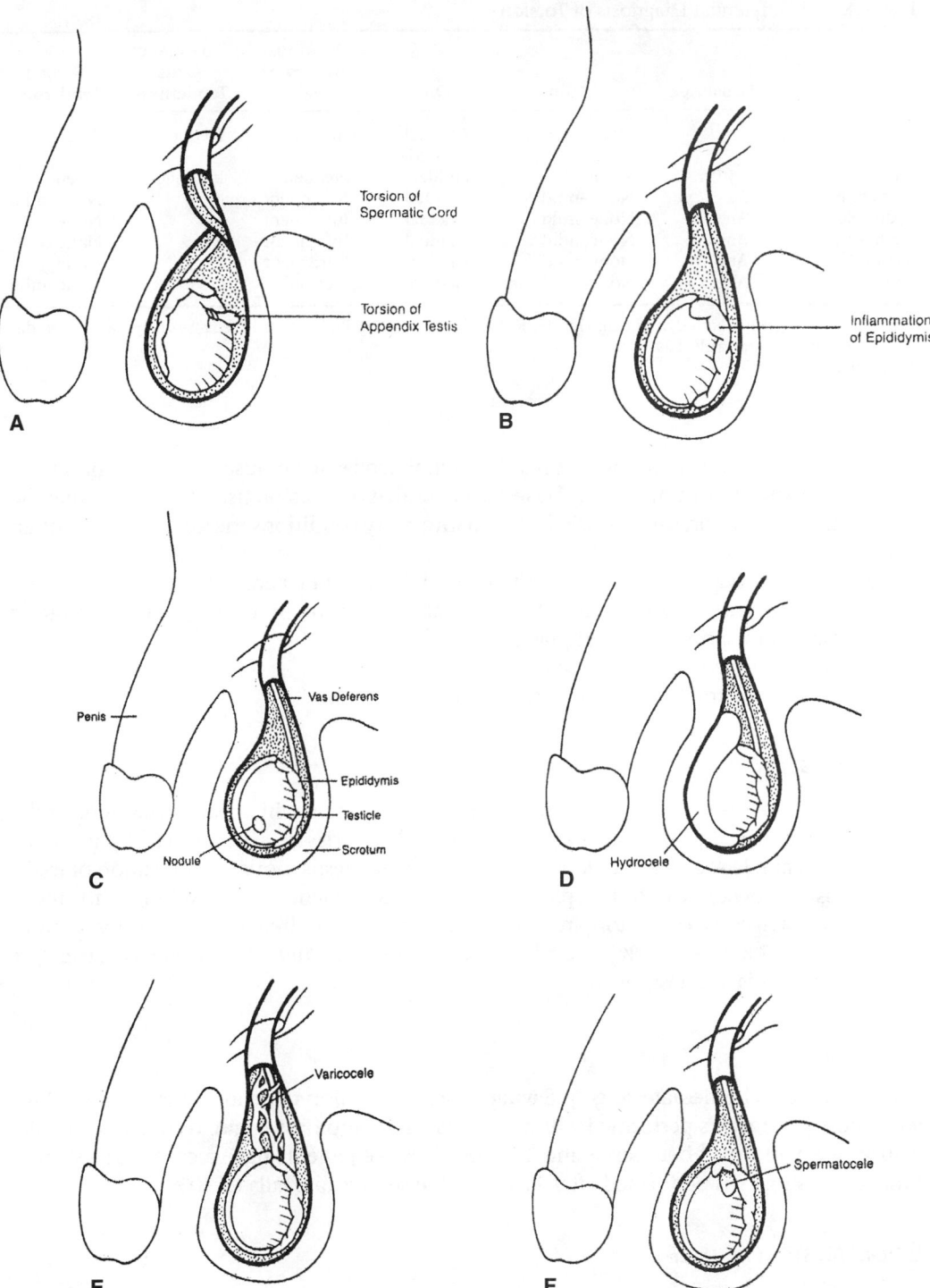

FIGURE 28.2. **A.** Torsions. **B.** Epididymitis. **C.** Testis tumor. **D.** Hydrocele. **E.** Varicocele. **F.** Spermatocele. (From Kapphahn C, Schlossberger N. Male reproductive health. I. Painful scrotal masses. Adolesc Health Update 1992;4[3]:1–8. II. Painless scrotal masses. Adolesc Health Update 1992;5[1]:1–8.)

TABLE 28.1.   Differential Diagnosis of Torsion

	Usual Age	Pain	Onset	Previous History of Pain	Spermatic Cord Tenderness	Scrotal Tenderness
Epididymitis	Any	Mild–severe	Gradual to sudden	Infrequent	Frequent	Severe
Torsion of testes	<30 yr	Severe	Sudden	Frequent	Infrequent	Severe
Testes tumor	18–32 yr	None–mild	Gradual	Infrequent	No	None–mild
Hydrocele	Any	None–mild	Gradual	Infrequent	No	None
Spermatocele	Any	None–mild	Gradual	Infrequent	No	None
Varicocele	Any	None–mild	Gradual	Infrequent	No	None
Hernia	Any	None–moderate	Gradual	Frequent	Frequent	None–mild

Adapted from Berger RE. Epididymitis. In: Holmes K, Mardh PA, Sparling PF, Wiesner PJ, eds. Sexually transmitted diseases. New York: McGraw-Hill, 1990.
*a*Nl, normal.

  b. Affected side is often higher than the contralateral side because of the elevation from the twisted spermatic cord. The testis that undergoes torsion usually twists so that the anterior portion turns medially. In inflammatory conditions the affected side is often lower.
  c. The epididymis, if palpable, is often out of the usual posterolateral location.
  d. The affected testis and often the contralateral testis lie in a horizontal plane rather than in the normal vertical plane.
  e. The cremasteric reflex is absent.
  f. Fever and scrotal redness are usually absent.

Diagnosis

The diagnosis of torsion should be suspected in any adolescent with a painful swelling of the scrotum. As outlined previously, helpful points in diagnosis are acute onset of pain, prior episodes of pain, lack of fever, lack of dysuria, high-riding testis, horizontal position of testis, and decreased flow on scan or Doppler study (Table 28.1). Generalized swelling of the testes is also more suggestive of torsion, in that it occurs much more frequently in torsion than in epididymitis (77% versus 28%). A urology consultation is an urgent necessity for a teenager whose diagnosis is in question.

Therapy

Therapy involves immediate surgery. Saving testicular function depends on early surgical intervention. If surgery is performed within 6 hours after symptoms begin, recovery is the rule; if surgery is performed between 6 and 12 hours, 70% of patients have recovery of testicular function. If surgery is performed after 12 hours, the success rate falls to 20%.

EPIDIDYMITIS (Fig. 28.2*B*)

Etiology

  1. *Chlamydia* is the most common causative organism.
  2. *Neisseria gonorrhoeae* is another frequent pathogen.
  3. Other pathogens are usually involved only if a history of genitourinary tract abnormality, insertive anal intercourse, or instrumentation is present.

Table 28.1.   *continued*

Transillu-mination	Decrease in Swelling	Fever	Location of Swelling	Urethritis, Pyuria, Bacteriuria	Scan (Update)	Doppler Ultrasound (Blood Flow)
No	No	Frequent	Posterior to testes	Yes	↑	↑
No	No	Infrequent	Testes	No	↓	↓
No	No	No	Testes	No	↑ or ↓	Nl[a]
Yes	No	No	Entire hemiscrotum	No	↓	Nl or ↓
Yes	No	No	Above testes	No	↓	Nl or ↓
No	Yes	No	"Bag of worms"	No	Nl or ↑	Nl
No	Yes	No	Above testes	No	Nl	Nl

Epidemiology

1. Uncommon in prepubertal males
2. Uncommon in non-sexually-active males or in those without a history of genitourinary tract abnormalities

Diagnosis

The diagnosis is suggested by the presentation of a sexually active teenager with subacute onset of epididymal swelling and tenderness, urethral discharge, dysuria, fever, and pyuria. Swelling of the epididymis alone is more common in epididymitis than with torsion of the testes (59% versus 15%). The evaluation should include an examination of urine, Gram stain of an endourethral swab specimen, gonorrheal and *Chlamydia* cultures, and urine culture (as necessary). In the absence of a urethral discharge, leukocytes from a Gram-stained endourethral swab specimen, or pyuria, an urgent urology consultation should be done for surgical exploration. If one of the preceding tests shows abnormal findings but the teen has any risk factors suggesting torsion (i.e., prepubertal teen, non-sexually-active teen, elevated or rotated testes, history of prior pain episodes, or acute onset with rapid progression), a scan or a Doppler sonogram should be performed. Orchitis may cause similar symptoms but usually without dysuria or urethral discharge. Mumps infections are the most common cause. Mumps orchitis is usually unilateral and occasionally occurs without a history of parotitis. Other viruses (e.g., adenovirus, Coxsackievirus, ECHO virus, Epstein-Barr virus) rarely cause orchitis.

Therapy

1. Scrotal support is needed.
2. Bed rest is therapeutic in the acute phase.
3. Ceftriaxone, 250 mg, is given intramuscularly once, and either doxycycline, 100 mg, is given orally twice a day for 10 days, or tetracycline, 500 mg, is given four times a day for 10 days. Alternative regimens include erythromycin base, stearate, or ethylsuccinate in doses listed for uncomplicated chlamydial infections. For patients more than 18 years of age, an alternative drug is ofloxacin, 300 mg b.i.d. for 10 days.
4. Lack of resolution requires referral to a urologist.

Testicular Tumors (Fig. 28.2C)

Etiology

Most testicular neoplasias are of germ-cell origin and are malignant. In prepubertal males, teratomas are most common, and in postpubertal males, seminomas are most common.

Other testicular tumors include embryonal cell carcinomas, choriocarcinomas, Sertoli's cell tumors, and Leydig's cell tumors.

Epidemiology

1. Testicular tumors are the most common solid tumor in males aged 15–35 years.
2. Incidence is 2.3 in 100,000 males.
3. The risk of a testicular tumor is increased 10–40 times in a teenager with a history of cryptorchidism.

Diagnosis

The diagnosis of tumor should be suspected in any male with a firm, painless mass associated with a testis, especially if the mass proves solid by transillumination or ultrasonography.

Therapy

Therapy involves a direct biopsy for confirmative diagnosis and cell type. Definitive therapy, though beyond the scope of this book, involves a coordinated effort among the urologist, the primary care specialist, and the oncologist.

HYDROCELE (Fig. 28.2*D*)

Etiology

Hydroceles arise through a defect in the processus vaginalis. The testis descends during the fetal period through a peritoneal sleeve called the processus vaginalis. If this sleeve remains fully open, an inguinal hernia will result. If a small opening remains, a hydrocele will form in the scrotum. If an opening remains but is closed distally before the scrotum, a hydrocele of the spermatic cord will form.

Diagnosis

A hydrocele should be suspected in a patient with a painless, soft, cystic, scrotal mass that is cystic on transillumination or ultrasonography. Hydroceles will often decrease in size by morning and increase in size by evening. The presence of a hydrocele should trigger the examiner to check for a possible underlying hernia, testicular tumor, or infection.

Therapy

Usually no therapy is required. Indications for treatment include:

1. Tense hydrocele that might reduce circulation to testis
2. A bulky mass that is uncomfortable and uncosmetic for the teenager (Definitive therapy involves resection of the parietal tunica vaginalis.)

VARICOCELE (Fig. 28.2*E*)

Etiology

A varicocele results from increased pressure and incompetent venous valves in the internal spermatic veins. The right internal spermatic vein enters the vena cava at an acute angle, so there is little back-flow pressure. However, the left internal spermatic vein enters the left renal vein at right angles, leading to increased back pressure.

Epidemiology

1. Common in the 10- to 20-year age group, with a prevalence of 5–15%.
2. Eighty-five percent of varicoceles occur on the left side, whereas 15% are bilateral.

Diagnosis

Varicoceles are detected in adolescents either on routine examination or on complaints of scrotal mass or ache. On examination there is a "bag of worms" appearance above the testes. The distention usually decreases when the patient lies down. If there is no decrease in size of a varicocele in the supine position, an intravenous pyelogram is indicated to eliminate the possibility of intra-abdominal disease.

Therapy

Kass et al. (1995) recommend varicocele repair in adolescents when

1. The results of semen analysis are abnormal
2. The volume of the left testis is at least 3 mL less than that of the right
3. The response of either luteinizing hormone or follicle-stimulating hormone to go-nadotropin-releasing hormone stimulation is supranormal
4. Bilaterally palpable varicoceles are detected
5. A large symptomatic varicocele is present

The earlier in life the varicocele appears, the higher the risk of testicular growth arrest; varicocelectomy during adolescence usually results in "catch-up growth" of the involved testis. Although varicoceles can cause a progressive loss of fertility during the reproductive years, more than 80% of men with varicoceles are fertile. Thus, although a preponderance of the literature supports a favorable effect of varicocelectomy on fertility, a definitive statement about which adolescents need surgery is impossible.

SPERMATOCELE (Fig. 28.2F)

A spermatocele is a painless, cystic mass containing sperm located in the upper portion of the epididymis. It is usually felt as a smooth, cystic sac located above and posterior to the testis. No therapy is indicated.

TESTICULAR SELF-EXAMINATION

Although females are commonly taught to self-examine their breasts, males are rarely taught testicular self-examination. In a study of young adult males, only 10% had been taught testicular self-examination (Goldenring and Purtell, 1984). Yet testicular cancer is the most common solid tumor in young adults. The recommendations for self-examination by the American Cancer Society are as follows:

1. Examine the testes during or after a hot bath or shower.
2. Examine each testicle with the fingers of both hands, using the index and middle fingers on the underside of the testicle and the thumbs on the top of the testicle.
3. Gently roll the testicle between the thumbs and fingers.

4. Be on the lookout for lumps, irregularities, change in size, or pain in the testicles.
5. The epididymis should not be mistaken for an abnormality.
6. If any abnormality such as a lump is found, it should be reported immediately.
7. Testicular self-examination should be performed once a month.

BIBLIOGRAPHY

Allen TD. Disorders of the male external genitalia. In: Kelalis PP, King LR, eds. Clinical pediatric urology. Philadelphia: WB Saunders, 1976.

Berger RE. Epididymitis. In: Holmes K, Mardh PA, Sparling PF, et al., eds. Sexually transmitted diseases. New York: McGraw-Hill, 1990.

Brothers LR. Blunt scrotal trauma: a review. Hosp Med 1985;21:61.

Centers for Disease Control and Prevention. 1993 sexually transmitted diseases: treatment guidelines. MMWR 1993;42(RR-14):1.

Chehval MJ, Purcell MH. Deterioration of semen parameters over time in men with untreated varicocele: evidence of progressive testicular damage. Fertil Steril 1992;57(1):174.

Colodny AH. Undescended testes: is surgery necessary? N Engl J Med 1986;314:510.

Corrales JG, Corbel L, Cipolla B, et al. Accuracy of ultrasound diagnosis after blunt testicular trauma. J Urol 1993;150:1834.

DeFazio J. Varicoceles repair and fertility. Ob-Gyn Clin Alert 1986;2:36.

Dewire DM, Begun FP, Lawson RK, et al. Color Doppler ultrasonography in the evaluation of the acute scrotum. J Urol 1992;147:89.

Docimo SG. The results of surgical therapy for cryptorchidism: a literature review and analysis. J Urol 1995;154:1148.

Gerscovich EO. High-resolution ultrasonography in the diagnosis of scrotal pathology. I. Normal scrotum and benign disease. J Clin Ultrasound 1993;21:355.

Gilchrist BF, Lobe TE. The acute groin in pediatrics. Clin Pediatr 1992;31:488.

Goldenring JM, Purtell E. Knowledge of testicular cancer risk and need for self-examination in college students: a call for equal time for men in teaching of early cancer detection techniques. Pediatrics 1984;74:1093.

Gorelick JI, Goldstein M. Loss of fertility in men with varicocele. Fertil Steril 1993;59(3):613.

Goroll AH, May LA, Mulley AG, eds. Evaluation of scrotal pain, masses, and swelling. In: Primary care medicine: office evaluation and management of the adult patient. Philadelphia: JB Lippincott, 1995.

Govan DE, Kessler R. Urologic problems in the adolescent male. In: Litt IF, ed. Symposium on adolescent medicine. Pediatr Clin North Am 1980;27:109.

Gutierrez CS. Cryptorchidism. West J Med 1995;163:67.

Hadziselimovic F, Herzog B, Jenny P. The chance for fertility in adolescent boys after corrective surgery for varicocele. J Urol 1995;154:731.

Harrison JH, Gittes RF, Perlmutter AD, et al. eds. Congenital anomalies of the testes. In: Campbell's urology. 4th ed. Philadelphia: WB Saunders, 1992.

Hoover DL. How I manage testicular injury. Physician Sportsmed 1986;14:127.

Horstman WG, Haluszka MM, Burkhard TK. Management of testicular masses incidentally discovered by ultrasound. J Urol 1994;151:1263.

Kapphahn C, Schlossberger N. Male reproductive health. I. Painful scrotal masses. Adolesc Health Update 1992a;4(3).

Kapphahn C, Schlossberger N. Male reproductive health. II. Painless scrotal masses. Adolesc Health Update 1992b;5(1).

Kass EJ, Freitas JE, Salisz JA, et al. Pituitary gonadal dysfunction in adolescents with varicocele. Urology 1993;42(2):179.

Kass EJ, Reitelman C. Adolescent varicocele. Urol Clin North Am 1995;22:151.

Klein BL, Ochsenschlager DW. Scrotal masses in children and adolescents: a review for the emergency physician. Pediatr Emerg Care 1993;9(6):351.

Laven JSE, Haans LCF, Mal WPTM, et al. Effects of varicocele treatment in adolescents: a randomized study. Fertil Steril 1992;58(4):756.

Lewis AG, Bukowski TP, Jarvis PD, et al. Evaluation of acute scrotum in the emergency department. J Pediatr Surg 1995;30:277.

Lund L, Rasmussen HH, Ernst E. Asymptomatic varicocele testis. Scand J Urol Nephrol 1993;27:395.

Lyon RP, Marshall S, Scott M. Varicocele in youth. West J Med 1983;138:832.

Maghnie M, Vanzulli A, Paesano P, et al. The accuracy of magnetic resonance imaging and ultrasonography compared with surgical findings in the localization of the undescended testis. Arch Pediatr Adolesc Med 1994;148:699.

McAleer IM, Packer MG, Kaplan GW, et al. Fertility index analysis in cryptorchidism. J Urol 1995;153:1255.

Neinstein LS, Goldenring JG. Pink pearly papules: an epidemiological study. J Pediatr 1984;105:594.

Neinstein LS, Shapiro J, Rabinowitz S, et al. Comfort of male adolescents during general and genital examination. J Pediatr 1989;115:494.

Pinto KJ, Kroovand RL, Jarow JP. Varicocele-related testicular atrophy and its predictive effect upon fertility. J Urol 1994;152(2 Pt 2):788.

Podesta ML, Gottlieb S, Medel R Jr, et al. Hormonal parameters and testicular volume in children and adolescents with unilateral varicocele: preoperative and postoperative findings. J Urol 1994;152(2 Pt 2): 794.

Pyorealea S, Huttunen NP, Uhari M. A review and meta-analysis of hormonal treatment of cryptorchidism. J Clin Endocrinol Metab 1995;80:2795.

Rabinowitz R, Hulbert WC Jr. Acute scrotal swelling. Urol Clin North Am 1995;22:101.

Rajfer J, Handelsman DJ, Swerdloff RS, et al. Hormonal therapy of cryptorchidism: a randomized, double-blind study comparing human chorionic gonadotropin and gonadotropin-releasing hormone. N Engl J Med 1986;314:466.

Rozanski TA, Bloom DA. The undescended testis. Theory and management. Urol Clin North Am 1995; 22:107.

Schlesinger MD, Wilets IF, Nagler HM. Treatment outcome after varicocelectomy: a critical analysis. Urol Clin North Am 1994;21(3):517.

Schulze KA, Pfister RR. Evaluating the undescended testis. Am Fam Physician 1985;31:133.

Sladkin KR. Overlooked anatomy: examining a boy's genitals. Emerg Med 1984;16:152.

Smith DR. Disorders of testis, scrotum, and spermatic cord. In: Smith, DR, ed. General urology. Los Altos, California: Lange Medical Publishers, 1992.

Stoller ML, Kogan BA, Hricak H. Spermatic cord torsion: diagnostic limitations. Pediatrics 1985;76:929.

United Kingdom Testicular Cancer Study Group. Aetiology of testicular cancer: association with congenital abnormalities, age at puberty, infertility, and exercise. United Kingdom Testicular Cancer Study Group. Br Med J 1994;308:1393.

Wilbert DM, Schaerfe CW, Stern WD, et al. Evaluation of the acute scrotum by color-coded Doppler ultrasonography. J Urol 1993;149:1475.

Witt MA, Lipshultz LI. Varicocele: a progressive or static lesion? Urology 1993;42(5):541.

SECTION VIII

Infectious Diseases

CHAPTER 29

Infectious Mononucleosis and *Mycoplasma pneumoniae*

INFECTIOUS MONONUCLEOSIS

Infectious mononucleosis (IM) is common in the adolescent and young adult years. IM is usually an acute, self-limited, benign lymphoproliferative disease caused by Epstein-Barr virus (EBV). IM is the most common clinical manifestation of EBV infection. EBV can also cause clinical disorders other than IM. In addition, mononucleosislike syndromes can be caused by other infections other than EBV.

Etiology

EBV is responsible for over 90% of mononucleosislike syndromes. The rest are caused by cytomegalovirus (CMV), toxoplasmosis, hepatitis viruses A and B, and adenovirus. EBV is usually contacted through saliva. The virus replicates in the lymphoreticular system, provoking an intense immunologic response usually involving lymph nodes, the spleen, the liver, and bone marrow. This immune response results in the clinical symptomatology.

EBV is a double-stranded DNA virus in the herpes family. The infection usually begins with viral replication in the nasopharyngeal epithelial cells and then spreads to B lymphocytes. These cells disseminate the infection throughout the lymphoreticular system. During this time there is a polyclonal B-cell proliferation and a vigorous T-cell response. In response to infected and transformed B cells, there is the appearance of atypical lymphocytes in the peripheral blood. These atypical cells represent primarily an expansion of the T-cell series, mainly cytotoxic or suppressor (CD8) cells. The time from initial acquisition of the virus to the appearance of large numbers of infected B cells in the peripheral circulation and symptoms is usually 30–50 days.

The immune response to EBV infection also leads to the formation of non-EBV-specific antibodies (heterophil antibodies) in addition to responses directed at several EBV-specific antigens. However, the major factor in controlling EBV and preventing EBV-induced lymphoproliferative disorders is a strong, cellular immune response.

During an acute infection, about 0.001% to 0.01% of circulating B cells are infected. Over 3–4 months, this declines to 0.00001%, which persists indefinitely. The EBV persists for life in both the B cells and salivary glands. About 70–90% of individuals shed virus until 8–24 weeks after resolution of the clinical disease. After this, 60–100% of normal asymptomatic EBV-seropositive individuals shed virus intermittently, with about 20–30% of individuals shedding virus at any one time. This percentage can be as high as 50% in immunosuppressed individuals.

Epidemiology

Prevalence Almost all humans are infected with EBV at some time. Most individuals in the world are infected in early childhood and have only inapparent or mild infections. This is associated with a lifelong latent infection and the potential for viral shedding at various times through life.

1. Age
   a. Developing countries: In developing countries, tropical areas, and other areas, including crowded areas in the United States, infection usually occurs early in life and is usually inapparent. Most children (>90%) under these circumstances seroconvert by age 6 years.
   b. Western Europe and the United States: Only 35–50% of children by age 5 are positive. A large group of adolescents and college-aged youth lack immunity. Thus, infections are quite common in individuals in high school and college. As many as 12% of susceptible college freshman become infected with EBV in their first year of college. The rate in adolescents is 320–370 cases per 100,000, which is eight times the overall rate in the population. In affected students 25–75% will develop clinical IM. Stress may be a risk factor for developing symptoms. IM prevalence in Western Europe and the United States peaks about 2 years earlier in girls (16 years compared to 18 years in boys).
2. Incubation period: 30–50 days
3. Sex and race: Equal prevalence
4. Season: No seasonal variation, except an increase in spring and fall among college students.
5. Contagiousness: Saliva is the main vehicle for transmission of EBV. Transmission requires direct and prolonged contact with infected oropharyngeal secretions. Kissing is an important modality of transmission in adolescents and young adults. IM does not occur in epidemics, as EBV has a low contagiousness in young adult populations and requires close personal contact. In families, about 10–40% of susceptible members will develop an EBV infection when exposed. EBV has also been found in the genital tracts of men and women. The role of this site in transmission is not yet defined; however, the possibility of sexual transmission may exist.

Clinical Manifestations

As mentioned previously, the majority of EBV infections in the world are either asymptomatic or associated with mild nonspecific symptoms such as diarrhea, fever, and rhinorrhea. Even in adolescents, where classic IM is common, the majority of EBV infections are subclinical.

The traditional hallmarks of IM include the triad of:

- Fever, malaise, lymph node enlargement, and tonsillopharyngitis
- Lymphocytosis with atypical lymphocytes
- Typical antibody response with presence of heterophil antibodies or EBV-specific antibodies

1. Incubation period: 30–50 days
2. Prodrome: 3–5 days of malaise, headache, anorexia, myalgia, and fatigue. This is followed usually by more severe symptoms and signs.
3. IM symptoms and signs: The common presentation includes fever, which may persist for several weeks. A prominent symptom is sore throat, which can be severe, including an exudative pharyngitis in up to 50% of individuals. Palatal petechiae may also be seen in the

throat. Anorexia with nausea and vomiting is common. Periorbital or facial edema may occur in about one-third of teens. Adenopathy is usually significant and is most commonly symmetric, with posterior cervical nodes more prominent than anterior cervical nodes. Splenomegaly may occur by the second week of illness with hepatomegaly being less common. About 10% of individuals will have a rash that may be either erythematous, maculopapular, morbilliform, urticarial, or erythema multiforme in appearance. A rash is especially common if ampicillin has been given (as high as 90%).

4. Prevalence of signs and symptoms

Symptoms	*Prevalence*
Malaise	90–100%
Anorexia	50–80%
Nausea	50–70%
Headache	40–70%
Cough	30–50%
Myalgia	12–30%
Chest pain	5–20%
Arthralgia	5–10%
Diarrhea	5–10%
Photophobia	5–10%
Abdominal pain	<5%

Signs	*Prevalence*
Adenopathy	85–100%
Fever	80–95%
Pharyngitis	65–85%
Tonsillitis	60%
Splenomegaly	50–60%
Bradycardia	35–50%
Hepatomegaly	15–25%
Palatal petechiae	25–35% (at junction of hard and soft palates)
Periorbital edema	25–35%
Liver or splenic tenderness	15–30%
Jaundice	5–10%
Rash (usually maculopapular)	3–15% (increased if adolescent receives ampicillin)
Pneumonitis	<3%

5. Patterns of presentation: Adolescents and young adults often present with one of three clinical forms predominating.
   a. Pharyngeal (anginose syndrome): The hallmark is an exudative tonsillitis with marked pharyngeal edema. Usually, the tonsillitis has an abrupt onset and high fever. In addition, the resolution in many individuals tends to be rapid, within 5–7 days. Cervical adenopathy in teens is generally symmetric, involving the posterior cervical chain to a greater degree than the anterior cervical chain. Sometimes these individuals are difficult to differentiate from individuals infected with group A β-hemolytic strep infections, especially since EBV and strep infections frequently coexist.
   b. Glandular: The adenopathy is prominent and out of proportion to their other symptoms such as pharyngitis and fever. Malaise is a significant symptom. Teens may be ill for 1–2 weeks or more before they seek medical attention.
   c. Febrile or systemic form: Prolonged fever and malaise without significant pharyngitis predominates. Lymphadenopathy occurs later in the illness. Anorexia, nausea, and vomiting may be severe.

6. Recovery: Almost all individuals with primary EBV infection recover without problems and develop a significant degree of long-lasting immunity. The acute symptoms usually resolve in 1–2 weeks, with the fatigue persisting longer.
7. Complications: Sometimes a complication of IM is the prominent clinical manifestation of the disease, and the classic symptoms either never appear or appear later in the course. Overall, the complication rate is about 1–2%. Complications include:

		Prevalence
a.	Neurological	1%
	Seizures	
	Facial or peripheral nerve palsies	
	Meningoencephalitis	
	Aseptic meningitis	
	Optic neuritis	
	Reye's syndrome	
	Coma	
	Transverse myelitis	
	Guillain-Barré syndrome	
	Acute psychosis	
	Acute cerebellar ataxia	
b.	Hematological	
	Hemolytic anemia (mild)	1.7–3%
	Thrombocytopenia purpura	Rare
	Coagulopathy	Rare
	Aplastic anemia	Rare
	Hemolytic-uremic syndrome	Rare
	Eosinophilia	Rare
c.	Cardiac	1.7–6%
	Pericarditis	
	Myocarditis	
	Electrocardiogram (ECG) changes	
d.	Splenic rupture	0.5%
e.	Pulmonary	
	Airway obstruction	Rare
	Pneumonitis	3–5%
	Pleural effusions	Rare
	Pulmonary hemorrhage	Rare
f.	Gastrointestinal	Rare
	Hepatitis with liver necrosis	
	Malabsorption	
g.	Dermatological	3–10%
	Dermatitis	
	Urticarial rash	
	Erythema multiforme	
h.	Renal	
	Glomerulonephritis	Rare
	Nephrotic syndrome	Rare
	Mild hematuria or proteinuria	Up to 13%
i.	Eye involvement	Rare
	Conjunctivitis	

	Prevalence
Episcleritis	
Uveitis	
j. Superimposed infections	
β-hemolytic streptococcal	Up to 33%
Staphylococcus aureus infections	
Mycoplasma pneumoniae	Up to 5%
k. Other	Uncommon
Bullous myringitis	
Orchitis	
Parotiditis	
Monarticular arthritis	

Specific Complications

1. Splenic rupture
   a. Frequency: About 1–2 per 1000 cases of IM
   b. Presentation: Abrupt pain in left upper quadrant radiating to the top of the left shoulder (Kehr's sign) and then followed by generalized abdominal pain, pleuritic chest pain, and signs and symptoms of hypovolemia. Splenic rupture occurs between the 4th and 21st day of symptomatic illness, with about 50% of cases occurring during the height of acute illness, and the other half in the early convalescent period. Splenic rupture may also be the first symptom of IM that brings a teen to medical attention. Less than 50% of individuals with splenic rupture had clinically apparent splenomegaly noted prior to the rupture. The majority of cases are also unrelated to a history of significant strain or trauma. Fatality is rare from this complication.
2. Airway obstruction
   a. An uncommon but life-threatening complication of IM related to massive lymphoid hyperplasia and mucosal edema. Corticosteroids have been used in an attempt to reduce the edema and hypertrophy of lymphoid tissue. If needed, tracheostomy or intubation can be performed.
3. Streptococcal pharyngitis
   a. Frequency: Coinfections occur in 2% to as many as 33% in some reports of individuals with IM.

Laboratory Diagnosis

1. Hematological abnormalities: The dramatic distinctive findings with IM are hematological. In general, there is an elevation of the white blood cell count in the range of 10,000–20,000/mm^3. A lymphocytosis is usually seen with greater than 50% of the leukocyte count being lymphocytes. This occurs secondary to the EBV activation of B lymphocytes, which causes a proliferation of T lymphocytes. In addition, at least 10% of the lymphocytes are atypical lymphocytes, which appear similar to large lymphoblasts with a vacuolated basophilic cytoplasm and appear indented by nearby erythrocytes. The atypical lymphocytes are either EBV-transformed B lymphocytes or usually activated suppressor or cytotoxic (CD8) T lymphocytes. These atypical lymphocytes can be seen in other viral infections such as CMV, human immunodeficiency virus (HIV), hepatitis, rubella, mumps rubeola, and toxoplasmosis but do not comprise over 10% of total leukocyte count except with EBV, CMV, and toxoplasmosis.

   Other common hematological abnormalities include a mild granulocytopenia and thrombocytopenia (usually in the range of 100,000–140,000/mm^3). Anemia is unusual.

Evidence of a mild hepatitis is present in about 90% of individuals including elevations in aminotransferases, alkaline phosphatase, and lactate dehydrogenase (LDH; about 2–3 times normal). Serum bilirubin is generally only in the 1–3 mg/dL range. Entirely normal findings from liver chemistries suggest a diagnosis other than primary EBV infection.

Frequency of hematological findings includes:

Lymphocytosis	95%
Atypical monocytosis	95%
Elevated liver function test results	80%
Hypergammaglobulinemia	80%
Thrombocytopenia	50%
Elevated bilirubin levels	40%
Cold agglutinins	30–80%

2. Serologic features
   a. Heterophil antibodies: The classic test for EBV-associated IM is the presence of heterophil antibodies. These tests detect immunoglobulin M (IgM) antibodies induced by EBV infections that cross-react with phylogenetically unrelated antigens (e.g., horse, sheep, or bovine erythrocytes). Although the presence of heterophil antibody is the hallmark of IM, it can be found in normal human serum in low titer, as well as higher titer in individuals with malignant diseases, in serum sickness, and in several other viruses. In addition, some patients with IM, especially children, are heterophil negative.

   To differentiate heterophil antibodies present during IM from those in normal serum or serum sickness, a preabsorption is performed with either guinea pig kidney or beef red blood cells (RBCs). Heterophil antibodies associated with IM agglutinate sheep and horse RBCs after preabsorption with guinea pig kidney, but not after preabsorption with bovine RBCs. This differential response is used in forming the heterophil screening tests for IM such as the Monospot and other slide and card tests. The tests are rapid, simple, and inexpensive. Tests such as the Monospot are highly sensitive (96–99%) in adolescents and young adults.

   Heterophil antibodies are detected during the first week of clinical infection (about 70% of individuals) but are maximal during the second and third weeks (85–95%). However, even in adolescents and young adults with EBV infection and classic IM, not all will develop heterophil antibodies and will therefore be Monospot negative. This is even more common in infants and young children. In children younger than 3 years old, the test results are rarely positive; in 3- to 8-year-olds the test results are positive in 50% of cases. Positivity for heterophil antibodies remains for weeks to months after an acute infection. In general, sheep and beef agglutination test results remain positive for about 3–6 months, whereas horse agglutination test results remain positive up to 18 months.

   Heterophil-negative mononucleosis syndrome describes those teens with mononucleosis-like symptoms but who are Monospot negative. They may have one of the following infections:
   — EBV (heterophil-negative individuals)
   — CMV
   — *Toxoplasma gondii*
   — Herpes virus 6
   — Adenovirus
   — HIV
   — Rubella

If EBV is suspected and the heterophil test results are negative, EBV-specific antibody tests can be performed.

b. Specific EBV titers: Antibody responses to several EBV antigens have been well studied. These include viral capsid antigen (VCA), early antigen (EA), and Epstein-Barr nuclear antigen (EBNA). These are usually measured by direct immunofluorescence while newer enzyme immunoassay techniques are being more carefully evaluated. Enzyme-linked immunosorbent assay (ELISA) techniques may eventually replace the indirect immunofluorescent tests. Figure 29.1 shows the characteristic EBV antibody responses to various EBV antigens. Table 29.1 shows the pattern of serologic testing in various EBV states.

— Viral capsid antigen (VCA): Antibodies against VCA are composed of both IgG and IgM. Antibody levels for both peak at about 3–4 weeks after the clinical onset of the disease. IgM declines rapidly and is undetectable by 3 months. IgG declines somewhat with time but persists for life. High persistent levels of IgG antibodies against VCA can indicate:

Remote EBV infection

Systemic lupus

Chronic renal failure

Burkitt's lymphoma or nasopharyngeal carcinoma

Leukemia

Sarcoidosis

Cancer

Acquired immunodeficiency syndrome (AIDS)

Hodgkin's lymphoma

Lymphoma

Rheumatoid arthritis

Immunodeficiency state

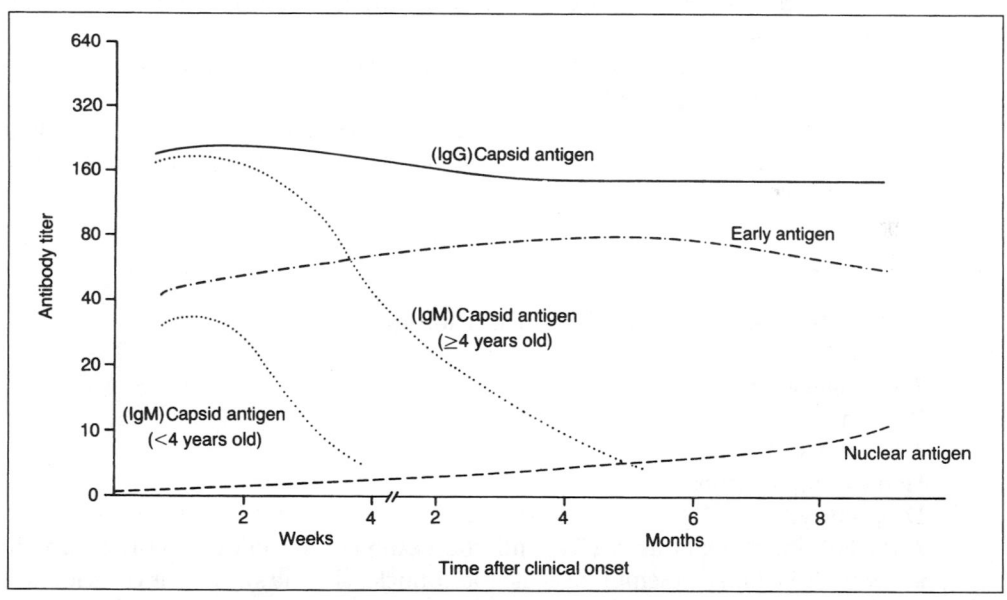

FIGURE 29.1. The evolution of antibodies to various Epstein-Barr virus (EBV) antigens in patients with infectious mononucleosis is shown above. The titers are geometric mean values expressed as reciprocals of the serum dilution. Immunoglobulin M (IgM) and IgG antibody responses to EBV capsid antigen develop during the acute phase, as does an IgG response to EBV early antigen in most cases. The IgG response lasts for life, but the IgM response is transient and shortest in very young children. Antibody response to nuclear antigen lasts for life and is typically quite late in onset. (From Sumaya CV. Epstein-Barr serologic testing: diagnostic indications and interpretations. Pediatr Infect Dis 1986;5:337–342.)

TABLE 29.1.   Patterns of Serology[a]

Type of Infection	Heterophil Antibody	VCA-IgG	VCA-IgM	Early Antigen		EBNA
				D-EA	R-EA	
Susceptible (nonimmune)	–	–	–	–	–	–
Acute primary infection	+	++	+	+	–	–
Remote past infection	–	+	–	–	–	+
Reactivated infection	+/–	+++	–	+	++	+/–

[a]D-EA, diffuse early antigen; EBNA, Epstein-Barr nuclear antigen; Ig, immunoglobulin; R-EA, restricted early antigen; VCA, viral capsid antigen.

— Early antigen (EA): Antibodies against EA are induced in 70–90% of individuals with acute EBV IM. The antibodies are produced very early in the infection and persist for 8–12 weeks. As many as 30% of individuals with past infections have positive titers for EA. EA antibodies have been divided into two patterns of staining (diffuse and restricted). Most adolescents and young adults with IM have antibodies against the D (diffuse) component.

— Nuclear antigen (EBNA): Antibodies against EBNA develop 2–3 months after the onset of infection and tend to persist indefinitely. Positive titers usually indicate an infection at least 1–2 months or longer in the past. Absent EBNA titers in patients with an EBV infection are associated with immunodeficiency states and rheumatoid arthritis.

— Diagnosis: Acute EBV IM syndrome is characterized (Table 29.1) by the presence of both IgM and IgG VCA and EA antibodies. Older and remote infections are characterized by the absence of IgM VCA antibodies and the appearance of IgG EBNA antibodies.

— EBV serology is best reserved for measurement in adolescents when:
  (1) Clinical IM is present and a heterophil test result is negative.
  (2) Clinical syndromes such as thrombocytopenia, pneumonia, or neurologic findings are present and the physician wishes to exclude the diagnosis of acute EBV disease.

Differential Diagnosis

1. Causes of EBV-negative mononucleosislike syndrome
   a. CMV
   b. *Toxoplasma gondii*
   c. Rubella
   d. Adenovirus
   e. Herpes simplex virus 6
   f. Drug side effects
   g. Acute HIV infection: Primary HIV-1 infection can present clinically as the abrupt onset of a febrile illness resembling acute mononucleosis. The symptoms coincide with high titers of culturable plasma viremia and antigenemia, which rapidly decrease with the emergence of detectable HIV-specific antibody and HIV-specific cytotoxic lymphocytes
2. Other considerations
   a. Group A β-hemolytic streptococcal pharyngitis
   b. Viral tonsillitis
   c. *M. pneumoniae*

    d. Vincent's angina
    e. Diphtheria
    f. Viral hepatitis
    g. Lymphoproliferative disorder or leukemia

Diagnosis

The diagnosis is based on the triad of:

1. Clinical symptoms: IM should be suspected in an adolescent with fatigue, fever, splenomegaly, adenopathy, and pharyngitis.
2. Abnormal white blood cell count: Patients will usually have:
   a. Relative lymphocytosis greater than 50%
   b. Absolute lymphocytosis greater than 4000 cells per milliliter
   c. Atypical mononuclear cell counts greater than 10–20% of the white blood cell count differential
      Atypical lymphocytes may be seen with other viral diseases such as rubella, rubeola, mumps, and acute viral hepatitis, but except for CMV infections and toxoplasmosis, such lymphocytes usually comprise less than 10% of total white blood cells.
3. Positive serology: Almost all adolescents with IM have positive heterophil antibodies. If a patient continues to be symptomatic and heterophil antibodies are negative, titers for EBV (including VCA and EBNA), CMV, and toxoplasmosis should be evaluated. If liver function test results are elevated, serology for hepatitis A, B, and C should be evaluated. A throat culture is indicated in patients with pharyngitis or tonsillitis.

    Chronic EBV Infections   In the vast majority of individuals lifelong significant immunity to EBV develops. There are rare individuals who have very high titers of EBV antibodies and have chronic, persistent active EBV infection, usually associated with an abnormal immune response to EBV. However, there is little evidence that EBV is associated with the chronic fatigue syndrome (see Chapter 34). EBV infections can also be associated with specific lymphoproliferative disorders in individuals with underlying abnormal immune responses. These include the virus-associated hemophagocytic syndrome (generalized histiocytic proliferation and hemophagocytosis), lymphomatoid granulomatosis, and the X-linked lymphoproliferative syndrome (XLP) in which affected males die of EBV disease sometimes in a matter of days. When EBV leaves the latent state and becomes chronically active, it can have a potential to trigger malignancies. Such EBV-associated malignancies include Burkitt's lymphoma, nasopharyngeal carcinoma, and thymic carcinoma.

Management

1. Quarantine: Absolutely not indicated
2. Antibiotics: In general, antibiotics serve no purpose; especially avoid ampicillin.
   If a secondary group A β-hemolytic streptococcal infection or *M. pneumoniae* infection occurs, then appropriate antibiotics are indicated.
3. Symptomatic care
   a. Rest as needed by the adolescent and in the acute phase: Teens should be aware that usually the acute symptoms resolve over 1–2 weeks with the fatigue lasting 2–4 weeks and sometimes longer.
   b. Administer analgesics for fever, arthralgias, and pharyngitis.
4. Athletic activity
   a. With splenomegaly or tender spleen: Restrict all athletics until resolved.

    b. Teens uninvolved in contact or strenuous sports: Light, nonimpact activities can be resumed after 21 days of illness if the teen feels ready. Full participation can be resumed about 1 month after onset of symptoms.

    c. Teens involved in strenuous training or contact sports: Easy training can be performed early as energy level dictates, but full participation in contact sports should be delayed at least 4–6 weeks. If there is a question of splenic enlargement, an ultrasound in these athletes could be used to assess and follow splenomegaly.

5. Steroids: The use of steroids should be avoided, if at all possible, in IM patients. Because of the latent nature of EBV, the potential for chronic or recrudescence of symptoms after steroid therapy use exists. Steroids may be needed if hemolysis, thrombocytopenia, airway obstruction, or neurological sequelae are life threatening. Steroids may also be considered for massive splenomegaly.

6. Future therapies: Acyclovir has good in vitro antiviral activity against EBV. However, in a placebo-controlled, double-blind study that used intravenous acyclovir, there were no significant differences in symptoms or laboratory parameters. Short-term suppression of viral shedding can be demonstrated, but significant clinical improvement is lacking. More data are needed before acyclovir could be recommended routinely for individuals with EBV IM.

MYCOPLASMA PNEUMONIAE

M. pneumoniae is a frequent cause of upper respiratory infections in adolescents and may account for 50% or more of pneumonias in teenagers.

Etiology

Mycoplasma and *Ureaplasma* species constitute the smallest free-living microorganisms. Over 50 species have been identified, including 10 in humans, of which three have proved to be pathogenic: *M. pneumoniae, M. hominis,* and *U. urealyticum.* These organisms have no cell walls and are thus resistant to β-lactam antimicrobials. They are similar in size to large viruses (about 100 nm).

Epidemiology

1. *M. pneumoniae* infections are most common in 5- to 9-year-old children and then in the 10- to 14-year-old age group. Although the number of cases of pneumonia secondary to *M. pneumoniae* decreases with age, the percentage of pneumonias secondary to this organism increases in older age groups. For example, in the early school-aged child, 9–16% of pneumonias are secondary to *M. pneumoniae;* in older children the percentage increases to 16–21%; and in college-aged individuals the percentage increases yet again to 30–50%. The organism causes about 20–30% of pneumonias in military recruits.

2. Epidemics tend to occur in fall and winter.

3. Epidemic spread is common among families, recruits in army bases, fraternities, and others in close surroundings.

4. Incubation period: 3 weeks

5. Risk of infection in other family members if one member is infected is about 65%.

Pathophysiology

M. pneumoniae infections are acquired via the respiratory route from small-particle aerosols or large droplets of secretions. *M. pneumoniae* adheres to respiratory epithelium and then causes cellular damage to the epithelium of bronchi and bronchioles. The organism also causes ciliostasis, which may lead to a prolonged cough. A variety of mechanisms have been suggested to explain the extrapulmonary complications, including metastatic infection, auto-antibodies and immune complexes, toxin production, hypercoagulability, and altered host immunity.

Clinical Manifestations

M. pneumoniae leads to an influenza-like respiratory illness with malaise, fever, and headache and usually causes upper respiratory tract and pulmonary infections.

Upper Respiratory Tract Infections   The majority of *M. pneumoniae* infections involve the upper respiratory tract. These can vary from mild infections with or without a pharyngitis to a severe bronchitis.

Pulmonary Infections   *M. pneumoniae* may account for 50% or more of pneumonias during adolescence.

Symptoms

1. Onset is gradual.
2. Malaise, fever, chills, and headache occur early in the course.
3. Cough: A cough develops 3–5 days after the onset. It usually starts as a nonproductive cough and may lead to the production of frothy white sputum. The cough may become paroxysmal. Occasionally, hemoptysis occurs.
4. Nausea, vomiting, and diarrhea may occur.
5. Chest pain, earache, and gastrointestinal complaints occur in about 25% of teenagers.
6. Coryza is an unusual manifestation.

The infection is usually mild and lasts about 2–4 weeks without treatment. Antibiotics can shorten the course.

Signs

1. Pharyngitis: 75%
2. Conjunctivitis: 50%
3. Lymphadenopathy: 25–50%
4. Chest: Lung findings are often minimal. If pneumonia is present, the teen may have isolated crackles or areas of wheezing over one of the lower lobes.

Complications

Nonrespiratory Infections and Complications   Nonrespiratory infections and complications usually occur 1–21 days after initial symptoms. One must use caution in the diagnosis of a *M. pneumoniae* infection in individuals with extrapulmonary manifestations and no respiratory tract symptoms.

1. Myringitis (may be bullous): 12%
2. Sinusitis
3. Musculoskeletal: Arthralgias, myalgias, arthritis. The arthritis is usually monoarticular or migratory and polyarticular.
4. Gastrointestinal: Gastroenteritis, hepatitis, pancreatitis

5. Dermatological: Most common are erythematous maculopapular lesions or vesicular exanthemas. Other rashes include vesicular-pustular, petechial, and urticarial. Erythema multiforme and Stevens-Johnson syndrome can occur.
6. Hematological: Hemolytic anemia, thrombocytopenia, or disseminated intravascular coagulopathy
7. Cardiovascular: Myocarditis, pericarditis, heart block, congestive heart failure, and acute myocardial infarction
8. Central nervous system: Meningitis, Guillain-Barré syndrome, cranial nerve involvement, transverse myelitis, focal encephalitis, cerebellar involvement, psychosis
9. Acute glomerulonephritis

Laboratory

1. White blood cell count: Occasionally, leukocytosis is present.
2. Chest x-ray examination: The chest x-ray examination may show a lobar or segmental infiltrate (lower lobes in 90% of patients). A reticular or interstitial infiltrate is often present, and occasionally, a pleural effusion occurs. The x-ray findings often appear worse than the clinical findings.
3. Cold agglutinins: Cold agglutinins are elevated to a titer of greater than 1:32 75% of the time. This test is nonspecific and may be elevated in patients with viral infections and in some noninfectious diseases such as hemolytic anemias.
4. Antibody titers: Both complement fixation titers and enzyme immunoassay (EIA) tests are available. A fourfold increase in titer is highly suggestive of a recent infection. Other technologies such as DNA probe techniques are under investigation.
5. Cultures: Cultures require about 3 weeks and are thus too slow to be of clinical use.

Differential Diagnosis

1. *Streptococcus pneumoniae*
2. Viral pneumonia
3. *Chlamydia pneumoniae:* Another relatively common, more recently discovered cause of pneumonia in adolescents and young adults. Seroprevalence studies in adult populations around the world suggest that more than 40% of adults have been previously infected. Usually starts with hoarseness and fever, respiratory tract symptoms may not appear for days. Infection with *C. pneumoniae* can trigger acute episodes of wheezing in children with asthma. Diagnosis is based on serologic testing, but *C. pneumoniae* specific testing is hard to obtain and requires acute and convalescent sera. Culture is more difficult than for *C. trachomatis,* and direct antigen detection does not appear to work well. Treatment is with erythromycin, tetracycline, doxycycline, or azithromycin. Some authorities prefer doxycycline or tetracycline if *C. pneumoniae* is the suspected cause of a pneumonia.
4. Legionella pneumonia: Accounts for about 1–3% of community-acquired pneumonias and up to one-fourth of "atypical" community-acquired pneumonias. Pneumonic illness usually begins abruptly with malaise, headache, myalgia, and weakness. About 24 hours later high fevers develop in over half of individuals. Nonproductive cough is most common. Other symptoms include pleuritic chest pain, dyspnea, diarrhea, nausea, vomiting, and abdominal pain. Physical findings are mild compared to radiographical findings. Complications may include lung abscess, hypotension, rhabdomyolysis, disseminated intravascular coagulation, thrombotic thrombocytopenic purpura, and renal failure. Other extrapulmonary infections related to bacteremia include pericarditis, myocarditis,

pyelonephritis, pancreatitis, sinusitis, and abscesses. Diagnosis is by culture, ELISA antibody tests, or indirect immunofluorescent antibody tests. A urine antigen test by radioimmunoassay (RIA) is also available. Drug of choice is erythromycin.

Less common causes of pneumonia in adolescents include tuberculosis infections and fungal infections. Other causes of pneumonia are rare in nonimmunosuppressed teenagers.

Diagnosis

The diagnosis of *Mycoplasma* infections involves a compatible symptom complex and a suspicion of the organism. Cold agglutinin test results are positive in 72–92% of patients with pneumonia after the first 1–2 weeks. The test is nonspecific but can be performed quickly, even at the teen's bedside. To perform the rapid test, add about 0.3–0.4 mL of blood to a standard laboratory collection tube containing 3.8% sodium citrate (blue-stoppered Protime [PT] tube). Place the tube in ice water for 15–30 minutes. Tilt on one side and examine for agglutination. The presence of coarse floccular agglutination is a positive test sign that correlates with a cold agglutinin titer of more than 1:64. About 66–85% of patients with a positive cold agglutinin test result will have *M. pneumoniae*. Complement fixation titers are more specific but require demonstration of a fourfold rise or fall in titer. ELISA techniques are becoming more commonly available to detect IgG and IgM antibodies, and DNA probe tests are also being developed.

Therapy

1. Antibiotics: Tetracycline 500 mg four times a day or erythromycin 500 mg four times a day; use either drug for 10 days. Azithromycin has also been used.
2. Decrease strenuous activity.

BIBLIOGRAPHY

Ali J. Spontaneous rupture of the spleen in patients with infectious mononucleosis. Can J Surg 1993;36:49.

Anikster Y, Glustein JZ, Weill M, et al. Extrapulmonary manifestations of *Mycoplasma pneumoniae* infections. Isr J Med Sci 1994;30:412.

Bailey RE. Diagnosis and treatment of infectious mononucleosis. Am Fam Physician 1994;49:879.

Block S, Hedrick J, Hammerschlag MR, et al. *Mycoplasma pneumoniae* and *Chlamydia pneumoniae* in pediatric community-acquired pneumonia: comparative efficacy and safety of clarithromycin vs. erythromycin ethylsuccinate. Pediatr Infect Dis J 1995;14:471.

Brandfonbrener A, Epstein A, Wu S, et al. Corticosteroid therapy in Epstein-Barr virus infection. Arch Intern Med 1986;146:337.

Brook I, de-Leyva F. Microbiology of tonsillar surfaces in infectious mononucleosis. Arch Pediatr Adolesc Med 1994;148:171.

Broughton RA. Infections due to *Mycoplasma pneumoniae* in childhood. Pediatr Infect Dis J 1986;5:71.

Buchwald D, Sullivan JL, Komaroff AL. Frequency of chronic active Epstein-Barr virus infection in a general medical practice. JAMA 1987;257:2303.

Cassell GH, Cole BC. Mycoplasmas as agents of human disease. N Engl J Med 1981;304:80.

Chetham MM, Roberts KB. Infectious mononucleosis in adolescents. Pediatr Ann 1991;20:206.

Connelly KP, DeWitt LD. Neurologic complications of infectious mononucleosis. Pediatr Neurol 1994;10:181.

Durbin WA, Sullivan JL. Epstein-Barr virus infection. Pediatr Rev 1994;15:63.

Emre U, Roblin PM, Gelling M. The association of *Chlamydia pneumoniae* infection and reactive airway disease in children. Arch Pediatr Adolesc Med 1994;148:727.

Evrard S, Mendoza-Burgos L, Mutter D, et al. Management of splenic rupture in infectious mononucleosis. Case report. Eur J Surg 1993;159:61.

Farber I, Wutzler P, Wohlrabe P. Serological diagnosis of infectious mononucleosis using three anti-Epstein-Barr virus recombinant ELISAs. J Virol Methods 1993;42:301.

Gan YJ, Sullivan JL, Sixbey JW. Detection of cell-free Epstein-Barr virus DNA in serum during acute infectious mononucleosis. J Infect Dis 1994;170:436.

Grayston JT, Aldous MB, Easton A, et al. Evidence that *Chlamydia pneumoniae* causes pneumonia and bronchitis. J Infect Dis 1993;168:1231.

Hammerschlag MR. Atypical pneumonias in children. Adv Pediatr Infect Dis 1995;10:1.

Hammond WP, Harlan JM, Steinberg SE. Severe neutropenia in infectious mononucleosis. West J Med 1979;131:92.

Holmes GP, Kaplan JE, Gantz NM, et al. Chronic fatigue syndrome: a working case definition. Ann Intern Med 1988;108:387.

Horwitz CA, Henle W, Henle G, et al. Heterophil-negative infectious mononucleosis and mononucleosis-like illness. Am J Med 1977;63:947.

Jarvis MR, Wasserman AL, Todd RD. Acute psychosis in a patient with Epstein-Barr virus infection. J Am Acad Child Adolesc Psychiatry 1990;29:468.

Johnson DH, Cunha BA. Atypical pneumonias. Clinical and extrapulmonary features of *Chlamydia, Mycoplasma,* and *Legionella* infections. Postgrad Med 1993; 93:69.

Kanegane H, Miyawaki T, Iwai K, et al. Acute thrombocytopenic purpura associated with primary Epstein-Barr virus infection. Acta Paediatr Jpn 1994;36:423.

Karppelin M, Hakkarainen K, Kleemola M, et al. Comparison of three serological methods for diagnosing *Mycoplasma pneumoniae* infection. J Clin Pathol 1993; 46:1120.

Leinonen M. Pathogenetic mechanisms and epidemiology of *Chlamydia pneumoniae.* Eur Heart J 1993; 14(suppl K):57.

Levine D, Tilton RC, Parry MF, et al. False positive EBNA IgM and IgG antibody tests for infectious mononucleosis in children. Pediatrics 1994;94:892.

Linderholm M, Boman J, Juto P, et al. Comparative evaluation of nine kits for rapid diagnosis of infectious mononucleosis and Epstein-Barr virus-specific serology. J Clin Microbiol 1994;32:259.

Murray HW, Masur H, Senterfit LB, et al. The protean manifestations of *Mycoplasma pneumoniae* infection in adults. Am J Med 1975;58:229.

Niederman JC. Chronicity of Epstein-Barr virus infection [Editorial]. Ann Intern Med 1985;102:119.

Niu MT, Stein DS, Schnittman SM. Primary human immunodeficiency virus type 1 infection: review of pathogenesis and early treatment intervention in humans and animal retrovirus infections. J Infect Dis 1993;168:1490.

Osamah H, Finkelstein R, Brook JG. Rhabdomyolysis complicating acute Epstein-Barr virus infection. Infection 1995;23:119.

Ostergaard L, Andersen PL. Etiology of community-acquired pneumonia. Evaluation by transtracheal aspiration, blood culture, or serology. Chest 1993;104: 1400.

Portnoy J, Ahronheim GA, Ghibu F, et al. Recovery of Epstein-Barr virus from genital ulcers. N Engl J Med 1984;311:966.

Rosner F, Grunwalk HW. Infectious mononucleosis and acute leukemia. JAMA 1981;246:1783.

Salmon P, Rademaker M. Erythema multiforme associated with an outbreak of *Mycoplasma pneumoniae* function. N Z Med J 1993;106:449.

Schooley RT, Carey RW, Miller G, et al. Chronic Epstein-Barr virus infection associated with fever and interstitial pneumonitis. Ann Intern Med 1986;104: 636.

Schreij G, Kuijpers RW, Pijpers E, et al. Unusual ocular symptoms and signs associated with infectious mononucleosis [Letter]. Lancet 1994;344:1302.

Straus SE. EB or not EB that is the question [Editorial]. JAMA 1987;257:2335.

Straus SE, Cohen JI, Tosato G, et al. Epstein-Barr virus infections: biology, pathogenesis, and management. Ann Intern Med 1993;118:45.

Straus SE, Dale JK, Tobi M, et al. Acyclovir treatment of the chronic fatigue syndrome: lack of efficacy in a placebo controlled trial. N Engl J Med 1988;319:1692.

Sue DY. Community-acquired pneumonia in adults. West J Med 1994;161:383.

Sumaya CV. Epstein-Barr virus serologic testing: diagnostic indications and interpretations. Pediatr Infect Dis 1986;5:337.

Sumaya CV. Interpreting serologic tests for suspected Epstein-Barr virus. Cont Intern Med 1990;October:12.

Sumaya CV. Mononucleosis in children: an update. Patient Care 1990;November 15:139.

Sumaya CV, Ench Y. Epstein-Barr virus infectious mononucleosis in children. I. Clinical and general laboratory findings. Pediatrics 1985a;75:1003.

Sumaya CV, Ench Y. Epstein-Barr virus infectious mononucleosis in children. II. Heterophil antibody and viral-specific responses. Pediatrics 1985b;75:1011.

Thacker WL, Talkington DF. Comparison of two rapid commercial tests with complement fixation for serologic diagnosis of *Mycoplasma pneumoniae* infections. J Clin Microbiol 1995;33:1212.

Thomas NH, Collins JE, Robb SA, et al. *Mycoplasma pneumoniae* infection and neurological disease. Arch Dis Child 1993;69:573.

Tobi M, Straus SE. Chronic Epstein-Barr virus disease: a workshop held by the National Institute of Allergy and Infectious Diseases. Ann Intern Med 1985;103:951.

Torg JS, Beer C, Bruno LA. Head trauma in football players with infectious mononucleosis. Physician Sportsmed 1980;8:107.

Wiedbrauk DL, Bassin S. Evaluation of five enzyme immunoassays for detection of immunoglobulin M antibodies to Epstein-Barr virus viral capsid antigens. J Clin Microbiol 1993;31:1339.

CHAPTER 30

Hepatitis

Wilbert H. Mason, Jr., and Lawrence S. Neinstein

ETIOLOGY

Hepatitis may be caused by viral infections such as hepatitis A virus; hepatitis B virus; non-A, non-B (NANB) hepatitis (or hepatitis C); delta virus; hepatitis E virus; Epstein-Barr virus; cytomegalovirus; or noninfectious causes such as hepatotoxins. This chapter primarily discusses hepatitis A, hepatitis B, and hepatitis C.

1. Hepatitis A: Hepatitis A is caused by a 27- to 28-nm, nonenveloped single-stranded RNA virus. The outer capsid is formed from three to four polypeptides that surround the inner RNA genome.
2. Hepatitis B: Hepatitis B is caused by a 42-nm diameter virus, with an outer lipid envelope surrounding the inner core containing the DNA genome (Fig. 30.1). Several components of this virus can be detected by electron microscopy.
   a. Dane particle: This is the whole 42-nm diameter virus.
   b. A 7-nm thick shell contains surface antigen (HBsAg).
   c. A 28-nm nucleocapsid: This central core contains the core antigen, HBcAg. The nuclear material is double-stranded DNA for 70% of its length and single-stranded DNA for 30% of its length.
   d. Peripheral blood also contains 20- to 22-nm spherical and tubular particles that contain HBsAg and represent excessive virus coat material.
3. NANB hepatitis: Most of these infections are caused by hepatitis C, a positive-stranded RNA molecule.
4. Delta virus: An HBsAg-coated 35- to 37-nm diameter particle that is a defective pathogen because it is dependent on the presence of hepatitis B to cause an infection.
5. Hepatitis E: Enterically transmitted NANB hepatitis in developing countries has been associated with an RNA virus that may be in the Calicivirus family.

EPIDEMIOLOGY

Table 30.1 outlines the epidemiology for hepatitis viruses. Following is a more detailed discussion.

Hepatitis A

Hepatitis A is primarily transmitted through a fecal-oral route such as by food handlers, poor hygiene, or contaminated shellfish. The virus is also frequently transmitted during oral-genital contact among homosexual males. Percutaneous or transfusion-related transmission is extremely rare. The virus is excreted in the stool before signs and symptoms develop. Viral ex-

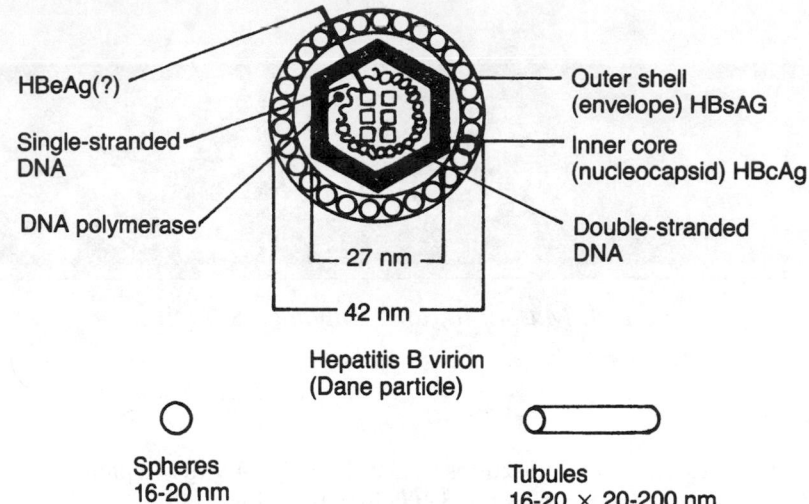

FIGURE 30.1.   Hepatitis B virion (*Dane particle*) and spherical and tubular HBsAg particles found in serum of infected persons. *HBcAg, HBeAg,* and *HBsAg:* hepatitis B core, e, and surface antigens, respectively. (From Kalser MH, Howard RB. Hepatic and pancreatic disorders. Postgrad Med 1986;79:199.)

TABLE 30.1.   Clinical and Epidemiological Comparison of Hepatitis Viruses

Characteristics	Hepatitis A	Hepatitis B	Hepatitis C	Hepatitis D	Hepatitis E
Transmission					
Usual	Enteric (fecal-oral)	Parenteral	Parenteral	Parenteral	Enteric
Alternative	Parenteral (rare)	Frequently non-parenteral (venereal, perinatal)	Venereal Perinatal	Venereal	Possibly parenteral
Distribution	Point-source outbreaks, random cases	Prevalent in young adults and urban populations	Posttransfusion hepatitis and random cases	Worldwide, not highly ende-mic in the United States	Primarily Asia, Africa, Mexico
Incubation period	15–50 days	45–160 days	49–63 days	Coinfection 45–60 days Superinfection 14–136 days	15–60 days
Onset	Acute	Often insidious	Insidious	Acute or insidious	Acute
Severity	Usually mild, often anicteric	More severe than hepatitis A; less often anicteric	Mild to moderate	Often severe or fulminant	Variable; severe in pregnancy
Chronic disease	None	90% of perinatal cases; 10% of adult cases	50–60% of cases	Yes	None
Carrier state	None	Yes	Yes	Yes	None
Case fatality rate	0–0.2%	0.3–15%	Unknown	Unknown	Unknown
Estimated inci-dence trend in the United States	Decreasing	Decreasing	Increasing	Unknown	Not endemic in the United States
Estimated proportion of acute hepatitis cases in the United States	~25%	~50%	~20%	Unknown	None

cretion usually disappears by the time jaundice appears, so that the most contagious period is early in the disease course. About 10–20% of individuals have evidence of prior infection by age 20 and about 50% by age 50 in the United States. In urban areas such as New York City, approximately 45% of residents have antibodies to hepatitis A, indicating prior infection.

Hepatitis B

Hepatitis B virus has been documented in almost all bodily secretions including tears, stools, saliva, blood, bile, breast milk, vaginal secretions, urine, sneeze droplets, and semen. Transmission occurs via percutaneous or permucosal routes, by infective blood or body fluids, through sexual contact, by contaminated needles, or during childbirth. Infection can also occur in settings of continuous close personal contact (such as institutions for persons with developmental disabilities or in households) presumably via inapparent or unnoticed contact of infective secretions with skin lesions or mucosal surfaces. Because of its parenteral and venereal transmission, the disease is prevalent in drug addicts, hemophiliacs, dialysis patients and workers, and the homosexual population. The Centers for Disease Control and Prevention in Atlanta estimate that 300,000 persons, primarily young adults, are infected with hepatitis B each year. About 15% of these will be in the 15–19 year age group. One-quarter of these individuals will become ill with jaundice, more than 10,000 patients will require hospitalization, and an average of 250 per year will die of fulminant disease. About 5–10% of infected individuals will become chronic carriers, and 25% of these carriers will develop chronic active hepatitis. There is an estimated pool of 1 million chronic carriers in the U.S. population. The overall incidence rate of hepatitis B has fallen every year since 1985, but the number of cases due to parenteral drug use and heterosexual activity has increased over the same period. At least 30% of patients with hepatitis B have no identifiable risk factor for their infection.

Non-A, Non-B or Hepatitis C Virus Hepatitis

NANB hepatitis is the leading cause of posttransfusion hepatitis, causing about 95% of such cases. Approximately 70% of acute NANB hepatitis is due to hepatitis C. The genome of this virus has been molecularly cloned and identified as a positive-stranded RNA molecule probably in the Flaviviridae family. A viral antibody test to hepatitis C virus (HCV) has been developed. Risk factors for hepatitis C include intravenous (IV) drug use, blood transfusion, contact with an infected family member, organ transplantation, and hemodialysis. The risk of infection with more than 6 units of transfused blood is 40–50% with paid donor blood and 6–10% with volunteer donor blood. This should decline with the use of blood screening for hepatitis C virus antibody (anti-HCV). Although 90% of posttransfusion hepatitis is due to hepatitis C, transfusions account for only 5–10% of new cases of hepatitis C. IV drug use is the most common risk factor reported in patients, but at least 40% of hepatitis C cases have no known risk factor. Chronic hepatitis develops in 50–60% of patients with hepatitis C infection.

Delta Hepatitis

Delta virus can only cause disease if hepatitis B virus is present. At least three clinical pictures can occur:

1. Acute hepatitis caused by a combination of both delta virus and hepatitis B virus (coinfection)
2. Acute hepatitis with delta virus acquisition in a chronic carrier of hepatitis B (superinfection)

3. Chronic infection with both delta virus and hepatitis B, leading to a more rapid progression in liver disease and higher mortality rate

The transmission of the virus is usually through a similar means, as in hepatitis B (blood or body fluids). Risk groups include IV drug users, male homosexuals, hemodialysis workers and patients, and recipients of blood products.

Hepatitis E

Hepatitis E is an enterically transmitted form of NANB viral hepatitis seen primarily in developing countries in central Asia and in Pakistan, Africa, and Mexico. It is caused by a single-stranded RNA virus which appears to be in the Calicivirus family. It has a variable presentation but is somewhat more severe than hepatitis A with fulminant hepatitis occurring in 2–5% overall but occurring in 20% of pregnant women. Although reported cases of hepatitis E have been identified in the United States, it is not endemically transmitted here, and therefore it will not be discussed further.

CLINICAL MANIFESTATIONS

Symptoms

Common early symptoms of viral hepatitis include fatigue, lassitude, anorexia, nausea, dark urine, drowsiness, low-grade fever, right upper abdominal discomfort, myalgias, and arthralgias. In hepatitis A approximately 20% of individuals have a history of diarrhea. In viral B hepatitis, immune complexes can lead to arthralgias, arthritis, and a rash. Much less commonly, extra-hepatic manifestations such as skin rash and arthralgias have been present with hepatitis A.

1. Arthritis: The arthritis of hepatitis B may precede the jaundice. The arthritis is usually a symmetrical polyarthritis affecting small joints. Larger joints may be affected, but the feet are usually spared.
2. Rash: The rash accompanying hepatitis B occurs in up to 50% of patients. The rash is usually urticarial in nature but may be maculopapular or petechial.

Signs

1. Icteric sclera
2. Tender liver or spleen
3. Splenomegaly: Occurs in 10% of cases
4. Arthritis
5. Skin rash

Laboratory Findings

1. Mild anemia
2. Relative lymphocytosis
3. Total bilirubin usually less than 15–20 mg/dL
4. Elevated serum transaminases
5. Mild elevation in serum alkaline phosphatase
6. Severe disease: Decreased serum albumin and prothrombin time
7. Hepatitis B arthritis: Decreased serum and joint complement. White blood cell (WBC) count in joint fluid ranges between 2000–90,000 WBC/mL.

Viral Antigens and Antibodies

To understand the clinical course and diagnosis of viral hepatitis, one must understand the various antigens and antibodies and their clinical significance.

1. Hepatitis A
   a. Immunoglobulin M anti–hepatitis A viral antibody (IgM anti-HAV): This antibody is detected early in the illness and remains detectable for approximately 2–3 months.
   b. Immunoglobulin G anti–hepatitis A viral antibody (IgG anti-HAV): This antibody rises more slowly and is persistent for years. It indicates a past infection and the presence of immunity to viral A hepatitis.
   c. Hepatitis A virus (HAV) (stool): This virus is usually present before the onset of clinical symptoms and is of little clinical utility.
2. Hepatitis B
   a. Hepatitis B virus (HBV): HBV is the etiologic agent of hepatitis B and is also known as Dane particle.
   b. Hepatitis surface antigen (HBsAg): This antigen becomes positive during the incubation period and disappears in most patients during the course of the clinical disease. However, in up to 10% of patients, this antigen may remain positive for life. A positive test result for HBsAg indicates either an acute hepatitis B infection or a chronic carrier state.
   c. Anti-hepatitis B surface antigen (anti-HBs): This antibody becomes positive usually months after the onset of the clinical disease. A positive blood test result indicates past infection. If acute hepatitis is present, the patient probably has hepatitis of another origin.
   d. Hepatitis core antigen (HBcAg): This antigen is not measurable in peripheral blood.
   e. Anti-hepatitis B core antigen (anti-HBc): This is the only serologic marker derived from core virion. It appears as HBsAg is falling and before anti-HBs appears. Anti-HBc can be fractionated into IgM and IgG components. This is extremely helpful in differentiating between acute and past infections. Anti-HBc (IgM) rises during clinical hepatitis, persists for 2–8 months, and then declines, whereas anti-HBc (IgG) rises at the same time to a much higher level and persists for a long time. The detection of anti-HBc (IgM) indicates an acute infection, whereas if only anti-HBc (IgG) is present, the illness must be of at least 6 months' duration. Anti-HBc may be the only test positive in some individuals during the window period after HBsAg has fallen and before anti-HBs has become positive.
   f. Hepatitis e antigen (HBeAg): The exact origin of e antigen is unknown. However, its presence, which usually comes during the incubation phase, correlates with increased DNA polymerase activity and increased Dane particles. Persistence of HBeAg beyond 10–12 weeks is probably indicative of a progression to a chronic carrier state. Persistent presence of HBeAg probably indicates:
      — A more active liver disease is present.
      — The chronic hepatitis B infection is in a relatively early stage.
      — The infection is in an active replicative stage, and the infectious viral particles are in the serum.
      — There is an increased risk of infection. The risk of infectivity in an "e" antigen, surface antigen–positive individual may be as high as 30,000 times the risk in an individual with just surface antigen positivity.
      About 10–15% of chronic carriers who are HBeAg positive will convert each year to negative with the development of anti-HBe titers. These individuals are generally less contagious and have less active liver disease. Conversely, an individual can have re-

activation of the disease, especially with immunosuppression, so that anti-HBe titers become negative and HBeAg becomes positive.

   g. Anti-hepatitis B "e" antigen (anti-HBeAg): This antibody indicates recent or remote infection. It usually indicates a low infectivity state.

3. Hepatitis C
   a. Tests for hepatitis C diagnosis have been evolving since 1990 and as yet are not as sensitive or specific as for hepatitis A or B.
   b. Enzyme-linked immunosorbent assay (ELISA) antibodies against antigens from the viral core region (nucleocapsid) and nonstructural and structural proteins can be measured in serum. The second generation ELISA test (ELISA-2) has enhanced sensitivity (80%) and specificity compared to the first generation test (ELISA-1). The lag time to positivity is also shorter (i.e., about 20 weeks). ELISA-2 is used as a screening test for hepatitis C. False-positive ELISA-2 tests are seen in volunteer blood donors without risk factors, autoimmune disease with hyperglobulinemia, acquired immunodeficiency syndrome (AIDS) patients, and patients with positive rheumatoid factors.
   c. Recombinant immunoblot assay (RIBA) is used as a confirmatory test for hepatitis C. RIBA detects antibodies to four HCV proteins. A positive RIBA-2 test indicates HCV viremia and therefore infectivity. Sensitivity is about 80% and lag time to positivity is about 20 weeks.
   d. Polymerase chain reaction (PCR) assays are the most sensitive and specific tests for HCV and detect viral RNA in serum within 1–2 weeks of exposure. They are not generally available and rates of false positivity and negativity require refinement. They are used to monitor response to therapy of hepatitis C.

4. Delta hepatitis
   a. Delta virus: Etiologic agent of delta hepatitis; may only cause infection in presence of hepatitis B.
   b. Delta antigen: Detectable in early acute delta infection.
   c. Delta antibody (anti-delta): Indicates past or present infection with delta virus. Current enzyme immunoassay (EIA) or radioimmunoassay (RIA) tests measure primarily IgG but also detect some IgM. Specific IgG and IgM tests are not currently clinically available for routine testing. The "gold standard" for diagnosis is liver biopsy with staining for hepatitis D antigen.

Course

1. Viral hepatitis A: The clinical course is summarized in Figure 30.2.
   a. Most patients are asymptomatic.
   b. Ninety-five percent of patients have a 4- to 6-week course.
   c. Stool isolates for HAV are the first positive finding.
   d. As IgM antibodies and liver enzymes rise, clinical symptoms appear.
   e. As clinical symptoms disappear and IgM antibodies fall, IgG antibodies rise.
   f. In rare instances, individuals can have a relapsing course lasting up to a year, which can cause confusion with other causes of chronic liver disease such as hepatitis B.

2. Viral hepatitis B: The clinical course of a typical case is summarized in Figure 30.3.
   a. HBsAg and HBeAg titers rise 4–8 weeks after exposure and 4–8 weeks before clinical symptoms appear.
   b. Liver transaminases rise, and clinical symptoms appear.
   c. HBsAg may peak and fall in uncomplicated cases or remain positive in chronic carriers.
   d. Anti-HBc titers rise as HBsAg titers fall.
   e. Anti-HBs appear weeks to months after HBsAg disappears.

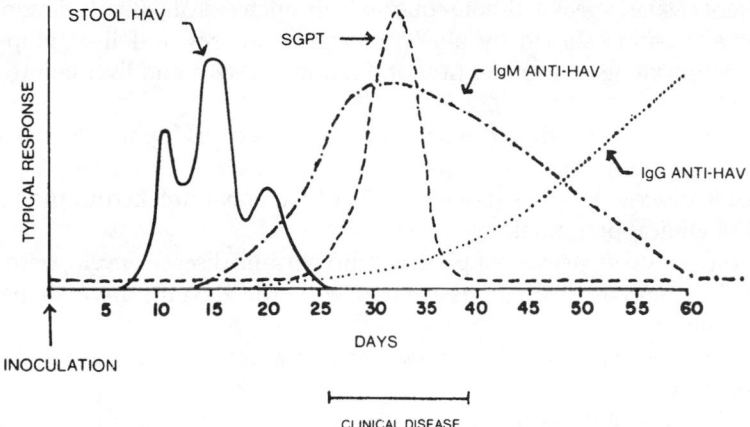

FIGURE 30.2.   Course of hepatitis A infection. (Adapted from Centers for Disease Control. Hepatitis Surveillance Report #42. June 1978.)

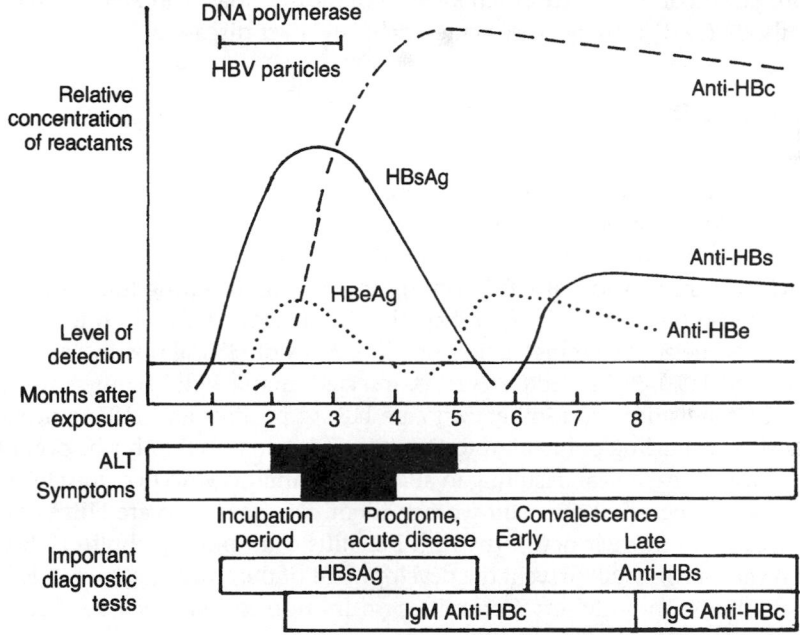

FIGURE 30.3.   Course of hepatitis B infection. Pattern of symptoms and serologic tests. *ALT,* alanine aminotransferase; *Anti-HBc,* hepatitis B core antibody; *Anti-HBe,* hepatitis B e antibody; *Anti-HBs,* hepatitis B surface antibody; *HBeAg,* hepatitis B e antigen; *HBsAg,* hepatitis B surface antigen; *HBV,* hepatitis B virus; *Ig,* immunoglobulin. (From Hollinger FB. Hepatitis markers. Guide to test selection. Diagnosis 1986;Aug:58.)

   f. A "window phase" exists where HBsAg may be negative before anti-HBs appears. During this phase, anti-HBc will be positive.
   g. Chronic phase
       — Ninety percent of patients with hepatitis B recover without sequelae.
       — Less than 1% develop fulminant hepatitis and die.
       — About 10% develop chronic liver disease: Seven percent of patients develop benign persistent hepatitis manifested mainly by elevated transaminases. These pa-

tients usually heal without sequelae. Three percent of patients develop chronic active hepatitis shown by abnormal transaminases and liver biopsy specimen. These patients may either heal or develop cirrhosis and liver failure.

3. Hepatitis C
   a. The clinical course varies from asymptomatic infection (up to 70%) to icteric hepatitis (25%) to fulminant failure (rare).
   b. Chronic disease develops in about 60% of patients unrelated to mode of transmission or clinical presentation.
   c. Ten to twenty-five percent of patients with chronic disease develop cirrhosis.
   d. HCV infection is strongly associated with the development of hepatocellular carcinoma.
   e. Serologic test results remain negative for several weeks after onset of disease.
4. Delta hepatitis
   a. Acute infection with both the delta virus and hepatitis B usually has a sequential expression with dual aminotransferase spikes. The interval between the first illness and the second is usually between 1.5 and 4 weeks (average, 2 weeks).
   b. Acute superinfection with delta virus in a chronic carrier of hepatitis B may be asymptomatic and only detected by an increase in transaminases and elevation of anti-delta antibody (IgM) or may cause acute or chronic liver disease.

CONSIDERATIONS DURING PREGNANCY

1. Hepatitis A
   a. There is no maternal-fetal transmission.
   b. Transmission can occur during delivery.
   c. Positive IgM antibodies in the infant indicate acute infection.
2. Hepatitis B: Transmission of HBV from mother to infant during the perinatal period is one of the most efficient modes of hepatitis B infection. This will often lead to severe long-term sequelae. The transmission rate to infants of HBsAg-positive and HBeAg-positive mothers is 70–90%, and 85–90% of infected infants will become chronic hepatitis B carriers. Infants born to mothers who are HBsAg positive and HBeAg negative have a lower risk of acquiring perinatal infection. An estimated 18,000 births occur to HBsAg-positive women each year, resulting in about 4000 infants who become chronic carriers. Prenatal screening of all pregnant women identifies those who are HBsAg positive and allows treatment of their newborns with hepatitis B immune globulin (HBIG) and hepatitis B vaccine that will prevent the development of the chronic carrier state in 85–95% of these infants. The Advisory Committee on Immunization Practices (Centers for Disease Control, 1991) advises the following:
   a. All pregnant women should be routinely tested for HBsAg during an early prenatal visit in each pregnancy. If the mother has a particularly high-risk behavior, an additional HBsAg test can be ordered later in the pregnancy. No other serologic hepatitis tests are necessary for maternal screening.
   b. If the woman was not screened prenatally, HBsAg testing should be done at the time of admission for delivery. If the mother is identified as HBsAg positive 1 month or more after giving birth, the infant should be tested for HBsAg. If the results are negative, the infant should be given HBIG and hepatitis B vaccine.
   c. Following all initial tests positive for HBsAg, a second test should be performed on the same specimen, followed by a confirmatory test using a neutralization assay. However, if the initial test was done during the hospitalization for delivery, initiation of treatment of the infant should not be delayed more than 24 hours for a second or confirmatory test.

TABLE 30.2. Recommended Doses of Currently Licensed Hepatitis B Vaccines

Group	Recombivax-HB[a]		Engerix-B[a]	
	Dose (μg)	(mL)	Dose (μg)	(mL)
Infants of HBsAg[b]-negative mothers and children <11 years	2.5	(0.25)	10	(0.5)
Infants of HBsAg-positive mothers; prevention of perinatal infection	5	(0.5)	10	(0.5)
Children and adolescents 11–19 years	5	(0.5)	10 or 20	(0.5) (1.0)
Adults >19 years	10	(1.0)	20	(1.0)
Dialysis patients and other immunocompromised persons	40	(1.0)[c]	40	(2.0)[d]

From Centers for Disease Control. Hepatitis B virus: a comprehensive strategy for eliminating transmission in the United States through universal childhood vaccination. Recommendations of the Immunization Practices Advisory Committee (ACIP). MMWR 1991;40(RR–13):1–25.
[a]Both vaccines are routinely administered in a three-dose series. Engerix-B has also been licensed for a four-dose series administered at 0, 1, 2, and 12 months.
[b]HBsAg, hepatitis B surface antigen.
[c]Special formulation.
[d]Two 1-mL doses administered at one site, in a four-dose schedule at 0, 1, 2, and 6 months.

    d. Infants born to HBsAg-positive mothers should receive HBIG (0.5 mL) intramuscularly once they are physiologically stable, preferably within 12 hours of birth. Hepatitis B vaccine should be administered intramuscularly at the appropriate infant dose. The first dose should be given concurrently with HBIG but at a different site. Subsequent doses should be given as recommended for the specific vaccine (Table 30.2). Testing infants for HBsAg and anti-HBs is recommended when the infants are 12–15 months of age to monitor the success or failure of therapy. If HBsAg is not detectable and anti-HBs is present, the children can be considered protected. HBIG and hepatitis B vaccination do not interfere with routine childhood vaccinations.

    e. Household members and sexual partners of hepatitis B carriers should be tested, and if susceptible, should receive hepatitis B vaccine.

    f. Obstetric and pediatric staff should be notified directly about HBsAg-positive mothers so that the neonates can receive therapy without delay after birth.

DIFFERENTIAL DIAGNOSIS

1. Drug-induced hepatitis
2. Alcoholic hepatitis
3. Toxic hepatitis
4. Viral hepatitis
   a. Hepatitis A virus
   b. Hepatitis B virus (with or without delta coinfection or superinfection)
   c. Hepatitis C
   d. Cytomegalovirus
   e. Epstein-Barr virus
   f. Varicella virus
   g. Rubella virus
   h. Coxsackie B virus
   i. Herpes simplex
   j. Echovirus
   k. Adenovirus
   l. Hepatitis E (acquired abroad)

TABLE 30.3. Interpretation of Hepatitis Antibody Test Results[a]

IgM Anti-HAV	HBsAg	Anti-HBc (IgM)	Anti-HBc (IgG)	Interpretation
+	–	–	–	Acute hepatitis A
–	+	–	–	Acute hepatitis B early state or chronic carrier with hepatitis of another origin
–	+	+	+	Acute hepatitis B
–	+	–	+	Chronic carrier state
–	–	+	+	Recent hepatitis B
–	–	–	–	Non-A, non-B hepatitis, other viruses, or other causes

[a]Anti-HAV, antibody to hepatitis A virus; anti-HBc, antibody to hepatitis B core antigen; HBsAg, hepatitis B surface antigen; Ig, immunoglobulin.

TABLE 30.4. Infectivity for Acute Hepatitis B Virus[a]

HBsAG	Anti-HBc	HBeAg	Anti-HBe	Infectivity
+	+	+	–	Acute infection or chronic carrier; very infectious
+	+	–	–	Acute or recent infection; possible chronic carrier state; moderately infectious
+	+	–	+	Recent infection or chronic carrier state; good prognosis; probably low infectivity

[a]Anti-HBc, antibody to hepatitis B core antigen; anti-HBe, antibody to hepatitis B e antigen; HBeAg, hepatitis B e antigen; HBsAg, hepatitis B surface antigen.

DIAGNOSIS

1. What causes acute hepatitis?
   a. Clinical history may suggest toxin, drug, or exposure to a source of hepatitis A, B, or C.
   b. Order IgM anti-HAV, HBsAg, anti-HBc, hepatitis C ELISA-2, and mononucleosis spot test. Table 30.3 provides an interpretation of results from the first three of these tests. Follow-up tests for hepatitis C are necessary because of long lag phase to seroconversion.
2. Acute hepatitis B: What is the infectivity of the patient? Table 30.4 summarizes the infectivity risk of acute hepatitis B virus.

THERAPY

Prevention

1. Disinfection
   a. Heat sterilization
      — Boiling in water at 100°C for 10 minutes
      — Steam autoclaving at 121°C and 15 pounds/inch³ for 15 minutes
      — Dry heat of 160°C for 2 hours
   b. Other presumed effective modalities
      — Sodium hypochlorite 2.5% for 30 minutes
      — Formalin 40% for 12 hours
      — Glutaraldehyde 2% for 10 hours
2. Prophylaxis (Centers for Disease Control, 1990, 1991; Immunization Practices Advisory Committee, 1987)

a. Hepatitis A pre-exposure prophylaxis: Pre-exposure prophylaxis for hepatits A includes human immune serum globulin (HISG) and hepatitis A vaccine.

— HISG: This has been the traditional and only pre-exposure prophylaxis for hepatitis A until recent years. The major group for whom pre-exposure prophylaxis is indicated is international travelers to endemic areas. Risk of infection in developing countries increases with duration of travel and is highest for those who live in or visit rural areas, trek in back country, or frequently eat or drink in settings of poor sanitation.

— Hepatitis A vaccine: The scope of prophylaxis changed with the introduction of a hepatitis A vaccine, which offers active immunization and thus longer and more effective protection than HISG. The vaccine (Havrix), an inactivated hepatitis A vaccine, was licensed by the Food and Drug Administration (FDA) in February 1995 for use in persons over 2 years old to prevent hepatitis A infections. The vaccine is licensed in both adult and pediatric formulations, with different dosages and administration schedules. Immunogenicity studies indicate that almost 100% of children, adolescents, and adults develop protective levels of antibody to hepatitis A virus after completing the vaccine series. Recipients of the vaccine have been followed for up to 4 years and still have protective levels of anti-HAV. Estimates suggest that protective levels can last at least 20 years. The vaccine can be administered simultaneously with other vaccines and toxoids including hepatitis B, diphtheria, tetanus, oral typhoid, cholera, Japanese encephalitis, rabies, and yellow fever without altering immunogenicity or adverse effects. However, if other vaccines are given simultaneously, they should be given at separate injection sites. If immune globulin is given at the same time as the first dose of vaccine, a lower antibody concentration is attained, but this is not thought to be clinically relevant.

Recommended dosing for Havrix (hepatitis A vaccine) includes:

Age (yr)	Dose (ELISA units)	Volume (mL)	No. Doses	Schedule (months)
2–18	360	0.5	3	0, 1, 6–12
>18	1440	1.0	2	0, 6–12

The following interim recommendations for the use of inactivated hepatitis A vaccine among international travelers is given by the Advisory Committee on Immunization Practices (ACIP) (MMWR, 1995):

a. All susceptible persons traveling to or working in countries with intermediate or high HAV endemicity (countries other than Australia, Canada, Japan, New Zealand, and countries in Western Europe and Scandinavia) should be vaccinated with hepatitis A vaccine or receive immunoglobulin (IG) before departure. Hepatitis A vaccine at the age-appropriate dose is preferred for persons who plan to travel repeatedly to or reside for long periods in these high-risk areas. IG is recommended for travelers aged more than 2 years.

b. After receiving the initial dose of hepatitis A vaccine, persons are considered to be protected for 4 weeks. For long-term protection, a second dose is needed 6–12 months later. For persons who will travel to high-risk areas less than 4 weeks after the initial vaccine dose, IG (0.02 mL per kg of body weight) should be administered simultaneously with the first dose of vaccine but at different injection sites.

c. Persons who are allergic to a vaccine component or otherwise elect not to receive vaccine should receive a single dose of IG (0.02 mL per kg of body weight), which provides effective protection against hepatitis A for up to 3 months. IG should be administered at 0.06 mL per kg of body weight and must be repeated if travel is for more than 5 months. Additional information about hepatitis A vaccine is available from the CDC's Hepatitis Branch, Division of Viral and Rickettsial Diseases, National Center for Infectious Diseases, 404-639-3048.

Other potential target populations include military personnel and day-care attendees. Hepatitis A vaccine may be recommended for all children after approval by the FDA and if a combination vaccine becomes available.

b. Hepatitis A postexposure prophylaxis:
— Agent: HISG
— Who: A serologic confirmation test for hepatitis A in the index case is recommended before consideration of prophylaxis in contacts. Serologic screening of contacts before giving HISG is not warranted because of cost and time considerations. Considerations for prophylaxis include:
  (1) Close personal contacts: Including household and sexual contacts of persons with hepatitis A, should receive HISG.
  (2) Day-care centers: For day-care centers or homes with children in diapers, immune globulin should be administered to all staff and attendees if one or more hepatitis A cases is recognized among children or employees, or if cases are recognized in two or more households of center attendees. In centers not enrolling children with diapers, only classroom contacts of an index case need be treated.
  (3) Schools: Routine administration of immune globulin is not indicated for pupils and teachers in contact with a patient. However, if an outbreak clearly exists, immune globulin may be given to those with close personal contact.
  (4) Institutions for custodial care: Because of crowded living conditions, prophylaxis is warranted during an outbreak of hepatitis to residents and staff with close contact with patients.
  (5) Hospitals: Routine immune globulin prophylaxis for hospital personnel is not indicated. Education should be stressed regarding sound hygienic practices and precautions regarding direct contact with potentially infective material. In outbreaks, prophylaxis of persons exposed to feces of infected patients may be indicated.
  (6) Offices and factories: Not indicated under usual office or factory conditions for persons exposed to fellow worker with hepatitis A
  (7) Common source exposure: Might be effective in preventing foodborne or waterborne hepatitis if exposure is recognized in time. However, HISG is not recommended for persons exposed to a common source after cases have begun to appear in those exposed, since the 2-week period during which HISG is effective will have passed.
— When: As soon as possible after exposure; immune serum globulin is helpful until about 6 days before onset of symptoms.
— Effectiveness: Decreases clinical disease in 80–95% of patients. Anicteric hepatitis is not prevented.
— Dose: 0.02 mL/kg
c. Hepatitis B pre-exposure prophylaxis: Two types of products are available for prophylaxis against hepatitis B. Hepatitis B vaccines provide active immunization against hepatitis B infection and are recommended for both pre-exposure and postexposure prophylaxis. HBIG provides temporary, passive protection and is indicated only in certain postexposure settings.

— HBIG: HBIG is prepared from plasma preselected to contain a high titer of anti-HBs. In the United States, HBIG has a titer greater than 1:100,000. Plasma used has been both screened for human immunodeficiency virus (HIV) antibodies and treated to inactivate and eliminate HIV from the final product. HBIG has not been shown to transmit HIV.

— Hepatitis B vaccine: There are now two types of hepatitis B vaccines licensed in the United States:

  (1) Plasma-derived vaccine (Heptavax-B): Heptavax B is a suspension of inactivated, alum-adsorbed, 22-nm surface antigen particles purified from human plasma. This vaccine was the first to become available for use in the United States in 1982. However, this vaccine is no longer being produced and is not available in the United States. In producing this vaccine, inactivation occurs with a threefold process that has been shown to inactivate all classes of viruses in human blood, including HIV.

  (2) Recombinant vaccines (Recombivax-HB and Engerix-B): These two vaccines are produced by introducing a plasmid containing the gene for HBsAg into baker's yeast. HBsAg is harvested, purified, and sterilized. These two vaccines have replaced plasma-derived vaccine.

— Indications for pre-exposure hepatitis B immunization: Prior strategy to prevent hepatitis B transmission in the United States rested on identification of mothers who were HBsAg carriers and prophylaxis of their newborn infants at birth and vaccination of persons who were in major risk groups for acquiring the infection. These efforts met with limited success because of an inability to identify all those at risk, lack of motivation on the part of certain at-risk individuals such as intravenous drug users, and failure to vaccinate susceptible household and sexual contacts. Therefore, a comprehensive strategy to eliminate transmission of HBV during infancy and childhood, as well as during adolescence and adulthood, was devised. This included:

  (1) Prenatal testing of pregnant women for HBsAg and immunoprophylaxis of their newborns and household contacts.

  (2) Universal immunization of all infants born to HBsAg-negative mothers. Recommended schedules for immunoprophylaxis to prevent perinatal transmission of hepatitis B and for vaccination of newborns are listed in Tables 30.5 and 30.6.

  (3) Immunization of certain adolescents and young adults: Adolescents at high risk of infection because of injecting drug use or multiple sexual partners should be immunized. Because adolescents and young adults are not easily identified with regard to high-risk behavior, universal immunization of all preadolescents, adolescents and young adults, and in particular those living in areas where high risk behavior is prevalent is recommended. The appropriate dose for age should be used (Table 30.2) and the 0-, 1-, and 6-month schedule is preferred.

  (4) Persons with occupational risk: The risk for health-care workers varies depending on exposure to blood or blood products. Higher risk individuals include individuals in training, medical technologists, operating room staff, phlebotomist, IV therapy nurses, surgeons, pathologists, oncologists, and hemodialysis staff. Other at-risk individuals include dental professionals, laboratory and blood bank technicians, emergency medical technicians, and morticians.

  (5) Persons with lifestyle risk

TABLE 30.5. Recommended Schedule of Hepatitis B Immunoprophylaxis to Prevent Perinatal Transmission of Hepatitis B Virus Infection

	Age of Infant
Infant born to mother known to be HBsAg[a] positive	
Vaccine dose[b]	
First	Birth (within 12 hours)
HBIG[c]	Birth (within 12 hours)
Second	1 month
Third	6 months[d]
Infant born to mother not screened for HBsAg	
Vaccine dose[e]	
First	Birth (within 12 hours)
HBIG[c]	If mother is found to be HBsAg positive, administer dose to infant as soon as possible, not later than 1 week after birth
Second	1–2 months[f]
Third	6 months[d]

From Centers for Disease Control. Hepatitis B virus: a comprehensive strategy for eliminating transmission in the United States through universal childhood vaccination. Recommendations of the Immunization Practices Advisory Committee (ACIP). MMWR 1991;40(RR–13):1–25.
[a]HBsAg, hepatitis B surface antigen.
[b]See Table 30.2 for appropriate vaccine dose.
[c]Hepatitis B immune globulin (HBIG): 0.5 mL administered intramuscularly at a site different from that used for vaccine.
[d]If four-dose schedule (Engerix-B) is used, the third dose is administered at 2 months of age and the fourth dose at 12–18 months.
[e]First dose, dose for infant of HBsAg-positive mother (see Table 30.2). If mother is found to be HBsAg negative, use appropriate dose from Table 30.6.
[f]Infants of women who are HBsAg negative can be vaccinated at 2 months of age.

TABLE 30.6. Recommended Schedules of Hepatitis B Vaccination for Infants Born to HBsAg[a]-Negative Mothers

Hepatitis B Vaccine	Age of Infant
Option 1	
Dose 1	Birth-before hospital discharge
Dose 2	1–2 months[b]
Dose 3	6–18 months[b]
Option 2	
Dose 1	1–2 months[b]
Dose 2	4 months[b]
Dose 3	6–18 months[b]

From Centers for Disease Control. Hepatitis B virus: a comprehensive strategy for eliminating transmission in the United States through universal childhood vaccination. Recommendations of the Immunization Practices Advisory Committee (ACIP). MMWR 1991;40(RR–13):1–25.
[a]HBsAg, Hepatitis B surface antigen.
[b]Hepatitis B vaccine can be administered simultaneously with diphtheria-tetanus-pertussis, *Haemophilus influenzae* type b conjugate, measles-mumps-rubella, and oral polio vaccines at the same visit.

(a) Heterosexual partners with multiple partners (more than one partner in preceding 6 months) or any sexually transmitted disease
(b) Clients and staff of institutions for mentally retarded individuals
(c) Homosexual and bisexual men
(d) Injecting drug users
(6) Special patient groups
(a) Hemodialysis patients
(b) Recipients of clotting factor concentrates

(7) Environmental risk factors
   (a) Household and sexual contacts of carriers
   (b) Adoptees from countries of high hepatitis B endemicity. These children should be screened for HBsAg. If the children are HBsAg positive, family members should be vaccinated.
   (c) Populations with high endemicity of hepatitis B infection. In the United States certain populations including Alaskan Natives, Pacific Islanders, and refugees from endemic areas are at high risk for infection during childhood. In these groups universal hepatitis B vaccination of infants is recommended to prevent disease transmission during childhood. Immigrants and refugees from endemic areas should be screened for hepatitis B. If a carrier is identified, all susceptible household contacts should be vaccinated.
   (d) Inmates of long-term correctional facilities
   (e) International travelers: Vaccination should be considered for those who plan to reside more than 6 months in an area with high levels of endemic hepatitis B infections and who will have close contact with the local population.
   (f) Other contacts of hepatitis B carriers: Persons in casual contact with carriers in settings such as schools and offices are at minimal risk of hepatitis B infection and vaccine is not routinely recommended.

— Immunogenicity and efficacy: When given in a three-dose series, both plasma-derived and recombinant vaccines induce protective antibodies (anti-HBs) in over 90% of healthy adults and more than 95% of infants, children, and adolescents from birth through 19 years of age. The deltoid (arm) muscle is the recommended site for the vaccination in adults and adolescents, as immunogenicity of the vaccine for adults is substantially lower when injections are given in the buttock. Hemodialysis patients and other immunocompromised persons in general develop a poorer response to the vaccines than healthy individuals and require a larger vaccine dose. The vaccine has been shown to be 80–95% effective in preventing infection or hepatitis among susceptible persons.

While protection during the first years is excellent, there is evidence that by 7 years 30–50% of individuals may develop low levels of antibodies, and 10–15% may have undetectable antibodies. However, protection against viremic infection and clinical disease appears to persist. Individuals less than 20 years of age seem to have a higher peak response and longer persistence of detectable levels of antibodies. Vaccination of carriers and immune individuals produces neither therapeutic nor adverse effects.

— Vaccine dosage (Table 30.2): Adults and older children: Primary vaccination includes three intramuscular doses of vaccine, with the second and third doses given 1 and 6 months after the first. Adults and adolescents should receive a full dose while children less than 11 years of age should receive half the full dose. An alternative schedule of four doses of vaccine given at 0, 1, 2, and 12 months has been approved for one vaccine for postexposure prophylaxis or for more rapid induction of immunity. For patients undergoing hemodialysis and for other immunosuppressed patients, higher vaccine doses or increased numbers of doses are required. The vaccine should be stored at 2–8°C but not frozen.

Data are not available on the safety of hepatitis vaccines for the developing fetus. However, because the vaccines contain only noninfectious HBsAg particles, there should be no risk to the fetus. Since hepatitis B may result in severe disease for the mother and chronic infection in the newborn, pregnancy or lactation should not be considered a contraindication to the use of the vaccine.

— Side effects: Seventeen percent of individuals experience soreness at site. Fifteen percent of individuals experience mild systemic symptoms including fever, headache, fatigue, and nausea. No potentially transmissible diseases, including HIV, have been reported.

— Prevaccination serologic screening: Screening for past infection is probably cost effective in groups with a prior high risk of infection (>20%), unless the cost of testing is extremely high. For groups with a low expected prevalence, such as health professionals in their training years, screening will not be cost effective. For routine screening, either anti-HBc or anti-HBs should be used. Anti-HBs will identify those previously infected, except carriers. Anti-HBc will identify all previously infected persons, both carriers and noncarriers. Kwan-Gett et al. (1994) evaluated prevaccination testing in preadolescents and adolescents. This study showed that no testing was the most cost-effective strategy. Prevaccination testing elevated costs by $2.9 million for every 100,000 patients and also lowered the rate of complete vaccination by 22% compared with vaccination without testing. Prevaccination testing was only cost effective when the seroprevalence of anti-HBs was greater than 40%.

— Postvaccination serology and revaccination: Testing for immunity is not recommended routinely but is advised for individuals who are expected to have a suboptimal response such as those who have received the vaccine in the buttock, persons over 50 years of age, and persons known to have HIV infection, or individuals whose subsequent management depends on knowing their immune status, such as dialysis patients and staff. When necessary, the testing should be done between 1 and 6 months after completion of the vaccine series.

— Testing of infants born to HBsAg-positive mothers who received immunoprophylaxis should be performed 3–9 months following completion of the vaccination series.

Revaccination in nonresponders produces adequate antibody in 15–25% after one additional dose and in 30–50% after three additional doses when the primary vaccination was given in the deltoid. If the primary vaccine was given in the buttock, revaccination in the arm induces adequate antibody in more than 75%. Revaccination should be considered for nonresponders who received the vaccine in the deltoid muscle and is recommended for nonresponders who received the primary vaccine in the buttock.

Long-term studies of children and adults suggest that immunologic memory lasts for at least 10 years and protects against chronic HBV infection even though antibody levels against HBsAg may become undetectable.

d. Hepatitis B postexposure prophylaxis: Prophylactic treatment to prevent hepatitis B infection after exposure should be considered in the following situations:

— Perinatal exposure of an infant born to an HBsAg-positive mother (see previous section, "Considerations during Pregnancy"). A regimen that combines one dose of HBIG at birth with the hepatitis B vaccine series started soon after birth is 85–95% effective. Regimens involving either multiple doses of HBIG alone or the vaccine series alone have 70–85% efficacy.

— Acute exposure to blood: Decision for prophylaxis depends on whether the source of the blood is available, the hepatitis status of the exposed person, and the status of the source. Following such exposure, a blood sample should be obtained from the person who was the source of the exposure and should be

TABLE 30.7.   Recommendations for Hepatitis B Prophylaxis Following Percutaneous Exposure

Exposed Person	Treatment When Source Is Found To Be		
	HBsAg Positive	HBsAg Negative	Unknown or Not Tested
Unvaccinated	Administer HBIG × 1[a] and initiate hepatitis B vaccine[b]	Initiate hepatitis B vaccine[b]	Initiate hepatitis B vaccine[b]
Previously vaccinated known responder	Test exposed person for anti-HBs 1. If adequate, no treatment 2. If inadequate, hepatitis B vaccine booster dose	No treatment	No treatment
Known nonresponder	HBIG × 2 or HBIG × 1, plus 1 dose of hepatitis B vaccine	No treatment	If known high-risk source, may treat as if source were HBsAg positive
Response unknown	Test exposed person for anti-HBs[c] 1. If inadequate, HBIG × 1 plus hepatitis B vaccine booster dose 2. If adequate, no treatment	No treatment	Test exposed person for anti-HBs[c] 1. If inadequate, hepatitis B vaccine booster dose 2. If adequate, no treatment

From Centers for Disease Control. Post-exposure prophylaxis for hepatitis B. Recommendations of the Immunization Practices Advisory Committee (ACIP). MMWR 1991;40(RR–13):21–24.
[a]Hepatitis B immune globulin (HBIG) dose 0.06 mL/kg intramuscularly.
[b]Hepatitis B vaccine dose (see Table 30.5).
[c]Adequate anti-HBs is ≥10 milli-international units.

tested for HBsAg. For greatest effectiveness, passive prophylaxis with HBIG, when indicated, should be given as soon as possible after exposure (the value beyond 7 days after exposure is unclear). A summary of recommendations is given in Table 30.7.

— Sexual contacts of HBsAg-positive individuals are at increased risk of infection, and HBIG is 75% effective in preventing such infections. Screening sexual partners for hepatitis antibodies (anti-HBc or anti-HBs) before treatment is recommended but should not delay treatment beyond 14 days after last exposure. Treatment consists of HBIG (0.06 mL/kg) followed by hepatitis vaccine series started at the same time if exposure continues.

— Household contacts of persons with acute infection: Not indicated unless there is exposure to blood of index case, such as sharing toothbrushes or razors. If indicated, treatment is with both HBIG and vaccine. If index patient becomes a carrier, all household contacts should receive hepatitis B vaccine. Treatment with HBIG and hepatitis B vaccine is also indicated for infants less than 12 months of age whose primary caregivers have an acute hepatitis B infection.

e. Delta hepatitis: Since delta hepatitis is dependent on hepatitis B for replication, prevention of hepatitis B infection suffices to prevent delta hepatitis. Exposures of individuals with known positivity for both delta hepatitis and hepatitis B should be treated exactly as such exposures to hepatitis B alone.

f. NANB hepatitis: Value of immune globulin against parenterally transmitted NANB hepatitis is unknown. It is reasonable to administer immune globulin (0.06 mL/kg) after percutaneous exposure to blood from a patient or after greater than 3 units of donor blood, especially if received from paid donors. There is no evidence that United States manufactured immune globulin will prevent enterically transmitted NANB hepatitis.

3. Hygiene

a. No sharing of razors, toothbrushes, food utensils, or towels.

   b. Careful personal hygiene; handwashing after patient contact.
   c. Careful handling of secretions of hepatitis B patient's saliva, blood, urine, including needle precautions.
   d. Hepatitis A: Isolate the patient until jaundice peaks; use stool precautions.

General Measures

1. Teenager should decrease physical activity level until he or she is feeling better.
2. Diet: There is no evidence that special diet affects the course of the disease. Have teenager eat as much as he or she can tolerate.
3. Adolescent should avoid alcoholic beverages until transaminases return to normal.
4. Adolescent should avoid oral contraceptives, steroids, and liver-toxic drugs.
5. Acetylcysteine is useful in acetaminophen-induced hepatitis.
6. Severe disease is indicated by:
   a. Total bilirubin greater than 25 mg/dL
   b. Elevated prothrombin time
   c. Albumin less than 2.5 g/dL
   d. Evidence of ascites, edema, or encephalopathy
   e. Transaminase levels greater than 2000 units/mL
7. Most teens with hepatitis can be managed at home. If the home environment is non-supportive or the disease activity particularly severe, hospitalization is indicated.
8. Follow the serum bilirubin and transaminases every week during the acute illness, then every 2–3 weeks as the teen improves and enzymes fall. Monitoring can be stopped when liver enzymes return to normal. In patients with chronic hepatitis B, enzymes should be continuously monitored but at less frequent intervals. Treatment of chronic hepatitis is beyond the scope of this book. In general, standard therapy for chronic hepatitis B and C remains interferon alfa-2b, although other agents may have potential. Overall, about 50% of patients respond initially to the treatment, but relapse rates can be high, particularly with hepatitis C (50% relapse rate).

COMPLICATIONS

1. Acute
   a. Pancreatitis
   b. Myocarditis
   c. Atypical pneumonia
   d. Aplastic anemia
   e. Transverse myelitis
   f. Glomerulonephritis
   g. Arthritis
2. Fulminant hepatitis
3. Chronic carrier state (HBsAg positive for more than 6 months)
4. Chronic hepatitis
   a. Chronic, persistent, benign hepatitis
   b. Chronic active hepatitis
      — Symptoms longer than 10 weeks
      — Sustained serum glutamic-oxaloacetic transaminase (SGOT) 10 times beyond normal or five times beyond normal with serum globulins two times beyond normal
      — Piecemeal necrosis and other abnormalities on liver biopsy

BIBLIOGRAPHY

Alter MJ. Review of serologic testing for hepatitis C virus infection and risk of posttransfusion hepatitis C. Arch Pathol Lab Med 1994;118:342.

Alter MJ, Margolis HS, Krawczynski K, et al. The natural history of community acquired hepatitis C in the United States. N Engl J Med 1992;327:1899.

Alter MJ, Sampliner RE. Hepatitis C: and miles to go before we sleep. N Engl J Med 1989;321:1538.

Babb RR. Chronic liver disease. The scope of causes and treatments. Postgrad Med 1992;91:89.

Balcarek DB, Bagley MR, Pass RF, et al. Safety and immunogenicity of an in-activated hepatitis A vaccine in preschool children. J Infect Dis 1995;171(suppl 1):S70.

Becherer PR. Viral hepatitis. What have we learned about risk factors and transmission? Postgrad Med 1995;98:65.

Bocke DJ. Hepatitis A revisited. Ann Intern Med 1986;105:960.

Brechot C. Polymerase chain reaction for the diagnosis of viral hepatitis B and C. Gut 1993;34:S39.

Bredfeldt JE. Hepatitis B virus: update on the spectrum of clinical infections and on prophylaxis. Postgrad Med 1985;78:71.

Brewer MA, Edwards KM, Decker MD. Who should receive hepatitis A vaccine? Pediatr Infect Dis J 1995;14:258.

Centers for Disease Control. Protection against viral hepatitis: Recommendations of the Immunization Practices Advisory Committee (ACIP). MMWR 1990;39:1.

Centers for Disease Control. Hepatitis B virus: a comprehensive strategy for eliminating transmission in the United States through universal childhood vaccination. Recommendations of the Immunization Practices Advisory Committee (ACIP). MMWR 1991;40(No. RR-13):1.

Centers for Disease Control and Prevention. Update: recommendations to prevent hepatitis B virus transmission—United States. JAMA 1995;274:603.

Centers for Disease Control and Prevention. Licensure of inactivated hepatitis A vaccine and recommendations for international travelers' use. JAMA 1995;274:603.

Clemens R, Safary A, Hepburn A, et al. Clinical experience with an inactivated hepatitis A vaccine. J Infect Dis 1995;171(suppl 1):S44.

Craven DE, Awdeh ZL, Kunches LM, et al. Nonresponsiveness to hepatitis B vaccine in health care workers: results of revaccination and genetic typings. Ann Intern Med 1986;105:356.

Czaja AJ. Chronic active hepatitis: the challenge for a new nomenclature. Ann Intern Med 1993;119:510.

Dana F, Becherer PR, Bacon BR. Hepatitis C virus. What recent studies can tell us. Postgrad Med 1994;95:121.

De Cock KM, Govindarajan S, Chin KP, et al. Delta hepatitis in the Los Angeles area: a report of 126 cases. Ann Intern Med 1986;105:108.

Dindzans VJ. Viral hepatitis: preexposure and postexposure. Postgrad Med 1992;92:43.

Foutch PG, Carey WD, Tabor E, et al. Concomitant hepatitis B surface antigen and antibody in thirteen patients. Ann Intern Med 1983;99:460.

Francis DP, Feorino PM, McDougal S, et al. The safety of the hepatitis B vaccine: inactivation of the AIDS virus during routine vaccine manufacture. JAMA 1986;256:869.

Frymoyer CL. Preventing the spread of viral hepatitis. Am Fam Physician 1993;48:1479.

Ganiats TG. Hepatitis B immunization for adolescents. West J Med 1995;163:70.

Gardner P, Schaffner W. Immunization of adults. N Engl J Med 1993;328:1252.

Gary GM, Gregory PB, Collins JA, et al. Gastroenterology. In: Rubenstein E, Federman E, eds. Scientific American medicine. New York: Scientific American, 1982.

Gershon AA. Present and future challenges of immunizations on the health of our patients. Pediatr Infect Dis J 1995;14:445.

Gindler J, Hadler SC, Strebel PM. Recommended childhood immunization schedule: United States—1995. Clin Pediatr 1995;34:66.

Gregorio GV, Mieli-Vergani G, Mowat AP. Viral hepatitis. Arch Dis Child 1994;70:343.

Hadler SC, Francis DP, Maynard JE, et al. Long-term immunogenicity and efficacy of hepatitis B vaccine in homosexual men. N Engl J Med 1986;315:209.

Hepatitis A vaccine. Med Lett Drugs Ther 1995;37:51.

Herrera JL. Serologic diagnosis of viral hepatitis. South Med J 1994;87:677.

Hess G. Virological and serological aspects of hepatitis B and the delta agent. Gut 1993;34:S1.

Hollinger FB. Hepatitis markers: guide to test selection. Diagnosis 1986;August:52.

Immunization Practices Advisory Committee. Update on hepatitis B prevention. Ann Intern Med 1987;107:353.

Innis BL, Snitbhan R, Kunasol P, et al. Protection against hepatitis A by an inactivated vaccine. JAMA 1994;271:1328.

Katkov WN, Dienstag JL. Hepatitis vaccines. Gastroenterol Clin North Am 1995;24:147.

Kumar ML, Dawson NV, McCullough AJ, et al. Should all pregnant women be screened for hepatitis B? Ann Intern Med 1987;107:273.

Kumar S, Pound DC. Serologic diagnosis of viral hepatitis. Postgrad Med 1992;92:55.

Kwan-Gett TS, Whitaker RC, Kempter KJ. A cost-effectiveness analysis of prevaccination testing for hepatitis B in adolescents and preadolescents. Arch Pediatr Adolesc Med 1994;148:915.

Lemon SM. Type A viral hepatitis: new developments in an old disease. N Engl J Med 1985;313:1059.

Lindsay KL. Management of chronic hepatitis in special populations. Am J Med 1994;96:57S.

Maddrey WC. Chronic hepatitis. Dis Mon 1993;39:53.

Maddrey WC. Chronic viral hepatitis: diagnosis and management. Hosp Pract 1994;29:117.

Mahoney FJ, Burkholder BT, Matson CC. Prevention of hepatitis B virus infection. Am Fam Physician 1993; 47:865.

Manns MP, Kruger M. Immunogenetics of chronic liver diseases. Gastroenterology 1994;106:1676.

Margolis HS. Prevention of acute and chronic liver disease through immunization: hepatitis B and beyond. J Infect Dis 1993;168:9.

Marlink RG. Hepatitis B vaccines: to switch or not to switch. JAMA 1987;257:2634.

MMWR. Licensure of inactivated hepatitis A vaccine and recommendations for use among international travelers. MMWR 1995;44:559.

Perrillo RP. The management of chronic hepatitis B. Am J Med 1994;96:34S.

Perrillo RP, Campbell CR, Strang S, et al. Immune globulin and hepatitis B immune globulin: prophylactic measures for intimate contacts exposed to acute type B hepatitis. Arch Intern Med 1984;144:81.

Petermann S, Ernest JM. Intrapartum hepatitis B screening. Am J Obstet Gynecol 1995;173:369.

Regenstein F. New approaches to the treatment of chronic viral hepatitis B and C. Am J Med 1994;96:47S.

Rosina F, Saracco G, Rizzetto M. Risk of post-transfusion infection with the hepatitis delta virus: a multi-center study. N Engl J Med 1985;312:1488.

Rubin RA, Falestiny M, Molet PF. Chronic hepatitis C: advances in diagnostic testing and therapy. Arch Intern Med 1994;154:387.

Sarver DK. Hepatitis in clinical practice 1. Hepatitis A and B. Postgrad Med 1986a;79.194.

Sarver DK. Hepatitis in clinical practice 2. Non-A, Non-B and delta hepatitis. Postgrad Med 1986b;79:218.

Schmilovitz-Weiss H, Levy M, Thompson N. Viral markers in the treatment of hepatitis B and C. Gut 1993;34:S26.

Sherlock DS. Chronic hepatitis C. Dis Mon 1994;40: 117.

Stevens CE, Taylor PE, Pindyck J, et al. Epidemiology of hepatitis C virus: a preliminary study in volunteer blood donors. JAMA 1990;263:49.

Szemuness W, Stevens CE, Harley EJ. Hepatitis B vaccine demonstration of efficacy in a controlled clinical trial in a high-risk population in the United States. N Engl J Med 1980;303:833.

Taswell HF. Viral hepatitis: diagnostic test using anti-HBc (IgM). Mayo Clin Proc 1985;60:488.

Trepo C, Zoulim F, Alonso C, et al. Diagnostic markers of viral hepatitis B and C. Gut 1993;34:S20.

Wagner G, Lavanchy D, Darioli R, et al. Simultaneous active and passive immunization against hepatitis A studied in a population of travelers. Vaccine 1993; 11:1027.

Weinstock HS, Bolan G, Moran JS, et al. Routine hepatitis B vaccination in a clinic for sexually transmitted diseases. Am J Public Health 1995;85:846.

Wright TL, Lau JY. Clinical aspects of hepatitis B virus infection. Lancet 1993;342:1340.

Van Dyke RW. Hepatitis B: what you should know about Dx, Rx, and prevention. Mod Med 1984;52: 154.

CHAPTER 31

HIV Infections and AIDS

Marvin E. Belzer and Lawrence S. Neinstein

Acquired immunodeficiency syndrome (AIDS) is one of the largest epidemics to hit modern society and the focal point of intense national and international debate. AIDS is the leading cause of death in men 25–44 years of age and of women 25–34 years of age and the leading cause of years of potential life lost in males aged 15–64. Worldwide, the World Health Organization (WHO) estimates that 50% of individuals infected with human immunodeficiency virus (HIV) contracted the virus before the age of 25. In the United States the National Institutes of Health (NIH) estimate that 25% contracted the virus before the age of 22.

Special issues are important to consider in relation to the adolescent population and infection with HIV, including a host of legal and ethical dilemmas regarding testing, disclosure of information, and consent for treatment in research protocols. For HIV-infected adolescents there is also the problem of availability of appropriate services and support groups.

Adolescents are in danger of contracting HIV because of their risky sexual behaviors, drug use, or both. Because a large group of adolescents are not yet infected but may be involved in high-risk behaviors, teens are a high-priority target group for preventive measures.

Information about HIV infection is developing rapidly. Several thousand articles are published yearly with information often quickly becoming outdated. This chapter includes a brief overview of HIV and AIDS, with a focus on considerations important in the adolescent. It is essential for the practicing physician to keep up to date—through the literature or continuing medical education courses—on the many aspects of HIV infections, including legal issues, diagnosis, evaluation, and treatment.

ETIOLOGY

The causative agent of AIDS is HIV, a retrovirus. This virus was isolated at both the NIH and the Pasteur Institute in Paris in 1983. HIV-1 is the cause of most cases of AIDS in the world. HIV-2, another retrovirus related to HIV-1, is found primarily in Central Africa. HIV-2 generally has much slower progression (20 years versus 5–10 years with HIV-1) but has a similar spectrum of disease.

EPIDEMIOLOGY

As of June 1995 there have been over 476,899 cases of AIDS reported to the Centers for Disease Control and Prevention (CDC). While only 2184 cases were in teens aged 13–19, approximately 20% of all cases are in 20- to 29-year-olds. With a median incubation of 7–10 years from HIV infection to AIDS, many of these cases in young adults were acquired as adolescents. Persons of color are dramatically overrepresented, making up 55% of all

TABLE 31.1.   HIV Infection Cases (not AIDS), by Sex, Age at Diagnosis, and Race/Ethnicity, Reported through June 1995, from States with Confidential HIV Infection Reporting

Age at Diagnosis (yr)	White, not Hispanic No. (%)	African-American, not Hispanic No. (%)	Hispanic No. (%)	Asian/Pacific Islander No. (%)	American Indian/ Alaska Native No. (%)	Total[a] No. (%)
Male						
Under 5	116 (0)	321 (1)	63 (2)	2 (1)	3 (1)	511 (1)
5–12	74 (0)	59 (0)	19 (1)	—	2 (1)	161 (0)
13–19	558 (2)	712 (3)	51 (2)	4 (3)	8 (3)	1,363 (2)
20–24	3,744 (15)	3,546 (14)	415 (13)	26 (17)	59 (19)	7,977 (14)
25–29	6,579 (26)	5,477 (21)	833 (25)	41 (28)	95 (30)	13,353 (24)
30–34	6,041 (24)	5,703 (22)	813 (24)	31 (21)	69 (22)	12,998 (23)
35–39	3,975 (16)	4,759 (19)	571 (17)	18 (12)	40 (13)	9,607 (17)
40–44	2,199 (9)	2,831 (11)	322 (10)	14 (9)	22 (7)	5,521 (10)
45–49	1,100 (4)	1,180 (5)	137 (4)	7 (5)	8 (3)	2,516 (4)
50–54	546 (2)	607 (2)	46 (1)	3 (2)	5 (2)	1,243 (2)
55–59	239 (1)	254 (1)	21 (1)	2 (1)	2 (1)	532 (1)
60–64	131 (1)	133 (1)	17 (1)	—	1 (0)	287 (1)
65 or older	116 (0)	123 (0)	11 (0)	1 (1)	—	268 (0)
Male subtotal	25,418 (100)	25,705 (100)	3,319 (100)	149 (100)	314 (100)	56,335 (100)
Female						
Under 5	115 (3)	291 (3)	85 (6)	2 (4)	6 (6)	491 (3)
5–12	21 (0)	51 (0)	16 (1)	1 (2)	1 (1)	93 (1)
13–19	252 (6)	930 (8)	52 (5)	1 (2)	10 (9)	1,264 (7)
20–24	816 (19)	1,924 (17)	149 (14)	10 (22)	19 (18)	2,960 (17)
25–29	1,047 (24)	2,462 (22)	271 (25)	16 (35)	18 (17)	3,888 (23)
30–34	931 (21)	2,406 (21)	255 (24)	9 (20)	20 (19)	3,689 (21)
35–39	590 (14)	1,678 (15)	122 (11)	1 (2)	22 (20)	2,452 (14)
40–44	264 (6)	883 (8)	80 (7)	3 (7)	9 (8)	1,264 (7)
45–49	158 (4)	332 (3)	35 (3)	2 (4)	2 (2)	546 (3)
50–54	53 (1)	148 (1)	15 (1)	1 (2)	1 (1)	222 (1)
55–59	45 (1)	100 (1)	13 (1)	—	—	160 (1)
60–64	22 (1)	50 (0)	5 (0)	—	—	79 (0)
65 or older	51 (1)	60 (1)	1 (0)	—	—	118 (1)
Female subtotal	4,365 (100)	11,315 (100)	1,079 (100)	46 (100)	108 (100)	17,226 (100)
TOTAL[b]	29,784	37,022	4,398	195	423	73,577

From Centers for Disease Control and Prevention. HIV/AIDS surveillance report. 1995;7(1):28.
[a]Includes 1,430 males and 313 females whose race/ethnicity is unknown.
[b]Includes 16 persons whose sex is unknown.

cases in youth aged 13–24. Table 31.1 shows HIV cases by sex, age at diagnosis, and race/ethnicity through June 1995. Table 31.2 shows AIDS cases by sex, age at diagnosis, and race/ethnicity through June 1995. Table 31.3 shows HIV cases in adolescents and adults under age 25 by sex and exposure category. Table 31.4 shows AIDS cases in adolescents and adults under age 25 by sex and exposure category. Table 31.5 shows AIDS cases and deaths from 1981 to 1995.

Males

For men 13–24, the primary modes of HIV transmission are men having sex with men (50–60%), injection drug use (5–10%), and men having sex with men and injection drug use (5–10%) (Tables 31.3 and 31.4). For males with AIDS, aged 13–19, 48% were infected by blood product transfusion, yet for males with HIV infection, the percent infected by blood product transfusion is much lower.

TABLE **31.2.**   AIDS Cases by Sex, Age at Diagnosis, and Race/Ethnicity, Reported through June 1995, United States

Age at Diagnosis (yr)	White, not Hispanic No. (%)	African-American, not Hispanic No. (%)	Hispanic No. (%)	Asian/ Pacific Islander No. (%)	American Indian/ Alaska Native No. (%)	Total[a] No. (%)
Male						
Under 5	401 (0)	1,593 (1)	630 (1)	15 (1)	9 (1)	2,651 (1)
5–12	288 (0)	270 (0)	193 (0)	8 (0)	1 (0)	761 (0)
13–19	649 (0)	468 (0)	288 (0)	18 (1)	13 (1)	1,437 (0)
20–24	6,054 (3)	4,641 (4)	2,735 (4)	99 (3)	48 (5)	13,599 (3)
25–29	29,889 (14)	16,854 (14)	10,851 (16)	384 (13)	210 (21)	58,268 (14)
30–34	49,941 (23)	27,096 (22)	16,750 (24)	646 (22)	272 (27)	94,836 (23)
35–39	47,371 (22)	28,321 (23)	15,311 (22)	630 (22)	199 (20)	91,986 (22)
40–44	34,274 (16)	20,518 (17)	10,332 (15)	509 (17)	142 (14)	65,883 (16)
45–49	20,271 (10)	10,877 (9)	5,608 (8)	281 (10)	63 (6)	37,156 (9)
50–54	10,900 (5)	5,863 (5)	2,923 (4)	154 (5)	30 (3)	19,899 (5)
55–59	6,082 (3)	3,236 (3)	1,677 (2)	90 (3)	15 (1)	11,128 (3)
60–64	3,514 (2)	1,746 (1)	908 (1)	42 (1)	11 (1)	6,230 (2)
65 or older	2,911 (1)	1,397 (1)	668 (1)	49 (2)	7 (1)	5,040 (1)
Male subtotal	212,545 (100)	122,880 (100)	68,874 (100)	2,925 (100)	1,020 (100)	408,874 (100)
Female						
Under 5	406 (3)	1,606 (4)	596 (4)	9 (3)	9 (5)	2,634 (4)
5–12	121 (1)	289 (1)	147 (1)	6 (2)	—	565 (1)
13–19	140 (1)	482 (1)	119 (1)	4 (1)	1 (1)	747 (1)
20–24	980 (6)	2,217 (6)	910 (6)	16 (5)	18 (10)	4,146 (5)
25–29	2,825 (18)	5,885 (16)	2,488 (18)	36 (11)	36 (20)	11,280 (17)
30–34	3,695 (23)	8,692 (23)	3,412 (24)	70 (21)	44 (24)	15,936 (23)
35–39	3,043 (19)	8,140 (22)	2,766 (20)	61 (18)	35 (19)	14,075 (21)
40–44	1,650 (11)	5,085 (14)	1,663 (12)	50 (15)	19 (10)	8,676 (13)
45–49	953 (6)	2,208 (6)	852 (6)	28 (8)	8 (4)	4,054 (6)
50–54	585 (4)	1,166 (3)	479 (3)	16 (5)	4 (2)	2,233 (3)
55–59	445 (3)	660 (2)	303 (2)	10 (3)	4 (2)	1,424 (2)
60–64	326 (2)	422 (1)	151 (1)	16 (5)	3 (2)	918 (1)
65 or older	748 (5)	415 (1)	150 (1)	18 (5)	1 (1)	1,333 (2)
Female subtotal	16,097 (100)	37,267 (100)	14,038 (100)	340 (100)	182 (100)	68,021 (100)
TOTAL[b]	228,644	160,148	82,910	3,265	1,202	476,899

From Centers for Disease Control and Prevention. HIV/AIDS surveillance report. 1995;7(1):13.
[a]Includes 630 males, 99 females, and 1 person of unknown sex whose race/ethnicity is unknown.
[b]Includes 4 persons whose sex is unknown.

Females

Women represent one of the fastest growing groups infected with HIV, with most in the reproductive-aged group. For women aged 13–24, 40–50% were infected by heterosexual contact and 22% by injection drug use (Tables 31.3 and 31.4).

Seroprevalence

There are no random seroprevalence studies for HIV in youth however there are several specific groups that do have data. In the Job Corps, a federally funded job training program for economically disadvantaged youth, the prevalence among 16- to 22-year-olds was 3.9/1000. The seroprevalence rates for young men in the Job Corps have decreased since 1988, while the rates among young women have approximately doubled since 1988 (Conway, 1991). Among over 1 million military recruits younger than 20 years old, the seroprevalence rate is 0.34/1000. In youth attending selected sexually transmitted disease

TABLE 31.3.   HIV Infection Cases (not AIDS) in Adolescents and Adults under Age 25, by Sex and Exposure Category, Reported July 1994 through June 1995, and Cumulative Totals through June 1995, from States with Confidential HIV Infection Reporting

	13–19 Yr		20–24 Yr	
	July 1994–June 1995	Cumulative Total	July 1994–June 1995	Cumulative Total
	No. (%)	No. (%)	No. (%)	No. (%)
Male exposure category				
Men who have sex with men	108 (46)	583 (43)	728 (53)	4,235 (53)
Injecting drug use	5 (2)	70 (5)	77 (6)	478 (6)
Men who have sex with men and inject drugs	7 (3)	82 (6)	59 (4)	530 (7)
Hemophilia/coagulation disorder	14 (6)	93 (7)	14 (1)	89 (1)
Heterosexual contact	9 (4)	90 (7)	84 (6)	428 (5)
Sex with an injecting drug user	1	17	24	93
Sex with person with hemophilia	1	2	—	1
Sex with transfusion recipient with HIV infection	—	1	1	4
Sex with HIV-infected person, risk not specified	7	70	59	330
Receipt of blood transfusion, blood components, or tissue	—	11 (1)	4 (0)	38 (0)
Risk not reported or identified[a]	91 (39)	434 (32)	401 (29)	2,179 (27)
Male subtotal	234 (100)	1,363 (100)	1,367 (100)	7,977 (100)
Female exposure category				
Injecting drug use	11 (4)	99 (8)	83 (12)	436 (15)
Hemophilia/coagulation disorder	—	—	—	1 (0)
Heterosexual contact	121 (40)	549 (43)	209 (30)	1,158 (39)
Sex with an injecting drug user	23	138	50	349
Sex with a bisexual male	6	41	22	128
Sex with person with hemophilia	2	10	7	26
Sex with transfusion recipient with HIV infection	2	4	2	11
Sex with HIV-infected person, risk not specified	88	356	128	644
Receipt of blood transfusion, blood components, or tissue	3 (1)	11 (1)	6 (1)	28 (1)
Risk not reported or identified	168 (55)	605 (48)	403 (57)	1,337 (45)
Female subtotal	303 (100)	1,264 (100)	701 (100)	2,960 (100)
TOTAL[b]	537	2,628	2,070	10,940

From Centers for Disease Control and Prevention. HIV/AIDS surveillance report. 1995;7(1):27.
[a]For HIV infection cases (not AIDS), "risk not reported or identified" refers primarily to persons whose mode of exposure was not reported and who have not been followed up to determine their mode of exposure, and to a smaller number of persons who are not reported with one of the exposures listed above after follow-up.
[b]Includes 4 persons whose sex is unknown.

(STD) clinics the rate is 11/1000. Sweeney et al. (1995) reviewed seroprevalence rates of HIV in American teenagers from January 1, 1990, through December 31, 1992, from 79,802 teenagers. The rates varied from 0.3% (range, 0–6.8%) in 33 correctional facilities, 0.5% (range, 0–3.5%) in 70 sexually transmitted disease clinics, and 1.1% (range, 0–4.1%) in five homeless youth centers. Most teenagers with risk information reported heterosexual activity as their only potential risk exposure to HIV-1. All these studies found that persons of color, people residing in large urban centers in the eastern and southeastern United States, and women are being disproportionately affected when comparing youth to adults. Still the highest rates are in young men who have sex with men and injection drug users.

TABLE 31.4.   AIDS Cases in Adolescents and Adults under Age 25, by Sex and Exposure Category, Reported July 1993 through June 1994, July 1994 through June 1995, and Cumulative Totals through June 1995, United States

	13–19 Yr			20–24 Yr		
	July 1993–June 1994	July 1994–June 1995	Cumulative Total	July 1993–June 1994	July 1994–June 1995	Cumulative Total
	No. (%)	No. (%)	No. (%)	No. (%)	No. (%)	No. (%)
Male exposure category						
Men who have sex with men	75 (29)	82 (32)	471 (33)	1,250 (60)	1,029 (60)	8,613 (63)
Injecting drug use	15 (6)	16 (6)	92 (6)	275 (13)	207 (12)	1,727 (13)
Men who have sex with men and inject drugs	10 (4)	10 (4)	68 (5)	178 (9)	112 (7)	1,486 (11)
Hemophilia/coagulation disorder	112 (43)	89 (35)	613 (43)	85 (4)	55 (3)	501 (4)
Heterosexual contact	10 (4)	10 (4)	36 (3)	95 (5)	108 (6)	456 (3)
Sex with an injecting drug user	3	1	13	26	37	196
Sex with person with hemophilia	—	1	1	—	—	1
Sex with transfusion recipient with HIV infection	—	—	—	2	2	11
Sex with HIV-infected person, risk not specified	7	8	22	67	69	248
Receipt of blood transfusion, blood components, or tissue	15 (6)	11 (4)	60 (4)	17 (1)	10 (1)	99 (1)
Risk not reported or identified	21 (8)	39 (15)	97 (7)	171 (8)	200 (12)	717 (5)
Male subtotal	258 (100)	257 (100)	1,437 (100)	2,071 (100)	1,721 (100)	13,599 (100)
Female exposure category						
Injecting drug use	18 (11)	14 (7)	122 (16)	223 (27)	183 (22)	1,351 (33)
Hemophilia/coagulation disorder	2 (1)	3 (2)	9 (1)	2 (0)	2 (0)	12 (0)
Heterosexual contact	93 (55)	89 (48)	397 (53)	455 (54)	423 (51)	2,093 (50)
Sex with injecting drug user	32	27	186	189	129	1,058
Sex with bisexual male	5	6	22	31	23	165
Sex with person with hemophilia	1	3	10	13	6	41
Sex with transfusion recipient with HIV infection	—	—	1	2	3	12
Sex with HIV-infected person, risk not specified	55	53	178	220	262	817
Receipt of blood transfusion, blood components, or tissue	7 (4)	13 (7)	57 (8)	12 (1)	10 (1)	98 (2)
Risk not reported or identified	49 (29)	68 (36)	162 (22)	149 (18)	209 (25)	592 (14)
Female subtotal	169 (100)	187 (100)	747 (100)	841 (100)	827 (100)	4,146 (100)
TOTAL	427	444	2,184	2,912	2,548	17,745

From Centers for Disease Control and Prevention. HIV/AIDS surveillance report. 1995;7(1):12.

Table 31.5. AIDS Cases, Case-Fatality Rates,[a] and Deaths by Half-Year and Age Group through June 1995, United States

Half-Year	Adults/Adolescents			Children <13 Yr		
	Cases Diagnosed during Interval	Case-Fatality Rate	Deaths Occurring during Interval	Cases Diagnosed during Interval	Case-Fatality Rate	Deaths Occurring during Interval
Before 1981	86	90.7	30	8	75.0	1
1981 Jan.–June	104	90.4	37	10	80.0	2
July–Dec.	203	92.1	83	6	83.3	6
1982 Jan.–June	428	93.2	151	15	93.3	10
July–Dec.	725	91.6	295	16	87.5	4
1983 Jan.–June	1,343	94.2	525	32	100.0	14
July–Dec.	1,700	94.2	945	44	90.9	16
1984 Jan.–June	2,667	93.6	1,423	52	88.5	26
July–Dec.	3,494	93.7	2,015	63	87.3	24
1985 Jan.–June	5,120	92.7	2,869	108	81.5	47
July–Dec.	6,529	93.1	3,973	137	85.4	72
1986 Jan.–June	8,647	92.1	5,185	143	83.2	68
July–Dec.	10,210	92.3	6,696	195	77.9	97
1987 Jan.–June	13,476	91.1	7,798	228	78.1	121
July–Dec.	14,860	89.4	8,233	269	73.6	171
1988 Jan.–June	17,283	87.5	9,671	262	68.3	137
July–Dec.	17,769	87.3	11,032	348	65.5	179
1989 Jan.–June	20,799	84.1	12,694	368	64.4	173
July–Dec.	21,131	82.8	14,592	345	67.5	194
1990 Jan.–June	23,901	80.0	14,995	386	60.6	193
July–Dec.	23,403	77.7	15,952	402	54.0	199
1991 Jan.–June	27,836	73.7	16,993	400	52.0	174
July–Dec.	29,924	69.3	18,861	389	48.1	218
1992 Jan.–June	36,048	61.3	19,247	473	44.4	190
July–Dec.	38,962	54.4	20,416	425	47.3	219
1993 Jan.–June	40,147	41.3	20,571	413	37.8	244
July–Dec.	32,818	34.0	21,503	396	36.9	254
1994 Jan.–June	32,090	24.2	22,091	345	26.7	271
July–Dec.	25,577	15.8	21,475	243	20.6	215
1995 Jan.–June	13,008	7.8	11,112	90	8.9	112
Total[b]	470,288	62.1	291,815	6,611	55.3	3,658

From Centers for Disease Control and Prevention. HIV/AIDS surveillance report. 1995;7(1):14.

[a]Case-fatality rates are calculated for each half-year by date of diagnosis. Each 6-month case-fatality rate is the number of deaths ever reported among cases diagnosed in that period (regardless of the year of death), divided by the number of total cases diagnosed in that period, multiplied by 100. For example, during the interval January through June 1982, AIDS was diagnosed in 428 adults/adolescents. Through June 1995, 399 of these 428 were reported as dead. Therefore, the case-fatality rate is 93.2 (399 divided by 428, multiplied by 100). The case-fatality rates shown here may be underestimates because of incomplete reporting of deaths. Reported deaths are not necessarily caused by HIV-related disease.

[b]Death totals include 352 adults/adolescents and 7 children known to have died, but whose dates of death are unknown.

HIV Staging

In 1993 the CDC expanded their AIDS definition criteria and changed their staging system (Table 31.6). The primary changes in definition included expanding the AIDS diagnosis to persons with a single CD4 count less than or equal to 200, pulmonary tuberculosis, recurrent bacterial pneumonias, and invasive cervical cancer.

Transmission

HIV can only be transmitted by the exchange of body fluids. Blood, semen, vaginal secretions, and breast milk are the only fluids documented to be associated with HIV infection.

TABLE 31.6.   1993 Revised Classification System for HIV Infection and Expanded AIDS Surveillance Case Definition for Adolescents and Adults

	Clinical Categories		
CD4+ T-cell categories	(A) Asymptomatic, Acute (Primary) HIV or PGL[a]	(B) Symptomatic, not (A) or (C) Conditions	(C) AIDS-Indicator Conditions
(1) ≥500/μL	A1	B1	C1
(2) 200–400/μL	A2	B2	C2
(3) <200/μL AIDS-indicator T-cell count	A3	B3	C3

Adapted from 1993 revised classification system for HIV infection and expanded surveillance case definition for AIDS among adolescents and adults. MMWR 1992;41:1.
[a]PGL, persistent generalized lymphadenopathy. Clinical category A includes acute (primary) HIV infection.
Conditions included in the 1993 AIDS Surveillance Case Definition (AIDS indicator conditions)

- Candidiasis of bronchi, trachea, or lungs
- Candidiasis, esophageal
- Cervical cancer, invasive
- Coccidioidomycosis, disseminated or extrapulmonary
- Cryptococcosis, extrapulmonary
- Cryptosporidiosis, chronic intestinal (>1 month's duration)
- Cytomegalovirus disease (other than liver, spleen or nodes)
- Cytomegalovirus retinitis (with loss of vision)
- Encephalopathy, HIV-related
- Herpes simplex: chronic ulcer(s) (>1 month's duration); or bronchitis, pneumonitis, or esophagitis
- Histoplasmosis, disseminated, or extrapulmonary
- Isosporiasis, chronic intestinal (>1 month's duration)
- Kaposi's sarcoma
- Lymphoma, Burkitt's (or equivalent term)
- Lymphoma, immunoblastic (or equivalent term)
- Lymphoma, primary, of brain
- *Mycobacterium avium* complex or *Mycobacterium kansasii*, disseminated or extrapulmonary
- *Mycobacterium tuberculosis*, any site (pulmonary or extrapulmonary)
- *Mycobacterium*, other species or unidentified species, disseminated or extrapulmonary
- *Pneumocystis carinii* pneumonia
- Pneumonia, recurrent
- Progressive multifocal leukoencephalopathy
- *Salmonella* septicemia, recurrent
- Toxoplasmosis of brain
- Wasting syndrome due to HIV infection

While HIV is found in saliva, tears, urine, and sweat, no case has been documented where these fluids have been implicated.

HIV is easily transmitted by the sharing of needles. The CDC has provided guidelines for the cleaning of needles with bleach. Because of the unreliability and frequent unacceptance of needle bleaching and unacceptance or inaccessibility of drug treatment, nearly all public health organizations support needle exchange. Here injection drug users can turn in dirty needles for clean ones while at the same time accessing condoms, bleach, and referral resources. Programs in San Francisco, California and New Haven, Connecticut, as well as others in the United States and Europe, have shown that injection drug use does not increase in the community or individual user where exchanges are available. Also HIV and other blood-borne disease transmission is markedly reduced with needle exchange.

Sexual transmission of HIV is thought to have a hierarchy of relative risk. Receptive anal intercourse without condoms is riskiest, followed by insertive anal intercourse and vaginal intercourse. Oral sex is less risky but has been shown to transmit HIV. Studies have shown that the proper and consistent use of latex condoms or dental dams can markedly reduce the risk for HIV transmission during sex.

The risk to health professionals with needle sticks from HIV-infected patients is estimated to be 1/200 to 1/500. Injuries involving injection of blood are much riskier than simple pricks. Double gloving while using needles will likely reduce the risk of transmission if a needle stick occurs on the covered hands. The role of the antiretroviral medication zidovudine (formerly AZT) after needle sticks is unclear, although most hospitals offer it. However, in a preliminary study from the CDC, AZT was found to be possibly helpful in reducing the risk of HIV infection to health-care workers after accidental needle stick with needles contaminated with an infected patient's blood (CDC, 1995). For the health-care workers in this study, the use of AZT decreased the risk 79%.

DEVELOPMENTAL ISSUES RELATED TO HIV INFECTIONS AND ADOLESCENTS

Although most of today's youth do not undergo extreme turmoil and distress in their teenage years, adolescence still provides many opportunities for risk for the teen with regards to HIV infections.

Cognitive and Emotional Development

Cognitive and emotional development factors that put teens at increased risk for AIDS include:

1. Greater experimentation and greater degree of influence by peer behaviors
2. Naïveté and lack of good judgment
3. Feelings of immortality and invulnerability
4. Ignorance of modes of AIDS transmission and prevention
5. Denial of personal risk
6. Identification with moral codes (i.e., those of peers) other than those of their parents

Some surveys indicate that adolescents do not believe that they are likely to become infected with HIV even if they are sexually active. In a study of Massachusetts adolescents, only 15% reported changing their sexual behaviors because of concern about AIDS. Of those who changed their behavior, only 20% selected effective methods such as condoms or abstinence.

Social, Behavioral, and Physiological Development

Adolescent behaviors that increase teens' risk for HIV infection include the following:

Sexual Activity A high percentage of adolescents engage in sexual intercourse, often without a barrier contraceptive or any contraceptive. In 1993, 53% of high school students reported that they have had intercourse (Centers for Disease Control [CDC], 1995). Teens in urban areas and particularly the inner city, group homes, and detention centers seem to have the earliest onset of sexual activity. As many as 27% of sexually active adolescent males and 12% of sexually active females had four or more sexual partners in the last month. Many adolescent males report having had at least one homosexual experience (17–37%). Only 52.8% of high school students reported using condoms at last sexual intercourse in the 1993 Youth Risk Behavior Survey (CDC, 1995).

Sexually Transmitted Diseases The high prevalence of sexually transmitted diseases in adolescents is an indicator both of high-risk behavior among teenagers and the lack of contraceptive or condom use. One in seven teens contracts a sexually transmitted disease annually. In the United States, adolescents have the highest rate of sexually transmitted diseases per sexually active individual (Hein, 1989a). In Central Africa the highest HIV rate is in 15- to 19-year-old females, demonstrating that HIV can heavily infect the adolescent population.

Illicit Drug Use Although there are no adequate national statistics on injection drug use among teenagers, estimates are that more than 200,000 high school students have used heroin. Millions of others have used cocaine, stimulants, or other opiates, all of which can be used intravenously. The 1993 through 1995 National Survey of High School Seniors (Johnston et al., 1995) have demonstrated an increase in drug use, reversing an over 10-year decline in previous years. This study also only includes adolescents in school. The high school dropout rate is as high as 40% or higher in urban areas, and it is probable that adolescent dropouts engage in the highest use of injected drugs. Teens may also be sharing needles in other ways, such as piercing ears, tattooing, or steroid use in teen athletes. Crack cocaine users appear to have an especially high rate of HIV infection. In addition, any drug use will impair a youth's ability to make good decisions concerning sexuality.

Runaway Behavior   About 1 million teenagers run away each year, with many of these involved in high-risk behaviors, including injection drug use and survival sex (sex for money, food, place to stay). AIDS-related risks are high but are often ignored in the context of the immediate crises of survival.

Physiological Factors   Adolescents may also be at increased risk of HIV infection from several physiological features, including:

1. Differences in the cervix of adolescents (more columnar epithelium)
2. Alterations of the vaginal pH as compared to adults
3. Differences in menstrual patterns (less ovulation, less progesterone, and thus less thick cervical mucus)

Family Relationships

Unresolved issues can lead to powerful conflicts between parents and adolescents. Sometimes the dysfunctional nature of the teen's family significantly increases the chances of the teen's involvement in high-risk behavior.

Levels of Risk

Not all adolescents present with the same risk profile. Hein (1989a) has described several levels of risk among adolescents:

1. Not at risk: Many adolescents are not at risk because they are either not involved in risk behaviors (i.e., sexual activity or injection drugs) or they are in a location without HIV infections.
2. Sexually active teens not yet exposed: This group may become at higher risk as the prevalence of HIV infection in adolescents increases.
3. High-risk teenagers: This group includes adolescents exposed to HIV-infected individuals, including homosexual contacts, injection drug users, or partners of either of these groups. Hein et al. (1995) examined the behavioral risk factors in HIV-infected adolescents compared to HIV-negative youth. HIV-positive adolescents were significantly more likely to be sexually abused, engage in anal sex and survival sex, have unprotected sex with casual partners, have had sex under the influence of drugs, have a sexually transmitted disease, use multiple drugs, and engage in multiple problem behaviors. HIV-positive females reported more oral or anal intercourse (or both) compared to HIV-negative females. HIV-positive males reported significantly higher rates of both insertive and receptive oral and anal intercourse than HIV-negative males.

PATHOPHYSIOLOGY

HIV initiates immune system dysfunction through the gradual decline in T helper (T_H) cells number and function. Most experts agree that HIV alone is sufficient to cause AIDS although many researchers continue to search for other cofactors like drugs and other infections that could hasten T_H cell decline.

While very little HIV can be found in the blood of recently infected persons, a great deal of HIV is found in lymph nodes. Early in infection, cellular and humoral immune responses appear to be effective in limiting viral replication. In perhaps 5–10% of individuals infected for over 10 years this immune response seems to keep HIV latent (these HIV-infected persons are often called "long-term survivors"). However, most individuals with HIV develop AIDS within 7–10 years.

How HIV causes T_H cell destruction is a focus of research. While HIV itself kills T_H cells this does not appear sufficient to explain the decline in T_H cells. Reviews on the pathogenesis of HIV can be found in the reference section (Levy, 1993; Weiss, 1993).

CLINICAL MANIFESTATIONS

The clinical spectrum of HIV infection ranges from healthy asymptomatic carriers to severely ill individuals with AIDS. The progression seems to be one way, although temporary periods of improved health can occur. It is difficult to predict how fast an individual will progress from one stage to another. Elevated levels of β_2-microglobulin, neopterin, P-24 antigen, and more recently HIV-RNA by polymerase chain reaction (PCR) predict more rapid development of illness. However, absolute CD4-positive lymphocyte count and percent closely parallel the clinical course.

Initial Infection

The first clinical evidence of infection is usually a mild mononucleosis-like syndrome. Seroconversion usually occurs between 6–24 weeks after the individual is infected. After initial infection the patient typically is asymptomatic for many years.

Early Manifestations of HIV Infection

Chronic lymphadenopathy
Unexplained weight loss
Oral candidiasis
Severe molluscum contagiosum
Seborrheic dermatitis
Isolated thrombocytopenia
Frequent tineas

Pruritic papular eruptions
Oral hairy leukoplakia
Chronic viral infections
Leukopenia
Exacerbations of psoriasis
Fatigue and malaise

Organ System Involvement

Pulmonary

1. Symptoms: Fever, dyspnea, nonproductive cough
2. Signs: Fever with minimal auscultatory findings
3. Organisms
   a. *Pneumocystis carinii* pneumonia (PCP): By far the most important common etiologic agent
   b. Cytomegalovirus (CMV)
   c. *Legionella* species
   d. *Mycobacterium avium-intracellulare* (MAI) or *Mycobacterium tuberculosis* (MTB)

   e. *Toxoplasma gondii*
   f. Blastomycosis
   g. *Histoplasma capsulatum*
   h. *Coccidioides immitis*
   i. *Nocardia*

Neurological   Major problems include primary HIV infection with its sequelae in the central nervous system (CNS), opportunistic infections, and cancers. The differential diagnosis of neurological problems can be broken down by symptom complex:

1. Meningitic signs and symptoms, including fever, headache, and focal neurological signs and symptoms
   a. CNS toxoplasmosis
   b. Progressive multifocal leukoencephalopathy
   c. Tuberculoma
   d. CMV meningoencephalitis
   e. Herpes simplex virus meningoencephalitis
   f. CNS lymphoma
   g. Cryptococcal meningitis
   h. Aseptic meningitis
2. Primary HIV meningitis: Progressive spinal cord syndrome with or without transverse myelitis. This is often associated with neurogenic bladder with flaccid motor weakness.
   a. Primary HIV
   b. Herpes simplex
   c. CMV
3. Mental status changes: Change in personality, loss of short-term memory, learning difficulties, and social isolation with or without seizures. Other common abnormalities include limb weakness, gait abnormalities, visual loss, and altered mental status. Most likely cause is HIV encephalopathy.
4. Peripheral neuropathy
   a. HIV infection
   b. Side effects of chemotherapy (vincristine, antiretrovirals)
5. Polymyopathy: Autoimmune phenomena

Gastrointestinal Syndromes   Gastrointestinal syndromes are usually manifested by profuse, watery diarrhea, abdominal pain, bloating, weight loss, and malabsorption.

1. Upper gastrointestinal tract disease is manifested mainly by dysphagia and hiccups
   a. Candida esophagitis
   b. CMV
   c. MAI or MTB
   d. Herpes esophagitis
   e. Kaposi's sarcoma (KS): Sarcoma derived from the endothelial cell of lymphatics in skin and mucosal surfaces
2. Lower gastrointestinal tract disease
   a. Abdominal pain without diarrhea
      — CMV
      — MTB or MAI
      — KS
      — *Cryptosporidium*
      — Abdominal lymphoma

   b. Diarrhea with or without cramps
      — Nonopportunistic infections including *Shigella, Campylobacter, Giardia, Entamoeba histolytica,* and *Blastocystis hominis*
      — *Cryptosporidium* or *Isospora belli*
      — *Clostridium*
      — Spruelike illness of unknown origin
3. Liver dysfunction: Liver function test results are often abnormal secondary to the wide array of systemic opportunistic organisms, neoplasias, and subsequent treatments used.

Rheumatological

1. Arthritis
   a. Reiter's syndrome and other reactive arthritides
   b. HIV-associated arthritis
   c. Psoriatic arthritis
   d. Septic arthritis caused by opportunistic organisms
2. Arthralgias
3. Myopathies
   a. Polymyositis
   b. Myositis ossificans
   c. Zidovudine-induced myositis
   d. Necrotizing, noninflammatory myopathy
   e. Infectious myositis with opportunistic organisms
4. Vasculitis
5. Sjögren's (sicca) syndrome
6. Autoimmune phenomena including antinuclear antibodies, antiplatelet antibodies, antilymphocyte antibodies, antigranulocyte antibodies, direct Coombs' test, immune complexes, rheumatoid factor, and cryoglobulins

Renal

1. Fluid and electrolyte abnormalities including hyponatremia
2. HIV-associated nephropathy
3. Nonglomerular renal lesions
   a. Disseminated infections
   b. Neoplasias
   c. Acute tubular necrosis
   d. Allergic interstitial nephritis
   e. Vascular including hemolytic-uremic syndrome

Skin and Mucosal Surfaces

1. KS
2. Oral or vaginal candidiasis
3. Gingivitis
4. Herpes zoster
5. Severe seborrheic dermatitis
6. Herpetic ulcerations
7. Oral hairy leukoplakia
8. Molluscum contagiosum
9. Syphilis

10. Dry skin
11. Extensive warts
12. Folliculitis

Retinal Problems

1. PCP
2. CMV retinitis
3. Reaction to HIV antigen itself
4. Toxoplasmosis
5. Syphilis

Hematological

1. Anemia
2. Leukopenia
3. Thrombocytopenia: Related to nonspecific deposition of complement and immune complexes on platelets and not antiplatelet immunoglobulin G (IgG), as in autoimmune thrombocytopenia purpura

Endocrine

1. Adrenal gland dysfunction secondary to opportunistic infections and KS: Drugs such as ketoconazole may also produce adrenal insufficiency.
2. Pituitary gland abnormalities: Syndrome of inappropriate antidiuretic hormone (SIADH) secondary to pulmonary or CNS infections or drugs
3. Testis: Hypogonadism secondary to hypothalamic deficiency associated with systemic illness or use of ketoconazole
4. Gynecomastia secondary to use of ketoconazole
5. Parathyroid: Hypocalcemia secondary to systemic illness or hypomagnesemia
6. Pancreatic islets: Hypoglycemia secondary to use of pentamidine, poor nutrition, or sepsis

Lymph Nodes   Generalized lymphadenopathy frequently develops in patients with HIV infection. With time the lymphadenopathy tends to diminish and is often a precursor to development of opportunistic infections. If one or more specific groups of nodes develops or expands rapidly, consider a lymphoma or KS. If hilar adenopathy develops, evaluate for a lymphoma.

Fever of Unknown Origin

1. Lymphoma
2. MAI or MTB: MAI and *Mycobacterium tuberculosis* cause disseminated disease in 25–50% of individuals with AIDS. MAI causes a nonspecific wasting syndrome with fever, malaise, anorexia, weight loss, weakness, night sweats, and diarrhea.
3. Any opportunistic infection

Common Infections with Important Alterations if Coinfected with HIV

1. Tuberculosis (TB): Tuberculosis and other mycobacteriosis have increased with the epidemic of HIV infection. HIV is an important risk factor for TB. It is also one of the few

respiratory diseases in HIV persons that is transmissible, curable, and preventable. In HIV patients, TB may present differently, with less apical pulmonary disease and more mediastinal, hilar lymphadenopathy, and extrapulmonary disease.

2. Syphilis: Several questions have arisen about how HIV alters the course of syphilis. While there have been no controlled studies, it appears that:
    a. Neurosyphilis may be more common in persons with HIV or AIDS.
    b. Some individuals with symptomatic syphilis may be serologically negative.
    c. Current treatments for infected patients may be inadequate in HIV-infected patients.

Indications for Cerebrospinal Fluid Examination in Patients with Syphilis

1. Syphilis at any stage with neurological or behavioral manifestations
2. Treatment failure
    a. Primary syphilis: Titer should decrease by two dilutions by 3 months and be seronegative by 1 year.
    b. Secondary syphilis: Titer should decrease by two dilutions by 6 months and be seronegative by 2 years.
3. Latent syphilis for over 1 year

TREATMENT OF SYPHILIS IN HIV-INFECTED PATIENTS

1. Syphilis of less than 1 year's duration
    a. Treatment recommended
        — Benzathine penicillin G 2.4 million units intramuscularly (IM)
    b. Unstudied alternatives
        — Benzathine penicillin G 2.4 million units IM weekly for 2–3 weeks
        — Doxycycline 100 mg b.i.d. for 14 days
2. Syphilis for over 1 year's duration
    a. Treatment recommended
        — Benzathine penicillin G 2.4 million units IM weekly for 3 weeks
    b. Unstudied alternatives
        — Above plus amoxicillin 2 g and probenecid 500 mg orally three times daily for 14 days (especially if patient refuses lumbar puncture)
        — Doxycycline 200 mg b.i.d. for 21 days orally
3. Neurosyphilis
    a. Treatment recommended
        — Aqueous crystalline penicillin G 2.4 million units IV every 4 hours for 10–14 days, OR
        — Aqueous procaine penicillin G 2.4 million units IM daily plus probenecid 500 mg orally q.i.d. for 10 days plus benzathine penicillin G 2.4 million units weekly for 3 weeks
    b. Unstudied alternatives
        — Ceftriaxone 1 g IM daily for 14 days

TESTING

Antibody Test

Most laboratories offer enzyme-linked immunosorbent assay (ELISA) screening with a confirmatory Western blot analysis for any blood specimen with two consecutive positive ELISA test results. A positive ELISA test result should never be reported to a patient as a positive test result for HIV. A positive Western blot has almost 100% specificity. Western blot tests can be indeterminate. This is common for patients in the window phase between acute infection and seroconversion. However, many patients with indeterminate tests will later test HIV negative by ELISA or Western blot. It is recommended that testing be repeated after 3 months for an indeterminate Western blot. Occasionally, laboratories use indirect immunofluorescent assay (IFA) as a confirmatory test, which also has over 99% specificity.

Other HIV Testing Techniques

1. Viral culture
2. P24 antigen: Results may be positive during acute HIV illness.
3. PCR

Consent and Confidentiality

Health-care practitioners must balance the protection of adolescents' rights against the amount of information needed to deliver proper care.

Individuals over 18 Years of Age Who Are Competent   These individuals must make an informed consent for HIV testing, which involves a dialogue of the risks and benefits of the test, the implications of the test, and alternatives to the test.

Individuals between 12 and 17   The laws vary widely from state to state. In many states the adolescent can and must give his or her own consent; however, as in any informed consent, the individual must be considered by the practitioner as competent to give an informed consent.

Individuals under 12 or Incompetent Adolescents   For these individuals a third party (parent or guardian) would authorize the testing. However, this may be restricted by state laws.

An increasing number of states have statutes governing HIV testing. Without such a statute, general laws regarding minors apply. In most states, adolescents can give their own consent for diagnosis and treatment of STD or contagious disease. It is not clear if HIV testing would fall under this category in states that do not declare AIDS to be a sexually transmitted disease. In some states adolescents are authorized to and must give their own consent. Generally, those adolescents who are judged to have the right to consent are considered to have the right to refuse testing and the right of confidentiality.

The physician should be aware of the current local laws regarding:

1. Consent for testing: Who can consent? What is the required informed consent? Are pretest and posttest counseling available?
2. Who can get the results of these tests?
3. Where can the test results be recorded?
4. Can results be disclosed to other involved individuals and under what circumstances?
5. What can be written in the chart regarding testing and test results?

To Whom Should HIV Testing Be Offered?

Teens whose behaviors put them at risk for HIV should be offered testing. Certain groups of youth are at very high risk:

1. Men who have sex with other men (youth in this group may not self-identify as gay or bisexual)
2. Youth who share needles (including tattooing, ear piercing, steroid injection, and recreational drugs)

3. Youth with partners from the above two groups
4. Youth who have had intercourse or shared needles with HIV-infected persons
5. Youth with sexually transmitted diseases
6. Pregnant or parenting youth
7. Sexually active youth from inner city or economically disadvantaged areas
8. Youth with multiple sexual partners
9. Recipients of blood transfusion prior to April 1985 in the United States; in some countries blood transfusions remain a risk factor

Other groups of youth who may benefit from testing:

1. Any sexually active youth
2. Youth with histories of sexual abuse
3. Youth with no apparent risk but seeking testing (they may not be able to confide risky behaviors or past sexual abuse)

Who Should Have HIV Testing Deferred?

1. Suicidal youth or youth who seriously state they would be suicidal if HIV positive
2. Intoxicated or drug-withdrawing youth
3. Severely mentally ill youth who cannot consent for testing

When Should Testing Be Repeated for Youth with Positive Confirmatory HIV Test Results?

1. Any youth desiring a second test
2. Any youth claiming to be HIV positive but with unreliable documentation (youth have falsely reported being HIV positive)
3. Extremely low-risk youth with a single positive test
4. Youth with normal T_H cells and only a single positive test in the past

Methods for HIV Testing

Anonymous   Youth are not identified by name but are given a number. Many youth prefer this method due to confidentiality issues, but it may lower the rate of return for posttest counseling or the rate of follow-up for early intervention or medical care if the adolescent is found to be HIV positive.

Confidential   Pretest and posttest counseling are done, and the results are part of the medical record. Normal laws regarding patient confidentiality still protect clients. Since the counselor or physician will likely know the patient's name and address, testers will be able to follow up with positive clients to ensure they receive adequate care.

Youth-Specific Testing   Many testing sites now have counselors (including peers) who are specifically trained to work with adolescents. The testing sites may be perceived as youth friendly, and the counselors may have more time for complete evaluations of risky behaviors and have knowledge of how to help youth change unhealthy behaviors. Often these youth-friendly sites are located where other services or activities are available (i.e., homeless shelters, free clinics, schools, recreational centers). Youth-specific testing should be recommended whenever possible because it can be an effective component of prevention education.

Pretest Counseling

Before testing, the adolescent should receive counseling regarding the nature of the test and the implications of both a negative and a positive test result. The teen must also give voluntary consent for the test, as well as be provided with any information on state or local laws that may affect disclosure of the test results. Pretest counseling could be assisted by means of videotape, printed material, or group lectures.

Good counseling skills are important to the success of the HIV-antibody testing process. This includes establishment of rapport with the teen and genuine, nonjudgmental concern and positive regard for the teen. The practitioner should allow the adolescent time to express feelings and reactions. Additional counseling or referral to specialized services should be done when necessary.

The American Medical Association (AMA) has developed guidelines on HIV blood test counseling (Rinaldi, 1988). Suggested essential parts of pretest counseling include:

1. Ask why the individual believes he or she should be tested.
2. Explain that AIDS is caused by a virus called HIV (human immunodeficiency virus) and that the virus infects the body and slowly damages the immune system.
3. Explain the modes of transmission:
   a. The virus is spread through the exchange of blood, semen, and vaginal secretions during sexual intercourse.
   b. HIV is spread through exchange of blood when syringes and injection drug needles are shared.
   c. Prior to 1985, when blood screening began, the virus was spread through blood transfusions. This risk has been minimal since 1985.
   d. Infected pregnant women can pass the virus to their unborn children (prenatally, perinatally, or through breast-feeding).
4. Explain that the test determines the presence or absence of antibodies to the virus. Estimates of the time between exposure and a positive test result are 6–12 weeks; however, the time from exposure to appearance of detectable antibodies may be longer. It is usually recommended that testing be conducted 3–6 months after presumed exposure. If a test is done immediately in anxious individuals, it should be repeated in 3–6 months.
5. Discuss the meaning of a positive and a negative test result. A positive test result means an individual has been infected and that certain behaviors can transmit the virus. A negative test result probably means no current infection but does not suggest future immunity. It is even possible that the individual has been infected but has not yet produced any antibodies.
6. Discuss the possibilities of false-positive and indeterminate results. An indeterminate result is a nondiagnostic band pattern on the Western blot confirmatory test. If this is the case, an alternative confirmatory test may be employed or testing repeated in 4–12 weeks.
7. Discuss sexual behavior and drug history or other risk behaviors. The practitioner should have taken a psychosocial history (e.g., a HEADSS inventory, see Chapter 3), which focuses on sexual behaviors, and a drug history. The physician should use frank, nonjudgmental questions and avoid technical jargon. The teen should be aware of why these questions are being asked. An introductory statement such as "To give you the best care I can, I need to ask some specific questions about your lifestyle and behaviors that relate to your health" is a good approach. This history should include:
   a. Prior history of STDs
   b. Current sexual practices and number of steady or nonsteady partners
   c. Past sexual practices

d. Regular sexual partners including any sex with male or female prostitutes, injection drug users, bisexual or homosexual males, or suspected or confirmed HIV-infected individuals
e. Regular sexual practices including:
— Penile-vaginal activity (use of condoms)
— Oral-genital activity (receptive, insertive, use of condoms)
— Anal-genital activity (receptive, insertive, ejaculation, bleeding, use of lubricants, use of condoms)
— Oral-anal activity (receptive, insertive)
— Mutual masturbation
f. Use and frequency of drugs including alcohol, marijuana, barbiturates, amphetamines and other stimulants, hallucinogens, cocaine, and heroin and other injected drugs
8. Discuss risk reduction techniques and safer sex:
a. Unprotected sex with partners who have AIDS or HIV or who engage in high-risk behaviors is dangerous and should be avoided.
b. The more sexual partners one has, the greater the risk of exposure. To lower the risk:
— Abstinence or mutual monogamy among partners known to be uninfected provides the surest protection against sexual transmission.
— The proper use of a latex condom during intercourse provides protection. Ideally a condom demonstration should be given.
— Sexual activities that could cause cuts or tears in the lining of the rectum, penis, or vagina should be avoided.
— Sex with male or female prostitutes should be avoided.
— Sharing needles or syringes with anyone should be avoided.
9. Discuss the difference between confidential and anonymous testing. Under certain conditions, confidentiality may be broken and information released with confidential testing. In anonymous testing, no identifying patient information is collected. Since laws differ from state to state and change rapidly, the practitioner must become familiar with current local regulations governing reporting and confidentiality. Laws may be particularly ambiguous as to how they pertain to adolescents.
10. Discuss possible stress between the time of testing and the teen's finding out the results.
11. Discuss potential negative social consequences of being tested seropositive. These could include effects on employment, housing, insurance, and personal relationships.
12. Obtain written consent for voluntary testing.
13. Make a follow-up appointment to discuss results.

Posttest Counseling

Posttest counseling should be given in person and should include:

1. Provide the results of test. This should be done in a direct manner at the beginning of the posttest session.
2. Allow the adolescent time to express feelings and reactions. If the test result is positive, it is important to give the adolescent hope, using information such as that only 7–10% of infected individuals actually become ill each year and that significant research and advances are occurring each month.
3. Assess the adolescent's understanding of the result. This is best assessed by asking the teen directly what the test result means to him or her. If negative, the teen should understand how to prevent future infection. If positive, the teen should understand how to avoid infecting others. The teen should also understand that although the virus is prob-

ably present for life, a positive antibody test does not mean one has AIDS. Antibody-positive adolescents should know:

a. Do not donate blood, semen, or body organs.
b. Employ safer sex practices.
c. Inform physicians and dentists of HIV status.
d. Encourage sexual partners and needle contacts to seek evaluation and testing.
e. No evidence exists that HIV is transmitted to family household members or to close contacts by routes other than sexual intercourse, exposure to infected blood, and perinatal transmission.
f. Household items may be shared by HIV-infected individuals and household members. Dishes and eating utensils should be routinely washed in hot water and a detergent. Personal hygiene items (i.e., razors and toothbrushes) should not be shared.
g. The HIV-seropositive individual's blood and other body fluids should be handled with care. Soiled clothes or linen should be washed with a detergent or bleach.
h. Bathroom facilities can be used by all household members.

4. Review routes of transmission.
5. Assess teen's emotional status and arrange for counseling follow-up when appropriate.
6. Assess risk behavior and work with the teen to promote a commitment to alter high-risk behaviors.
7. Recommend medical follow-up and other support services when appropriate.

MANAGEMENT OF HIV-INFECTED ADOLESCENTS

Initial Assessment

History and Physical Examination   The history and physical examination should stress:

1. Prior exposure to diseases that are likely to reactivate in individuals with HIV, including TB, syphilis, herpes genitalis, herpes zoster, or CMV
2. Number of children, ages, and health status
3. Injection drug use history and history of alcohol and other drug use
4. Travel history to find out about possible exposure to fungal infections that are endemic in certain areas such as histoplasmosis, coccidioidomycosis, or blastomycosis
5. Sexual history
6. Prior immunizations
7. A review of systems should focus particularly on:
   a. Systemic: Anorexia, weight loss, fevers, night sweats
   b. Skin: Pruritus, rashes, pigmented lesions
   c. Lymphatics: Increased size of lymph nodes
   d. Head, eyes, ears, nose, and throat: Headache, change in vision, sinus congestion
   e. Cardiopulmonary: Cough, dyspnea
   f. Gastrointestinal: Dysphagia, abdominal pain, diarrhea
   g. Musculoskeletal: Myalgias, arthralgias
   h. Neurological: Memory loss, neuralgias, motor weakness, depression, headache
8. Careful measurement of weight at each visit
9. Careful examination particularly focusing on:
   a. Skin: Seborrhea, folliculitis, KS lesions, psoriasis, tinea, herpetic lesions, molluscum contagiosum
   b. Eye: Visual acuity and fields, cotton-wool and hemorrhagic exudates on fundoscopic examination

    c. Mouth: Hairy leukoplakia (white plaques along lateral aspect of tongue), thrush, oral ulcers, KS lesions

    d. Lymphatics: Asymmetric, tender, enlarged nodes, particularly posterior cervical, axillary, and epitrochlear

    e. Cardiopulmonary: Rales, murmurs (in injection drug users)

    f. Gastrointestinal: Hepatosplenomegaly

    g. Rectal: Perianal herpes, condyloma, fissures, proctitis

    h. Neurological: Focal findings, altered mental status

Laboratory Evaluation   Initial assessment should include:

1. Complete blood count (CBC; for anemia, leukopenia, or pancytopenia)
2. Platelet count
3. Chemistry panel (looking for hypergammaglobulinemia, hypoalbuminemia, hypocholesterolemia, increased liver enzymes, or decreased renal function)
4. Urinalysis
5. T4 helper or inducer lymphocyte cell count (CD4+ cell count and percent)
6. Purified protein derivative of tuberculin (PPD) skin test
7. Multiple skin anergy screening
8. Serology for toxoplasmosis, syphilis, and hepatitis B
9. Chest x-ray examination if anergic or positive PPD
10. Tests for gonorrhea and chlamydia infections if HIV was acquired sexually
11. Pap smear and rubella serology in women

Vaccinations

1. Influenza: Should be given annually to all HIV-infected individuals.
2. Pneumococcal: Should be given once in previously unimmunized individuals.
3. *Haemophilus influenzae* (Hib): Consider giving this to all patients although cost-effectiveness has not been studied.
4. Hepatitis B: Recommended for all patients without evidence of hepatitis B immunity or chronic infection.
5. Measles-Mumps-Rubella (MMR): All patients should have received two MMR vaccinations in their lifetime. MMR is considered safe in patients with HIV.
6. Tetanus-Diphtheria: Same as if uninfected.
7. Polio: Patients requiring primary or booster immunizations should only receive the inactive form (inactivated poliovirus [IPV] not oral poliovirus vaccine [OPV]).
8. Chickenpox (Varicella): Chickenpox vaccination is now available for children and adults. At present there are no recommendations for its use in HIV-infected individuals. The vaccine is not advised for use in those with acquired or primary immunodeficiencies.

Follow-up

Patients should have their medical and social needs assessed at least every 3 months. These appointments should focus on signs and symptoms of disease progression, coping skills, and secondary prevention education. Secondary prevention focuses on preventing the spread of HIV to others but also prevents unwanted pregnancy and STDs that are commonly seen in youth. Follow-up should include:

1. CBC with platelet count and CD4 count every 3–6 months
2. Optional β_2-microglobulin, P-24 antigen neopterin or quantitative HIV RNA by PCR to evaluate for risk of progression
3. Chemistry panel every 6–12 months

4. PPD and controls yearly
5. Chest x-ray examination if anergic
6. VDRL or rapid plasma reagin (RPR) yearly
7. Toxoplasmosis IgG yearly if previously negative (may be cost effective to defer until CD4 less than or equal to 200 cells/mL)
8. Pap smear every 6–12 months in women
9. Regular discussion of safe(r) sex and family planning
10. Discussion of partner notification as needed
11. Discussion of nutrition, exercise, disease progression, medication options, potential clinical trials
12. Regular evaluation of emotional status
13. Focused interval history and physical examination, concentrating on illnesses common for the patient's stage of illness

Common Psychosocial Problems

1. Depression and suicidal ideation
2. Substance abuse
3. Self-blame
4. Social isolation: Including family and peers
5. Unsafe sex
6. Sexual identity
7. Homelessness
8. Survival sex
9. Denial

The cornerstone to good care is the availability of a strong primary care team including physician, nurse, social worker, psychologist or psychiatrist, nutritionist, substance abuse counselor, and medical subspecialists as needed. Coordinating the team to focus on the *patient's identified needs* will improve compliance and facilitate normal adolescent development.

Travel

Visiting regions outside one's normal community can expose an individual to many pathogens. In developing countries opportunities for exposure to enteric pathogens including *Cryptosporidium* and *Isospora* increase. Risk for certain respiratory infections like coccidioidomycosis, histoplasmosis, and TB also increase in many developing countries and in certain geographic regions of the United States. The CDC offer an international travelers' hotline (404-332-4555). Patients planning significant travel should discuss preventive strategies with their physician.

1. Avoid contaminated food and drink (i.e., tap water).
2. Receive appropriate immunizations.
3. Extended travel should be accompanied by appropriate medications and phone numbers of emergency care.
4. Seek medical attention promptly if fever, diarrhea, or other illness occurs both during and after travel.

Sports Participation

When Ervin "Magic" Johnson announced he was infected with HIV, many questions surrounding the advisability of vigorous exercise occurred. To date there have been no studies documenting a positive or negative impact of exercise on HIV. Currently, we recommend using common sense in guiding the youth on sports participation.

There have been no documented cases of HIV transmission during athletic participation. We would not withhold a youth from competitive sports (even full contact like wrestling or football) solely on HIV status. The principal risks athletes have for acquiring HIV are related to off-the-field settings (Mast et al., 1995). However, all participants (HIV infected or uninfected) should not compete when open wounds occur, and universal precautions should always be followed when bleeding occurs.

Evaluation of Specific Syndromes

Pulmonary (Cough or Shortness of Breath)

1. If CD4 count is less than or equal to 200 cells/mL or CD4 percent is less than or equal to 20% the patient requires:
   a. Chest x-ray examination: Look for interstitial infiltrates or other infiltrates
   b. Arterial blood gas (ABG) for hypoxemia
   c. Induced sputum for PCP
   d. Consider gallium scan or bronchoscopy for PCP evaluation
2. In patients with CD4 count higher than 200 cells/mL and CD4 percent higher than 20% it is unlikely to be PCP:
   a. Consider evaluation for bronchitis, sinusitis, TB, and bacterial pneumonia
   b. Chest x-ray examination or sinus films
   c. Subsequent PPD and controls
   d. Sputum for culture and sensitivity (C & S), acid-fast bacillus (AFB)

Fever   Evaluation in patients with severe immunosuppression (CD4 <200 cells/mL) but lack of specific organ system signs or symptoms should include the following:

1. Chest x-ray examination: Interstitial infiltrates are consistent with PCP, *Mycobacterium avium* complex (MAC), CMV; focal infiltrates are consistent with TB, bacterial pneumonia
2. CBC: Anemia is common in MAC
3. Chemistry panel: Elevated lactate dehydrogenase (LDH) is common with PCP, elevated alkaline phosphatase is common in MAC
4. Blood cultures for bacteria, virus (CMV), fungus, and AFB
5. Serum cryptococcal antigen

If fever persists and above is inconclusive consider:

1. Lumbar puncture: May pick up cryptococcal infection
2. Bone marrow biopsy: May pick up disseminated MAC, CMV, or fungus
3. Ophthalmology consult: Looking for CMV
4. Body computed tomography (CT): Looking for lymphoma
5. Sinus films

In patients with mild immunosuppression (CD4 counts are 200–500 cells/mL)

1. Look for common illnesses: Viral or bacterial
2. Consider looking for TB, sinusitis, pneumonia

In patients with minimal immune suppression (CD4 count >500 cells/mL) avoid costly workups unless conservative evaluation fails.

Diarrhea

Patients with Severe Immunodeficiency (CD4 Count <200 cells/mL)

1. If diarrhea is mild, consider empiric treatment with diphenoxylate (Lomotil) or loperamide (Imodium).

2. If diarrhea is severe, check stool for ova and parasites (O & P), C & S, *Cryptosporidium* and *Isospora*.
3. If above is inconclusive, consider colonoscopy looking for CMV, MAC, and *Isospora*.

Patients without Severe Immunodeficiency

1. Usually self-limited and one should avoid costly evaluations.
2. Consider stool O & P, bacterial C & S if patient is sexually active, homeless, or had recent foreign travel.

Neurological (New Headaches, Seizures, Focal Neurologic Signs)

Patients with Severe Immunodeficiency (CD4 Count <200 cells/mL)

1. Emergency CT or magnetic resonance imaging (MRI) of head: Multiple enhancing ring lesions are usually indicative of toxoplasmosis. Primary CNS lymphoma is also common.
2. Lumbar puncture for cell count, protein, cryptococcal antigen, Gram's stain, routine AFB, and fungal cultures, VDRL

Dysphagia

1. If oral thrush is present, consider empiric treatment for *Candida* organisms with fluconazole or ketoconazole.
2. If there is no oral thrush or above empiric treatment fails, try endoscopy with evaluations for fungus, CMV, and herpes simplex virus (HSV).

Prophylaxis

Prophylaxis is one of the most important ways patients with severe immunosuppression can maintain their health. Great advances in primary and secondary prophylaxis have been made in recent years and are summarized in the following outlines. Of interest, we have found that adolescents comply with and tolerate prophylactic medications much better than antiretrovirals and may have more benefit in terms of quality of life.

Primary Prophylaxis

1. Pneumocystis: Initiate when CD4 count is less than or equal to 200 cells/mL or CD4 percent is less than or equal to 20%.
   a. Drug of choice: Trimethoprim-sulfamethoxazole double strength tablet daily or three times weekly
   b. Alternatives: Dapsone 50–100 mg orally per day (check for glucose-6-phosphate dehydrogenase [G6PD] deficiency prior to using); nebulized pentamidine 150 mg every 2 weeks or 300 mg every 4 weeks via Respirguard II nebulizer (May be method of choice in noncompliant youth.)
2. Tuberculosis: Initiate in teens who are PPD positive or who are anergic but come from populations at high risk for exposure (i.e., born in developing country, history of homelessness, or history of substance abuse).
   a. Drug of choice: Isoniazid (INH) 300 mg daily for at least 1 year
   b. Alternative: Rifampin 600 mg daily for at least 1 year
3. *Mycobacterium avium* complex: Initiate when CD4 counts are less than or equal to 100 cells/mL

    a. Drug of choice: Rifabutin 300 mg daily

    b. Alternative: Clarithromycin 500 mg one to two times daily (However, resistance seems to develop quickly.)

4. Candida and cryptococcus: *Experimental*

    a. Drug of choice: Fluconazole 100 mg daily; Consider in patients with no history of severe fungal infections but CD4 counts less than or equal to 100 cells/mL.

Secondary Prophylaxis

1. Herpes simplex: Initiate in patients with frequent or severe outbreaks.

    a. Treatment of choice: Acyclovir 400 mg b.i.d. minimum (This in combination with zidovudine has been shown to prolong survival in patients with HIV and HSV.)

    b. Alternative: Foscarnet IV

2. Cryptococcal meningitis

    a. Treatment of choice: Lifelong oral fluconazole 200 mg daily

    b. Alternative: Amphotericin B 1 mg/kg weekly

3. Candidiasis: Consider in patients with recurrent esophagitis, vaginitis, or pharyngitis.

    a. Treatment of choice: Fluconazole 100 mg/week to 100 mg daily

    b. Alternative: Ketoconazole 200 mg daily (less effective than fluconazole but also less expensive); Nystatin 500,000 units five times daily for oral thrush; clotrimazole troches 10 mg five times daily for oral thrush

4. Toxoplasmosis

    a. Treatment of choice: Pyrimethamine 25–50 mg daily plus sulfadiazine 0.5–1 g four times daily plus folinic acid 5 mg daily

    b. Alternative: Pyrimethamine 25–50 mg daily plus clindamycin 300–450 mg t.i.d. to q.i.d. plus folinic acid 5 mg daily

Antiretroviral Therapy

Currently there are six antiretrovirals available, but this number should increase soon. Azidothymidine (AZT, old name; zidovudine [ZDV], new name), didanosine (DDI), zalcitabine (DDC), stavudine (D4T), and lamivudine (3TC) are all nucleoside analog reverse transcriptase inhibitors and reduce viral replication. The newest medication released is sanguinavir, which is an inhibitor of HIV protease. After years of initiating patients on ZDV monotherapy, recent data from the AIDS Clinical Trials (ACTC) Study 175 demonstrated that combination therapy with ZDV and either DDI or DDC is superior to monotherapy with ZDV or DDI. Initial evidence also suggests that triple therapy with ZDV, 3TC, and a protease inhibitor may come close to complete viral suppression. Important caveats for use in youth include frequent noncompliance, especially as the frequency of dosing increases. The author's experience is that use of fear tactics or pressure does not improve compliance. Instead use gentle guidance, thorough explanations of benefits and side effects, and patience. In more immunocompromised patients (i.e., CD4 counts <200 cells/mL) consider starting prophylactic medications prior to antiretrovirals. For patients interested in aggressive treatment, consider referral to an AIDS Clinical Trial Group (ACTG) or Community Program for Clinical Research on AIDS (CPCRA). For information on experimental protocols call 1-800-Trials-A.

    For pregnant teens the use of zidovudine both prenatally and perinatally has demonstrated a marked reduction in mother-to-child transmission of HIV. Connor et al. (1994) in pregnant women with mildly symptomatic HIV disease and no prior treatment with antiretroviral drugs during pregnancy found that a regimen of zidovudine given antepartum and intrapartum to the mother and newborn for 6 weeks reduced the risk of maternal-infant HIV transmission by approximately two-thirds.

With the availability of six antiretrovirals, there are no comprehensive studies of all possible combinations on which to base firm recommendations for treatment. However, we suggest the following guidelines:

1. For symptomatic patients or patients with CD4 cells less than 500 cells/mL, we recommend starting antiretroviral therapy with any of the following combinations:
   a. ZDV plus DDI
   b. ZDV plus 3TC
   c. ZDV plus DDC
   d. DDI plus D4T
2. For patients with new symptoms (including a new opportunistic infection), a fall in CD4 count by 25–50% on a given regimen or medication intolerance, consider changing to a new combination with two or more novel medications (the exception is that 3TC-naive patients may benefit from a combination of ZDV and 3TC), regardless of previous ZDV use.
3. For patients with poor compliance, consider monotherapy with D4T. While not strongly advised, monotherapy with ZDV, DDI, or DDC can be considered, but monotherapy with 3TC or saguinavir should never be used because of the rapid development of resistance.
4. Although little is known about saguinavir combination therapy, it should be considered in patients who have failed other regimens or show rapid CD4 cell decline.
5. There is much promise in using combination drugs including ZDV, 3TC, and one of the new protease inhibitors. Newer protease inhibitors including indinavir and ritonavir may prove even more potent than saguinavir, the first in this class to be approved.

Antiretroviral Dosing and Toxicity

1. AZT
   a. Initial dose is 100 mg t.i.d. Increase to 200 mg t.i.d. as tolerated. Alternative dosing includes 100 mg five times per day or 300 mg b.i.d. or 100 mg t.i.d. in patients unable to tolerate higher doses.
   b. Early toxicity includes headache, nausea, myalgias, and insomnia and usually resolve in the first few weeks of therapy.
   c. Late effects include bone marrow suppression, myopathy, rashes, and nail discoloration.
2. DDI
   a. Dosing: Greater than or equal to 60 kg two 100-mg tablets on empty stomach b.i.d.; less than or equal to 60 kg one 100-mg tablet and one 25-mg tablet on empty stomach b.i.d.
   b. Toxicity: Pancreatitis, peripheral neuropathy, gastrointestinal intolerance, rash
3. DDC
   a. Dosing: 0.75 mg t.i.d. as monotherapy; 0.375 mg t.i.d. in combination therapy is frequently used.
   b. Toxicity: Includes pancreatitis, peripheral neuropathy, hepatitis, rash and oral ulcers
4. D4T
   a. Dosing: Greater than or equal to 60 kg 40 mg b.i.d.; less than or equal to 60 kg 30 mg b.i.d.
   b. Toxicity: Peripheral neuropathy, elevated transaminases
5. 3TC
   a. Dosing: 150 mg b.i.d. (use only in combination with ZDV)
   b. Toxicity: Headache, nausea, malaise, nasal symptoms, diarrhea, and neuropathy

6. Saguinavir
   a. Dosing: Three 200-mg capsules t.i.d. taken within 2 hours after a full meal
   b. Toxicity: Elevated transaminases

Future Antiviral Therapy

1. Protease inhibitors: This class of antiviral medication has been found to be extremely potent in reducing HIV viral load. However, resistance to this class of medication has occurred quickly and must be overcome before it will be clinically useful.
2. Nonnucleoside reverse transcriptase inhibitors: Clinical trials are currently evaluating the efficacy of this class of antiviral agents.
3. Vaccines: Thus far vaccine has not proved beneficial, but studies continue.
4. Gene therapy: This is another area of research but it is unlikely that this form of therapy will be available in the near future.

Prognosis

1. Twenty percent to 30% of those infected with HIV develop AIDS or illness within 5 years. According to the San Francisco City Clinic Cohort Study, the mean time period from infection with HIV until AIDS (opportunistic infection or neoplasm) is 9.8 years.
2. Mortality: Fifty-six percent of all AIDS patients and 85% of those diagnosed before 1986 are reported to have died. Due to incomplete reporting of deaths, the actual case fatality rate is higher. The San Francisco City Clinic Cohort Study group shows an average survival after diagnosis of AIDS of 15 months. However, these data pertain only to a cohort of gay men.
3. Prognostic indicators of disease progression:
   a. Low or declining absolute CD4+ cell counts: Cell counts of over 500 cells/mL are a good sign, whereas cell counts under 200 are associated with a very poor prognosis and severe immunodeficiency. For those individuals with a CD4+ lymphocyte count less than 200 cells/mL, 31% will develop an opportunistic infection or neoplasm within 1 year and 84% within 4 years. The CD4+ lymphocyte count is the best single predictor of prognosis to AIDS (Fahey et al., 1990).
   b. Increased serum β_2-microglobulin level
   c. Neopterin (a product of stimulated macrophages)
   d. HIV P-24 antigenemia: This has little predictive value over CD4+ lymphocyte counts.
   e. Rising levels of HIV by PCR
   f. Anemia
   g. Increased erythrocyte sedimentation rate (ESR)
   h. Anergy

Prevention

1. Education: Until a vaccine is found, health education and counseling are the main tools to reduce the risk of infection. Appropriate educational interventional goals for adolescents include:
   a. Reducing misinformation and panic among teens
   b. Helping to reduce high-risk behavior, including recommendations to decrease sexual activity, numbers of partners, and experimentation with drugs
   c. Increasing the use of condoms in adolescents having intercourse
   AIDS education needs to be conducted at schools, religious organizations, youth organizations, medical facilities, and in meetings with parents. Such programs should include information about:
   — Epidemiology of AIDS
   — Myths about AIDS
   — Sexual transmission and prevention, including abstinence, safer sex, and condom use

— Transmission through needles and drug use prevention
— AIDS and pregnancy
— Testing and counseling
— Biology of AIDS
— Medical aspects of AIDS
— Peer pressure and dating skills
— Community resources

It is important to offer AIDS education in language that the adolescent can under-stand. The information must be simple, accurate, and direct.

Many youths are not at school and thus are not reachable through school programs. Street youth service workers who have regular contact with these teens may be effective AIDS educators. Involving peers in the education process can also be helpful.

2. Networks of youth-serving agencies: Task forces on adolescent AIDS representing health education and social service agencies need to be developed further.
3. Development of educational materials: The CDC have established a central clearing-house for existing materials (see "Resources" list at end of this chapter).
4. Survey tools of attitudes, knowledge, and beliefs among adolescents must be developed and standardized.
5. Condom distribution must be improved.
6. Studies of the incidence, prevalence, and natural history of HIV infections must be conducted.
7. Ethical and legal guidelines need evaluation for youth.
8. Particular subpopulations of adolescents such as gay youth and heterosexual youth en-gaging in homosexual intercourse and injection drug use are at increased risk for AIDS and may derive greater benefit from prevention programs than many teenagers and adults.
9. A comprehensive system of care should be developed for seropositive youth. Counseling is a core component of this care, as well as resources for meeting basic survival needs.

Recommendations for Primary Care Physicians

Primary care practitioners should:

1. Obtain a sexual history and perform counseling on safer sexual behaviors.
2. Be able to perform pretest and posttest HIV antibody counseling.
3. Be able to manage asymptomatic individuals with HIV infections.
4. Know how to evaluate common AIDS-related symptoms such as fever, lymphadenopa-thy, headache, and diarrhea.
5. Be able to identify which patients will require referral to subspecialists (e.g., individuals with KS and CMV retinitis).
6. Be familiar with community resources for adolescents with HIV infections.

Controlling Transmission   Blood and body fluid precautions should be consistently used for all patients, as medical history and examination cannot reliably identify all patients infected with HIV.

RESOURCES

Selected National HIV Resources

National Pediatric Resource Center
15 South 9th Street
Newark, NJ 07107
201-268-8251
800-362-0071
FAX 201-485-2753

Magic Johnson Foundation
1888 Century Plaza East, Suite 310
Los Angeles, CA 90067
310-785-0201
FAX 310-785-0131

Peer Education Program of Los Angeles
(PEP-LA)
5410 Wilshire Boulevard, Suite 203
Los Angeles, CA 90036
213-937-0766

AIDS Project Los Angeles
1313 North Vine Street
Los Angeles, CA 90028
213-993-1600
FAX 213-993-1598

AIDS Policy Center
910 17th Street, NW, Suite 422
Washington, DC 20006
202-785-3564
FAX 202-785-3579

Advocates for Youth
a. Media Project
3733 Motor Avenue, Suite 204
Los Angeles, CA 90034
310-559-5700
FAX 310-559-5784
b. National Office
1012 14th Street, NW, Suite 1200
Washington, DC 20005

AIDS Hotline United States Public Health
Services
800-342-2437
800-344-7432—in Spanish
800-243-7889—for hearing impaired

HIV Information Network
FAX NEWSLETTER
University of Alabama School of Medicine
FAX 212-481-8534

National Center for Youth Law
Adolescent Health Care Project
114 Sansome Street, Suite 900
San Francisco, CA 94104
415-543-3307
FAX 415-956-9024

National AIDS Information Clearinghouse
800-458-5231

Project AHEAD (Youth Newsletter, support
groups, speakers bureau)
1242 Market Street, 3rd Floor
San Francisco, CA 94102
415-487-5777
FAX 415-487-5771

Western AIDS Education, Training Center
For help with a clinical HIV problem,
call 800-933-3413

World Health Organization, Appropriate
Health Resources & Technologies Action
Group
Essential AIDS Information Resources
For catalog:
CH 1211 Geneva 27, Switzerland
Telephone +41-22-791-4652

Gay and Lesbian Community Services Center—Youth Services
213-993-7400

Educational Resources

ETR Associates—800-321-4407
Has comprehensive Health Education Re-
sources for K–12. Includes HIV or AIDS,
STD, Drugs, Family Life Education, and
Reproductive Health

Project SNAPP: Skills & Knowledge for
AIDS & Pregnancy Prevention
An 8-session curriculum and video for
middle school students.
Division of Adolescent Medicine
Childrens Hospital Los Angeles
Published by ETR Associates
800-321-4407

CDC National AIDS Clearinghouse
Has lists of HIV or AIDS materials
800-458-5231

At Risk Resources
800-99-Youth

Advocates for Youth
Has fact sheets on youth sexuality including HIV or AIDS and many educational
materials
202-347-5700

Churchhill Films—*AIDS: What Everyone
Needs to Know*—Video (3rd edition)
800-334-7830

Reality Check—Video for Youth by Youth
Project AHEAD
415-487-5777

Alfred Higgins Production, Inc. (Video)
Teens At Risk: Breaking the Immortality Myth
818-762-3300

San Francisco Study Center (Video)
Between Friends
415-626-1650

BIBLIOGRAPHY

AIDS and adolescents: exploring the challenge: J Adolesc Health Care 1989;10(3, suppl).

American Academy of Pediatrics. AAP statement on adolescents and HIV. American Academy of Pediatrics [News]. Am Fam Physician 1993;48:346.

American College of Physicians and Infectious Diseases Society of America. Human immunodeficiency virus infection. Ann Intern Med 1994;120:310.

American Medical Association. HIV early intervention: physician guidelines. 2nd ed. Chicago: American Medical Association, 1994.

Anderson MM, Morris RE. HIV and adolescents. Pediatr Ann 1993;22:436.

Barnes PF, Le HQ, Davidson PT. Tuberculosis in patients with HIV infection. Med Clin North Am 1993; 77:1369.

Berger JR, Kaszovitz B, Post JD, et al. Progressive multifocal leukoencephalopathy associated with human immunodeficiency virus infection: A review of the literature with a report of sixteen cases. Ann Intern Med 1987;107:78.

Boette SA, Finkelstein DM, Spector SA, et al. A randomized trial of three antipneumocystis agents in patients with advanced human immunodeficiency virus infection. N Engl J Med 1995;332:693.

Bozzette SA, Finkelstein DM, Spector SA, et al. A randomized trial of three antipneumocystis agents in patients with advanced human immunodeficiency virus infection. N Engl J Med 1995;332:693.

Braun L. Role of human immunodeficiency virus infection in the pathogenesis of human papillomavirus-associated cervical neoplasia. Am J Pathol 1994;144: 209.

Brown LK, Schultz JR, Gragg RA. HIV-infected adolescents with hemophilia: adaptation and coping. The Hemophilia Behavioral Intervention Evaluation Project. Pediatrics 1995;96:459.

Burke DS, Brundage JF, Goldenbaum M, et al. Human immunodeficiency virus infections in teenagers. Seroprevalence among applicants for US military service. JAMA 1990;263:2074.

Calabrese LH, Kelley D. AIDS and athletes. Physician Sportsmed 1989;17:127.

Cao Y, Qin L, Zhang L, et al. Virologic and immunologic characterization of long-term survivors of human immunodeficiency virus type 1 infection. N Engl J Med 1995;332:201.

Center for Health Promotion and Education, Centers for Disease Control. Guidelines for effective school health education to prevent the spread of AIDS. J School Health 1988;58:142.

Centers for Disease Control. Revision of the CDC surveillance case definition for acquired immunodeficiency syndrome. MMWR 1987;36 (suppl 1S):3S.

Centers for Disease Control. HIV-related beliefs, knowledge, and behaviors among high school students. MMWR 1988;37:717.

Centers for Disease Control. Guidelines for prevention of transmission of human immunodeficiency virus and hepatitis B virus to health-care and public-safety workers. MMWR 1989a;38:1.

Centers for Disease Control. Tuberculosis and human immunodeficiency virus infection: recommendations of the Advisory Committee for the Elimination of Tuberculosis. MMWR 1989b;38:236.

Centers for Disease Control. Update: acquired immunodeficiency syndrome United States, 1981–1988. MMWR 1989c;38:229.

Centers for Disease Control. Recommendations of the US Public Health Service Task Force on the use of zidovudine to reduce perinatal transmission of human immunodeficiency virus [43:RR–11, 1994]. N Engl J Med 1994;320:1458.

Centers for Disease Control. HIV/AIDS surveillance report: mid-year edition. Atlanta: US Department of Health and Human Services, June 1994.

Centers for Disease Control. Trends in sexual risk behavior among high school students—United States, 1990, 1991, 1993. MMWR 1995;44:124.

Centers for Disease Control. Case-control study of HIV seroconversion in health-care workers after percutaneous exposure to HIV-infected. MMWR 1995;44: 929.

Chaisson RE, Keruly JC, Moore RD. Race, sex, drug use, and progression of human immunodeficiency virus disease. N Engl J Med 1995;333:751.

Chapel T, Lezin N, Zaro S. Final report. Assessment for HIV counseling and testing: relevant issues for women and adolescents. Submitted to Centers for Disease Control, November 30, 1992. Macro International Inc.

Chariot P, Ruet E, Authier FJ, et al. Acute rhabdomyolysis in patients infected by human immunodeficiency virus. Neurology 1994;44:1692.

Chu QD, Medeiros LJ, Fisher AE, et al. Thrombotic thrombocytopenic purpura and HIV infection. Southern Med J 1995;88:82.

Committee on School Health, American Academy of Pediatrics. Acquired immunodeficiency syndrome education in schools. Pediatrics 1988;82:278.

Concorde Coordinating Committee. Concorde: MRC/ANRS randomised double-blind controlled trial of immediate and deferred zidovudine in symptom-free HIV infection. Lancet 1994;343:871.

Connor EM, Sperling RS, Gelber R, et al. Reduction of maternal-infant transmission of human immunodeficiency virus type 1 with zidovudine treatment. N Engl J Med 1994;331:1173.

Consortium for Retrovirus Serology Standardization. Serological diagnosis of human immunodeficiency virus infection by Western blot testing. JAMA 1988; 260:674.

Conway GA, Epstein MR, Hayman CR, et al. Trends in HIV prevalence among disadvantaged youth: survey results from a National Job Training Program, 1988 through 1992. JAMA 1991;265:1709.

Coodley GO. A checklist for evaluation of HIV-infected patients. Postgrad Med 1993;93:101.

Dangelo LJ. Adolescents and HIV infection: a clinician's perspective. Acta Paediatr 1994;400:88S.

Daul CB, DeShazo RD, Andes WA. Human immunodeficiency virus infection in hemophiliac patients. Am J Med 1988;84:801.

Detmer WM, Lu FG. Neuropsychiatric complications of AIDS: a literature review. Int J Psychiatry 1986;16:21.

English A. AIDS testing and epidemiology for youth. Recommendation of the work group. J Adolesc Health Care 1989;10:52(S).

Eron JJ, Benott SL, Jemsek J, et al. Treatment with lamivudine, zidovudine or both in HIV positive patients with 200 to 500 CD4+ cells per cubic millimeter. N Engl J Med 1995;333:1662.

Fahey JL, Taylor JMG, Detels R, et al. The prognostic value of cellular and serologic markers in infection with human immunodeficiency virus type 1. N Engl J Med 1990;322:166.

Fallon J, Eddy J, Wiener L, et al. Medical progress: human immunodeficiency virus infection in children. J Pediatr 1989;114:1.

Feldblum PJ, Fortney JA. Condoms, spermicides, and the transmission of human immunodeficiency virus: a review of the literature. Am J Public Health 1988;78:52.

Finck BK, Katz MH, Hernandez SR. The care of asymptomatic HIV-infected patients. West J Med 1989;151: 464.

Fischl MA, Richman DD, Hansen N, et al. The safety and efficacy of zidovudine (AZT) in the treatment of subjects with mildly symptomatic human immunodeficiency virus type 1 (HIV) infection. Ann Intern Med 1990;112:727.

Fleming DW, Cochi SL, Steece RS, et al. Acquired immunodeficiency syndrome in low-incidence areas. How safe is unsafe sex? JAMA 1987;258:785.

Futterman D, Hein K, Kunins H. Treating the HIV-positive adolescent. Contemp Pediatr 1993;55.

Futterman D, Hein K, Reuben N, et al. Human immunodeficiency virus-infected adolescents: the first 50 patients in a New York City program. Pediatrics 1993;91:730.

Gallant JE, Moore RD, Chaisson RE. Prophylaxis for opportunistic infections in patients with HIV infection. Ann Intern Med 1994;120:932.

Gayle HD, D'Angelo LJ. Epidemiology of acquired immunodeficiency syndrome and human immunodeficiency virus infection in adolescents. Pediatr Infect Dis J 1991;10:322.

Glassock RJ. Human immunodeficiency virus (HIV) infection and the kidney. Ann Intern Med 1990;112:35.

Goldschmidt RH, Dong BJ. Current report—HIV treatment of AIDS and HIV-related conditions—1994. J Am Board Fam Pract 1994;7:155.

Gordon SM, Eaton ME, George R, et al. The response of symptomatic neurosyphilis to high-dose intravenous penicillin G in patients with human immunodeficiency virus infection. N Engl J Med 1994; 331:1469.

Gostin LO. Public health strategies for confronting AIDS: legislative and regulatory policy in the United States. JAMA 1989;261:1621.

Grant I, Atkinson H, Hesselink JR, et al. Evidence for early central nervous system involvement in the acquired immunodeficiency syndrome (AIDS) and other human immunodeficiency virus (HIV) infections: studies with neuropsychologic testing and magnetic resonance imaging. Ann Intern Med 1987;107:828.

Grinspoon SK, Bilezikian JP. HIV disease and the endocrine system. N Engl J Med 1992;327:1360.

Haverkos HW, Edelman R. The epidemiology of acquired immunodeficiency syndrome among heterosexuals. JAMA 1988;260:1922.

Hayman C, Peterson L, Miller C. HIV infection in underprivileged teenagers: update from the Job Corps [Abstract]. Sixth International Conference on AIDS, San Francisco, 1990.

Hein K. AIDS in adolescents: a rationale for concern. NY State J Med 1987;87:290.

Hein K. AIDS in adolescence: a rationale for concern. Washington DC: Council on Adolescent Development of The Carnegie Corporation, October 1988a:145.

Hein K. AIDS in adolescence: exploring the challenge. Paper prepared for National Invitational Conference on AIDS in Adolescence, New York, March 27–28, 1988b.

Hein K. AIDS in adolescents: exploring the challenge. J Adolesc Health Care 1989a;10:10S.

Hein K. Commentary on adolescent acquired immunodeficiency syndrome: the next wave of the human immunodeficiency virus epidemic? J Pediatr 1989b; 114:144.

Hein K, Dell R, Futterman D, et al. Pediatrics: comparison of HIV+ and HIV− adolescents: risk factors and psychosocial determinants. Pediatrics 1995;95:96.

Hein K, Hurst M. Human immunodeficiency virus infection in adolescence: a rationale for concern. Adolesc Pediatr Gynecol 1988;1:73.

Hirsch MS, D'Aquila RT. Therapy for human immunodeficiency virus infection. New Engl J Med 1993; 328:1686.

HIV Early Care: AMA Physician Guidelines. Chicago: American Medical Association, 1990.

Ho DD, Pomerantz RJ, Kaplan JC. Pathogenesis of infection with human immunodeficiency virus. N Engl J Med 1987;317:278.

Holtgrave DR, Qualls NL, Curran JW, et al. An overview of the effectiveness and efficiency of HIV prevention programs. Public Health Rep 1995;110:134.

Hoth DF, Bolognesi DP, Corey L, et al. HIV vaccine development: a progress report. Ann Intern Med 1994; 121:603.

Imagawa DT, Lee MH, Wolinsky SM, et al. Human immunodeficiency virus type 1 infection in homosexual men who remain seronegative for prolonged periods. J Adolesc Health Care 1988;9:84.

Jaffe LR, Seehaus M, Wagner C, et al. Anal intercourse and knowledge of acquired immunodeficiency syndrome among minority-group female adolescents. J Pediatr 1988;112:1005.

Jaffe LR, Wortman RN. The fear of AIDS: guidelines to the counseling and HTLV-III antibody screening of adolescents. J Adolesc Health Care 1988;9:84.

Johns D, Tierney M, Felsenstein D. Alteration in the natural history of neurosyphilis by concurrent infection with the human immunodeficiency virus. N Engl J Med 1987;316:1569.

Johnston LD, O'Malley PM, Bachman JG. National Survey of American High School Seniors, [Press release]. Ann Arbor: News and Information Services, University of Michigan, 1995.

Jones JL, Hanson DL, Chu SY, et al. Surveillance of AIDS-defining conditions in the United States. Adult/Adolescent Spectrum of HIV Disease Project Group. AIDS 1994;8:1489.

Kaye BR. Rheumatologic manifestations of infection with human immunodeficiency virus (HIV). Ann Intern Med 1989;111:158.

Kaplan ME, Schonberg SK. HIV in adolescents. Clin Perinatol 1994;21:75.

Keusch GT, Thea DM. Malnutrition in AIDS. Med Clin North Am 1993;77:795.

Kipke MD, O'Connor S, Palmer R, et al. Street youth in Los Angeles. Profile of a group at high risk for human immunodeficiency virus infection. Arch Pediatr Adolesc Med 1995;149:513.

Laine L, Bonacini M. Esophageal disease in human immunodeficiency virus infection. Arch Intern Med 1994;154:1577.

Lane HC, Laughon BE, Falloon J, et al. NIH conference: recent advances in the management of AIDS-related opportunistic infections. Ann Intern Med 1994;120:945.

Legg JJ. Women and HIV. J Am Board Fam Pract 1993;6:367.

Lemp GF, Payne SF, Rutherford GW, et al. Projections of AIDS morbidity and mortality in San Francisco. JAMA 1990;263:1497.

Levine C, Bayer, R. The ethics of screening for early intervention in HIV disease. Am J Public Health 1989;79:1661.

Levy JA. The transmission of HIV and factors influencing progression to AIDS. Am J Med 1993;95:86.

Lifson AR. Do alternate modes for transmission of human immunodeficiency virus exist? A review. JAMA 1988;259:1353.

Lindegren ML, Hanson C, Miller K, et al. Epidemiology of human immunodeficiency virus infection in adolescents, United States. Pediatr Infect Dis J 1994;13:525.

Main DS, Iverson DC, McGloin J, et al. Preventing HIV infection among adolescents: evaluation of a school-based education program. Prev Med 1994;23:409.

Markovitz DM. Infection with the human immunodeficiency virus type 2. Ann Intern Med 1993;118:211.

Marzuk PM, Teirney H, Tardiff K, et al. Increased risk of suicide in persons with AIDS. JAMA 1988;259:1333.

Masci JR. Primary and ambulatory care of the HIV-infected adult. St. Louis, Missouri: Mosby Year Book, 1992.

Mast EE, Goodman RA, Bond WW, et al. Transmission of blood-borne pathogens during sports: risk and prevention. Ann Intern Med 1995;122:283.

McLeod GX, Hammer SM. Zidovudine: five years later. Ann Intern Med 1992;117:487.

Medical News and Perspectives. When sports and HIV share the bill, smart money goes on common sense. JAMA 1992;267:1311.

Mellors JW, Kingsley LA, Rinaldo CR Jr, et al. Quantitation of HIV-1 RNA in plasma predicts outcome after seroconversion. Ann Intern Med 1995;122:573.

Melton GB. Ethical and legal issues in research and intervention. J Adolesc Health Care 1989;10:36S.

Miller L, Downer A. AIDS: what you and your friends need to know: a lesson plan for adolescents. J School Health 1988;58:137.

Millstein SG, Moscicki AB, Broering JM. Female adolescents at high, moderate, and low risk of exposure to HIV: differences in knowledge, beliefs, and behavior. J Adolesc Health Care 1994;15:133.

Minkoff HL. Care of pregnant women infected with human immunodeficiency virus. JAMA 1987;258:2714.

Moscicki AB, Millstein SG, Broering J, et al. Risks of human immunodeficiency virus infection among adolescents attending three diverse clinics. J Pediatr 1993;122:813.

Moss N. Behavioral risks for HIV in adolescents. Acta Paediatr 1994;400:81S.

Neuzil KM. Pharmacologic therapy for human immunodeficiency virus infection: a review. Am J Med Sci 1994;307:368.

Nicholas SW, Spondheimer DL, Willoughby AD, et al. Human immunodeficiency virus infection in childhood, adolescence, and pregnancy: a status report and national research agenda. Pediatrics 1989;83:293.

Niu MT, Stein DS, Schnittman SM. Primary human immunodeficiency virus type 1 infection: review of pathogenesis and early treatment intervention in humans and animal retrovirus infections. J Infect Dis 1993;168:1490.

O'Connor PG, Selwyn PA, Schottenfeld RS. Medical care for injection-drug users with human immunodeficiency virus infection. N Engl J Med 1994;331:450.

Oliva G, Rutherford G, Grossman M, et al. Guidelines for the control of human immunodeficiency virus infection in adolescents. West J Med 1988;148:586.

Oliva G, Shalwitz J, Back A, et al. The case for blind HIV seroprevalence testing in adolescents: making the case for resource allocation. Abstracts of the 5th Annual National Pediatrics AIDS Conference. Los Angeles, September 1989.

Pantaleo G, Graziosi C, Fauci AS. The immunopathogenesis of human immunodeficiency virus infection. N Engl J Med 1993;328:327.

Peckham C, Gibb D. Mother-to-child transmission of the human immunodeficiency virus. N Engl J Med 1995;333:298.

Pennbridge JN, Belzer ME, Schneir AS, et al. AIDS: a complete guide to psychosocial intervention. In: Land H, ed. Adolescents, HIV and AIDS, Milwaukee, Wisconsin: Family Service of America, 1992:169–186.

Phair J, Munoz A, Detels R, et al. The risk of *Pneumocystis carinii* pneumonia among men infected with human immunodeficiency virus type 1. N Engl J Med 1990;322:161.

Powderly WG, Findelstein DM, Feinberg J. A randomized trial comparing fluconazole with clotrimazole troches for the prevention of fungal infections in patients with advanced human immunodeficiency virus infection. N Engl J Med 1995;332:700.

Rawitscher LA, Saitz R, Friedman LS. Adolescents' preferences regarding human immunodeficiency virus (HIV)-related physician counseling and HIV testing. Pediatrics 1995;96:52.

Remafedi GJ. Preventing the sexual transmission of AIDS during adolescence. J Adolesc Health Care 1988;9:139.

Rinaldi RC. HIV blood test counseling: AMA physician guidelines. Chicago: American Medical Association, 1988.

Rotheram-Borus MJ, Koopman C, Haignere C, et al. Reducing HIV sexual risk behaviors among runaway adolescents. JAMA 1991;266:1237.

Sachs MK, Dickinson GM. Intestinal infections in patients with AIDS. Postgrad Med 1989;85:309.

Sande MA, Carpenter CC, Cobbs C, et al. Antiretroviral therapy for adult HIV-infected patients. Recommendations from a state-of-the-art conference. National Institute of Allergy and Infectious Diseases State-of-the-Art Panel on Anti-Retroviral Therapy for Adult HIV-Infected Patients [see comments]. JAMA 1993; 270:2583.

Sellers DE, McGraw SA, McKinlay JB. Does the promotion and distribution of condoms increase teen sexual activity? Evidence from an HIV prevention program for Latino youth. Am J Public Health 1994;84: 1952.

Sewell DD, Jeste DV, Atkinson JH. HIV-associated psychosis: a study of 20 cases. San Diego HIV Neurobehavioral Research Center Group. Am J Psychiatry 1994;151:237.

Sherer R. Physician use of the HIV antibody test. The need for consent, counseling, confidentiality, and caution. JAMA 1988;259:264.

Simpson DM, Tagliati M. Neurologic manifestations of HIV infection. Ann Intern Med 1994;121:769.

Smith GH. Treatment of infections in the patient with acquired immunodeficiency syndrome. Arch Intern Med 1994;154:949.

Smith PD, Quinn TC, Strober W, et al. Gastrointestinal infections in AIDS. Ann Intern Med 1992;116:63.

Society for Adolescent Medicine: HIV infection and AIDS in adolescents. A position paper of the Society for Adolescent Medicine. J Adolesc Health Care 1994;15:427.

Stamm WE, Handsfield HH, Rompalo AM, et al. The association between genital ulcer disease and acquisition of HIV infection in homosexual men. JAMA 1988;260:1429.

Stone HD, Appel RG. Human immunodeficiency virus-associated nephropathy: current concepts. Am J Med Sci 1994;307:212.

Stricof RL, Novick LF, Kennedy JT. HIV-1 seroprevalence in facilities for runaway and homeless adolescents in four states [Abstract]. Sixth International Conference on AIDS, San Francisco, 1990.

Strunin L, Hingson R. Acquired immunodeficiency syndrome and adolescents: knowledge, beliefs, attitudes, and behaviors. Pediatrics 1987;79:825.

Sweeney P, Lindegren ML, Buehler JW, et al. Teenagers at risk of human immunodeficiency virus type 1 infection. Results from seroprevalence surveys in the United States. Arch Pediatr Adolesc Med 1995;149: 521.

US Department of Health and Human Services. HIV/AIDS Surveillance Report through December 1993, vol. 5, no. 4.

Varghese GK, Crane LR. Evaluation and treatment of HIV-related illnesses in the emergency department. Ann Emerg Med 1994;24:503.

Vermund SH, Hein K, Cary J. Heterosexually acquired AIDS in NYC adolescents. Pediatr Res 1988;23: 207A.

Volberding PA, Lagakos SW, Koch MA, et al. Zidovudine in asymptomatic human immunodeficiency virus infection: a controlled trial in persons with fewer than 500 CD4-positive cells per cubic millimeter. N Engl J Med 1990;322:941.

Wang CY, Snow JL, Su WP. Lymphoma associated with human immunodeficiency virus infection. Mayo Clin Proc 1995;70:665.

Weiss RA. How does HIV cause AIDS? Science 1993; 260:1273.

Wendell DA, Onorato IM, McCray E, et al. Youth at risk: sex, drugs and human immunodeficiency virus. Am J Dis Child 1992;146:76.

Wilfert CM, Wilson C, Luzuriaga K, et al. Pathogenesis of pediatric human immunodeficiency virus type 1 infection. J Infect Dis 1994;170:286.

Wood AJ. Prevention and treatment of pneumocystis pneumonia. N Engl J Med 1992;327:1853.

Eating Disorders

CHAPTER 32

Obesity

Richard MacKenzie and Lawrence S. Neinstein

Obesity is a common problem among adolescents. It is a disorder in which the psychobiological cues for eating are discordant with energy requirements. Adolescents in general eat a diet that is high in saturated fats and low in calcium and iron. Both genetic and environmental factors contribute to obesity and overweight problems. Endocrine etiologic factors are unusual in adolescents. The prevalence of obesity and overweight in American teenagers ranges from 16–22%, depending primarily on sex, race, family history, and physical activity.

DEFINITION

Overweight and *obesity* are defined as either body weight or excess body fat above an arbitrary standard often defined in relation to height. However, both of these conditions are difficult to define in the adolescent age group because of the difficulty in measuring body fat and the variable height with age. At present there is no generally well-accepted objective definition of obesity for children or adolescents. Definitions of obesity have varied and have included the following indices.

1. Percentile weight for age: Body weight 20% over ideal body weight (IBW) is considered to be obese. However, this measure does not take into account height.
2. Weight (W) for height (H): The National Center for Health Service chart stops at 120 pounds and 59 inches. Above this range the curve is inaccurate and depends on age.
3. Weight-for-height percentiles for age: The percentiles are probably accurate but charts are based on data from the 1960s. Criteria often used for body weight in relation to IBW include:

90–110% of IBW	normal
111–120% IBW	overweight
>120% IBW	obesity
>200% IBW	morbid obesity
80–85% IBW	mild malnutrition
70–80% IBW	moderate malnutrition
<70% IBW	severe manutrition

Weight in kilograms for youth 12–17 by sex and height are available in Tables 32.1 through 32.6 from National Center for Health Statistics data.

Example: 14-year-old male, 156 cm and 50 kg. Look at Table 32.3 and 50th percentile for range of 155 – 159.9 = 46.1 kg. 50 kg/46.1 kg = 1.085 kg. Multiply by 100 for percent of IBW = 108.5% of IBW.

TABLE 32.1.   Weight in Kilograms of Youths Aged 12 Years at Last Birthday by Sex and Height Group, United States, 1966–1970[a]

Sex and Height	n	N	$\overline{X}$	s	s_2	5th	10th	25th	50th	75th	90th	95th
						\multicolumn{7}{c}{Percentile}
Male									\multicolumn{4}{c}{*In kilograms*}
Under 130 cm	5	15										
130.0–134.9 cm	4	8										
135.0–139.9 cm	34	111	32.50	3.741	0.727	26.6	27.6	30.2	31.6	34.7	37.7	39.4
140.0–144.9 cm	80	241	34.28	3.635	0.601	28.1	30.0	31.8	34.1	36.5	38.6	40.7
145.0–149.9 cm	123	386	39.27	6.243	0.615	32.1	33.2	35.7	38.2	40.9	46.1	52.5
150.0–154.9 cm	156	513	42.90	6.314	0.480	34.9	36.1	38.2	42.1	46.0	51.6	56.3
155.0–159.9 cm	135	432	47.35	7.551	0.769	38.3	39.4	41.9	46.2	50.5	57.4	61.9
160.0–164.9 cm	65	201	50.82	8.735	1.388	42.1	42.7	44.9	48.4	56.0	61.1	67.1
165.0–169.9 cm	29	88	55.75	8.811	2.031	43.3	46.4	49.0	54.4	59.9	68.3	76.6
170.0–174.9 cm	8	21	62.37	4.503	1.993	54.0	58.1	60.1	61.0	66.0	69.1	69.5
175.0–179.9 cm	3	10										
180.0–184.9 cm	1	2										
185.0–189.9 cm												
190.0–194.9 cm												
195.0 cm and over												
Female												
Under 130 cm												
130.0–134.9 cm	3	10										
135.0–139.9 cm	12	44	29.41	3.372	0.914	25.0	25.0	26.4	28.9	32.1	34.1	34.2
140.0–144.9 cm	32	116	38.30	7.314	1.194	28.8	30.6	33.3	36.8	41.4	49.2	55.1
145.0–149.9 cm	72	258	39.78	6.205	0.975	31.8	32.8	35.5	38.5	42.8	48.3	50.6
150.0–154.9 cm	147	517	44.00	7.421	0.677	34.4	35.8	38.9	42.8	47.4	52.9	57.4
155.0–159.9 cm	144	525	48.74	8.369	0.714	37.9	39.2	43.0	46.8	53.8	60.7	63.5
160.0–164.9 cm	95	336	53.06	8.010	0.658	42.5	43.9	47.2	51.1	57.2	65.6	69.6
165.0–169.9 cm	31	117	54.89	7.022	1.384	43.9	47.1	50.4	53.1	59.7	64.5	71.3
170.0–174.9 cm	11	42	63.66	14.501	6.214	48.7	50.1	50.8	56.7	82.2	86.0	86.1
175.0–179.9 cm												
180.0–184.9 cm												
185.0–189.9 cm												
190.0–194.9 cm												
195.0 cm and over												

From Hergenroeder AC, Phillips S. Advising teenagers and young adults about weight gain and loss through exercise and diet: practical advice for the physician. In: Shenker IR, ed. Monographs in clinical pediatrics: adolescent medicine. Switzerland: Harwood Academic Publishers, 1994. Adapted from US Vital and Health Statistics [Series 11, No 124]. Baltimore: National Center for Health Statistics.
[a]n, sample size; N, estimated number of youths in population in thousands; $\overline{X}$, mean; s, standard deviation; s_2, standard error of the mean.

For youth 18 and over a rough estimate of IBW is as follows:

Females: IBW (pounds) = 100 pounds + 5 pounds for every inch over 5 feet of height
Males: IBW (pounds) = 106 pounds + 6 pounds for every inch over 5 feet of height

4. Quetelet's or body mass index (BMI): Body weight in kilograms is divided by height in meters^2. The formula is accurate in adults, but accuracy in children and adolescents is variable primarily due to their rapid growth and development and the differential deposition of adipose tissue with linear growth. The Expert Committee on Clinical Guidelines for Overweight in Adolescent Preventive Services (Himes and Dietz, 1994) recommended using a BMI greater than the 95th percentile for age and sex to be considered obese (see Table 6.2).
5. The ponderal index $(ht/(wt)^{1/3})$ overestimates obesity when compared with measures of body fat.
6. Body fat measurements: Total body fat can be measured indirectly by determining total body water, lean body mass, and body density; estimating body volume by water and gas

TABLE 32.2.   Weight in Kilograms of Youths Aged 13 Years at Last Birthday by Sex and Height Group, United States, 1966–1970[a]

Sex and Height	n	N	$\overline{X}$	s	s_2	5th	10th	25th	50th	75th	90th	95th
						Percentile						
Male								*In kilograms*				
Under 130 cm	2	5										
130.0–134.9 cm	6	25										
135.0–139.9 cm	18	56	32.62	5.624	7.716	27.2	27.6	28.9	31.0	34.9	43.1	43.2
140.0–144.9 cm	65	204	36.54	5.852	1.607	30.0	30.5	32.1	36.1	39.2	41.7	53.2
145.0–149.9 cm	99	312	39.03	5.270	0.662	32.4	33.9	36.1	37.9	41.2	44.5	56.4
150.0–154.9 cm	131	421	42.58	6.724	0.865	34.8	36.2	37.9	41.0	45.5	49.4	61.0
155.0–159.9 cm	125	393	47.27	7.482	0.717	37.8	39.2	41.7	45.8	51.1	58.7	61.7
160.0–164.9 cm	91	285	53.01	9.324	0.916	41.5	43.7	46.9	50.4	58.2	64.4	72.5
165.0–169.9 cm	63	215	55.92	8.560	0.833	46.3	47.5	49.3	53.6	59.4	69.0	75.0
170.0–174.9 cm	19	68	62.01	10.362	1.033	51.2	51.6	53.7	60.1	67.0	76.0	85.0
175.0–179.9 cm	5	15	67.92	12.085	3.428	56.3	57.9	60.1	63.3	70.3	88.3	89.0
180.0–184.9 cm												
185.0–189.9 cm												
190.0–194.9 cm												
195.0 cm and over												
Female												
Under 130 cm												
130.0–134.9 cm	1	3										
135.0–139.9 cm												
140.0–144.9 cm	15	51	37.13	7.317	2.259	26.6	27.5	30.5	36.7	40.1	44.5	56.1
145.0–149.9 cm	47	165	42.23	6.880	0.888	34.7	35.6	38.2	40.5	44.2	53.6	57.6
150.0–154.9 cm	98	329	44.32	7.029	0.787	35.6	36.5	39.2	42.9	47.3	53.7	57.9
155.0–159.9 cm	152	499	49.75	8.757	0.699	39.1	39.9	43.8	48.4	53.8	61.0	65.9
160.0–164.9 cm	156	515	53.16	8.399	0.522	41.2	43.9	47.7	52.2	57.0	63.8	68.5
165.0–169.9 cm	86	284	58.17	9.125	0.921	46.2	47.4	52.2	58.1	61.5	69.3	76.2
170.0–174.9 cm	24	87	58.11	13.209	2.343	46.2	47.1	48.4	52.9	65.3	68.6	96.8
175.0–179.9 cm												
180.0–184.9 cm												
185.0–189.9 cm												
190.0–194.9 cm												
195.0 cm and over												

From Hergenroeder AC, Phillips S. Advising teenagers and young adults about weight gain and loss through exercise and diet: practical advice for the physician. In: Shenker IR, ed. Monographs in clinical pediatrics: adolescent medicine. Switzerland: Harwood Academic Publishers, 1994. Adapted from US Vital and Health Statistics [Series 11, No 124]. Baltimore: National Center for Health Statistics.
[a]n, sample size; N, estimated number of youths in population in thousands; $\overline{X}$, mean; s, standard deviation; s_2, standard error of the mean.

displacement; or establishing total body fat using xenon, krypton, or cyclopropane. However, these are impractical in a clinical setting. Another method used to estimate percent body fat has been skinfold thickness. Measurement of either triceps and calf skinfold thickness or triceps and subscapular skinfold thickness has been used. Slaughter et al. (1988) have advocated using the following equation to estimate percent body fat:

Males: % body fat = 0.735 (triceps + calf) + 1.0
Females: % body fat = 0.610 (triceps + calf) + 5.1

Another index uses the regional distribution of body fat. The ratio of abdominal or waist circumference to the hip or gluteal circumference generates an index that correlates well with future obesity-related health risk. Abdominal fat is characteristic of males (android distribution), while hip fat (gynoid distribution) is characteristic of females.

7. In general, methods that use just height and weight are cheap and easy but do not include a consideration of regional body fat distribution. Skinfold measurements are also cheap

Table 32.3. Weight in Kilograms of Youths Aged 14 Years at Last Birthday by Sex and Height Group, United States, 1966–1970[a]

| Sex and Height | n | N | $\overline{X}$ | s | s_2 | Percentile | | | | | | |
						5th	10th	25th	50th	75th	90th	95th
Male						*In kilograms*						
Under 130 cm												
130.0–134.9 cm												
135.0–139.9 cm	2	7										
140.0–144.9 cm	3	13										
145.0–149.9 cm	11	42	40.51	1.829	0.644	36.9	38.6	39.6	40.6	42.0	42.5	42.7
150.0–154.9 cm	45	135	43.63	6.277	1.182	36.2	37.0	39.0	41.4	48.0	51.7	55.3
155.0–159.9 cm	83	261	47.42	7.822	0.872	37.7	38.7	41.8	46.1	51.2	58.0	62.7
160.0–164.9 cm	96	299	52.28	6.785	0.584	42.5	44.0	47.5	52.1	56.3	61.5	65.1
165.0–169.9 cm	134	432	58.07	9.416	1.054	47.7	49.3	51.6	55.4	62.3	70.6	75.7
170.0–174.9 cm	144	435	62.37	11.516	1.095	49.7	51.0	55.0	59.4	65.6	79.2	86.3
175.0–179.9 cm	71	228	65.54	9.704	1.306	50.9	55.1	58.5	64.7	69.9	74.5	84.0
180.0–184.9 cm	25	81	72.44	13.014	2.298	59.6	60.0	65.1	69.4	77.0	83.0	94.3
185.0–189.9 cm	3	9										
190.0–194.9 cm	1	3										
195.0 cm and over												
Female												
Under 130 cm												
130.0–134.9 cm												
135.0–139.9 cm	1	2										
140.0–144.9 cm	2	6										
145.0–149.9 cm	17	52	42.00	5.879	1.683	32.0	35.3	36.3	42.3	47.5	49.5	51.1
150.0–154.9 cm	64	196	48.26	6.797	0.926	37.7	39.2	42.5	47.9	53.3	55.9	58.8
155.0–159.9 cm	157	508	51.35	7.705	0.520	41.2	43.4	46.3	49.6	55.6	62.2	64.3
160.0–164.9 cm	186	603	54.59	8.810	0.707	43.0	45.0	48.4	53.0	59.7	66.7	70.7
165.0–169.9 cm	114	372	58.46	10.185	0.955	45.9	47.5	52.1	56.8	61.8	70.5	76.4
170.0–174.9 cm	36	121	64.37	15.821	2.814	49.2	52.1	56.2	59.8	70.5	72.9	99.4
175.0–179.9 cm	7	28	61.33	5.496	2.620	51.7	52.0	57.7	59.8	64.6	70.2	70.6
180.0–184.9 cm	2	7										
185.0–189.9 cm												
190.0–194.9 cm												
195.0 cm and over												

From Hergenroeder AC, Phillips S. Advising teenagers and young adults about weight gain and loss through exercise and diet: practical advice for the physician. In: Shenker IR, ed. Monographs in clinical pediatrics: adolescent medicine. Switzerland: Harwood Academic Publishers, 1994. Adapted from US Vital and Health Statistics [Series 11, No 124]. Baltimore: National Center for Health Statistics.
[a]n, sample size; N, estimated number of youths in population in thousands; $\overline{X}$, mean; s, standard deviation; s_2, standard error of the mean.

and easy but can be inaccurate. Simple portable office ultrasound instruments that increase the accuracy of measuring fat thickness by removing interobserver variance are now available. Other methods using immersion in water or isotopes are more expensive, more difficult, and although accurate for total body fat, do not map regional body fat distribution.

Pubertal Changes

1. Effects of puberty on body composition: During adolescence lean body mass increases in both sexes. The increase is greater in males, owing to a greater increase in skeletal muscle. The maximum increase in muscle mass occurs around the time of peak height velocity (PHV) in both sexes, while the maximum fat deposition occurs 2 years before PHV. However, in females significant fat deposition continues throughout puberty.
2. Effects of obesity on puberty

TABLE 32.4.   Weight in Kilograms of Youths Aged 15 Years at Last Birthday by Sex and Height Group, United States, 1966–1970[a]

Sex and Height	n	N	$\overline{X}$	s	s_2	Percentile 5th	10th	25th	50th	75th	90th	95th
Male							*In kilograms*					
Under 130 cm												
130.0–134.9 cm												
135.0–139.9 cm												
140.0–144.9 cm												
145.0–149.9 cm	1	2										
150.0–154.9 cm	10	30	45.72	8.582	3.550	35.7	39.2	42.6	44.7	46.0	48.7	76.1
155.0–159.9 cm	34	99	52.81	10.552	1.695	40.3	43.1	46.7	49.2	56.7	69.6	76.3
160.0–164.9 cm	71	206	53.01	8.417	0.986	42.7	44.1	46.9	51.5	56.3	65.3	68.8
165.0–169.9 cm	132	404	57.72	8.503	0.819	48.0	48.8	53.1	56.4	61.3	67.1	73.3
170.0–174.9 cm	176	574	62.88	8.464	0.633	51.6	53.4	56.7	61.9	67.2	72.9	78.1
175.0–179.9 cm	118	374	65.80	9.457	1.045	53.1	55.6	59.7	64.3	69.5	80.2	89.2
180.0–184.9 cm	51	144	72.00	11.928	1.724	54.6	60.3	64.4	70.2	78.4	84.4	96.6
185.0–189.9 cm	14	48	74.21	15.035	5.200	58.3	58.5	62.9	70.7	84.6	92.4	110.8
190.0–194.9 cm	6	15	83.39	16.431	10.332	66.4	66.7	69.6	73.8	103.0	105.7	106.2
195.0 cm and over												
Female												
Under 130 cm												
130.0–134.9 cm												
135.0–139.9 cm												
140.0–144.9 cm	2	5										
145.0–149.9 cm	15	51	47.91	7.875	3.623	36.0	39.4	42.1	45.4	52.7	55.7	66.3
150.0–154.9 cm	69	242	49.69	8.895	1.190	39.1	40.6	44.3	48.1	52.8	60.5	68.3
155.0–159.9 cm	111	400	51.52	8.473	0.934	41.4	43.5	46.3	50.8	55.1	59.8	65.2
160.0–164.9 cm	137	509	57.03	10.828	0.875	45.1	47.3	50.2	55.0	60.2	71.7	77.7
165.0–169.9 cm	109	398	60.71	10.357	1.053	47.5	49.3	55.1	58.4	65.7	74.1	81.0
170.0–174.9 cm	49	188	65.27	10.730	1.880	49.7	53.6	57.2	61.2	71.6	85.3	86.4
175.0–179.9 cm	7	23	63.30	8.872	4.807	49.7	49.9	53.8	62.4	71.1	71.9	79.2
180.0–184.9 cm	3	26										
185.0–189.9 cm	1	3										
190.0–194.9 cm												
195.0 cm and over												

From Hergenroeder AC, Phillips S. Advising teenagers and young adults about weight gain and loss through exercise and diet: practical advice for the physician. In: Shenker IR, ed. Monographs in clinical pediatrics: adolescent medicine. Switzerland: Harwood Academic Publishers, 1994. Adapted from US Vital and Health Statistics [Series 11, No 124]. Baltimore: National Center for Health Statistics.
[a]n, sample size; N, estimated number of youths in population in thousands; $\overline{X}$, mean; s, standard deviation; s_2, standard error of the mean.

a. Obese adolescents tend to be taller and larger in skeletal mass and more advanced in skeletal development. A short, obese preadolescent or early adolescent may be a "red flag" for endocrine disease.

b. Obese female adolescents tend to have earlier sexual maturation and menarche. Maturation of the hypothalamic-pituitary-ovarian axis has been hypothesized to be related to total body fat (Frisch hypothesis).

c. Obese adolescents have a higher average hematocrit.

d. Menstrual irregularities: Aromatization of androgens to estrogen occurs in adipose tissue in the female and is a significant source of extragonadal estrogen. Thus, excessive body weight, through its effect on estrogen metabolism, may lead to suppression of follicle-stimulating hormone (FSH) and sensitization of the pituitary gland to release gonadotropin-releasing hormone, with a resultant increase in luteinizing hormone (LH). The resultant changes in FSH and LH can stimulate androstenedione

TABLE 32.5.   Weight in Kilograms of Youths Aged 16 Years at Last Birthday by Sex and Height Group, United States, 1966–1970[a]

Sex and Height	n	N	$\overline{X}$	s	s_2	Percentile 5th	10th	25th	50th	75th	90th	95th
Male						*In kilograms*						
Under 130 cm												
130.0–134.9 cm												
135.0–139.9 cm												
140.0–144.9 cm												
145.0–149.9 cm												
150.0–154.9 cm	4	12										
155.0–159.9 cm	11	33	49.89	7.323	3.572	42.0	42.2	44.7	46.8	54.4	59.8	67.2
160.0–164.9 cm	32	108	53.09	6.459	1.273	44.2	44.9	48.2	51.4	58.0	60.9	66.1
165.0–169.9 cm	87	275	59.39	9.178	0.981	48.5	49.8	52.7	58.0	63.9	69.3	75.9
170.0–174.9 cm	166	552	62.66	7.556	0.629	51.6	53.8	57.5	61.6	67.1	73.1	78.0
175.0–179.9 cm	149	511	67.33	9.018	0.856	56.3	58.2	61.0	65.4	72.5	80.1	83.8
180.0–184.9 cm	72	227	72.38	12.485	1.993	58.3	59.3	64.4	68.9	76.5	90.2	96.9
185.0–189.9 cm	29	95	81.06	14.268	3.265	63.7	66.6	69.7	78.4	90.3	97.0	111.4
190.0–194.9 cm	3	10										
195.0 cm and over	2	7										
Female												
Under 130 cm												
130.0–134.9 cm												
135.0–139.9 cm												
140.0–144.9 cm	2	5										
145.0–149.9 cm	10	33	52.58	8.198	3.191	43.9	44.1	44.9	51.0	54.5	72.0	72.1
150.0–154.9 cm	57	178	51.79	10.457	1.053	41.4	42.0	45.8	48.9	54.1	61.5	83.3
155.0–159.9 cm	117	354	53.20	7.766	0.734	44.0	45.6	48.4	51.6	56.4	61.9	69.0
160.0–164.9 cm	160	547	57.71	11.129	1.246	46.1	47.3	51.5	55.5	61.2	69.5	75.1
165.0–169.9 cm	122	450	61.72	11.998	0.802	47.1	48.8	53.3	59.1	67.3	78.7	86.7
170.0–174.9 cm	53	170	63.61	8.734	1.126	52.9	53.6	58.1	62.1	66.8	73.8	84.2
175.0–179.9 cm	14	45	72.55	15.012	5.224	58.6	58.8	61.7	65.9	80.6	99.1	105.5
180.0–184.9 cm	1	2										
185.0–189.9 cm												
190.0–194.9 cm												
195.0 cm and over												

From Hergenroeder AC, Phillips S. Advising teenagers and young adults about weight gain and loss through exercise and diet: practical advice for the physician. In: Shenker IR, ed. Monographs in clinical pediatrics: adolescent medicine. Switzerland: Harwood Academic Publishers, 1994. Adapted from US Vital and Health Statistics [Series 11, No 124]. Baltimore: National Center for Health Statistics.
[a]n, sample size; N, estimated number of youths in population in thousands; $\overline{X}$, mean; s, standard deviation; s_2, standard error of the mean.

and testosterone production in the ovary and can be associated with anovulatory cycles and heavy menstrual flow.

ETIOLOGY

Although many theories have been advanced, the cause of obesity is still unclear. Obesity is a multifactorial chronic disease. Clearly a number of subtypes of obesity exist. Recent evidence points to a significant genetic component with certain subtypes. At some future time obesity may be divided into different disease classifications with therapies tailored to match the underlying cause. At present, only 5% of obese children and adolescents have an underlying specific cause identified. This includes about 3% with endocrine problems (hypothyroidism, Cushing's syndrome, hypogonadism) and 2% with rare syndromes (Prader-Willi, Laurence-Moon-Biedl, Fröhlich's, Alström's, Kallmann's).

TABLE 32.6. Weight in Kilograms of Youths Aged 17 Years at Last Birthday by Sex and Height Group, United States, 1966–1970[a]

Sex and Height	n	N	X̄	s	s_2	5th	10th	25th	50th	75th	90th	95th
						In kilograms						
Male												
Under 130 cm												
130.0–134.9 cm												
135.0–139.9 cm												
140.0–144.9 cm												
145.0–149.9 cm												
150.0–154.9 cm	1	3										
155.0–159.9 cm	11	39	54.63	9.397	3.414	43.8	46.4	48.2	49.7	57.8	69.9	73.2
160.0–164.9 cm	25	81	57.75	6.503	1.355	49.7	51.1	52.5	56.9	61.6	70.1	70.8
165.0–169.9 cm	63	248	62.57	8.344	1.224	50.2	53.2	56.4	61.5	66.9	72.7	77.3
170.0–174.9 cm	115	396	67.06	11.163	0.704	53.3	55.5	59.5	64.6	71.9	80.9	91.6
175.0–179.9 cm	151	537	68.37	9.907	0.831	56.9	58.9	61.5	66.5	73.6	79.4	88.4
180.0–184.9 cm	80	297	73.31	12.454	1.335	59.6	61.0	61.1	71.2	78.4	91.8	102.7
185.0–189.9 cm	36	133	76.03	9.171	1.301	62.4	66.3	70.5	75.3	80.8	90.3	92.9
190.0–194.9 cm	7	25	81.40	10.985	7.588	62.9	62.9	67.8	87.3	90.3	90.6	90.6
195.0 cm and over												
Female												
Under 130 cm												
130.0–134.9 cm												
135.0–139.9 cm												
140.0–144.9 cm	2	5										
145.0–149.9 cm	8	26	43.49	3.939	1.604	38.6	38.8	40.1	45.1	45.7	51.1	51.2
150.0–154.9 cm	43	151	49.96	6.508	0.827	41.6	42.3	44.6	48.9	53.5	59.2	64.1
155.0–159.9 cm	103	385	54.71	9.903	0.775	44.4	45.5	48.7	53.2	57.7	61.6	76.2
160.0–164.9 cm	133	506	57.79	10.620	1.028	46.8	48.0	50.2	55.4	61.5	72.3	83.3
165.0–169.9 cm	116	433	60.63	10.117	1.182	47.9	50.3	55.1	59.3	65.1	69.4	71.6
170.0–174.9 cm	51	186	62.18	9.132	1.407	-50.6	52.9	55.5	60.2	65.7	76.1	82.7
175.0–179.9 cm	12	47	65.76	8.405	2.229	54.9	56.7	60.1	61.7	75.2	75.9	83.0
180.0–184.9 cm	1	2										
185.0–189.9 cm												
190.0–194.9 cm												
195.0 cm and over												

From Hergenroeder AC, Phillips S. Advising teenagers and young adults about weight gain and loss through exercise and diet: practical advice for the physician. In: Shenker IR, ed. Monographs in clinical pediatrics: adolescent medicine. Switzerland: Harwood Academic Publishers, 1994. Adapted from US Vital and Health Statistics [Series 11, No 124]. Baltimore: National Center for Health Statistics.
[a]n, sample size; N, estimated number of youths in population in thousands; X̄, mean; s, standard deviation; s_2, standard error of the mean.

INFLUENCING FACTORS

Familial or Genetic

1. There is an increased incidence of obesity in people with obese parents. In one study of Swedish twins, if one parent was obese, there was a 30% risk, if both parents, a 70% risk. Despite the genetic implications, these findings may also be partially environmentally influenced.
2. Stunkard et al. (1990) found a high correlation of BMI between twins, even when reared apart.
3. Stunkard et al. (1986) also demonstrated that there was a strong relationship between the weight class of adoptees and the BMI of their biological parents and no relationship between the weight class of the adoptees and the BMI of their adoptive parents.
4. West et al. (1994) have linked dietary obesity in mice to specific chromosomal loci.

Fat Cell Theory

Fat cells multiply at three stages of life: gestation, first year of life, and adolescence. The fat cell theory suggests that fat cells gained early in life and during puberty cannot be lost, but only reduced in size. It suggests that overfeeding during the first year of life and during puberty is critical to the development of obesity. In obese adolescents there is an increased proliferation of the fat cells as compared to normal weight adolescents.

Activity and Energy Expenditure

There are conflicting reports regarding energy expenditure in obese individuals. Obese individuals filmed in time-lapse photography seem to move less than normal weight individuals. Although some studies show no evidence to implicate a decrease in energy utilization in overweight individuals, Ravussin et al. (1988) found that the rate of energy expenditure was lower in obese individuals and that these rates of expenditure seem to cluster in families. Dietz (1993), drawing from longitudinal data collected in the National Health and Nutrition Examination Survey (NHANES), states that the most powerful predictor of the development of obesity in adolescence is the time a child 6–11 years of age spends viewing television, even when controlling for other known variables associated with childhood obesity. However, DuRant et al. (1994) could not find a relationship between television watching and body composition, and Robinson et al. (1993) only found a weak relationship between television and obesity.

Leibel et al. (1995) demonstrated that maintenance of a body weight 10% or more below initial weight was associated with a mean reduction in total energy expenditure in both obese and nonobese individuals. In addition, maintenance of body weight 10% or more above usual weight was associated with an increase in total body energy expenditure in both obese and nonobese individuals.

Calories

Caloric intake is variably elevated in obese adolescents and is dependent on where they eat. In one study obese adolescent boys ingested more calories at school than at home as compared to their lean counterparts. Retrospective diet histories tend to underreport caloric intake.

Behavior

Obese patients often exhibit the following behaviors:

- Eating fast
- Skipping breakfast and lunch and ingesting the majority of their calories at night
- Eating when not *hungry* but when food is available or when their *appetite* is stimulated by environmental cues
- Eating when depressed or anxious
- Eating that is associated with other activities such as television
- Underestimating the total number of calories ingested
- Overindulging in 'fast foods'

Central Regulation Theory

The central regulation theory suggests that the hunger or satiety center in the hypothalamus in obese individuals may not function properly in suppressing appetite. The energy-regulating system, operating at a high set point, gives rise to a predetermined body weight.

Psychological Theory

Psychological theories of obesity contend that obese individuals are depressed or anxious and use eating as a means to alter their mood.

Body Image Theory

The body image theory holds that some obese adolescents have a distorted and fat body image. According to this theory, one cannot achieve weight change until one has visualized and become comfortable with a smaller body image.

Hormonal Theory

A hormone named leptin has recently been discovered that appears to play a role in obesity in some instances. This hormone has induced significant weight reduction, decrease in appetite, and increase in activity in mice. The hormone has not been studied in humans. Leptin appears to play a role in monitoring and controlling body fat and energy balance. In mice, there appears to be a defective gene that does not allow for proper feedback for leptin production.

To varying degrees, probably all of these play a role in adolescent obesity. The extent to which each plays a role is unique to each adolescent.

EPIDEMIOLOGY

1. Comparison of the skinfold data from the 1963–1965 National Health Examination Survey with the data collected from 1976 to 1980 reveals a 54% increase in the prevalence of obesity among children 11 years of age and a 39% increase among children aged 12–17 (Gortmaker et al., 1987). There was even a greater increase in the prevalence of superobesity (skinfold ≥95th percentile) in 6- to 11-year-olds (98%) and 12- to 17-year-olds (64%).
2. Data are available in adults aged 20 through 74 years examined in each of the four national surveys during 1960–1962 (the first National Health Examination Survey [NHES I]), 1971–1974 (the first National Health and Nutrition Examination Survey [NHANES I]), 1976–1980 (NHANES II), and 1988–1991 (NHANES III phase 1). In the period 1988–1991, 33.4% of U.S. adults 20 years of age or older were estimated to be overweight. There was a dramatic increase from prior studies in all race and sex groups. Overweight prevalence increased 8% between the 1976–1980 and 1988–1991 surveys. In addition, during this period the mean body index increased from 25.3 to 26.3 and the mean body weight increased 3.6 kg. In the NHANES III study, 20% of boys and 22% of girls aged 12–19 were overweight based on measures of BMI. This compared to 15% for both boys and girls in the NHANES II (1976–1980) survey.
3. A study of Boston high school students by Johnson et al. (1956) found:
   a. Among females, there was a 12.9% prevalence of obesity.
   b. Among males, there was a 9.5% prevalence of obesity.
4. A 10-state nutrition survey by Garn and Clark (1976) found:
   a. Among females, 12% had triceps skinfold measurements greater than the 95th percentile.
   b. Among males, 11% had triceps skinfold measurements greater than the 95th percentile.
5. Sixty percent to 70% of obese adolescents are female.
6. Eighty percent to 85% of obese adolescents will be obese adults. Odds against attaining IBW:

    a. If obese at age 12, the odds are 4:1 against attaining ideal body weight.

    b. After adolescence, the odds are 28:1 against attaining ideal body weight.

7. Weight loss practices among U.S. adolescents: In a national study, Serdula et al. (1993) found that 44% of female students and 15% of male students reported that they were trying to lose weight. Students had used the following weight control methods in the 7 days preceding the survey: exercise (51% of female students and 30% of male students), skipping meals (49% and 18%), taking diet pills (4% and 2%), and vomiting (3% and 1%).

INFLUENCE OF OBESITY ON HEALTH

Future medical problems are rarely a concern to the obese adolescent, who is more preoccupied with the psychosocial aspects of obesity. The obese adolescent who becomes an obese adult will have more severe obesity than those adults whose obesity began in adulthood. A 50-year follow-up study of obese adolescents showed that the mortality and morbidity from cardiovascular disease was significantly increased compared with their lean counterparts (Must et al., 1992). Moreover, the influence of adolescent obesity on adult morbidity and mortality was independent of the effects of adolescent obesity on adult weight. Despite this, controversy still exists over how much obesity actually alters health and whether the psychological consequences of obesity may exceed the physical consequences.

1. Hypertension: Obesity is associated in some adolescents with elevated blood pressure, although most do not become hypertensive.

    a. The NHANES showed a 2.9 times higher prevalence of hypertension in overweight as opposed to nonoverweight adults. (National Institutes of Health [NIH] Consensus Development Panel, 1985).

    b. The Framingham study (Kannel et al., 1967) demonstrated a tenfold increase in hypertension in people more than or equal to 20% overweight.

    c. Several studies indicate only a tenuous relationship and suggest that differences in blood pressure relate more to salt restriction in low-calorie diets than to weight loss itself.

2. Cerebrovascular disease: A positive relationship exists between obesity and cerebrovascular disease in adults, as demonstrated in the Evans County Prospective Study (Heyden et al., 1971). Males overweight by age 20 and gaining 30 pounds or more thereafter had three times more cerebrovascular disease than thin males who did not gain any weight.

3. Cardiovascular disease: Divergent results have been found. Some studies show little correlation between obesity and coronary artery disease. The Framingham study demonstrated obesity to be independent of other risk factors, and Salel et al. (1974) showed that the most prevalent risk factor in young patients with coronary artery disease was obesity. Other studies indicate that the distribution of fat deposits may be a better predictor of coronary artery disease than the degree of obesity (i.e., excess abdominal fat, android obesity, is more related to disease than are fat deposits in the thigh or gluteal areas). Increased central body fat correlates with other risk factors of hypertension and dyslipoproteinemia that are related to precursor atherosclerotic plagues in children and adolescents. More recently, Must et al. (1992) demonstrated an increase in mortality in adult males and females related to obesity as adolescents, and Lee et al. (1993) demonstrated an increase in cardiovascular mortality rates in males related to obesity. Obesity can also result in alteration in cardiac structure and function even in the absence of systemic hypertension and underlying organic heart disease. Increased total blood volume can create a high cardiac output state leading to ventricular dilation and hypertrophy of the left and sometimes right ventricle.

4. Serum lipids: Cholesterol and triglycerides are related to weight in a linear fashion. In addition, the more one weighs, the lower are the protective high-density lipoprotein (HDL) levels. The NHANES demonstrated that the incidence of hypercholesterolemia in a young overweight group was 2.1 times that of the nonoverweight group (Denke et al., 1994; NIH Health Consensus Development Panel, 1985).

5. Diabetes mellitus: There exists a positive correlation of obesity with an increased risk of non-insulin-dependent (type II) diabetes. Obesity also increases the insulin needs of insulin-dependent diabetics.

6. Cancer: Obese males have higher mortality rates of colon, rectal, and prostate cancer than do nonobese males. Obese females have higher mortality rates from cancer of the gallbladder, biliary passages, breast, uterus, and ovaries.

7. Gallbladder disease: Increased cholesterol production and thus biliary excretion increases the risk of gallstone disease. In one study obese women between 20 and 30 years old had a sixfold increase in the risk of developing gallbladder disease.

8. Skeletal deformity and arthritis: Late-onset tibia vara characterized by inhibited growth of the medial portion of the proximal tibial growth plate has been well documented in obese African-American adolescents. Clinical presentation is one of a progressive asymptomatic bowleg deformity that is often masked by the obesity itself. The incidence of gout and osteoarthritis in weight-bearing joints in adults is associated with overweight during adolescence and young adulthood.

9. Psychological problems: Adolescents are less likely to be affected or concerned with the medical complications of obesity than they are with psychosocial concerns and problems. Psychosocial problems of obesity include:

    a. Poor body image: Especially important during adolescent years and can be significantly altered by obesity. Significant gender differences exist with females being more sensitive. Body image also correlates with parents' weight for height status.

    b. Social isolation: Can be related to fears of rejection and nonacceptance by peers of the same or opposite sex. Gortmaker et al. (1993) in a 7-year follow-up study of 16- to 24-year-olds found that obese females completed fewer years of school, were less likely to be married, had lower household incomes, and had higher rates of household poverty than women who had not been overweight. Males that had been overweight were less likely to be married but there was no impact on earnings. Sargent and Blanchflower (1994) also examined the relationship between obesity and wage earnings as an adult and found an inverse relationship for obese females. This relationship was not found in obese males.

    c. Low self-esteem: Living in a world in which who you are is so much determined by how you look, obese adolescents may feel like failures. They may have a tendency to self-deprecate. Sense of failure is often reinforced by their inability to lose weight. However, in a prospective study examining the relationship between BMI and self-esteem, Rumpel and Harris (1994) found no relationship.

    d. Depression: The preceding three factors may all be interrelated in a downward spiral of feelings of rejection, isolation, and depression, leading to more inactivity and more eating.

THERAPY

Therapy for obesity is a challenge for both the health-care provider and patient at any age. Young adolescents are often harder to treat than older adolescents because less motivation is present. In general, treatment focuses on control rather than cure, as is so often the case with chronic medical conditions. When is it appropriate to recommend weight reduction? Certainly, adolescents with morbid obesity (those with twice normal weight or greater than 100 pounds overweight) are at significant risk and should lose weight. Without other risk factors, obesity becomes clinically significant at approximately 20–30% over ideal weight for sex and height. At this point, mortality from obesity exceeds normal levels. In adolescents with special circumstances such as non-insulin-dependent diabetes mellitus, hypertension, and hypercholesterolemia, weight loss may be recommended in even milder degrees of obesity. It must be kept in mind that weight loss during the growth spurt may have undesirable metabolic effects. There is a need for further studies on medical problems associated with dieting in growing adolescents. At present, no medical therapy promises the majority of individuals long-term significant weight reduction.

Anorexigenic Drugs (Sympathomimetic Drugs, Diuretics, or Hormones)

Anorexigenic drugs include schedule II drugs such as methamphetamine hydrochloride, schedule III drugs such as phendimetrazine tartrate and benzphetamine hydrochloride, and schedule IV drugs including diethylpropion hydrochloride (Tenuate), fenfluramine hydrochloride (Pondimin), mazindol (Sanorex and Mazanor), and phentermine (Fastin and Ionamin). Most of the currently available appetite-suppressant drugs act on noradrenergic and possibly dopaminergic receptors to produce satiety. A smaller number increase excess neuronal serotonin levels by blocking serotonin reuptake or by increasing its release. Of these drugs that produce loss of appetite, one, fenfluramine, has received renewed attention for appetite control. Its effect seems to be more than just decreasing caloric intake. It decreases meal size, preferred foods, the rate at which meals are eaten, and possibly stress-induced eating. All appetite-suppressant drugs produce significantly greater weight loss than does placebo in most adult studies. Weight loss can be sustained for up to 36 months. Net weight loss, compared with placebo, ranges from 2 to 10 kg. However, after terminating drug treatment weight regain occurs, demonstrating that these drugs do not work when not taken. Overall, long-term results are dependent not only on the natural history of the specific weight disorder but also the use of adjunctive methods. Without adjunctive methods weight regain is common (Pfohl et al., 1994). Stahl and Imperiale (1993) review the efficacy and safety of fenfluramine in adults. To date no studies have shown efficacy in adolescents.

Abuse is a problem with amphetamine, methamphetamine, and benzphetamine, whereas other drugs such as the fenfluramines have minimal or no potential for abuse.

Diets

A change in eating habits is an essential part of weight loss. Reducing caloric intake below expenditure is associated with weight loss and a change in body composition. However, a diet alone is rarely successful in achieving permanent weight loss. Predicting weight loss for an individual teenager based on caloric intake is difficult and can vary widely. In general, the heavier the adolescent, the faster will be the weight loss. The type of caloric restriction should be well planned and should take into account present food types, eating habits, situation-dependent eating, and family and racial preferences. Inasmuch as growth and development is often at its peak, there must always be good nutritional balance.

Approximate energy needs in the postpubertal adolescent:

males = 900 + 10 × (wt in kg) × activity factor
females = 800 + 7 × (wt in kg) × activity factor
activity factor = low activity level = 1.2
moderate activity level = 1.4
high activity level = 1.6

The energy requirement for each extra kilogram of body weight increases approximately 22 kcal. Thus, an adolescent who weighs 20 kg over another will need 440 extra kcal to maintain that weight.

1. Low-carbohydrate diets: A high-fat, low-carbohydrate diet can cause ketosis and dehydration.
2. Very low calorie diets: When first introduced these diets often contained less than 400 kcal/day and used low-quality protein supplements, resulting in deaths usually due to cardiac arrhythmias. More recent very low calorie diets usually contain 400–800 kcal/day and high-quality protein, as well as carbohydrate and adequate quantities of potassium, magnesium, vitamins, and minerals. These have not been associated with significant arrhythmias. Wadden (1993) reviewed recent studies of the treatment of obesity with moderate and severe caloric restriction. Patients treated in randomized trials using a conventional 1200 kcal/day reducing diet, combined with behavior modification, lost approximately 8.5 kg in 20 weeks. One year later, they regained approximately two-thirds of this weight loss. Patients treated under medical supervision using a very low calorie diet (400–800 kcal/day) lost approximately 20 kg in 12–16 weeks. About one-half to two-thirds of this loss was maintained in the following year. Both dietary interventions were associated with increasing weight regain over time. The National Task Force on the Prevention and Treatment of Obesity (1993) also reviewed studies from 1966 through 1992 on very low calorie diets. In these studies weight loss averaged 1.5–2.5 kg/week with a total loss after 12–16 weeks averaging 20 kg. These diets averaged 800 kcal/day compared to standard low-calorie diets of 1200 kcal/day, which led to weight losses of 0.4–0.5 kg/day. There is little evidence that intakes of less than 800 kcal/day result in better weight losses. Intake of at least 1 g/kg of IBW per day of protein of high biologic value appears to be important in helping to preserve lean body mass. Serious complications of modern very low calorie diets are unusual. Long-term maintenance of weight lost with these diets is not very satisfactory and is no better than with other forms of obesity treatment. Incorporation of behavioral therapy and physical activity seems to improve maintenance. The very low caloric diets are contraindicated in pregnant women, lactating females, and adolescents who are still growing. They should be limited to individuals over 18 who are moderately (60–99% overweight) or morbidly (100% or more overweight) obese.
3. Liquid formula diets such as Metrecal and Slender: These diets tend to be monotonous, boring, and constipating.
4. Prolonged fasting: Defined as an intake of less than 200 kcal. Starvation diets are associated with significant metabolic abnormalities and a high recurrence of weight gain after termination of the diet. Fasting is not a recommended therapy.
5. Special food combinations such as steak and grapefruit: These diets tend to be monotonous, unbalanced, or expensive and in follow-up studies are found to be no more efficacious that a calorie-restricted balanced diet.
6. A balanced weight reduction diet should contain the following:
   a. Foods from all five food groups (milk, meat, bread, fruits, and vegetables)
   b. Instructions to eat at least three meals per day
   c. Instructions to eat less food or calories than previously
   d. Instructions on ways of preparing low-calorie foods and of substituting high-calorie foods with less calories

Behavior Modification

Some success has been reported with the use of behavioral modification for weight reduction. This approach has been reviewed by Penich et al. (1971), Stunkard et al. (1970), and Foreyt and Kondo (1984). These programs usually contain several components:

1. Contract or reward system for weight loss
2. An initial food diary that contains items such as time spent eating, place, hunger rating, mood, other activity done while eating, food consumed, and amount
3. Change current behavior through eating awareness and a food diary:
   a. Eat three to five regular meals instead of gorging at dinner and evening.
   b. At mealtimes, eat favorite dish first.
   c. "Just eat the icing off the cake." For calorie-dense foods, just eat that part that is liked the most (eat only the chocolate chips, rather than the whole cookie)
   d. Eat defensively, avoid the junk.
   e. Eat more slowly, allow the body to signal when it is full.
   f. Do not keep "weakness" foods available or easily accessible.
   g. Eat only where eating is meant to occur (e.g., at the dinner table, in restaurants).
   h. Do not watch television while eating.
   i. Do not eat on the go; sit down to eat.
   j. Learn to differentiate between appetite and hunger.
   k. Eat only when hungry and not just when food is available.
   l. Have a breakout activity when out of control or when eating is related to depression, anxiety, or unhappiness.
   m. Be honest about lapses in control.

Two books designed for teenage use that advocate behavior changes include:

Slim Chance in a Fat World—Behavioral Control of Obesity by B. Davis and R. Stuart (Champaign, Illinois: Research Press, 1978)

For Teenagers Only—Change Your Habits to Change Your Shape by J. Ikeda (Palo Alto, California: Bull Publishing, 1978)

Exercise

Every weight reduction program should include an increase in physical activity. This can include:

1. Changes in regular activity such as walking instead of using the bus: Using stairs instead of elevators; walking to the television set instead of using a remote control (when combined with other exercises, even minor increases in activity can make a difference overall)
2. An exercise prescription
3. Participation in a regular physical exercise program

Groups

Group participation as part of the weight loss program is often beneficial. A group supplies the following:

1. Encouragement and support
2. Opportunity for release of feelings
3. Opportunity for peer contacts and acceptance

Group participation can be in the form of a diet group such as Teenage Obesity Programs (TOPS), Overeaters Anonymous, Weight Watchers, or a group that is part of a more comprehensive weight reduction program, such as that described in:

Shapedown by Laurel Mellin (available from Balboa Publishing, 583 Tenth Avenue, San Francisco, CA 94118)

However, the practitioner must keep in mind that groups have very high attrition rates of between 40% and 70%.

Gastrointestinal Procedures

Gastrointestinal procedures are rarely indicated in adolescents and young adults and reserved for those who are superobese or have significant medical complication of their obesity (pickwickian syndrome, skeletal deformity, arthritis). Success is dependent on the experience of the medical-surgical team and the avoidance of metabolic complications. Rand and Macgregor (1994) reviewed 34 adolescents aged 11–19 undergoing surgery for obesity. While weight loss and psychosocial adjustment were significant, the patients reported poor compliance with exercise and dietary instructions and also did not follow through with the intake of vitamin B_{12}, multivitamin supplements, and calcium as directed. Procedures available include:

1. Gastric balloon
2. Vertical banded gastroplasty
3. Gastric bypass procedure
4. Biliary-pancreatic bypass procedure

PREVENTION

1. During pregnancy
   a. Maintain a moderate weight gain in last trimester.
2. During infancy and childhood
   a. Breast-feed in first year of life.
   b. Delay cereals until 3–4 months of age.
   c. Be sensitive to the deceleration of growth at $1\frac{1}{2}$ years of age so as not to exceed the child's decreased demands.
3. During puberty and adolescence
   a. Encourage careful nutritional practices in early puberty when there is again an increase in fat cells.
   b. Encourage a lifestyle of activity and participation rather than one of inactivity and observation through role modeling. Discourage television viewing and other sedentary pastimes.

BIBLIOGRAPHY

A summary of the workshop on child and adolescent obesity: what, how, and who? Crit Rev Food Sci Nutr 1993;33:287.

Alpert MA, Hashimi MW. Obesity and the heart. Am J Med Sci 1993;306:117.

Atkinson RL, Hubbard VS. Report on the NIH Workshop on Pharmacologic Treatment of Obesity. Am J Clin Nutr 1994;60:153.

Bray GA. Use and abuse of appetite-suppressant drugs in the treatment of obesity. Ann Intern Med 1993; 119:707.

Bray GA, Gray DS. Obesity, Part I. Pathogenesis. West J Med 1988;149:429.

Bray GA, Gray DS. Obesity, Part II. Treatment. West J Med 1988;149:555.

Brownell KD, Rodin J. The dieting maelstrom—is it possible and advisable to lose weight? Am Psychol 1994;49(9):781.

Brownell K, Stunkard A. Behavioral treatment of obesity in children. Am J Dis Child 1978;132:403.

Bullen BA, Reed RB, Mayer J. Physical activity of obese and non-obese adolescent girls appraised by motion picture sampling. Am J Clin Nutr 1964;14:211.

Canadian Task Force on the Periodic Health Examination. Periodic health examination, 1994 update: 1. Obesity in childhood. Can Med Assoc J 1994;15:871.

Committee to Develop Criteria for Evaluating the Outcomes of Approaches to Prevent and Treat Obesity Food and Nutrition Board, Institute of Medicine, National Academy of Sciences. Summary: weighing the options—criteria for evaluating weight-management programs. J Am Diet Assoc 1995;95:96.

Consensus Development Conference Panel. Gastrointestinal surgery for severe obesity. Ann Intern Med 1991;115:956.

Council on Scientific Affairs. Treatment of obesity in adults. JAMA 1988;260:2547.

Davis B, Stuart R. Slim chance in a fat world—behavioral control of obesity. Champaign, Illinois: Research Press, 1978.

Denke MA, Sempos CT, Grundy SM. Excess body weight. An under-recognized contributor to dyslipidemia in white American women. Arch Intern Med 1994;154:401.

Dietz WH. Therapeutic strategies in childhood obesity. Horm Res 1993;39:86.

DuRant RH, Baranowski T, Johnson M, et al. The relationship among television watching, physical activity, and body composition of young children. Pediatrics 1994;94:449.

Edwards K. An index for assessing weight change in children: weight/height ratios. J Appl Behav Anal 1978;11:421.

Flegal KM. Defining obesity in children and adolescents: epidemiologic approaches. Crit Rev Food Sci Nutr 1993;33:307.

Foreyt JP, Kondo AT. Advances in behavioral treatment of obesity. Prog Behav Modif 1984;16:231.

Garn SM, Clark DC. Trends in fatness and the origins of obesity. Pediatrics 1976;57:443.

Gortmaker SL, Dietz WH Jr, Sobol AM, et al. Increasing pediatric obesity in the United States. Am J Dis Child 1987;141:535.

Gortmaker SL, Must A, Perrin JM, et al. Social and economic consequences of overweight in adolescence and young adulthood. N Engl J Med 1993;329:1008.

Gross I, Wheeler M, Hess K. The treatment of obesity in adolescents using behavioral self-control. Clin Pediatr (Phila) 1976;15:920.

Henderson RC. Tibia vara: a complication of adolescent obesity. Pediatrics 1992;121:482.

Hergenroeder AC, Phillips S. Advising teenagers and young adults about weight gain and loss through exercise and diet: practical advice for the physician. In: Shenker IR, ed. Monographs in clinical pediatrics: adolescent medicine. Switzerland: Harwood Academic Publishers, 1994:133–136.

Heyden S, Hames CG, Bartel A, et al. Weight and weight history in relation to cerebrovascular and ischemic heart disease. Arch Intern Med 1971;128:956.

Himes JH, Dietz WD. Guidelines for overweight in adolescent preventive services: recommendations from an expert committee. Am J Clin Nutr 1994;59:307.

Hubert HB, Feinleib M, McNamara PM, et al. Obesity as an independent risk factor for cardiovascular disease: a 26 year follow-up of participants in the Framingham Heart Study. Circulation 1983;67:968.

Huse DM, Branes LA, Colligan RC, et al. The challenge of obesity in childhood. I. Incidence, prevalence, and staging. Mayo Clin Proc 1982;57:279.

Ikeda J. For teenagers only—change your habits to change your shape. Palo Alto, California: Bull Publishing, 1978.

Janz KF, Nielsen DH, Cassady SL, et al. Cross-validation of the Slaughter skinfold equations for children and adolescents. Med Sci Sports Exerc 1993;25:1070.

Johnson ML, Burke BS, Mayer J. The prevalence and incidence of obesity in cross-section of elementary and secondary school children. Am J Clin Nutr 1956;4:23.

Kannel WB, Brand N, Skinner JJ Jr, et al. Relationship of adiposity to blood pressure and development of hypertension: Framingham study. Ann Intern Med 1967;67:48.

Keesey RE. The body-weight set point: what can you tell your patients? Postgrad Med 1988;83:114.

Keesey RE, Powley TL. The regulation of body weight. Ann U Rev Psychol 1986;37:109.

Kerndt PR, Naughton JL, Driscoll CE, et al. Fasting: the history, pathophysiology, and complications. West J Med 1982;137:379.

Keys A, Fidanza F, Karvonen M, et al. Indices of relative weight and obesity. J Chronic Dis 1972;25:329.

Kuczmarski RJ, Flegal KM, Campbell SM, et al. Increasing prevalence of overweight among US adults. The National Health and Nutrition Examination Surveys, 1960 to 1991. JAMA 1994;272:205.

Lee IM, Manson JE, Hennekens CH, et al. Body weight and mortality. A 27-year follow-up of middle-aged men. JAMA 1993;270:2823.

Leibel RL, Rosenbaum M, Hirsch J. Changes in energy expenditure resulting from altered body weight. N Engl J Med 1995;332:621.

MacMahon SW, Wilcken EEL, MacDonald GJ. The effect of weight reduction on left ventricular mass: a randomized controlled trial in young, overweight hypertensive patients. N Engl J Med 1986;314:334.

Mallick MJ. Health hazards of obesity and weight control in children: a review of the literature. Am J Public Health 1983;73:78.

Mann G. The influence of obesity on health, parts 1 and 2. N Engl J Med 1974;291:178, 226.

Manson JE, Stampfer MJ, Hennekens CH, et al. Body weight and longevity: a reassessment. JAMA 1987;257:353.

Melnyk MG, Weinstein E. Preventing obesity in black women by targeting adolescents: a literature review. J Am Diet Assoc 1994;94:536.

Messerli FH. Cardiopathy of obesity: a not-so-Victorian disease. N Engl J Med 1986;314:378.

Morley JE, Levine AS. Appetite regulation: modern concepts offering food for thought. Postgrad Med 1985;77:42.

Must A, Jacques PF, Dallal GE, et al. Long-term morbidity and mortality of overweight adolescents. A follow-up of the Harvard growth study of 1922–1935. 1992;327:1350.

National Institutes of Health Consensus Development Panel on the Health Implications of Obesity. Health implications of obesity. Ann Intern Med 1985;103: 147.

National Institutes of Health Technology Assessment Conference. Methods for voluntary weight loss and control. Ann Intern Med 1993;119:641.

National Task Force on the Prevention and Treatment of Obesity. Very low-calorie diets. JAMA 1993;270: 967.

Noach EL. Appetite regulation by serotoninergic mechanisms and effects of d-fenfluramine. Neth J Med 1994;45:123.

Paige DM. Obesity in childhood and adolescence. Postgrad Med 1986;79:233.

Penich S, Filion R, Fox S, et al. Behavior modification in the treatment of obesity. Psychosom Med 1971; 33:49.

Pfohl M, Luft D, Blomberg I, et al. Long-term changes of body weight and cardiovascular risk factors after weight reduction with group therapy and dexfenfluramine. Int J Obes 1994;18:391.

Rand CS, Macgregor AM. Adolescents having obesity surgery: a 6-year follow-up. South Med J 1994;87: 1208.

Ravussin E, Lillioja S, Knowler WC, et al. Reduced rate of energy expenditure as a risk factor for body-weight gain. N Engl J Med 1988;318:467.

Revicki DA, Israel RG. Relationship between body mass indices and measures of body adiposity. Am J Public Health 1986;76:992.

Roberts SB, Savage J, Coward WA, et al. Energy expenditure and intake in infants born to lean and overweight mothers. N Engl J Med 1988;318:461.

Robison JI, Hoerr SL, Petersmarck KA, et al. Redefining success in obesity intervention: the new paradigm. J Am Diet Assoc 1995;95:422.

Robinson TN. Defining obesity in children and adolescents: clinical approaches. Crit Rev Food Sci Nutr 1993;33:313.

Robinson TN, Hammer LD, Killen JD, et al. Does television viewing increase obesity and reduce physical activity? Cross-sectional and longitudinal analyses among adolescent girls. Pediatrics 1993;91:273.

Rocchini AP. Adolescent obesity and hypertension. Pediatr Clin North Am 1993;40:81.

Rosenblatt E. Weight-loss programs: pluses and minuses of commercial and self-help groups. Postgrad Med 1988;83:137.

Rumpel C, Harris TB. The influence of weight on adolescent self-esteem. J Psychosom Res 1994;38:547.

Salel A, Riggs K, Mason D, et al. The importance of type IV hyperlipoproteinemia as a predisposing factor in coronary artery disease. Am J Med 1974;57:897.

Sargent JD, Blanchflower DG. Obesity and stature in adolescence and earnings in young adulthood. Analysis of a British birth cohort. Arch Pediatr Adolesc Med 1994;148:681.

Schapira DV, Clark RA, Wolff PA, et al. Visceral obesity and breast cancer risk. Cancer 1994;74:632.

Serdula MK, Collins ME, Williamson DF, et al. Weight control practices of US adolescents and adults. Ann Intern Med 1993;119:667.

Simopoulos AP, Van Itallie TB. Body weight, health, and longevity. Ann Intern Med 1984;100:285.

Sims EAH, Berchtold P. Obesity and hypertension: mechanisms and implications for management. JAMA 1982;247:49.

Slaughter MH, Lohman TG, Boileau RA, et al. Skinfold equations for estimation of body fatness in children and youth. Hum Biol 1988;60:709.

Stahl KA, Imperiale TF. An overview of the efficacy and safety of fenfluramine and mazindol in the treatment of obesity. Arch Fam Med 1993;2:1033.

Sterner TG, Burke EJ. Body fat assessment: a comparison of visual estimation and skinfold techniques. Phys Sportsmed 1986;14:101.

Stunkard A. New theories for eating disorders. Behavior modification of obesity and anorexia nervosa. Arch Gen Psychiatry 1972;26:391.

Stunkard A, Levine H, Fox S. The management of obesity. Arch Intern Med 1970;125:1067.

Stunkard A, Mendelson M. Obesity and the body image, parts 1 and 2. Am J Psychiatry 1967;123:1296, 1443.

Stunkard AJ, Harris JR, Pedersen NL, et al. The bodymass index of twins who have been reared apart. N Engl J Med 1990;322:1483.

Stunkard AJ, Sorensen TIA, Hanis C, et al. An adoption study of human obesity. N Engl J Med 1986;314: 193.

Suskind RM, Sothern MS, Farris RP, et al. Recent advances in the treatment of childhood obesity. Ann NY Acad Sci 1993;699:181.

Tienboon P, Rutishauser IH, Wahlqvist ML. Adolescents' perception of body weight and parents' weight for height status. J Adolesc Health 1994;15:263.

Van Itallie TB. Bad news and good news about obesity. N Engl J Med 1986;314:239.

Volkmar FR, Stunkard AJ, Woolston J, et al. High attrition rates in commercial weight reduction programs. Arch Intern Med 1981;141:426.

Wadden TA. Treatment of obesity by moderate and severe calorie restriction. Results of clinical research trials. Ann Intern Med 1993;119:688.

Wadden TA, Stunkard AJ, Brownell KD. Very low calorie diets: their efficacy, safety, and future. Ann Intern Med 1983;99:675.

West DB, Goudey-Lefevre J, York B, et al. Dietary obesity linked to genetic loci on chromosomes 9 and 15 in a polygenic mouse model. J Clin Invest 1994;94: 1410.

White EM, Wilson AC, Greene SA, et al. Body mass index percentile charts to assess fatness of British children. Arch Dis Child 1995;72:38.

Williamson DF, Pamuk ER. The association between weight loss and increased longevity. A review of the evidence. Ann Intern Med 1993;119:731.

CHAPTER 33
Anorexia Nervosa and Bulimia

Richard MacKenzie and Lawrence S. Neinstein

ANOREXIA NERVOSA

Anorexia nervosa is an eating disorder primarily affecting young women. It is best thought of as a malingestion syndrome as compared to a malabsorption or maldigestion syndrome. It is characterized by a self-induced weight loss; various psychological disturbances including distorted body image, fear of obesity, active pursuit of thinness, and a loss of recognition of a number of body enteroreceptive sensations; and secondary physiological abnormalities. For the health-care provider, few patients arouse as much compassion, confusion, and frustration as those with anorexia nervosa. Anorexia nervosa must be distinguished from:

- Weight preoccupied: Individuals who are constantly aware of body weight, often driven by employment or internal self-concept. There is not a loss of control or lack of enteroceptive awareness. However these young people are at risk for a DSM IV (*Diagnostic and Statistical Manual of Mental Disorders*, 4th ed.) classifiable eating disorder.
- Food faddism: Individuals become preoccupied with the type of food rather than the amount. Food faddism often may be an associated characteristic or early sign of a restrictive eating disorder.
- Fat phobia: With the increased awareness of food content through labeling of food products, individuals are avoiding and restricting diet for health reasons. Done without nutritional guidance, deficiencies and malnutrition may develop. Fat phobia may be seen as an early indicator of a restrictive eating disorder.
- Finicky eater: An individual eats only a small amount of food or certain types of food but in adequate quantities to maintain a body weight usually less than the 10th percentile. There is no pursuit of thinness or distorted body image, and the individual is usually as well adjusted as peers.

Etiology

The exact cause of anorexia nervosa is unknown. In the 18th and 19th centuries, anorexia nervosa was described as "nervous consumption." In the early 20th century, the disease was ascribed to pituitary failure. In the 1930s and 1940s, the disease was distinguished from organic pituitary disease, and from the 1940s to the 1960s, psychoanalytical theory provided the stimulus for research on the condition. Theorists attributed anorexia nervosa to unconscious fantasies regarding oral impregnation. It was speculated that the weight loss alleviated the young woman's fear of sexual development and responsibility. In the 1960s and 1970s knowledge was gained in regard to the perceptual disturbances of anorectic individuals, their family dynamics, and their hypothalamic disturbances. Most authorities currently attribute many of the behaviors, physical signs, and symptoms of the condition to malnutrition.

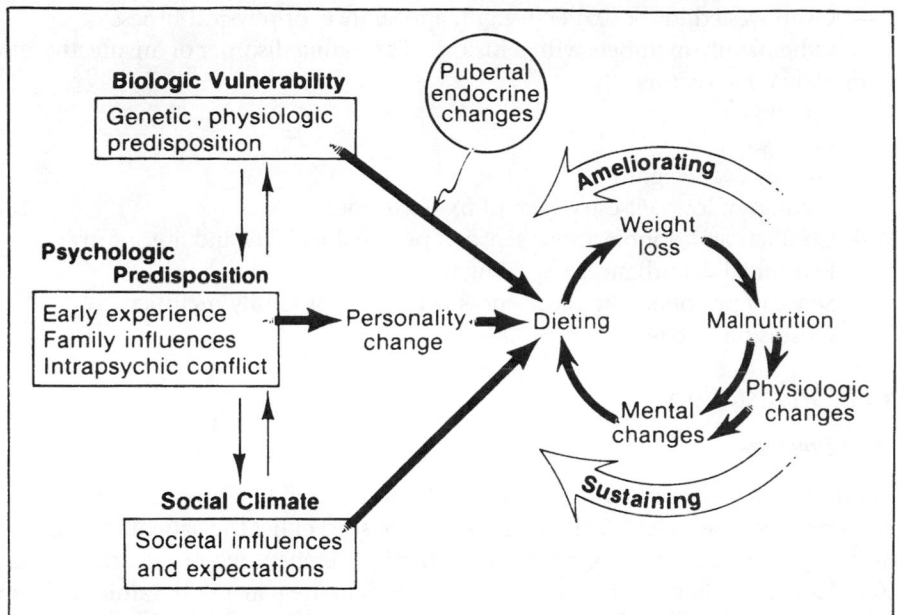

FIGURE 33.1.   Biopsychosocial model for anorexia nervosa. (From Lucas AR. Toward the understanding of anorexia nervosa as a disease entity. Mayo Clin Proc 1981;56:254.)

No doubt a combination of biological, psychological, and social factors underlies the cause of anorexia nervosa. A good model is provided by Lucas (1981) and is diagrammed in Figure 33.1. The figure demonstrates how biological vulnerability, family problems, and emotional problems can combine in a given social climate to cause the typical dieting of anorectic individuals. This weight loss, in turn, leads to malnutrition, which contributes to the physical and emotional changes of the anorectic patient and perpetuates a vicious cycle.

Epidemiology

1. Incidence: The worldwide incidence of anorexia nervosa is 1 per 100,000; however, the incidence among white, pubertal females in Western countries may be as high as 1 per 200. A survey of girls in private schools in England revealed an incidence of 1 per 100. The incidence seems to have doubled in the past two decades.
2. Sex: Anorexia nervosa generally occurs in females, with a sex distribution of approximately 9–10:1.
3. Age: The mean age of onset is 13.75 years. However, the age range is from about 10 years to 25 years.
4. Risk factors: Katz (1985) has identified cultural, familial, and individual risk factors that predispose an individual to anorexia nervosa. These include:
   a. Cultural risk factors
      — Equating thinness with both beauty and happiness
      — Emphasis on self and body
      — Capability of disseminating these values and styles through visual media
   b. Family risk factors
      — Achievement oriented
      — Intrusive, enmeshed, overprotective, rigid, and unable to resolve conflicts
      — Frugal with support, nurturance, and encouragement

— Overinvested in food, diet, weight, appearance, or physical fitness
— Other family members with a history of an eating disorder or an affective disorder
c. Individual risk factors
— Female
— Adolescent
— Slightly overweight
— Feelings of low self-esteem or of ineffectiveness
— Conflicts and doubts about sense of personal identity and autonomy
— Perceptual disturbances regarding body
— Sense of personal competitiveness with peers or family members
— Obsessional style

Clinical Manifestations

Typical Presentation

1. Pinpoint onset: Often anorexia nervosa can be pinpointed to a precise time when the patient decided to lose weight. This is often in response to either the patient feeling too fat or to a critical comment on his or her figure by family members, teacher, coach, or peers. The onset of anorexia often precedes or follows changes in the patient's or family's life, such as recent growth and development, menarche, parental divorce, or a death in the family.
2. Relentless pursuit of thinness: Weight loss is achieved easily, as the patient is reinforced by initial positive comments from parents and peers who admire the patient's will power. In addition, the behavior is reinforced by physiological adaptations within the central nervous system (CNS), and the patient loses control over eating. Weight loss continues due to the difficulty the individual has in overcoming these physiological adaptations and the accompanying distortions of body and body cues that accompany the starving state.
3. Food faddism and rituals: Eating behaviors change. Rituals appear that may take the form of breaking food into smaller and smaller portions, hiding food, secretly throwing food away or hiding it as if it had been ingested, or eating the low-calorie foods (e.g., salad with vinegar and no oil, diet frozen foods, diet soft drinks). These rituals are largely due to a starving brain and are reversed with attainment of improved nutrition.
4. Interest in paraeating behaviors: Although eating less, the typical individual with anorexia will develop or maintain an interest in food by cooking and preparing food for others, vegetable gardening, collecting recipes, and setting the dinner table.
5. Increased physical activity: While the individual with anorexia loses weight, the activity level often increases. Young people with anorexia nervosa will often jog, run up and down stairs, or do floor exercises or calisthenics in an effort to expend energy and control body configuration.
6. Purge behaviors: Some patients with anorexia discover that purge behaviors facilitate and expedite weight loss. Purge may take the form of catharsis, diuresis, or emesis.
7. Family characteristics: Families are generally white, middle-to-upper class, and described as "perfect families" in their communities. In recent years, families with less characteristic family patterns have become more common. Parenting style tends to encourage enmeshment, be overprotective and inflexible, and fail to resolve conflicts.
8. Disagreements and conflict: There is a strong sense of "right and wrong" often to the point of not accepting individual differences.
9. School behavior: Young people with anorexia nervosa usually have average to above-average intelligence and are described as excellent students and as overachievers.
10. Peer contacts: Young people with anorexia nervosa usually will withdraw from their classmates and friends. This reflects an attempt to minimize contact with criticizing or

teasing peers. It is also a manifestation of their low self-esteem and somewhat restricted social skills.

11. Lack of concern: Despite continued weight loss there is often a lack of concern for their increasingly emaciated appearance.
12. Food as a battleground: As the weight loss persists, food becomes the central topic of discussion and arguments in the family. This situation worsens as the parents become more concerned and frustrated with their child's weight loss, and the patient becomes more stubborn and set in his or her behavior.

Presenting Symptoms

1. Weight loss
2. Amenorrhea: Almost 100% prevalence. In 25% of anorectic patients the amenorrhea precedes the weight loss; in about 50% the amenorrhea occurs at about the same time as the weight loss; and in about 25% the amenorrhea occurs after substantial weight loss. Persistence of amenorrhea despite effective weight gain usually signifies persistence of psychological or social factors that contributed to the problem initially.
3. Hyperactivity
4. Constipation: This is secondary to both dietary factors and a lack of response to the usual enteroceptive cues to defecation.
5. Postural dizziness
6. Social isolation or depression
7. Hair loss
8. Yellow skin
9. Preoccupation with food
10. Abdominal bloating, discomfort, and pain
11. Cold intolerance
12. Epigastric pain, nausea, and vomiting
13. Fatigue, muscle weakness, and cramps

Presenting Physical Signs   Most of the signs in anorexia nervosa are related to the weight loss and have been reported in starvation states:

1. Decreased weight and cachexia
2. Decreased temperature
3. Bradycardia: No increase with exercise
4. Hypotension often with significant postural changes
5. Acrocyanosis
6. Edema
7. Dry skin with hyperkeratotic areas (dirty skin)
8. Cold extremities
9. Yellowish discoloration of the skin
10. Nail changes: Pitting, ridging
11. Increased lanugo hair
12. Superior mesenteric artery syndrome
13. Systolic murmur sometimes associated with mitral valve prolapse
14. Short stature: Nussbaum, Baird, et al. (1985) noted that 76% of their adolescents with anorexia nervosa were under the 50th percentile in height.

Patients with anorexia nervosa will often present wearing bulky pants and sweaters in an attempt to conceal their weight loss.

Presentation in Young Adolescents and Children   Atkins and Silber (1993) reviewed cases of anorexia nervosa in children aged 7–12. Their findings showed that the youngest ones had a diagnostic delay, a high severity of illness, and positive response to intensive treatment and there was a high incidence of family psychiatric history. Some of these children also presented with a personality disorder, and another group with features of the "vulnerable child syndrome."

Presentation in Males   Olivardia et al. (1995) reviewed eating disorders in males. Although less common in males than in females, males with eating disorders closely resemble females with eating disorders. Siegel et al. (1995) suggested that there may be a higher proportion of male adolescents with anorexia nervosa with medical abnormalities due to difficulties in establishing the diagnosis and the delay in seeking medical treatment.

Laboratory Features   Laboratory findings in anorectic patients can include:

1. Endocrine: The hormonal changes in the anorectic patient are most likely related to severe weight loss and are partially beneficial in preserving energy.
   a. Thyroid
      — Thyrotropin: Normal
      — Thyroxine (T_4): Normal or slightly low
      — 3,5,3'-Triiodothyronine (T_3): Often low, probably representing increased conversion of T_4 to reverse T_3
      — The thyroid changes represent adaptation to starvation and will reverse with weight gain.
   b. Growth hormone: Normal or high levels
      — Decreased somatomedin
   c. Prolactin: Normal levels
   d. Gonadotropins
      — Basal levels of luteinizing hormone (LH) and follicle-stimulating hormone (FSH): Usually low or low-normal levels
      — Twenty-four hour LH pattern: Usually similar to prepuberty or early adolescence, with constant low levels and no spikes or occasional nocturnal spikes
      — FSH and LH response to gonadotropin-releasing hormone (GnRH): Often a severely blunted response to GnRH, especially if weight loss is severe
   e. Sex steroids
      — Estradiol: Low in females
      — Testosterone: Low in males
   f. Cortisol: Normal secretion on stimulation. Basal levels are normal or occasionally slightly high. A decreased response of adrenocorticotropic hormone (ACTH) to corticotropin-releasing hormone has been noted (Gold et al., 1986). This resolves by 6 months after weight gain has occurred. This abnormality of ACTH response is not found in individuals with bulimia with normal weight.
   g. Other hypothalamic disturbances: Hypothermia and partial diabetes insipidus in some anorectic patients
2. Chemistry
   a. Increased blood urea nitrogen (BUN)
   b. Mildly increased serum glutamic-oxaloacetic transaminase (SGOT) and serum glutamic-pyruvic transaminase (SGPT) levels
   c. Hypophosphatemia
   d. Depressed serum magnesium and calcium
   e. Increased cholesterol

    f. Increased serum carotene in 15–40% of anorectic patients, low sensitivity but high specificity

    g. Decreased vitamin A

    h. Decreased serum zinc and copper

3. Hematological

    a. Leukopenia: May be relative lymphocytosis

    b. Anemia: A late finding

    c. Thrombocytopenia

    d. Decreased serum complement C3 (but normal C4) and granulocyte killing defect; no evidence for increased susceptibility to bacterial infection

    e. Decreased erythrocyte sedimentation rate (ESR; less than 4 mm/hr)

4. Cardiac

    a. Electrocardiogram: Bradycardia, low-voltage changes, T-wave inversions, and occasional ST segment depression

    b. Decreased cardiac size and left ventricular wall thickness

    c. Increased prevalence of mitral valve prolapse (Johnson et al., 1986)

5. Gastrointestinal

    a. Upper gastrointestinal tract series: Usually normal findings, with occasional hypomotility

    b. Barium enema: Normal

    c. Fecal fat: Normal

6. Renal and metabolic

    a. Decreased glomerular filtration rate

    b. Elevated BUN

    c. Decreased maximum concentration ability

    d. Chloride-responsive metabolic alkalosis

Psychosocial Features   The anorectic patient can be characterized by several psychological, behavioral, and perceptual features, including:

1. Psychological

    a. No predominant psychiatric diagnosis

    b. Lowered self-esteem

    c. Features of depression, anxiety, and obsessional thoughts

    d. Perfectionistic attitude

    e. Social anxiety and withdrawal

    f. Overachieving

2. Perceptual

    a. Disturbed body image: Overestimation, especially of face and torso sizes

    b. Misperception of physical sensations: Distorted hunger awareness and denial of fatigue

    c. Sense of ineffectiveness: Feelings of being controlled by, rather than controlling, the environment

3. Behavioral

    a. Preoccupation with food

    b. Hyperactivity

    c. Willful weight loss

    d. Vomiting and laxative abuse

    e. Decreased sexual interest

4. Family: The families of anorectic patients generally enjoy academic, social, and economic success and lack obvious problems. Many of the families stress intellectual and physical

appearances rather than emotional concerns. Often, there has been a lack of communication among family members other than factual information. While appearing calm on the surface, the families often have problems of:

a. Rigidity
b. Conflict resolution
c. Overprotectiveness
d. Lack of privacy within the family
e. Development of overly strong ties within certain segments of the family

Diagnosis and Assessment

The diagnosis of anorexia nervosa should be suspected in any adolescent with unexplained weight loss, hyperactivity, and food avoidance. Other possible causes such as Crohn's disease, early pregnancy, sarcoidosis, tuberculosis, cystic fibrosis, brain tumors, and depression should be explored.

Diagnostic and Statistical Manual of Mental Disorders *Criteria*   The diagnosis of anorexia is based not only on the absence of a defined organic cause but also on the presence of certain characteristics. The American Psychiatric Association's *Diagnostic and Statistical Manual of Mental Disorders* (1993) criteria for anorexia nervosa include:

1. Refusal to maintain body weight over a minimal normal weight for age and height (e.g., weight loss leading to maintenance of body weight less than 85% of that expected; or failure to make expected weight gain during period of growth, leading to body weight less than 85% of that expected).
2. Intense fear of gaining weight or becoming fat, even though underweight.
3. Disturbance in the way in which one's body weight, size, or shape is experienced, undue influence of body weight or shape on self-evaluation, or denial of the seriousness of the current low body weight.
4. In postmenarchal females, absence of at least three consecutive menstrual cycles when otherwise expected to occur (primary or secondary amenorrhea).

Two types are defined:

1. Restricting type: During the current episode the person has not regularly engaged in binge-eating or purging behavior
2. Binge-eating or purging type: During the current episode the person has regularly engaged in binge-eating or purging behavior.

Evaluation   The evaluation of the anorectic patient should include a comprehensive history and physical examination. Questions regarding eating and weight control behavior that may be helpful include:

1. How does the teen handle weight control?
2. How much does the teen want to weigh?
3. How often does the teen weigh himself or herself?
4. Is the teen a compulsive exerciser?
5. Is there any purging behavior such as vomiting, laxative abuse, diuretic use, ipecac use, or use of diet pills?
6. What is the teen's self-image (fat or thin), and is there any area that is seen as particularly ugly such as buttocks or thighs?

Several instruments have been developed to aid in the diagnosis of eating disorders and the differentiation of anorexia from bulimia nervosa. These include:

1. EAT: A rating scale that attempts to distinguish patients with anorexia nervosa from weight preoccupied and otherwise normal college females
2. EDI: Used to predict the emergence of an eating disorder in a high-risk group
3. BITE: Used to measure the symptoms and severity of bulimia

The signs and symptoms of anorexia nervosa as previously outlined should be sought, as well as those suggestive of an organic process. Organic diseases that could be confused with anorexia nervosa include:

Hyperthyroidism or hypothyroidism
Malabsorptive states
Inflammatory bowel disease
Diabetes mellitus
Brain tumors especially of the fourth ventricle
Collagen vascular disease
Addison's disease

In addition, an effort should be made to look for behavioral, perceptual, and family changes as outlined in previous sections. The laboratory evaluation should include:

1. Complete blood count and platelet count
2. ESR
3. BUN and creatinine
4. Urinalysis
5. Serum electrolytes and liver function tests
6. Serum calcium and phosphate
7. Serum albumin
8. Carotene
9. T_4
10. Chest x-ray

Optional

1. Stools for occult blood and fat
2. Upper gastrointestinal tract series and small bowel series
3. Barium enema
4. Computed tomography (CT) or magnetic resonance imaging (MRI) of the head

Nutritional Assessment   The nutritional assessment should include weight, height, triceps, skinfold, and midarm circumference. Monitoring the percentage of body fat is helpful in the ongoing evaluation of adolescents with anorexia. The percentage of body fat can be calculated from skinfold thickness measurements or approximated from the following formulas:

total body water = −10.313 + [0.252 × (weight in kg)] + [0.154 × (height in cm)]
lean body mass = total body water ÷ 0.72
body fat = body weight − lean body mass
% body fat = (body fat ÷ body weight) × 100

Most menarchal females have at least 17% of body weight as fat, and most ovulatory females have at least 22% of body weight as fat.

Treatment

Many therapies have been attempted in anorectic patients, including psychotherapy, behavioral therapy, drug therapy, hyperalimentation, and family therapy. The important issues in therapy are correction of malnutrition and associated psychological symptoms of starvation. Concomitantly, work should begin on the resolution of the psychological dysfunction within the patient and family. Failure to address these issues on both a short-term and a long-term basis will lead to failure of the therapy. The intervention should be divided into several stages:

1. Diagnosis: The first critical step is to make a correct diagnosis and inform the patient and the family of the problem and the plan for treatment.
2. Repletion of nutritional stores: This is important, as many of the patient's physical and emotional problems may center around malnutrition. If the adolescent is in physical danger with hypovolemia and hypotension, if the home situation is unstable, or if the patient and family are in extreme crisis, the adolescent should be admitted for at least a short-term hospitalization. The goals for this hospitalization should be weight gain and institution of a cognitive approach to psychotherapy. Attempts should be made to achieve weight gain through the oral route, if possible. Behavioral contracts have been helpful (Figs. 33.2 through 33.4 are examples of contracts), but these should only be used in conjunction with the ongoing cognitive work. If cardiac arrhythmias occur without electrolyte disturbances, if the patient is listless, or if oral therapy fails, nutrition should be repleted by the safest method available. This can be done by nasogastric tube or intravenous hyperalimentation.
3. Long-term therapy: After discharge from the hospital or after initial evaluation and diagnosis, long-term therapy should be begun. This is best achieved through both individual and family sessions. Goals should be to encourage self-control through self-definition and to elevate self-esteem. A contract may also be of value for outpatients. An example of such a contract is given in Figure 33.4. Particularly in those teens with anorexia nervosa with a significant depression, antidepressants may be of value. An excellent discussion of the family dynamics involved in these sessions is found in *Psychosomatic Families: Anorexia Nervosa in Context* by S. Minuchin, B.L. Roseman, and L. Baker (Cambridge, Massachusetts: Harvard University Press, 1978). Additional information and referral sources can be obtained from the National Association of Anorexia Nervosa and Associated Disorders, Box 271, Highland Park, IL 60035.

Complications

1. Cardiovascular
   a. Adaptations to starvation: Sinus bradycardia, sinus arrhythmia, and hypotension
   b. Ventricular dysrhythmias
   c. Reduced myocardial contractility
   d. Prolonged QT intervals
   e. Sudden death probably secondary to arrhythmias
   f. Heart muscle damage secondary to ipecac abuse
   g. Mitral valve prolapse
2. Renal
   a. Increased BUN
   b. Decreased glomerular filtration rate
   c. Renal calculi
   d. Edema
   e. Hypokalemia secondary to diuretics
   f. Renal concentrating defect

Contract for _____[Name]_____

Step 1 — Nasogastric tube and intravenous feedings.
[Agreement weight] — Room on 5-East. Stay in room. No TV, phone calls, mail, visitors,
_____ work experience, free-time ward activities, or eating in cafeteria.

Step 2 — Nasogastric feedings.
— Room on Rehabilitation Unit. Stay in room except for meals in
dome area (1 hour).
— No TV, visitors, mail, phone calls, work experience, free-time ward
_____ activities, or meals in cafeteria.

Step 3 — Stay in room except for meals.
— No TV, visitors, mail, phone calls, work experience, free-time ward
activities, or meals in cafeteria.
_____ — Initiate Sustacal (or equivalent) 8 oz three times a day.

Step 4 — May watch TV.
— No visitors, mail, phone calls, work experience, or free-time ward
activities.
_____ — Sustacal 8 oz three times a day.

Step 5 — Receive mail and send out mail.
— No visitors, phone calls, work experience, free-time ward activi-
ties, or meals in cafeteria.
_____ — Continue Sustacal 8 oz three times a day.

Step 6 — May eat in cafeteria.
— Telephone calls: Two outgoing calls per day for 20 minutes per
call. No incoming calls.
— Free-time ward activities.
— No work experience.
_____ — Continue Sustacal 8 oz twice a day.

Step 7 — Two visitors per day for 1 hour: Patient's choice.
— Telephone calls: Two outgoing calls for 20 minutes per call.
— Work experience.
_____ — Continue Sustacal 8 oz once a day.

Step 8 — Visitors.
— Unlimited telephone calls (outgoing and incoming).
_____ — Discontinue Sustacal.

Step 9 — Visitors.
_____ — Out-of-hospital pass 4 hours per week.

Step 10 _____ — 48-hour pass.

Step 11 _____ — Discharge home for office care.

FIGURE 33.2.   Sample contract for inpatient with anorexia nervosa. A weight for each step should be negotiated between the teenager and practitioner.

3. Gastrointestinal
   a. Delayed gastric emptying
   b. Superior mesenteric artery syndrome
   c. Constipation
   d. Elevated liver enzyme levels
   e. Gastric dilation
   f. Necrotizing colitis
4. With purging behaviors
   a. Pancreatitis
   b. Parotid gland enlargement
   c. Esophagitis

AGREEMENT

Name _____   Date _____

I currently weigh _____ .

Our mutual goal is for me to gain weight and change eating habits to improve my physical health and sense of control. I agree to the step-wise method as outlined. With each gain, I will obtain a greater opportunity to maintain control and make my own choices.

My weight goal is _____ .

I will begin at step _____ and if I remain on the same level for more than _____ without weight increase, I will automatically drop down one level (i.e., step 6 to step 5).

Agreement in effect from _____ to _____ .

_____
(Patient)

_____
(Physician)

FIGURE 33.3.   Management of anorexia nervosa: Sample contract.

    d. Mallory-Weiss lesions
    e. Hypokalemia secondary to laxative abuse
    f. Paralytic ileus secondary to laxative abuse
    g. Cathartic colon
5. Hematological
    a. Anemia
    b. Leukopenia
    c. Thrombocytopenia
6. Endocrine or metabolic
    a. Elevated cholesterol
    b. Amenorrhea
    c. Osteoporosis: Females with anorexia nervosa have been found to have lower bone mineral densities (BMD) than menstruating females with normal body weights. In young females with amenorrhea associated with weight loss, BMD loss will be occurring soon after the amenorrhea develops. The BMD in adolescents with anorexia nervosa can increase as the individual recovers from anorexia nervosa and may start to increase even before menses returns. Females who recover from anorexia nervosa at a young age (<15 years of age) can have normal total body BMD, but regional

Initial weight:
Initial height:
Goal weight:

—————————

Visits clinic twice weekly until ————— lb
Visits clinic weekly until ————— lb
Visits clinic every 2 weeks until ————— lb
Visits clinic once a month until ————— lb
Visits clinic every 3 months for 1 year after ————— lb reached
— Hospitalization if weight or physical state does not improve over a 4-week period.
— No cooking or kitchen work until ————— lb
— No ballet until ————— lb
— No gymnastics until ————— lb
— No participation in physical education classes at school until ————— lb

—————————————————————
(Patient)

—————————————————————
(Physician)

FIGURE 33.4.   Sample outpatient contract for adolescent with anorexia nervosa.

(lumbar spine and femoral neck) BMD may remain low (Hergenroeder, 1995). The longer the anorexia nervosa persists, the less likely it is that the BMD will return to normal. Hormonal supplementation for females with anorexia nervosa has not been well documented to significantly increase bone density. Seeman et al. (1992) found that the risk of lower BMD was greatest in women with anorexia nervosa and primary amenorrhea. This study also suggested that women with anorexia nervosa who had received oral contraceptives had BMD that were greater than those receiving no contraceptives but lower than a control population.

   d. Decreased somatomedin C
   e. Short stature
   f. Partial diabetes insipidus
   g. Abnormal temperature regulation
   h. Hypercarotenemia
   i. Metabolic alkalosis
   j. Hyponatremia
   k. Hypokalemia
   l. Decreased magnesium with resultant muscle cramps, weakness, and restlessness
7. Neuromuscular
   a. Generalized muscle weakness
   b. Seizures secondary to metabolic abnormalities

    c. Peripheral neuropathies
    d. Myopathy secondary to ipecac abuse
    e. Syncope in absence of orthostatic hypotension
    f. Diplopia
    g. Movement disorders

8. Correlates of sudden death
    a. Prolonged QT interval
    b. Decreased serum phosphate
    c. Ipecac myopathy
    d. Weight loss more than or equal to 35% ideal body weight
    e. Suicide

9. Dental
    a. Complications of vomiting include:
      — Dental and enamel erosions from vomiting
      — Caries and periodontal disease
    b. Recommendations for dental care in adolescents with a history of vomiting include:
      — Topical fluoride therapy daily
      — Alkaline mouth rinse after vomiting
      — No toothbrushing after vomiting, as this increases risk of dental damage
      — Vigorous oral hygienic measures maintained

10. Pulmonary
    a. Aspiration pneumonia secondary to vomiting
    b. Pneumomediastinum secondary to vomiting

Prognosis

Studies regarding prognosis of anorexia nervosa are often marred by lack of proper diagnosis criteria, failure of adequate follow-up, or inadequate information at follow-up. Hsu (1980) reviewed 16 studies of the outcome of anorexia nervosa between 1954 and 1980, and Herzog et al. (1988) reviewed 33 studies up to 1986. Other recent studies of prognosis include Gillbert et al. (1994) and Steinhausen and Seidel (1993). Following are some of the findings:

1. Mortality: The mortality rate ranged from 0–22%, with the majority of the studies having mortality rates of less than 4%.
2. Nutritional: At follow-up, 22–79% were within normal limits for weight, 15–43% were 11–21% below normal, 2–10% were overweight.
3. Menses: Thirty-eight percent to 95% of anorectic patients were menstruating at follow-up.
4. Eating difficulties: Fifteen percent to 82% were eating normally at follow-up, 23–67% had restricted food intake, 11–50% were still vomiting or abusing laxatives.
5. Psychological disturbances: Psychiatric disturbances were common in follow-up studies. Depressive symptoms were common; 24–45% had anxiety in meeting people; 13–44% had obsessive-compulsive features; and many also had a definite or probable affective disorder. Estimates of good or satisfactory psychosocial functioning ranged from 22–73%. Twenty-five percent to 55% of patients with anorexia nervosa go on to become bulimic.
6. Psychosexual disturbances: Twenty percent of anorectic patients had abnormal attitudes and behavior. Fear of pregnancy was not uncommon.
7. Psychosocial: The majority of anorectic patients were engaged in full-time employment, with good work attendance. Social anxiety was common, and many had problems with their families.

In conclusion, the anorectic patient's weight seems to respond best to therapy; menstrual function responds less well to therapy; and psychological readjustment has the worst prognosis. Certain factors seem to relate to a good prognosis or poor prognosis, while other factors have no effect:

1. Good prognosis
   a. High educational achievement
   b. Early age of onset
   c. Good educational adjustment
   d. Improvement in body image after weight gain
   e. Good initial ego strength
   f. Supportive family
2. Poor prognosis
   a. Late age of onset
   b. Continued overestimation of body size
   c. Premorbid obesity
   d. Self-induced vomiting or bulimia
   e. Laxative abuse
   f. Low social class
   g. Long duration of illness
   h. Disturbed parental relationship
   i. Males
   j. Marriage
   k. Marked depression, obsessional behavior, or somatic complaints
3. No effect
   a. Premorbid personality type
   b. Hyperactivity
   c. Degree of weight loss
   d. Pharmacotherapy

Anorexia nervosa appears to have lower recovery rates than that of bulimia.

BULIMIA

Bulimia is an eating disorder characterized by binge eating coupled with behavior intended to promote weight loss such as self-induced vomiting, laxative abuse, excessive exercise, and prolonged fasting. Some feel that both bulimia and anorexia nervosa are on a continuum. Differentiation is a mute point theoretically, but for the physician the behavior governs the treatment. With bulimia, the profound emaciation associated with anorexia is not present, and most individuals have a normal weight. The individual with bulimia is usually quite aware that the eating pattern is abnormal. Although many patients with anorexia nervosa have bingeing or purging behaviors, bulimia is classified as a unique disease in the *Diagnostic and Statistical Manual of Mental Disorders* (DSM; American Psychiatric Association, 1993).

Epidemiology

1. Onset: Onset is usually during late adolescence or early adulthood, although the age range may be from 13 to 58 years.
2. Sex: Ninety percent to 95% are female, although recently a reported increased prevalence in males, especially those who must weight qualify for interscholastic events (e.g., wrestlers).

3. Prevalence: Estimates are that approximately 1–3% of young females in Western industrialized countries have bulimia. In a recent survey by Schotte and Stunkard (1987) of college students, 1.3% of females and 0.1% of males were classified as bulimic, based on the DSM-III or DSM-III-R (the revision of DSM-III) classifications. Their conclusion was that bulimic behavior is common, but that clinically significant bulimia is not as common as many people fear. Zuckerman et al. (1986), using DSM-III criteria, found a 4% prevalence of bulimia in college women and 0.4% in college men. Symptoms of bulimia, including bingeing and purging behavior, were found to be more common than this. For example, 23% of the females and 14% of the males reported binges at least once each week, and 23% of the women and 9% of the men used one of the following methods of weight control: dieting, vomiting, laxatives, or diuretics.
4. Alcohol and substance abuse: This type of problem is not an uncommon association in individuals with bulimia, especially obese binge eaters. It usually occurs later in the course of the disease.
5. There is an increased prevalence of a major affective disorder in individuals with bulimia.

Clinical Manifestations

The DSM-IV diagnostic criteria for bulimia are as follows:

1. Recurrent episodes of binge eating (rapid consumption of a large amount of food in a discrete period of time, usually less than 2 hours)
2. A sense of lack of control over eating during the episode (i.e., a fear of not being able to stop eating)
3. A regular cycle of self-induced vomiting, use of laxatives, or rigorous dieting or fasting to counteract the effects of binge eating
4. A minimum average of two binge-eating episodes per week for at least 3 months

Two types identified:

1. Purging type: Individual regularly indulges in self-induced vomiting or abuse of laxatives, diuretics, or enemas.
2. Nonpurging type: Individual uses other inappropriate compensatory behaviors such as fasting or excessive exercise but not purge.

Binge Episodes   The most important clinical feature is the binge episode, with the self-perceived loss of control of eating. This results in a panic over gaining weight and purge behavior. The bulimic episodes often start following a period of pressure to lose weight. This might occur when the adolescent is involved with an activity such as ballet, cheerleading, gymnastics, or running. Any weight loss that occurs is often accompanied by feelings of inadequacy, depression, or low self-esteem. This may lead to binge-eating episodes, usually when the adolescent is alone. The binge leads to increased feelings of loss of control, shame, and fear. The teen may try to resolve these feelings by purging. This may then lead to a recurrent cycle of binge-purging in an attempt to manage feelings of depression and anxiety. Initially, the binge-purge activity may be infrequent, but with time it increases to daily or even several times a day. The binge often occurs following a short period of starvation, typically in the afternoon after having skipped breakfast or lunch. It may begin with an after-school snack. Characteristics of the binge eating include:

1. Food is eaten fast and often swallowed without chewing.
2. The quantity of food eaten is large and usually of high caloric value.

3. The individual often experiences anxiety, guilt, and depression over the eating episodes.
4. The binge episodes often occur alone and secretively.
5. The binge may have a frenzied quality, with consumption of food occurring in an anxious manner.

Signs and symptoms may be minimal but can include:

Symptoms

1. Swelling of hands and feet
2. Weakness and fatigue
3. Headaches
4. Abdominal fullness
5. Nausea

Signs

1. Skin changes: Primarily on the dorsum of the hand related to self-induced vomiting; may include elongated superficial ulceration to hyperpigmentation, calluses, or scarring
2. Enlargement of the salivary glands, particularly the parotid glands; usually bilateral and painless
3. Dental erosions: Usually occurs in the lingual, palatal, and posterior occlusal surfaces of the teeth

Table 33.1 contrasts anorexia nervosa with bulimia.

Evaluation

Evaluation includes complete history and physical examination. Laboratory screening includes complete blood count, electrolytes, BUN and creatinine, glucose, calcium, electrolytes, calcium and phosphate, serum amylase (to confirm vomiting), electrocardiogram with rhythm strip, and possibly urine samples to detect laxative or diuretic abuse.

TABLE 33.1. Anorexia Nervosa Versus Bulimia

Area	Anorexia Nervosa	Bulimia
Epidemiology	90% female	Same
	Increased prevalence of eating disorders and depression in families	Same
	Onset early- to mid-adolescence	Slightly older onset
	Prevalence <1%	Prevalence 1–4% and even higher for bulemic behavior
Psychopathology	High prevalence of personality disorders:	Same
	Often feelings of guilt and self-blame	Same
	More obsessional	More histrionic
	Less aware of distress	More aware of psychological distress
Weight loss	>25% weight loss	Usually normal weight; may have slight gain or loss
Behavior	Perfectionistic, immature	May have wide variety of behavioral abnormalities such as stealing, drug use, promiscuity
Social patterns	Regressed and isolated social pattern	Same
Menses	Absent	Usually absent or irregular

Treatment

The treatment principles include:

1. Do not emphasize purging as the primary target symptom: The focus should be on decreasing the bulimic eating. With a decrease in bulimic eating, a decrease in the need to purge will follow. Eating three normal meals a day should be encouraged.
2. Encourage the adolescent to avoid those foods that trigger a binge such as ice cream or baked goods.
3. Treat the depression that often accompanies bulimia.
4. Have the adolescent participate in individual psychotherapy with or without family therapy, depending on the adolescent's current involvement with the family.
5. Encourage the adolescent to exercise in moderation: Moderate exercise can be used as a modality for weight control rather than purging. However, it bears repeating that the exercise should be kept in moderation.
6. Antidepressants: Some studies have demonstrated a positive effect of use of antidepressants for controlling bulimia. Usually, the more stimulant, appetite-suppressant antidepressants, such as the selective serotonin reuptake inhibitors or tricyclics, are recommended.
7. Groups and self-help organizations may be of benefit to some individuals.
8. If the individual has used diuretics, a low-salt diet may be of benefit, as there may be some fluid retention rebound when use of diuretics is discontinued.
9. If the individual has abused laxatives, bran may help the resultant constipation.
10. Referral for dental consultation for those teens with dental damage secondary to vomiting.

Complications

The complications of bulimia are the same as those related to purging behaviors listed earlier in this chapter for anorexia nervosa.

Prognosis

Herzog et al. (1988) reviewed seven studies on the outcome of bulimia. Results included:

1. Mortality: None
2. Weight: Most studies reported normal body weights at follow-up.
3. Menses: No data available
4. Eating behavior: Twenty-nine percent to 87% were having binge-eating behaviors; 28–77% reported at least one induced vomiting episode; 3–13% reported laxative abuse.
5. Psychologic state: Fifteen percent to 36% reported depression.

BIBLIOGRAPHY

Agras WS. Eating disorders: management of obesity, bulimia, and anorexia nervosa. New York: Pergamon Press, 1987.

American Psychiatric Association. Diagnostic and statistical manual of mental disorders. 4th ed. Washington DC: American Psychiatric Association, 1993.

Anderson AE. Anorexia nervosa and bulimia: a spectrum of eating disorders. J Adolesc Health Care 1983;4:15.

Arroyo D, Tonkin R. Adolescents with bulimic and nonbulimic eating disorders. J Adolesc Health Care 1985;6:21.

Atkins DM, Silber TJ. Clinical spectrum of anorexia nervosa in children. J Dev Behav Pediatr 1993;14:211.

Baran SA, Weltzin TE, Kaye WH. Low discharge weight and outcome in anorexia nervosa. Am J Psychiatry 1995;152:1070.

Beumont PJ, Russell JD, Touyz SW. Treatment of anorexia nervosa. Lancet 1993;341:1635.

Birmingham CL, Goldner EM, Bakan R. Controlled trial of zinc supplementation in anorexia nervosa. Int J Eat Disord 1994;15:251.

Bowers TK, Eckert E. Leukopenia in anorexia nervosa: lack of increased risk of infection. Arch Intern Med 1978;138:1520.

Boyar RM, Katz J, Finkelstein JW et al. Anorexia nervosa: immaturity of the 24 hour luteinizing hormone secretory pattern. N Engl J Med 1974;291:861.

Brown S, Bonifazi DZ. An overview of anorexia and bulimia nervosa, and the impact of eating disorders on the oral cavity. Compendium 1993;14:1596.

Brownell KD, Rodin J. The dieting maelstrom—is it possible and advisable to lose weight? Am Psychol 1994;49:781.

Bruch H. Eating disorders: obesity and anorexia nervosa. New York: Basic Books, 1973.

Bruch H. Perils of behavior modification in treatment of anorexia nervosa. JAMA 1974;230:1419.

Bruch H. Psychological antecedents of anorexia nervosa. In: Vigersky RD, ed. Anorexia nervosa, 10th ed. New York: Raven Press, 1977.

Bruch H. The golden cage: the enigma of anorexia nervosa. Cambridge, Massachusetts: Harvard University Press, 1978.

Bruch H. Anorexia nervosa: therapy and theory. Am J Psychiatry 1982;139:1531.

Burket RC, Hodgin JD. Factors predicting reluctance to seek treatment in patients with eating disorders. South Med J 1993;86:529.

Casper RC, Eckert ED, Halmi K, et al. Bulimia: its incidence and clinical importance in patients with anorexia nervosa. Arch Gen Psychiatry 1980;37:1030.

Comerci GD: Eating disorders: anorexia and bulimia. In: Levine MD, Carey WB, Crocker AC, eds. Developmental-behavioral pediatrics, 2nd ed. Philadelphia: WB Saunders, 1992.

Connors ME, Morse W. Sexual abuse and eating disorders: a review. Int J Eat Disord 1993;13:1.

Crisp AH, Palmer RL, Kalucy RS. How common is anorexia nervosa? A prevalence study. Br J Psychiatry 1976;128:549.

Crow SJ, Mitchell JE. Rational therapy of eating disorders. Drugs 1994;48:372.

de-Simone G, Scalfi L, Galderisi M. Cardiac abnormalities in young women with anorexia nervosa. Br Heart J 1994;71:287.

Drewnowski A, Hopkins SA, Kessler RC. The prevalence of bulimia nervosa in the U.S. college student population. Am J Public Health 1988;78:1322.

Drossman DA, Ontjes DA, Heizer WD. Anorexia nervosa. Gastroenterology 1979;77:1115.

DuPont RL. Bulimia: a modern epidemic among adolescents. Pediatr Ann 1984;13:908.

Edwards KI. Obesity, anorexia, and bulimia. Med Clin North Am 1993;77:899.

Fairburn CG, Norman PA, Welch SL, et al. A prospective study of outcome in bulimia nervosa and the long-term effects of three psychological treatments. Arch Gen Psychiatry 1995;52:304.

Feighner JP, Robins E, Guze SB, et al. Diagnostic criteria for use in psychiatric research. Arch Gen Psychiatry 1972;26:57.

Fosson A, Knibbs J, Bryant-Waugh R, et al. Early onset anorexia nervosa. Arch Dis Child 1987;62:114.

Frank DL, Walton BE. Pregnancy and eating disorders: a review and clinical implications. Int J Eat Disord 1993;13:41.

Garfinkel PE, Garner DM. Anorexia nervosa: a multidimensional perspective. New York: Brunner/Mazel, 1982.

Garfinkel PE, Garner DM, eds.The role of drug treatments for eating disorders. New York: Brunner/Mazel, 1987.

Garfinkel PE, Moldofsky H, Garner DM. The heterogeneity of anorexia nervosa: bulimia as a distinct subgroup. Arch Gen Psychiatry 1980;37:1036.

Garner DM, Garfinkel PE, eds. Diagnostic issues in anorexia nervosa and bulimia nervosa. New York: Brunner/Mazel, 1988.

Gillbert IC, Rastam M, Gillberg C. Anorexia nervosa outcome: six-year controlled longitudinal study of 51 cases including a population cohort. J Am Acad Child Adolesc Psychiatry 1994;33:729.

Gold PW, Gwirtsman H, Avgerinos PC, et al. Abnormal hypothalamic-pituitary-adrenal function in anorexia nervosa: pathophysiologic mechanisms in underweight and weight-corrected patients. N Engl J Med 1986;314:1335.

Gold PW, Kaye W, Robertson GL, Ebert M. Abnormalities in plasma and cerebrospinal-fluid arginine vasopressin in patients with anorexia nervosa. N Engl J Med 1983;308:1117.

Goldbloom DS, Olmstead MP. Pharmacotherapy of bulimia nervosa with fluoxetine: assessment of clinically significant attitudinal change. Am J Psychiatry 1993;150:770.

Golden NH, Shenker IR. Amenorrhea in anorexia nervosa. Neuroendocrine control of hypothalamic dysfunction. Int J Eat Disord 1994;16:53.

Hall RCW, Hoffman R, Stickney SK. Bulimia: managing a complicated disorder. Female Patient 1986;11:24.

Halmi K, Brodlan G, Loney J. Prognosis in anorexia nervosa. Ann Intern Med 1973;78:907.

Health and Public Policy Committee, American College of Physicians. Eating disorders: anorexia nervosa and bulimia. Ann Intern Med 1986;105:790.

Heebink DM, Sunday SR, Halmi KA. Anorexia nervosa and bulimia nervosa in adolescence: effects of age and menstrual status on psychological variables. J Am Acad Child Adolesc Psychiatry 1995;34:378.

Herzog DB. Pharmacotherapy of anorexia nervosa and bulimia. Pediatr Ann 1984;13:915.

Herzog DB. Eating disorders. N Engl J Med 1985;313:295.

Herzog DB, Keller MB, Lavori PW. Outcome in anorexia nervosa and bulimia nervosa: a review of the literature. J Nerv Ment Dis 1988;176:131.

Herzog DB, Sacks NR, Keller MB, et al. Patterns and predictors of recovery in anorexia nervosa and bulimia nervosa. J Am Acad Child Adolesc Psychiatry 1993;32:835.

Hoffman L, Halmi K. Psychopharmacology in the treatment of anorexia nervosa and bulimia nervosa. Psychiatr Clin North Am 1993;16:767.

Hsu LK. Outcome of anorexia nervosa: a review of the literature. Arch Gen Psychiatry 1980;37:1041.

Hsu LKG. The treatment of anorexia nervosa. Am J Psychiatry 1986;143:573.

Hsu LK, Crisp AH, Harding B. Outcome of anorexia nervosa. Lancet 1979;1:60.

Isner JM, Roberts WC, Heymsfield SB, et al. Anorexia nervosa and sudden death. Ann Intern Med 1985; 102:49.

Johnson GL, Humphries LL, Shirley PB, et al. Mitral valve prolapse in patients with anorexia nervosa and bulimia. Arch Intern Med 1986;146:1525.

Johnson GL, Sansone RA, Chewning M. Good reasons why young women would develop anorexia nervosa: the adaptive context. Pediatr Ann 1992;21:731.

Katz, JL. Some reflections on the nature of the eating disorders: on the need for humility. Int J Eat Disord 1985;4:617.

Katz RL, Keen CL, Lit IF, et al. Zinc deficiency in anorexia nervosa. J Adolesc Health Care 1987;8:400.

Klibanski A, Biller BM, Schoenfeld DA, et al. The effects of estrogen administration on trabecular bone loss in young women with anorexia nervosa. J Clin Endocrinol Metab 1995;80:898.

Kreipe RE, Harris PJ. Myocardial impairment resulting from eating disorders. Pediatr Ann 1992;12:760.

Lucas AR. Toward the understanding of anorexia nervosa as a disease entity. Mayo Clin Proc 1981;56: 254.

Lucas AR, Beard CM, O'Fallon WM, et al. Anorexia nervosa in Rochester, Minnesota: a 45 year study. Mayo Clin Proc 1988;63:433.

Maloney MJ, Farrell MK. Treatment of severe weight loss in anorexia nervosa with hyperalimentation and psychotherapy. Am J Psychiatry 1980;137:310.

Mickley DW. Evaluating common eating disorders. Ten questions to ask your patient. Female Patient 1988; 13:33.

Milner MR, McAnarney ER, Klish WJ. Metabolic abnormalities in adolescent patients with anorexia nervosa. J Adolesc Health Care 1985;6:191.

Minuchin S, Roseman BL, Baker L. Psychosomatic families: anorexia nervosa in context. Cambridge, Massachusetts: Harvard University Press, 1978.

Mitchell JE, Seim HC, Colon E, et al. Medical complications and medical management of bulimia. Ann Intern Med 1987;107:71.

Moodie DS, Salcedo E. Cardiac function in adolescents and young adults with anorexia nervosa. J Adolesc Health Care 1983;4:9.

Newman MM, Halmi KA. The endocrinology of anorexia nervosa and bulimia nervosa. Endocrinol Metab Clin North Am 1988;17:195.

Nussbaum M, Baird D, Sonnenblick M, et al. Short stature in anorexia nervosa patients. J Adolesc Health Care 1985;6:453.

Nussbaum M, Shenker IR, Baird D, et al. Follow-up investigation in patients with anorexia nervosa. J Pediatr 1985;106:835.

Olivardia R, Pope HG Jr, Mangweth B, et al. Eating disorders in college men. Am J Psychiatry 1995;152:1279.

Palla B, Litt IF. Medical complications of eating disorders in adolescents. Pediatrics 1988;81:613.

Palmer EP, Guay AT. Reversible myopathy secondary to abuse of ipecac in patients with major eating disorders. N Engl J Med 1985;313:1457.

Patchell RA, Fellows HA, Humphries LL. Neurologic complications of anorexia nervosa. Acta Neurol Scand 1994;89:111.

Peterson DS, Barkmeier WW. Oral signs of frequent vomiting in anorexia. Am Fam Physician 1983;27: 199.

Price WA. Pharmacologic management of eating disorders. Am Fam Physician 1988;37:157.

Pyle RL, Mitchell JE, Eckert ED. The incidence of bulimia in freshmen college students. Int J Eat Disord 1983;2:75.

Rigotti NA, Nussbaum SR, Herzog DB, et al. Osteoporosis in women with anorexia nervosa. N Engl J Med 1984;311:1601.

Rock CL, Curran-Celentano J. Nutritional disorder of anorexia nervosa: a review. Int J Eat Disord 1994;15: 187.

Robin AL, Siegel PT, Koepke T, et al. Family therapy versus individual therapy for adolescent females with anorexia nervosa. J Dev Behav Pediatr 1994;15:111.

Sakka S, Hurst P, Khawaja H. Anorexia nervosa and necrotizing colitis: case report and review of the literature. Postgrad Med J 1994;70:823.

Schork E, Eckert ED, Halmi KA. The relationship between psychopathology, eating disorder diagnosis, and clinical outcome at 10-year follow-up in anorexia nervosa. Compr Psychiatry 1994;35:113.

Schotte DE, Stunkard AJ. Bulimia vs. bulimic behaviors on a college campus. JAMA 1987;258:1213.

Schwabe AD, Lippe BM, Chang J. Anorexia nervosa: UCLA conference. Ann Intern Med 1981;94:371.

Seeman E, Szmukler GI, Formica C. Osteoporosis in anorexia nervosa: the influence of peak bone density, bone loss, oral contraceptive use, and exercise. J Bone Miner Res 1992;7:1467.

Sharp CW, Freeman CP. The medical complications of anorexia nervosa. Br J Psychiatry 1993;162:452.

Sherman P, Leslie K, Goldberg E, et al. Hypercarotenemia and transaminitis in female adolescents with eating disorders: a prospective, controlled study. J Adolesc Health 1994;15:205.

Siddiqui A, Ramsay B, Leonard J. The cutaneous signs of eating disorders. Acta Derm Venereol 1994;74:68.

Siegel JH, Hardoff D, Golden NH, et al. Medical complications in male adolescents with anorexia nervosa. J Adolesc Health 1995;16:448.

Solanto MV, Jacobson MS, Heller L, et al. Rate of weight gain of inpatients with anorexia nervosa under two behavioral contracts. Pediatrics 1994;93:989.

Steinhaursen HC. Treatment and outcome of adolescent anorexia nervosa. Horm Res 1995;43:168.

Steinhausen HC, Seidel R. Outcome in adolescent eating disorders. Int J Eat Disord 1993;14:487.

Sullivan PF. Mortality in anorexia nervosa. Am J Psychiatry 1995;152:1073.

Thiel A, Broocks A, Ohlmeier M, et al. Obsessive-complusive disorder among patients with anorexia nervosa and bulimia nervosa. Am J Psychiatry 1995;152:72.

Touyz SW, Liew VP, Tseng P, et al. Oral and dental complications in dieting disorders. Int J Eat Disord 1993;14:341.

Trygstad O, Foss I, Edminson PD, et al. A urinary anorexigenic peptide. Chromatographic patterns of urinary peptides in anorexia nervosa. Acta Endocrinol (Copenh) 1978;89:196.

Vigersky RA, Loriaux L, Anderson AE, et al. Delayed pituitary hormone response to LRF and TRF in patients with anorexia nervosa and with secondary amenorrhea associated with simple weight loss. J Clin Endocrinol Metab 1976;43:893.

Warren MR, Vande Weile RL. Clinical and metabolic features of anorexia nervosa. Am J Obstet Gynecol 1973;117:435.

Warren SE, Steinberg S. Acid base and electrolyte disturbances in anorexia nervosa. Am J Psychiatry 1979;136:415.

Yager J. Psychosocial treatments for eating disorders. Psychiatry 1994;57:153.

Yates A. Current perspectives on the eating disorders. J Am Acad Child Adolesc Psychiatry 1989;28(Part 1):813 and 1990;29(Part 2):1.

Yates A. Biologic considerations in the etiology of eating disorders. Pediatr Ann 1992;21:739.

Zuckerman DM, Colby A, Ware NC, et al. The prevalence of bulimia among college students. Am J Public Health 1986;76:1135.

For Adolescents, Parents, and Teachers

Bruch H. The golden cage. The enigma of anorexia nervosa. Cambridge, Massachusetts: Harvard University Press, 1978.

Crisp AH. Anorexia nervosa. Let me be. New York: Grune & Stratton, 1980.

Hautzig D. Second star to the right. New York: Greenwillow, 1981.

Levenkron S. The best little girl in the world. New York: Contemporary Books, 1978.

Levenkron S. Treating and overcoming anorexia nervosa. New York: Charles Scribner's Sons, 1982.

Liu A. Solitaire. New York: Harper & Row, 1980.

Sacker IM, Zimmer MA. Dying to be thin. Understanding and defeating anorexia nervosa and bulimia. A practical lifesaving guide. New York: Warner Books, 1987.

Miscellaneous Medical Disorders

CHAPTER 34
Fatigue

Marvin E. Belzer and Lawrence S. Neinstein

Adolescents have abundant energy, so a complaint of fatigue needs to be taken seriously, especially if the complaint originates with the adolescent and not his or her parents. Parents commonly complain of their tired or fatigued teen. Such complaints may reflect overly high expectations by the parents, adolescent-parent conflicts, or organic illness. Most fatigue in adolescents is nonorganic in origin, representing a reaction to stress, anxiety, conflict, or depression. However, most adolescents complaining of tiredness are asking for help, either in the form of "I think something's wrong with me—tell me about it" or "I'm scared or anxious—help me."

CAUSES OF FATIGUE

Psychological Causes

In adolescents, psychological causes are responsible for 80–90% or more of fatigue that is unrelated to too much activity and too little sleep. Such fatigue may stem from:

1. Depression
2. Anxiety
3. Stressful situations

Physiological Causes

Physiological causes, another common factor in fatigue, may relate to:

1. Inadequate sleep
2. Dieting
3. Too much activity
4. Pregnancy

Organic Causes

Organic causes of fatigue are infrequent during adolescence. Such fatigue may result from:

1. Drugs: Antihistamines, sedatives, tetracycline, alcohol, anticonvulsants, oral contraceptives, and steroids
2. Infections
   a. Infectious mononucleosis
   b. Viral hepatitis

    c. Influenza

    d. *Mycoplasma* pneumonia

    e. Human immunodeficiency virus (HIV) infections and acquired immunodeficiency syndrome (AIDS)

    f. Tuberculosis

    g. Brucellosis

    h. Parasitic infections

    i. Bacterial endocarditis

    j. Lyme disease

3. Allergies
4. Anemia
5. Neoplasm
6. Renal failure
7. Connective tissue disease
   a. Fibromyalgia
   b. Polymyositis
   c. Systemic lupus
8. Inflammatory bowel disease
9. Congenital heart disease
10. Endocrine-related causes
    a. Hypothyroidism
    b. Hypoglycemia
    c. Addison's disease
    d. Diabetes mellitus
    e. Hyperparathyroidism
    f. Hypopituitarism
    g. Cushing's syndrome
11. Liver failure
12. Heavy-metal intoxication
13. Chronic fatigue syndrome

EVALUATION

History

1. Careful review of systems, with evaluation for medical conditions causing fatigue
2. Medical history: Evidence of organic disease
3. Thorough history of peer relationships, school attitude and performance, and family situation; history of depression or other psychiatric disorders
4. Diet and sleep history
5. Alcohol and substance-abuse history
6. Medical history; history of use of over-the-counter medications
7. History of daily activities
8. History suggestive of emotional fatigue
   a. Fatigue that is present on arising and stays the same or lessens throughout the day
   b. Fatigue that is unchanged despite adequate sleep
   c. Frequent changes in level of fatigue throughout the day
   d. Fatigue that is worse at home or in certain situations
   e. History of conflict with parents, peer problems, sex problems, boredom, or anxiety
   f. Other signs of depression: Acting-out behavior, insomnia, apathy, social withdrawal

    g. Other signs of anxiety: Headache, abdominal pain, palpitations, chest pains

    h. Fatigue unassociated with other symptoms

9. History suggestive of organic cause

    a. Fatigue that increases during the day

    b. Fatigue that decreases with rest

    c. History of fever, weight loss, night sweats, lymphadenopathy, change in bowel movements, drug use, arthritis, skin changes, or any symptoms consistent with endocrinopathy, infection, or a neoplastic problem

Physical Examination

Fatigue associated with nonorganic causes is usually accompanied by a normal physical examination. Important areas to examine include:

1. General appearance: Evidence of chronic illness
2. Height and weight
3. Lymph nodes: Evidence of adenopathy
4. Thyroid gland: Presence of goiter
5. Cardiac: Evidence of abnormal heart murmur
6. Abdomen: Hepatosplenomegaly
7. Extremities: Evidence of arthritis
8. Sexual maturity rating: Puberty advance normal or not
9. Mental status examination to identify abnormalities in mood, intellectual function, memory, and personality—in particular, signs of depression or anxiety

Laboratory Tests

    Screening Evaluation   Many adolescents will not require any laboratory tests; the diagnosis of psychological fatigue will be evident after history taking and physical examination. If there is a question of the diagnosis, screening evaluation should include:

1. Urinalysis
2. Complete blood cell count with differential cell count
3. Mononucleosis test
4. Erythrocyte sedimentation rate

    Additional Tests   A more extensive evaluation for the teen with severe, prolonged fatigue would include, in addition:

1. Thyrotropin and adjusted thyroxine (T_4) determinations
2. Chest x-ray examination
3. Tuberculosis skin test
4. Fasting blood sugar test
5. Electrocardiography
6. Liver function tests
7. Serum electrolytes
8. Creatinine and blood urea nitrogen (BUN) values
9. Calcium and phosphorus concentrations
10. Total bilirubin concentration; alkaline phosphatase and liver aminotransferase activity
11. Creatine kinase activity
12. Antinuclear antibody measurement
13. HIV antibody measurement

No other additional tests, including neuroimaging studies, have been shown to be helpful in investigating chronic fatigue unless the history, physical examination, or initial laboratory findings suggest a specific disorder.

Chronic Fatigue Syndrome

Chronic fatigue syndrome (CFS) is a clinically defined syndrome (see case definition from the Centers for Disease Control and Prevention [CDC], below) that is characterized by severe, disabling fatigue and a combination of symptoms highlighted by self-reported impairments in concentration and short-term memory, musculoskeletal pain, and sleep disturbances. Diagnosis includes the exclusion of other medical and psychiatric causes of chronic fatigue symptoms. At the present time there are no specific signs or diagnostic tests for this condition. In addition, no definitive treatment exists. Some individuals improve with time, but many will remain functionally impaired for several years.

Etiology

Clinicians frequently have strong opinions regarding the organic versus the psychological cause of CFS. Though originally linked to Epstein-Barr virus and later to other viruses such as human herpes virus 6, cytomegalovirus, Coxsackievirus, and human T-cell lymphotrophic viruses (non-HIV type 1), CFS has not been consistently linked to any single virus. More recent studies have focused on immunological abnormalities in patients with CFS including chronic immune system activation and T-lymphocyte dysfunction, with abnormalities of natural killer cell function, mitogen stimulation, and lymphocyte phenotype. In addition, abnormalities in the central nervous system have been theorized as causes of the fatigue symptoms. These changes have included abnormalities in cerebral perfusion, hypothalamic function, and neurotransmitter regulation. At present the pathogenesis of symptoms remains a mystery.

Bates et al. (1995) studied laboratory abnormalities in 597 patients who met the CDC or Australian case definition of CFS. The major abnormalities found were immunologic; however, each lacked sufficient sensitivity to be a diagnostic test and none have proven specificity in evaluating other organic and psychiatric conditions that can produce fatigue. The most notable abnormalities in this study were elevated immune complexes or elevated IgG levels in 48% of cases who underwent both tests compared to only 6% in control subjects.

Cytokine interleukin-1 has also been of theoretical interest for several years. Elevated serum levels of interleukin-1 have been found in many patients with CFS (Cotton, 1991). The highest levels have been found in patients who have been the most disabled.

CFS is relatively rare in adolescents and has a slight female preponderance. Regardless of the cause, CFS can cause severe and prolonged morbidity and requires aggressive treatment to minimize disability.

Diagnosis

The elements of the CDC case definition are listed below. It is unclear how these criteria, designed for adult populations, apply to youth. The hallmarks of CFS in youth include:

1. A prodromal illness
2. Severe fatigue for at least 6 months
3. Exacerbation of fatigue with exercise
4. Somatic complaints such as headache, sore throat, swollen lymph nodes, myalgias, arthralgias, and fever (Table 34.1)

TABLE 34.1. Frequency of Symptoms and Signs in Patients with Chronic Fatigue Syndrome

Symptoms and Signs	Frequency (%)	Symptoms and Signs	Frequency (%)
Fatigue	100	Nocturia	50–60
Low-grade fever	60–95	Nausea	50–60
Myalgias	20–95	Dizziness	30–50
Sleep disorder	15–85	Arthralgias	40–50
Impaired cognition	50–85	Tachycardia	40–50
Depression	70–85	Dry eyes	30–40
Headache	35–85	Dry mouth	30–40
Pharyngitis	50–75	Diarrhea	30–40
Anxiety	50–70	Anorexia	30–40
Muscle weakness	40–70	Cough	30–40
Postexertional malaise	50–60	Digital swelling	30–40
Worsening of premenstrual symptoms	50–60	Night sweats	30–40
Stiffness	50–60	Painful lymph nodes	30–40
Visual blurring	50–60	Rash	30–40

Adapted from Komaroff AL, Buchwald D. Symptoms and signs of chronic fatigue syndrome. Rev Infect Dis 1991;13:59.

5. Neuropsychiatric complaints, especially difficulty in concentrating and depression
6. No preexisting psychiatric illness

A diagnostic study should generally be initiated to exclude organic illnesses as described in the preceding section on fatigue. Currently it is not advisable to order viral serological tests (other than a test for HIV-1, as indicated), immunological tests, neuroimaging scans, or serological testing for *Candida albicans* in patients who may have CFS. A psychological assessment to exclude a preexisting psychiatric illness is strongly advised. Depression occurring after the onset of CFS does not exclude the diagnosis of CFS.

CDC Case Definition The CDC (Holmes et al., 1988) has made a case definition for the chronic fatigue syndrome. An individual must fulfill both major criteria and the following minor criteria: 6 of the 11 symptom criteria and 2 or more of the physical criteria; or 8 or more of the 11 symptom criteria. These criteria do not appear to define a distinct group of cases; thus there has been significant discussion that they need revision. Better criteria and evaluation standards are needed because many individuals with chronic fatigue have received either an inadequate or excessive medical evaluation.

Major Criteria

1. New onset of persistent or relapsing debilitating fatigue in a person with no previous history of similar symptoms, which does not resolve with bed rest, and which is severe enough to reduce or impair daily activity to less than 50% for a period of at least 6 months
2. Exclusion (after thorough evaluation) of other clinical conditions that could cause these symptoms, such as autoimmune disease; localized infection, chronic or subacute bacterial disease, fungal disease, and parasitic disease; disease related to human immunodeficiency virus infection; chronic psychiatric disease; chronic inflammatory disease; neuromuscular disease; endocrine disease; drug dependency or abuse; and side effects of a medication or other toxic agents

Minor Criteria

SYMPTOM CRITERIA

1. Mild fever
2. Sore throat

3. Painful lymph nodes in anterior or posterior cervical or axillary distribution
4. Unexplained generalized muscle weakness
5. Muscle discomfort or myalgia
6. Prolonged generalized fatigue after levels of exercise previously tolerated
7. Generalized headaches
8. Migratory arthralgia without joint swelling or redness
9. Neuropsychological complaints such as photophobia, transient visual scotomata, excessive irritability, confusion, inability to concentrate, depression
10. Sleep disturbance
11. Main symptom complex developed during the course of a few hours to a few days

PHYSICAL CRITERIA   Physical criteria must be documented by a physician on at least two occasions, at least 1 month apart.

1. Low-grade fever: Oral temperature between 37.6°C and 38.6°C
2. Nonexudative pharyngitis
3. Palpable or tender anterior or posterior cervical or axillary lymph nodes

Treatment

1. Reassurance: Adolescents need to know that they do not have a life-threatening illness. Though CFS typically has a prolonged course (2–5 years), most cases will eventually lessen in severity or resolve. Parents also need reassurance and guidance. Frustration with this illness frequently leads to "physician shopping," expensive evaluations, and the use of unproved and potentially dangerous treatments. Parents should be strongly advised to help their child continue in school and to avoid home study programs. Attending school reduces deconditioning and social isolation.
2. Medications: Trials of low-dose therapy with antidepressants such as fluoxetine (Prozac), 10–20 mg, sertraline (Zoloft), 25–50 mg, and doxepin (Sinequan), 10–30 mg, have been anecdotally reported to improve patients sense of well-being. A diagnosis of a major depression requires that psychiatric care be given and may require the use of full-dose antidepressant therapy. Youth with pain caused by headaches or myalgias may benefit from anti-inflammatory agents. The use of narcotic analgesics is inadvisable in the treatment of chronic pain.
3. Psychotherapy: Youth with CFS frequently have a reactive depression and need support in dealing with the frustrations of a prolonged illness. Patients will typically have trouble in coping with typical adolescent issues such as separation/individuation, peer relationships, body image, and school performance, as well as with chronic pain and fatigue.
4. Physical therapy: With the typical exacerbation of symptoms seen with exercise, many youth become severely deconditioned. A program of gentle exercise with gradual increases is advisable and may best be implemented with the assistance of a physical therapist. Severely affected youth who are bedridden may benefit from an inpatient rehabilitation program. Case reports from Great Britain and Canada focus on a joint psychiatric and rehabilitation approach and report success.

Prognosis

Very little is known about the natural course of CFS in youth. Smith et al. (1991) studied 15 youth thought to have CFS and reported that at telephone follow-up 13–32 months after evaluation, 4 were completely well, 4 markedly improved, and 7 unimproved or worse. Studies of adults suggest that some individuals improve with time, but most remain functionally impaired for several years (Wilson et al., 1994).

The CDC has a hot-line number (404-332-4555) for information on CFS. In addition, the Chronic Fatigue and Immune Dysfunction Syndrome Association of America has information for patients and families. For immediate assistance, call 900-896-2343 (toll call). To receive information by mail, call 800-442-3437.

BIBLIOGRAPHY

Bates DW, Buchwald D, Lee J. Clinical laboratory test findings in patients with chronic fatigue syndrome. Arch Intern Med 1995;155:97.

Bates DW, Schmitt W, Buchwald D, et al. Prevalence of fatigue and chronic fatigue syndrome in a primary care practice. Arch Intern Med 1993;153:2759.

Bell DS. Chronic fatigue syndrome update. Postgrad Med 1994;96:73.

Calabrese L, Danao T, Camara E, et al. Chronic fatigue syndrome. Am Fam Physician 1992;45:1205.

Carter BD, Edwards JF, Kronenberger WG, et al. Case control study of chronic fatigue in pediatric patients. Pediatrics 1995;95:179.

Centers for Disease Control. The chronic fatigue syndrome [Information pamphlet MSA32]. Atlanta, Georgia: U.S. Department of Health and Human Services, January 1990.

Cho WK, Stollerman GH. Chronic fatigue syndrome. Hosp Pract 1992;September 15:221.

Cotton P. Treatment proposed for chronic fatigue syndrome: research continues to compile data on disorder. JAMA 1991;266:2667.

Epstein KR. The chronically fatigued patient. Med Clin North Am 1995;79:315.

Friedman HH. Problem-oriented medical diagnosis. Boston: Little, Brown, 1981:1.

Fukuda K, Straus SE, Hickie I, et al. The chronic fatigue syndrome: a comprehensive approach to its definition and study. Ann Intern Med 1994;121:953.

Gantz NM. An update on chronic fatigue syndrome. Contemp Intern Med 1992;April:53.

Goldenberg DL. Fibromyalgia, chronic fatigue syndrom, and myofascial pain syndrom. Curr Opin Rheumatol 1995;7:127.

Goodnick PJ, Sandoval R. Psychotropic treatment of chronic fatigue syndrome and related disorders. J Clin Psychiatry 1993;54:13.

Goroll AH, May LA, Mulley AG, eds. Evaluation of chronic fatigue. In: Primary care medicine. Philadelphia: JB Lippincott, 1995.

Hayden SP. A practical approach to chronic fatigue syndrome. Cleve Clin J Med 1991;58:116.

Hoffmann AD, Greydanus DE, eds. Emotional problems with physical manifestations. In: Adolescent medicine. Norwalk, Connecticut: Appleton & Lange, 1989.

Holmes GP, Kaplan JE, Gantz NM, et al. Chronic fatigue syndrome: a working case definition. Ann Intern Med 1988;108:387.

Katon W. Chronic fatigue syndrome criteria. Arch Intern Med 1992;152:1604.

Khan AS, Heneine WM, Chapman LE, et al. Assessment of a retrovirus sequence and other possible risk factors for the chronic fatigue syndrome. Ann Intern Med 1993;118:241.

Landay AL, Jessop C, Lennette ET, et al. Chronic fatigue syndrome: clinical condition associated with immune activation. Lancet 1991;338:707.

Levine PH, Jacobson S, Pocinki AG, et al. Clinical, epidemiologic, and virologic studies in four clusters of the chronic fatigue syndrome. Arch Intern Med 1992;152:1611.

Manu P, Lane TJ, Matthews DA. The frequency of the chronic fatigue syndrome in patients with symptoms of persistent fatigue. Ann Intern Med 1988;109:554.

McKenzie R, Straus SE. Chronic fatigue syndrom. Adv Intern Med 1995;40:119.

Melnick A. When an adolescent is tired all the time. Consultant 1981;July:150.

Peterson PK, Shepard J, Macres M, et al. A controlled trial of intravenous IgG in chronic fatigue syndrome. Am J Med 1990;89:554.

Ruffin MT, Cohen M. Evaluation and management of fatiue. Am Fam Physician 1994;50:625.

Schluederberg A, Straus SE, Peterson P, et al. Chronic fatigue syndrome research: definition and medical outcome assessment [NIH conference]. Ann Intern Med 1992;117:325.

Shafran SD. The chronic fatigue syndrome. Am J Med 1991;90:730.

Smith MS, Mitchell J, Corey L, et al. Chronic fatigue in adolescents. Pediatrics 1991;88:195.

Strickland MC. Depression, chronic fatigue syndrome, and the adolescent. Primary Care 1991;18:259.

Vereker MI. Chronic fatigue syndrome: a joint pediatric-psychiatric approach. Arch Dis Child 1992;67:550.

Wachsmuth JR, MacMillan HL. Effective treatment for an adolescent with chronic fatigue syndrome. Clinical Pediatrics 1991;30:488.

Walford GA, MacNelson W, McCluskey PR. Fatigue, depression, and social adjustment in chronic fatigue syndrome. Arch Dis Child 1993;68:384.

Wilson A, Hickie I, Lloyd A, et al. Longitudinal study of outcome of chronic fatigue syndrome. Br Med J 1994;308:756.

CHAPTER 35

Chronic, Recurrent Abdominal Pain

Dan W. Thomas and Lawrence S. Neinstein

Chronic recurrent abdominal pain is a frequent complaint of teenagers and young adults, and treatment efforts can lead to intense frustration among both patients and health-care practitioners. The condition is usually defined as three or more separate episodes of pain during a 3-month period. It often interferes with normal daily activities or performance. In most cases (approximately 95%) of recurrent abdominal pain in adolescents, no organic abnormality is found.

EPIDEMIOLOGY

In a study by Oster (1972) of patients 6–19 years of age, the prevalence of recurrent abdominal pain was as follows:

1. Males: 12.1%
2. Females: 16.7%
3. Peak prevalence occurred at age 9 (21% male, 30% females)
4. Prevalence by age 16–17 was approximately 5% of all adolescents

DIFFERENTIAL DIAGNOSIS AND CLINICAL MANIFESTATIONS

The following conditions are listed in approximate order of occurrence during adolescence.

Functional Pain

Most recurrent abdominal pain in adolescents is nonorganic and is related to everyday stress.

1. Pain character: Nonspecific periumbilical, crampy, or dull pain. It often occurs two to four times a week. There is usually no radiation. In about 75% of patients, the pain lasts less than 3 hours. The pain is most often unrelated to eating, bowel movements, or physical activity, and does not awaken the patient from sleep. Stool retention is frequent.
2. Family history of abdominal pain is common.
3. Relationship exists between pain and periods of stress. School and family problems are commonly associated stress factors.
4. Associated symptoms are common:
   a. Nausea: Up to 50%
   b. Vomiting: 19–66%
   c. Headaches: 4–50%

    d. Fatigue: 45%
    e. Dizziness: 25%
    f. Diarrhea: 4–24%
    g. Loose stools: 10–20%

Irritable Bowel Syndrome

1. Onset is usually during late adolescence or young adulthood.
2. Prevalence in females is two times more common than in males.
3. Pain is colicky in nature and is located in the hypogastrium or the left lower quadrant of the abdomen. Pain increases with food intake and decreases with bowel movements.
4. Pain is often associated with diarrhea, constipation with pellet-like stools, or both.
5. Symptoms increase with stress.
6. The cause probably relates to a dysfunctional colon with increased dysfunctional muscular contractions.
7. Considered a variant of functional chronic abdominal pain.

Lactose Intolerance

Lactose intolerance is associated with crampy abdominal pain, diarrhea, flatulence, and belching. It is common in African-American, Asian, Hispanic, and Jewish persons.

Gynecological Conditions

1. Pelvic inflammatory disease
2. Ectopic pregnancy
3. Mittelschmerz
4. Endometriosis
5. Torsion or ruptured ovarian cyst

Musculoskeletal Pain

Costochondritis, myositis, or abdominal wall muscle strain may be the cause of abdominal pain.

Capsular Distension or Inflammation

1. Hepatitis, hepatomegaly, Fitz-Hugh and Curtis syndrome
2. Splenomegaly

Gastrointestinal Infections

Giardiasis, in particular, may mimic psychogenic pain. Individuals with giardiasis may complain of subacute or chronic abdominal pain with bloating, as well as flatulence with or without diarrhea.

Referred Pain

Referred pain may be a result of involvement of the lower lobes of the lung (i.e., pneumonia). An uncommon source of referred pain is from spinal cord tumors (Neinstein, 1989).

Mucosal Ulceration

1. Peptic ulcer disease: The typical pain of this disease is midepigastric burning pain occurring 1–3 hours after meals or at night. Pain decreases with the ingestion of food or antacids. The younger the patient, the more atypical the pain; approximately 50% of adolescents will have the classic pain pattern. Peptic ulcers are frequently associated with *Helicobacter pylori* gastritis.
2. Inflammatory bowel disease: This disease is manifested by:
   a. Poor growth
   b. Anemia and elevated erythrocyte sedimentation rate
   c. Bloody stools
   d. Systemic symptoms: arthritis, iritis, hepatitis, erythema nodosum
   e. Abnormal findings on radiographical contrast studies

Obstructed Viscus

1. Bowel obstruction, caused by adhesions or volvulus, may be present.
2. Biliary tract obstruction can result in recurrent episodes of epigastric and right upper quadrant abdominal pain, often with nausea and tenderness of the right upper quadrant of the abdomen. Most adolescents with gallbladder stones have one of the following risk factors: use of oral contraceptives, recent pregnancy, family history, or obesity. In adolescents, gallstones are seldom found to be associated with hemolysis, diabetes mellitus, or congenital biliary tract defects (Adye and Ryan, 1983). Another risk group for gallstones in this age group are teens receiving parenteral nutrition. A common complication in children and adolescents with gallstones is pancreatitis (8%) (Reif et al., 1991).
3. Ureter obstruction, caused by kidney stones, results in colicky pain, often radiating to the groin.

Systemic Conditions

1. Diabetic ketoacidosis
2. Sickle cell crisis
3. Hereditary angioneurotic edema
4. Polyarteritis
5. Hemolytic-uremic syndrome
6. Lead intoxication
7. Porphyria

Pancreatitis

Pancreatitis is typified by midepigastric pain radiating to the back and associated with nausea and vomiting.

DIAGNOSIS

The organic nature of abdominal pain is usually suggested by the history, physical examination findings, and results of simple screening laboratory tests.

History

1. Pain description: Location, intensity, character, chronology, aggravating and alleviating factors, and associated signs and symptoms. The diagnosis of functional pain should not

be made on the basis of exclusion alone but should be made in association with a history of stress, anxiety, or depression.

    a. Characteristics of functional pain include:
- Poorly described periumbilical discomfort
- Variable location
- Does not awaken teen from sleep
- Often exacerbated by stress
- May have been present for months or years before teen sought medical assistance
- Rarely associated with significant weight loss
- May have other associated systemic symptoms but they are usually not consistent with disease process

    b. Characteristics of organic abdominal pain include:
- Well localized pain
- Location that usually remains constant
- May awaken teen from sleep
- May be precipitated by foods
- Onset usually relatively acute
- Bloody stools
- Bilious emesis
- May be associated with weight loss or other systemic symptoms that are more consistent with disease process such as arthritis/arthralgias, recurrent fevers

2. Family history: Relevant features of the family history include:

    a. History of abdominal pain

    b. History of metabolic or hematological problems: porphyria, diabetes, or sickle cell anemia

    c. Family function and stress

3. Current stresses and relationship to pain: Common stressors for precipitating abdominal pain include:

    a. Home
- Parental arguments, separation, or divorce
- Illness or abdominal pain in family member
- Loss of family member
- Move to another location

    b. Peers
- Loss of friends
- Teasing by friends
- Pressures by friends

    c. School
- Change of school
- School failure
- Pressure in school
- Teacher-pupil problems

4. Pain diary: It is usually helpful to have the teen keep a diary of the pain pattern for a 1- to 3-week period, including timing, severity, and precipitating factors.

Physical Examination

Functional abdominal pain is usually associated with normal findings on physical examination or mild midepigastric tenderness without rebound. Mild lower left colon or rectosigmoid tenderness can be found. Signs of organic disease include:

1. Lack of growth: Evidence of weight loss, short stature, decreased growth, or delayed puberty—often early signs of organic disease
2. Hepatosplenomegaly
3. Abdominal masses
4. Perianal area: Fistulas or abscesses
5. Pelvic examination: Ovarian masses, adnexal tenderness

Laboratory Tests

1. Primary screening tests
   a. Complete blood cell count
   b. Erythrocyte sedimentation rate
   c. Urinalysis with or without culture
   d. Chemistry profile with liver function tests
   e. Stool samples obtained for evidence of occult blood, ova and parasites, and stool *Giardia* antigen screening test
   f. Stool α_1-antitrypsin test (screening test for protein-losing enteropathy)
   g. Plain film of the abdomen
   h. *H. pylori* antibody titer
2. Secondary tests, performed if history indicates need
   a. Sigmoidoscopy and biopsy: If evidence of bleeding, abnormal gastrointestinal films, or elevated erythrocyte sedimentation rate
   b. Barium enema
   c. Upper gastrointestinal (GI) tract x-ray series and small-bowel follow-through
   d. Endoscopy of the upper GI tract
   e. Intravenous pyelogram or renal ultrasonography: If renal abnormalities are detected
   f. Serum amylase and lipase: If pancreatitis is suspected
   g. Abdominal ultrasonography: If ovarian mass or gallstones are suspected
   h. Technetium Tc 99m iminodiacetic acid scan: Useful in diagnosing acute cholecystitis
   i. Sickle cell screening: For African-American patients
   j. Urine porphyrins: If unusual, recurrent, severe abdominal pain exists, especially in association with an abnormal mental status
   k. Lactose tolerance test

The diagnosis of functional abdominal pain depends on symptoms related to stress or life events, a history that is nonsuggestive of organic disease, and normal findings on physical examination and screening laboratory tests. A family history of functional abdominal problems such as irritable bowel syndrome, or "spastic colitis," is supportive evidence. Some adolescents seem to have benign abdominal pain without any evidence of organic problems or psychological stresses.

Approach to Evaluation

After a careful history and physical examination have revealed no obvious organic source, the practitioner should explain to the teen that an evaluation is being done to check for many possibilities, including organic and stress-related causes. This is a good time to explain that real symptoms, including pain, can result from feelings. A good example is blushing—a physiological response to the feeling of embarrassment. At this point the teen should be asked to keep a pain diary, screening laboratory tests should be performed, and a follow-up appointment should be scheduled in 1–3 weeks.

TABLE 35.1.   Examples of High-Fiber Foods

Food	Amount	Plant Fiber (g)
Bran cereal	$^1/_2$ cup	33.1
Popcorn	3 cups	15.5
Wheat cereal	$^3/_4$ cup	13.1
Cornflakes	$^3/_4$ cup	11.0
Rye bread	1 slice	10.8
Graham crackers	2 crackers	10.1
Pinto beans	$^1/_2$ cup	10.0
Peas	$^1/_2$ cup	7.8

THERAPY

Therapy for functional recurrent abdominal pain includes counseling and dietary changes.

Counseling

Counseling consists of reassuring the adolescent and family that the pain is real but that no physical or organic problem exists. Reassurance is given that the adolescent is physically healthy and can continue with all activities. The practitioner should stress that the pain is not "in the adolescent's head" but is a real manifestation of stress. If the teen is missing school, the family and school nurse should help to keep the teen in school. If the pain becomes severe, the teen should report to the nursing office and be referred to the practitioner's office for an examination. The relationship of stress and gastrointestinal distress should be reexplained. Stress-reduction techniques can be offered. If significant depression, anxiety, or family problems are uncovered, the teen and family should be referred for further counseling.

Silverberg (1991) examined chronic abdominal pain in adolescents and found that response to treatment was better in males who had signs and symptoms for less than 6 months and was relatively poor in adolescents with complaints for 2 years.

Fiber Diet

If constipation, diarrhea, or irritable colon is suspected, a high-fiber diet is helpful. Foods high in fiber are listed in Table 35.1. If such foods are unsuccessful, 1 teaspoon of psyllium seed (Metamucil) in orange juice, one to three times a day, can be used. In some individuals, if gas or flatulence is a significant complaint, particularly in Asian, African-American, and Jewish teenagers, a trial of a lactose-free diet may be indicated.

BIBLIOGRAPHY

Adye B, Ryan JA Jr. Cholecystitis in teenage girls. West J Med 1983;139:471.

Aiges H, Daum F. Crohn's disease in children and adolescents. Curr Concepts Gastroenterol 1983;8:22.

Alperstein G, Daum F. Management of inflammatory bowel disease in children and adolescents. Practical Gastroenterology 1982;6:26.

Apley J. The child with abdominal pains. 2nd ed. London: Blackwell Scientific Publications, 1975.

Apley J, Naish N. Recurrent abdominal pains: a field survey of 1,000 schoolchildren. Arch Dis Child 1958; 33:165.

Barr RG, Levine MD, Wilkinson H, et al. Chronic and occult stool retention. Clin Pediatr 1979;18:674–686.

Buchta RM, Bell L. Chronic fibrosing pancreatitis in a 12-year-old female. J Adolesc Health 1991;12:395.

Drumm B, Rhoads JM, Stringer DA, et al. Peptic ulcer disease in children: etiology, clinical findings, and clinical course. Pediatrics 1988;82:410–414.

Eulalia RY, Cheng MD. Cholecystitis and cholelithiasis in children and adolescents. J Natl Med Assoc 1986; 78:1073.

Farrell MK. Abdominal pain. Pediatrics 1984;74(suppl): 955.

Feldman W, McGrath P, Hodgson C, et al. The use of dietary fiber in the management of simple, childhood, idiopathic, recurrent, abdominal pain. Am J Dis Child 1985;139:1216–1218.

Galler JR, Neustein S, Walker WA. Clinical aspects of recurrent abdominal pain in children. Adv Pediatr 1980;27:31.

Garber J, Zeman J, Walker LS. Recurrent abdominal pain in children: psychiatric diagnoses and parental psychopathology. J Am Acad Child Adolesc Psychiatry 1990;29:648.

Greene JW, Walker LS, Hickson G, Thompson J. Stressful life events and somatic complaints in adolescents. Pediatrics 1985;75:19–22.

Konzen KM, Perrault J, Moir C, et al. Long-term follow-up of young patients with chronic hereditary or idiopathic pancreatitis. Mayo Clin Proc 1993;68:449.

Krishnamurthy GT. Acute cholecystitis: the diagnostic role for current imaging tests. West J Med 1982;137:87.

Lebenthal E. Recurrent abdominal pain in childhood. Am J Dis Child 1980;134:347.

Lennard-Jones JE. Current concepts: functional gastrointestinal disorders. N Engl J Med 1983;308:432.

Li BUK. Recurrent abdominal pain in childhood: an approach to common disorders. Compr Ther 1987;13:46–53.

Liebman WM. Recurrent abdominal pain in children. Clin Pediatr 1978;17:149.

Lynn RB, Friedman LS. Irritable bowel syndrome. Managing the patient with abdominal pain and altered bowel habits. Med Clin North Am 1995;79:373.

Magni G, Pierri M, Donzelli F. Recurrent abdominal pain in children: a long-term follow-up. Eur J Pediatr 1987;146:72–74.

McGrath PJ, Feldman W. Clinical approach to recurrent abdominal pain in children. J Dev Behav Pediatr 1986;7:56–61.

McGrath PJ, Goodman JT, Firestone P, Shipman R, Peters S. Recurrent abdominal pain: a psychogenic disorder? Arch Dis Child 1983;58:888.

Mews C, Sinatra F. Abdominal pain. In: Wyllie R, Hyams JS, eds. Pediatric gastrointestinal disease. Philadelphia: WB Saunders, 1993:177–186.

Neinstein LS. Abdominal and flank pain as presenting symptoms of schwannoma. J Adolesc Health Care 1989;10:143.

Oster J. Recurrent abdominal pain, headache, and limb pains in children and adolescents. Pediatrics 1972; 50:429.

Pineiro-Carrero VM, Andres JM, Davis RH, et al. Abnormal gastroduodenal motility in children and adolescents with recurrent functional abdominal pain. J Pediatr 1988;113:820–825.

Poole SR. Recurrent abdominal pain in childhood and adolescence. Am Fam Physician 1984;30:131.

Rappaport L. Recurrent abdominal pain: theories and pragmatics. Pediatrician 1989;16:78–84.

Reif S, Sloven DG, Lebenthal E. Gallstones in children: characterization by age, etiology, and outcome. Am J Dis Child 1991;145:105.

Rosenberg AJ. Recurrent abdominal pain in children. Drug Therapy 1982;July:161.

Shimada A, Takano M. [Irritable bowel syndrome in adolescence]. Jpn J Clin Med 1992;50:2729.

Silverberg M. Chronic abdominal pain in adolescents. Pediatr Ann 1991;20:179.

Stickler CG, Murphy DB. Recurrent abdominal pain. Am J Dis Child 1979;133:486.

Talley NJ, Phillips SF. Non-ulcer dyspepsia: potential causes and pathophysiology. Ann Intern Med 1988; 108:865–879.

Thomas DW, Sinatra FR, Merritt RJ. Fecal alpha-1-antitrypsin excretion in young people with Crohn's disease. J Pediatr Gastroenterol Nutr 1983;2:491–496.

Walker LS, Garber J, Greene JW. Somatization symptoms in pediatric abdominal pain patients: relation to chronicity of abdominal pain and parent somatization. J Abnorm Child Psychol 1991;19:379.

CHAPTER 36

Chest Pain

Chest pain in teenagers, although a common complaint, is rarely indicative of a serious problem. However, the symptom may be alarming to the adolescent, especially when there is a family history of cardiac disease. Nationwide there are as many as 650,000 visits for chest pain per year for individuals ages 10–21. This complaint is exceeded in frequency only by headaches and abdominal pain. The potential impact can be enormous, because two-thirds of these adolescents decrease their normal activity and 40% miss school.

DIFFERENTIAL DIAGNOSIS

Within each subgroup of the causes that follow, causes are listed in the approximate order of their frequency in the adolescent age group. The most common causes of chest pain in teenagers are idiopathic, anxiety related, and musculoskeletal problems. Two studies examining the frequency of various causes of chest pain in adolescents found the following:

1. Pantell and Goodman (1983)
   a. Musculoskeletal: 31%
   b. Hyperventilation: 20%
   c. Idiopathic: 39%
2. Selbst et al. (1988) (N = 132)
   a. Idiopathic: 26%
   b. Functional: 22%
   c. Musculoskeletal: 15%
   d. Costochondritis: 125%
   e. Gastrointestinal abnormalities: 8%

Musculoskeletal Causes

Musculoskeletal causes account for almost one-third of chest pain cases in adolescents (Pantell and Goodman, 1983). In general, musculoskeletal pain is a well-localized, sharp, nagging pain. The onset is often insidious. Movement and breathing often increase the intensity of the pain.

1. Stitch: A common cause of chest pain, manifested by a fleeting 30-second to several-minute jabbing or sticking pain, usually well localized to the left sternal border or cardiac apex. The pain varies in frequency and has a sudden onset. The pain often occurs at rest and is increased with deep breathing and by bending over. The cause is unknown.
2. Muscle strain: Strain of the chest-wall muscles after exercise or lifting can result in chest pain. Localized tenderness is frequently present. Movement of the arms and chest often increases the pain. Prolonged coughing can also lead to muscle strain.

3. Costochrondritis: May account for as many as 79% of chest pain cases in adolescents (Brown, 1981). Costochondral pain is usually a well-localized pain with local tenderness, usually anywhere from the second through the sixth ribs of the anterior chest wall. The pain is more often unilateral and in multiple locations. The pain may radiate to the back or abdomen. Actual swelling is not characteristic. Deep breathing may increase the pain. The clue to the diagnosis is tenderness over the involved articulations at the costochrondral junction. Costochondritis may be preceded by an upper respiratory tract infection or by exercise.

4. Rib or chest-wall trauma: Trauma can result in rib fractures or muscle contusions, resulting in localized chest pain.

5. Gynecomastia: Pubertal gynecomastia may be associated with tenderness and pain overlying the breast tissue.

6. Tietze's syndrome: A rare cause of costochrondral pain is associated with a tender solitary swelling or nodule, usually located at the second or third costal cartilage. The swelling is typically unilateral, with either a sudden or a gradual onset. The pain may persist from days to months or longer. The pain is often increased with breathing and movements.

7. Metastatic disease of bone: This is an uncommon cause of chest pain in adolescents.

8. Slipping rib syndrome: This is an unusual cause of lower chest pain. This syndrome is caused by the slipping of the 8th, 9th, or 10th rib on the immediately superior rib. These three ribs do not attach to the sternum. A tear in the connecting fibrous tissue between these two ribs can allow for this slippage. The pain is sharp, stabbing, and located in the upper portion of the abdomen or at the inferior costal margin. It is usually insidious in onset and unilateral. Occasionally a click is heard with movements. The pain can be reproduced by hooking the fingers under the ribs and pulling anteriorly.

Anxiety

Adolescents under stress, with or without hyperventilation, may describe a tightness or heaviness of the chest. Anxiety may also induce intermittent sharp, knifelike pains or persistent precordial aching unrelated to effort. Hyperventilation may lead to light-headedness, shortness of breath, tachycardia, and syncope.

Pleuropulmonary Causes

Most pulmonary causes of pain in adolescents are associated with other symptoms such as cough, fever, pain on inspiration, and fatigue. The pain associated with pleural pulmonary causes is usually more diffuse and difficult to describe.

1. Cough: Persistent cough is a frequent cause of chest pain.

2. Asthma: Asthma is another relatively common cause of chest pain.

3. Pneumonia: Pneumonia, especially when the infection involves the pleura, can give rise to pleuritic chest pain.

4. Pleurodynia: Infections associated with Coxsackie B virus often lead to pleuritic chest pain. The onset often follows a typical viral prodrome.

5. Spontaneous pneumothorax: Symptoms include an acute onset of pleuritic chest pain and dyspnea. Those individuals with cystic fibrosis, asthma, or Marfan's syndrome are at increased risk of having this complication. Cocaine inhalation can also induce a pneumothorax or pneumomediastinum.

6. Pulmonary embolism: A pulmonary embolism can give rise to the acute onset of dyspnea and chest pain. This is an uncommon problem in teenagers, unless predisposing factors exist, such as obesity, immobilization, or use of oral contraceptives (high-dose estrogen).

7. Pulmonary hypertension: This is a rare cause of chest pain in adolescents.

Cardiac Causes

Pain related to cardiac disease is one of the less common causes of chest pain in adolescents. The pain is often associated with exertion. Other symptoms may include syncope, palpitation, and dizziness.

1. Mitral valve prolapse: This condition is often associated with exertional or nonexertional chest pain. However, the pain may also be associated with gastroesophageal sources. Woolf et al. (1991) found that 14 of 17 adolescents with mitral valve prolapse and chest pain had abnormal findings on esophageal study.
2. Pericarditis: Infections, especially viral infections, can cause pericarditis leading to chest pain. Pericardial pain is usually sharp and is aggravated by respiratory motion, yawning, or swallowing. Sitting up and leaning forward often lessen the pain. Distant heart sounds, a friction rub, tachycardia, and a recent viral infection suggest pericarditis.
3. Arrhythmias: Supraventricular tachycardias and premature ventricular contractions can cause palpitations and chest pain.
4. Aortic outlet obstruction: Severe aortic stenosis or asymmetric septal hypertrophy can cause chest pain. Characteristic physical findings are present.
5. Ischemic heart disease: Ischemic heart pain is almost nonexistent in the adolescent age group. Unless there are predisposing factors, such as prolonged hypertension, a strong family history, severe hyperlipidemia, or local arteritis, ischemic heart disease is unlikely.
6. Dissecting aortic aneurysm: Dissecting aortic aneurysm is an extremely rare problem during adolescence, except with a predisposing condition such as Marfan's syndrome.

Gastrointestinal Causes

Numerous gastrointestinal disorders can cause substernal chest pain. However, these conditions are uncommon among teenagers. Included in this group are:

1. Esophageal spasm and reflux
2. Peptic ulcer disease
3. Cholecystitis
4. Pancreatitis

DIAGNOSIS

History

A careful history is the most effective means of determining the cause of chest pain in adolescents. The history should include questions regarding:

1. Pain
   a. Quality: A localized sharp, aching pain suggests localized chest wall pain, whereas a deep, gnawing pain suggests a visceral cause.
   b. Location: Pain in the T1-T4 dermatome distribution is often referred from the myocardium, pericardium, aorta, or esophagus. Pain in the T5-T6 distribution can be from the diaphragm, gallbladder, pancreas, duodenum, or stomach. This pain may also be referred to the back and right scapulas.
   c. Timing: Brief pain often has a musculoskeletal or chest-wall origin. A deep, long pain often suggests a visceral origin.
   d. Precipitating and alleviating factors: Substernal pain increasing with exertion and lying down suggests reflux or esophagitis. Pain decreasing with antacids suggests ulcer disease. Pain increasing with breathing, cough, or movement suggests pleural or chest-

wall pain. Pain increasing with stress suggests hyperventilation or anxiety. Pain that increases at night or awakens the adolescent during the night suggests an organic cause.

   e. Onset: Patients with acute onset of chest pain are more likely to have an organic disease.

2. Recent activity: This includes activity that could cause chest-wall strain, such as lifting weights, exercising, or performing household chores.
3. Recent trauma: Has the adolescent been injured recently?
4. Recent infections or systemic illness: Are there any systemic illnesses such as lupus erythematosus or asthma that could contribute to the chest pain? Has there been persistent cough or vomiting that could contribute to the chest pain?
5. Medications or drugs. Are there any medications that could account for the chest pain? Is the teen using cocaine?
6. Any associated symptoms: Persistent cough or vomiting could contribute to chest pain. Is there associated light-headedness, oral parethesias, or tingling in the extremeties, suggesting hyperventilation syndrome?
7. Recent stress: A thorough psychosocial evaluation is important.

Physical Examination

1. General state: Is there evidence of anxiety or hyperventilation?
2. Vital signs: Is there evidence of tachypnea, tachycardia, or fever?
3. Chest wall: Examine the adolescent for focal tenderness or swelling along the ribs and intercostal spaces. The individual sternocostal and costocostal junctions may need to be palpated. Are there any palpable signs of subcutaneous air?
4. Cardiopulmonary examination: In a careful cardiopulmonary examination, the practitioner looks for:
   a. Absent breath sounds: Pneumothorax
   b. Rales: Pneumonia or pulmonary embolism
   c. Pleural rub: Pleurodynia, pleurisy, or pulmonary embolism
   d. Cardiac friction rub: Pericarditis
   e. Midsystolic click, late-systolic murmur: Mitral valve prolapse
   f. Evidence of other cardiac lesions: For example, aortic stenosis

Laboratory Tests

Most adolescents require no evaluation other than history taking and physical examination. In general, unless these findings are highly suggestive of a specific organic cause, the laboratory is usually not helpful in diagnosing chest pain. An electrocardiogram and chest x-ray film almost always show no abnormalities. However, if other conditions such as pneumothorax, pneumonia, pulmonary embolism, or pericarditis are suspected, then further tests are ordered as indicated. These may include:

1. Pneumothorax: Chest x-ray study
2. Pneumonia: Chest x-ray study
3. Pulmonary embolism: Chest x-ray study and lung scan
4. Pericarditis or mitral valve prolapse: Electrocardiography and echocardiography
5. Cocaine use: Drug screen

THERAPY

It is rare that chest pain is life-threatening in adolescents and necessitates immediate intervention. Because the diagnosis is usually based on the history and the physical examination findings, adolescents rarely need referral to a subspecialist. In most instances the adolescent needs reassurance that he or she does not have a significant cardiac problem and, in addition, an explanation of the cause of the pain. Therapy depends on the specific diagnosis.

1. Musculoskeletal pain
   a. Reassurance
   b. Analgesics: Nonsteroidal anti-inflammatory agents
2. Pleurodynia: Analgesics
3. Pneumothorax:
   a. Partial pneumothorax in healthy adolescents: May be well tolerated and managed with rest.
   b. Major pneumothorax: Immediate insertion of chest tube to allow reexpansion of the lung; alternatively, a small opening in the chest wall with a large-bore needle as an emergency, temporary measure
4. Pneumonia: Appropriate antibiotics
5. Pulmonary embolism: Anticoagulation
6. Pericarditis: Analgesics
7. Mitral valve prolapse:
   a. Reassurance
   b. Severe chest pain or chest pain associated with arrhythmias: Possible benefit from propranolol or another β-blocker
8. Anxiety
   a. Reassurance
   b. Stress-reduction techniques

BIBLIOGRAPHY

Berezin S, Medow MS, Glassman M, et al. Chest pain of gastrointestinal origin. Arch Dis Child 1988;63:1457.

Branch WT Jr, McNeil BJ. Analysis of the differential diagnosis and assessment of pleuritic chest pain in young adults. Am J Med 1983;75:671.

Brenner JI, Berman MA. Chest pain in childhood and adolescence. J Adolesc Health Care 1983;3:271.

Brown RT. Costochrondritis in adolescents. J Adolesc Health Care 1981;1:198.

Brown RT. Recurrent chest pain in adolescents. Pediatr Ann 1991;20:194.

Coleman WL. Recurrent chest pain in children. Pediatr Clin North Am 1984;31:1007.

Fam AG, Smythe HA. Musculoskeletal chest wall pain. Can Med Assoc J 1985;133:379.

Feinstein RA, Daniel WA Jr. Chronic chest pain in children and adolescents. Pediatr Ann 1986;15:685.

Goroll AH, May LA, Mulley AG. Evaluation of chest pain. In: Goroll AH, ed. Primary care medicine. Philadelphia: JB Lippincott, 1987.

Jonides L, Rudy C, Walsh S. Chest pain in a young athlete. J Pediatr Health Care 1995;9:87.

Kaden GG, Shenker IR, Gootman N. Chest pain in adolescents. J Adolesc Health 1991;12:251.

Kayser HL. Tietze's syndrome: a literature review. Am J Med 1956;21:982.

Pantel RH, Goodman BW. Adolescent chest pain: a prospective study. Pediatrics 1983;71:881.

Porter GE. Slipping rib syndrome: an infrequently recognized entity in children—a report of three cases and review of the literature. Pediatrics 1985;76:810.

Selbst SM. Chest pain in children. Pediatrics 1985;75:1068.

Selbst SM. Chest pain in children. Am Fam Physician 1990;41:179.

Selbst SM, Ruddy RM, Clark BJ, et al. Pediatric chest pain: a prospective study. Pediatrics 1988;82:319.

Tunaoglu FS, Olgunturk R, Akcabay S, et al. Chest pain in children referred to a cardiology clinic. Pediatr Cardiol 1995;16:69.

Weiner MD, Putman CE. Pain in the chest in a user of cocaine. JAMA 1987;258:2087.

Woolf PK, Gewitz MH, Berezin S, et al. Noncardiac chest pain in adolescents and children with mitral valve prolapse. J Adolesc Health 1991;12:257.

Woodward GA, Selbst SM. Chest pain secondary to cocaine use. Pediatr Emerg Care 1987;3:153.

CHAPTER 37

Reiter's Syndrome

Reiter's syndrome is characterized by arthritis, urethritis, conjunctivitis, and mucocutaneous lesions.

ETIOLOGY

The exact cause of Reiter's syndrome is unknown. However, it is probably a reactive arthritis occurring after certain enteric and venereal infections. Suspected agents include *Shigella flexneri, Campylobacter, Yersinia enterocolitica, Salmonella,* and certain venereal agents, including *Chlamydia trachomatis* and *Ureaplasma urealyticum.* Horowitz et al. (1994) found *U. urealyticum* in 74% of patients with Reiter's syndrome, in comparison with 14% of control subjects. Others have found that *C. trachomatis* may be the most common pathogen associated with this syndrome. Persons with the histocompatibility antigen HLA-B27 are at greatly increased risk of having Reiter's syndrome.

EPIDEMIOLOGY

1. Age: The majority of affected individuals are 18–40 years old; however, Reiter's syndrome has been reported in patients as young as 2 years old.
2. Sex: Male/female ratio is 20:1, although prevalence in females may be higher than was previously believed.

CLINICAL MANIFESTATIONS

1. Urethritis
   a. Often first symptom
   b. Most often scanty and serous but may be profuse and purulent
2. Conjunctivitis
   a. Usually bilateral, mild, and fleeting but may be severe and purulent
   b. Other eye abnormalities: Anterior uveitis (iridocyclitis), corneal ulcerations, episcleritis, optic and retrobulbar neuritis, and panophthalmia.
3. Arthritis
   a. Usually begins 1–3 weeks after symptoms start as an asymmetrical oligoarticular arthritis of large weight-bearing joints, especially ankles and knees
   b. Other common problems: Achilles tendonitis and lumbar or sacral spondylitis
4. Mucocutaneous lesions
   a. Balanitis: Circinate or diffuse
   b. Mouth: Superficial painless ulcerations on tongue, palate, pharynx, and buccal mucosa; possible geographic tongue

    c. Skin: Keratoderma blennorrhagicum
      — Usually occurs 4–6 weeks after onset of urethritis, with small red to yellow or brown vesicles or papules that are usually firm and nontender and that may become confluent
      — May mimic psoriasis
    d. Nails: Onycholysis, subungual keratosis
    e. Vulva: Rarely, erythematous, crusted plaques on the vulva, as well as cervical lesions (Edwards and Hansen, 1992)
5. Cardiac abnormalities: Pericarditis, myocarditis, aortic insufficiency, and conduction abnormalities; electrocardiogram probably needed for evaluation for cardiac abnormalities and as a baseline
6. Neurological abnormalities: Rare manifestation but includes peripheral neuropathy, transient hemiplegia, meningoencephalitis, and cranial nerve palsies
7. Systemic abnormalities: Fever, fatigue, anorexia, and weight loss

Presentation in Children and Younger Adolescents

Cuttica et al. (1992) reviewed the clinical manifestations of Reiter's in children and younger adolescents. There was often a history of a diarrheal illness before the onset of Reiter's syndrome in 69% of younger adolescents and children. The most common manifestation in this younger group was arthritis. However, 15–25% of this group initially had only urethritis or conjunctivitis. The arthritis usually involved the lower limbs (96%); the pattern was pauciarticular (69%) in most, polyarticular in 27%, and monoarticular in one case (4%). More than half of this younger group (58%) had a complete remission; the rest had a sustained or fluctuating course. Half of the males had balanitis.

ASSOCIATION WITH ACQUIRED IMMUNODEFICIENCY SYNDROME

Reiter's syndrome has been found to occur also in association with human immunodeficiency virus (HIV) infection (Altman et al., 1994). Rheumatic manifestions in general are more common in HIV-infected individuals, with arthralgias reported in 45%, arthritis in 10%, and Reiter's syndrome in 8% (Medina-Rodriguez et al., 1993). In HIV-infected individuals, the course of Reiter's syndrome appears to be more severe, progressive, and refractory to treatment. The role of HIV in the pathogenesis of Reiter's syndrome is still under investigation.

COURSE

Reiter's syndrome is usually thought of as a self-limited disease lasting 6 weeks to 6 months. However, a study by Fox et al. (1979) of 131 patients with a mean follow-up of 5.6 years showed that 83% of patients had disease activity with arthritis or synovitis at some time during the follow-up period; 22% had annoying symptoms; 34% had sustained disease activity; 16% had had to change jobs; and 11% were unemployable.

DIAGNOSIS

Proposed criteria for diagnosis by the Arthritis Foundation (Willkens et al., 1982) include an episode of peripheral arthritis lasting longer than 1 month, in association with urethritis or cervicitis. However, certainly an individual with two or three of the following would have to be strongly considered for a diagnosis of Reiter's syndrome: arthritis, urethritis, conjunctivitis, balanitis, oral mucosa ulcers, and keratoderma blennorrhagicum.

Laboratory Tests

There are no specific tests; nonspecific findings include:

1. Mild normocytic, normochromic anemia
2. Elevated erythrocyte sedimentation rate (often >100 mm/hr)
3. HLA-B27: Present in 63–93% of patients
4. X-ray studies
   a. Sacroiliac joint changes
   b. Calcaneal spurs
   c. Nonmarginal vertebral syndesmophytes
   d. Demineralization of bone

Differential Diagnosis

1. For a comparison of Reiter's syndrome with other seronegative spondyloarthropathies, see Table 37.1.
2. In a comparison of cases of Reiter's syndrome after various stimuli, the following have been noted:
   a. Reiter's syndrome after infection with Yersinia has the highest percentage of patients in whom arthritis develops (33% versus 1–3% for other stimuli).
   b. The male/female ratio is highest for Reiter's syndrome after a sexually transmitted disease (28:1).
   c. Development of the full triad is most common after *Shigella*-induced Reiter's syndrome.

TABLE 37.1.   Comparison of Reiter's Syndrome With Other Seronegative Spondyloarthropathies During Initial Attack[a]

Signs or Symptoms	RS (%)	AS (%)	SNRA (%)	PsA (%)	GcA (%)
Arthritis	99	100	100	100	100
Tendinitis	25	12	7	6	23
Back pain	40	12	0	4	8
Polyarticular	81	29	68	84	54
Monoarticular	14	8	30	15	30
Urethritis	85	4	0	0	38
Conjunctivitis	57	20	0	4	0
Mucous membrane lesions	1	0	0	2	12
Skin lesions	49	2	0	96	54
Multiple locations	21	2	—	90	54
Nail changes	9	0	—	67	0
Balanitis	39	0	—	2	0
Diarrhea	14	4	0	0	4
CNS involvement	1	2	0	0	0
Fever	37	2	6	4	50
Weight loss	38	4	9	12	0
Acute attack	77	25	32	19	100
Duration of initial attack					
<1 wk	0	2	4	2	42
1 wk–1 month	1	7	4	0	46
>1 month	99	91	92	98	12
Family history of arthritis	13	33	29	30	0
HLA-B27 present	86	97	33	47	0

Adapted from Willkens RF, Arnett FC, Bitter T, et al. Reiter's syndrome. Bull Rheum Dis 1982;32:31.
[a]RS, Reiter's syndrome; AS, ankylosing spondylitis; SNRA, seronegative rheumatoid arthritis; PsA, psoriatic arthritis; GcA, gonococcal arthritis.

d. The period from initial infection to symptoms varies from 10 days after *Campylobacter* infection to 18 days after *Shigella* infection.
e. The duration of symptoms is approximately equal in all the groups listed in Table 37.1, with the mean duration between 18 and 19.5 weeks.

THERAPY

1. No specific therapy
2. Anti-inflammatory agents (e.g., nonsteroidal anti-inflammatory agents)
3. Tetracycline or doxycycline for initial short-term role
4. Ophthalmology referral for individuals with eye involvement

BIBLIOGRAPHY

Altman EM, Enteno LV, Mahal M, et al. AIDS-associated Reiter's syndrome. Ann Allergy 1994;72:307.

Arnett FC. Seronegative spondyloarthropathies. Bull Rheum Dis 1987;37:1.

Braverman PK, Strasburger VC. Sexually transmitted diseases. Clin Pediatr 1994;33:26.

Calin A. Spondyloarthropathies. In: Rubenstein E & Federman D, eds. Scientific American medicine. New York: Scientific American, 1986.

Cuttica RJ, Scheines EJ, Garay SM, et al. Juvenile-onset Reiter's syndrome: a retrospective study of 26 patients. Clin Exp Rheumatol 1992;10:285.

Deer T, Rosencrance JG, Chillag SA. Cardiac conduction manifestations of Reiter's syndrome. South Med J 1991;84:799.

Deesmchok U, Tumrasvin T. Clinical comparison of patients with ankylosing spondylitis, Reiter's syndrome and psoriatic arthritis. J Med Assoc Thai 1993;76:61.

Edwards L, Hansen RC. Reiter's syndrome of the vulva: the psoriasis spectrum. Arch Dermatol 1992;128:811.

Fox R, Calin A, Gerber RC, et al. The chronicity of symptoms and disability in Reiter's syndrome. Ann Intern Med 1979;91:190.

Horowitz S, Horowitz J, Taylor-Robinson D, et al. *Ureaplasma urealyticum* in Reiter's syndrome. J Rheumatol 1994;21:877.

Keat A. Reiter's syndrome and reactive arthritis in perspective. N Engl J Med 1983;309:1606.

Medina-Rodriguez F, Guzman C, Jara LJ, et al. Rheumatic manifestations in human immunodeficiency virus positive and negative individuals: a study of 2 populations with similar risk factors. J Rheumatol 1993;20:1880.

Osial TA Jr, Cash JM, Eisenbeis CH Jr. Arthritis-associated syndromes. Primary Care 1993;20:857.

Peterson MC. Rheumatic manifestations of *Campylobacter jejuni* and *C. fetus* infections in adults. Scand J Rheumatol 1994;23:167.

Rahman MU, Hudson AP, Schumahcer HR Jr. *Chlamydia* and Reiter's syndrome. Rheum Dis Clin North Am 1992;18:67.

Rosenbaum JT. Acute anterior uveitis and spondyloarthropathies. Rheum Dis Clin North Am 1992;18:143.

Rosenberg AM, Petty RE. Reiter's disease in children. Am J Dis Child 1979;133:394.

Rossen RM, Goodman DJ, Harrison DC. A-V conduction disturbances in Reiter's syndrome. Am J Med 1975;58:280.

In: Schumacher HR Jr, ed. Reiter's syndrome. Primer on the rheumatic diseases. 9th ed. Atlanta: Arthritis Foundation, 1988.

Silveira LH, Gutierrez F, Scopelitis E, et al. *Chlamydia*-induced reactive arthritis. Rheum Dis Clin North Am 1993;19:351.

Thomas DG, Roberton DM. Reiter's syndrome in an adolescent girl. Acta Paediatr 1994;83:339.

Willkens RF, Arnett FC, Bitter T, et al. Reiter's syndrome. Bull Rheum Dis 1982;32:31.

CHAPTER 38

Noninflammatory Rheumatism
Fibromyalgia and Reflex Sympathetic Dystrophy

Bram Bernstein

Muscle and joint complaints are a relatively common problem among adolescents and young adults. The two musculoskeletal pain conditions discussed in this chapter may occur during the adolescent or young adult period and have been particularly frustrating for practitioners to diagnose and treat. In some individuals, fibromyalgia may overlap with chronic fatigue syndrome.

FIBROMYALGIA

The fibromyalgia syndrome (FMS), formerly termed fibrositis, is a disorder characterized by diffuse musculoskeletal pain and the presence of characteristic tender points. Although a common disorder in adults, affecting as many as three to six million Americans, the syndrome is infrequently diagnosed in children and adolescents. Nevertheless, 28% of adults with FMS reported pain symptoms beginning in childhood, especially during the teen years.

Although few studies address FMS in the adolescent population, available data suggest that musculoskeletal and nonmusculoskeletal symptoms, as well as the psychological characteristics, are similar to those in older populations. FMS is usually found in otherwise healthy patients, but it may occur in association with underlying musculoskeletal diseases, such as juvenile rheumatoid arthritis (JRA), which result in abnormal stress on muscles. In fact, a significant number of individuals with lupus erythematosus and rheumatoid arthritis also have fibromyalgia. Children and adolescents with FMS are often referred to a pediatric rheumatologist to rule out diseases such as JRA or systemic lupus erythematosus, sometimes because of a falsely positive antinuclear antibody test result.

There is evidence that emotional factors may play a role in many childhood and adolescent cases. Concomitant medical and psychiatric disorders, such as migraine, irritable bowel syndrome, chronic fatigue syndrome, mood disorders, and panic disorder, are frequently present. In addition, a high prevalence of major depression and bipolar disorder has been reported in relatives and in FMS patients themselves, suggesting a possible association between FMS and affective disorders. However, although the prevalence of major depression in individuals with FMS is double that of the general population, the majority of patients with fibromyalgia do not currently have major depression.

Diagnosis

The diagnosis of FMS requires a history of widespread pain (meaning pain on both the left and right sides of the body and above and below the waist), present for at least 3 months, and the presence of tenderness at 11 or more of 18 specific tender points (Fig. 38.1) (American College of Rheumatology, 1990 criteria). Axial skeletal pain (cervical vertebrae, anterior portion of the chest, thoracic vertebrae or low region of the back) must also be present. The 18 identified tender points are generally in areas where muscles attach to ligaments or bone. When testing for pain at these sites, the practitioner should apply just enough pressure—about 4 kg—to blanch his or her thumbnail. In true FMS, the teen should feel pain, not just tenderness. In addition to the criteria noted above, many patients have concomitant symptoms, which include:

1. Sleep disturbance, usually nonrefreshing sleep
2. Generalized fatigue of 3 months' duration or longer
3. Subjective swelling, numbness, or tingling of extremities

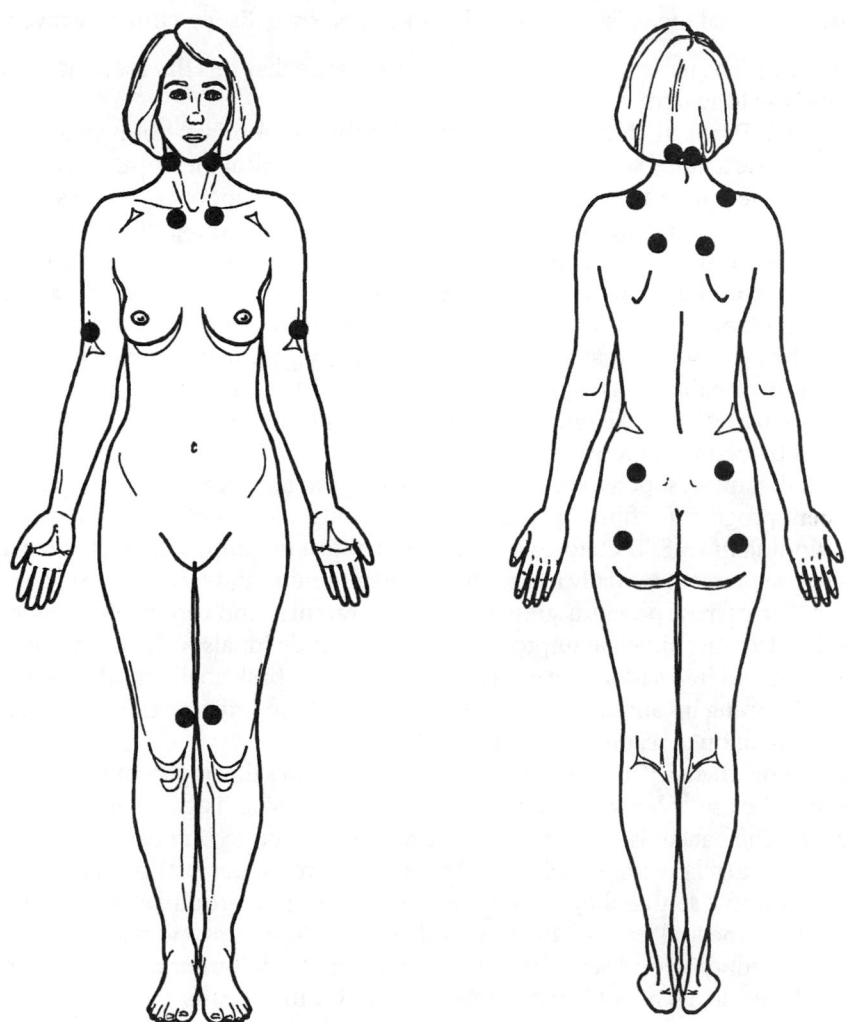

FIGURE 38.1.   Locations of tender points in fibromyalgia.

4. Chronic headaches
5. Irritable bowel syndrome
6. Temporomandibular joint syndrome

In contrast to reflex sympathetic dystrophy, objective physical changes are not seen. A sleep history is an important part of the history taking because sleep disorders are often associated with fibromyalgia. Possible sleep disorders include disturbed sleep, sleep deprivation, nonrefreshing sleep, and sleep apnea.

Management

Comprehensive and effective treatment of teens with FMS should include the entire family. Most experts agree that FMS is a chronic condition associated in many individuals with a depressed mood and with high levels of stress. With a few exceptions, treatment is usually carried out in the outpatient setting. The treatment program should address both the emotional and the physical aspects of the condition by combining the efforts of physician, nurse, physical and occupational therapists, and social worker, and by enlisting family involvement.

1. Reassurance: The patient and family need reassurance that this disease is not destructive and that the long-term outlook is good.
2. Evaluation: The teen should be examined by the appropriate team members, which might include a nurse, social worker or psychologist, physical therapist, and occupational therapist. The nurse can help educate the teen and family about FMS. The social worker can evaluate the teen and the family to assess possible psychological stress factors or disorders. The social worker can also provide teen and family support or counseling and can arrange for community mental health referral if indicated. Both nurse and social worker can emphasize the importance of participation in normal activities and advise the parents on how to avoid situations in which secondary gain may result from the patient's complaints of pain. Teens with FMS may also need to learn to pace themselves better. Certain activities may take longer than formerly, and strenuous activities may need to be followed by periods of more restful activity.
3. Physical therapy: A supervised, systematic exercise program is a critical component of the treatment program for fibromyalgia. Deconditioning because of physical inactivity is the usual finding in FMS. Therefore the physical therapist develops a graduated reconditioning exercise program for daily use at home. Strengthening and flexibility exercises are prescribed. The exercise program stresses postural awareness and correction of poor posture, as well as activities aimed at improving endurance. Individuals with fibromyalgia should probably avoid impact-loading exercises (e.g., jogging, basketball, or other activities that involve jumping up and down). Better exercises include walking, riding on a stationary cycle, walking on a treadmill, or swimming.
4. Occupational therapy: The occupational therapist assesses the impact of FMS on the teen's daily life. The use of body mechanics during typical activities is evaluated and modified if necessary. The patient is instructed in the use of relaxation techniques. Myofascial release may be used to relieve trigger points, and patients (as well as parents) are taught to use these releases at home so that they can take an active role in the treatment and reduce dependence on the medical team. With these modalities, muscle stress and pain can be decreased and overall function and sense of well-being improved. Most important, the patient will begin to develop a sense of having some control over the disease.
5. Medications
   a. Tricyclic antidepressants: Antidepressants such as amitriptyline (Elavil) are often useful in low doses (10–25 mg at bedtime) to treat the commonly associated sleep dis-

turbance. The drug produces an atropine-like effect and therefore may cause dryness of the mouth and other mucous membranes. These small doses (much lower than those used to treat depression) are usually well tolerated.

   b. Nonsteroidal anti-inflammatory drugs: May be helpful for periods of acute severe pain but generally not very helpful for the chronic pain of fibromyalgia.

   c. Corticosteroids: Have not been shown to be effective and in general should be avoided.

6. Support groups: Sometimes having teens or their parents link up with support groups can be helpful. Sources of information, education, and support on fibromyalgia include:

National Fibromyalgia Research Association, Inc.
Box 500
Salem, OR 97308

Fibromyalgia Network
Box 31750
Tucson, AZ 85751-1750
602-290-5508
Publishes quarterly newsletter for patients and other publications, including:
- *Fibromyalgia Syndrome: A Patient's Guide*
- *Coping With Fibromyalgia*
- *Fibromyalgia Syndrome and Chronic Fatigue Syndrome in Young People: A Guide for Parents*

American Fibromyalgia Syndrome Association
Box 9699
Bakersfield, CA 93389
805-663-1137

Arthritis Foundation
Box 19000
Atlanta, GA 30326
800-283-7800

REFLEX SYMPATHETIC DYSTROPHY

Reflex sympathetic (neurovascular) dystrophy (RSD) is a noninflammatory musculoskeletal pain syndrome that includes a syndrome of pain, hyperesthesia, vasomotor disturbances and dystrophic changes. The pathophysiology of this disorder is not well understood but is thought to be related to abnormal activity in the sympathetic nervous system. Underrecognized in the pediatric age groups, RSD is most common in adolescent girls but can occur in younger children and in either sex. Although the outlook is better in adolescents than in adults, RSD can produce long-term disability and eventually trophic changes, resulting in permanent damage to the extremity.

Predisposing Factors

1. Personality factors: Personality factors seem to predispose individuals to the syndrome. Characteristically, adolescents with RSD are overachievers. They *seem* to be "perfect children from perfect families." Secondary gain (perhaps a respite from responsibilities) is often operative.
2. Trauma: The classic case of RSD follows a history of trauma to the involved area; however, many cases occur without such history. Trauma may include burns, contusions, frac-

tures, lacerations, nerve injury, and sprains and strains. Trauma may account for as many as 30% of the cases.

3. Neurological factors: These factors include multiple sclerosis, peripheral neuropathy, tumors, and cerebrovascular accidents.

4. Other precipitating factors: Local cold injury, and revascularization of an ischemic injury. The precipitating factor in RSD is frequently trivial and the pain response out of proportion to the injury.

Clinical Manifestations

RSD is characterized by complaints of severe extremity pain and inability to use the extremity. Most characteristic is an exquisite tenderness to the lightest touch. Many of these patients cannot tolerate so much as the weight of a sheet on the involved area. Objective changes caused by vasomotor instability produce swelling, blotchiness or bluish discoloration, reduced skin temperature, and decreased pulsations. Perspiration may be decreased or sometimes increased in the involved area. Pain is present in 98% of cases, decreased range of motion in 77%, swelling in 62%, and vasomotor changes in 47%. Early changes usually involve burning or aching pain, edema, and hyperthermia or hypothermia. Trophic skin changes, hair loss, and osteoporosis come later. Flexion contractures may also occur at a late stage. The definitive diagnosis of RSD is usually based on distal extremity pain, vasomotor instability, and extremity swelling.

Laboratory Findings

1. Bone scan: A bone scan may reveal reduced blood flow; however, a normal scan does not rule out RSD.

2. X-ray studies: In long-standing cases there may be radiological signs of a patchy osteoporosis (Sudeck's atrophy), especially with patchy demineralization of the epiphyses and the short bones of the hands and feet.

Differential Diagnosis

1. Chronic arterial insufficiency: Pulses absent (present in RSD)
2. Raynaud's disease: Aggravated by cold (RSD especially aggravated by exercise)
3. Phlebothrombosis: No associated neurological changes
4. Rheumatic disorders such as lupus erythematosus (RSD usually associated with normal erythrocyte sedimentation rate and no elevation in autoimmune antibody concentration)
5. Localized infections (no leukocytosis or fever in RSD)

Management

Treatment should be aimed at improving function, rather than primarily at pain control. Treatment outcome is improved if initiated early. In RSD, pain in general is not amenable to direct therapeutic intervention. Furthermore, experience has demonstrated that as function improves, pain tends to diminish. The basic therapeutic approach, therefore, is to treat with a combination of physical therapy and psychological counseling. *Extremities should not be immobilized.* Physical therapy fosters use of the involved extremity, and psychological counseling is aimed at helping the adolescent to deal with underlying feelings and conflicts in more appropriate ways. It should be emphasized to teens that the more they use the involved extremity, the quicker the extremity is going to get better; conversely, disuse will worsen the condition. When the teen complains of pain, the practitioner should listen and then move on to deal with other issues as soon as possible.

1. Discussion of disease and prognosis: Treatment begins with discussing the diagnosis and its implications with the patient and parents in a clear, straightforward manner. As soon as the diagnosis is established, they should be so informed in definite terms. The important role that emotional factors may play in disease etiology should be explained. The fact that the prognosis is good with treatment should be emphasized. This is the time to set the stage for ongoing psychotherapy. In our experience, helping the family deal with the emotional aspects of the disease is crucial to the achievement of an excellent outcome. Although the prognosis for short-term improvement with physical therapy alone is good, without psychological intervention it is common for RSD to recur or another psychosomatic illness to ensue.

2. Medications
   a. Steroids and sympathetic blockers: The adult literature reports that some patients benefit from corticosteroids, ganglionic blocking agents, and chemical sympathetic blockers. Our experience is that these modes of treatment generally produce short-lived or no benefit and may be associated with adverse effects. Furthermore, they may divert the adolescent from dealing with underlying psychological issues. Except when emotional factors are not implicated, these forms of therapy should be avoided.
   b. Nonsteroidal anti-inflammatory drugs: These drugs can play a role in the initial treatment of pain, but the major emphasis should be on improving function, which seems to lessen pain.
   c. Phenoxybenzamine: This adrenergic (α-receptor) blocker has been helpful in some of the more classic cases of RSD caused by obvious trauma.

3. Inpatient management in a rehabilitation center: In mild cases, outpatient management may suffice. When symptoms are more severe and long-standing, however, admission to a rehabilitation center is indicated.
   a. Diagnosis, prognosis, and treatment plan: The diagnosis and its implications, both physical and emotional, must be explained to the patient and family. At this time the goal of treatment is established. A typical example of a "discharge goal" for the adolescent with lower extremity involvement might be to walk for a reasonable distance, wearing shoes and socks, with no more than a minimal limp. Prosthetic devices and aids, such as wheelchairs, crutches, and braces, are quickly withdrawn. Patients are permitted to receive mild analgesics, such as acetaminophen, but they are advised that drugs are not likely to provide major pain relief.
   b. Weekly conferences: A weekly conference of multidisciplinary team members is held to review the patient's progress and to set a series of objectives for the week. These objectives, usually exercises consisting of use of the involved extremity, must be quantifiable and sufficiently challenging so that the teen will have to work diligently to accomplish them by the end of the week. At the same time, they must be realistic and attainable. We tell the teen and family that the week begins on Monday and ends on Sunday. If the weekly objective is achieved earlier than the end of the week (e.g., on Friday), the teen may have a weekend pass. If not, we say to the teen: "That's okay! But, of course, the work must continue until the objective is met"; thus no pass is given. In this way we attempt to avoid having the teen interpret not receiving a pass as punishment.
   c. Role of the therapeutic team members
      — Physician: The physician sets the overall direction of the patient's management, determines the discharge goal, conducts team meetings, regularly examines the

patient, and communicates with the patient and his or her parents. The physician may need to play the role of "bad guy" when appropriate.

— Nurse: The registered nurse plays a central role in the day-to-day coordination of the patient's care. These tasks include scheduling weekly team meetings; presenting and explaining weekly objectives to the teen; and checking on the teen's progress in meeting these objectives and his or her eligibility for weekend pass. The nurse is responsible for reporting 24-hour daily nursing observations of patient actions and interactions to the team members. Most important, the nurse has a special role to fulfill in establishing a trust relationship with the patient. This includes providing emotional support by encouraging the teenager to talk about feelings and express anger *in appropriate ways*, listening to the teen's complaints of pain and providing support to the family.

— Physical therapist: The physical therapist provides weight-bearing exercises for the involved extremity. Desensitization techniques, such as vigorous toweling or immersion in contrast baths, are used. Atrophied muscles are strengthened and endurance is improved. Throughout this process, choices are permitted within limits (i.e., a "win-win" situation is set up in such a way that the teen attains his or her objectives while at the same time being allowed a certain amount of control over the treatment regimen. For example, the teen may be given the choice of vigorously toweling the involved extremity for a longer period, or having the therapist do so for a shorter period. This fosters assertiveness, a trait frequently lacking in these adolescents. Throughout the process, the therapist uses a firm but nonpunitive approach.

— Occupational therapist: Adolescents with RSD are often overachievers. Clearly, being an overachiever carries with it a psychological "price." Therefore the occupational therapist (OT) evaluates the teen's capabilities and the psychological costs involved in reaching their own or the family's expectations. If these expectations are not appropriate, they need to be modified. The OT's role extends to facilitating age-appropriate activities and interactions. The OT provides opportunities for the teen to make choices and to exercise age-appropriate independence. In adolescents with RSD, upper extremity involvement is less common than lower extremity involvement. When the former is present, however, the OT provides tasks requiring hand and arm use in much the same way as the PT does for the lower extremities.

— The parents: The parents form a vital component of the therapeutic team. Without their active participation, recovery tends to be slower and relapses are more common. Both mother and father should be enlisted as full members of the team. We encourage both to participate with their teenager in the exercise program. We instruct the parents to "cheer the patient on" but to avoid negative statements about the activity. For example, when the teen is working out on the stationary bicycle, the parent might do the same on another bicycle.

— Social worker or psychologist: The role of this team member is crucial in terms of the long-term outlook. His or her first task is to evaluate patient and family psychosocial dynamics. The experience of this therapeutic team member in dealing with many RSD cases has proved to be an extremely valuable asset; patients with RSD, when previously evaluated elsewhere, may have been informed they had no psychological problems. Our studies, in contrast, have established a high frequency of subtle family conflict, difficulty in expressing anger, and enmeshment with the mother. The father, on the other hand, is frequently viewed by teen and mother as powerful but remote. Although the patient may be the family member with symptoms, RSD can usually be seen as a family disorder, and family therapy may be highly desirable.

The treatment program outlined above has evolved in our institution for many years. It has proved to be highly effective in returning the great majority of patients to normal functioning, with a very low rate of disease recurrence.

BIBLIOGRAPHY

Fibromyalgia

Bennett RM. Fibromyalgia and the facts: sense or nonsense. Rheum Dis Clin North Am 1993a;19:45.

Bennett RM. A multidisciplinary approach to treating fibromyalgia. In: Avery H, Masker H, eds. Progress in fibromyalgia and myofascial pain. New York: Elsevier Science Publishers, 1993b:393–410.

Bennett RM. Fibromyalgia: the commonest cause of widespread pain. Compr Ther 1995;21:269.

Bennett RM, McCain GA. Coping successfully with fibromyalgia. Patient Care 1995;March 15:29.

Bohr TW. Fibromyalgia syndrome and myofascial pain syndrome. Do they exist? Neurol Clin 1995;13:365.

Boissevain MD, McCain GA. Toward an integrated understanding of fibromyalgia syndrome. I. Medical and pathophysiological aspects. Pain 1991;45:227.

Buchwald D, Garrity D. Comparison of patients with chronic fatigue syndrome, fibromyalgia, and multiple chemical sensitivities. Arch Intern Med 1994;154:2049.

Buskila D, Press J, Gedalia A, et al. Assessment of nonarticular tenderness and prevalence of fibromyalgia in children. J Rheumatol 1993;20:368.

Carette S, Bell MJ, Reynolds WJ, et al. Comparison of amitriptyline, cyclobenzaprine, and placebo in the treatment of fibromyalgia: a randomized, double-blind clinical trial [see Comments]. Arthritis Rheum 1994;37:32.

Clauw DJ. Fibromyalgia: more than just a musculoskeletal disease. Am Fam Physician 1995;52:843.

Doherty M, Jones A. ABC of rheumatology: fibromyalgia syndrome. Br Med J 1995;310:386.

Goldenberg DL. Fibromyalgia, chronic fatigue syndrome, and myofascial pain syndrome. Curr Opin Rheumatol 1995;7:127.

Hudson JI, Goldenberg DL, Pope HG Jr, et al. Comorbidity of fibromyalgia with medical and psychiatric disorders. Am J Med 1992;92:363.

Hudson JI, Hudson MS, Pliner LF, et al. Fibromyalgia and major affective disorder: a controlled phenomenology and family history study. Am J Psychiatry 1985;142:441.

Littlejohn GO. A database for fibromyalgia. Rheum Dis Clin North Am 1995;21:527.

Middleton GD, McFarlin JE, Lipsky PE. The prevalence and clinical impact of fibromyalgia in systemic lupus erythematosus. Arthritis Rheum 1994;37:1181.

Wolfe F. When to diagnose fibromyalgia. Rheum Dis Clin North Am 1994;20:485.

Wolfe F, Ross K, Anderson J, et al. The prevalence and characteristics of fibromyalgia in the general population. Arthritis Rheum 1995;38:19.

Wolfe F, Smythe HA, Yunus MB, et al. The American College of Rheumatology 1990 criteria for the classification of fibromyalgia: report of the multicenter criteria committee. Arthritis Rheum 1990;33:160.

Wortmann RL. Searching for the cause of fibromyalgia: is there a defect in energy metabolism [Editorial]? Arthritis Rheum 1994;37:790.

Yunus MB, Masi AT. Juvenile primary fibromyalgia syndrome: a clinical study of thirty-three patients and matched normal controls. Arthritis Rheum 1985;28:138.

Reflex Sympathetic Dystrophy

Barrett J. Reflex sympathetic dystrophy: recognizing a cause of chronic pain. Physician and Sportsmedicine 1995;23:51.

Bernstein BH, Singsen BH, Kent JT, et al. Reflex neurovascular dystrophy in childhood. J Pediatr 1978;93:211.

Koman LA, Barden A, Smith BP, et al. Reflex sympathetic dystrophy in an adolescent. Foot Ankle 1993;14:273.

Kozin F. Reflex sympathetic dystrophy syndrome: a review. Clin Exp Rheumatol 1992;10:401.

Lynch ME. Psychological aspects of reflex sympathetic dystrophy: a review of the adults and paediatric literature. Pain 1992;49:337.

Malleson PN, Al-Matar M, Petty RE. Idiopathic musculoskeletal pain syndromes in children. J Rheumatol 1992;19:1786.

Schwartzman RJ, McLellan TL. Reflex sympathetic dystrophy: a review. Arch Neurol 1987;44:555.

Sherry DD, Weisman MA. Psychologic aspects of childhood reflex neurovascular dystrophy. Pediatrics 1988;81:572.

Silber TJ, Massoud M. Reflex sympathetic dystrophy syndrome in children and adolescents: report of 18 cases and review of the literature. Am J Dis Child 1988;142:1325.

Smith DL, Campbell SM. Reflex sympathetic dystrophy syndrome: diagnosis and management. West J Med 1987;147:342.

Veldman PH, Reynen HM, Arntz IE, et al. Signs and symptoms of reflex sympathetic dystrophy: prospective study of 829 patients. Lancet 1993;342:1012.

CHAPTER 39

Toxic Shock Syndrome

Lawrence S. Neinstein and Wilbert H. Mason, Jr.

Toxic shock syndrome (TSS) is an acute, multisystem, potentially lethal disease, predominantly affecting menstruating females. Forty-two percent of cases have occurred in girls between 11 and 19 years of age. The syndrome was first described in 1978 and peaked in incidence in 1980, with national attention given to its association with tampons. However, the disease has not disappeared, and cases continue to be reported throughout the United States.

ETIOLOGY

TSS is thought to be associated with TSS toxin type 1 (TSST-1), sometimes known as staphylococcal enterotoxin F. This toxin has been recovered from 90% of *Staphylococcus aureus* strains in TSS associated with menstruation cases and from 60% of *S. aureus* strains associated with nonmenstruation cases.

Approximately 9% of females will have *S. aureus* organisms that can be cultured from secretions of the labia or vagina. Approximately 10% of these strains will produce TSST-1. During menstruation, there is probably an enhancement in growth of these organisms because of menstrual blood and fluid. The release of these toxins is presumed to be enhanced by microabrasions caused by tampons and, in particular, by superabsorbent tampons. This toxin can affect multiple systems of the body, either directly or through the hypoperfusion that can result from the toxin's effect on the vascular system.

Epidemiology

1. Incidence: The incidence peaked in 1980 at between 0.25 and 2 in 100,000 persons in the general population and between 2 and 14.4 in 100,000 in the menstruating female population. Since the removal of highly absorbent tampons from the market, the incidence of menstrual TSS has decreased to 1.0 in 100,000; the rate in the general population is about 0.10 in 100,000. In 1980, 91% of TSS cases were associated with menstruation. In 1988, menstrual cases fell to 55%.
2. Age: Forty-two percent of TSS cases have occurred in females younger than 19 years of age. The peak incidence is in girls 16–17 years of age.
3. Sex: Ninety percent of cases have occurred in females.
4. Race: Ninety-eight percent of cases among menstruating females have been in white females; while there is no racial predilection for cases not involving menstruation.
5. Risk factors
   a. Tampons: Ninety-nine percent of females with TSS associated with menstruation use tampons. Risk increases with the degree of absorbency of the tampon, and the overall risk ratio for TSS is 32.8 when tampon users are compared with those not using tampons.

b. Menstruation: Ninety-five percent of TSS cases in females occur at or near the time of menses.

c. Non-menstruation-associated cases: These cases seem to be associated with either skin infections, surgical wound infections, traumatic injuries, or postpartum infections. Rare cases have been associated with diaphragm use, sponge use, or influenza infection. Rosen et al. (1993) reported on one case that occurred after a loop electrosurgical excision procedure.

CLINICAL MANIFESTATIONS

TSS is a multisystem disease with a wide range of signs and symptoms. Acute illness may start with a prodrome, including malaise, headaches, myalgias, fatigue, vomiting, and watery diarrhea. The acute illness characteristically has an acute onset with or without the prodrome and includes:

1. High fever, with a temperature higher than 38.9°C
2. Rash: Usually begining as diffuse erythema similar to sunburn, with a blanching macular erythema that may be particularly prominent around the perineum and inner aspect of the thighs. Around day 5 to 12, the rash develops fine, dandrufflike desquamation around the face, trunk, and extremities. Afterward, a full-thickness peeling of the palms and soles occurs.
3. Gastrointestinal symptoms
   a. Vomiting and watery diarrhea develop in 90% of individuals.
   b. Generalized abdominal pain and tenderness are common.
   c. A decrease in bowel sounds is common.
4. Musculoskeletal symptoms
   a. Myalgias: 88–100%
   b. Arthralgias
   c. Sterile knee effusions
5. Renal symptoms: Occur in at least 80% of cases
   a. Azotemia
   b. Sterile pyuria
   c. Hematuria
   d. Proteinuria
6. Neurological symptoms
   a. Headaches
   b. Somnolence
   c. Disorientation
   d. Hysteria
   e. Confusion
   f. Agitation
   g. Photophobia
   h. Paresthesias
   i. Seizures
   j. Meningeal signs
7. Cardiovascular symptoms
   a. Hypotension
   b. Tachycardia
   c. Nonspecific ST-T segment changes
   d. Premature ventricular contractions

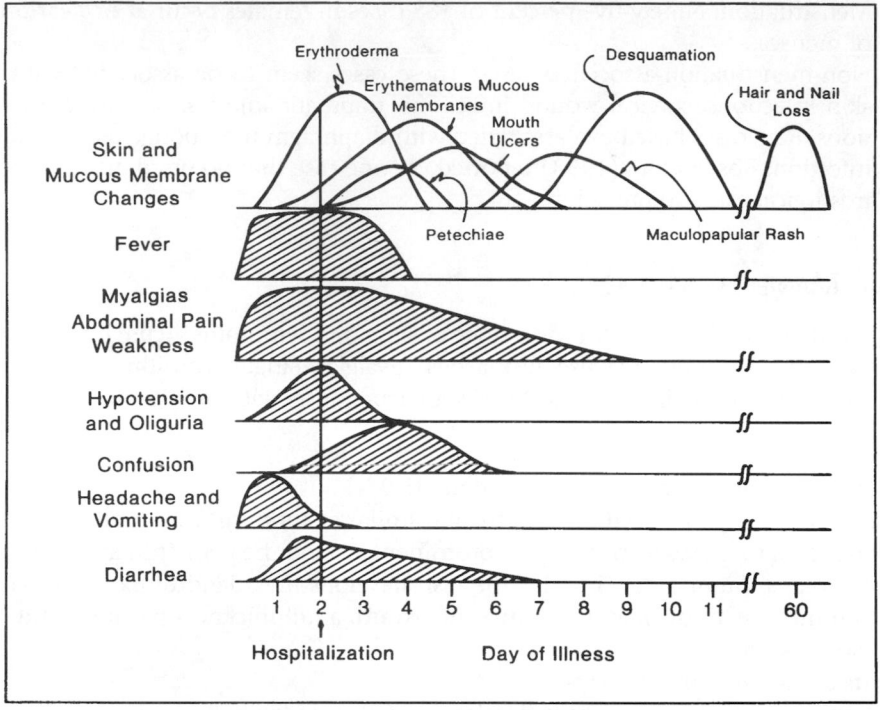

FIGURE **39.1.** Course of major systemic, skin, and mucous membrane manifestations of toxic shock syndrome. (From Chesney PJ, Davis JP, Purdy WK, et al. Clinical manifestations of toxic shock syndrome. JAMA 1981;246:743.

    e. First-degree heart block
    f. Pericarditis
  8. Pulmonary symptoms
    a. Hypoxemia: oxygen tension often less than 60 mm Hg
    b. Possible adult respiratory distress syndrome
  9. Gynecological symptoms
    a. Hyperemia of external genitalia
    b. Punctate pustules or ulcers of vagina
    c. Vaginal discharge
    d. Adnexal tenderness

The course of the illness is outlined in Figure 39.1.

DIFFERENTIAL DIAGNOSIS

NOTE: An asterisk (*) denotes that the entry is a primary consideration in the differential diagnosis.

Exanthemas

  1. Kawasaki disease (mucocutaneous lymph node syndrome)*
    a. Usual age: Less than 10 years

    b. Usually no abdominal pain
    c. Usually no shock
    d. Usually no myalgias
    e. Usually no thrombocytopenia
    f. Usually more significant adenopathy
    g. Associated with coronary aneurysms in some cases
2. Streptococcal scarlet fever*
    a. Uncommon after 10 years of age
    b. Usually follows upper respiratory tract infection with recovery of group A streptococci from pharynx
    c. Usually has characteristic sandpaper rash
3. Streptococcal toxic shock–like syndrome*
4. Group A streptococci: Occasionally the cause of a syndrome similar to TSS
    a. Pain: Most common initial symptom, usually of an extremity
    b. Evidence of localized soft tissue infection: 80% of patients
    c. Necrotizing fasciitis or myositis: Often evolves from soft-tissue infection
5. Staphylococcal scarlet fever*
6. Rocky Mountain spotted fever*: Presence of febrile agglutinins for *Proteus* strains OX-19 and OX-2
7. Leptospirosis*
8. Meningococcemia and other septicemias*
9. Erythema multiforme
10. Stevens-Johnson syndrome
11. Rubeola* and rubella
12. Systemic lupus erythematosus

Gastrointestinal Disorders

1. Gastroenteritis
2. Staphylococcal food poisoning
3. Appendicitis and other causes of acute abdominal conditions

Other Disorders

1. Acute pyelonephritis*
2. Septic shock*
3. Hemolytic-uremic syndrome
4. Tularemia
5. Pelvic inflammatory disease
6. Rhabdomyolysis

DIAGNOSIS

Diagnosis is based on clinical manifestations as already outlined, laboratory abnormalities as outlined next, negative results on culture of specimens from the throat and cerebrospinal fluid (CSF), and negative serologic findings for Rocky Mountain spotted fever, leptospirosis, and rubeola.

Laboratory Abnormalities (adapted from Tofte and Williams, 1982)

	Prevalence
Decreased calcium concentration	83%
Pyuria	81%
Decreased serum concentration of protein	81%
Decreased albumin concentration	76%
Leukocytosis with bands	72%
Elevated bilirubin concentration	68%
Elevated aspartate aminotransferase (AST) and alanine aminotransferase (ALT) activity	65%
Elevated prothrombin time	64%
Elevated blood urea nitrogen (BUN) and creatinine concentrations	61%
Elevated creatine kinase activity	53%
Decreased hemoglobin level	50%
Decreased serum concentration of phosphorus	50%
Decreased platelet count	25%

Case Definition

The Centers for Disease Control and Prevention case definition for TSS includes (Wager, 1983):

1. Fever (temperature >38.9°C)
2. Rash (diffuse macular erythroderma)
3. Desquamation: 1–2 weeks after onset of illness, particularly of palms and soles
4. Hypotension (systolic blood pressure <90 mm Hg for adults or <5th percentile by age for children less than 16 years of age, or orthostatic syncope)
5. Involvement of three or more of the following:
    a. Gastrointestinal tract: Vomiting or diarrhea at onset of illness
    b. Muscles: Severe myalgia or creatine phosphokinase activity at twice the normal level
    c. Mucous membranes: Vaginal, oropharyngeal, or conjunctival hyperemia
    d. Renal system: BUN or creatinine concentrations two times normal, or more than 5 leukocytes per high-power field in the absence of a urinary tract infection
    e. Hepatic system: Total bilirubin concentration and AST and ALT activity two times normal
    f. Blood: Platelet count less than100,000 mm³
    g. Central nervous system: Disorientation or alterations in consciousness without focal neurological signs when fever and hypotension are absent
6. Negative results on the following tests, if obtained:
    a. Cultures of blood, throat, or CSF specimens, except for *S. aureus* in the blood
    b. Serologic tests for Rocky Mountain spotted fever, leptospirosis, or measles
        Initial evaluation should include complete history and physical examination, especially a pelvic examination. Specimens of blood, vaginal secretions, wound exudate, oropharyngeal secretions, and CSF (if indicated) should be obtained for culture. In addition, the following should be performed: a complete blood cell count; urinalysis; measurements of electrolytes, BUN or creatinine, serum calcium, phosphate, and albumin, AST and ALT activity, bilirubin, prothrombin and partial thromboplastin times; and chest radiography and electrocardiography. Serum should also be stored for serologic tests.

THERAPY

1. Remove tampons or other objects from the vagina and drain any wounds.
2. Give supportive therapy, including intravenous fluids; often 8–12 L/day is required.
3. Carefully monitor, including with the use of a Foley catheter and a Swan-Ganz pulmonary artery catheter if needed.
4. Give antibiotics, including coverage for both penicillin-sensitive and penicillin-resistant *S. aureus.* Before diagnosis is made and culture results are known, broad-spectrum coverage is recommended.
5. Monitor cardiac, respiratory, renal, hepatic, central nervous system, and metabolic function.
6. Corticosteroids have been recommended by some practitioners (Todd et al., 1984), though no prospective studies demonstrate efficacy in the treatment of TSS.

Intravenously administered immune globulin has high levels of antibody to TSST-1 and has proved effective in an animal model (Melish et al., 1989); it is reportedly widely used in the United Kingdom to treat TSS. Barry et al. (1992) reported on one case in which immune globulin was used to treat toxic streptococcal syndrome; it appeared to be highly effective.

COMPLICATIONS AND PROGNOSIS

Although most patients recover, there is a 2–4% mortality rate, which is even higher for males (12.2%). Recurrent episodes occur in as many as 30% of individuals; however, cases recur only in menstruating females. Although recovery is usually complete, there are reports of long-term renal abnormalities, gangrene of fingers and toes, and neurologic sequelae such as peripheral neuropathies and decreased memory. For prevention of the disease and of recurrences, it is recommended that:

1. Individuals with a history of TSS no longer use tampons.
2. Females without a history of TSS should use tampons only when menstrual flow is heavy, should not use them continuously, and should avoid nighttime use and superabsorbent tampons.
3. Females should wash their hands before changing a tampon.

BIBLIOGRAPHY

Barry W, Hudgins L, Donta ST, et al. Intravenous immunoglobulin therapy for toxic shock syndrome. JAMA 1992;267:3315.

Berkley SF, Hightower AW, Broome CV, et al. The relationship of tampon characteristics to menstrual toxic shock syndrome. JAMA 1987;258:917.

Centers for Disease Control. Reduced menstrual toxic shock syndrome—United States. MMWR 1990;39:421.

Centers for Disease Control: CDC defines group A streptococcal toxic shock syndrome. Am Fam Physician 1993;47:1643.

Chesney PJ, Davis JP, Purdy WK, et al. Clinical manifestations of toxic shock syndrome. JAMA 1981;246:741.

Cowan RK, Maretns MG. Toxic shock syndrome mimicking pelvic inflammatory disease presumably resulting from tattoo. South Med J 1993;86:1427.

Davis JP, Chesney J, Wand PJ, et al. Toxic-shock syndrome: epidemiologic features, recurrence, risk factors, and prevention. N Engl J Med 1980;303:1430.

Garbe PL, Arko RJ, Reingold AL, et al. *Staphylococcus aureus* isolates from patients with nonmenstrual toxic shock syndrome: evidence for additional toxins. JAMA 1985;253:2538.

Litt IF. Toxic shock syndrome: an adolescent disease. J Adolesc Health Care 1983;4:270.

MacDonald KL, Osterholm MT, Hedberg CW, et al. Toxic shock syndrome: a newly recognized complication of influenza and influenza-like illness. JAMA 1987;257:1053.

Markowitz LE, Hightower AW, Broome CV, et al. Toxic shock syndrome: evaluation of national surveillance data using a hospital discharge survey. JAMA 1987; 258:75.

McGregor JA, Todd JK. Toxic shock syndrome: still a threat. The Female Patient 1987;12:32.

Melish ME, Murata S, Fukunaga C, et al. Corticosteroid and immunoglobulin therapy in toxic shock syndrome. Rev Infect Dis 1989;11(suppl 1):S332.

Raab MG, O'Brien M, Hayes JM, et al. Postoperative toxic shock syndrome. Am J Orthop 1995;24:130.

Rosen DJ, Margolin ML, Menashe Y, et al. Toxic shock syndrome after loop electrosurgical excision procedure. Am J Obstet Gynecol 1993;169:202.

Sagraves R. Menstrual toxic shock syndrome. Am Pharm 1995;NS35:12.

Shands KN, Schmid GP, Dan BB, et al. Toxic-shock syndrome in menstruating women: association with tampon use and *Staphylococcus aureus* and clinical features in 52 cases. N Engl J Med 1980;303:1436.

Stevens DL, Tanner MH, Winship J, et al. Severe group A streptococcal infections associated with a toxic shock–like syndrome and scarlet fever toxin A. N Engl J Med 1989;321:1.

Strausbaugh LJ. Toxic shock syndrome: are you recognizing its changing presentations? Postgrad Med 1993;94:107.

Tanner MH, Pierce BJ, Hale DC. Toxic shock syndrome. West J Med 1981;134:477.

Todd JK, Ressman M, Caston SA, et al. Corticosteroid therapy for patients with toxic shock syndrome. JAMA 1984;252:3399.

Tofte RW, Williams DN. Toxic shock syndrome: clinical and laboratory features in 15 patients. Ann Intern Med 1981;94:149.

Tofte RW, Williams DN. Clinical and laboratory manifestations of toxic shock syndrome. Ann Intern Med 1982;96:843.

Wager GP. Toxic shock syndrome: a review. Am J Obstet Gynecol 1983;146:93.

Wolf JE, Rabinowitz LG. Streptococcal toxic shock–like syndrome. Arch Dermatol 1995;131:73.

Sexuality and Family Planning

CHAPTER 40

Adolescent Sexuality

Lawrence S. Neinstein and Martin M. Anderson

Adolescents are often sexually active, a reality that parents, doctors, and adolescents themselves are not always comfortable addressing. A practitioner who approaches the topic of teenage sexuality by focusing solely on possible outcomes related to the sexual act itself, such as pregnancy and sexually transmitted diseases, ignores the reality that all teenagers are sexual beings whether or not they are sexually active. In fact, sexual behavior does not start during adolescence or adulthood, but with childhood sexual curiosity. During adolescence there is a sudden upsurge of curiosity and interest in one's own body and the bodies of one's peers. Even very young adolescents are interested in "how things work" and are exposed to a wide range of sexual topics through friends, school, and the media. Although problems arise during adolescence from lack of information, more confusion and difficulties stem from inexperience with sexuality and lack of decision-making skills. It is essential for health-care providers caring for adolescents to understand sexuality during the teenage period and to be familiar with ways to deal with teenagers' questions, feelings, and problems. This chapter provides an overview of adolescent sexuality and methods by which the professional can better deal with adolescent sexuality.

ADOLESCENT SEXUAL DEVELOPMENT

Preadolescence

During the preadolescent period, biological sex based on chromosomes, gonads, and hormones is determined. In addition, gender identity or sense of masculinity and femininity is established. Characteristics of preadolescent sexual development include:

1. A low physical and mental investment in sexuality exists.
2. Collecting of information and myths about sexuality from friends, school, and family is common.
3. Physical appearance is prepubertal.

Early Adolescence

Characteristics of sexual development in early adolescence include:

1. Physical maturation starts.
2. Extreme concern and curiosity exists about one's own body and that of one's peers.
3. Sexual fantasies are common and may serve as a source of guilt.
4. Masturbation begins during this period and may be accompanied by guilt.

627

5. Sexual activities are usually nonphysical. Early adolescents are often highly content with nonsexual interactions such as telephone calls to peers.

Middle Adolescence

Sexual development in middle adolescence is characterized by:

1. Full physical maturation is attained and menstruation begins in females.
2. Sexual energy is at a high level, with more emphasis on physical contact.
3. Sexual behavior is of an exploring and exploiting nature.
4. Dating and petting are common, and casual relationships with both noncoital and coital contact are prevalent.
5. Denial of consequences of sexual behavior is typical.

Late Adolescence

Sexual development in late adolescence is characterized by:

1. Full physical and sociolegal maturation.
2. Sexual behavior becomes more expressive and less exploitative.
3. Intimate sharing relationships may develop.

As already outlined here, adolescent sexuality is an important developmental process and cannot be reduced merely to outcomes such as pregnancy and intercourse. Adolescents are struggling with their identity and issues such as:

1. How do I know I'm ready for sex?
2. What is important in a relationship?
3. How do I say no?
4. How do I deal with anger, rejection, and loneliness?

Adolescents are involved with sexual activity because of peer pressure, to experience affection, to feel grown up, to experience closeness, for experimentation, and because it feels good.

SEXUAL BEHAVIOR

Differences have occurred in society in the past 50–100 years that have influenced sexual behaviors. In 1890, the interval for women between puberty and marriage was 7.2 years compared to 11.8 years in 1988 for women and 12.5 years for men. Other societal changes have influenced adolescent behaviors including higher divorce rates, urbanization and crowdedness, ethnic diversity, and racial and ethnic tensions. Overall, however, most teens still have values that reflect their parent's goals including valuing education, marriage, family life, and religious commitment. Although statistics on sexual behavior do not summarize adolescent sexuality, the health-care provider can use this data to develop a framework of normal adolescent behavior.

1. Masturbation
   a. Prevalence (Sorenson, 1973)
      — Males: Sixty percent to 90% have masturbated during adolescence.
      — Females: About 40% have masturbated during adolescence.
      Leitenberg et al. (1993) more recently examined masturbation behavior among university students. Results showed that men still masturbate much more than women.

TABLE 40.1.   Frequency of Masturbation in Adolescents

Frequency of Masturbation (per month)	All (%)	Males (%)	Females (%)
1–2 times	30	21	43
3–4 times	29	36	18
5–10 times	23	21	27
11–19 times	11	12	9
>20 times	7	10	3
TOTAL	100	100	100

Adapted from Sorenson RC. Adolescent sexuality in contemporary America. New York: World Publishing, 1973.

TABLE 40.2.   Age of First Masturbation Experience in Adolescents

Age of First Masturbation	All (%)	Males (%)	Females (%)
10 years or under	20	12	33
11 years	11	12	8
12 years	14	15	13
13 years	29	36	16
14 years	18	17	19
15–19 years	8	8	9
TOTAL	100	100	100

Adapted from Sorenson RC. Adolescent sexuality in contemporary America. New York: World Publishing, 1973.

Twice as many men as women had ever masturbated and the men who masturbated did so three times more frequently during early adolescence and young adulthood than the women who masturbated during these same age periods. There was no relationship found between masturbation during preadolescence or early adolescence and intercourse experience, sexual satisfaction, sexual arousal, or sexual difficulties in relationships during young adulthood.

    b. Frequency (Table 40.1)
    c. Age of first masturbation experience (Table 40.2)

2. Petting (Hass, 1979)
    a. Percentage of boys who have touched a girl's breast:
       — By age 13: 48%
       — By age 15: 73%
       — By age 18: 90%
    b. Percentage of girls who had their breast touched by a boy by age 17–19: 91%

3. Oral sex
    a. Prevalence (Moscicki, 1993)
       — Fellatio: Males 79%, females 70%
       — Cunnilingus: Males 59%, females 78%
    b. Age at first experience of oral sex (Table 40.3)

4. Anal intercourse (heterosexual)
    a. Prevalence
       — Females: 20–25% (Jaffe et al., 1988; Moscicki, 1993)
       — Males: 23–27% (Moscicki, 1993; Pendergrast et al., 1992)

5. Sexual intercourse: Of 29 million teenagers aged 12 and up, approximately 12 million (7 million males and 5 million females) are sexually active, this includes about 50% of women and three-fourths of men by their 18th birthday. However, most teens do not initiate sexual intercourse as early as most adults believe. In addition, all teenagers are not

Table 40.3.   Age of Teenagers' First Experience with Oral Sex

Age of First Experience	Fellatio		Cunnilingus	
	Males (%)	Females (%)	Males (%)	Females (%)
By age 13	8	4	11	5
By age 16	35	34	36	37

Adapted from Hass A. Teenage sexuality—a survey of teenage sexual behavior. Los Angeles: Pinnacle Books, 1979.

Table 40.4.   Percentage of Adolescents 12–19 Having Sexual Intercourse, 1988

Age	Never Had Intercourse (%)	Ever Had Intercourse (%)
12	91	9
13	84	16
14	77	23
15	70	30
16	58	42
17	41	59
18	29	71
19	18	82

Adapted from Alan Guttmacher Institute. Sex and America's teenagers. New York: Alan Guttmacher Institute, 1994 using data from 1990 Youth Risk Behavior Survey; Alan Guttmacher Institute's tabulations of data from 1988 National Survey of Family Growth; Sonenstein FL, Pleck JH, Ku LC. Sexual activity, condom use and AIDS awareness among adolescent males. Family Planning Perspectives 1989;21:152, and Hollman FW. Estimates of the population of the United States by age, sex, and race. Current population reports [Series P–25, No 1095]. Washington, DC: US Bureau of the Census, 1993.

Table 40.5.   Percentage of Never-Married Metropolitan-Area Teens Ever Having Had Sexual Intercourse, by Age and Sex, 1988

Age	Male (%)	Female (%)
15	33	27
16	50	34
17	66	52
18	72	70
19	86	78

Male data: Sonenstein FL, Pleck JH, Ku LC. Sexual activity, condom use, and AIDS awareness among adolescent males. Fam Plann Perspect 1989;21:152. *Female data:* National Survey of Family Growth. Hyattsville, Maryland: National Center for Health Statistics, 1988.

sexually active. Most younger teens are not sexually experienced and over 20% of adolescents do not have sexual intercourse at all during the teenage years.
  a. Sexual activity rates
    — The percentage of sexual intercourse for teens 12–19 is shown in Table 40.4.
    — The percentage of sexually active adolescents by age and sex is shown in Table 40.5.
    — Selected sexual behaviors by age is shown in Table 40.6.
    — The percentage of sexually active adolescents by grade and sex is shown in Table 40.7.
    — The percentage of sexually active high school students by sex and race is shown in Table 40.8.
    — The percentage of teenagers ever having intercourse by age, in six countries, is shown in Figure 40.1.
  b. Trend in sexual activity rates: The trend of sexual activity among never-married adolescents from 1971 to 1988 is shown in Tables 40.9 and 40.10. Table 40.11 demonstrates the percentage of women and men who have had intercourse by age 18 from

TABLE 40.6.   Percentage of Persons Aged 12–21 Years Who Engaged in Selected Sexual Behaviors, by Age Group—United States, Youth Risk Behavior Survey, National Health Interview Survey, 1992

Behavior	Age Group			
	12–13 (%)	14–17 (%)	18–21 (%)	Total (%)
Ever had sexual intercourse	([a])	43.4	81.7	63.0
Sexual intercourse with ≥4 sex partners	([a])	13.3	41.3	27.6
Used condom during most recent sexual intercourse	([a])	58.5	36.9	43.5

Adapted from US Department of Health and Human Health Services. Health risk behaviors among persons aged 12–21 years—United States, 1992. MMWR 1994;43:231.
[a]Respondents aged 12–13 were not asked this question.

TABLE 40.7.   Percentage of High School Students Reporting Having Had Sexual Intercourse by Sex and Grade—United States, 1993

Grade	Female (%)	Male (%)	Total (%)
9th	31.6	43.5	37.7
10th	44.9	47.4	46.1
11th	55.1	59.5	57.5
12th	66.3	70.2	68.3
TOTAL	50.2	55.6	53.0

Adapted from Youth Risk Behavior Surveillance—United States, 1993. MMWR 1995;44(SS-1):1.

TABLE 40.8.   Percentage of High School Students Reporting Having Had Sexual Intercourse by Sex and Race—United States, 1993

Race or Ethnicity	Female (%)	Male (%)	Total (%)
White, non-Hispanic	47.4	49.3	48.4
African-American	70.4	89.2	79.7
Hispanic	48.3	63.5	56.0

Adapted from Youth Risk Behavior Surveillance—United States, 1993. MMWR 1995;44(SS-1):1.

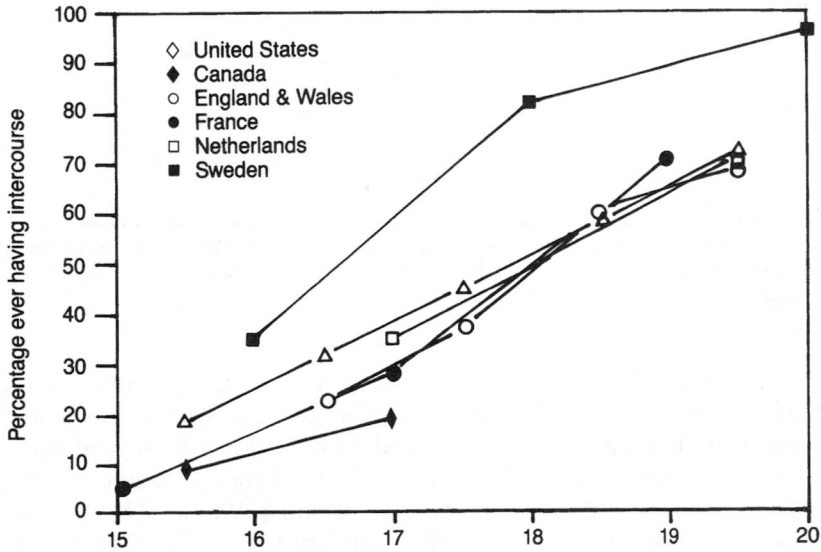

FIGURE 40.1.   Percentage of teenagers every having had intercourse, by age, in six countries. (Reproduced with permission from Hatcher RA, et al. Contraceptive technology 1988–1989. New York: Irvington Publishers, 1988.)

Table 40.9. Trends in Percentage of U.S. Never-Married Metropolitan-Area 15- to 19-Year-Old Females Ever Sexually Active

	1971 (%)	1976 (%)	1979 (%)	1982 (%)	1988 (%)
Total	30	43	50	45	53
White	26	38	47	43	52
African-American	54	66	66	54	60

Adapted from Hofferth SL, et al. Premarital sexual activity among US teenage women over the past three decades. Fam Plann Perspect 1987;19:46; and National Survey of Family Growth. Hyattsville, Maryland: National Center for Health Statistics, 1988.
Note: Data calculated from 1971, 1976, and 1979 National Surveys of Young Women and 1982 and 1988 National Surveys of Family Growth.

Table 40.10. Trends in Percentage of U.S. Never-Married Metropolitan-Area Teenage Males Ever Sexually Active, by Race and Age

	1979 (%)	1988 (%)
Total[a]	66	76
Non–African-American	65	73
African-American	71	88
15	NA	33
16	NA	50
17	56	66
18	66	72
19	78	86

Sonenstein FL, Pleck JH, Ku LC. Sexual activity, condom use, and AIDS awareness among adolescent males. Fam Plann Perspect 1989;21:152.
[a]Ages 17–19.

Table 40.11. Percentage of U.S. Women and Men Who Have Had Intercourse by Age 18

Year of 18th Birthday	Intercourse by Age 18	
	Men (%)	Women (%)
1956–1958	([a])	27
1959–1961	([a])	31
1962–1964	([a])	31
1965–1967	([a])	31
1968–1970	55	35
1971–1973	61	45
1974–1976	64	47
1977–1979	64	47
1980–1982	63	51
1983–1985	64	52
1986–1988	73	56

Adapted from Alan Guttmacher Institute (AGI). Sex and America's teenagers, New York: Alan Guttmacher Institute, 1994, using data adapted by AGI from tabulations from the 1982 National Survey of Family Growth, 1988 National Survey of Family Growth, and the 1991 National Survey of Men.
[a]Not available.

1956 to 1988. Other recent data of trends of sexual activity among high school students from 1990 to 1992 from the Youth Risk Behavior Study is shown in Table 5.18. These data obtained from the 1982 and 1988 National Surveys of Family Growth (Pratt et al., 1984); the 1979 and 1988 National Surveys of Adolescent Males; the 1971, 1976, and 1979 National Surveys of Young Women (Zelnick and Kantner, 1980); the 1991 National Survey of Men; and the Centers for Disease Control (CDC) Youth Risk Behavior Surveys suggest that sexual activity rates among teens in the United States increased in the 1970s and 1980s (Tables 40.9 through 40.11).

Koffi-Blanchard et al. (1994) have reported on trends in the past 20 years in Switzerland among youth 16–20 in an attempt to explore the influence of AIDS concerns on sexual behavior. They found that the the percentage of sexually active 17-year-olds increased in the last 20 years for girls from 33% to 46% and for boys of the same age, from 23% to 51%. The increase took place before 1987, and since then, the proportion of sexually active young people has not changed.

  c. Characteristics of teens who have been sexually active (Table 40.12)

    — Race: Differences in rates of sexual activity have been reported based on race and ethnicity with 50% of African-American men indicating they have had sex by age 15 but Hispanic and white men not reporting this level of sexual activity until they are nearly 17. Half of African-American women report having had intercourse by age 16.5, which is about 1 year earlier than white and Hispanic women.

    — Family income: Poor and low-income teenagers are more likely to be sexually experienced than adolescents from higher income families, although rates are at 50% or above in all three groups.

    — Other risk behaviors: Adolescents who engage in other high-risk behavior such as drinking and drug use are more likely than others to be sexually experienced (Table 40.13).

  d. Number of partners: Adolescents do not have as many partners as many adults might believe. In fact, among the unmarried adolescents, adolescents are less likely than older unmarried individuals to have more than one partner in a 3-month period. For example, 8% of sexually active unmarried women 15–17 had more than one sex partner in the last 3 months compared to 12% of women 25–29. Younger women are more likely than older women to have more than one sexual partner in a short time period because most younger women are unmarried (Alan Guttmacher Institute, 1994).

    — Half of sexually experienced young women wait almost 18 months between the time they first have intercourse and the time they have a second sexual partner. In another 25%, the waiting period is almost 2 years (Alan Guttmacher Institute, 1994).

    — Young age: Women who begin sexual activity at a young age are more likely to more quickly move on to another second partner.

TABLE 40.12. Sexual Activity among Adolescent U.S. Females Aged 15–19 Based on Race, Income, Religion, or Location

	Sexually Active Females Aged 15–19 (%)
Race	
African-American	61
Hispanic	49
White	52
Income	
Poor	60
Low income	53
Higher income	50
Religion	
Roman Catholic	48
Fundamentalist Protestant	55
Other	54
Protestant	60
Location	
Urban	53
Rural	53

Adapted from Alan Guttmacher Institute (AGI). Sex and America's teenagers, New York: Alan Guttmacher Institute, 1994, using data from Forrest JD, Singh S. The sexual and reproductive behavior of American women 1982–1988, Fam Plann Perspect 1990;22:206; and from AGI tabulations of data from the 1988 National Survey of Family Growth.

Table 40.13.   Risk Taking Behaviors and Sexual Activity Rates among Young U.S. Teens, 1990

Risk Taking Behaviors	14- to 15-Year-Olds Who Have Had Intercourse (%)
Alcohol	
None	26
Some	43
Regular	66
Cigarettes	
None	31
Some	55
Regular	69
Marijuana	
None	36
Some	68
Regular	87

Adapted from Alan Guttmacher Institute, Sex and America's teenagers. New York: Alan Guttmacher Institute, 1994, using data from 1990 Youth Risk Behavior Survey.

— Sexually experienced female adolescents: Of sexually experienced women aged 15–17, 55% have had two or more partners with 13% having had sex with at least six men. By their early 20s, 71% of women who are sexually experienced have had more than one partner, and 21% have had six or more partners.

— Sexually experienced male adolescents: Sexually experienced young men on average report having had more sexual partners since first intercourse than young women of similar ages.

— Swiss youth: Koffi-Blanchard et al. (1994) in their study of Swiss youth found that in 1992, 28% of girls and 23% of boys aged 17–20 years had had more than four sexual partners. There had been no changes in these percentages since 1987.

e. Contraceptive use: Most at-risk teens who are sexually active use a contraceptive method at least some of the time, with about two-thirds of adolescents using some method, usually the male condom, the first time. About 72–84% of teenage women use a method of contraception on an ongoing basis. Contraceptive use among adolescent females at first intercourse has risen from 48% in 1982 to 65% in 1988 (Alan Guttmacher Institute, 1994). Overall, contraceptive pill use increases with age, while condom use declines. Overall, adolescents use contraceptives about as effectively as adults, with both groups making mistakes. More frequent contraceptive use is associated with higher age, white race, and higher income. Despite increasing contraceptive use, 40% of teens still delay seeking medical services for contraception during the first year after they begin intercourse.

Koffi-Blanchard et al. (1994) in their study of Swiss youth also found that the use of contraception during the first sexual intercourse has become more frequent. In girls aged 16–20 years it rose from 47% in 1976 to 76% in 1992; in boys it increased from 50% in 1976 to 76% in 1992. For 17- to 20-year-olds, condom use with an occasional sexual partner rose from 16% in 1987 to 69% in 1992.

f. Reported place of first intercourse (Table 40.14): This data is from an older study and may be different in current adolescents.

g. Reasons for having intercourse, according to females (Sorenson, 1973):
— Mutual consent: 60–85%
— Go along with boyfriend: 13–28%
— Boyfriend could not say no: 5–12%
— Boyfriend will leave for another girl: 2–6%
— Other girls doing "it": 2–3%

TABLE 40.14.   Place of First Intercourse among U.S. Adolescents

Place of First Intercourse	All (%)	Females (%)	Males (%)
In the teenager's home	19	21	18
In a friend's home	10	9	10
In an automobile	20	16	24
In the girl or boy's home	20	19	21
In a motel	2	0	5
Outdoors	20	26	13
Other	9	9	9
TOTAL	100	100	100

Adapted from Sorenson RC. Adolescent sexuality in contemporary America. New York: World Publishing, 1973.

TABLE 40.15.   U.S. Adolescents' Reaction to Their First Intercourse

Reaction to First Intercourse	All (%)	Males (%)	Females (%)
Excited	37	46	26
Afraid	37	17	63
Happy	35	42	26
Satisfied	33	43	20
Thrilled	30	43	13
Curious	26	23	30
Joyful	23	31	12
Mature	23	29	14
Fulfilled	20	29	8
Worried	20	9	35
Guilty	17	3	36
Embarrassed	17	7	31
Tired	15	15	14
Relieved	14	19	8
Sorry	12	1	25
Hurt	11	0	25
Powerful	9	15	1
Foolish	8	7	9
Used	7	0	16
Disappointed	6	3	10
Felt raped	3	0	6

Adapted from Sorenson RC. Adolescent sexuality in contemporary America. New York: World Publishing, 1973.

h. Adolescents' reactions to their first intercourse (Table 40.15).
i. Orgasm (Hass, 1979): The percentage of sexually active teenage females who have had an orgasm:
   — Yes: 42%
   — No: 25%
   — I am not sure: 33%
6. Unwanted sexual experiences
   a. The percentage of students in grades 8–11 reporting unwanted sexual comments or actions is shown in Table 40.16.
   b. Six out of 10 students in grades 8–11 reported that they have subjected someone else at school to unwanted sexual comments or actions (Alan Guttmacher Institute, 1994).
   c. Nonvoluntary sexual intercourse: Sexual intercourse in young adolescents in particular may not be voluntary. Data presented by the Alan Guttmacher Institute indicates that about 74% of women who had intercourse before age 14 and 60% of those who

TABLE 40.16.   Percentage of U.S. Students in Grades 8–11 Reporting Unwanted Sexual Comments or Actions, 1993

Race or Ethnicity	Female	Male
African-American	84	81
Hispanic	82	69
White	87	75

Adapted from Alan Guttmacher Institute. Sex and America's teenagers. New York: Alan Guttmacher Institute, 1994.

TABLE 40.17.   Percentage of Sexually Experienced U.S. Females Aged 19 and Younger with History of Involuntary Intercourse

Age at First Intercourse	Involuntary Intercourse Only (%)	Both Voluntary and Involuntary Intercourse (%)	Voluntary Intercourse Only (%)
13 and younger	61	13	26
14 and younger	43	17	40
15 and younger	26	14	60
16 and younger	10	14	76
17 and younger	5	13	82
18 and younger	3	12	85
19 and younger	1	14	85

Adapted from Alan Guttmacher Institute. Sex and America's teenagers. New York: Alan guttmacher Institute, 1994, using data from Moore KA, Nord CW, Peterson JL. 1987 National Survey of Children, Fam Plann Perspect 1989;21:110.

had sex before age 15 report having had sex involuntarily (Alan Guttmacher Institute, 1994; Table 40.17). In 1987, 7% of sexually experienced young people aged 18–22 reported that they had been forced to have sex against their will at least once.

WHY IS ADOLESCENT SEXUALITY A CONCERN?

Assuming adolescent sexuality is part of a natural development, why is it a focus of so much attention and concern? The following are some explanations for this dichotomy:

1. Opposing views of sexuality: Inherent in the problem of adolescent sexuality are the differing attitudes about sexuality expressed by adolescents and the community. Predominant views among adolescents are that sex is justified as physical pleasure or as new experience; that it is an index of maturity; that it reflects peer-group conformity; that it represents a challenge to parents or to society; and that it offers an escape from pressures. The adolescent's parents or the community, on the other hand, often view sex among teenagers as a crime, a sin, or a sickness.
2. Body-mind gap: Although the age of physical maturity has progressively declined over the past 200 years, the age of economic independence and marriage has increased. This widening gap of perhaps 1–15 years or more must be filled with some form of developing sexuality for the adolescent. The enlarging time period of adolescent sexuality and society's inability to deal with the issue compound the problems of teenagers' sexuality.
3. Lack of communication: Numerous studies reveal that about two-thirds or more of adolescents cannot communicate with their parents about sex. Many parents assume that their teenagers do not want to talk about sex, when in fact many adolescents wish they could talk with their parents about sex. This miscommunication furthers misunderstanding and lack of trust.
4. Media: The media, including radio, movies, and television, promote an unrealistic image of sexual behavior, one based primarily on violence rather than love. Such an image leads to further adolescent confusion about sexuality.

5. Peer pressure: Adolescents find increasing pressures from their peers to be sexual, a pressure that represents a formidable struggle for many adolescents.

6. Developmental stage: A typical characteristic of early and middle adolescent development, as discussed earlier in Chapter 2, is a sense of immortality, with resultant risk-taking behavior. Adolescents thus often react without a full sense of the potential consequences of their actions. Caught between peer values, parental values, the image of sex portrayed by the media, and their own developing values, adolescents frequently act impulsively, engaging in sexual intercourse without being prepared mentally for it and thus avoiding "premeditated" sex. The resultant guilt that many adolescents feel can become a barrier to development of healthy attitudes about sex.

7. Sex education: Most sex education courses, if available, stress reproductive function and menstruation. Although it is important for teenagers to be informed in these areas, adolescents also need help in decision-making skills and in dealing with their feelings, fears, and relationships.

RECOMMENDATIONS

Several suggestions to help adolescents better deal with their sexuality include:

1. Parental or counselor skills
   a. Trying to understand adolescent attitudes about sex can be frustrating, leading to feelings of anger on the part of the parent or counselor. Communication is enhanced if the parent or counselor tempers his or her own response and tries to listen to and appreciate the adolescent's feelings and concerns regarding sexuality. Parents must be made aware that although adolescents have control over their own sexual behavior, parents can exert a strong positive influence, not through moralizing, lecturing, or invasion of privacy, but through helping the adolescent in his or her decision-making process.
   b. Timing: Because sexuality begins in childhood, it is important to treat sexuality as a natural part of life from birth onward. Given this perspective, it is much less awkward to have discussions about sexuality when children grow up.
   c. Education: Adolescents should be informed and knowledgeable—with the aid of parents, school, or community resources—in the following areas:
      — Basic reproductive anatomy and physiology
      — Basic sexual functioning, including common sexual myths and alternatives to intercourse
      — The health consequences of sexual intercourse
      — The relationship between having sex, using birth control, getting pregnant, and being a parent
      — The similarities and differences between male and female roles
      — The range of human relationships
      — The components of decision making
      — The importance of self-esteem and of respecting one's choices
      — Available resources to utilize to answer concerns, questions, or problems
      Parents need education in the following areas:
      — The similarities and differences between parent and adolescent roles
      — The role of sexuality in adolescent growth and development
      — Basic sexual functioning
      — How differences in values affect decision making
      — The similarities and differences in male and female roles during adolescence
      — The role of self-esteem in parent-adolescent relationships

d. Do not joke: Adolescents are uncomfortable about sexuality, and joking about the subject only heightens their discomfort.

e. Admit personal discomfort: Adolescents respect honesty, and this approach will often allow for additional trust between the adolescent and the parent or counselor.

f. Resources: Be informed about available books, pamphlets, and other resources in regard to adolescent sexuality. Some valuable references and organizations are listed in the Appendix II to this book.

g. Privacy: Respect the adolescent's privacy. Although allowing the adolescent to feel comfortable about discussing sexuality, it is important not to pry into details.

2. Community resources

a. Sex education: Schools need to incorporate a curriculum on sex education that, in addition to including facts, stresses concepts of sexual responsibility and sexual decision making.

b. Family-planning clinics: Increased availability of family-planning clinics that serve adolescents is essential.

c. Professional education: It is crucial that physicians and other professionals continue to be educated regarding adolescent sexuality, resultant problems, and helpful resources.

3. Contraceptive technology: Development of a safe, effective, easy-to-use contraceptive that would complement the adolescent's active lifestyle is needed.

BIBLIOGRAPHY

Alan Guttmacher Institute. Sex and America's teenagers. New York: Alan Guttmacher Institute, 1994.

Alan Guttmacher Institute. Teenage pregnancy: the problem that hasn't gone away. New York: Alan Guttmacher Institute, 1981.

Braverman PK, Strasburger VC. Adolescent sexuality: Part 2. Contraception. Clin Pediatr (Phila) 1993;32: 725.

Braverman PK, Strasburger VC. Adolescent sexuality: Part 4. The practitioner's role. Clin Pediatr (Phila) 1994;33:100.

Committee on Communications, American Academy of Pediatrics. Sexuality, contraception, and the media. Pediatrics 1995;95:298.

Deisher RW. Adolescent sexuality. J Curr Adolesc Med 1980;2:41.

Forrest JD, Singh S. The sexual and reproductive behavior of American women 1982–1988. Fam Plann Perspect 1990;22:206.

Gordon S, Scales P, Everly K. The sexual adolescent: communicating with teenagers about sex. Belmont, Massachusetts: Duxbury Press, 1979.

Haka-Ikse K, Mian M. Sexuality in children. Pediatr Rev 1993;14:401.

Hass A. Teenage sexuality: a survey of teenage sexual behavior. Los Angeles: Pinnacle Books, 1979.

Hatcher RA, Guest F, Stewart F, et al. Contraceptive technology, 1988–1989. New York: Irvington Publishers, 1988.

Hayes C, ed. Risking the future: adolescent sexuality, pregnancy, and childbearing, vol 1. Washington DC: National Academy Press, 1987.

Hofferth SL, Kahn JR, Baldwin W. Premarital sexual activity among US teenage women over the past three decades. Fam Plann Perspect 1987;19:46.

Hollman FW. Estimates of the population of the United States by age, sex, and race. Current population reports [Series P–25, No 1095]. Washington, DC: US Bureau of the Census, 1993.

Jaffe LR, Seehaus M, Wagner C, et al. Anal intercourse and knowledge of acquired immunodeficiency syndrome among minority group female adolescents. J Pediatr 1988;112:1007.

Jones EF, Forrest JD, Goldman N, et al. Teenage pregnancy in developed countries: determinants and policy implications. Fam Plann Perspect 1985; 17:53.

Koffi-Blanchard MC, Dubois-Arber F, Michaud PA, et al. Has the age of onset of sexual activity in youths changed in the time of AIDS? Literature review 1972–1992. Schweiz Med Wochenschr 1994;124: 1047.

Kreutner A, Hollingsworth DR, eds. Adolescent sexuality. In: Adolescent obstetrics and gynecology. Chicago: Year Book Medical Publishers, 1978.

Langdell JI. Adolescent sexual preoccupations. Medical Aspects of Human Sexuality 1980;14:90.

Leitenberg H, Detzer MJ, Srebnik D. Gender differences in masturbation and the relation of masturbation experience in preadolescence and/or early adolescence to sexual behavior and sexual adjustment in young adulthood. Arch Sex Behav 1993;22:87.

Moore K, Wenk D, Hofferth S. Statistical appendix. In: Hofferth S, Hayes C, eds. Risking the future: adolescent sexuality, pregnancy, and childbearing, vol. 2. Washington DC: National Academy Press, 1987.

Moore KA, Nord CW, Peterson JL. Nonvoluntary sexual activity among adolescents. Fam Plann Perspect 1989; 21(3):110.

Moore KA, Nord CW, and Peterson JL. Nonvoluntary sexual activity among adolescents. Fam Plann Perspect 1989;21:110.

Moscicki AB, Millstein SG, Broering J, et al. Risks of human immunodeficiency virus infection among adolescents attending three diverse clinics. J Pediatr 1993;122(5, Part 1):813.

Pendergrast RA Jr, DuRang RH, Gaillard GL. Attitudinal and behavioral correlates of condom use in urban adolescent males. J Adolesc Health Care 1992;13:133.

Physicians' symposium: Adolescent sexuality, Parts 1 and 2. Transitions (June 15; August 15): 1980.

Pratt W, Mosher W, Horn M. Understanding US fertility: findings from the National Survey of Family Growth, Cycle III. Popul Bull 1984;39:1.

Selected behaviors that increase risk for HIV infection, other sexually transmitted diseases, and unintended pregnancy among high school students —United States, 1991. MMWR 1992;41(50):945.

Sexual behavior among high school students—United States, 1990. 1992;40(51–52);885.

Sonenstein FL, Pleck JH, Ku LC. Sexual activity, condom use, and AIDS awareness among adolescent males. Fam Plann Perspect 1989;21:152.

Sorenson RC. Adolescent sexuality in contemporary America. New York: World Publishing, 1973.

Stout JW, Kirby D. The effects of sexuality education on adolescent sexual activity. Pediatr Ann 1993;22: 120.

US Department of Health and Human Services. A decision-making approach to sex education: a curriculum guide and implementation manual for a model program with adolescents and parents. Washington DC: US Government Printing Office, 1979.

Van de Polder J. Why parents' sexual warnings to adolescents backfire. Medical Aspects of Human Sexuality 78, April 1980.

White SD, DeBlassie RR. Adolescent sexual behavior. Adolescence 1992;27:183.

Zelnick M, Kantner J. Sexual activity, contraceptive use, and pregnancy in the first months of intercourse. Fam Plann Perspect 1979;11:215.

Zelnick M, Kantner JF. Sexual activity, contraceptive use and pregnancy among metropolitan-area teenagers: 1971–1979. Fam Plann Perspect 1980;12:230.

CHAPTER 41

Homosexuality

Eric Cohen and Lawrence S. Neinstein

Homosexuality, an emotionally charged issue, is a difficult topic to deal with not only for the adolescent but also for his or her family and physician. The health-care provider should be equipped to deal with both the anxieties of adolescents with a strong homosexual orientation and the fears of heterosexual adolescents who are involved in homosexual experimentation. Practitioners must also be prepared to counsel concerned parents as they attempt to deal with their complex fears and guilts over the sexual orientation of their child. If the health-care provider is unable to handle homosexual issues because of personal beliefs, he or she should at least be prepared to refer the adolescent to an appropriate resource. This chapter discusses homosexuality and specific related medical and psychological concerns. Important features of counseling both homosexual teens and their parents are outlined. Homosexuality is a long-term developmental issue, and simple avoidance of it during adolescence will not alleviate the associated medical or psychosocial problems.

The removal of homosexuality as a behavioral disorder from the American Psychiatric Association's *Diagnostic and Statistical Manual of Mental Disorders,* third edition, (DSM III) in 1980 signaled a readjustment to the approach to understanding and managing homosexual teens and their parents. There are no data from scientific studies to justify the unequal treatment of homosexual people or their exclusion from any group.

The need for health-care provider involvement is suggested in both the 1983 and 1993 Committee Paper of the American Academy of Pediatrics. The American Academy of Pediatrics recognizes the physicians' responsibility to provide health care for homosexual adolescents and for those young people struggling with problems of sexual expression. In an era where sexually transmitted diseases (STDs) are among the most significant risks to adolescent morbidity and mortality, it is incumbent on the health-care provider to become familiar with issues surrounding the care of homosexual youth.

GENERAL CONSIDERATIONS

There is no precise definition of homosexuality. Definitions include:

1. "A persistent pattern of homosexual arousal accompanied by a persistent pattern of absent or weak heterosexual arousal" (Spitzer, 1981).
2. A person with a persistent erotic attraction, as an adult, to a member of the same sex and who usually, but not always, engages in a sexual relationship with them.

As opposed to a homosexual, a transvestite is an individual who derives pleasure (sometimes but not always erotic) by dressing in the clothing of the opposite sex. A transsexual is an individual who believes that the body he or she was born with does not match the sex he or she prefers to be. Neither the transvestite nor the transsexual teenager should be assumed to be homosexual.

The word *gay,* meaning homosexual, entered into common usage in the late sixties and was associated with the gay rights movement. Today, the term *gay* usually refers to males (but can refer to females), and the term *lesbian* always refers to females.

Sexual orientation refers to a person's potential to respond erotically to either or both sexes. Important considerations in sexual development include:

1. Sexual orientation is probably a continuum. Kinsey et al. (1948a, 1948b) developed a 7-point scale for rating sexual behavior based on psychological reactions and overt sexual practices. A "0" is a person who is exclusively heterosexual, while a "6" is a person who is exclusively homosexual. The other numbers represent people on a continuum of degrees of homosexual and heterosexual fantasy and behavior.

2. Most children and adolescents will at some time experiment with sexual play with their same-sex friends. For most of these adolescents, this genital "play" appears to be part of a developmental process leading to a heterosexual identity. Some of these teens may experience confusion and panic. A small subset of these adolescents do have the sense that their experimentation has deeper meaning. These adolescents are aware from an early age that their feelings set them apart from their peers. They are aware that they must suppress outwardly, inwardly, or both the expression of these feelings. An even smaller subset of this group do clearly identify themselves as homosexual and have an integrated identity consisting of a homosexual peer group. These homosexual teenagers are often referred to as teens who are "out."

3. Although sexual orientation usually becomes defined in the preadolescent years, expression of that orientation is often suppressed until early adulthood and sometimes not expressed at all. Sexual experimentation during adolescence can be seen as a behavior to help confirm the teen's sexual orientation.

4. Sexual behavior during early adolescence may or may not parallel the direction of adult sexual expression. Some adolescents, particularly young girls, may display mainly same-sex sexual behavior (petting and kissing) but have predominantly heterosexual orientation. On the other hand, some adolescents may hide their "true" homosexual tendencies with heterosexual activity.

5. Some heterosexual adolescents will engage in homosexual behavior under certain circumstances where the environment creates opportunities for same-sex sexual experimentation. Examples of these situations are incarcerated teenagers, adolescents in boarding schools or summer camps, and persons in the military. Most of these individuals will revert to heterosexual behavior when their environment changes.

PREVALENCE

1. Males
   a. Kinsey et al. (1948b) found that 37% of males have had some homosexual experience *resulting in orgasm* between adolescence and old age. *Eight percent* of males are more or less exclusively homosexual for at least 3 years between the ages of 16 and 55 and 4% of males are exclusively homosexual throughout their lives.
   b. Sorenson (1973) found that 17% of male respondents 16–19 years of age reported some homosexual activity.
   c. The 1970 Kinsey National Opinion Research Center (NORC) survey (Fay et al., 1989) indicated that a minimum of 20.3% of adult males had sexual contact to orgasm with another male at some time in their life. Roughly 90% of these contacts began

before the age of 19. It should be remembered that these estimates are likely under-reported.

d. In a recent review of a wide variety of U.S. studies, Seidman and Rieder (1994) estimate that 2% of men are exclusively homosexual and 3% are bisexual.

2. Females: Statistics on female homosexual activity are more difficult to obtain, since more female homosexuals keep their sexual preferences private. However, most studies indicate prevalence in females of about 50% of those listed for males.

3. Remafedi's 1987 study of 29 gay adolescent males reported the following:

a. Thirty-one percent were attracted to men during childhood, and the rest were aware of their attraction to men in mid-adolescence (11–16 years of age).

b. The mean age of self-identification was 14.

c. Most identified themselves as homosexual based on their persistent attraction to men or sexual experiences with men.

4. Saghir et al. (1969) found that 77% of gay males had developed preadolescent homosexual attachments and 86% had engaged in homosexual activity by the age of 15.

5. A l993 study by Rotheram-Borus notes that the average age of first sex was considerably younger for gay males when compared with their heterosexual counterparts (12.7 versus 15.7).

ETIOLOGY AND ACQUISITION OF HOMOSEXUAL IDENTITY

Issues regarding the development, etiology, and meaning of adolescent homosexual behavior and orientation have not been adequately investigated. A growing body of literature pertains to this issue, some of which is referred to in this section. Confusion about sexual orientation is common among teens. Most youths who experiment with same-sex erotica do not adopt a homosexual lifestyle. The various influences of genetics, prenatal hormonal levels, and environment have been proposed either alone or in combination to affect sexual orientation. Following is a brief summary of the major theories of the development of a homosexual identity.

Genetic Theory

Homosexual behavior at some level of frequency exists in many if not all cultures. Ford and Beach (1951) proposed that homosexual orientation is not universally well-documented because of cultural taboos. Human behavioral research based on family and twin studies of homosexuality support a biological foundation for sexual orientation. The occurrence of homosexuality in family pedigrees generally exceeds the incidence of homosexuality in society at large. Twin studies by Kallmann (1952a, 1952b, 1960) and Heston and Shields (1968) support the idea that there is considerably higher concordance for homosexuality among monozygotic twins (as high as 50%) and dizygotic twins. Considerable methodological problems exist with these studies, principally the low number of twin pairs studied.

Hamer et al. (1993) found possible evidence of a gene that influences homosexual orientation in males contained on the X chromosome. Thirty-three of 40 homosexual pairs of siblings were found to be concordant for five markers in the distal region of the X chromosome. The remaining seven were discordant at one or more of these loci.

Hormonal Theory

Kolodny et al. (1971, 1972) were leading proponents of an etiology of homosexuality determined by different levels of sex hormones. Based on current research by Gartrell (1982) and

Friedman and Downey (1993), the testosterone theory appears invalid. Prenatal hormonal effects of estrogen and luteinizing hormone (LH) gained popularity with Dorner and colleagues (Dorner, 1977a, 1977b; Dorner et al., 1975), Money (1988) and recently challenged by Gooren et al. (1990). Controversy continues to exist regarding the exact influences of gonadotropin on sexual dimorphism and resultant behavioral sequelae.

Psychoanalytical Theory

The primary etiologic effects leading to adolescent homosexuality appear repeatedly in the psychoanalytical literature. In general, according to Ovesey and Woods (1980), such theories view individuals as driven from normal heterosexuality to homosexuality by the "intrusion of fear arising in response to unconscious fantasies generated by unconscious conflicts."

Combination Theories

Kallmann (1960) combined the biological and psychoanalytical theories and proposed that a balance of genes effects the development of the neuropsychological mechanism that influences an individual's object relations during the sexual developmental period. An imbalance in genetic coding changes these neuropsychological influences and results in a predisposition to homosexuality.

Social Process Theory

This theory maintains that homosexuality is a learned deviance and emphasizes the external world's impact on sexual behavior. Such pressures may include being labeled (either by self or others) as gay or pubertal maturation (between the ages of 8–13) resulting in increased sex drive. These pressures, when combined with a concomitant inaccessibility of heterosexual outlet, may lead to homosexual behavior. Further pressure may occur in these situations when there are opportunities for same-sex stimulation, such as in all-boys' or all-girls' schools. In other words biological puberty is accompanied by sexual drives that initially are more or less undirected; with a rich same-sex exposure and unavailability of the opposite sex, these drives can lead to "homosocial" bonding and homosexual activity.

Brain Differences

Unreplicated reports have been published about several differences in the brain of homosexual men, including an increased size of the superchiasmatic nucleus of the hypothalamus, decreased size of the third anterior interstitial nucleus, and increased size of the anterior commissure (Allen and Gorski, 1992; LeVay, 1991; Swaab and Hofman, 1991). Most researchers agree that biological factors play some role in the creation of a homosexual identity, and while it is possible that anatomical brain differences might be involved, the current research is inconclusive.

Very probably, each of these theories acts to a greater or lesser extent to determine homosexual orientation. According to Savin-Williams (1988), whatever the cause, "the pre-gay and gay adolescent who is confronting the truthfulness and inevitability of her or his `unusual' orientation needs a perspective that will lead to a nonjudgemental presentation of facts."

Stages of Acquisition of Homosexual Identity

Troiden (1979, 1988) has outlined the following four stages in the acquisition of homosexual identity:

1. Stage I: Sensitization. In Stage I the child feels a sense of being different, without understanding the reason for these feelings. By early adolescence there may be awareness of a different sexual orientation, including feelings and behaviors that would be considered homosexual.
2. Stage II: Identity confusion. In Stage II the individual may use various defenses to try to ignore any homosexual impulses and activity or regard them as a passing phase. In mid-adolescence there may be same-sex arousal and limited same-sex experiences, followed by periods of guilt and withdrawal.
3. Stage III: Identity assumption. In Stage III, which may not come until adulthood, if ever, individuals self-identify themselves as homosexual.
4. Stage IV: Commitment. In Stage IV the individual experiences satisfaction, self-acceptance, and an unwillingness to alter sexual identity.

Troiden identifies average ages for typical events in the coming out process:

	Male (Age)	Female (Age)
Same-sex interest	13	14–16
First same-sex activity	15	20
First same-sex love relationship	21–24	22–23
Disclosure to nonhomosexuals	23–28	28

Paroski (1987) evaluated 121 male and female homosexual adolescents regarding their acquisition of homosexual identity. An approximate 18-month process was described:

1. Realization of same-sex desire
2. Guilt and shame for these feelings
3. Attempts to change to heterosexuality through altering behavior and fantasy
4. Failure to alter sexual orientation, with the subsequent development of poor self-esteem
5. Investigation into homosexual lifestyle through various methods including sexual activity
6. Acceptance and development of positive homosexual identity

HOMOPHOBIA

Weinberg (1992) reports that the term *homophobia* was coined in 1967 to signify an irrationally negative attitude toward homosexuals. In the United States, Greenberg (1988) reports that two particularly prominent influences foster homophobia: religious fundamentalism and heterosexism, the belief that heterosexuality is inherently morally superior. Although there has been some improvement in the level of tolerance afforded homosexuals, a majority of respondents in a 1987 poll indicated that they would prefer not to work around homosexual people. Homophobia is also present in the medical community. Numerous authors, have reported such negative attitudes in physicians, medical students, nurses, and mental health practitioners. The wish to avoid contact with male homosexuals has intensified since the AIDS epidemic began.

MEDICAL CONCERNS

This section focuses on the medical concerns of male gay adolescents. Gay female adolescents have no specific organic medical problems that are related specifically to their sexual orientation.

The major medical concerns specific to homosexual male patients are:

1. Sexually transmitted diseases
2. Traumatic injuries relating to sexual intercourse
3. Psychological problems relating to poor adjustment to a homosexual identity

Sexually Transmitted Diseases in Gay Youth

There is an epidemic of STDs among the male homosexual population, due to multiple partners, high prevalence of asymptomatic carriers of STDs, and anonymity of sexual contacts and resultant difficulty in contact treatment. Although some progress has been made in the adult homosexual community with regard to increased use of barrier methods (condoms), the adolescent population as yet does not seem to have responded to the same degree.

History   In evaluating the gay adolescent for medical problems, the practitioner must first be able to get correct information regarding the teen's sexual practices. The health-care provider must do three things in approaching this sensitive part of the history.

1. Establish confidentiality: The provider must first establish confidentiality. If the laws of a particular state do not specifically disallow confidential health care to teens, then it is recommended to start the interview by assuring the adolescent that all information gathered will be kept in confidence (unless the adolescent is a danger to himself or others).
2. Establish a "need to know": Tell the adolescent that there will be some personal questions asked, and that although the teen does not have to answer the questions, an honest response will help the practitioner give the best care possible.
3. Ask questions in a nonjudgmental fashion: This maximizes the likelihood of an honest response. An example might be:
    a. "Have you begun to have sexual relations (making love?)"
    b. "Are these relations with men, women, or both?"
4. Inquire into specific sexual practices: The health-care provider must investigate the adolescent's specific types of sexual practices. Such knowledge may help to determine the adolescent's risk for STDs and may direct investigation to unconventional areas of sexual contact. It also provides an opportunity to provide education regarding prevention of STDs. Specific questions should be directed toward:
    a. Fellatio: Active or passive
    b. Anal intercourse: Inserter or insertee
    c. Anilingus (rim or scat): Active or passive
    d. Multiple sexual partners
    e. Frequency of sexual contact
    f. Use of condoms
    g. Prior history of STDs
    h. Human immunodeficiency virus (HIV) status (if known)

It may become necessary to ask questions about the use of sex toys (dildos) or manual anal manipulation with fingers or fist (fisting) if there is evidence of anal trauma in the male homosexual. It is not advised to ask these questions routinely.

Documentation   In gathering this information, documentation must be considered carefully. Access to the adolescent's chart by health professionals, allied health-care workers, insurance companies, the courts, and parents carries certain legal and ethical ramifications. The health-care provider must consider himself or herself as a patient advocate, protecting confidentiality. The practitioner must also be aware of state laws governing documentation. With increasing prevalence of HIV in adolescents and the possible devastating social consequences, practitioners must be very careful if documenting HIV status and other HIV risk factors (such as gay or anal sex) in an accessible part of the patient's chart. This issue is discussed more completely in Chapter 31.

Sexually Transmitted Disease Screening   Not all homosexual males need a full STD workup. If the history indicates that the teen is either not sexually active or is sexually active with one partner who is also monogamous and he is using appropriate barrier methods, a simple routine physical examination and routine syphilis serology would be adequate. The practitioner's judgment of the reliability of the teen's history should also be considered. If a question of veracity exists, it may be wise to simply offer "routine" STD screening.

Appropriate screening of the sexually active gay male adolescent with any risk factors as outlined in the section on specific sexual questions would include the following physical examination and laboratory studies.

Physical Examination   Close attention should be paid to:

1. The lymphatic system, looking for evidence of lymphadenopathy
2. The skin, looking for rashes
3. The anus, examining for trauma or an STD
4. The throat, looking for rashes and STDs
5. The genitalia, looking for discharge or lesions

Laboratory Studies

1. Gonorrhea culture
2. Chlamydia testing: DNA probe, direct fluorescent antibody (DFA) assay or culture. These should be done on all appropriate sites of sexual contact.
3. Syphilis serology
4. Hepatitis B surface antigen and antibody
5. HIV screening: This is a controversial area at present. Many authorities recommend routine screening in sexually active gay males. This position is becoming increasingly advocated with the development of treatment for asymptomatic HIV-positive individuals. Others do not routinely recommend testing because of the fear of discriminatory practices and infringement of civil rights of those who do test positive. This is a sensitive area, and whether the test is ordered or not must be accompanied by considerable health education. The practitioner is reminded here of the difference between recommending, suggesting, and discussing. Discussion about the advisability of an HIV test can always be done if the practitioner feels knowledgeable enough to deal with the issue. Suggesting and recommending have increasingly directive meanings. Since the HIV test may have far-reaching effects on the adolescent's life, practitioners must be sure to fully explain the possible consequences to the adolescent and to allow the adolescent to decide whether or not to have the test, rather than making it a physician-directed decision.

Specific Sexually Transmitted Diseases or Conditions

Anal Disease   Anal problems include:

1. Anorectal trauma secondary to anal intercourse, or use of foreign objects for anal intercourse resulting in anal fissures
2. Foreign body lodging in the anus secondary to use during anal intercourse
3. Proctitis and inflammation of perianal area secondary to allergies caused by contactants such as lubricants and infectious agents
4. Pruritus ani secondary to oil-based lubricants and blockage of anal pores leading to inflammation

5. Anal condylomata secondary to sexual transmission of human papilloma virus during anal intercourse: Anal warts can and often are found in both the external and internal anal canals. Warts do not usually occur in the rectum.
6. Hematochezia secondary to anal lacerations secondary to anal intercourse, fisting, or use of sex toys
7. Anal ulcers secondary to herpes (usually seen in crops and are painful) or syphilis (usually only one and painless)
8. Anal discharge secondary to bacterial STDs.

In a study by Sohn and Ribilotti (1977) the following prevalences of problems were found in 260 homosexual males with rectal complaints:

	(%)
Warts	51.5
Hemorrhoids	16.5
Proctitis (nonspecific)	12.0
Fistulas	11.5
Abscesses	6.9
Fissures	6.9
Amebiasis	6.5
Pruritus ani	6.0
Polyps	5.4
Hepatitis	5.4
Rectal dyspareunia	5.0
Gonorrhea	3.1
Syphilis	2.7
Trauma	2.7
Shigellosis	2.3
Ulcers	1.9
Lymphogranuloma venereum	1.2

Another study by Quinn et al. (1983) showed the polymicrobial nature of intestinal infections in homosexual males (Table 41.1).

All homosexually active teenagers who admit to being sexually active with males and who engage in passive (insertee) anal intercourse without the regular use of condoms should

TABLE 41.1.   Causative Agents of Intestinal Infections in Homosexual Males

Anorectal or Intestinal Pathogens	Symptomatic Males (N = 119)		Asymptomatic Males (N = 75)	
	No.	%	No.	%
Neisseria gonorrhoeae	37	31	17	23
Herpes simplex virus	23	19	3	4
Chlamydia trachomatis	12	10	4	5
Treponema pallidum	6	5	1	1
Entamoeba histolytica	20	29	6	25
Giardia lamblia	10	14	1	4
Campylobacter jejuni or fetus	8	7	2	3
Shigella flexneri	3	3	1	1
Clostridium difficile cytotoxin	3	3	1	1
Enterovirus	3	3	1	1
Any of the above	95	80	29	39

Adapted from Quinn TC, et al. The polymicrobial origin of intestinal infections in homosexual men. N Engl J Med 1983; 309:576.

be examined and tested for anal gonorrhea and chlamydia and have blood taken for syphilis serology. The evaluation of the rectum and anus in a symptomatic teen should include proctoscopy, gonorrhea, and chlamydia tests; stool for routine culture and ova and parasites; and syphilis serology. Treatment is directed at the etiological agent.

Anorectal Gonorrhea

1. Clinical manifestations: Sixty-six percent of patients are asymptomatic, 2–5% have clinical proctitis, and 30% have nonspecific symptoms; acute proctitis rectal burning, tenesmus, and mucopurulent anal discharge.
2. Differential diagnosis: Inflammatory bowel disease; amebiasis; chlamydial proctitis; contact dermatitis or proctitis (allergic proctitis); giardiasis; lymphogranuloma venereum; syphilis; and chancroid
3. Complications: Abscess formation, strictures, fistulas, chronic fissures
4. Diagnosis: Proctoscopy, Gram's stain (only helpful if Gram-negative intracellular diplococci are found), and gonorrhea culture. Culture or DNA probe test may be obtained by proctoscopy or blindly. A cotton-tipped swab is inserted 1 inch into the rectum and moved from side to side for approximately 10 seconds. It is then plated directly on modified Thayer-Martin agar or placed in a transport container for testing by culture or DNA probe. The sample should be taken before use of lubricants, due to their bacteriostatic properties.
5. Treatment: Ceftriaxone 125 mg intramuscularly (IM) at one time OR cefixime 400 mg orally in a single dose *or* ciprofloxacin 500 mg orally in a single dose OR ofloxacin 400 mg orally in a single dose. PLUS: A regimen effective against possible coinfection with *Chlamydia trachomatis* such as either azithromycin 1 g in a single dose or doxycycline 100 mg orally two times a day for 7 days.
   a. All the above regimens appear to cure more than 95% of anal and genital infections.
   b. Cefixime has the advantage of a one-time oral dose. The serum levels are not as high as with ceftriaxone nor as sustained. Its effectiveness against incubating syphilis is not known.
   c. Ciprofloxacin has been used at both 250- and 500-mg doses, but the 500-mg dose is recommended due to problems with decreasing susceptibility to some quinolones.
   d. Quinolones are contraindicated for pregnant or nursing women and for persons under 18 years of age.
   e. 125 mg of ceftriaxone appears to be as effective as 250 mg and no ceftriaxone-resistant strains of *Neisseria gonorrhoeae* have been reported.

Pharyngeal Gonorrhea   Homosexually active teens who are engaging in fellatio should be tested by culture or DNA probe for gonorrhea routinely.

1. Prevalence: Three percent to 5% asymptomatic carrier rate
2. Clinical manifestations: Ranges from asymptomatic state with normal-appearing pharynx to exudative pharyngitis
3. Differential diagnosis: Infectious mononucleosis; streptococcal pharyngitis; viral pharyngitis
4. Treatment: Use either ceftriaxone 125 mg IM once or ciprofloxacin 500 mg orally in a single dose. Cotreatment for possible chlamydia genital infection is also a good idea. Ciprofloxacin is not recommended in growing individuals.

Syphilis   Prior to the AIDS era, syphilis in gay males accounted for approximately 50% of cases among males. In the AIDS era, during which condom use has increased substantially among homosexual males, current epidemiological data show an increase in the percentage

of syphilis cases among heterosexual males. Diagnosing the primary lesion may be difficult, because in the anal area it may not be seen or felt. Syphilitic lesions are generally painless. Rectal syphilis can, however, cause pain, and the lesion can appear atypical, resembling a carcinoma with shaggy borders. A syphilis serology is recommended every 3–6 months for homosexual males with multiple sex partners.

There is evidence that infection with HIV may alter infections with syphilis. This has led to cases of HIV-positive individuals either not responding to traditional therapy or having accelerated courses of syphilis. There have also been reports of patients with HIV infections and evidence of syphilis who have negative syphilis serology. HIV-positive adolescents with syphilis require careful evaluation for late and unusual manifestations of syphilis, including cerebrospinal fluid evaluation. These individuals may also need more aggressive penicillin therapy.

Hepatitis   There is a high prevalence of hepatitis B in the homosexual community. Homosexual males have a 37–51% prevalence of hepatitis B antibodies and a 5.6% prevalence of the antigen. The prevalence in the heterosexual population for antibody is 3.5% and 0.9% for antigen. It is recommended that those gay teens with negative test results for hepatitis B surface or core antibody receive hepatitis B vaccine. Prevalence of hepatitis A is 30% in homosexual males.

Cytomegalovirus   It is estimated that each year up to 80% of homosexual males who are engaging in sex with multiple partners will acquire cytomegalovirus. This infection is largely asymptomatic but may lead to a severe mononucleosislike illness, particularly in the immune-suppressed HIV-positive teen. However, the presence of a severe mononucleosislike illness in a gay adolescent does not mean the teen is HIV positive.

Enteric Infections   Teenagers who engage in unprotected passive anal sex and who engage in active anilingus run a higher risk of contracting various enteric pathogens. Pathogens include but are not limited to *Entamoeba histolytica, Giardia lamblia, Shigella, N. gonorrhoeae, Treponema pallidum,* syphilis, *C. trachomatis,* human papillomavirus (warts), and herpes simplex virus. These can also occur in females with a history of rectal intercourse.

Condyloma Acuminatum (Venereal Warts)   Venereal warts are common both on the penis and on the rectal area.

External Warts   External warts are best treated with podophyllin, trichloracetic acid, or a combination of both. Practitioners should be careful to coat the noninvolved mucosal surfaces or skin surfaces with petroleum jelly so that the chemical will not burn the healthy tissue. Podophyllin at a strength of between 25% and 50% is applied to the wart and left to dry. The patient is instructed to wash the podophyllin off in 6–8 hours following treatment. Podophyllin and trichloracetic acid often require multiple treatments. Electrocautery is another method of treatment that is being used. If the warts are easily accessible, infiltration with 1% xylocaine without epinephrine, followed by cautery of the wart, may resolve the problem in one treatment. This should be done carefully, as electrocautery can lead to disfigurement, scarring, and perforations. Where lasers are available, this may be the treatment of choice.

Rectal Warts   These can be treated through an anoscope with topical application of podophyllin. Patients with internal warts are often referred to specialist physicians for treatment with surgery or lasers. In early studies (Eron et al., 1986) therapy with intralesional injections of interferon alfa 0.1 mL of 1:1000 solution injected directly into the base of the wart three times a week for 3 weeks has proven effective.

Herpes Simplex Herpes simplex infections of the penis or rectum can occur in homosexual males. Rectal lesions have a typical appearance of multiple shaggy-bordered erythematous punched-out ulcers that are painful to the touch and may cause a nonspecific proctitis. Lesions on the penis may appear in their early forms as multiple crops of blisters, which then ulcerate and are identical to the rectal lesions. Findings associated with herpes simplex proctitis include fever, difficulty with urination or defecation, sacral paresthesias, inguinal adenopathy, severe anorectal pain, tenesmus, constipation, perianal ulcerations and the presence of diffuse ulcerations or vesicular or pustular lesions in the distal 5 cm of the rectum. Treatment for herpes simplex is outlined in Chapter 65.

Acquired Immunodeficiency Syndrome Acquired immunodeficiency syndrome (AIDS) is discussed in Chapter 31. Although all teens need to be informed about AIDS, it is especially important in the homosexually active adolescent. A discussion should take place between the practitioner and the homosexual adolescent about HIV testing. Practitioners are advised to become comfortable with this issue and to be knowledgeable about the ramifications of HIV testing within their geopolitical setting. Use of a condom for all forms of intercourse should be encouraged among all sexually active teens, but particularly in the homosexually active male. The adolescent should be informed of safer sexual practices, including:

1. Limitation of numbers of sexual partners (monogamy is the safest).
2. Avoidance of sexual practices involving the exchange of body fluids such as blood or semen, which includes unprotected anal sex (active or passive), oral sex (active or passive), and anilingus (active).
3. Awareness of the danger of sharing needles and that if needles must be used, the needles should be clean, fresh from a sealed pack, or flushed with household bleach and then water.
4. Importance of using latex, not natural lambskin, condoms, as the latter have been shown to be potentially porous.
5. If lubricants are used, water-based products rather than oil-soluble ones should be used, as the latter can deteriorate the latex in condoms, as well as being a factor in pruritus ani.

Counseling Issues

According to Gonsiorek (1988) the majority of gay and lesbian youth, given the opportunity to develop within a supportive environment, present no more serious mental health problems than the general adolescent population. It is the effect of homophobia that may cause teens to feel guilt and shame and to develop psychological problems. Reported psychological problems related to poor adjustment to homosexual identity include:

1. Suicide: In their 1992 study of suicide amongst youths, Prenzlauer et al. reported a disproportionately high rate of homosexuals represented in their study population. Ramafedi findings were similar, with 41% of 147 gay teens studied reporting having attempted suicide. Youths consistently list fears over "coming out" and internalized homophobia (self-loathing) as causes for suicide attempts.
2. Alcoholism and substance abuse: An increased frequency of alcoholism among lesbians when compared to heterosexual women has been reported. Similar trends exist with males, but the association is not as strong. The major criticism of these studies is that subjects were recruited in gay-lesbian bars and therefore may have skewed the frequencies.

More current and better designed studies are needed to define the frequency and severity of drug and alcohol problems amongst gay and lesbian youth.

Counseling the Concerned Teen

1. The health-care provider must first clearly state that the teen's sexual preference has no bearing on how he or she feels about them. The adolescent may fear that the physician may reject their "differentness," adopting the perceived societal homophobia. Acceptance sets the tone for developing an atmosphere of trust. Health-care providers have an obligation to help their homosexual teens preserve and build self-esteem and avoid or deal with anxiety or depression.

2. The teen should be told that homosexuality is a nonpathological variation along the continuum of normal sexual orientation, and that sexual orientation is probably established early in childhood. Discussing this may serve to alleviate guilt. The teen should understand that homosexuality is not simply a problem of making a wrong "choice," as choice is rarely, if ever, a factor. Along these lines, using the word preference implies choice and should be avoided when referring to sexual orientation.

3. In discussing the teen's sexual orientation, the adolescent should be informed that attempts to change sexual orientation have generally been unsuccessful over time. Data on long-term outcome of various "treatments" is sparse. Haldeman's 1991 review of outcomes of therapy showed that, at least among men who never had experienced sexual attraction to women, that replacement of homosexual fantasies with heterosexual ones was not possible. Such attempts at change may contribute to guilt, low self-esteem, and psychological problems. If, however, the adolescent and not the parent is requesting help with changing, the health-care practitioner should respond to this with an appropriate referral to an experienced, nonbiased psychological clinician.

4. It is important not to minimize the adolescent's concerns regarding sexual orientation. Stating "It's just a phase" may actually intensify the teen's confusion.

5. Discussing homosexuality with teens will not make them homosexual, in much the same way as discussing suicide will not make them suicidal. As with suicide, discussion of concerns regarding sexual orientation may actually alleviate anxiety.

6. There is no need to have teens decide on their sexual orientation quickly. Assuring them that their sexual orientation will emerge in time may take some of the urgency out of the question "Am I or am I not?"

7. For the male: Whether or not he is concerned about his sexual orientation, it is of paramount importance to deliver accurate, clear, frank, specific information regarding safer sexual practices and AIDS risk-reduction techniques. This is probably the single most important reason today for knowing a male teen's sexual practices.

Counseling the Unconcerned Teen

Not all homosexual teens are concerned about their orientation. If comfortable with their sex lives, the same general information as just presented should be given. Whether the adolescent is concerned or not, it remains important for practitioners to discuss safer sexual practices with the gay male teen.

Counseling Concerned Parents

Telljohann and Price (1993) found in a study of homosexual youth that 42% of the females and 30% of the males indicated that their families responded in a negative manner toward them because of their sexual orientation. Only about one-fourth of the students claimed they were able to talk with school counselors about the issue. Less than one in five students could identify someone who had been supportive of them. Some suggestions for parents include:

1. The parent(s) of a homosexual teen may feel any combination of anger, fear, shame, guilt, and grief. The health-care provider must try to find out which parental feelings predominate and why. Only then can the parent be helped to deal with each of these feelings.
2. Parents may feel that they did something to cause the homosexuality. Mothers may worry about events that occurred while they were pregnant or they may be concerned about being overbearing, raising, in the case of a male, a "momma's boy." Fathers whose boys are a concern may feel that they were not around enough to provide adequate role modeling. The converse is true of parents of lesbian teens. These fears should be put to rest. As this chapter has pointed out, the origins of homosexuality are far from that simple.
3. Parents need correct information about homosexuality. The points outlined in the section on counseling the concerned teen may be equally useful in counseling his or her parents.
4. Parents should be told that not every emotional problem manifested by a teen is a result of his or her homosexuality. Homosexual teens have the same problems as the general adolescent population.
5. Parents should be encouraged to question society's dichotomous belief that homosexuality is bad and that heterosexuality is good.
6. Religious beliefs should be explored and appropriate counsel sought if possible.
7. AIDS should be discussed with parents, particularly if the teen is male. Today, parents make automatic connections between homosexuality and AIDS.
8. Counseling of parents can be supplemented by referring them to parent support groups like Parents and Friends of Lesbians and Gays (P-FLAG). The national headquarters is located at:

Federation of Parents and Friends of Lesbians and Gays
1101 14th Street NW, Suite 1030
Washington DC, 20005
202-638-4200
FAX: 202-638-0243

Another resource, the Gay and Lesbian Community Services Center in Los Angeles, offers counseling, medical services, vocational counseling, legal services, information and referral for housing, and a youth department. The center's address is:

Gay and Lesbian Community Services Center
1625 North Schrader Boulevard
Los Angeles, CA 90028-9998
213-993-7400

9. Finally, the most important point to emphasize to concerned parents is that the gay adolescent who has disclosed to them his or her sexual orientation is the same teen who sat before them prior to the disclosure. This adolescent's main need has been, is, and will always be love and acceptance.

BIBLIOGRAPHY

Allen LS, Gorski RA. Sexual orientation and the size of the anterior commissure in the human brain. Proc Natl Acad Sci USA 1992;89:7199.

American Academy of Pediatrics, Committee on Adolescence. Homosexuality and adolescence. Pediatrics 1983;72:249.

American Academy of Pediatrics, Committee on Adolescence. Hhomosexuality and adolescence. Pediatrics 1993;92:631.

Billy JO, Tanfer K, Grady WR, et al. The sexual behavior of men in the United States. Fam Plann Perspect 1993;25:52.

Borhek MV. Helping gay and lesbian adolescents and their families: a mother's perspective. J Adolesc Health Care 1988;9:123.

Coleman E. Developmental stages of the coming out process. J Homosex 1982;7:31.

Deisher R, Robinson G, Boyer D. The adolescent female and male prostitute. Pediatr Ann 1982;11:819.

Diamond M. Homosexualtiy and bisexuality in different populations. Arch Sex Behav 1993;22:291.

Dorner G. Hormone dependent differentiation, maturation, and function of the brain and sexual behavior. Endocrinologie 1977a;69:306.

Dorner G. Hormones, brain differentiation, and fundamental processes of life. J Steroid Biochem 1977b; 8:531.

Dorner G, Rohde W, Stahl F. A neuroendocrine predisposition for homosexuality in men. Arch Sex Behav 1975;4:1.

Downey JI. Sexual orientation issues in adolescent girls. Women's Health Issues 1994;4:67.

Eron LJ, Judson F, Tucker S, et al. Interferon therapy for condylomata acuminata. N Engl J Med 1986;315: 1059.

Fay RE, Turner CF, Klassen AD, et al. Prevention and pattern of same-gender sexual contact among men. Science 1989;243:338.

Ford CS, Beach FA. Patterns of sexual behavior. New York: Harper & Row, 1951.

Friedman RC, Downey J. Neurobiology and sexual orientation: current relationships. J Neuropsychiatry Clin Neurosci 1993;5:131.

Friedman RC, Downey JI. Homosexuality 1994;331:923.

Gartrell NK. Hormones and homosexuality. In: Homosexuality: social, psychological, and biological issues. Paul W, Weinrich JD, Gonsiorek JC, and Hotvedt ME, eds. Beverly Hills, California: Sage, 1982.

Gonsiorek JC. An introduction to mental health issues and homosexuality. Am Behav Sci 1982;25:367.

Gonsiorek JC. Mental health issues of gay and lesbian adolescents. J Adolesc Health Care 1988;9:114.

Goodell SE, Quinn TC, Mkrtichian E, et al. Herpes simplex virus proctitis in homosexual men: clinical, sigmoidoscopic, and histopathological features. N Engl J Med 1983;308:868.

Gooren L, Fliers E, Courtney K. Biological determinants of sexual orientation. Annu Rev Sex Res 1990;175:96.

Greenberg DF. The construction of homosexuality. Chicago: University of Chicago Press, 1988.

Haldeman DC. Sexual orientation conversion therapy for gay men and lesbians: a scientific examination. In: Gonsiorek JC, Weinrich JD, eds. Homosexuality: research implications for public policy. Newbury Park, California: Sage 1991:149–161.

Hamer DH, Hu S, Magnuson VL, et al. A linkage between DNA markers on the X chromosome and male sexual orientation. Science 1993;261:321.

Handsfield HH, Schwebke J. Trends in sexually transmitted diseases in homosexually active men in King County, Washington, 1980–1990. Sex Transm Dis 1990;17:211.

Hendin H. Suicide among homosexual youth. Am J Psychiatry 1992;149:1416.

Herek GM. Stigma, prejudice, and violence against lesbians and gay men. In: Gonsiiorek JC, Weinrich JD, eds. Homosexuality: research implications for public policy. Newbury Park, California: Sage, 1991:60–80.

Heston LL, Shields J. Homosexuality in twins: A family study and a registry study. Arch Gen Psychiatry 1968; 18:149.

Kallmann FJ. Comparative twin study on the genetic aspects of male homosexuality. J Nerv Ment Dis 1952a;115:283.

Kallmann FJ. Twin and sibship study of overt male homosexuality. Am J Hum Genet 1952b;4:136.

Kallmann FJ. Discussion of homosexuality and heterosexuality in identical twins. Psychosom Med 1960; 22:258.

Kinsey AC, Pomeroy WB, Martin CE. Sexual behavior in the human female. Philadelphia: WB Saunders, 1948a.

Kinsey AC, Pomeroy WB, Martin CE. Sexual behavior in the human male. Philadelphia: WB Saunders, 1948b.

Kolodny R, Jacobs LS, Masters WH. Plasma gonadotrophins and prolactin in male homosexuals. Lancet 1972;2:18.

Kolodny R, Masters W, Hendry J. Plasma, testosterone, and semen analysis in male homosexuals. N Engl J Med 1971;285:1170.

Leaman TL. The lesbian patient, Part II. When she is your patient. Female Patient 1987;12:12.

LeVay S. A difference in hypothalamic structure between heterosexual and homosexual men. Science 1991;253:1034.

Markel EK, Havens RF, Kuritsubo RA. Intestinal parasitic infections in homosexual men at a San Francisco health fair. West J Med 1983;139:177.

Martin AD. Learning to hide: the socialization of the gay adolescent. Adolesc Psychiatry 1982;10:52.

Mintz L, Drew L, Miner RC, et al. Cytomegalovirus infections in homosexual men: An epidemiological study. Ann Intern Med 1983;99:326.

Money J. Gay, straight and in-between: the sexology of erotic orientation. New York: Oxford University Press, 1988.

Money J. Genetic and chromosomal aspects of homosexual etiology. In: Marmor J, ed. Homosexual behavior: a modern reappraisel New York: Basic Books, 1980.

Neinstein LS, Cohen E. Homosexuality in adolescents. In: Gellis SS, Kagan BM, eds. Current pediatric therapy. 14th ed. Philadelphia: WB Saunders, 1993.

Ostrow DG. Homosexual behavior and sexually transmitted diseases. In Holmes KK, Mardh PA, Sparling

PF, and Wiesner PJ eds. Sexually transmitted diseases, 2nd ed. New York: McGraw-Hill Information Services Company, 1990.

Ovesey L, Woods SM. Pseudohomosexuality and homosexuality in men: psychodynamics as a guide to treatment. In: Marmor J, ed. Homosexual behavior: a modern appraisal. New York: Basic Books, 1980: 325–341.

Owen WF. Medical problems of the homosexual adolescent. J Adolesc Health Care 1985;6:278.

Paroski P. Health-care delivery and the concerns of gay and lesbian adolescents. J Adolesc Health Care 1987; 8:188.

Phillips SC, Mildvan D, William DC, et al. Sexual transmission of enteric protozoa and helminths in a venereal-disease-clinic population. N Engl J Med 1981;305:603.

Pillard RC, Poumadere JI, Carretta RA. Is homosexuality familial? A review, some data, and a suggestion. Arch Sex Behav 1981;10:465.

Prenzlauer S, Drescher J, Winshel R. Suicide among homosexual youth. Am J Psychiatry 1992;149:1416.

Quinn TC, Goodell SE, Fennell C, et al. Infections with *Campylobacter jejuni* and *Campylobacter*-like organisms in homosexual men. Ann Intern Med 1984; 101:187.

Quinn TC, Stamm WE, Goodell SE. The polymicrobial origin of intestinal infections in homosexual men. N Engl J Med 1983;309:576.

Reik M. Counseling the parents of teenage homosexuals. Sexual Medicine Today 1982;(March):20.

Remafedi GJ. Adolescent homosexuality: issues for pediatricians. Clin Pediatr 1985;24:481.

Remafedi GJ. Adolescent homosexuality: psychosocial and medical implications. Pediatrics 1987a;79:331.

Remafedi GJ. Homosexual youth: a challenge to contemporary society. JAMA 1987b;258:222.

Remafedi GJ. Male homosexuality: the adolescents' perspective. Pediatrics 1987c;79:326.

Remafedi G, Blum R. Working with gay and lesbian adolescents. Pediatr Ann 1986;15:773.

Remafedi G, Farrow JA, Deisher RW. Risk factors for attempting suicide in gay and bisexual youth. Pediatrics 1991;87:869.

Robinson LS, Dalton R. Homosexuality in adolescence. Medical Aspects of Human Sexuality 1986;(June): 106.

Roesler T, Deisher RW. Youthful male homosexuality. JAMA 1972;219:1018.

Saghir MT, Robins E, Walbian B. Homosexuality. Arch Gen Psychiatry 1969;21:219.

Savin-Williams RC. Theoretical perspectives accounting for adolescent homosexuality. J Adolesc Health Care 1988;9:95.

Seidman SN, Reider RO. A review of sexual behavior in the United States. Am J Psychiatry 1994;151:330.

Smith S, McClaugherty LO. Adolescent homosexuality: a primary care perspective. Am Fam Physician 1993; 48:33.

Sohn N, Ribilotti JG. The gay bowel syndrome. Am J Gastroenterol 1977;67:487.

Sorenson RC. Adolescent sexuality in contemporary America. New York: World Publishing, 1973:285–293.

Spitzer RL. The diagnostic status of homosexuality in DSM III: a reformulation of the issues. Am J Psychiatry 1981;138:210.

Stewart DS. The homosexual adolescent and the pediatrician. California Pediatrician 1988;(Spring):15.

Swaab DF, Hofman MA. An enlarged suprachiasmatic nucleus in homosexual men. Brain Res 1991;537:141.

Telljohann Sk, Price JH. A qualitative examination of adolescent homosexuals' life experiences: ramifications for secondary school personnel. J Homosex 1993;26:41.

Troiden RR. Becoming homosexual: a model of gay identity acquisition. Psychiatry 1979;42:362.

Troiden RR. Homosexual identity development. J Adolesc Health Care 1988;9:105.

Weinberg GH. Society and the healthy homosexual. New York: St. Martin's Press, 1992.

Fiction for Teens and Parents

Ages 6–12

Harris RH. It's perfectly normal. Cambridge, Massachusetts: Candlewick, 1994. (Book about sexuality and growing up with nonjudgmental section on homosexuality and includes same-sex couples in its illustrations.)

Salat C. Living in secret. New York: Bantam, 1993. (Eleven-year-old Amelia runs away with her mother and her mother's lover when her father will not let them be together.)

Ages 12 and Up

Bauer MD, ed. Am I blue? Coming out from the silence. New York: Harper Collins, 1994. (Collection of stories featuring gay characters by popular young adult writers.)

Koertge R. The Arizona kid. Boston: Bantam Doubleday Dell, 1988. (Boy-meets-girl stories, with an unselfconscious portrait of the main character's gay uncle.)

McClain LJ. No big deal. New York: Lodestar, 1994. (Thirteen-year-old girl is forced into action when her mother joins a campaign to get her favorite teacher fired because of rumors that he's gay.)

Nelson T. Earthshine. New York: Orchard, 1994. (Twelve-year-old Slim narrates the story of her life with her father and his lover during the last few months before the lover's death.)

Older Teens

Clark D. Loving someone gay. Berkeley, California: Celestial Arts, 1991.

Fricke A. Reflections of a rock lobster. Boston: Alyson Publishing, 1981. (Story of a teenage boy who takes his lover to the prom.)

Heron A. Two teenagers in twenty, writings by gay and lesbian youth. Boston: Alyson Publications, 1994.

Kerr ME. Is that you Miss Blue? New York: Harper & Row, 1975. (Teenage gay love story.)

Marcus E. Is it a choice? Answers to the 300 most frequently asked questions about gays and lesbians. San Francisco: Harper Collins, 1993.

Warren PN. Fancy dancer. New York: Morrow Publishing, 1976.

Warren PN. Front runner. New York: Bantam Books, 1975.

Parents

Fairchild B, Hayward N. Now that you know: what every parent should know about homosexuality. San Diego: Harcourt Brace, 1989.

CHAPTER 42

Teenage Pregnancy

Lawrence S. Neinstein, Susan J. Rabinovitz, and Arlene Schneir

Teenage pregnancy is a major public health concern for adolescents, health-care providers, and society. This chapter discusses the scope of the problem, factors contributing to adolescent pregnancy, associated difficulties for teen parents and their children, and the role of the practitioner in counseling and management.

SCOPE OF THE PROBLEM

Information from a variety of sources describes the scope and seriousness of the problem of adolescent pregnancy and illustrates current trends in this area.

1. Annually more than one million teenage girls become pregnant, the overwhelming majority unintentionally (Henshaw, 1993). In 1990, the most recent year for which data are available, an estimated 1,040,000 females under age 20 became pregnant (Alan Guttmacher Institute, 1994). Among all the 15- to 19-year age group in the United States, 12% become pregnant each year, and among those who had had sexual intercourse 21% become pregnant. Of all births in the United States, 12% are to adolescents, with 4% to those under age 18 and 8% to 18- and 19-year-olds (Alan Guttmacher Institute, 1994).

2. Pregnancy rates: Among all females 15–19, the pregnancy rates have gone up 23% from 95/1000 in 1972 to 117/1000 in 1990 (Fig. 42.1). Significantly, however, the rates for sexually experienced teens in this age group have declined 19% over these years from 254/1000 to 207/1000. This is an encouraging indicator that sexually experienced adolescents are using contraceptives more effectively. The overall pregnancy rate has increased because of the increasing proportion of teens who have had intercourse over the past two decades.

   Pregnancies per 1000 sexually experienced women in 1990 in the United States were:

14 and younger	93
15–17	184
18–19	222
20–24	233

3. Birthrates: For the first time after a 15-year decline, birthrates among both all teens and sexually experienced teens have begun to rise. In the years between 1960 and 1986 the birthrate for all females 15–19 and sexually experienced females decreased (Fig. 42.2). However, since 1987 the U.S. birthrate for both these groups has increased slightly (Alan Guttmacher Institute, 1994) due to the decrease in the abortion rates. Since 1988 the proportion of teenage pregnancies ending in birth rather than abortion has risen from 54% to about 60%. This increase in births followed a significant decline from 76% in 1972 to 55% in 1979.

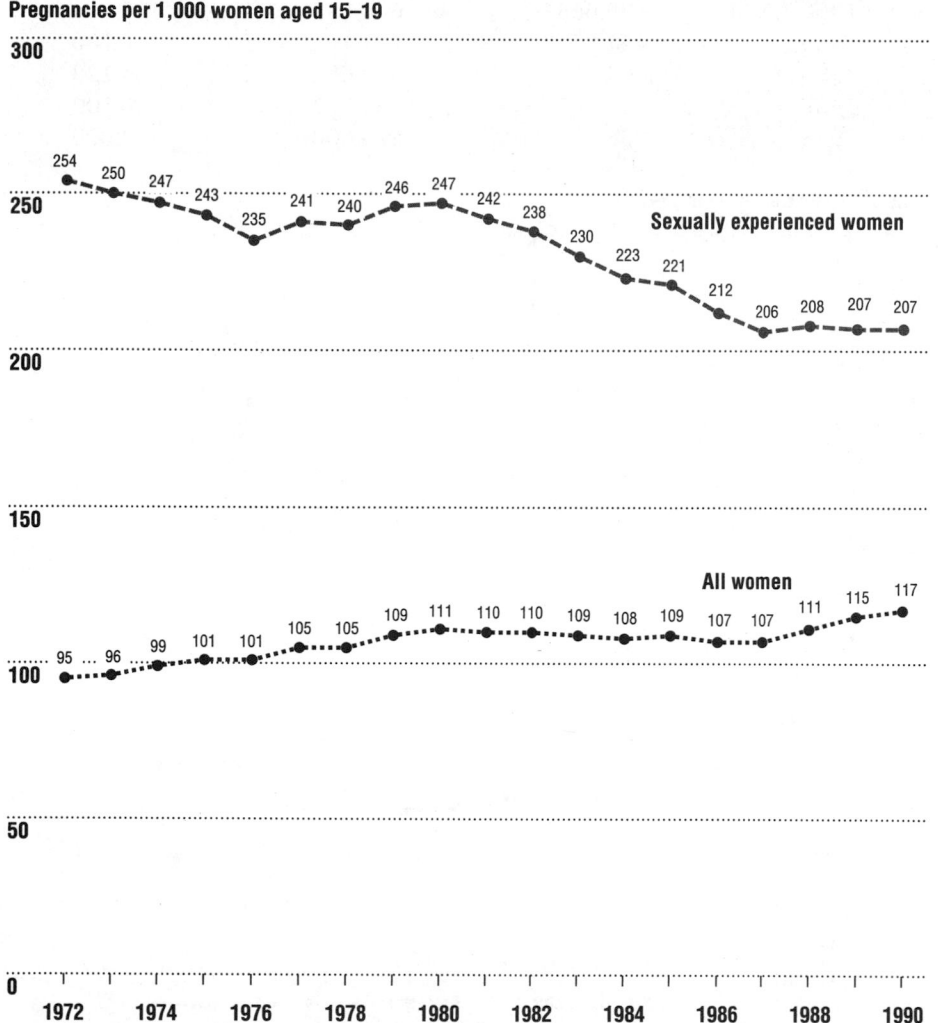

FIGURE 42.1.   Decline and rise in pregnancy rates. Over the last two decades the pregnancy rate among teenage women who have had intercourse has declined; however, since proportionately more adolescents are having intercourse, the pregnancy rate among all teenage women has increased. *Notes.* Pregnancy: Pregnancies are defined as the sum of births, abortions, and miscarriages. Miscarriages are estimated as 20% of births and 10% of abortions. Sexually experienced women: The sexually experienced population was estimated by interpolating from sexual behavior data for 1971, 1976, 1982, and 1988. Data were extrapolated for 1989 and 1990 using the 1982–1988 trend. *Information sources.* Births, 1972–1990: National Center for Health Statistics. Advance report of final natality statistics. Monthly Vital Statistics Report 1974–1993;23–41(suppl) Abortions, 1973–1988: Henshaw SK, Van Vort J, eds. Abortion factbook, 1992 edition: readings, trends, and state and local data to 1988. New York: AGI, 1992:1972–1973; Abortions, 1972, 1989–1990: Henshaw SK, US teenage pregnancy statistics. New York: AGI, 1993. Sexual experience data: Jones EF et al. Teenage pregnancy in industrialized countries. New Haven and London: Yale University Press, 1986:47; Forrest JD, Singh S. The sexual and reproductive behavior of American women, 1982–1988. Fam Plann Perspect 1990;22:207–208. From Alan Guttmacher Institute. Sex and America's teenagers. New York: Alan Guttmacher Institute, 1994.

The following statistics compare total pregnancies, births, and elective abortions between the years 1960 and 1988 in teenage females aged 15–19.

Year	Total Pregnancies	Total Births	Total Abortions
1960	839,663	644,708	150,000
1980	1,151,851	552,161	444,780
1984	1,004,859	469,682	401,128
1987	984,544	462,312	390,700
1988	988,000	478,000	393,000

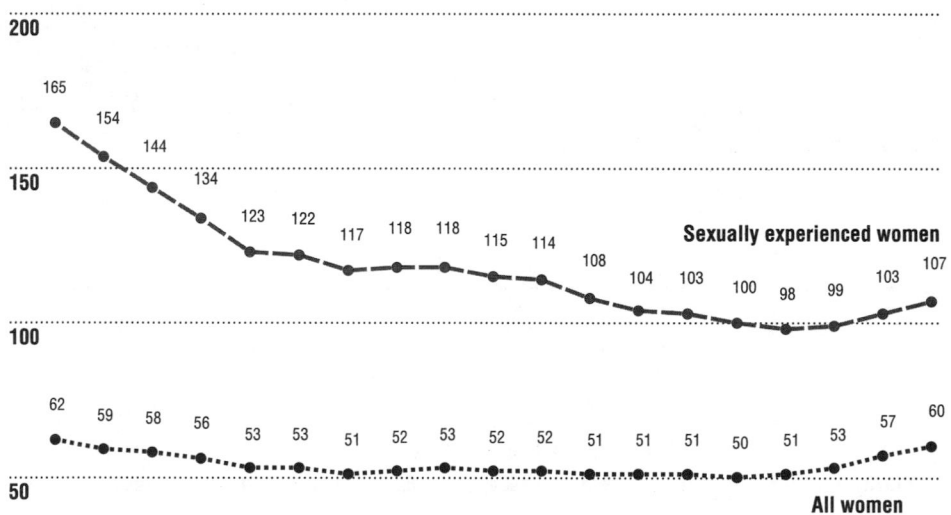

FIGURE 42.2. Birthrates rising. After a 15-year decline among sexually experienced teenagers, birthrates among both sexually experienced and all teenage women have begun to go up. *Notes.* Sexually experienced women: The sexually experienced population was estimated by interpolating from data for 1971, 1976, 1982, and 1988. To estimate sexual activity after 1988, data were extrapolated for 1989 and 1990 using the 1982–1988 trend. *Information sources.* National Center for Health Statistics. Advance report of final natality statistics, 1991. Monthly Vital Statistics Report 1993;42(3, suppl):20. Sexual experience: Jones EF, et al. Teenage pregnancy in industrialized countries, New Haven and London: Yale University Press, 1986:47; Forrest JD, Singh S. The sexual and reproductive behavior of American women, 1982–1988. Fam Plann Perspect 1990;22:207–208. From Alan Guttmacher Institute. Sex and America's teenagers. New York: Alan Guttmacher Institute, 1994.

4. Unintended pregnancies: About 85% of adolescent pregnancies are unintended. However, 55% of pregnancies among older women are also unintended. Teens account for only about one-fourth of all unintended pregnancies annually. Pregnancies among white teens and teens from families with higher incomes are more likely to be unintended. Hispanic teens are more likely than African-American youth or non-Hispanic white youth to have either wanted to get pregnant or not cared if they became pregnant (Alan Guttmacher Institute, 1994).

5. Abortion rates: Abortion rates among sexually experienced teens have decreased since 1980 from about 95/1000 to 72/1000 per year (Fig. 42.3). Teens account for about one-

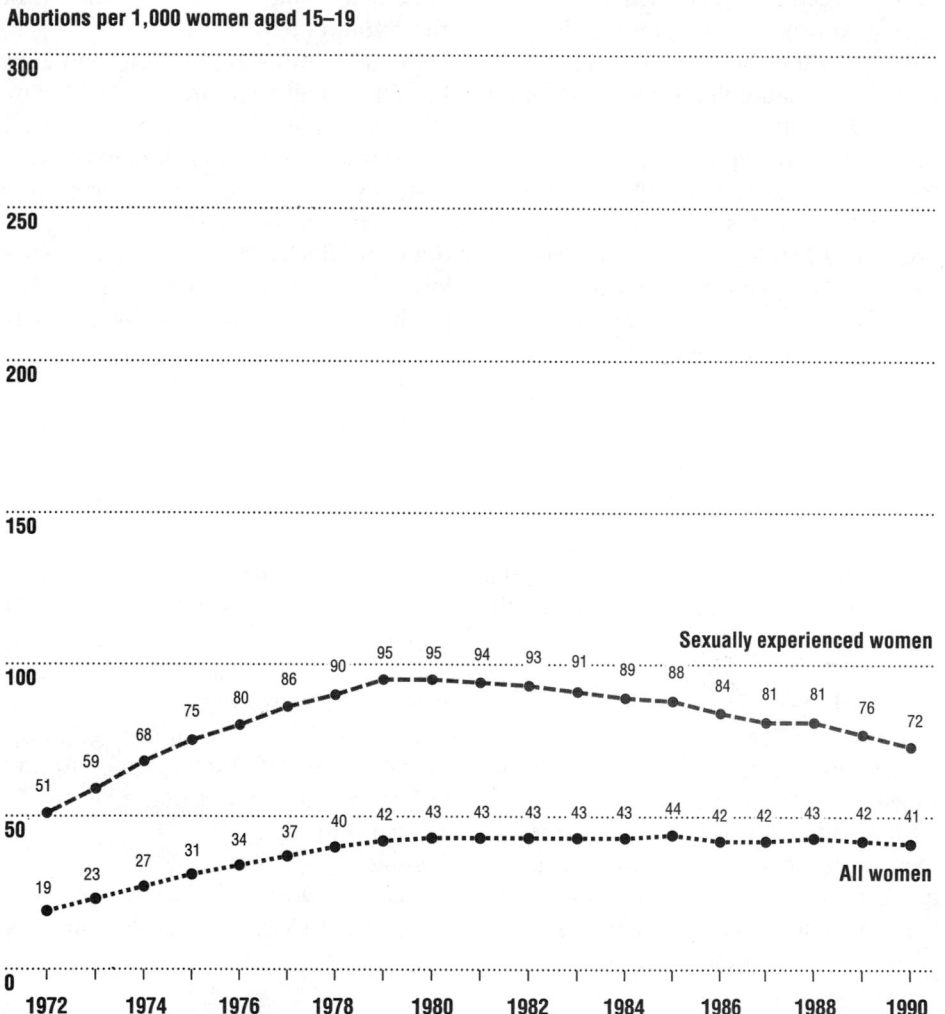

Abortions per 1,000 women aged 15–19

FIGURE 42.3.   Decline in teenage abortion rates. Since the late 1970s, the abortion rate has declined among sexually experienced teenagers. *Notes.* Sexually experienced women: The sexually experienced population was estimated by interpolating from data for 1971, 1976, 1982, and 1988. To estimate sexual activity after 1988, data were extrapolated for 1989 and 1990 using the 1982–1988 trend. *Information sources.* Abortions, 1973–1988: Henshaw SK, Van Vort J, eds. Abortion factbook, 1992 edition: readings, trends, and state and local data to 1988. New York: AGI, 1992:172–173; Abortions, 1972, 1989–1990: Henshaw SK. US teenage pregnancy statistics. New York: AGI, 1993. Sexually experienced women: Jones EF, et al. Teenage pregnancy in industrialized countries. New Haven and London: Yale University Press, 1986: Forrest JD, Singh S. The sexual and reproductive behavior of American women, 1982–1988. Fam Plann Perspect 1990;22:207–208. From Alan Guttmacher Institute. Sex and America's teenagers. New York: Alan Guttmacher Institute, 1994.

quarter of abortions in the United States. The majority of unintended pregnancies in teens (53%) end in abortion. Other correlates to a pregnant teen having an abortion include:
   a. Higher income status
   b. Parents with more education
   c. White teens
   d. A younger partner

Overall, 6/10 unmarried teens under the age 18 have involved one or both of their parents with the abortion process (Alan Guttmacher Institute, 1994).

6. Adoption: Placing a baby for adoption has become an unpopular choice, with the rates decreasing from 19% of white teens in 1972 to 3% in 1982–1988. Adoption has never been a common choice among African-American youth (1%).

7. Out-of-wedlock births: The total number of nonmarital births to teens less than 20 years of age has quadrupled since 1960 for a total of 69% of all teen births in 1991. Among teens 15–17 the rate of out-of-wedlock births has risen dramatically. In 1960–1964, 59% of the teens giving birth in this age group were unmarried, with 26% marrying during pregnancy, leading to a 33% out-of-wedlock rate. By 1985–1989, 92% of first births to 15- to 17-year-olds occurred among unmarried teens, with only 11% marrying during pregnancy, leading to an 81% prevalence of out-of-wedlock births (Alan Guttmacher Institute, 1994). However, as nonmarital childbearing becomes more common among older U.S. women, the proportion of all nonmarital births accounted for by teens has declined (Moore and Snyder, 1994).

   Out-of-wedlock births (Alan Guttmacher Institute, 1994):

First Births of Women Aged 15–17	*1960–1964*	*1985–1989*
Nonmarital birth	33%	81%
Legitimated birth	26%	11%
Marital birth	41%	8%

8. Outcomes: Of the 1,040,000 teen pregnancies in 1990, 51% delivered, 35% aborted, and 14% miscarried (Alan Guttmacher Institute, 1994). Table 42.1 reviews outcome of teen pregnancies based on marital status.

9. The United States has the highest teenage pregnancy, abortion, and childbirth rates among all Western countries; our pregnancy rate for those under age 15 is five times that of most other Western countries (Hardy, 1988). For the 15- to 19-year-old age group the United States pregnancy rate is 97/1000 compared to 40/1000 in Canada, 46/1000 in England, and 10/1000 in Japan. Sexual activity rates among teens in the United States rank about in the middle of rates for industrialized countries.

10. Demographics of teen pregnancy and related issues
   a. Age: Of teen pregnancies about two-thirds occur in women 18–20. Among sexually experienced teens, about 9% of 14-year-olds, 18% of 15- to 17-year-olds, and 22% of 18- to 19-year-olds become pregnant each year.

Table 42.1. Pregnancy Outcomes among Married Women 19 and Younger

	Overall group (1990) (1,040,000)	Married (1988)[a] (180,000)	Unmarried (1988)[a] (716,000)
Miscarriage	14%		
Abortion	35%	17%	50%
Intended birth	14%	33%	43%
Unintended birth	37%	50%	7%

Adapted from Alan Guttmacher Institute. Sex and America's teenagers. New York: Alan Guttmacher Institute, 1994.
[a]Does not include miscarriages.

b. Race and ethnicity: The birthrate for teens 15–19 in the United States is highest among African-Americans; however, the recent increase in the teen birth rate has been particularly large among Hispanic youth (Moore and Snyder, 1994). About 19% of all African-American teens aged 15–19 become pregnant each year compared to 13% for Hispanics and 8% for non-Hispanic white teens.

c. Timing: One-fifth of all premarital pregnancies occur within the first month after commencing sexual intercourse; one-half occur in the first 6 months (Zelnick and Kantner, 1980). Approximately 1 in 15 teenagers who experience a premarital pregnancy become pregnant again within a year (Grimes, 1994).

d. Income: Poorer teens are more likely to get pregnant than teens from families with higher incomes.

e. Male partners: Male partners of teens becoming pregnant are generally older. Only 26% of men involved in the pregnancies among women under age 18 are a similar age, with 35% being 18–19 and 39% at least age 20.

11. Demographics of teen births and related issues

a. Births by age and race: There are large differences in birthrates among teens depending on race and ethnicity (Birthrates/1000 teens, 1990) (Alan Guttmacher Institute, 1994):

Age	White	Hispanic	African-American
15–17	23	65	84
18–19	72	148	163
20–24	98	181	165

b. Births based by income: Poor and low-income teens accounted for 83% of women 15–19 who gave birth in 1988 while comprising only 38% of all women in that age group. About 60% of teens who become mothers are living in poverty at the time of giving birth, with about 60% of those who give birth having their delivery fees covered by public funds.

c. Location: About three-quarters of pregnant youth under 18 live with one or both of their parents, with 60% still living at home even after giving birth.

d. Repeat births: Nineteen percent of teens who become mothers between 15 and 17 and 25% of those who become mothers between 18 and 19 have a second child within 2 years.

FACTORS CONTRIBUTING TO TEENAGE PREGNANCY

Multiple factors contribute to adolescent pregnancy and childbearing. Some relate to developmental processes and others to familial and societal influences. Attempts to isolate a unifying trait among pregnant adolescent females have failed; there is no unique profile common to most pregnant teenagers. However, some studies suggest that one or more of the following social, environmental, or psychological characteristics may be present:

1. Poverty
2. Low self-esteem
3. Poor academic achievement
4. Poor familial relationships
5. History of family violence, substance abuse, physical or sexual abuse, and neglect
6. Familial or cultural acceptance of adolescent childbearing

Information regarding some specific contributing factors is provided below:

1. Early puberty: Since the turn of the century, the average age of menarche has decreased approximately 3 months per decade (Stevens-Simon, 1992), from about 16–17 years in

the late 19th century to 12.4 years at present (Jaskiewicz and McAnarney, 1994). This earlier physical maturation has widened the gap between reproductive capacity and cognitive and emotional maturation and has increased the risk of unintended pregnancy in this age group.

2. Use of contraception: While most sexually experienced teens use contraception (72% of 15- to 17-year-old women and 84% of 18- to 19-year-old women, many teens do not use contraception each time they have intercourse. Teenage women's contraceptive use at first intercourse rose from 48% in 1982 to 65% in 1988. However, current contraceptive use declined slightly among sexually experienced teens between 1988 and 1990 from 61% to 58%, and the proportion of sexually experienced teens who were sexually active in the past month without using contraception increased from 8% to 22%. In addition, only 40% of teens go for medical contraceptive services within the first year after they begin intercourse. Older teens are more likely to use contraception at first intercourse than younger teens. Sixty percent of males older than 18 when initiating sexual activity used contraception compared with only about one-third of boys who were younger than 15 years old when they became sexually active (Hayes, 1987).

3. Early sexual activity: The high rate of teen pregnancy reflects a growing trend in the United States in which adolescents are engaging in sexual intercourse at younger ages. According to the 1990 Centers for Disease Control and Prevention National School-Based Youth Risk Behavior Survey, nearly one-third of ninth grade girls and nearly one-half of ninth grade boys reported having sexual intercourse (Grimes, 1994). The age of sexual debut for out-of-school youth such as dropouts and homeless youth and youth in urban centers is often reported to be much lower; these youth also report more lifetime sexual partners (Centers for Disease Control, 1994).

4. Media: Young people are inundated with sexual images and messages in advertising and entertainment. TV shows and movies are filled with sexual activity and innuendo but offer few role models demonstrating responsible sexual behavior. American adolescents view approximately 14,000 sexual references on TV each year, yet only 165 refer to topics such as sex education, sexually transmitted disease, birth control, or abortion (Harris, 1988).

5. Developmental issues: Many developmental characteristics of adolescents, particularly of younger teens, interfere with decision making regarding sexual activity and the successful use of contraceptives. These include a limited ability to plan for the future or to foresee the consequences of their actions and a sense of personal invulnerability.

6. Barriers to contraceptive use: Many environmental, social, and psychological barriers interfere with decision making regarding sexual activity and contraception among teens. Significant obstacles to successful contraception include:
   a. Inaccurate information: Many teens have misinformation regarding conception and reproduction. Among other myths, many mistakenly believe that they are too young to get pregnant or that pregnancy cannot occur the first time they have intercourse.
   b. Accessibility: Many young people want to prevent pregnancy but:
      — They lack information regarding available methods.
      — They do not know about their legal rights to care.
      — They do not know where to obtain contraceptives.
      — They have concerns regarding confidentiality.
      — They have concerns regarding cost.
      — Services are often not offered at times that meet the needs of young people.
      — They lack transportation to services.
   c. Contraceptive acceptability: Teens may seek out contraceptive services but are often:
      — Fearful of specific methods and perceived side effects (especially the possibility of cancer and weight gain they assume to be associated with oral contraceptives)

— Concerned about contraceptive use affecting their future fertility
— Embarrassed over the acquisition or use of the method
— Concerned that the method might interfere with pleasure

d. Partner issues: Many young people are interested in contraception but are often unable to discuss contraception with their partners or their partners refuse to use available methods.

e. Religious beliefs: Teens may become involved in sexual activity despite religious beliefs prohibiting premarital sexual activity and contraception but may not be able to seek contraceptive services.

f. Intended pregnancy: Some young women do not protect themselves from pregnancy because of a desire to have a baby. This desire may emerge from a need to:
— Solidify their relationship with their partner or please their partner
— Have someone to love and take care of
— Change their status in their family or assert their independence
— Rebel against their family
— Escape from an abusive home environment by cementing a relationship with another family or by creating their own new family
— Establish their fertility

7. Provider problems: Acquiring contraceptive services can be difficult for young people because:

a. Clinicians may not address sexuality and contraceptive use with their adolescent patients who may be too embarrassed to initiate the discussion themselves.

b. Some providers are unwilling to prescribe contraceptives for their patients without parental knowledge or consent.

c. Many providers are overtly judgmental about sexual activity among their young patients, which discourages disclosure and discussion of sexual involvement and prohibits dispensing of appropriate education and birth control methods.

CONSEQUENCES OF ADOLESCENT PARENTHOOD

Maternal Problems

1. Increased health risks: Most recent studies suggest that the majority of the negative maternal health consequences associated with teenage childbearing are due to socioeconomic factors, prepregnancy health status, and health behaviors rather than to the physiological effects of age. However, the following risks have been implicated:

a. Teenagers 17 and under have a higher than average risk of pregnancy-related anemia, hypertension, cervical trauma, and premature delivery (National Commission to Prevent Infant Mortality, 1988).

b. The mortality rate for mothers under 15 is 60% greater than for women in their 20s. (National Commission to Prevent Infant Mortality, 1988).

c. Despite controlling for marital status, educational level, and prenatal care, young teenage mothers 13–17 had significantly higher risk than mothers who were 20–24 for bearing low–birth weight, premature, and small for gestational age infants. However, this study only included white teens in the state of Utah (Fraser et al., 1995).

2. Education: Teenage mothers complete less education than their peers who delay childbearing.

a. More than two-thirds of the adolescents who have their first child before age 15 and more than half of those whose first birth is between the ages of 15 and 17 years do not complete high school with their peers.

      b. Educational status is one of the most accurate indicators of eventual employment and economic self-sufficiency.

      c. Studies show that 70% of all adolescent girls who become mothers do finish high school by the time they are 35–39, compared with over 90% of women who first become mothers after adolescence.

3. Unemployment
   a. Teenage parents are more likely than those who delay childbearing to have low status, low-paying jobs, or to be unemployed (Alan Guttmacher Institute, 1981).
   b. Studies have shown that some of the employment and income differences between early and late childbearers diminish somewhat over time (Hayes, 1987).
4. Welfare: Teen parenthood is associated with socioeconomic disadvantage.
   a. An estimated 53% of funds of the Aid to Families with Dependent Children (AFDC) budget was expended on families in which the mother was a teenager when her first child was born (Alan Guttmacher Institute, 1994).
   b. As teenage mothers get older, however, many move off public assistance. A recent follow-up study of teenage mothers found that a substantial majority finished high school, found regular employment, and achieved economic independence (Furstenberg et al., 1987).
5. Marriage
   a. Teen marriages have a higher rate of divorce. The younger a couple is when they marry, the more likely they are to divorce (Alan Guttmacher Institute, 1994).
   b. Teens who marry because of pregnancy are three times more likely to divorce than women who have children in their twenties (McCarthy and Menken, 1979).
6. Number of subsequent children: Teenage mothers have more children.
   a. Trussell and Menken (1978) reported that the younger a female is at her first pregnancy, the more children she will have, and the closer spaced they will be.
   b. Keeve et al. (1969) reported that 60% of girls who delivered before the age of 17 were pregnant again before the age of 19. In the United States, 19% of adolescents who become mothers between 15 and 17 and 25% of those between 18 and 19 have a second child within 2 years.

Infant Outcome and Problems

1. Birth weight: As compared to mothers in their twenties, the risk of low–birth weight babies is increased two times among mothers less than 15 years of age; 1.5 times among mothers aged 15–17 years; and 1.3 times among mothers 18–19 years old. Part or all of this risk may relate to inadequate prenatal care and nutrition, as well as to other health-compromising behaviors among pregnant adolescents.
2. Infant mortality: The risk of a baby dying in the first year of life increases as the age of the mother decreases below 20 years. Almost 6% of first babies born to girls under 15 years old die in their first year, a rate 2.4 times higher than for babies born to women in their early twenties. Again, part of this mortality may relate to other health and environmental factors, rather than to the age of the mother.
3. Cognitive and social emotional development: Some studies show that the cognitive development of a child is influenced by the age of the mother, even after controlling for the effects of socioeconomic status (Hatcher et al., 1994). However, the difference is small. Studies examining the relationship between maternal age and social-emotional development have been inconclusive (Hatcher et al., 1994). Some studies report no differences between social-emotional behavior and maternal age. Other studies suggest children of teenage mothers are less responsive, less expressive, and have lower self-esteem and trust

(Phipps-Yonas, 1980). However, in these studies maternal age was shown to have much less influence than the socioeconomic variables (Hatcher et al., 1994).

In conclusion, the full complement of risks associated with adolescent childbearing are not fully understood. It is clear that at least some problems are related to lack of adequate prenatal care, lack of postnatal care, and inadequate education in parenting. However, there is also evidence to suggest that the optimum time of pregnancy for maternal and fetal health is after adolescence. Some excellent reviews of teenage pregnancy are Phipps-Yonas (1980), Alan Guttmacher Institute (1981, 1989a, 1989b, 1994), Hayes (1987), and Lancaster and Hamburg (1986).

THE ROLE OF THE PRACTITIONER

Pregnancy in an adolescent can be a crisis for the teen and her family. The practitioner is in a unique position to offer guidance and support during this time. Opportunities for intervention include:

1. Diagnosis of pregnancy and facilitated decision-making
2. Service planning and referrals
3. Management of pregnancy, if the teen chooses to continue the pregnancy
4. Preparation for parenthood, if the teen chooses to raise the child
5. Family planning and safer sex education

DIAGNOSIS OF PREGNANCY

Most young women delay seeking reproductive health care until months after they become sexually active. Often, it is the fear of pregnancy that prompts these young women to seek family planning and gynecological health-care services for the first time. It is important for the practitioner to consider that any female adolescent patient may have concerns about pregnancy even if they are not expressed. Sexuality and contraception should be explored in any complete evaluation of an adolescent. The patient interview should be structured to obtain an accurate sexual history and related concerns.

Practitioners should keep in mind the following considerations when conducting the adolescent interview:

1. The adolescent should be seen alone to allow for more complete questioning and more honest disclosure.
2. If there is any concern about pregnancy, the practitioner should offer a pregnancy test even if the teen denies recent sexual activity.
3. Once pregnancy test results are known, it is often difficult for a teen to discuss her feelings regarding an unexplained pregnancy. Therefore, practitioners should briefly assess her desire to be pregnant and her perceived options, prior to conducting the test.

CLINICAL PRESENTATION AND MEDICAL DIAGNOSIS

1. Common presentations
   a. Typical symptoms
      — Secondary amenorrhea
      — Breast tenderness or fullness
      — Morning nausea
      — Weight gain

    b. Distracting complaints: Often an adolescent will be primarily concerned about pregnancy but will mask this concern by presenting with an alternate major complaint such as:
   - Fatigue or nausea
   - Weight change
   - Abdominal pain
   - Request for a complete checkup
   - Late period
   - Request for contraception

2. Physical examination
   a. Enlarged uterus
   b. Cervical cyanosis
   c. Soft cervix

3. Laboratory tests: Following is information on the three major types of pregnancy tests for use in the clinic or office. (For a more complete description, please refer to Hatcher et al., 1994 & 1996):
   a. Immunometric tests
      - Immunometric tests are the most commonly used and recommended office tests because of accuracy, speed, early diagnosis, and versatility.
      - They are based on enzyme-linked immunosorbent assay (ELISA) design.
      - Test results are positive in 98% of women within 7 days after implantation.
      - Test results are specific for the β subunit for human chorionic gonadotropin (hCG); cross-reaction with other hormones is not a problem.
      - The test provides qualitative (yes or no) results comparable with radioimmunoassay (RIA) tests but at less cost.
      - Table 42.2 displays a sample of commonly used immunometric tests.
   b. Quantitative β-hCG RIA
      - Accurate quantitative results are reliable within 7 days after fertilization.
      - Radioisotopes are required to conduct test, and this limits the test's use in offices or small clinics.
      - Serial test specimens can be used in evaluation of ectopic pregnancy, impending miscarriage, possible retained placental fragments, or molar pregnancies.
   c. Agglutination inhibition slide tests
      - Slide tests are inexpensive and have been widely used for the last 15 years.
      - Because most slide tests are not specific for the β subunit of hCG, cross-reactions are possible.

TABLE 42.2. Common Immunometric Tests

Name (Manufacturer)	Sensitivity (mIU/mL)[a]	Time Required	Steps and Comments
Clearview hCG (Wompole)	50	5 min	1 step/urine
Icon II hCG (Hybritech)	20	5 min	5 steps/serum
	25	4 min	5 steps/urine
Surall hCG (Kodak)	30	2 min	2–3 steps/serum
	30	1 min	2–3 steps/urine
	50	1 min	2–3 steps/urine
Testpack plus hCG (Abbott)	50	5 min	1 step/urine

Adapted from Hatcher RA, Trussell J, Stewart F, et. al. Contraceptive technology. 16th revised ed. New York: Irvington Publishers, 1994.
[a]Sensitivity specified as the lower limit of reliable hCG detection in product literature. Test results may be positive at lower hCG levels in some cases.

— Slide tests are only appropriate for confirming pregnancy when the gestation is between 6 and 16 weeks. hCG levels in early or later pregnancy may be below the level required.
— The tests are not appropriate to rule out pregnancy.

ALTERNATIVES FOR PREGNANT ADOLESCENTS

Decision Making

The adolescent will require a supportive listener, often a physician or counselor, who can help her make a decision about the pregnancy. Many factors, including age, attitudes, support, race, ethnicity, culture, education, and socioeconomic status, may have an impact on this decision. Physicians or counselors should keep in mind the following considerations in this regard:

1. The adolescent should be aware that the decision about the pregnancy and its resolution is hers.
2. The adolescent should be encouraged to explore all options and to express all her feelings, both positive and negative, about the pregnancy.
3. The male partner should be included in the discussion, if appropriate. This, however, should be left to the discretion of the pregnant teen.
4. As part of the decision-making process, specific information regarding perinatal health care, abortion procedures, and adoption and foster care alternatives should be explained.
5. Appropriate resources and plans for follow-up care should be provided. Practitioners should become familiar with the resources in their community.
6. Practitioners who are not comfortable with or whose practice does not allow sufficient time for pregnancy counseling should refer pregnant patients to a local clinic that provides nondirective, nonjudgmental pregnancy counseling services.

ABORTION

The majority of unintended pregnancies among teenagers end in abortion (Alan Guttmacher Institute, 1994). Adolescents who have abortions most often cite young age and low income as the reasons for choosing this option.

When a teen chooses abortion, it is important for her to identify a supportive person to accompany her to the procedure or support her through this process. This person may be a parent, partner, friend, or caring adult.

Practitioners must know their specific state's laws that govern minor access to abortion services. Although abortion was legalized in the United States in 1973, many states restrict minor access to abortion services and require either parental consent or notification. Although most of these states have a mechanism to bypass parental consent through a judicial process, teens are often uninformed of their rights and ill equipped to negotiate the judicial system alone. Furthermore, most states prohibit the use of public funds or facilities for abortion services, thereby reducing access for low-income teens. Practitioners who are not familiar with their state's laws should refer teens to a local Planned Parenthood or other appropriate facility for assistance.

Abortion Methods

First Trimester

1. Surgical methods: In the United States the most common abortion procedures are:
   a. Vacuum aspiration

— The most widely used abortion procedure
— Relatively simple technique requiring small cervical dilation
— May be performed with local anesthesia
— Can be done in an office through 14 weeks' gestation.

b. Dilation and evacuation (D & E)
— D & E requires more dilation than aspiration method.
— Laminaria or other osmotic dilators are often inserted before the procedure to gradually dilate the cervix. This may be a 1- to 2-day procedure.
— D & E is commonly used for procedures between 13 and 16 weeks, although many clinicians use this procedure up through 20+ weeks.
— Paracervical or general anesthesia is used prior to evacuating the uterus.

2. Medical methods: There are no routinely available medical methods of first trimester abortion available in the United States. Mifepristone (RU 486), used in combination with prostaglandins, is used in Europe and other countries for effective early abortion. In addition, studies have been conducted in the United States with methotrexate and misoprostol indicating a 96% success rate without side effects (Hausknecht, 1995).

Second Trimester

1. Surgical methods: D & E procedures are the most common type of second trimester abortion in the United States due to the fact that they are safer, faster, and less expensive than existing medical methods.
2. Medical methods: Currently there are three medical methods available in the United States. However, in 1989 these represented only 10% of all abortions (Hatcher et al., 1994). Methods include:
a. Hypertonic saline instillation
b. Hypertonic urea instillation
c. Prostaglandin E_2 suppository

Abortion Risks and Complications

1. Mortality
a. The mortality for all women is 0.5 deaths per 100,000 from curettage, 3.7 deaths per 100,000 from D & E, and 7.1 deaths per 100,000 from intrauterine instillation.
b. Mortality increases with length of gestation (Table 42.3).
c. Although studies have shown teens to have the lowest risk of all age groups for abortion-related mortality, their increased use of second-trimester abortions exposes them to a higher risk of complications.

Table 42.3.   Abortion Mortality Rates, United States

Weeks of Gestation	Mortality Rate per 100,000 (1972–1987)
≤8	0.4
9–10	0.8
11–12	1.4
13–15	2.9
16–20	9.3
>21	12.0

Adapted from Hatcher RA, Trussell J, Stewart F, et al. Contraceptive Technology, 16th revised ed. New York: Irvington Publishers, 1994.

2. Complications: The two primary factors that influence morbidity are gestational age and abortion technique. An additional factor is choice of anesthetic. The five most serious postabortion problems are:
    a. Infection: This can be minimized by preprocedure diagnosis and treatment of gonorrhea, chlamydia, and cervicitis and by the use of prophylactic antibiotics. Infection due to retained products of conception requires antibiotic treatment and an additional procedure.
    b. Intrauterine blood clots
    c. Cervical or uterine trauma: Women under the age of 17 have an increased risk of cervical injury. Use of laminaria and skillful technique lowers the risk considerably.
    d. Bleeding
    e. Failed abortion
3. Long-term postabortion implications
    a. Medical: Data relating to long-term complications of abortion do not show major risks from the most common methods. However, there may be a risk of subsequent adverse reproductive outcomes with multiple-induced abortions (Hogue et al., 1982).
    b. Psychological: Although some studies report that teens may consider abortion to be a stressful experience, these symptoms are often short-lived and can be mitigated with support before, during, and after the procedure (Ashton, 1980; Biro et al., 1986). In a prospective study of 360 black teenage women from urban family planning clinics, Zabin et al. (1989) found that those adolescents having a therapeutic abortion were more likely to remain in school and were better off economically than those continuing their pregnancy or those having a negative pregnancy test. Those teens who terminated their pregnancy experienced no greater levels of stress or anxiety and were no more likely to have psychological problems 2 years later. The teens obtaining an abortion were also less likely to experience a subsequent pregnancy than either of the other two groups.

ADOPTION

As single parenthood has become less stigmatized, the likelihood that a teen will place her baby for adoption has declined dramatically. Almost all of the decline has occurred in adoption rates among white women, with adoption rates decreasing from 19% of white teens in 1972 to 3% in 1982–1988 (Alan Guttmacher Institute, 1994). Historically, African-American young women have rarely chosen adoption. As the adoption process has changed with open adoption and private adoption becoming available, more young women may consider this choice. Adoption should be presented during the initial pregnancy counseling and reconsidered, as appropriate, during pregnancy and the early postpartum period. Practitioners should be familiar with adoption counseling and placement resources in their community, including both public and private agencies.

PARENTHOOD

Ninety-four percent of unmarried pregnant teens who do not miscarry or have an abortion, choose parenthood. The practitioner has a unique role in the management of adolescent pregnancy and in preparing these young women and their families for the responsibilities of parenthood. Attention should be focused on evaluating the potential for involvement on the part of the father. The practitioner may provide or refer for quality perinatal health care, health education, and parent education. It is important to identify and use existing community resources that provide comprehensive support and care to pregnant and parenting adolescents.

MANAGEMENT OF ADOLESCENT PREGNANCY

Pregnant adolescents, because of increased maternal and fetal risks, require special prenatal management. Practitioners should note that young women are at risk for inadequate care, and therefore they should make special efforts to ensure early linkages with prenatal providers. Pregnant teenagers are twice as likely, when compared to all pregnant women, to receive no prenatal care or care initiated only at the third trimester. Twelve percent of all teenagers (12–19 years old) and more than 20% of those younger than age 15 receive only third-trimester care or no care at all prior to delivery.

Following is a brief guide for the practitioner in important areas of prenatal care for the adolescent patient.

1. Initial evaluation: Initial evaluation should include a thorough history, including both a family history of chronic illness and personal medical history. A drug history, especially for tobacco, alcohol, and illicit substances, is important. (See the review of drugs and pregnancy at the end of this section.) A thorough and sensitive discussion regarding the pregnant teen's and her partner's risk for human immunodeficiency virus (HIV) infection should be initiated. (Appropriate referrals for pretest counseling and testing should be provided.) Due to young people's reluctance to disclose sensitive information during an initial visit, practitioners should continue to assess a teen's risk status throughout her pregnancy. A complete physical examination and pelvic examination should be performed. Laboratory evaluation should include:
   a. Complete blood count
   b. Urinalysis
   c. Blood type and group
   d. Screening syphilis serology (VDRL)
   e. Sickle cell test in black patients
   f. Tay-Sachs test for patients of Mediterranean or Jewish heritage
   g. Rubella titer
   h. Pap smear
   i. Gonococcal culture
   j. *Chlamydia* culture or screening test
   k. Hepatitis B serology
   l. HIV antibody counseling and testing should be offered
2. Topics to be covered on successive visits include:
   a. Physiology of pregnancy
   b. Maternal nutrition
   c. Substance abuse
   d. Sexually transmitted diseases and HIV infection
   e. Discussion and referral to a prepared childbirth class
   f. Childbirth
   g. Breast-feeding and infant nutrition
   h. Infant care and infant development
   i. Contraception and sexuality
   j. Postdelivery care needs
3. Nutrition: General recommendations include:
   a. Ideal weight gain should range from 25 pounds for an overweight teen to 40 pounds for an underweight teen.
   b. Daily caloric needs increase from 2200 to 2500 kcal/day. Adolescents 11–14 years old require 2700 kcal/day (Gutierrez and King, 1993).

    c. The teen should be advised against dieting during pregnancy.

    d. A prenatal vitamin supplement should be prescribed.

    e. Additional iron is required if iron deficiency is diagnosed.

    f. Adolescents consuming less than 600 mg of calcium per day should be given a calcium supplement.

4. Prenatal visits: Pregnant adolescents should be seen as early as possible in their pregnancy. Thereafter, they should be seen every 2–4 weeks, depending on their risk status, until the 8th month; they should be seen every 2 weeks in the 8th month and weekly thereafter.

5. Psychosocial aspects: It is essential to consider that the pregnant teenager's acceptance of the pregnancy and her relationship with her parents or the father of the child may change during the course of the pregnancy. It is important to monitor the teen's psychosocial needs and to intervene appropriately.

6. Medications and pregnancy: Medication should be avoided when possible during pregnancy. The following is a list of commonly used drugs and their effects during pregnancy:

Adrenocortical steroids	Low incidence of cleft palate suspected
Amphetamines	May cause malformations
Antacids	May cause malformations; avoid in early pregnancy
Antibiotics	
Acyclovir	Safety not established; use only under strong indications
Aminoglycosides	Possible eighth nerve toxicity in fetus
Cephalosporins	Probably safe
Clindamycin	None known; caution advised
Erythromycin	Considered safe
Erythromycin estolate	Risk of cholestatic hepatitis in mother; avoid during pregnancy
Isoniazid	Embryotoxic in animals; caution advised
Metronidazole	May affect chromosomes; avoid during pregnancy if possible, particularly in first trimester
Penicillins	Considered safe
Spectinomycin	Probably safe
Sulfonamides	Hemolysis in newborns with glucose-6-phosphate dehydrogenase (G6PD) deficiency and increased risk of kernicterus in newborns; avoid at term
Tetracycline	Congenital limb abnormalities, cataracts, inhibition of bone growth in fetus, discoloration of fetal teeth; avoid during pregnancy
Trimethoprim	Folate antagonism in fetus; potentially teratogenic; avoid during pregnancy
Anticonvulsants	
Carbamazepine (Tegretol)	Effects unknown; questionable association with facial dysmorphism, hypoplasia of fingers or toenails, spina bifida and congenital heart disease
Diazepam (Valium)	Possible risk of cleft lip without cleft palate
Ethosuximide (Zarontin)	Low teratogenic potential
Phenobarbital	Possible increase in learning difficulties

Phenytoin (Dilantin)	Developmental disturbances appear lower than previously reported and anomalies may be genetically linked to epilepsy; hypertelorism and digital hypoplasia reported in higher frequency with use of phenytoin; other problems more questionable, including intrauterine growth retardation, mental retardation, and developmental delay; craniofacial abnormalities including depressed nasal bridge, ptosis, inner epicanthal folds, and ocular hypertelorism; limb abnormalities (digital and limb hypoplasia); cardiac defects; and hernias
Valproic acid	Teratogenic in rodents; increased risk of spina bifida if used in first trimester
Antidepressants	Conflicting reports
Antihistamines Diphenhydramine	Suspicious of higher rate of cleft palate
Aspirin	Association with hydrocephalus, congenital heart disease, and hip dislocation; conflicting reports
Bronchodilators Aminophylline	No current evidence of abnormalities
Phenothiazines	Cleft palate, hypospadias, microcephaly, syndactyly, cardiac malformations, club foot
Retinoic acid	Severe teratogenic effects causing craniofacial, cardiac, and thymic malformations

7. The chronically ill adolescent: Pregnancy in chronically ill adolescents presents specific challenges and requires coordination with their specialty care providers. Each illness is associated with specific risks. For an overview of the relationship between chronic illness and pregnancy see Neinstein (1994).
8. Substance use or abuse: Due to the serious consequence of substance use for both the mother and the baby, a thorough assessment of drug use history and current practices is necessary at pregnancy diagnosis and throughout the prenatal period. Although prepregnancy substance use is high in adolescents, particularly among inner-city youth, one large epidemiological study found that adolescents were more likely than adult women to stop alcohol and drug use once pregnancy was confirmed (Hall et al., 1993). Studies suggest that adolescents also decrease substance use postpartum (Hall et al., 1993). The following is a list of common substances and their effects during pregnancy:

Alcohol	Fetal alcohol syndrome including prenatal and postnatal growth retardation; facial dysmorphogenesis (microcephaly, short palpebral fissures, cleft palate, and micrognathia); abnormalities of the central nervous system including mental retardation; also increased risk of cardiac defects, joint abnormalities, hepatic fibrosis, and learning difficulties
Amphetamines	May cause malformations
Cocaine	Increased risk of spontaneous abortion and premature delivery; neurobehavioral deficits in the newborn, increased prevalence of abruptio placentae; increased risk of genital and urinary tract defects including prune belly syndrome, hypospadias, and hydronephrosis; increased reports of other congenital defects

Heroin	Intrauterine growth retardation, neonatal abstinence syndrome; increased risk of hepatitis, HIV, and other infections in the mother
Lysergic acid diethylamide (LSD)	Increased risk of congenital abnormalities including hydrocephalus, spina bifida, and myelomeningocele
Marijuana	Potentially mutagenic; questionable increased risk of birth defects
Nicotine	Impaired growth; increased risk of spontaneous abortion

9. HIV disease: Practitioners should offer HIV counseling and testing to all pregnant teens. Education regarding the risks of perinatal transmission should also be provided. Pregnant women infected with HIV should be referred for appropriate treatment and supportive services. Some women found to be infected may choose to terminate their pregnancy once their HIV status is known. Others will want access to specialized care designed to manage their infection and reduce their risk of perinatal transmission. Due to the risks of HIV transmission through breast milk, breast-feeding is not recommended for HIV-infected women.

10. Battering: Battering often starts or becomes worse during pregnancy. Studies suggest that 8% of all pregnant women are battered (Helton, 1990). Prenatal risk assessment should include specific questions regarding family and partner violence. Practitioners must be knowledgeable about domestic violence reporting laws in their state and should be familiar with community resources.

ADDITIONAL PREGNANCIES

Data suggest that although many young women can overcome the obstacles to completing their education and obtaining employment when they have only one child, these tasks become significantly more difficult with each additional pregnancy (Alan Guttmacher Institute, 1994). This makes the prevention of additional adolescent pregnancies as important as the prevention of first adolescent pregnancies (Stevens-Simon, 1992).

The role of the practitioner in the prevention of subsequent adolescent pregnancies is critical. However, the mere prescription of a birth control method following delivery is not adequate. Extended postpartum care and patient teaching that addresses both the new tasks of parenthood and the ongoing developmental needs of the adolescent is important. This can best be accomplished in coordination with comprehensive support programs that help these young women plan their families, education, and careers.

THE MALE ADOLESCENT

The role of the male adolescent in teenage pregnancy has not been well studied, and the needs and concerns of young men have often been overlooked by service providers.

Involvement in Pregnancy

1. Only 26% of the men involved in the pregnancies of women under age 18 are estimated to have been that young: 35% are aged 18–19, and 39% are at least 20 (Alan Guttmacher Institute, 1994). These figures suggest that adolescent men are less likely than adolescent women to be involved in a pregnancy.

2. Due to the frequency with which there may be a significant age difference between a pregnant adolescent and her partner, practitioners must be familiar with mandatory reporting requirements for sex between minors and adults.

3. Practitioners must be sensitive to the relationship between the adolescent female and her partner. Although there may be legitimate concerns about the teen father's commitment to his partner and child, many young fathers are interested in providing emotional and financial support but lack the skills to do so. Practitioners should assess the potential for positive male involvement and support the young man in this role.

Involvement in Parenthood

1. In 1987 at least 105,000 teenage boys became fathers (National Center for Health Statistics, 1989). A 1984 study documented that 7% of all young men reported having fathered a child while a teenager (Marsiglio, 1987).
2. One study showed that 84% of the fathers of children born to adolescent mothers live apart from their children (Hardy et al., 1989).
3. Only one-third of these fathers report visiting their children at least once a week 1 year after the child's birth (Hardy et al., 1989).
4. In 1984 only 42% of all males aged 20–24 earned enough to support a family of three above the poverty line (Childrens Defense Fund, 1987).

Impact on Young Men

1. Many young men who become fathers during adolescence do not graduate from high school. Males who have no children or who waited until after 20 to become a parent have a dropout rate of 14.1%. This compares to a dropout rate of 40.7% among young males aged 11–17 and unmarried at the birth of a child and 61.5% among similarly aged males who were married at the birth of a child (Marsiglio, 1987).
2. Studies indicate that teenage fatherhood is likely to be repeated from one generation to the next.

BIBLIOGRAPHY

Alan Guttmacher Institute. Teenage pregnancy: the problem that hasn't gone away. New York: Alan Guttmacher Institute, 1981.

Alan Guttmacher Institute. United States and cross-national trends in teenage sexuality and fertility behavior. New York: Unpublished data, 1986.

Alan Guttmacher Institute. Teenage pregnancy in the United States: the scope of the problem and state responses. New York: Alan Guttmacher Institute, 1989a.

Alan Guttmacher Institute. The Alan Guttmacher reports on teenage pregnancy. New York: Alan Guttmacher Institute, 1989b.

Alan Guttmacher Institute. Private communication from Susan Tew. New York: Alan Guttmacher Institute, 1990.

Alan Guttmacher Institute. Sex and America's teenagers. New York: Alan Guttmacher Institute, 1994.

Alexander CS, Greyer B. Adolescent pregnancy occurrence and consequences, Pediatr Ann 1993;22:2.

Ashton JR. The psychosocial outcome of induced abortion. Br J Obstet Gynaecol 1980;87:1115.

Baldwin W, Cain V. The children of teenage parents. Fam Plann Perspect 1980;12:34.

Biro FM, Wildey LS, Hillard PJ, et al. Acute and long term consequences of adolescents who choose abortion. Pediatr Ann 1986;15:667.

Blumberg BD, Golbus MS. Psychologic sequelae of elective abortion. West J Med 1975;123:188.

Breuner CC, Farrow JA. Pregnant teens in prison. Prevalence, management, and consequences. West J Med 1995;162:328.

Carruth BR. Smoking and pregnancy outcome of adolescents. J Adolesc Health Care 1981;2:115.

Centers for Disease Control. Teenage pregnancy and birth rates—United States, 1990. MMWR 1993;42:733.

Centers for Disease Control. Health risk behaviors among adolescents who do and do not attend school—US, 1992. MMWR 1994;43(8):129–132.

Centers for Disease Control. Abortion surveillance: preliminary data—United States, 1992. JAMA, 1995;273:371.

Chasnoff IJ, Burns WJ, Schnoll SH, et al. Cocaine use in pregnancy. N Engl J Med 1985;313:666.

Childrens Defense Fund. Declining earnings of young men: their relation to poverty, teen pregnancy, and family formation. May 1987.

Childrens Defense Fund. Adolescent and young adult fathers: problems and solutions. May 1988.

Chow AW, Jewesson PJ. Use and safety of antimicrobial agents during pregnancy. West J Med 1987;146:761.

Cox JE, Bithoney WG. Fathers of children born to adolescent mothers. Predictors of contact with their children at 2 years. Arch Pediatr Adolesc Med 1995;149:962.

Elster, AB, and Roberts, D. The financial impact of a comprehensive adolescent pregnancy program on a university hospital. J Adolesc Health Care 1986;6:17.

Evans J, Selstad G, Welcher W. Teenagers: fertility control behavior and attitudes before and after abortion, childbearing, or negative pregnancy test. Fam Plann Perspect 1976;8:192.

Felice ME, Shragg P, James M, et al. Clinical observations of Mexican-American, Caucasian, and Black pregnant teenagers. J Adolesc Health Care 1986;7: 305.

Felice ME, Shragg P, James M, et al. Psychosocial aspects of Mexican-American, Caucasian, and Black teenage pregnancy. J Adolesc Health Care 1987;8:330.

Finkel M, Finkel D. Male adolescent contraceptive utilization. Adolescence 1978;13:413.

Finkelstein JW, Finkelstein JA, Christie M, et al. Teenage pregnancy and parenthood: outcomes for mother and child. J Adolesc Health Care 1982;3:1.

Flanagan PJ, McGrath MM, Meyer EC, et al. Adolescent development and transitions to motherhood. Pediatrics 1995;96:273.

Fraser AM, Brockert LE, Ward RH. Association of young maternal age with adverse reproductive outcomes. N Engl J Med. 1995;332:1113.

Furstenberg FF Jr, Brooks-Gunn J, et al. Adolescent mothers in later life. New York: Cambridge University Press, 1987.

Garn SM, Petzold AS. Characteristics of the mother and child in teenage pregnancy. Am J Dis Child 1983; 137:365.

Giblin PT, Poland ML, Sachs BA. Effects of social supports on attitudes and health behaviors of pregnant adolescents. J Adolesc Health Care 1987;8:273.

Grimes DA. The contraception report, adolescent pregnancy prevention programs. 1994;5(2):4-5.

Gutierrez Y, King JC. Nutrition during teenage pregnancy. Pediatr Ann 1993;22:2.

Hall JA, Henggler SW, Felice ME. Adolescent substance use during pregnancy. J Pediatr Psychol 1993;18(2): 265-271.

Hardy JB. Preventing adolescent pregnancy: counseling teens and their parents. Medical Aspects of Human Sexuality 1987;(July):32.

Hardy JB. Premature sexual activity, pregnancy, and sexually transmitted diseases: the pediatrician's role as counselor. Pediatr Rev 1988;10:69-76.

Hardy JB, Duggan AK. Teenage fathers and the fathers of infants of urban, teenage mothers. Am J Public Health 1988;78:919.

Hardy JB, Duggan AK, Masnyk K, et al. Fathers of children born to young urban mother. Fam Plann Perspect 1989;21(4):159-163, 187.

Hardy JB, King TM, Repke J. The Johns Hopkins adolescent pregnancy program: an evaluation. Obstet Gynecol 1987;69:300.

Harris L, et al. Sexual material on American network television during the 1987-88 season. New York: Planned Parenthood Federation of America, 1988.

Hatcher RA, Trussell J, Stewart F, et al. Contraceptive technology. 16th and 17th revised eds. New York: Irvington Publishers, 1994 & 1996.

Hausknecht RU. Methotrexate and misoprostol to terminate early pregnancy. N Engl J Med 1995;333: 537.

Hayes CD, ed. Risking the future: adolescent sexuality, pregnancy, and childbearing, vol 1. Washington DC: National Academy Press, 1987.

Helton AS. Women and children, some thoughts on pregnancy, teenagers and family violence. Summit on Crimes Against Women. Background Paper, Houston, September 18, 1990.

Henshaw SK, Van Vort J. Teenage abortion, birth and pregnancy statistics: an update. Fam Plann Perspectives 1989;21:85.

Henshaw S. US teenage pregnancy statistics. New York: AGI, 1993.

Hill LM. Effects of drugs and chemicals on the fetus and newborn, part II. Mayo Clin Proc 1984;59:755.

Hofferth SL, Hayes CD, eds. Risking the future: adolescent pregnancy and childbearing. Working papers and statistical appendixes, vol 2. Washington DC: National Academy Press, 1987.

Hogue CJ, Cates W, Tietze C. Effects of induced abortion on subsequent reproduction. Epidemiol Rev 1982;4:66.

Jaskiewicz JA, McAnarney ER. Pregnancy during adolescence. Pediatr Rev 1994;15(1):32-38.

Jones EF, Forrest DJ, Goldman N, et al. Teenage pregnancy in developed countries: determinants and policy implications. Fam Plann Perspect 1985;17:53.

Kaunitz AM, Grimes DA, Kaunitz KK. A physician's guide to adoption. JAMA 1987;258:3537.

Keeve J, Schlesinger ER, Wight BW, et al. Fertility experience of juvenile girls in a community-wide ten-year study. Am J Publ Health 1969;59:2185.

Kinard EM, Reinherz H. Behavioral and emotional functioning in children of adolescent mothers. Am J Orthopsychiatry 1984;54:578.

Klerman LV. Adolescent pregnancy and parenting: controversies of the past and lessons of the future. J Adolesc Health 1993;14:553-561.

Lancaster JB, Hamburg BA. School-age pregnancy and parenthood: biosocial dimensions. New York: De Gruyter, 1986.

Leland NL, Petersen DJ, Braddock M, et al. Variations in pregnancy outcomes by race among 10-14-year-old mothers in the United States. Public Health Rep 1995;110:53.

Leppert PC, Namerow PB, Barker D. Pregnancy outcomes among adolescent and older women receiving comprehensive prenatal care. J Adolesc Health Care 1987;7:112.

Levin AA, Schoenbaum SC, Monson RR. Association of induced abortion with subsequent pregnancy loss. JAMA 1980;243:2495.

MacGregor SN, Keith LG. Substance abuse in pregnancy—A practical management plan. Female Patient 1989;14:49.

Madden JD, Payne TF, Miller S. Maternal cocaine abuse and effect on the newborn. Pediatrics 1986;77:209.

Makinson C. The health consequences of teenage fertility. Fam Plann Perspect 1985;17:133.

Marsiglio W. Adolescent fathers in the US: their initial living arrangements, marital experience and educational outcomes. Fam Plann Perspect 1987;19:247.

McCarthy J, Menken J. Marriage, remarriage, marital disruption, and age at first birth. Fam Plann Perspect 1979;11:21.

Moore KA, Snyder NO. Facts at a glance, Child Trends. Washington DC: 1994.

Moss NE. Effects of father-daughter contact on use of pregnancy services by Mexican, Mexican-American, and Anglo adolescents. J Adolesc Health Care 1987; 8:419.

Mott FL, Marsiglio W. Early childbearing and completion of high school. Fam Plann Perspect 1985;17:234.

National Center for Health Statistics. Advance report of final natality statistics. Monthly Vital Statistics Report 1983;32(9).

National Center for Health Statistics. Advance report of final natality statistics. Monthly Vital Statistics Report 1984;33(6).

National Center for Health Statistics. Advance report of final natality statistics, 1987. Monthly Vital Statistics Report 1989;(suppl, June).

National Commission to Prevent Infant Mortality. Death before life: the tragedy of infant mortality: appendix. Washington DC: 1988.

Neeson JD, Patterson KA, Mercer RT, et al. Pregnancy outcome for adolescents receiving prenatal care by nurse practitioners in extended roles. J Adolesc Health Care 1983;4:94.

Neinstein, LSN. Issues in reproductive management. New York: Thieme Medical Publishers, 1994.

Nelson KG, Key D, Fletcher JK, et al. The teen-tot clinic: an alternative to traditional care for infants of teenaged mothers. J Adolesc Health Care 1982;3:19.

Paul EW, Schaap P. Legal rights and responsibilities of pregnant teenagers and their children. In: Stuart IR, Wells CF, eds. Pregnancy in adolescence: needs, problems, and management. New York: Van Nostrand Reinhold, 1981.

Peplow PV. RU486 combined with PGE1 analog in voluntary termination of early pregnancy—a comparison of recent findings with gemeprost or misoprostol. Contraception 1994;50:69.

Phipps-Yonas S. Teenager pregnancy and motherhood—a review of the literature. Am J Orthopsychiatry 1980;50:403.

Reis J. Teenage pregnancy and parenthood in Illinois. J Adolesc Health Care 1987;8:177.

Repke JT. Adolescent pregnancy: can we solve the problem. Mayo Clin Proc 1990;65:1152–1154.

Scholl TO, Decker E, Karp RJ, et al. Early adolescent pregnancy: a comparative study of pregnancy outcome in young adolescents and mature women. J Adolesc Health Care 1984;5:167.

Segal S, Anyan WR, Cohen SN, et al. Anticonvulsants and pregnancy. Pediatrics 1979;63:331.

Shiono PH, Klebanoff MA, Rhoads GG. Smoking and drinking during pregnancy. JAMA 1986;255:82.

Stevens-Simon C. Recent developments in adolescent pregnancy. Curr Prob Pediatr 1992;22(7):295–301.

Trussell J, Menken J. Early childbearing and subsequent fertility. Fam Plann Perspect 1978;10:209.

Ulmann A, Silvestre L. RU486: the French experience. Hum Reprod 1994;9:126.

Zabin LS, Hirsch MB, Emerson MR. When urban adolescents choose abortion: effects on education, psychological status, and subsequent pregnancy. Fam Plann Perspect 1989;21:248.

Zabin LS, Smith EA, Hirsch MB, et al. Evaluation of a school and clinic based primary pregnancy prevention program for urban teenagers. Fam Plann Perspect 1986;18:119.

Zelnik M, Kantner JF. Sexual and contraceptive experience of young unmarried women in the United States, 1976 and 1971. Fam Plann Perspect 1977; 9:55.

Zelnik M, Kantner JE. Sexual activity, contraceptive use, and pregnancy among metropolitan area teenagers: 1971–1979. Fam Plann Perspect 1980;12:230.

CHAPTER 43

Contraception

Lawrence S. Neinstein and Anita Nelson

Adolescent sexual activity has increased steadily over the last century, reflecting earlier onset of menarche as well as changing social conditions, although in more recent years sexual activity appears to have plateaued (Alan Guttmacher Institute, 1994; Centers for Disease Control [CDC], 1992). CDC surveys estimate that 5% of 13-year-old males have been sexually active and that by age 19 the average American male has had 5.11 partners. Adolescent women have also increased in their sexual activity: 31% have been sexually active by their freshman year in high school, and 56% have been by their 18th birthday. Overall, 10.4 million of the 17.5 million teens in the 15- to 19-year-old group in 1988 were sexually experienced (Alan Guttmacher Institute, 1994). In the 1992 CDC Youth Behavior Risk Survey, about 43% of adolescents between 14 and 17 had indicated a history of prior sexual intercourse, and about 82% of 18- to 21-year-old adolescents and young adults had a history of prior sexual intercourse. The forces underlying these trends have been outlined in Chapter 40 and the impacts on teenage pregnancy are detailed in Chapter 42.

The trends in sexuality among American adolescents mirror similar trends in teenagers in many developed countries. However, there the similarity ends. The unintended pregnancy rates in developed European countries are 50–85% lower than in the United States due to our lack of societal consensus about birth control, especially when considering adolescents.

Despite this lack of consensus, contraceptive use by adolescents increased dramatically in response to concerns about sexually transmitted disease (STD) transmission in the mid-1980s. Two-thirds of adolescents now report using some form of birth control at the time of first intercourse, usually a male condom, but there are still significant delays in obtaining medical assistance for contraception. Most young women are sexually active for months before they seek medical attention; only 40% seek medical contraceptive services within 12 months after they begin intercourse.

Most sexually active adolescents today in the United States are using contraceptives on an ongoing basis. Recent surveys show that 72% of sexually active 15- to 17-year-olds and 84% of 18- to 19-year-olds use some method of birth control. The success rate of sexually active never-married adolescents in avoiding pregnancy with pill or condom use is roughly equal to that of married 20- to 24-year-olds.

The ideal contraceptive for adolescents would be safe, effective, reversible, inexpensive, convenient, private, and have few side effects. In the following chapters, each of the major methods of birth control is analyzed using this list as a yardstick. Overall, however, several important generalizations must be recognized:

1. Every method of contraception for adolescents is safer than pregnancy.
2. There is no ideal contraceptive method. Every decision about birth control is a compromise.

3. In the absence of an ideal contraceptive, the goal of health-care providers is to have as rich an array of contraceptive choices available to meet the individual needs of patients, respecting their religious and cultural beliefs, and medical conditions.
4. Sexually active adolescents who face two risks (STDs and unintended pregnancy) are candidates for two interventions: one method for STD risk reduction (condoms, safer sex practices) and another to effectively reduce pregnancy (usually hormonal contraception).
5. Compliance with contraception depends on motivation, which, in turn, depends on patient education and understanding. Age-appropriate counseling and patient education is crucial.
6. Noncontraceptive benefits offered by birth control methods should be considered when selecting methods.
7. Adolescents with chronic medical problems have a more complex decision in determining the balance between risk and benefits.

To effectively impact on the unintended pregnancy, health providers must be familiar with each of the methods of birth control and should closely analyze their practices to ensure teens' effective access to those methods. This chapter provides an overview of efficacy and safety of reversible contraceptives, a discussion of the key elements needed to ensure access and to integrate family planning services into comprehensive care, and a summary highlighting the special contraceptive needs of adolescents with chronic medical problems. Subsequent chapters discuss specific contraceptive techniques in detail.

Contraceptive Efficacy

The measure of the effectiveness of a method of contraception is its failure rate. Even though a wide range of failure rates has been developed for each method estimating failure rates with perfect use, user failure, and method failure, the clinically appropriate estimate of efficacy is

Table 43.1. First-Year Failure Rates by Contraceptive Method

	Women Experiencing Pregnancy (%)	
	Typical Use	Perfect Use
Implant	0.09	0.09
Injectable	0.3	0.3
IUD		
Copper T380A	0.7	0.6
Progesterone T	2.0	1.5
Oral contraceptive		
Combined	2.5–6.0	0.1
Progestin-only	3.0–10.0	0.5
Male condom	12.0	3.0
Diaphragm with spermicide	16.0–18.0	6.0
Cervical cap	17.4	6.0
Withdrawal	19.0	4.0
Periodic abstinence	20.0	
Calendar "rhythm"		9.0
Cervical mucus		3.0
Symptothermal		2.0
Spermicides	21.0	6.0
Female condom	21.0–26.0	5.0
No method	85.0	85.0

FDA labeled rates noted are adapted from Hatcher RA, Trussell J, Stewart F, et al. Contraceptive technology, 16th revised ed. New York: Irvington Publishers, 1994 and Jones EF, Forrest JD. Contraceptive failure rates based on 1988 NSFG. Fam Plann Perspect 1992;24(1):12.

the *typical failure rate*. This is the number that best reflects the pregnancy rate in actual use by the average patient. Other estimates, such as perfect use failure rates, may provide motivation to encourage patient compliance but should not be routinely quoted as realistic estimates. While precise estimates of efficacy may vary, the following tables are provided to give a basis for patient counseling and insight into factors that affect outcome. Table 43.1 summarizes for each birth control method the typical failure rates and the perfect use failure rates. Table 43.2 estimates the range failure rates for adolescents compared to averages for all users where differences exist. Table 43.3 shows the profound influence income and marital status have on failure rates.

As a general rule adolescents have an extremely distorted estimate of contraceptive efficacy. For many of the younger teens, the concept of probabilities is difficult to comprehend. They tend to think of risk as an all-or-nothing proposition. Some teens who are told

TABLE 43.2.   Estimates of Highest and Lowest Age-Specific Failure Rates

	Age	Lowest	Highest
Implants	15–44	0.05	0.5
Injectables	15–44	0.3	0.4
Intrauterine devices[a]	15–19	2.2	6.3
	15–44	2.5	4.5
Oral contraceptives	15–19	8.0	18.1
	15–44	3.8	8.7
Condom	15–19	11.4	19.3
	15–44	9.8	18.5
Diaphragm or cervical cap	15–19	10.6	35.5
	15–44	12.0	38.9
Withdrawal	15–44	14.7	27.8
Spermicides	15–19	29.7	35.0
	15–44	21.6	25.6
Periodic abstinence	15–19	25.1	34.1
	15–44	13.8	19.2

Adapted from Alan Guttmacher Institute. Preventing pregnancy, protecting health: a new look at birth control choice in the United States. New York: Alan Guttmacher Institute, 1991.
[a]Mixture of intrauterine devices.

TABLE 43.3.   First-Year Contraceptive Failure Rates by Income, Age, and Marital Status

	Failure Rate	
Marital Status, Income, and Age	Pill	Condom
Never married, <200% of poverty		
<20	12.9	27.3
20–24	15.0	31.1
25–29	12.8	27.0
Ever married, <200% of poverty		
<20	26.8	51.3
20–24	14.0	29.3
25–29	8.8	19.0
Never married, ≥200% of poverty		
<20	5.9	13.2
20–24	6.9	15.2
25–29	5.9	13.0
Ever married, ≥200% of poverty		
<20	12.9	
20–24	6.4	14.2
25–29	4.0	6.9

Adapted from Jones EF, Forrest JD. Contraceptive failure rates based on the 1988 NSFG. Fam Plann Perspect 1992;24(1):12.

that they will become pregnant if they engage in intercourse are genuinely surprised after a few short months that they have not conceived. However, misunderstanding about efficacy is pervasive and extends beyond probability concepts. The American College of Obstetricians and Gynecologists (ACOG, 1994) commissioned Gallop to survey patient attitudes in 1985 and 1993; these surveys clearly reveal misconceptions about contraceptive risk and benefits by all age groups. Over 40% of those surveyed estimated the first-year failure rate of the birth control pill to be in excess of 10%; 23% thought the failure rate was at least 20%. Combining the teenager's underestimating the efficacy of existing methods of birth control with the teen's intrinsic sense of invulnerability result in a high level of unintended pregnancy.

CONTRACEPTIVE SAFETY

The message practitioners must provide to all sexually active adolescents and those contemplating coitus is that all methods of birth control are safer for a young woman's health than pregnancy. Only abstinence is truly safe, but every method of birth control significantly reduces the health hazards compared to the real health hazards associated with pregnancy. Table 43.4 provides estimates by age of the risk of mortality per 100,000 women using various methods of contraception. It should be noted that much of the "risk" associated with each of the methods represents the hazards caused by pregnancy, which result from contraceptive failure.

Despite the proven safety of contraception, patient concerns about contraceptive safety are widespread. In the 1993 Gallop poll of attitudes toward use of contraceptives, nearly two-thirds of Americans incorrectly reported that taking birth control pills was at least as hazardous to health as pregnancy (ACOG, 1994). The wide discrepancy between observed clinical safety of contraceptives and public perception is in part fostered by the techniques used to measure contraceptive efficacy in Food and Drug Administration (FDA) trials. The default option to contraception is always assumed to be abstinence. Benefits for contraception never accrue for maternal deaths prevented. Instead, the side effects of the method are tallied and stand alone with no benefits to counterbalance them in the patient's eyes.

Adolescents are particularly vulnerable to misinformation. Often they count on peer group members for advice. But even when teens consult adult authorities, those experts may not be well informed. Surveys of school sex education teachers demonstrate serious lack of information. When true-false questions were administered to over 1300 sex education teachers, only 72% answered correctly that having a baby was a greater risk for a teenager than taking the pill; only 30% knew that the statement "Pill use by teenagers may have a detrimental effect on later fertility" was false; and only 23% correctly said that the statement "Pill use should be stopped periodically to give the body a rest" was false.

TABLE 43.4.   Risk of Death by Contraceptive Method and Age

Method of Control and Outcome	Age					
	15–19	20–24	25–29	30–34	35–39	40–44
No fertility control methods	7.0	7.4	9.1	14.8	25.7	28.2
Oral contraceptives nonsmokers	0.3	0.5	0.9	1.9	13.8	31.6
Oral contraceptives smokers	2.2	3.4	6.6	13.5	51.1	117.2
Intrauterine device	0.8	0.8	1.0	1.0	1.0	1.4
Condom	1.1	1.6	0.7	0.2	0.3	0.4
Diaphragm or spermicide	1.9	1.2	1.2	1.3	2.2	2.8
Periodic abstinence	2.5	1.6	1.6	1.7	2.9	3.6

Adapted from Ory HW. Mortality associated with fertility and fertility control—1983. Fam Plann Perspect 1983;15:57-63.

ACCESS TO CONTRACEPTIVE SERVICES AS PART OF COMPREHENSIVE HEALTH CARE

Adolescent patients are confronted with several challenges in accessing contraceptive services, which can be classified into the following groups of concerns:

1. Access to low cost medical services: Adolescents often have limited discretionary income. Even low-cost medical services can be prohibitively expensive for them. Lack of familiarity with large managed care systems can functionally limit access. Once in a system, the teen must find providers to address their issues. Adolescents often wish to discuss issues of sexuality and contraception with their providers but are reluctant to introduce the subjects themselves. This reluctance, as well as a provider's hesitancy, results in a wide discrepancy between what teens want to discuss and what they do discuss with their primary health-care physicians (Table 43.5).

2. Access to confidential services: Health-care providers are pledged to maintain patient confidentiality but are faced with several special challenges with adolescent patients. The wishes of the patients and their parents may conflict; this causes extreme frustration, especially when the parents are paying for the patient's care. Any failure to disclose information to the parents can result in the loss of the patient from the practice. As adults and parents themselves, providers may feel sympathetic to the parents' desire to have complete access to information about their children. Finally, even if the provider were immune to all these pressures personally, the insurance billing system often discloses facts about services provided to the teen, which seriously compromises confidentiality. The bill for pregnancy testing destroys confidentiality for the teen who had not told her parents she was sexually active. Providers trapped in such situations may have to refer their patients to settings where confidentiality can be better preserved, such as free or low-cost family planning clinics.

3. Access to age-appropriate services: Modern media have profoundly impacted adolescent attitudes toward sex and adolescents' communication or learning styles. Estimates are that the average teen witnesses 14,000 instances of sexual behavior on television each year. This visualization may not have increased the accuracy of the teen's database on sexuality and its risks, but it increases the teen's curiosity and expectations and significantly influences behavior.

    The medium itself has also transformed adolescent learning styles. Attention spans have been constricted to the 45-second sound bite. In the age of MTV, written handouts may have very limited educational benefit. If written materials are used, they must be corrected for age-appropriate literacy and for short reader attention spans. Furthermore, since many adolescents may not have confided in their parents that they are sexually active, written materials found in their possession might be incriminating. Videotapes

TABLE 43.5.   Adolescents' Desires to Discuss Sexuality Issues versus Actual Discussion with Physicians

Topic	Teens Wanting to Discuss (%)	Actual Physician Discussion (%)
Sexually transmitted diseases	70	18
Contraception	66	22
Menstruation	55	47
Sexual functioning	53	24
Sexual characteristic	50	23
Sexual abuse	36	6

Adapted from Malus M, LaChauce PA, Lamy L, et al. Priorities in adolescent health care: the teenager's viewpoint. J Fam Pract 1987;25:159–162; and Braverman PK, Strasburger VC. Contraception. Clin Pediatr 1993;32(12):725–734.

played in the office prior to the provider interaction are quite helpful, as are individual counseling sessions with nursing staff trained in dealing with teens. Peer counselors are also effective adjuncts in outreach programs and in practice settings.

In providing contraceptive services to adolescents it is crucial to remember that adolescents are not just younger versions of adults. They are in transition to adulthood and progress through different developmental stages with different thought processes over time. While each adolescent progresses through the stages at different rates, there are some generalizations that are helpful in providing counseling.

Adolescents aged 12–14 are in early adolescence. Traditionally, they struggle for autonomy, identify with same-sex peer groups, and are preoccupied with body image. They are very concrete thinkers and somewhat self-centered. Effective communication tools for those teens are very concrete (rather than abstract), written in pictographic style (rather than tables or graphs), and clearly deal with issues that most concern these patients (such as weight gain and acne).

Adolescents aged 15–17 are strongly attached to their peer groups and have concerns with appeal to the opposite sex. Often they are risk takers and view themselves as invincible. They have a strong urge to prove their autonomy. A health-care system that is perceived by teens as an authority figure trying to control them because the providers *tell* them what to do or *threaten* them with an unfavorable outcome, runs the risk of inciting rebellion in the adolescent. It is crucial to have the teenager (and possibly his peers) identify with the health-care message to ensure compliance and success. Peer counseling (if carefully selected) can be effective with this age group.

Older adolescents aged 18 and 19 often have achieved more adult abstract reasoning and respond well to more traditional counseling approaches.

4. Access to teen-friendly services: Most adolescents do not get out of school until late in the afternoon and may have difficulty keeping appointments during the usual office hours, particularly if they have limited access to transportation and are trying to maintain privacy. Late afternoon or early evening office hours or weekend availability can enhance adolescent access to services. Privacy needs may also limit the times and ways that the teen can interact with a health-care provider. The adolescent who calls from a pay phone to ask about a contraceptive side effect cannot be put on hold and cannot be called back later when the provider is between patients. One successful arrangement is to identify someone on the staff to answer such calls and arrange the staff person's lunch hour around the teen's schedule. Since the teen interacts with all members of the staff, each should be selected and trained to be responsive to teens and their special needs.

5. Access to broader community-based programs: Each of the access issues listed above is relevant at the individual provider level. To make even more impact on adolescent pregnancy rates and teenage sexuality, demonstration projects have shown us that broader community-based programs are needed. One recent study of a comprehensive project that increased teen awareness of and accessibility to family planning services was provided in a large metropolitan area in Philadelphia. Two years later, there was no detectable change in teen pregnancy rates, contraceptive use, or understanding. On the other hand, a program that involved media, local clergy, and schools and emphasized decision making, communication skills, self-esteem enhancement, and human reproduction in a section of South Carolina county saw the pregnancy rate for 14- to 17-year-old women fall from 67 per 1000 to 25 per 1000. After removal of key providers and support elements, the pregnancy rate rose again. Other studies using peer counseling in schools and nurse practitioner counselors in off-campus sites have also been successful, but a coordinated effort that focuses on the root causes of teen sexuality has even more leverage.

The practitioner must be aware of whether his or her own office or clinic hours and setup are conducive to adolescent health-care needs. In addition, the practitioner should be aware of available sources of referral for services such as contraception, STD treatment, and therapeutic abortions.

GENERAL CONSIDERATIONS IN METHOD SELECTION

In counseling adolescent patients it is crucial to determine their knowledge base, motivations, and personal characteristics and conditions:

1. Knowledge base: Adolescents can be very embarrassed to describe their own understanding of sexual activity and contraception when directly questioned. Reflective questions such as "What would you tell a friend who was thinking about having sex?" can be richly revealing about teen attitudes and understanding.
2. Motivation: Effective counseling of teens to aid them in selecting birth control methods requires that the provider know:
   a. What is the teen's sexual history?
   b. How important is it to the teen to avoid pregnancy, and what is the teen's perception of the risks of pregnancy?
   c. What is the teen's understanding about STD risks?
   d. What is the teen's relationship with her or his partner(s), and what does the teen believe her or his partner's childbearing plans are?
   e. What concerns does the teen have about contraception in general and any of the methods offered?
   f. How much control does the teen have over sexual activity and contraceptive use?
   g. How would the teen react to contraceptive side effects?
3. Personal characteristics and conditions: The living conditions and personal characteristics of the teen (particularly the young woman) profoundly influence the selection and use of a contraceptive.
   a. How strong is the teen's self-esteem? Her upward mobility?
   b. Does she have siblings or friends who have been sexually active, used birth control, or become pregnant?
   c. Will it be possible to integrate any given method into the teen's lifestyle (private space for birth control pills, access to condoms)?
   d. What is the frequency of intercourse? Is it anticipatable?
   e. Is the teen able to discuss or negotiate with the partner(s)?
   f. Is the teen comfortable touching genitals?

RECOMMENDED CONTRACEPTIVE METHODS FOR TEENS

The most frequently recommended methods of contraception for adolescents include:

1. Condoms and spermicides
2. Oral contraceptives
3. Injectable progestins
4. Long-acting contraceptive implants

Regardless of the method used, the teen should use a latex condom for every act of intercourse to protect against STDs. Each of these methods and the advantages and disadvantages are discussed in depth in the next several chapters, but a summary follows below.

Condoms plus spermicides are recommended for first intercourse, sporadic intercourse, and for females who cannot tolerate or use hormones. Oral contraceptives (plus condoms) are useful for adolescents who would like regular menstrual cycles, can remember to take a pill every day, and can use estrogen. Injectable progestins (plus condoms) are useful for teens who want the convenience of not remembering a daily pill (or who have a contraindication to estrogen) but do not mind having irregular menses or amenorrhea. The long-acting contraceptive implants (plus condoms) are useful for those teens who want the maximum amount of protection and convenience, do not want a pregnancy for at least several years, and do not mind irregular menses. Emergency postcoital contraception should be more widely available for teens to prevent many unwanted pregnancies. However, it is a method that should be followed with a more ongoing method of contraception.

The following methods are not frequently used in adolescents but could be used in highly selected teens: intrauterine devices (IUDs), diaphragms, and cervical caps.

CONTRACEPTIVE CONSIDERATIONS IN ADOLESCENTS WITH CHRONIC ILLNESSES OR DISABILITY

As many as 10–20% of all children and adolescents experience a chronic illness or disability by age 20. Sexuality issues, including the contraceptive needs in this group of patients, are often forgotten by health professionals. When contraception is discussed, accurate advice is often difficult to obtain. Most information about the effects of each of the methods of birth control is based on experience with healthy subjects. As a result, theoretical concerns and small scale studies have an exaggerated impact on "knowledge" about the safety of birth control methods for patients with medical problems. Often lost in concern for possible adverse impacts that contraceptive methods may have is consideration of the problems that would result from pregnancy. Providers must strike a balance between these two risks.

Outstanding references are now available detailing the impacts of contraceptive methods on a wide array of medical conditions based on comprehensive review of the literature (Neinstein, 1994) or from expert consensus conferences (Grimes et al., 1993). The following attempts to summarize the concerns and conclusions of those authors for a select subset of diseases most likely to be found in the adolescent population.

Cardiac or Thromboembolic Disease

Hypertension, Thromboembolic Disease

1. Patients with mild or well-controlled hypertension may be considered for low-dose combination oral contraceptives or progestin-only methods (implant, injections, minipill), particularly in the absence of other risk factors such as smoking, diabetes, hyperlipidemia, or obesity. Selection of a particular method should also consider the method's impacts on lipid profile, glucose tolerance, and weight.
2. Progestin-only methods (implant, injections, minipill) may be used in patients with history of thromboembolic disease or pulmonary embolism despite warnings on package labeling. Contraceptives containing estrogen would be contraindicated in patients with any of these thrombotic histories unless the patients are anticoagulated.
3. IUDs may be used if the patient is otherwise an IUD candidate.
4. Barrier and natural family planning (NFP) methods are associated with higher failure rates and, if selected, must be fastidiously used.
5. For severely affected patients in whom pregnancy could be life- threatening, sterilization should be offered. Those with progressive disease might consider early childbearing with subsequent sterilization.

Significant Valvular Disease

1. Oral contraceptives and injections provide ovulation suppression and reduce the risk of internal hemorrhage associated with monthly oocyte extrusion in anticoagulated patients. Nonanticoagulated patients with significant valvular disease should not be offered oral contraceptives.
2. Progestin-only methods (implants, injections, and minipills) must be evaluated for their effects on fluid retention but often are quite useful.
3. IUD use may be feasible, but appropriate American Heart Association antibiotic prophylaxis must be used at insertion and removal. The IUD's effects on menstrual flow should be considered, since anticoagulation itself increases menorrhagia.
4. Barrier methods do not directly affect cardiac disorders but may be associated with unacceptably high failure rates, which could present a health hazard to the adolescent.

Neurological Disease

Epilepsy

1. Oral contraceptives do not have a clinical impact on the frequency or intensity of seizures despite the theoretical concern that estrogen lowers seizure threshold and increases spike amplitude. Balancing the estrogen in the pill is the progestin, which has opposite effects. More significant are the interactions between anticonvulsants and sex steroids. Virtually all anticonvulsants (except valproic acid) increase cytochrome P-450 activity and increase the metabolic clearance of the sex steroids. Therefore, the use of triphasic and ultra low dose oral contraceptive formulations should be avoided; the lowest dose that should be used is 35 µg of ethinyl estradiol. If breakthrough bleeding persists for more than 3 months on the 35-µg dose, a higher dose pill (50 µg) should be considered. Estrogen may speed the metabolism of anticonvulsants, and serum levels should be rechecked after initiation of oral contraceptives.
2. Anticonvulsants that increase the clearance of the already low doses of levonorgestrel from the Norplant System significantly increase the system's first-year failure rates to 20%. The Norplant device should be avoided in these individuals.
3. Medroxyprogesterone acetate (DMPA; (Depo-Provera) is an outstanding choice for teens with seizure disorders, since progestins themselves are weak anticonvulsants. The circulating levels of DMPA are sufficiently high as to be unaffected by increased cytochrome P-450 activity. Furthermore, ultimate amenorrhea associated with injections can be helpful to women suffering anticonvulsant-induced hypermenorrhea.
4. IUDs are extremely effective for appropriate candidates (parous women in stable, mutually monogamous relationships) but the impact of copper-containing IUDs on menstrual flow should be considered. Progestin IUDs may also be used.
5. Barrier methods and NFP have higher failure rates. The teratogenicity of anticonvulsants makes these a less attractive choice.

Headaches The concern with the use of combination pills in women with migraine headaches centers on estrogen's impact on coagulation factors and the possibility that, in the face of severe vasoconstriction, increased coagulation factors will predispose vulnerable patients to thrombus formation and stroke. Patients with underlying migraine headaches with neurologic prodromes (auras) are not candidates for combined oral contraceptives. Other migraine patients may well be candidates for all forms of hormonal contraception, but they should be closely followed to ensure there is no worsening of the intensity or frequency of the migraines, especially those receiving estrogen-containing preparations.

All hormonal methods of birth control have been associated with increased complaints of headaches. If headaches are severe and not responsive to over-the-counter therapies, the hormonal contraceptive may need to be discontinued. Implant users who experience new onset or significant worsening of headaches should undergo fundoscopic examination to rule out papilledema associated with pseudotumor cerebri. If papilledema is discovered, the implants should be removed.

IUDs, barriers, and NFP have no impacts on headaches.

Pulmonary Disease

Asthma   Some theoretical concern has been raised about estrogen effect on mucus production and progestin's thickening of it, but studies fail to find any consistent association between oral contraceptive use and asthma attacks. Only minimal drug-drug interactions exist between asthma medication and hormonal methods of contraception, but patients using medications hepatically cleared should have the levels rechecked after starting to use oral contraceptives, especially if there is a suspicion of clinical deterioration. Decreased clearance of aminophylline may require a reduction in dose by about 30%, depending on the strength of the oral contraceptive used. Other methods of birth control have no impact on asthma. However, patients using steroids have reduced ability to fight infection and are not candidates for IUDs.

Cystic Fibrosis   The major potential side effect that exists with oral contraceptives and individuals with cystic fibrosis involves the effect of progesterone on mucus. Progesterone causes thick cervical mucus, and this same effect could lead to thick bronchial mucus. A preliminary study by Fitzpatrick et al. (1984) suggests that oral contraceptives may not exacerbate pulmonary disease. However, oral contraceptives should be used with extreme caution in teens with cystic fibrosis until further studies indicate that they are safe in such patients.

Gastrointestinal Disease

Inflammatory Bowel Disease   If disease is active or malabsorption exists, oral contraceptive pill use is not appropriate. Parenteral hormonal methods (implants and injections) bypass the enteric absorption problems and can therefore be used. In teens with stable quiescent inflammatory bowel disease, oral contraceptives can be used with caution under close monitoring for possible impact on disease activity. IUDs would be feasible in appropriate candidates unless the patient is immunocompromised by steroid use. Barrier methods and NFP are not contraindicated, but enthusiasm for them is tempered by their higher pregnancy rates.

Hepatitis   Contraceptive steroids alter hepatocellular function and rely on hepatic metabolism for clearance. Hormonal methods are contraindicated during active liver disease or cirrhosis. Following a bout of acute hepatitis, liver function test results should be normalizing before initiating hormonal contraceptives. IUDs may be acceptable in appropriately selected teens unless the hepatitis was sexually transmitted. Barrier methods and NFP are not contraindicated. Patients with hepatitis B should be tested for continued infectious status with surface antigen. Sex partners should be tested and, if not immune, should be vaccinated. Male condoms should be added until partner immunity is established.

Endocrine Disease

Diabetes Mellitus   There has been a dramatic change in contraceptive practices for women with diabetes in the last decade due to an increased appreciation of the safety of low-dose oral contraceptives in this high-risk population.

1. Development of diabetes mellitus: Older studies of patients using oral contraceptives demonstrated an increased risk of developing reversible glucose intolerance. However, more recent studies, including the Royal College of General Practitioners' study (Hannaford and Kay, 1989), demonstrate no evidence of an increased risk of glucose intolerance among healthy current users of modern formulations. Even among women with previous history of gestational diabetes, Kjos et al. (1990) found no difference in glucose tolerance between women with recent gestational diabetes who were assigned to different low-dose oral contraceptives and to nonhormonal contraceptive methods. Their conversion to overt diabetes was not accelerated by the use of oral contraceptives. Skouby et al. (1984) found a decrease in insulin sensitivity in women with histories of gestational diabetes, but not of sufficient magnitude to alter glucose tolerance as measured by serum glucose or insulin levels.

2. Glucose control in women with diabetes mellitus: For women with diabetes, studies have also examined the effect of oral contraceptives on glucose control. Skouby et al. (1984) compared the metabolic effects of four oral contraceptive formulations in insulin-dependent diabetic women. They found no differences in fasting glucose, 24-hour insulin requirements, glycosylated hemoglobin, low-density lipoprotein (LDL) cholesterol or the high-density lipoprotein (HDL) cholesterol–to–total cholesterol ratio between each treatment group. Steel and Duncan (1978) evaluated insulin-dependent women taking a combination low-dose oral contraceptive. There were no problems in maintaining glucose control; 81% required no changes in insulin at all. Glycemic control does not seem to be a major problem in insulin-dependent women taking combination oral contraceptives.

3. Progestin-only pills: Progestin-only pills have lower doses of progestin and have an even lower impact on glucose tolerance. Steel and Duncan (1978) found no changes in insulin requirements in 45 insulin-dependent women using norethindrone 0.35 mg/day. However, there is a higher failure rate with progestin-only oral contraceptives, and they do not offer the estrogen-related noncontraceptive benefits of the combination pill.

4. Other hormonal methods: The impact of other hormonal methods of birth control on glucose tolerance has not been studied in diabetic women. Implants have been found to have very minimal effect on glucose tolerance in normal subjects. During clinical trials, patients demonstrated no change in fasting blood sugar levels or in 2-hour postglucose tolerance test levels when tested prior to capsule placement and after 2 years of use. The 1-hour test value of the 2-hour glucose tolerance test did show slight elevation. Progestin injections have a more profound impact on glucose tolerance test results, affecting both insulin and glucose levels, although all values stayed within normal ranges in nondiabetic subjects. While these changes in normal subjects may have clinical relevance for overt diabetics, the benefits of ease and efficacy of the injections may outweigh the risks associated with changes in glucose levels or increased insulin dosages.

5. Effect on cardiovascular disease: Another critical issue for diabetics is the impact of contraceptives on cardiovascular disease. Oral contraceptives have been thought to affect coronary artery disease via several potentially conflicting mechanisms. Considerable interest has been focused on the impacts oral contraceptives have on lipoprotein profiles. Estrogen is known to increase HDL cholesterol and triglycerides and lower LDL cholesterol. Progestins (androgen derivatives) in oral contraceptives have had an opposite ef-

fect by lowering HDL and raising LDL. Some progestins (desogestrel, norgestimate) have been developed to minimize their androgenicity; others have minimal effect (norethindrone). Dosage also influences the net balance between estrogen and progestin effect of any formulation. Two studies evaluating insulin-dependent diabetic women taking oral contraceptives failed to find significant changes in lipoproteins or HDL fractions. Implants have essentially neutral impacts on lipoproteins, but progestin-only injections may depress HDL and increase LDL.

There are no prospective studies showing a significant increase in cardiac and cerebrovascular complications in diabetic women using oral contraceptives. Studies of oral conceptives' effect on retinopathy and hypertension are conflicting, but the conflict may be due to the different strength formulations studied. The Royal College of General Practitioners' study (Hannaford and Kay, 1989) demonstrated a direct relationship between the amount of progestin in oral contraceptives and the incidence of major vascular disease. Two recent studies indicate no change in cardiovascular risk profile (Petersen et al, 1994) or renal or retinal complications (Garg et al., 1994) in diabetic women taking oral contraceptives.

It is now understood that the lipids play only a minor role in estimating the influence oral contraceptives have on cardiovascular disease. The older model of the pill inducing progressively worsening atherosclerotic plaques as a result of adverse lipid effects has been abandoned due to the lack of epidemiological support for it. Exusers of pills have no higher risk of coronary artery disease than never users. There is no duration of pill use relationship with risk for coronary artery disease. Animal models using monkeys have shown a disassociation between lipid values and atherosclerotic plaque size in coronary arteries (Clarkson et al., 1990). Studies in Puget Sound (Porter et al., 1987), Walnut Creek (Ramcharan et al., 1981), and Finland (Hirvonen and Idānpāān-Heikkilā, 1990) all show decreased risk of death from cardiovascular disease in oral contraceptive users compared to nonusers, even in the older age groups. These benefits are thought to be mediated by estrogen impact. Progestin-only methods have not been studied as closely but in clinical trials did not seem to increase the risk of cardiovascular disease.

6. IUD use: For several decades, IUDs were the method of choice for diabetics. For a short time, the FDA labeling on the Copper T380A IUD listed diabetes as a contraindication, fearing immunosuppression. Today most labeling has been changed, and diabetic women can again be considered for IUD use if they are in stable, mutually monogamous relationships.

7. Barrier methods: Barrier methods offer risk reduction from STDs, which could be more difficult to successfully treat in diabetic patients and should be considered an adjunct for every woman at risk for STDs. However, the relatively high failure rates of barrier methods used by themselves for pregnancy prevention must be considered. Similarly, NFP should be reserved only for those patients with personal beliefs or other concerns preventing them from using other more effective methods.

8. Adolescents with diabetes mellitus: Adolescents with diabetes mellitus are a particularly important subgroup. Fennoy (1989) found that they were at higher risk than expected to become pregnant at a time when their glucose control was often at its worse. Adolescents are also less likely to have developed vascular complications than older diabetics and may be the best to use low-dose birth control pills. The presence of additional risk factors for cardiovascular disease (such as smoking or hypertension) requires careful reevaluation of the risk-benefit ratio for oral contraceptive use. Implants may be attractive due to their glucose and lipid neutrality. Progestin injections add privacy to the element of convenience but have more notable deleterious impacts of glucose control and lipid profile, which necessitates careful consideration of benefits and risks. All diabetics using hormonal methods of birth control require ongoing monitoring.

Thyroid Disease   There have been no reports of complications in individuals with thyroid disease who are using oral contraceptives. Oral contraceptives do increase thyroid-binding globulin and thus cause an increase in total thyroxine. However, adjusted thyroxine levels and free thyroxine levels are normal.

Oligomenorrhea and Amenorrhea   The cause of menstrual irregularity should be identified, since it may require therapy (e.g., hypothyroidism, prolactinoma) or may profoundly influence contraceptive choices (e.g., polycystic ovary syndrome, lactational amenorrhea, exercise-induced amenorrhea). For example, women with exercise-induced amenorrhea may require estrogen supplementation to prevent osteoporosis, in which case combination oral contraceptives may be ideal. Women with a long history of oligomenorrhea have a higher prevalence of infertility and must be reminded that although oral contraceptives will regulate menses when the pills are used, the patient's menstrual irregularities will return after cessation of the pills. The pills will not influence their long-term fertility when they are stopped. Timing of method initiation may present some challenges for other methods. The only method that might be impossible for women with irregular menses to use is NFP.

Hematological Disorders

Iron Deficiency Anemia   Hormonal methods of birth control can be helpful for patients with iron deficiency anemia, since they tend to limit menstrual flow. Long-term use of progestin injections usually results in amenorrhea, which is extremely attractive to patients with anemia. Copper-bearing IUDs should be discouraged in the face of severe anemia, but progesterone IUDs may be used, since they do not increase menstrual blood loss. Barrier methods and NFP have no direct effects on anemia.

Hemorrhagic Disorders   Hormonal methods of birth control are excellent choices for patients with hemorrhagic disorders. They tend to diminish the menorrhagia many women with hemorrhagic disorders suffer by limiting or eliminating menstrual flow. Oral contraceptives and progestin injections also suppress ovarian function and decrease the ever-present risk of hemorrhage with ovulation. There are several reports of progestational compounds lessening bleeding tendencies in patients with factor X deficiency or von Willebrand's disease (Neinstein, 1994).

Sickle Cell Hemoglobinopathies   Earlier concerns that estrogen-containing oral contraceptives might worsen sickling episodes have been diminished by clinical experience and the realization that estrogen's effects on the coagulation cascade is mediated via the extrinsic pathway, and it does not increase sickling. Progestin-only methods are also excellent choices. In particular, injections are very popular with sickle cell anemia patients because of the decrease in bleeding and also the sense of enhanced well-being they engender. Copper-bearing IUDs tend to induce heavier menstrual bleeding and could aggravate problems of anemia. Barrier methods and NFP would have no deleterious effects.

Oncology

Concerns among teens with tumors may be twofold: (*a*) effects of pregnancy or contraception on the tumor and (*b*) effects of the treatment of the tumor on pregnancy and fertility.

1. Effects of treatment on fertility: Byrne et al. (1987) indicate that radiation therapy directed below the diaphragm depressed fertility in males and females by about 25%.

Chemotherapy with alkylating agents with or without radiation to sites below the diaphragm was associated with a 60% fertility in males. In females there was no apparent effect with chemotherapy when used alone and a mild fertility deficit when combined with radiation below the diaphragm. Age also is a factor in that chemotherapy in prepubertal individuals seems to cause less damage than to individuals receiving chemotherapy after puberty. Radiation and chemotherapy have also been reported to cause fetal wastage and malformations. It is recommended that pregnancy be avoided until 1 year after successful chemotherapy.

2. Effects of hormones or pregnancy on tumor: No evidence exists that pregnancy or oral contraceptives have an adverse effect on nonhormonal-dependent tumors. Adolescents with such tumors should use an effective contraceptive and should time pregnancy based on therapy schedule, severity of disease, prognosis, and preference of the patient.

Psychiatric Disease and Mental Retardation

Mentally ill adolescents often have their family planning needs overlooked or their sexuality is seen as acting out or a manifestation of their underlying disease. Once recognized as having contraceptive needs, these patients may have difficulty providing informed consent or in effectively using a contraceptive method. Many mentally ill patients, even in adolescence, have dual diagnoses, such as substance abuse and mental illness (often depression) or epilepsy. Barrier methods may provide needed reduction of risk of STDs but may not be consistently used by these patients. IUDs are usually not appropriate because these patients often are in unstable relationships. Hormonal methods may be preferable with the following caveats:

1. Depression may be exacerbated by any of the hormonal methods. Patients with severe depression, especially with suicidal ideation, are not candidates for hormone methods. Others with more mild disease may be considered for hormonal methods but must be closely monitored for signs or symptoms of deterioration.
2. Women who are also treated for convulsive disorders must have that problem factored into method selection (see above).
3. Institutionalized patients or those who are in stable settings may benefit from daily oral contraceptives. However, those whose living arrangements are less secure (such as the homeless) may not be able to comply with a daily regimen and will benefit from long-acting agents.
4. Severely afflicted paranoid patients may not accept implants.
5. Mentally retarded adolescents: Mentally retarded patients also require special consideration. Sexual education is often neglected in these patients, leading to unprotected exploration. Many are vulnerable to exploitation. Since the introduction of modern birth control methods in the mid-1950s, the birthrate of mentally retarded women has increased compared to the decrease seen in other women. The provider faces both legal questions and practical problems in trying to assess the patient's understanding of alternative methods and ability to apply the selected method effectively. Hormonal contraceptives usually do not encounter any medical contraindications, but long-term compliance with contraceptives in noncontrolled environments is very low. In a study of mentally retarded female adolescents (Chamberlain et al., 1984), there was only a 32% 1-year continuation rate with oral contraceptives. Satisfaction was highest with injectable contraception. Implants require patient cooperation for insertion and removal without general anesthesia. Severely retarded patients may not be able to comply. Injections offer effective intermediate-term contraception and usually the additional benefit of ultimate amenorrhea. IUDs may have

application in patients able to check strings each month and who are in stable, mutually monogamous relationships. Barrier methods and NFP have no adverse effects on women who are mentally retarded but the severely compromised patient may not be capable of understanding how to use the methods.

Connective Tissue Disease

Systemic Lupus Erythematosus   Systemic lupus erythematosus (SLE) has been closely related to hormones. The strong bias in the female-to-male ratio and the relative frequency of flares during pregnancy raise concerns for the use of estrogen-containing hormonal contraceptives. Although only small scale studies, usually without control groups, have been conducted, many authorities would caution against the use of combination oral contraceptives in patients with SLE or limit their use cautiously to women with very mild lupus with no hypertension or vascular involvement. Progestin-only methods appear safe in most women with lupus; in studies to date there have been no significant differences in numbers of episodes of active SLE in progestin users versus controls. Care should be taken to minimize infection risk with insertion if implants are selected. Some SLE patients experience depression; this must be considered when choosing a hormonal method. IUDs are not recommended because SLE patients are immunocompromised. Barrier methods have the least number of associated side effects and offer STD risk reduction; however, they have high rates of pregnancy, which can pose serious hazards to the woman with SLE. NFP similarly has no direct adverse effects, but is associated with a relatively higher failure rate.

Rheumatoid Arthritis   Hormonal contraceptive methods are excellent choices for women with rheumatoid arthritis. Some studies have suggested that oral contraceptives may reduce the risk of developing this disease, but there is little evidence they will reduce the severity of existing disease. The IUD may be used by women able to check monthly for strings except for those using steroids or other immunosuppressive therapy. Barrier methods are not contraindicated, but female barrier methods may not be appropriate for women with severe disabilities of their hands or hips.

Renal Disease

Hemodialysis   Most adolescents with chronic renal failure are infertile secondary to hypothalamic-pituitary dysfunction. During dialysis therapy some women resume normal ovulatory function. For those adolescents with menstrual function, contraception is an important issue. The major contraindications to oral contraceptive use in these adolescents would be hypertension or thromboembolic complications. Progestin-only methods are effective alternatives, even for those with prior thromboembolic problems or stable hypertension. Levels of progestin from injections are adequate for patients undergoing hemodialysis. IUDs would be contraindicated due to anemia and immunocompromise associated with renal failure. Barrier methods are not contraindicated but may be associated with unacceptably high failure rates. NFP methods are difficult to use in the face of irregular menstruation.

Transplantation   Ovulation and fertility often return within 6 months of a successful renal transplant. Information regarding oral contraceptive use in adolescents with a renal transplant is very limited. In teens with no significant hypertension, low-dose oral contraceptives or the minipill could be used with extreme caution. Other methods can be used as outlined above.

Postpartum and Breast-feeding Teens

1. Starting contraception: In postpartum teens ovulation can occur before the first menstrual cycle. Women who fully breast-feed should begin contraception by the third postpartum month, while other breast-feeding women should begin at least by 3–6 weeks postpartum.
2. Non-breast-feeding women: In non-breast-feeding women combination pills can be started between the third and fourth postpartum week. Progestin-only methods may be started immediately postpartum. Lubricated condoms should be used before other methods can be started and may alleviate problems associated with postpartum vaginal dryness.
3. Breast-feeding women: Combination oral contraceptives should be avoided until either the infant is weaned or until about 6 months postpartum. The concern with estrogen is in reducing breast milk production and not any effect on the baby. The progestin-only oral contraceptive can be started soon after pregnancy. The Norplant implant and DMPA can be used 6 weeks postpartum, although some authorities advocate its use immediately postpartum. The IUD can be inserted 6–8 weeks postpartum after the uterus has completely involuted.

TABLE 43.6.   Drugs Reported To Be Possibly Associated with Reduced Oral Contraceptive Efficacy

Drug	Documentation	Management Taking Medication ≤1 Week	Taking Medication >1 Week
Antibiotics			
Rifampin	Established	Use backup method while taking drug and for 2 weeks thereafter	Switch to a norhormonal method
Tetracycline	Minimal	None	None, or may increase oral contraceptive dose with spotting
Penicillins Chloramphenicol Cephalosporins Sulfonamides Nitrofurantoin	Contradictory	Available evidence suggests no change, could use backup method until 1 week after discontinuation of antibiotics	Conservative approach is to use backup method for 1 month; some sources advocate an alternative contraceptive
Griseofulvin	Strongly suspected	Usually used for over 1 week	Either switch to nonhormonal method or use oral contraceptive with 50 µg of estrogen
Anticonvulsants Phenytoin Phenobarbital Carbamazine Ethosuximide Primidone	Strongly suspected	Use backup method until 2 weeks after discontinuation of medication	Either switch to nonhormonal method or use oral contraceptive with 50 µg of estrogen; DMPA can also be used

Adapted from Neinstein LS. Issues in reproductive management. New York: Thieme Medical Publishers, 1994.

TABLE 43.7.   Drugs Reported To Be Possibly Associated with Enhanced Oral Contraceptive Efficacy or Increased Side Effects

Drug	Effect
Vitamin C	1 g daily increases ethinyl estradiol blood levels by 50%
Co-trimoxazole	Increased ethinyl estradiol levels, norgestrel nor affected

Adapted from Neinstein LS. Issues in reproductive management. New York: Thieme Medical Publishers, 1994.

TABLE **43.8.**   Drugs Reported To Have Altered Effects when Used with Oral Contraceptives

Interacting Drug	Adverse Effect	Recommendations
Acetaminophen	Possible decreased pain-relieving effect	Monitor pain-relieving response
Anticoagulants (oral	Decreased anticoagulant effect	Use alternative contraception
Antidepressants (Elavil, Norpramin, Tofranil, and others)	Possible increased antidepressant effect	Monitor antidepressant concentration
Benzodiazepine tranquilizers (Ativan, Librium, Serax, Tranxene, Valium, Xanax and others)	Possible increased or decreased drug effect	Use with caution
β-Blockers	Possible increased β-blocker effect	Monitor cardiovascular response
Corticosteroids	Possible increased corticosteroid toxicity	Relationship not established
Meperidine	Increased analgesic effect	Smaller dose may be required
Theophylline	Increased theophylline effect	Monitor theophylline concentration

HIV Infection   As HIV infections in women and heterosexual transmission of HIV infections are increasing, contraceptive concerns of HIV-infected women become an increasing need. Fertility rates are not affected by HIV infection or AIDS. HIV-infected individuals who choose to continue to be sexually active require maximal protection from pregnancy, from STDs, and from spreading the virus. Hormonal contraceptives appear safe in these individuals along with the use of condoms. While there has been the theoretical concern of oral contraceptives enhancing the shedding of virus from infected women, there is currently no evidence that supports this concern. The IUD would not be recommended because of the possibility of increased bleeding or abrasions of the penis. Both of these could lead to an increased risk of HIV transmission. Male condoms are key to reducing spread of the virus.

Medication Interactions   Medication interactions are shown in Tables 43.6, 43.7, and 43.8. For a more complete discussion see Neinstein (1994).

BIBLIOGRAPHY

Adler NE, Kegeles SM, Irwin CE Jr, et al. Adolescent contraceptive behavior: an assessment of decision process. J Pediatr 1990;116:463.

Alan Guttmacher Institute. Preventing pregnancy, protecting health: a new look at birth control choice in the United States. New York: Alan Guttmacher Institute, 1994.

American College of Obstetricians and Gynecologists, Office of Public Information. Poll shows women still skeptical of contraceptive safety. ACOG new release, January, 1994.

Alan Guttmacher Institute. Sex and America's teenagers. New York: Alan Guttmacher Institute, 1994.

Beach RK. Contraception for adolescents: part 1 and 2. Adolescent health update, vol 7. American Academy of Pediatrics, 1994 & 1995.

Braverman PK, Strasburger VC. Contraception. Clin Pediatr 1993;32:725–734.

Brown RT, Cromer BA, Fisher R. Adolescent sexuality and issues in contraception. Obstet Gynecol 1992; 19(1):177.

Bluestein D, Starling ME. Helping pregnant teenagers. West J Med 1994;161:140.

Byrne J, Mulvihill JJ, Myers MH, et al. Effects of treatment on fertility in long-term survivors of childhood or adolescent cancer. N Engl J Med 1987;317: 1315.

Centers for Disease Control. Sexual behavior among high school students, United States, 1990. MMWR 1992;40:885.

Chamberlain A, Rauh J, Passer A, et al. Issues in fertility control for mentally retarded female adolescents. Pediatrics 1984;73:445.

Clarkson TB, Shively CA, Morgan TM, et al. Oral contraception and coronary artery atherosclerosis of cynomolgus monkeys. Obstet Gynecol 1990;75:217.

Corson SL, Davis AJ, Derman RJ, et al. Clinical challenge: effects of OCs on disease states. Int J Fertil 1994;39(suppl 3):132.

Davis AJ. Contraceptive choices: the adolescent years. Dialogues in Contraception. 1995;4:1.

Diamond MP, Greene JW, Thompson JM, et al. Interaction of anticonvulsants and oral contraceptives in epileptic adolescents. Contraception 1985;31(6):623.

Fennoy I. Contraception and adolescent diabetes. Health Educ (Wash) 1989;20:21.

Fitzpatrick SB, Stockes DC, Rosenstein BJ, et al. Use of oral contraceptives in women with cystic fibrosis. Chest 1984;86:863.

Forrest JD, Singh S. The sexual and reproductive behavior of American women 1982–1988. Fam Plann Perspect 1990;22(5):206.

Forrest JD. Epidemiology of unintended pregnancy and contraceptive use. Am J Obstet Gynecol 1994;170:1485.

Garg SK, Chase HP, Marshall G. Oral contraceptives and renal and retinal complications in young women with insulin-dependent diabetes mellitus. JAMA 1994;271:1099.

Goldenring JM, Cohen E. Getting into adolescent heads. Contemp Pediatr 1988;July:75–90.

Gordon DE. Formal operational thinking: the role of cognitive-developmental processes in adult decision-making about pregnancy and contraception. Am J Orthopsychiatry 1990;60(3):346.

Greydaul DE, Lonchamp D. Contraception in the adolescent. Med Clin North Am 1990;74(5):1205.

Grimes DA. The morbidity and mortality of pregnancy: still risky business. Am J Obstet Gynecol 1994;170:1489.

Grimes DA, Mishell DR Jr, Speroff L. Contraceptive choices for women with medical problems. Am J Obstet Gynecol 1993;168:1979.

Hannaford PC, Kay CR. Oral contraceptive and diabetes mellitus. Br Med J 1989;299:1315–1316.

Hatcher RA, Trussell J, Stewart F, et al. Contraceptive technology, 16th revised ed. New York: Irvington Publishers, 1994.

Hirvonen E, Idänpään-Heikkilä J. Cardiovascular deaths among women under 40 years of age using low-dose estrogen contraceptives and intrauterine devices in Finland from 1975–1984. Am J Obstet Gynecol 1990;163:281.

Hughes ME, Furstenberg FF Jr, Teitler JO. The impact of an increase in family planning services on the teenage population of Philadelphia. Fam Plann Perspect 1995;27(2):60.

Kay CR. The RCGP oral contraceptive study. Clin Obstet Gynecol 1984;11:759.

Kjos SL, Shoupe D, Douyan S, et al. Effect of low-dose oral contraceptives on carbohydrate and lipid metabolism in women with recent gestational diabetes: results of a controlled, randomized, prospective study. Am J Obstet Gynecol 1990;163:1822.

Klein JBE, Moss SE, Klein R. Oral contraceptives in women with diabetes. Diabetes Care 1990;13:895.

Koo HP, Dunterman GH, George C, et al. Reducing adolescent pregnancy through a school- and community-based intervention: Denmore SC, revisited. Fam Plann Perspect 1994;26:206.

Loriaux DL, Wild RA. Contraceptive choices for women with endocrine complications. Am J Obstet Gynecol 1993;168:2021.

Mastroianni L Jr, Robinson JC. Hassle-free methods of contraception. Patient Care 1995;(March 15):46.

Mosher WD, McNalley JW. Contraceptive use at first premarital intercourse: United States 1965–1988. Fam Plann Perspect 1991;23(3):108.

Neinstein LS. Issues in reproductive management. New York: Thieme Medical Publishers, 1994.

Neinstein LS, Katz B. Contraceptive use in the chronically ill adolescent female. Part I. J Adolesc Health Care 1986;7:123.

Petersen KR, Skouby SO, Sidelmann J, et al. Effects of contraceptive steroids on cardiovascular risk factors in women with insulin-dependent diabetes mellitus. Am J Obstet Gynecol 1994;171:400.

Porter JB, Jick H, Walker AM. Mortality among oral contraceptive users. Obstet Gynecol 1987;70:29.

Quigley C, Cowell C, Jimenez M, et al. Normal or early development of puberty despite gonadal damage in children treated for acute lymphoblastic leukemia. N Engl J Med 1989;321:143.

Radberg T, Gustafson A, Dryten A, et al. Oral contraception in diabetic women: diabetes control, serum and high density lipoprotein lipids during low-dose progestogen, combined oestrogen/progestogen and non-hormonal contraception. Acta Endocrinol (Copenh) 1981;98:246.

Ramcharan S, Pellegrin FA, Ray RM, et al. The Walnut Creek Contraceptive Drug Study: a comprehensive study of the side effects of oral contraception. Vol. III. An interim report: a comparison of disease occurrence leading to hospitalization or death in users and nonusers of oral contraceptives. National Institutes of Health Publication No. 81–54, Jan., 1981.

Shoupe D, Bopp B. Contraceptive options for the gestational diabetic woman. Int J Fertil 1991;(suppl 2):80.

Skouby SO, Andersen O, Kuhl C. Oral contraceptives and insulin receptor binding in normal women and those with previous gestation diabetes. Am J Obstet Gynecol 1984;155:802.

Skouby SO, Molsted-Pedersen L, Kuehl C, et al. Oral contraceptives in diabetic women: metabolic effects of four compounds with different estrogen/progestogen profiles. Fertil Steril 1986;46:858.

Spellacy WN, Newton RE, Buhi WC, et al. Lipid and carbohydrate metabolic studies after one year of megestrol acetate treatment. Fertil Steril 1976;27:157.

Steel JM, Duncan LJP. Serious complications of oral contraception in insulin-dependent diabetics. Contraception 1978;17:291.

Sulak PJ, Haney AF. Unwanted pregnancies: understanding contraceptive use and benefits in adolescents and older women. Am J Obstet Gynecol 1993;168:2042.

Trussell J, Leveque JA, Koenig JD, et al. The economic value of contraception: a comparison of 15 methods. Am J Public Health 1995;85:494.

Wynn V, Adams PW, Godsland I, et al. Comparison of effects of different combined oral-contraceptive formulations on carbohydrate and lipid metabolism. Lancet 1979;1:1045.

Yeshurun D, Barak C, Blumensohn R, et al. A comparison of plasma cholesterol, triglycerides and high density lipoprotein cholesterol levels in women using contraceptive pills and a control group. Gynecol Obstet Invest 1984;18:169.

CHAPTER 44

Oral Contraceptives

Anita Nelson and Lawrence S. Neinstein

Oral contraceptives (OCs) are the most widely used method of reversible birth control in the United States. With more than 35 years of successful use in this country, considerable professional confidence has developed in the safety and efficacy of OCs and a growing appreciation is building among health-care providers for their extensive noncontraceptive benefits. However, public understanding of these issues lags considerably. A 1993 American College of Obstetricians and Gynecologists' (ACOG) Gallup poll found that 65% of Americans incorrectly believed that the pill was at least as hazardous to a woman's health as pregnancy; 58% could not name one noncontraceptive benefit of the pill. These public perceptions directly influence patient compliance and continuation rates. Much of this misinformation results from a confusion between the effects of earlier pills and the more modern formulations. A brief review of the history of the pill can be instructive in clarifying these issues.

HISTORY

In 1960 the U.S. Food and Drug Administration (FDA) approved the birth control pill for contraception. The first pill approved was called Enovid, which contained 150 mg of estrogen (mestranol) and 10 mg of progestin (norethynodrel). By the time the pill was approved in this country, physicians in Europe had several years of experience with virtually unrestricted use of these high-dose pills and were soon to gain a few years experience with pills with slightly lower doses. By 1967 reports from the Royal College of General Practitioners, in particular, began to emerge linking pill use with deep venous thrombosis, pulmonary emboli, stroke, and myocardial infarction (MI). Within a very short period, follow-up studies reported that the risk of serious complications was markedly increased in older women and indicated there was a duration of use risk with OC use. From these studies came the advice that women over 35–40 be prohibited from OC use and the idea that prolonged OC use should be discouraged—that the body should be periodically given a "rest" from sex steroids. It has taken decades to conclusively demonstrate that these findings and advice were flawed. Early in the history of OC pills, no restrictions were placed on the patients who were pill candidates. Women with uncontrolled hypertension or histories of MI or thrombotic disorders routinely used these high-dose pills. Since the incidence of many of these disorders increases with age, older women tended to have a higher incidence of serious complications with OC use. The duration of use that was reported in the early studies is now understood to have been a dose response. English women in 1967 who had used OCs for several years had, perforce, been taking high-dose pills because lower dose ones were not introduced overseas until early in the 1960s. Women who had been using pills for shorter periods of time had been given the newer, lower dose pills. The problems the "longer users" were having should have been attributed to the higher dose pills they were using.

Current Formulations

Since those early studies the doses of both the estrogen and the progestin components of the pills have been dramatically reduced without significantly sacrificing efficacy. All pills with more than 50 µg of estrogen have been removed from the market. Modern OCs routinely have only about one-third the estrogen content of the original pill. The hormones available for use in the pill include:

1. Estrogen component: All combination oral contraceptives contain one of two synthetic estrogens-mestranol or ethinyl estradiol, as diagrammed in Figure 44.1. These two estrogens differ by only a methyl group at the C-3 site. Mestranol must be hepatically activated

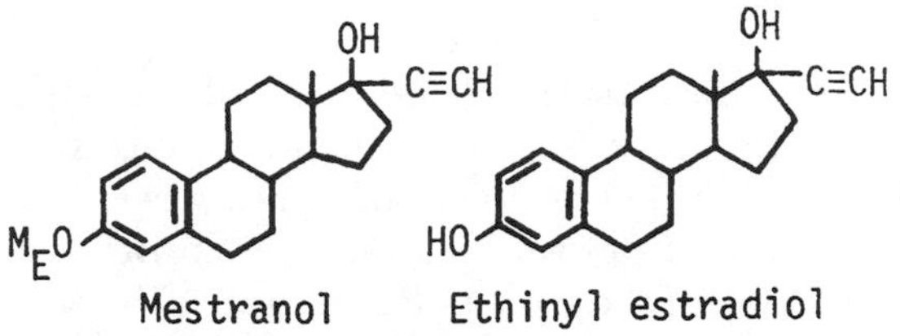

Figure 44.1.   Synthetic estrogens in combination oral contraceptives.

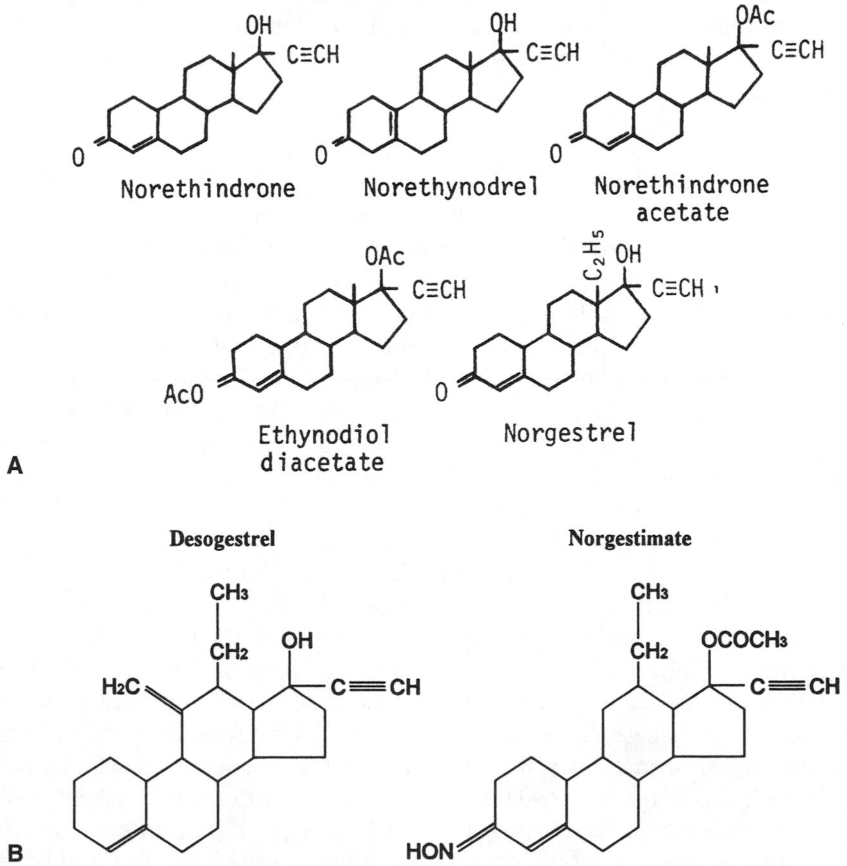

Figure 44.2.   Progestins in combination oral contraceptives.

into ethinyl estradiol. In rodents, ethinyl estradiol is 1.5–2.0 times as potent as mestranol. The difference is less in humans and depends on how completely mestranol is converted to ethinyl estradiol. The majority of combination pills prescribed today contain 30–35 μg of ethinyl estradiol, although a few formulations are available with 20 μg of ethinyl estradiol.

2. Progestin component: All combination pills have one of seven synthetic progestins: norethindrone, norethynodrel, norethindrone acetate, ethynodiol diacetate, norgestrel-levonorgestrel, norgestimate, and desogestrel. All are derived from testosterone and produce both progestational and androgenic effects. In many instances the latter can be interpreted as antiestrogenic. Figure 44.2 diagrams these progestins and Table 44.1 outlines their characteristics.

A wide range of formulations has been developed to attempt to meet the needs of a broad range of women with individual sensitivities to the sex hormone formulations, combinations, and strengths. There are three classes of OC pills today:

1. Monophasic pills: Each active ingredient pill has the same dose of estrogen and progestin. Placebo pills are often added to cycle packs to enable the patient to remember to start the next cycle pack.
2. Multiphasic packets (biphasic or triphasic): The active ingredient pills vary in strength in the estrogen and progestin components throughout the 21-day cycle. Seven placebo pills are included in the 28-day packet.
3. Progestin-only or minipill: The pill is composed of small doses of a progestin. No estrogen is included in the active pills. No placebo pills are included.

TABLE 44.1. Characteristics of Sex Hormones in Combination Oral Contraceptives

Class Compound	Progestational Activity[a]	Estrogenic Activity[b]	Androgenic Activity[c]	Endometrial Activity[d]
Progestins[e]				
19-Nortestosterone progestins				
Estrane				
Norethindrone	1.0	1.0	1.0	1.0
Norethindrone acetate	1.2	1.5	1.6	0.4
Ethynodiol diacetate	1.4	3.4	0.6	0.4
5(10)-Estrane				
Norethynodrel	0.8	8.3	0	0
Gonane				
Levonorgestrel	5.3	0	8.3	5.1
Norgestrel	2.6	0	4.2	2.6
Norgestimate	1.3	0	1.9	1.2
Desogestrel	9.0	0	3.4	8.7
Estrogens[f]				
Ethinyl estradiol	0	100	0	0
Mestranol	0	67	0	0

Adapted from Dickey RP. Managing contraceptive pill patients, 8th ed. Durant, Oklahoma: Essential Medical Information Systems, 1994:130–131.
[a]Based on amount required to induce vacuoles in human endometrium. Desogestrel, gestodene, levonorgestrel, and norgestimate based on oral stimulation of endometrium in immature estrogen-primed rabbits relative to levonorgestrel = 5.3.
[b]Comparative potency based on oral rat vaginal epithelium assay (norethindrone = 0.25 when ethinyl estradiol = 100).
[c]Comparative potency (oral) based on rat ventral prostate assay (norethindrone = 1.0 when methyltestosterone = 50) (Levonorgestrel and desogestrel relative to norethindrone = 1.0) (Norgestimate, relative to levonorgestrel = 8.3) and (gestodene relative to levonorgestrel = 8.3).
[d]Based on estimation of amount required to suppress bleeding for 20 days in 50% of women.
[e]Calculated on the basis of norethindrone = 1.0 in activity.
[f]Calculated on the basis of ethinyl estradiol = 100 in activity.

TABLE 44.2. Oral Contraceptive Formulations

Name	Estrogen	Amount (μg)	Number of Days	Progestin	Amount (mg)	Number of Days
Monophasic combination oral contraceptives						
Brevicon, Modicon Nelova 0.5/35E	Ethinyl estradiol	35	21	Norethindrone	0.5	21
Demulen	Ethinyl estradiol	50	21	Ethynodiol diacetate	1	21
Demulen 1/35	Ethinyl estradiol	35	21	Ethynodiol diacetate	1	21
Desogen, Ortho-Cept	Ethinyl estradiol	30	21	Desogestrel	0.15	21
Genora 1/35, Nelova 1/35E, Norethin 1/35 E, Norinyl 1 + 35, Ortho-Novum 1-35	Ethinyl estradiol	35	21	Norethindrone	1	21
Genora 1/50, Norethin 1/50 M, Norinyl 1/50, Ortho-Novum 1/50	Mestranol	50	21	Norethindrone	1	21
Levlen, Nordette	Ethinyl estradiol	30	21	Levonorgestrel	0.15	21
Loestrin 1.5/30	Ethinyl estradiol	30	21	Norethindrone acetate	1.5	21
Loestrin 1/20	Ethinyl estradiol	20	21	Norethindrone acetate	1	21
Lo/Ovral	Ethinyl estradiol	30	21	Norgestrel	0.3	21
Norlestrin 1/50	Ethinyl estradiol	50	21	Norethindrone acetate	1	21
Ortho-Cyclen	Ethinyl estradiol	35	21	Norgestimate	0.25	21
Ovcon-35	Ethinyl estradiol	35	21	Norethindrone	0.4	21
Ovcon-50	Ethinyl estradiol	50	21	Norethindrone	1	21
Ovral	Ethinyl estradiol	50	21	Norgestrel	0.5	21
Multiphasic combination oral contraceptives						
Jenest-28	Ethinyl estradiol	35	21	Norethindrone	0.5	7
					1.0	14
Ortho-Novum 7/7/7	Ethinyl estradiol	35	21	Norethindrone	0.5	7
					0.75	7
					1.0	7
Ortho-Novum 10/11	Ethinyl estradiol	35	21	Norethindrone	0.5	10
					1.0	11
Ortho Tri-Cyclen	Ethinyl estradiol	35	21	Norgestimate	0.180	7
					0.215	7
					0.250	7
Tri-Levlen, Triphasil	Ethinyl estradiol	30	6	Levonorgestrel	0.05	6
		40	5		0.075	5
		30	10		0.125	10
Tri-Norinyl	Ethinyl estradiol	35	21	Norethindrone	0.5	7
					1.0	9
					0.5	5
Progestin-only oral contraceptives						
Micronor, Nor-Q.D.	None	0		Norethindrone	0.35	21
Ovrette	None	0		Norgestrel	0.075	21

Adapted from Dickey RP. Managing contraceptive pill patients, 8th ed. Durant, Oklahoma: Essential Medical Information Systems, 1994:132–134.

Table 44.2 presents the hormonal components of each of the pill formulations currently available.

EFFICACY

The typical first-year failure rate is 2.5–3.0% in all age groups, with the perfect use rate of 0.1%. The failure rate in users younger than 22 years of age is 4.7%; in those aged 15–19 it is quoted to be 8.0–18.1%. Of significant concern is the high discontinuance rate with the pill (25–50% over 1 year), mostly due to nonmedical reasons.

One other point should be made in regard to effectiveness. Serum hormonal levels persist for several days after stopping the combination pill, so pregnancies may be more often a consequence of starting pills late after menses than of missing one pill during the middle of the cycle.

MECHANISMS OF ACTION

1. Thickening of cervical mucus: The progestin component produces a thick, viscid, scanty mucus that is hostile to sperm penetration. This is the single most important action of all hormonal methods of contraception.
2. Inhibition of ovulation: All hormonal methods suppress hypothalamic release of gonadotropin-releasing hormone (GnRH) pulses and directly affect the pituitary gland, reducing its follicle-stimulating hormone (FSH) and luteinizing hormone (LH) secretion. The progestin-only pill has such low dose that ovulation is inhibited in only a fraction of cycles. The combination pill, containing estrogen and a higher dose of progestin, suppresses ovulation in 95–98% of cycles by inhibiting the LH surge. FSH levels with the combination pill are decreased to 70% of normal; LH levels are only 20% of levels found in women who are not taking OCs.
3. Endometrial changes: The presence of a progestin early in the cycle results in a thin endometrium with atrophic glands and minimal glycogen stores, which is not suitable for implantation.
4. Slowed tubal motility: The progestin in the pill slows tubal motility and disrupts the carefully orchestrated sequence of events necessary for successful fertilization and impregnation.

METABOLIC IMPACTS

Figure 44.3 reviews metabolic effects of the estrogen and progestin component of OCs.

	Estrogens	Progestins
Protein	▲Globulins	None
CHO	None	Insulin Resistance: ▲ Insulin ▼ Glucose Tol.
Lipids	▲ HDL-Chol ▼ LDL-Chol	▼HDL-Chol ▲LDL-Chol
Electrolytes	Na retention	Na retention

FIGURE 44.3. Metabolic effects of oral contraceptives. *CHO*, carbohydrate; *HDL-Chol*, high-density lipoprotein cholesterol; *LDL-Chol*, low-density lipoprotein cholesterol; *Tol.*, tolerance.

Hepatic Synthesis

Coagulation Factors   Factors associated with the extrinsic pathway of the cascade (fibrogen, factors I, V, VII, VIII, and X) are uniformly increased by estrogen-containing birth control pills in proportion to their estrogen dose. Balancing this increase in virtually all women is a compensatory increase in fibrinolytic factors, much as is found in pregnancy. Some women, such as those with protein S or C deficiencies, are unable to compensate for the increase in clotting factors and may be subject to an increased risk for thromboembolic problems. The overall relative risk of thrombolytic effects is between 2.6 and 4.0; the absolute incidence of venous thrombosis is 15 per 100,000 for most of the low-dose formulations. Pills containing the progestins desogestrel or gestodene may be associated with venous thrombosis at a rate of 30 per 100,000 (World Health Organization, 1995). Venous thrombosis in pregnancy rates are about 60 per 100,000. Recent studies have found no increased risk of stroke with OC use. The recommendation to stop OC use 1 month prior to any scheduled surgery has been tempered to reflect modern surgical practices. OC use may not need to be interrupted if the patient is not expected to require prolonged postoperative bed rest.

Binding Globulins   Estrogen increases hepatic synthesis of carrier proteins such as albumin, sex hormone–binding globulin (SHBG), thyroxine-binding globulin (TBG), and corticosteroid-binding globulin (CBG), which has impacts on the interpretation of laboratory tests but also has clinical implications. Increased levels of SHBG bind more free testosterone and reduce androgen-related problems such as hirsutism and acne. The effect of the progestin depends on its androgenicity and dose; more androgenic formulations may blunt this increase in hepatic synthesis.

Angiotensinogen   The estrogen in the combination birth control pill increases hepatic production of renin, which then is serially converted to angiotensinogen, which in turn can cause reversible hypertension in selected patients. Angiotensinogen sensitivity is difficult to predict. Even women with histories of pregnancy-induced hypertension are not at increased risk for developing elevated blood pressures while using OCs. However, women who have experienced hypertension with OC use have high recurrence risk.

Lipid Metabolism

Estrogen increases total cholesterol, high-density lipoprotein (HDL) cholesterol, and triglycerides while it decreases low-density lipoprotein (LDL) cholesterol. The androgenic component of the progestin has the opposite effect. The net impact on lipids, therefore, depends on the composition of the pill. The newer progestins, designed to have greater selectivity for progestin receptors, have less of an androgenic impact. In combination with estrogen, they may cause no change in HDL or LDL but may cause an increase in "fluffy" triglycerides, which many lipid experts claim are not conducive to plaque formation. Older progestins at lower doses similarly have minimal impacts on lipid metabolism. At higher doses some of the older, more potent progestins have a slightly adverse impact on HDL-LDL ratios. Whether these alterations should be translated into concerns about increased risks for cardiovascular disease is not clear, but patients with dyslipidemias should be offered appropriate formulations and monitored.

Glucose Metabolism

Both of the sex steroids have been implicated in influencing glucose metabolism: estrogen may suppress insulin response; progestins can increase peripheral insulin resistance. At

TABLE 44.3.   Laboratory Tests and Potential Alteration[a]

Group	Increased	Decreased
Carbohydrate metabolism	Fasting blood sugar and 2-hr pp Insulin	Glucose tolerance
Hematological and coagulation	Coagulation factors II, VII, XIII, IX, X, XII Fibrinogen Leukocyte count PTT, PT Plasminogen Platelet count, platelet aggregation, platelet adhesiveness	Antithrombin III Hematocrit PT
Lipid metabolism	Cholesterol, lipoproteins HDL increased by estrogen Triglycerides	HDL decreased by progestins
Liver function and gastrointestinal tests	Alkaline phosphatase Bilirubin, SGOT, SGPT, GGT Protoporphyrin, coproporphyrin excretion (urine)	Haptoglobin Urobilinogen excretion (urine)
Metals	Copper and ceruloplasmin Iron, iron-binding capacity and transferrin	Magnesium Zinc
Thyroid function	Thyroid-binding globulin T_4	Free thyroxin
Vitamins	Vitamin A	Folate Vitamins B_6, B_{12} Vitamin C
Other hormones and enzymes	Adolesterone Angiotensinogen Angiotensin I and II Cortisol Growth hormone Testosterone	Estradiol FSH, LH 17-hydroxycorticosteroids Renin
Miscellaneous	α_1-antitrypsin Antinuclear antibody Lactate Sodium	Albumin Calcium Immunoglobulin A, G, M

[a]FSH, follicle-stimulating hormone; GGT, γ-glutamyltransferase; HDL, high-density lipoprotein; LH, luteinizing hormone; PT, prothrombin time; PTT, partial thromboplastin time; SGOT, serum glutamic-oxaloacetic transaminase; SGPT, serum glutamic-pyruvic transaminase.

higher hormonal doses older formulations of birth control pills were noted to cause a deterioration of glucose tolerance test in a minority of patients. Most studies have found that modern formulations with lower hormonal doses cause no impairment in glucose tolerance in euglycemic women. In a prospective study of women with histories of gestational diabetes using low-dose estrogenic OC pills, Kjos et al. (1990) reported no acceleration to overt diabetes compared to women using nonhormonal contraceptives.

Impacts on Laboratory Tests

Changes in laboratory tests among pill users are listed in Table 44.3.

CONTRAINDICATIONS (FROM LABELING)

1. History of cholestatic jaundice, heart attack, stroke, deep venous thrombosis, pulmonary embolism, or retinal thrombosis
2. Known or suspected cancer of breast, endometrium, cervix, or vagina
3. Hepatic tumors (benign or malignant)
4. Angina pectoris

5. Unexplained vaginal bleeding
6. Jaundice
7. Known or suspected pregnancy

NOTE: Clinical exceptions to the above list:

1. Women who are currently anticoagulated after deep venous thrombosis (DVT) or pulmonary embolism (PE) may be candidates for OC use.
2. Women with non-estrogen-dependent tumors, such as cervical tumors, may benefit from OCs during evaluation and treatment.
3. Once the cause of vaginal bleeding is established, OCs can be used.

Rᴇʟᴀᴛɪᴠᴇ Cᴏɴᴛʀᴀɪɴᴅɪᴄᴀᴛɪᴏɴs (ғʀᴏᴍ Lᴀʙᴇʟɪɴɢ)

Relative contraindications include a personal or family history of:

1. Breast nodules, fibrocystic disease of the breast, an abnormal breast x-ray examination or mammogram results
2. Diabetes
3. Elevated cholesterol or triglycerides
4. Migraine or other headaches
5. Epilepsy
6. Mental depression
7. Gallbladder, heart, or kidney disease
8. Scanty or irregular menstrual periods

NOTE: Clinical exceptions to the above list: Many of the relative contraindications have been more fully dealt with in Chapter 43. However, others deserve mention here.

1. A family history of noncancerous breast abnormalities is only tangentially related to any risk for OC use in patients. The only requirement is to attempt to rule out a breast cancer in the patient. OCs are known to help reduce the risk of fibrocystic breast changes and are often selected as a birth control method to help control those symptoms. Women with family histories of breast cancer are at higher risk of developing breast cancer themselves, but OC use does not further increase this risk.
2. A history of scanty or irregular menses deserves evaluation before OC use masks the problem and therefore delays the diagnosis of a potentially serious problem, such as hypothyroidism. Women with irregular menses due to known causes, such as polycystic ovary syndrome (PCOS) or exercise amenorrhea, actually benefit greatly from regular cycling induced by OCs.

Dʀᴜɢ Iɴᴛᴇʀᴀᴄᴛɪᴏɴs

1. Decreased contraceptive effect
   a. By inducing liver enzymes (barbiturates, phenytoin [Dilantin], and rifampin)
   b. By decreasing gastrointestinal absorption (Ampicillin, penicillin, and neomycin)
      Patients combining the preceding drugs (in *a* or *b*) with OCs should watch for breakthrough bleeding as a possible sign of decreased estrogen effect. If bleeding is noted, patients should use another contraceptive device while continuing to use both drugs or increase the estrogen dose.
2. Tricyclic antidepressants: Effect of tricyclic antidepressants may be increased by OCs, owing to liver enzyme inhibition.

HEALTH ISSUES

A summary of the serious side effects traditionally associated with OC use is displayed on Table 44.4 with both relative risks and an estimate of absolute risk. These estimates are based on a mixture of newer and *older* formulations, as well as *different age groups*. More specific information is provided below about selected issues.

Thromboembolism

As outlined above the increased clotting factors induced by estrogen-containing OCs can induce a functionally hypercoagulable state if there is no counterbalancing increase in thrombolytic factors. The incidence of this has dramatically dropped with decreasing levels of estrogen in the pill (Table 44.5). In healthy teens and young women with no altering medical factors, there appears to be only a slight risk of thromboembolism with current OC preparations. The risk may also vary by progestin formulation. As previously mentioned, desogestrel- and gestodene-containing pills may have a twofold risk of thromboembolism compared to pills containing other progestins. However, even if this concern was fully confirmed, the risk is still 50% of the risk of thromboembolism during pregnancy.

Cardiovascular Disease

There has been a fundamental change in understanding about the mechanisms by which OC could be linked to MI in high-risk patients. Previously, it had been thought that the androgenicity of the progestin induced atherosclerotic plaque formation, which increased cardiovascular disease. This atherosclerotic hypothesis was abandoned after it was observed that:

TABLE 44.4. Medical Complications of Oral Contraceptive Use

Adverse Effects	Relative Risk	Absolute Risk
Cholelithiasis	2x	1:1250
Myocardial infarction (smokers >35)	3x	1:5000
Thrombophlebitis	3x	1:10,000
Thromboembolism	4x	1:30,000
Stroke	3x	1:30,000
Hepatic adenoma	500x	1:50,000
Mild hypertension	2–3x	<1:20

Courtesy Paul Brenner, MD, University of Southern California.

TABLE 44.5. Ratio of Observed to Expected Outcomes by Estrogen Dose in the United Kingdom (1974–1977)

Outcome	Ethinyl Estradiol Dose	
	50 µg	30 µg
Venous deaths	1.40	0.65
Nonvenous deaths	1.52	0.53
Ischemic heart disease	1.48	0.54
Stroke	1.20	0.80

Adapted from Meade TW, Greenberg C, Thompson SG. Progestins and cardiovascular reactions associated with oral contraceptives and a comparison of the safety of 50- and 30-µg estrogen preparations. Br Med J 1980;280:1157.

1. Former OC users had no higher risk of MI than never users of OCs. If the effects were due to adverse lipid profiles, past users should have established irreversible plaque and experienced increased long-term MI risk.
2. There is no duration-of-use relationship between OC use and MI risk. Plaque formation is progressive. If the pill were implicated, it would have been expected that the longer the use, the higher the MI rate.
3. Cynomolgus monkeys given relatively androgenic OC pills and atherosclerotic diets demonstrated a deterioration of their serum lipids but at necropsy were found to have less plaque than was found in control animals.

Currently, it is thought that any risk of cardiovascular disease in OC users results from arterial thrombosis not atherosclerosis.

Overall, however, it is clear that for healthy, nonsmoking women, the use of OCs does not appear to increase the risk for MI. Ischemic heart disease in OC users in the United Kingdom dropped in women using low-dose OCs. Three large scale controlled studies have demonstrated no increased risk of heart attacks or death from MI in OC users under age 45 compared to controls and a significantly increased risk of developing cardiovascular disease while using OCs occurs only in women with other risk factors. For example, in the 6-year Puget Sound study (Porter et al., 1987) of 10,000 healthy OC users and 30,000 healthy controls aged 15–44, there were no heart attacks among OC users and only one in the controls. Only one OC user and 14 controls had strokes. The Finnish study (Hirvonen and Idänpään-Heikkilä, 1990) of low-dose OC users versus controls found a relative risk of 0.2 for deaths from cardiovascular disease in OC users.

There are clearly identified groups with higher risk for MI with combined birth control pill use. Smokers at all ages have increased risks for cardiovascular disease when they use OCs, but those synergistic effects do not become clinically significant until women are 35–40 years old. Even though teens have a relative risk of over 2.0 for MIs if they smoke and use OCs, the absolute risk of that event is still so small as to be overwhelmed by their risk of dying from pregnancy or pregnancy-related complications. In addition to older women who smoke, women with current uncontrolled hypertension or renal compromise (due to diabetes, systemic lupus erythematosus [SLE]) or with histories of pulmonary emboli, deep venous thrombosis, MI, or stroke should not be offered combination OCs. Fortunately, few adolescents have such medical problems.

Hypertension

Approximately 3% of OC pill users experience increased blood pressure while using birth control pills. The incidence is related to the estrogen content of the pill. Blood pressure changes are thought to be caused by an angiotensinogen sensitivity and are usually reversible within 3 months. If the hypertension does not spontaneously resolve, then other causes must be considered.

Liver-Gallbladder Impacts

1. Cholelithiasis: A doubling of the risk of gallstones has been suggested by several prospective and retrospective studies. Although the risk is more impressive in higher dose pills, it is still apparent in the lower dose formulations. Cholelithiasis is secondary to increased cholesterol saturation and stasis. The risk appears to be concentrated in a few short-term users who may be prone to gallbladder disease.
2. Cholestatic jaundice is very rare, but it has been reported as a result of OC pill use.
3. Pruritus similar to that seen in pregnancy may develop with OC use.

IMPACT OF ORAL CONTRACEPTIVE PILLS ON NEOPLASIA

The single largest concern women voice about OC use is the risk of cancer. Nearly one-third of all women believe OCs cause cancer, but only 7% believe that OC use can decrease ovarian cancer and endometrial cancer. Table 44.6 summarizes the current data about OC use and neoplasia. A few of the more pertinent neoplasms for adolescents are discussed below.

Leiomyoma

Historically, there has been concern that OC use might stimulate leiomyoma growth, since leiomyoma (fibroids) are known to be estrogen-sensitive tumors. However, progesterone down-regulates the estrogen receptors on endometrial and myometrial cells. Since OCs are progestin dominant, their net effect on fibroids is marginal. Friedman and Thomas (1995) followed OC users with fibroids for 1 year, compared them to controls with fibroids, and found no increase in uterine size during OC use. In addition, the progestin impact on the endometrium significantly reduced menstrual blood loss.

Endometrial Hyperplasia and Cancer

Epidemiologic data are very persuasive that use of combination OC pills significantly reduces the risk of endometrial hyperplasia and cancer by preventing unopposed estrogen stimulation. Ever users have at least a 40% reduction in the risk of endometrial cancer; this protection persists for at least 15 years beyond the last use of OCs. For this reason it is important to offer teens with oligomenorrhea hormonal methods to provide predictable bleeding and reduce their risk of endometrial cancer later in life.

Ovarian Epithelial Carcinoma

By suppressing "incessant ovulation" OCs significantly reduce the risk of ovarian cancer. Epidemiologic studies show that the longer a woman uses OCs, the more significant is this reduction. Ever users have nearly a 40% reduction; women who have used OCs for 10 or more years have an 80% reduction in risk. This protection persists for 15 years after OC discontinuation.

TABLE 44.6.   Oral Contraceptives and Neoplasms

Type of Neoplasm	Oral Contraceptive Effect		
	Protective	Neutral	Adverse
Ovarian cysts	X	X	
Benign breast disease	X		
Liver adenoma	X	X	X
Leiomyoma	?	X	
Prolactinoma		X	
Cervical dysplasia			X
Breast cancer		?	?
Cervical cancer		?	?
Endometrial cancer	X		
Ovarian cancer	X		
Hepatic carcinoma		X	
Gestational trophoblastic disease		X	

Summary courtesy of Paul Brenner, MD, University of Southern California.

Cervical Cancer

Studies linking OC use and cervical cancer have been confounded by design flaws and biases, including inappropriate control groups. Some studies have suggested that women using OCs for more than 5 years have an increased risk of developing cervical carcinoma, even after controlling for known cervical cancer risk factors; other studies have failed to confirm this. Studies by the U.S. Centers for Disease Control and Prevention (CDC) in Puerto Rico with appropriate controls did find an increase in cervical dysplasia in OC users, which is physiologically plausible since estrogen everts the cervix and exposes more of the metaplastic cells to possible human papilloma virus (HPV) infection (see Chapter 65). However, OC users do not require more intensive or frequent cervical screening than the routine screening advocated by risk factor analysis.

Breast Cancer

In contrast to the obvious benefits OCs have on reducing endometrial and ovarian cancer, their impact on breast cancer has been more controversial. Estrogen is known to stimulate glandular cell division; progesterone stimulates ductal mitosis. In humans, there is no evidence that either hormone can initiate the development of cancer from normal breast tissue.

Epidemiological studies of present and past OC users have presented conflicting results, but virtually all the risk ratios for breast cancer calculated in these studies cluster around 1.0 or their confidence intervals include 1.0, indicating no statistically significant increased risk. One particular exception is the Pike et al. study (1983), which found an unequivocal increase in breast cancer in a very special subgroup of women under age 25 who used OCs with a high dose of certain gestagens (such as those used in the 1960s) for more than 5 years. In that same study, however, no increased risk of developing breast cancer was found in a group of similar women using lower dose OCs.

The CDC's Cancer and Steroid Hormone (CASH) study has reviewed its extensive database looking for various associations between OC use and breast cancer (CDC, 1983). They have reported no increased risk in breast cancer overall with OC use. Importantly, they have investigated several high-risk groups and found that OC use does not increase breast cancer in the following important subgroups:

1. Women with family history of breast cancer
2. Women with and without benign breast disease
3. Women who started using OCs before their first pregnancy

Therefore, denying an adolescent hormonal contraceptives because of a family history of breast cancer or because she has physiologic nodularities is not appropriate. A WHO study of 5000 women also found no increased risk with duration of OC use. In fact, the risk dropped over time.

The CDC study mentioned above also reported a paradoxical age-specific difference in OC impacts on breast cancer. In women aged 25–35 it was found that OC use could increase breast cancer cases by 2–3 cases per 100,000; but in women over 50 who had been OC users there would be 30 fewer cases per 100,000. While the finding does raise interesting questions of cancer potentiation versus resistance, it is a moot point today because there are no tools to predict which groups of women will benefit and which will not. Until more data are available, it is important to share with patients that there is no conclusive evidence that OCs increase a woman's risk of breast cancer.

Advantages

1. Safe, effective contraception
2. Relatively easy method (once a day)

3. Taken at time independent of coitus
4. Rapidly reversible method
5. Decreases menstrual bleeding and cramping
6. Decreases iron deficiency anemia
7. Eliminates Mittelschmerz
8. Decreases risk of functional ovarian cysts
9. Decreases benign breast disease, especially fibrocystic breast changes
10. Reduces acne and hirsutism
11. Decreases incidence of salpingitis (pelvic inflammatory disease [PID]) even though cervicitis risks may be higher
12. Permits women to adjust when they menstruate, to avoid conflicts with athletic meets or other important dates
13. Decreases lifetime risk of endometrial and ovarian cancer

DISADVANTAGES

1. Requires daily administration
2. Side effects (see below)
3. Requires counseling on safer sex practices
4. Post–pill use amenorrhea

SIDE EFFECTS

As described earlier, the sex hormones in OCs have various degrees of progestational, estrogenic, antiestrogenic, and androgenic activity. These differences are important to understand, especially in responding to side effects. Both the estrogen and progestin components affect various female organ systems differently, and the impacts of the relative potencies vary from individual to individual.

Side effects associated with the use of OCs are often a result of the pharmacological dose of hormone or of hormonal imbalances. Many side effects are temporally self-limited and will resolve spontaneously in the first few cycles, but sometimes they require a change of pill formulation. When these side effects arise, it is important to analyze them by the constituent hormonal effects. Additional changes result from interactions between the constituent hormones. For some problems, there are at least two possible approaches: either to increase one component or to decrease the other (Table 44.7).

Management of Common Side Effects

1. Breakthrough bleeding: Initially as many as 30–40% of women experience irregular spotting or bleeding. Most will resolve within 3 months. Treatment for persistent spotting in the face of appropriate pill use depends on the timing or spotting within the woman's cycle (Table 44.8).
2. Acne, hirsutism, or noncyclic generalized weight gain: Usually due to relative increase in free androgens. Approaches include:
   a. Increase estrogen content, which will increase sex hormone–binding globulin and reduce unbound testosterone levels.
   b. Decrease progestin dose or switch to less androgenic progestin content.
3. Chloasma or melasma is due to estrogen stimulation of melanocytes. Suggestion: Decrease estrogen content.

TABLE 44.7. Side Effects of Combination Oral Contraceptives

Estrogen-Related	Progestin-Related	
Estrogenic	Progestogenic	Androgenic
Nausea and vomiting	Fatigue	Noncyclic weight gain
Edema, leg cramps	Depression	Oily skin
Bloating	Bloating	Hirsutism
Cervical ectropion	Mastalgia	Acne
Visual changes or vascular headaches	Increased breast size	Increased appetite
Telangiectasia	Venous dilation, pelvic congestion	Changes in libido
Cyclic weight gain	Oligomenorrhea, amenorrhea, vaginal spotting	Decreased breast size
Irritability	Cholestatic jaundice	
Clear vaginal discharge	Pruritus	
Cystic breast changes		
Chloasma, hyperpigmentation		
Hypermenorrhea (menorrhagia)		

TABLE 44.8. Management of Breakthrough Bleeding

Spotting Time	Cause	Hormone Change	Timing
Premenstrual spotting	Lack of progestin	Increase progestin	In last week of active pills
Postmenstrual spotting	Lack of estrogen or excess progestin	Increase estrogen or decrease progestin	At beginning of cycle
Midcycle spotting	Lack of estrogen or progestin	Increase estrogen or progestin	Midcycle or throughout cycle

INCREASING ADOLESCENT COMPLIANCE

Adolescent compliance with contraceptive methods is often suboptimal. Health-care providers must remember that adult compliance is far from perfect. In one San Francisco study, less than 20% of women took pills every day at approximately the same time for 8 months. Many factors play important roles in compliance; the desire of teens for independence and seeming invincibility decreases their motivation to use contraception. The unpredictability and frequent disruptions in their relationships cause them to frequently stop contraception. Misinformation about OC impacts and effectiveness also reduce compliance (Table 44.9).

To enhance compliance, experts have suggested several measures:

1. Emphasize the noncontraceptive benefits of oral contraceptives.
2. Demonstrate concretely how to use pills.
3. Have the patients explicitly discuss their concerns about pill use so that they can be assuaged. Widespread myths about the danger of OCs abound and can magnify the significance of a minor side effect.
4. Help the teen plan for crucial logistics: Where to store the pills (school lockers don't work on weekends!), how to remember to take them each day (placing them by makeup or pierced earring holder works better than locating them near toothpaste).
5. Always use 28-day packs so teens do not have to remember when to restart taking their pills.
6. Start an adolescent on monophasic pills to reduce the chance of escape ovulation if she neglects to take a pill early in the cycle.
7. Consider starting pills immediately if pregnancy can be ruled out to simplify instructions. (Use barrier method as back-up for first cycle.)

Special considerations in adolescents:

1. When to start: Ideally a teen would have at least three to six regular periods before starting the pill. However, if a young teen is sexually active, the risks of pregnancy exceed

those of the risks of taking hormonal contraceptives, even if she has not had any regular cycles yet. There is no evidence that the early use of OCs leads to epiphyseal closure, as this is well on the way when a teen begins to first menstruate.

2. After a therapeutic abortion, the pill should be started immediately to prevent ovulation. After a pregnancy, 2 weeks should be allowed before starting, due to the risk of thromboembolism.

3. If the teen has very irregular cycles, she should be informed that her cycles are likely to be irregular when the pills are stopped, and that her menses may not return for some time after discontinuation. However, there is no evidence that the teen's fertility rates would be any lower than if she never used the pill. If an adolescent or young woman wishes to conceive and has been highly irregular before using birth control pills, she should discontinue use about 1 year before the planned pregnancy, to allow time for menses and ovulation to return.

4. Initial examination
   a. History: Menses, sexually transmitted diseases (STDs), history of problems that relate to the contraindications for use of the pill, and sexual and family history
   b. Physical examination: Thyroid examination, breast examination, abdominal examination, pelvic examination, weight and blood pressure
   c. Laboratory tests: Pap smear. Screening for *Chlamydia* and gonorrhea are recommended for every sexually active teen. Other tests such as urinalysis for protein and glucose are helpful but not required.

5. Follow-up
   a. See the teenager at 1 month and again at 3 months after starting the pill and then every 6 months. The visit after 1 month is important, especially in younger teens, as some teenagers discontinue the pill during the first month due to minor side effects.
   b. Check blood pressure and weight every 6–12 months.
   c. Perform breast and pelvic examination every 12 months.

A sample set of instructions for using birth control pills is shown in Figure 44.4.

TABLE 44.9.   Myths Associated with Oral Contraceptive Use

Myth	Response
Pills cause cancer.	Number one concern
Pills increase fertility.	Highly concerned
Pills cause birth defects. Need to stop pills 3–6 months before conception.	51%
The body needs a "rest" from the pills every few years.	56%
Young women shouldn't use pills, because it will stunt their growth.	

AMA Harris Survey. American women's attitudes toward reproductive health. Presented in New York, May 18, 1995.

INSTRUCTIONS FOR USING BIRTH CONTROL PILLS

Combined birth control pills contain two female hormones, estrogen and progestin. They work by stopping ovulation (egg release) each month. If there is no egg to meet a sperm, there is no pregnancy.

Remember: Birth control pills prevent pregnancy; they provide no barrier against sexually transmitted diseases (STDs) or from human immunodeficiency virus (HIV) and acquired immunodeficiency syndrome (AIDS). Therefore, in addition to taking the pill throughout your cycle, use a condom every time you have intercourse.

FIGURE 44.4.   Sample instruction sheet. (Adapted from Hatcher RA, Trussell J, Stewart F, et al. Contraceptive technology, 16th revised ed. New York: Irvington Publishers, 1994.)   *Figure continued on following page.*

First month: Use a backup method of birth control (such as condoms or foam) with your first packet of pills, since the pills may not fully protect you from pregnancy during the first cycle. This is probably not needed if you start your pills on the first day of your period.

TAKING YOUR BIRTH CONTROL PILLS CORRECTLY

You may start taking your pills in one of several different schedules. This could include:

1. Starting your first pack on the first day of your period
2. Starting your first pack on the first Sunday after your period begins
3. Starting your first pack today if you are certain that you are not pregnant

Always read the package insert: The package insert gives additional detailed information about pill benefits and risks.

1. Take one pill a day each day at about the same time until you have taken all the pills in one cycle package. Try to associate taking your pills with some regularly scheduled activity, like going to bed or washing in the morning. If you experience any nausea, you may want to try taking them before bedtime.
2. If you are using a 28-day pack, begin a new pack immediately. If you are taking a 21-day pack, stop taking the pills for 1 week, then start your new pack.
3. If you experience bleeding between periods, try to take the pills at the same time every day. If this occurs for two or more cycles, call your doctor. Never stop taking your pills before checking with your doctor. This is an easy way to get pregnant.
4. Check your pack of pills each morning to be sure you took your pill for the preceding day.
5. Other medications: The effectiveness of birth control pills may be decreased slightly by a number of drugs that affect the liver. Be sure to tell you doctor if you are using rifampin, phenytoin (Dilantin), carbamazepine, ampicillin, or tetracycline.

IF YOU FORGET TO TAKE THE PILLS

If you forget to take your pill at the regular time, take it as soon as you remember.

If You Miss One Pill

If you do not remember to take the pill until the next day, take the forgotten pill as soon as you remember, and then take that day's pill at the regular time. You probably won't get pregnant. Just to be sure, you could use your backup method of protection for 7 days after the missed pill.

If You Miss Two Pills

Take two pills on the day you remember and two pills on the next day. *Example:* You forget your pills on Tuesday and Wednesday evenings but remember Thursday morning. Take two pills on Thursday as soon as you remember and two pills on Friday. Then continue with one pill a day. *Important!* Be sure to use a backup method of birth control for the rest of the cycle. You may have some spotting during the month.

If You Miss Three Pills

If you miss three pills, you will probably begin your period. Throw away your old pack of pills and start a new pack of pills the same way you begin the first (i.e., Sunday or immediately). *Important!* Be sure to use a backup method of birth control until you have been back on the pill for 7 days.

If the only pills you missed are from the fourth week of a 28-day pack, just throw away the missed pills and continue taking the pills from your current package of pills on schedule. The pills in the fourth week do not contain hormones, so missing these pills does not increase your risk for pregnancy at all.

If you have diarrhea or vomiting, use your backup method of birth control until your next period. Start using a backup method on your first day of diarrhea or vomiting. If nausea continues, see you clinician, doctor, nurse, or physician assistant.

Figure 44.4.   *continued*

BIBLIOGRAPHY

ACOG Technical Bulletin. Hormonal contraception. 1994;198.

ACOG issues report on hormonal contraception. Am Fam Physician 1995;51:543.

Archer DF. Clinical and metabolic features of desogestrel: a new oral contraceptive preparation. Am J Obstet Gynecol 1994;170:1550.

Berenson AB, Wiemann CM. Use of levonorgestrel implants versus oral contraceptives in adolescence: a case-control study. Am J Obstet Gynecol 1995;172:1128.

Brill K, Schnitker J, Albring M. Clinical experience with a modern low-dose gestodene-containing oral contraceptive in adolescents. Adv Contracept 1994;10:237.

Bringer J. Norgestimate: a clinical overview of a new progestin. Am J Obstet Gynecol 1992;166:1969.

Burkman RT. Noncontraceptive effects of hormonal contraceptives: bone mass, sexually transmitted disease and pelvic inflammatory disease, cardiovascular disease, menstrual function, and future fertility. Am J Obstet Gynecol 1994;170:1569.

Burkman RT Jr. Oral contraceptives: an update. Hosp Pract 1995;30:85.

Centers for Disease Control. OC use and the risk of breast cancer in young women. MMWR 1984;22:353.

Centers for Disease Control, Cancer and Steroid Hormone Study. Long-term oral contraceptive use and the risk of breast cancer. JAMA 1983;249:1591.

Clarkson TB, Shively CA, Morgan TM, et al. Oral contraceptives and coronary artery atherosclerosis of cynomolgus monkeys. Obstet Gynecol 1990;75:217.

Colditz GA. Oral contraceptive use and mortality during 12 years of follow-up: the Nurses' Health Study. Ann Intern Med 1994;120:821.

Collins DC. Sex hormone receptor binding, progestin selectivity, and the new oral contraceptives. Am J Obstet Gynecol 1994;170:1508.

Cromer BA, Smith RD, Blair JM, et al. A prospective study of adolescents who choose among levonorgestrel implant (Norplant), medroxyprogesterone acetate (Depo-Provera), or the combined oral contraceptive pill as contraception. Pediatrics 1994;94:687.

Davis, AJ. The role of hormonal contraception in adolescents. Am J Obstet Gynecol 1994;170:1581.

Derman R. Selecting an oral contraceptive. Female Patient 1994;19:25.

Duchin SE, Ledger WJ, Schulze RJ, et al. OCs: risks, benefits, guidelines. Patient Care 89 1989;(March):30.

Dunson TR, McLaurin VL, Israngkura B, et al. A comparative study of two low-dose combined oral contraceptives: results from a multicenter trial. Contraception 1993;48:109.

Eatmon TM, Huff PS. The new progestins: the pill with no side effects? Contraceptive Technology 1994;(March):38.

Emans SJ, Grace E, Woods ER, et al. Adolescent compliance with the use of oral contraceptives. JAMA 1987;257:3377.

Friedman AJ, Thomas PP. Does low-dose combination oral contraceptive use affect uterine size or menstrual flow in premenopausal women with leiomyoma? Obstet Gynecol 1995;85:631.

Godsland IF, Crook D. Update on the metabolic effects of steroidal contraceptives and their relationship to cardiovascular disease risk. Am J Obstet Gynecol 1994;170:1528.

Gold MA. New progestins oral contraceptives and the female condom. Pediatr Ann 1995;24:211.

Goldzieher JW. Are low-dose oral contraceptives safer and better? Am J Obstet Gynecol 1994;171:587.

Hirvonen F, Idänpään-Heikkilä J. Cardiovascular deaths among women under 40 years of age using low-dose estrogen contraceptives and intrauterine devices in Finland from 1975–1984. Am J Obstet Gynecol 1990;163:281.

Kjos SL, Shoupe D, Douyan S, et al. Effect of low-dose oral contraceptives on carbohydrate and lipid metabolism in women with recent gestational diabetes: results of a controlled, randomized, prospective study. Am J Obstet Gynecol 1990;163:1822.

Lobo RA, Stanczyk FZ. New knowledge in the physiology of hormonal contraceptives. Am J Obstet Gynecol 1994;170:1499.

Meade TW, Greenberg C, Thompson SG. Progestins and cardiovascular reactions associated with oral contraceptives and a comparison of the safety of 50- and 30-µg estrogen preparations. Br Med J 1980;280:1157.

Mishell DR Jr. Non-contraceptive health benefits of oral steroidal contraceptives. Am J Obstet Gynecol 1982;142:809.

Mishell DR Jr. Update on oral contraceptives. Drug Therapy 1989;(April):118.

Nakajima ST. The new progestins. West J Med 1994;161:163.

New Zealand Contraception and Health Study Group. Risk of cervical dysplasia in users of oral contraceptives, intrauterine devices or depo-medroxyprogesterone acetate. Contraception 1994;50:431.

Oakley D, Sereika S, Bogue EL. Oral contraceptive pill use after an initial visit to a family planning clinic. Fam Plann Perspect 1991;23:150.

Peterson, HB, Lee NC. The health effects of oral contraceptives: misperceptions, controversies, and continuing good news. Clin Obstet Gynecol 1989;32:339.

Pike MC, Henderson BE, Krailo MD, et al. Breast cancer in young women and use of oral contraceptives: possible modifying effect of formulation and age at use. Lancet 1983;2:926.

Porter JB, Jick H, Walker AM. Mortality among oral contraceptive users. Obstet Gynecol 1987;70:29.

Reubinoff BE, Gurbstein A, Meirow D. Effects of low-dose estrogen oral contraceptives on weight, body composition, and fat distribution in young women. Fertil Steril 1995;63:516.

Robinson GE. Low-dose combined oral contraceptives. Br J Obstet Gynaecol 1994;101:1036.

Robinson JC, Plichta S, Weisman CS, et al. Dysmenorrhea and use of oral contraceptives in adolescent women attending a family planning clinic. Am J Obstet Gynecol 1992;166:578.

Runnebaum B. The androgenicity of oral contraceptives: the young patient's concerns. Int J Fertil 1992; 37:211.

Schlesselman JJ. Net effect of oral contraceptive use on the risk of cancer in women in the United States. Obstet Gynecol. 1995;85:793.

Shoupe D. New progestins—clinical experiences: gestodene. Am J Obstet Gynecol 1994;170:1562.

Speroff L, DeCherney A. Evaluation of a new generation of oral contraceptives. The Advisory Board for the New Progestins. Obstet Gynecol 1993;81: 1034.

Stewart DL. The new oral contraceptives: understanding the pharmacology. Female Patient 1993;18:69.

Thomas DB. The WHO collaborative study of neoplasia and steroid contraceptives: the influence of combined oral contraceptives on risk of neoplasms in developing and developed countries. Contraception 1991;43:695.

Trussell J, Leveque JA, Koenig JD, et al. The economic value of contraception: a comparison of 15 methods. Am J Public Health 1995;85:494.

Weisberg E. Prescribing oral contraceptives. Drugs 1995;49:224.

Weiss N. Third-generation oral contraceptives: how risky? Lancet 1995;346:1570.

White MM, McGregor JA. Update on oral contraceptives. Phys Assist 1992;(January):66.

Woods ER, Grace E, Havens KK, et al. Contraceptive compliance with levonorgestrel triphasic and a norethindrone monophasic oral contraceptive in adolescent patients. Am J Obstet Gynecol 1992;166:901.

World Health Organization Collaborative Study of Cardiovascular Disease and Steroid Hormone Contraception. Venous thromboembolic disease and combined oral contraceptives; results of international multicentre case-control study. Lancet 1995;346:1575.

World Health Organization Collaborative Study of Cardiovascular Disease and Steroid Hormone Contraception. Effect of different progestagens in low-oestrogen oral contraceptives on venous thromboembolic disease. Lancet 1995;346:1582.

World Health Organization Collaborative Study of Cardiovascular Disease and Steroid Hormone Contraception. Risk of idiopathic cardiovascular death and nonfatal venous thromboembolism in women using oral contraceptives with differing progestagen components. Lancet 1995;346:1589.

CHAPTER 45

Intrauterine Devices

Lawrence S. Neinstein and Anita Nelson

The intrauterine device (IUD) is a safe, effective long-term method of birth control for appropriately selected patients. The recommended IUD user is a parous woman who is in a stable, mutually monogamous relationship, and has no history of pelvic inflammatory disease. These features are designed to ensure she has no obvious risk for acquiring a sexually transmitted disease (STD). It is also important to note that IUD candidates need *not* have completed their families but should be interested in avoiding pregnancy for at least one to several years (depending on the type of IUD being contemplated). While many adolescents fail to meet these criteria, there are some teens and young adults for whom the IUD is an ideal method. Older studies have shown that an adolescent's acceptance of IUD is adequate; 72% of users in a 1980 study expressed satisfaction. While this is relatively high for teens, it is markedly lower than the 98% satisfaction rating all IUD users expressed in a 1991 contraceptive survey.

COMMON MISCONCEPTIONS ABOUT INTRAUTERINE DEVICES

The IUD is tremendously underutilized by all age groups in the United States compared to its usage in other developed countries. A great deal of this underutilization can be traced to the following *misconceptions* regarding IUD usage:

1. The IUD causes pelvic inflammatory disease (PID): PID risk seems to be concentrated in women with unstable relationships. Women in stable relationships have only a temporary increase in their risk of infection. The risk is confined to the first few months but particularly the first 20 days after insertion, reflecting inoculation of the endometrium at the time of insertion, either by contamination during insertion or poor patient selection (Farley et al., 1992). After that critical time period, the rates of PID in IUD users blend with the background rate of sexually active users of nonbarrier methods. Furthermore, there is no increase in PID risk with long-term use. These data emphasize the importance of screening patients for vaginal and cervical infections before insertion and of using fastidious sterile technique with insertion. A second important set of conclusions would be that (*a*) the longer the IUD can be used, the lower the infectious risk and that (*b*) the more frequently it requires removal and reinsertion, the higher the infectious sequelae.

2. The IUD is an abortifacient: While the mechanism of action for each IUD is incompletely understood, the evidence, as outlined below, is clear that each type of IUD acts as a contraceptive.

3. All IUDs increase the risk of ectopic pregnancy: Experience with the Copper T380A has conclusively demonstrated that ParaGard reduces a user's risk of all pregnancies, including ectopic pregnancy. The progesterone IUD (Progestasert) does not reduce a woman's risk for ectopic pregnancy, although it significantly reduces the overall pregnancy rate.

4. The IUD causes lawsuits: Historically, this has certainly been true. The litigation over the Dalkon Shield caused the demise of AJ Robins Company, Inc. However, recent experience with the modern IUDs, patient selection, and more complete consent forms has completely changed the medicolegal environment. Since the introduction of the Copper T380A IUD in 1988, no lawsuits have been brought against the IUD.

5. The IUD is expensive: Studies have clearly demonstrated that the Copper T380A IUD is the most cost effective method of birth control. Trussell et al., (1995) found that over a 5-year period the Copper T380A IUD costs only $205–$498 and saves $14,122 in reproductive health care costs when compared to using no method of birth control.

6. The IUD reduces future fertility: Early studies that caused alarm about the possible association between IUD use and infertility actually showed that in *low-risk* IUD users tubal infertility was not increased. In later prospective, controlled studies of IUD users, the fertility of women after IUD removal has been shown to be comparable to the general population; within 48 months of IUD removal, 91.5% of the nulligravida women and 95.7% of the gravid women had conceived. Wilson (1989) found there was no difference in the first-year rates of the fertility, ectopic pregnancy, miscarriage, or preterm delivery rates for women who had asked to have IUDs removed to conceive compared to women who had IUDs removed because of complications.

Types of Intrauterine Devices

Two different designs of IUDs are currently available in this country: the T380A copper-bearing IUD (ParaGard) and the progesterone-releasing IUD (Progestasert). Each provides effective and safe birth control and has to overcome the similar misconceptions about IUD use, but each has sufficiently different individual characteristics to warrant separate discussion.

ParaGard (Copper T380A) Intrauterine Device

1. Description of device: The Copper T380A is composed of a polyethylene body, enhanced with coils of copper wire on the stem and collars of solid copper on each of the transverse arms, totaling 380 mm^2 of copper. Monofilament strings are threaded through the bulb at the end of the stem. The stem contains barium sulfate to make it radiopaque. The Copper T380A IUD is approved by the Food and Drug Administration (FDA) for 10 years of continuous usage. The IUD is traditionally inserted on menses to exclude the possibility of pregnancy, but can be inserted at any time in the cycle if the patient is not pregnant. Postpartum insertion is best done after uterine involution is complete.

2. Effectiveness: The typical first-year failure rate of the Copper T380A IUD is between 0.7–0.8% with a 10-year cumulative failure rate of 2.1%. This 10-year failure rate is lower than the typical first-year failure rate with oral contraceptives.

3. Mechanism of action: The IUD does not work as an abortifacient; it does not interrupt an established pregnancy. Uterine flushing studies have demonstrated that the IUD acts prior to the time the blastocyst arrives in the uterine cavity. Alvarez et al. (1988) have shown that there are no normally developing fertilized ova to be found in the fallopian tubes of IUD users. The copper in the IUD interferes with sperm transport and capacitation. So the best description of the mechanism of action of the Copper T380A IUD is that it functions as a spermicide. There is an absolute decrease in the number and motility of sperm found in IUD users. Fertilization may also be impeded by the increased prostaglandin levels in the peritoneal fluid. The clinical significance of the inflammatory changes induced in the endometrium is unknown.

4. Contraindications: The Copper T380A should not be inserted when one or more of the following conditions exists:

    a. Pregnancy or suspicion of pregnancy
    b. Abnormalities of the uterus resulting in distortion of the uterine cavity
    c. Acute PID or a history of PID
    d. Postpartum endometritis or infected abortion in the past 3 months
    e. Known or suspected uterine or cervical malignancy, including unresolved, abnormal results from Pap smear
    f. Genital bleeding of unknown cause
    g. Untreated acute cervicitis or vaginitis, including bacterial vaginosis, until infection is controlled
    h. Presence of diagnosed Wilson's disease
    i. Known allergy to copper
    j. Patient or her partner has multiple sexual partners
    k. Conditions associated with increased susceptibility to infections with micro-organisms: Such conditions include, but are not limited to, leukemia, acquired immunodeficiency syndrome (AIDS), intravenous (IV) drug abuse, and long-term corticosteroid therapy.
    l. Genital actinomycosis
    m. A previously inserted IUD that has not been removed
    n. Uterine size less than 6 cm or greater than 9 cm on sounding

5. Relative contraindications
    a. Anemia
    b. Menorrhagia
    c. Severe dysmenorrhea

6. Advantages
    a. Extremely effective form of contraception
    b. Decreased risk of ectopic pregnancy
    c. Convenient method (only requires monthly string checks to confirm its presence)
    d. Private method: The IUD is not detectable by parents and often unnoticed by partner.
    e. Immediately reversible by practitioner removal

7. Disadvantages
    a. Available only through medical providers: Professional assistance is required for insertion and removal, and trained providers are limited but increasing in number.
    b. Available only for low-risk women
    c. Provides no protection against STDs and may increase risks of complication of STDs if contracted (e.g., PID)
    d. Increases menstrual flow and cramping
    e. Occasional side effects (see below)
    f. Relatively high initial costs

8. Side effects
    a. Increased menstrual bleeding and cramping: Copper T380A IUDs typically increase menstrual blood loss by at least 35%, and concomitant dysmenorrhea can result. Treatment with nonsteroidal anti-inflammatory drugs (NSAIDs) readily reverses this increase; however, patients must initiate NSAID usage in anticipation of menses or at the beginning of the flow to effectively block prostaglandin formation. An isolated episode of increased or untimely bleeding or cramping may indicate partial expulsion or failure and requires prompt medical evaluation.
    b. IUD Expulsion: Average first-year expulsion rates range from 2–10%, with the average at 5.7%. Rates are increased if insertion is accomplished during the days of heavy menstrual flow and minimized if insertion is done after the eleventh cycle day. Other risk factors for expulsion include young user age, menorrhagia, and severe dysmenorrhea prior to Copper T380A insertion.

c. Perforation or embedment: The partial or total uterine perforation is a rare event with the Copper T380A IUD, averaging 1 per 1000. Rates are increased in a woman whose uterus is not fully involuted postpartum, who is lactating, or whose uterus is markedly retroverted. The most important predictive variable, however, is the experience of the inserter. Embedment of the Copper T380A in the endometrium or myometrium can cause a difficult removal and may require hysteroscopically guided or surgical removal.

Progestasert Intrauterine Device

1. Description of device: The Progestasert (Progesterone T) IUD measures 36 mm in length and 32 mm in width and is composed of a vertical ethylene vinyl acetate copolymer filled with 38 mg progesterone and enough barium sulfate to make it visible on x-ray examination. The arms are inert and help stabilize the device within the uterine cavity. Blue-black double strings attach at the base of the stem. The device releases progesterone at a rate of 65 g per day and has an approved life of 12 months.
2. Efficacy: The typical failure rate for the Progestasert IUD is 2.0%, although the perfect use failure rates are only 1.5%. The rate of ectopic pregnancy is not decreased by the Progestasert IUD and may even be slightly increased.
3. Mechanism of action: The Progestasert IUD works as a local application of progesterone, thickening cervical mucus to prohibit sperm penetration and inducing atrophic changes in the endometrium. There is virtually no systemic increase in progesterone.
4. Contraindications: Contraindications for the Progestasert are similar to those of the Copper T380A IUD except that there is no contraindication for patients with Wilson's disease or copper allergy. The upper limit of uterine size is 9 cm for Copper T380A but 10 cm for Progestasert. Anemia and menorrhagia are not contraindications for Progestasert because the progesterone-containing IUD does not increase menstrual flow.
5. Advantages
   a. Highly effective method of birth control
   b. Convenient method (requires only monthly monitoring of strings to verify its presence)
   c. Private method
   d. Immediately reversible when removed
   e. Compared to Copper T380A—no increase in cramping or bleeding and may be used in women with larger uteri
6. Disadvantages
   a. Menstrual changes: Spotting and amenorrhea increase.
   b. Annual changing is required, which increases costs and risk of infection (compared to Copper T380A IUD).
   c. Otherwise, disadvantages are similar to copper IUD.
7. Side effects: Progesterone IUD expulsion and perforation are roughly equivalent to the copper devices. The embedment rates may be slightly lower for Progestasert IUDs because they must be changed annually.

USE IN ADOLESCENTS

Diaz et al. (1993) compared the clinical performance of 995 parous adolescents using a copper IUD with a cohort of paired controls 10 years older of the same parity. While the pregnancy rates, expulsion rates, and removal rates were higher in adolescents, the ranges were within those reported in the literature for the IUD. Removal rates for infections were few and not significantly different from rates for older women. Overall, the performance was similar or better than other reversible methods in this age group. Thus, in the appropriate adolescent or young adult (parous women in a monogamous relationship) an IUD should be considered along with other methods.

PREGNANCY WITH AN INTRAUTERINE DEVICE IN PLACE

Pregnancies in current IUD users are rare. When an IUD is in place and a pregnancy occurs, spontaneous abortions are common, occurring in about 50% of women. It is recommended that the IUD be removed as soon as possible if the strings are visible in the vagina. Removal reduces the risk of spontaneous abortion by about 50%, or to a 25% rate. If a women elects to keep the IUD, she should be counseled about the increased risk of premature labor and delivery, low birth weight, and stillbirth. If the strings are not visible, there is no reason to attempt to remove the IUD. The risk of birth defects is not increased. If a teen elects to abort, the IUD can be removed at the time of the procedure.

GUIDELINES TO PATIENTS

Following is a suggested format for informing teens about IUDs.

1. What is an IUD?
   The IUD (intrauterine device) is a small plastic device that is placed in the uterus (womb).
2. How does the IUD work?
   The IUD appears to work by preventing fertilization. The copper in copper IUDs probably has an antisperm effect.
3. How effective are IUDs?
   IUDs are among the most effective forms of birth control. For every 100 women using the copper IUD less than one per year will become pregnant. With the progesterone IUD about two to three women per year will become pregnant.
4. Are there different types of IUDs?
   In the United States today there are two types of IUDs available. One contains copper and the other contains a hormone called progesterone. Both are shaped like the letter T and are about $1^1/_4$ inches tall. Each IUD has a thread or tail on the end, which allows the woman to check that the IUD is in place and also makes it easier for the doctor to remove the IUD.
   The copper IUD has copper sleeves on the arms and copper wire coiled around the stem. The cooper IUD can be left in place and is effective for up to 10 years. The progesterone device has a hollow stem that contains the natural hormone progesterone, which is slowly continuously released into the uterus and acts locally. This type of IUD must be replaced once a year.
5. Are there side effects?
   With the copper IUD the most common side effects are increased menstrual flow and cramps, which can be relieved by the use of an over-the-counter pain medication such as ibuprofen. These side effects lessen after the first few months. Spotting or bleeding may also occur between menstrual periods with the progesterone IUD, although total blood loss and dysmenorrhea (painful periods) are reduced.
6. Are IUDs safe?
   IUDs are a safe and effective method of birth control when used in the appropriate individuals. They should be used in women who have had children and who have only

one long-term sexual partner. Women at risk for an STD (sexually transmitted disease) should not select the IUD. This is important because the IUD does not protect against STDs and can increase a woman's risk of having an STD or uterine infection and becoming infertile if her partner has an STD or if she has multiple partners.

7. What are the benefits of an IUD?

   IUDs are a safe, effective, easy-to-use, and less expensive form of contraception. There is no need to remember to use the method every day or with every act of sex. *However, the IUD does not protect against STDs. If you may be at risk for STDs, use a latex condom to help protect yourself against infection.*

Remember:

1. Check for the string of the IUD frequently during the first months and at least after each period thereafter.
2. If you ever have fever, pelvic pain, severe cramping, unusual vaginal bleeding, or foul vaginal discharge, contact your doctor immediately. These may be signs of a serious infection or a warning that you are losing your IUD.
3. If you miss a menstrual period, contact your doctor immediately.
4. Do not remove the IUD yourself or pull on the strings.
5. If you have any problems or questions call the clinic.

BIBLIOGRAPHY

Alvarez R, Brache V, Fernandez F, et al. New insights on the mode of action of intrauterine devices in women. Fertil Steril 1988;49(5):768.

Bromham DR. Intrauterine contraceptive devices—a reappraisal. Br Med Bull 1993;49:100.

Contraceptive Technology Update. Third-generation IUDs have fewer complications. Contraceptive Technology Update 1992;(February):23.

Cramer DW, et al. Tubal infertility and the intrauterine device. N Engl J Med 1985;12:941.

Diaz J, Neto AMP, Bahamondes L, et al. Performance of the Copper T 200 in parous adolescents: are copper IUDs suitable for these women? Contraception 1993;48:23.

Farley TM, Rosenberg MS, Rowe PJ, et al. Intrauterine devices and pelvic inflammatory disease: an international perspective. Lancet 1992;339(8796):785.

Farr G, Rivera R. Interactions between intrauterine contraceptive device use and breast-feeding status at time of intrauterine contraceptive device insertion: analysis of TCu-380A acceptors in developing countries. Am J Obstet Gynecol 1992;167(1):144.

Forrest, JD. Acceptability of IUDs in the United States. Paper presented at: A new look at IUDs—advancing contraceptive choices. New York, March 27–28, 1992.

Franks AL, Beral V, Cates W, et al. Contraception and ectopic pregnancy rates. Am J Obstet Gynecol 1990; 163:1120.

Hatcher RA, Trussell J, Stewart F, et al. Contraceptive technology, 16th revised ed. New York: Irvington Publishers, 1994:347.

Heartwell SF, Schlesselman S. Risk of uterine perforation among users of intrauterine devices. Obstet Gynecol 1983;61:31.

Kulig JW, Raugh JL, Burket RL, et al. Experience with the Copper 7 intrauterine device in an adolescent population. J Pediatr 1980;96(4):746.

Lee NC, Rubino GL, Borueki R. The intrauterine device and pelvic inflammatory disease revisited: new results for the women's health study. Obstet Gynecol 1988;72(1):1.

Mishell D Jr, Roy S. Copper intrauterine contraceptive device event rates following insertion 4 to 8 weeks postpartum. Am J Obstet Gynecol 1982;143:29.

Ortho Pharmaceutical Corporation. Annual birth control study. Raritan, New Jersey: Ortho Pharmaceutical Corporation, 1991.

Ortiz ME, Croyatto HB. The mode of action of IUDs. Contraception 1987;36(1):37.

Pollack AE, Girvin S. When should an IUD be removed and replaced? Medical Aspects of Human Sexuality 1992;26:46.

Sivin I. IUDs are contraceptives, not abortifacients: a comment on research and belief. Stud Fam Plann 1989;20(6–1):355.

Sivin I. Dose- and age-dependent ectopic pregnancy risks with intrauterine contraception. Obstet Gynecol 1991;78:291.

Sivin I, Schmidt F. Effectiveness of IUDs: a review. Contraception 1987;36:55.

Skjeldestad F, Bratt H. Fertility after complicated and non-complicated use of IUDs. A controlled prospective study. Adv Contracept 1988;4:179.

Speroff L, Darney P. A clinical guide for contraception. Baltimore: Williams & Wilkins, 1992;161.

Tatum HJ. Clinical aspects of intrauterine contraception: 1976. Contraception 1977;28:16.

Trussell J, Leveque A, Koenig JD, et al. Economic value of contraception: a comparison of 15 methods. Am J Public Health 1995;85:494.

White MK, Ory HW, Rooks JB, et al. Intrauterine device termination rates and the menstrual cycle day of insertion. Obstet Gynecol 1980;55(2):220.

Wilson JC. A prospective New Zealand study of fertility after removal of copper intrauterine contraceptive devices for contraception and because of complications: a four year study. Am J Obstet Gynecol 1989;160:391.

World Health Organization (WHO) Scientific Group. Mechanisms of action, safety, and efficacy of intrauterine devices. WHO Technical Report 753, 1987.

Zhang J, Chi I-C, Feldblum PJ, et al. Risk factors for Copper T IUD expulsion: an epidemiologic analysis. Contraception 1992;46(5):427.

CHAPTER 46

Barrier Contraceptives

Lawrence S. Neinstein and Anita Nelson

Barrier contraceptives are agents that kill sperm or block their movement toward the cervical os. Barrier contraceptives are available in a wide variety of designs, including male and female condoms, diaphragms, cervical cap, and vaginal spermicides. In general, they have higher failure rates but fewer systemic side effects than other contraceptives. Barrier methods also offer some sexually transmitted disease (STD) risk reduction. Many barriers are available over the counter and improve adolescent access to birth control. The high user failure rate of barrier methods could be considerably lowered if they were used more consistently and if they were combined with the use of emergency contraception (see Chapter 47).

MALE CONDOMS

Male condoms (Fig. 46.1) are the oldest and most reliable male method of contraception and are the second most popular method of birth control in the United States. Overall, teen condom use tends to be greatest at the time of sexual debut; 29% of sexually experienced 15- to 17-year-olds use this as their primary contraception. That number declines to 24% among 18- to 19-year olds. At last intercourse 58.5% of 14- to 17-year-olds used condoms compared to 36.9% at age 18–21. The reverse trend is seen in Hispanic teens, whose condom usage increases with age. Condom use has improved among adolescents, increasing from 46.2% of adolescents at most recent sexual intercourse in 1991 to 52.8% in 1992. Condoms are very cost effective for episodic intercourse, which is often found among teens. For long-term use, however, the condom's higher failure rate drives its overall cost much higher.

The human immunodeficiency virus (HIV) epidemic has heightened public awareness and acceptance of condoms. A significant degree of STD protection is afforded by latex condoms, which are impermeable to *Chlamydia trachomatis*, *Neisseria gonorrhoeae*, herpes simplex virus, cytomegalovirus, hepatitis B virus, and human papilloma virus. Millions of women use condoms in conjunction with other methods (sterilization, birth control pills, foam) to capture this STD risk reduction benefit.

Types of Male Condoms

More than 100 brands of condoms available in the United States provide a wide range of choices in sizes, shapes, thicknesses, lubricants, and design features to trap the ejaculate. Three different materials are used in manufacturing condoms; latex dominates the market (99%), while skin condoms and polyurethane together account for less than 1%. Condoms are available in three sizes, but most condoms are 170 mm long and 50 mm wide. The thickness ranges from 0.03–0.10 mm. Condom shapes vary (they can be straight-sided or contoured), as do their textures (smooth or ribbed). Condoms are lubricated internally and ex-

THE MALE CONDOM (RUBBER)

The condom is a sheath of rubber shaped to fit snugly over the erect penis. It acts as a barrier between the penis and vagina to prevent the transmission of semen into the vagina during intercourse. It also represents the most effective contraceptive device in reducing the risk of sexually transmitted diseases (STDs). It can also be used with other contraceptive methods such as pills, intrauterine devices (IUDs), Depo-Provera shots, and Norplant implant devices to add protection against STDs. If used every time and correctly with each act of intercourse, the condom is 97% effective as a method of birth control. By using contraceptive foam with condoms, the effectiveness is increased to 99%.

INSTRUCTIONS TO PATIENTS

Condoms must be used with every sex act.
  How to use the condom:

1. The condom should be put on the erect penis (by either partner) before the penis is put in the vagina or comes in contact with the woman's genital area.
2. The package should be opened carefully to avoid tearing a hole in the condom with a fingernail.
3. The condom rim should be unrolled all the way to the bottom of the erect penis. If the condom was unrolled incorrectly (backward), it should be removed and thrown away, starting with a new condom. This will prevent any pre-ejaculatory fluid that may contain sperm or STDs from coming in contact with your partner.
4. Leave about $\frac{1}{2}$ inch of empty space at the tip of the condom. This will collect the semen so the condom does not burst. You may buy condoms that already have nipple tips to hold the semen.
5. Adequate lubrication is important before penetration. Condoms come lubricated. For extra lubrication, you can use products such as water, K-Y jelly, or spermicidal creams, jellies, foam, or suppositories. Do not use oil-based products such as petroleum jelly, massage oil, baby oil, or cold creams, as this can cause the latex of the condom to deteriorate.
6. Condoms will stay good for about 2 years if stored away from heat. Do not keep your condoms in your wallet for a long time period, as body heat can cause deterioration of the rubber.
7. If you feel the condom slipping off during intercourse, stop and check the condom. If the condom is torn or has come off in the vagina, insert contraceptive foam or jelly immediately. Also replace the damaged condom with a new condom before continuing intercourse. If no spermicidal product is available, wash both the penis and the vagina with soap and water to minimize any risk of infection. Do not douche, as this may force sperm and bacteria into the uterus.
8. When the male withdraws the penis soon after ejaculation, the rim of the condom should be held so the condom does not fall off in the vagina.
9. When the penis is away from the partner's genitals, the condom can be removed and thrown away. Condoms should not be reused for either oral, vaginal, or anal intercourse.

FIGURE 46.1. Sample instruction sheet for condoms. (Courtesy Teenage Health Center, Childrens Hospital of Los Angeles.) *Figure continued on following page.*

ternally by a wide range of materials: silicones, spermicides, or water-based surgical gels. Other features are intended to make them more aesthetically appealing with a wide array of colors and scents. The richness in choices of condoms permits flexibility in selection and is intended to increase user compliance. The natural skin condoms afford nearly equal pregnancy protection but do not reduce STD risks.

  The newer polyurethane male condoms that have recently been introduced into the United States have many attractive features. They are nonbiodegradable and require less fas-

Side Effects

A very few individuals have had an allergic reaction to the rubber in condoms. If this occurs, polyurethane condoms can be used. The major complaint with condoms is of reduction of sensitivity and of pleasure. Lubricated condoms may resolve this problem.

Advantages

1. Effective if used properly and with every sexual act
2. No health risks
3. Can be purchased at a drugstore without a prescription
4. Effective in reducing the risk of contracting an STD, including human immunodeficiency virus (HIV)
5. Can be put on by male or female and incorporated into foreplay

Disadvantages

1. May decrease sensitivity for the male
2. May interrupt sexual activity
3. May break or slip off in the vagina, possibly causing pregnancy

Following are do's and don'ts related to condom use.

Do's	Don'ts
Do buy latex, reservoir-tipped condoms.	**Don't** buy condoms made of any other material.
Do check expiration date.	**Don't** buy outdated condoms.
Do store in cool dry place.	**Don't** store in glove compartment.
	Don't store in hip wallet for long periods of time.
Do roll condom on penis as soon as penis is hard.	**Don't** wait until you are ready to enter your partner; it may be too late. Drops of semen may come out before ejaculation.
Do leave ¼ to ½ inch extra space at tip if the condom has no nipple.	**Don't** twist, bite, or prick condom with a pin.
Do hold condom at the rim when removing condom.	**Don't** let penis go soft inside partner, as condom may fall out inside of partner.
	Don't allow semen to spill on your hands, body, or an open wound. Wash hands if contact occurs.

Fɪɢᴜʀᴇ **46.1.**   *continued*

tidious handling prior to use. They are not susceptible to damage by petroleum-based lubricants. The polyurethane male condoms transmit heat and may be more pleasurable to use. They lack the latex antigens that cause allergic reaction. Although the polyurethane itself is a stronger material than latex, the thinness of the new condoms may reduce that benefit. Questions still remain about the breakage rates of polyurethane condoms at different thicknesses and the associated pregnancy rates and STD protection afforded by these new thin condoms. Studies are ongoing to more accurately quantify these risks. Until better analysis has been completed, the thin polyurethane male condom may best be reserved for couples who cannot tolerate latex products.

A review of the individual types of condoms and reliability has been outlined in *Consumer Reports*, 1995.

Mechanism of Action

Condoms are latex (rubber-based), processed collagenous tissue, or polyurethane sheaths that fit over the erect penis and block transmission of semen. Condoms with spermicidal agents (e.g., nonoxynol) also work by killing sperm within the condom.

Effectiveness

The latex male condom is the most effective barrier method available. The typical first-year failure rate with the latex male condom is 12%, with failure rates ranging from as low as 2% for perfect use to as high as 51.3% for use by ever-married teens with incomes less than 200% of the federal poverty level. The most critical variable in predicting efficacy is consistent utilization, followed closely by proper technique.

Keys to Improving Condom Success

1. Teach patients to keep condoms handy at all times (and places) and to:
   a. Incorporate condom placement into the lovemaking process, when the penis is flaccid, if possible, but certainly prior to any genital contact. (The pre-ejaculatory semen contains few sperm, but STD spread may occur early. Furthermore, the teen's ability to arrest sexual activity to place the condom is markedly diminished after genital contact.) Condom placement practice with models during office visits can be very helpful for inexperienced users.
   b. Open the packaging carefully. Any foil edges shearing across the condom may tear into the latex.
   c. Correctly place the condom. Allow slack at the top of condoms with no reservoir; more snugly fit those provided with ejaculatory reservoir once erection is complete. Squeeze the air out of the reservoir areas.
   d. Use only water-based lubricants or spermicides to reduce vaginal friction against the latex condom, which could compromise its structural integrity. Explicitly admonish patients to avoid petroleum-based products such as Vaseline, baby oils, and lotions. (Over 50% of current condom users are unaware that they should avoid those products.) Petroleum can react with the latex in seconds and undermine the strength of the condom. Within a minute, microscopic tears may develop and become large enough to permit the passage of virus.
   e. After ejaculation, firmly grasp the rim of the condom at the base of the penis and carefully withdraw the unit while the penis is still firm. Any delays in removal can result in spillage and loss of protection.
   f. Inspect the condom for signs of breakage or spillage.
   g. Be prepared with fast-acting spermicide should the condom break or spill.
   h. Use emergency contraception as needed (see Chapter 47).
2. Be responsive to patient complaints and apprehension.
   a. For the young woman who is unsure her partner will use condoms, role play with her different scenarios until she believes she has the ability to discuss the issue with her partner and persuade him to use condoms.
   b. If the male partner complains of constriction or blunted sensation, recommend one of the following strategies:
      — Try a larger condom size. Three sizes are currently available.
      — Try a different condom style. Condoms with reservoirs at the side are available to reduce glans pressure and purportedly enhance stimulation. Ridged condoms are also designed to increase sensation.

— Advise the couple to place a second condom over the first one after it has been well lubricated. The friction between the condoms may enhance male sensation. It also reduces the impact of breakage problems.

Advantages

1. Readily available: Condoms may be purchased in drug stores, mail order houses, or vending machines or obtained in family planning clinics or school clinics without prescriptions.
2. Relatively inexpensive: Sometimes they are even free from clinics!
3. Portable: Condoms can be easily carried in wallet, purse, or other vehicle to be available whenever the need arises.
4. Male participation: Even though over half of condoms are purchased by women today, they are still used by men.
5. Visible proof of protection: Couples can get reasonably accurate feedback that protection was offered by observing ejaculate contained in condom.
6. Significant reduction in risk of STDs including HIV and cervical dysplasia: Hatcher et al. (1994) estimate that simultaneous use of a condom and spermicide is 99.9% effective in reducing the risk of STD transmission per act of vaginal intercourse. A recent study of seroconversion of the unaffected partners who engaged in heterosexual behavior with their HIV-positive partners highlights the effectiveness of condoms. There was an 82% conversion rate among couples not using condoms and only a 17% conversion rate among condom users.

Disadvantages

1. Requires placement with each act of intercourse
2. May interrupt lovemaking
3. Requires male's cooperation: Women cannot enforce male condom usage.
4. Higher pregnancy rates than hormonal contraceptive methods or intrauterine devices (IUDs)
5. May diminish pleasure of intercourse
   a. Blunts sensation for man
   b. Results in less vigorous intercourse due to fear that the condom may break or slip
   c. Requires prompt withdrawal
   d. May increase vaginal irritation in women, especially those with inadequate or low adequate lubrication
   e. Poorly transmits heat (latex condoms)
6. May encourage unsafe sex practices (e.g., multiple sex partners) by inappropriately decreasing adolescent's sense of STD vulnerability

Side Effects of Male Condoms

An increasing percentage of the population is developing allergies to latex antigens. Estimates are that in 2–4% of couples using foam and condoms one or more partners has an allergic reaction. This number may be lower in the teen population with less previous exposure to latex.

Uses of Male Condoms

Contraceptive Uses

1. As a primary method of birth control alone or in conjunction with spermicides
2. As a backup method of contraception during a partner's first cycle of pills or whenever two or more consecutive pills have been missed
3. As a barrier method used in fertility awareness methods during vulnerable days

Noncontraceptive Uses

1. Reduce transmission of STDs
2. Blunt sensation and treat premature ejaculation
3. Reduce cervical antisperm antibody titers in women with associated infertility
4. Reduce allergic reaction in women with sensitivity to sperm

IMPROVING BARRIER UTILIZATION

Dozens of excellent studies have been conducted to identify factors that predict consistent use of barrier methods, variables that would predict poor utilization, and ways to design interventions that might improve barrier utilization. Most such research has focused on condom usage. Given the vital role barriers play in slowing the spread of STDs, answers to these questions are desperately needed. Unfortunately, studies show that solutions will not be easy to achieve.

There are profound differences in condom use by gender (Brown et al., 1992; Leland and Barton, 1992) with adolescent women reporting far less use of condoms than adolescent men. (This reflects not only safer sex practices of gay men, but also the profound role older men play in adolescent female activity.) A perceived risk of STD or HIV is associated with higher condom usage and also intentions to use condoms in the future (Brown et al., 1992; Donald et al., 1994; Orr and Langefeld, 1993). However, several studies show that many of those at clearly increased risk for STDs have little appreciation for their vulnerability. A common finding of virtually all studies is that condom usage is increased when adolescents believe that their peers use condoms and that condoms can prevent STDs, when they can talk to their partner about risks, when they have easy access to a supply of condoms, and when they carry condoms with them (Joffe and Radius, 1993). Condom use is decreased when risky sexual behavior is just one of a cluster of risky health behaviors (smoking, substance abuse) or other lifestyle risks (violence). Substantial societal changes apparently will be needed to address these issues. Putting condoms in open containers may be necessary to provide adolescent access to condoms but is clearly not sufficient to assure the condom's usage.

FEMALE CONDOMS

The only female condom (Fig. 46.2) currently available in the United States is the Reality female condom. The device is a thin polyurethane sheath measuring 17 cm in length and 7.8 cm in width. It contains two flexible polyurethane rings. One ring is anchored to the base of the device and remains outside the vagina. The inner ring is loose within the sheath; it is pivoted along the axis of the vagina, used to introduce the device as a diaphragm, and then rotated at the top of the vault to stabilize the device. The female condom provides a barrier along the length of the vagina and partially covers the introitus. It is lined internally with a silicone-based "dry" lubricant and may be combined with vaginal spermicides to enhance efficacy. It should never be combined with use of the latex male condom.

Efficacy

The female condom underwent 6-month clinical trials, during which time a 12.5% failure rate was observed in typical use in the United States. This rate has been annualized, by adjusting for various factors, to a 21–25% typical first-year failure rate. Perfect use rates are considerably lower (2.2–2.6% failure in 6 months), reflecting perhaps the difficulty users experienced using this method. Its efficacy in STD protection has not been tested, but is assumed to parallel its pregnancy rates.

THE FEMALE CONDOM

What is the female condom?
The female condom is a thin, soft, loose-fitting pouch with two flexible rings at either end. One ring helps hold the device in place inside the woman's vagina over the end of the womb (cervix), while the other ring rests outside the vagina.

Outer ring lies against the labia

Inner ring is used for insertion; helps hold female condom in place

How does it work?

The female condom is made of polyurethane, a type of plastic. The plastic condom covers the inside of the vagina, cervix, and perineum (outer lips). The device acts as a barrier to help prevent pregnancy and the transmission of germs that can cause sexually transmitted diseases (STDs), including human immunodeficiency virus (HIV) and acquired immunodeficiency syndrome (AIDS). The device can be inserted by the woman up to 8 hours before sex.

How to insert the female condom

1. Find a comfortable position. You may want to stand up with one foot on a chair, squat with knees apart, or lie down with legs bent and knees apart.
2. Hold the female condom with the open end hanging down. Squeez the inner ring with your thumb and middle finger.
3. Holding the inner ring squeezed together, insert the ring into the vagina and push the inner ring and pouch into the vagina past the pubic bone.
4. When properly inserted, the outer ring will hang down slightly outside the vagina. During intercourse, when the penis enters the vagina, the slack will lessen.

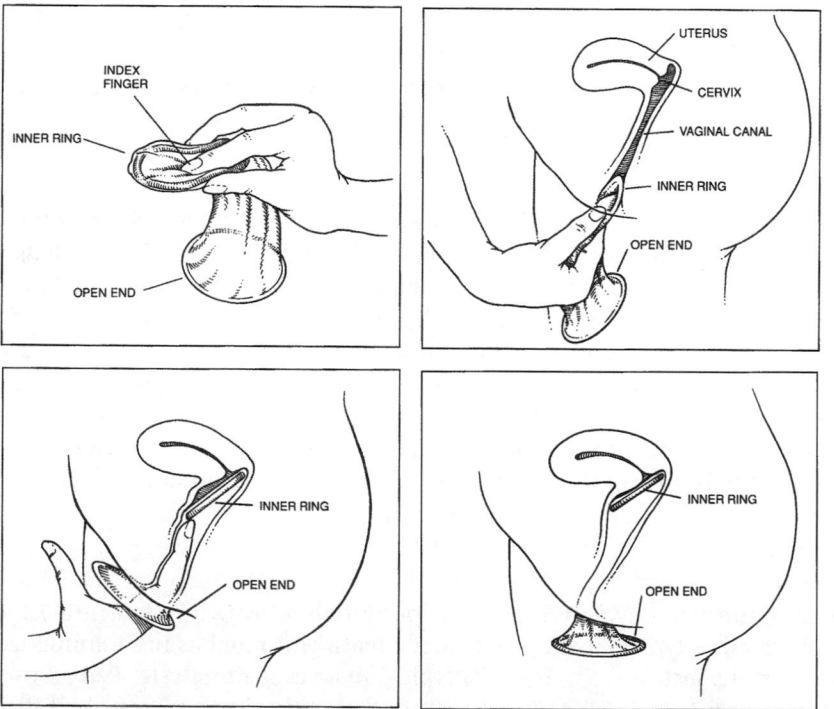

FIGURE 46.2. The female condom.

Remember:

The female condom may be hard to hold or slippery at first. Before you use one for the first time during sex, practice inserting one to get used to it. Take your time. Be sure to insert the condom straight into the vagina without twisting the pouch.

During Sex

1. It's helpful to use your hand to guide the penis into the vagina inside the female condom.
2. The ring may move from side to side or up and down during intercourse. This is OK.
3. If the female condom seems to be sticking to and moving with the penis rather than resting in the vagina, stop and add more lubricant to the inside of the device (near the outer ring) or to the penis.

How to remove the female condom after intercourse

1. Squeeze and twist the outer ring to keep the sperm inside the pouch.
2. Pull the female condom out gently.
3. Throw the condom away in the garbage. Do not flush down the toilet.
4. Do not wash out and use again.

Special Reminders

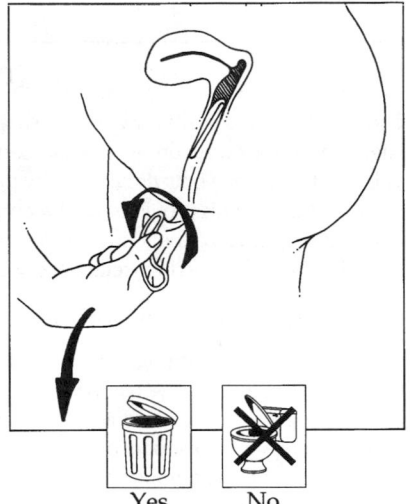

Yes   No

- Use a new female condom with every act of intercourse.
- Use it every time you have intercourse.
- Read and follow the directions carefully.
- Do not use a male and female condom at the same time.
- Be careful not to tear the condom with fingernails or sharp objects.
- Use enough lubricant.

Latex condoms for men are highly effective at preventing STDs, including HIV infection (AIDS), if used properly. If your partner refuses to use a male latex condom, use a female condom to help protect yourself and your partner.

FIGURE 46.2. *continued*

Advantages and Disadvantages

The female condom is available over the counter in single size disposable units, which are more expensive than the male condom. Users inexperienced with diaphragm insertion may find it difficult to insert. The package instructions say correct placement may be difficult in the first or second try due to the device's lubrication. The female condom may be inserted up to 8 hours prior to intercourse to permit a relaxed insertion. The consumer is warned not to tear the sheath with her fingernails or other sharp objects. The penis must be guided in place by the woman, at least with the first few uses, and the couple is to remain attentive throughout coitus to the position of the outer ring to ensure that it does not ride up or get pushed into the vagina. The male partner must ensure that there is no adhesion of his penis to the device, which increases the breakage rate. The relative complexity of the device, its low typical efficacy rate, and the lack of evidence demonstrating reduction in STD risk make the female condom a second choice after the male latex condom. However, the female condom may make an important contribution for women whose partners refuse to use male latex condoms. For adolescents, extensive education and hands-on practice may be needed to assure correct use of the female condom.

Diaphragm

The diaphragm (Fig. 46.3) is a rubber latex shield on a flexible rim, which when introduced into the vagina, extends from the posterior fornix to the anterior vaginal wall to completely cover the cervix. It is intended to be used with contraceptive gel to add spermicidal activity. The diaphragm must be professionally fitted and is available only by prescription.

Types of Diaphragms   Diaphragms are available in sizes ranging from 50–105 mm in 5-mm increments and in four styles, which vary primarily by the construction of the rim or the seal.

DIAPHRAGM

The diaphragm is a shallow, dome-shaped cup made of soft rubber. It is inserted into the vagina and placed securely over the cervix. It must be used with spermicidal cream or jelly. The diaphragm prevents pregnancy by providing a barrier between the sperm and uterus. Additional protection is provided by the contraceptive cream or jelly, which kills the sperm cells. The diaphragm is 97% effective as a method of birth control if it has been fitted properly by your doctor and is used correctly every time you have sex.

INSTRUCTIONS TO PATIENTS

Before use, check diaphragm for tears or holes by holding it up to a bright light and stretching the rubber slightly. Always use with contraceptive cream or jelly and never use with petroleum jelly. To apply contraceptive jelly or cream, hold the diaphragm with the dome down (like a cup). Squeeze a tablespoon of cream or jelly into the dome and spread it around the dome and onto the rim with your finger.

To insert your diaphragm, press the edges of the diaphragm together with one hand. With your other hand, spread the lips of your vagina and insert the diaphragm into your vagina. This can be done standing with one foot propped up (i.e., on the toilet seat), squatting, or lying on your back. Push the diaphragm downward and back along the back wall of your vagina as far as it will go. Then tuck the front rim up along the roof of your vagina behind the pubic bone.

To check the placement of your diaphragm use your index finger to make sure the cervix is completely covered by the soft rubber dome and that the front rim of the diaphragm is snugly in place behind your pubic bone. (The cervix will feel soft and spongy like the tip of your nose.) The spermicidal cream (inside the dome of the diaphragm) should be next to your cervix. When properly placed, the diaphragm will neither cause discomfort nor interfere with sex.

The diaphragm and contraceptive cream or jelly can be inserted up to 6 hours before intercourse. If 6 hours have passed since insertion and the time intercourse occurs, insert an applicator full of jelly or cream into your vagina without removing the diaphragm.

A new application of spermicidal cream or jelly is necessary with each additional act of intercourse. Do not remove the diaphragm. Use the plastic applicator to insert the jelly or cream in front of the diaphragm.

The diaphragm must be left in place for *6 to 8 hours* after the last time your have intercourse. Do not douche during that time. After the 6- to 8-hour period, the diaphragm can be removed whenever it is convenient. If you anticipate intercourse again, you may wash the diaphragm, apply new spermicide, and reinsert it. It should be removed and washed at least once every 24 hours. Remember: Do not remove diaphragm until at least 6 hours have passed after intercourse.

FIGURE 46.3.   Sample instruction sheet for diaphragms. (Courtesy Teenage Health Center, Childrens Hospital of Los Angeles.)

TO REMOVE THE DIAPHRAGM

To remove the diaphragm, place your index finger behind the front rim of the diaphragm and pull down and out. Sometimes squatting and pushing with your abdominal muscles (i.e., bearing down as though you were having a bowel movement), helps to hook your finger behind the diaphragm.

After use, the diaphragm should be washed with soap and water, rinsed thoroughly, and dried with a towel. Store it in its plastic container. You may dust it with cornstarch. Do not use talcum, perfumed powder, Vaseline, baby oil, or contraceptive foam, as they may damage the diaphragm. Inspect the diaphragm (especially around the rim) for holes or defects.

SIDE EFFECTS

Occasionally, the spermicidal cream or jelly has been found to be irritating. Changing to another brand should resolve the problem. Some patients have reported bladder symptoms or urinary tract infections with use of the diaphragm. These difficulties are often resolved by changing to a smaller size or to another rim type of diaphragm. Rare cases of toxic shock syndrome have been reported in users of the diaphragm. Therefore, avoid leaving the diaphragm in longer than 24 hours, and contact your physician if you have:
* Fever over 38.3°C (101°F)
* Diarrhea
* Vomiting
* Muscle aches
* Rash (sunburnlike)

ADVANTAGES

1. Effective and safe
2. Can be worn during your period to hold back menstrual flow during intercourse
3. Can be inserted by partner and incorporated into foreplay

DISADVANTAGES

1. Some women find it difficult to insert, inconvenient, or messy.
2. If you have any problems or questions, please feel free to call the Teenage Health Center at [phone number].

FIGURE 46.3.   *continued*

1. Flat-spring rim: Thin, delicate rim with gentle spring action that is more comfortable for women with firm vaginal wall tone. A plastic diaphragm introducer may be used.
2. Coil-spring rim: Sturdier rim that folds flat for insertion with no arc. It is suitable for a woman with average muscle tone and pubic arch angle. A plastic diaphragm introducer may be used, if needed.
3. Arcing spring rim: A very sturdy rim that folds for insertion but springs open to stabilize the device's position within the vagina. It is designed for universal use, but is uniquely good for vaginas with limited muscle tone. There are two versions: one that folds only in one direction and another that is flexible in all directions.
4. Wide seal rim: Has flexible flange attached to inner edge of the rim to hold spermicide in place and to maintain a better seal. It is available with arcing spring and coil-spring rims.

Contraindications to Use

1. History of toxic shock syndrome
2. Allergy to rubber or spermicidal agents

3. Recent pregnancy, prior to renormalization of anatomy
4. Inability of patient to correctly insert and remove diaphragm

Effectiveness

Typical failure rates in general usage vary between 16–18%. Perfect use failure rate is estimated to be 6%. Women who are more successful users of diaphragms are usually older, comfortable touching their genitals, and able to anticipate coitus; but adolescents certainly can be taught to be effective diaphragm users.

Tips to Improve Success of Method   Correct fitting of device (see below).

1. Detailed, hands-on instruction for patient education (see below)
2. Careful monitoring of diaphragm between uses to identify any defects (see below)
3. Careful selection of patient
   a. Offer only to motivated woman willing to touch her genitals and to use device with every act of intercourse.
   b. Avoid offering to women with markedly anteverted or retroverted uteri (diaphragm tends to dislodge).
   c. Discourage coital positions that compromise stability of diaphragm, particularly the female superior position.

Correct Fitting of Diaphragm   A diaphragm must be fitted properly to be effective. To determine correct size, a pelvic examination is conducted, measuring the diagonal length of the vaginal canal from the posterior aspect of the symphysis pubis to the posterior vaginal fornix. The physician can do this by:

1. Inserting the second and third fingers deep in the vagina until the tip of the middle finger touches the posterior vaginal wall, then
2. Marking the point at which the second finger touches the symphysis pubis with the thumb, then
3. Withdrawing the hand and placing the diaphragm on the tip of the third finger and the opposite rim in front of the thumb to measure the correct size.
4. An alternative method is a trial of increasing sizes of diaphragm rims by inserting them one at a time and ambulating the patient. The correct size is one size smaller than the first one perceived by the patient. For example, starting at size 60 and increasing the sizes until the patient perceives pressure with a size 70 would suggest that a size 65 would be appropriate for her. This would be confirmed by examining the patient with the diaphragm in place. The diaphragm should touch the lateral vaginal walls, cover the cervix, and fit snugly between the posterior vaginal fornix and behind the symphysis pubis. It is essential to remember that a diaphragm that is too large may buckle and that a diaphragm that is too small may slip out of place. The health-care provider should appreciate that the adolescent may be tense during initial fitting, causing the fitting of a smaller diaphragm than would be required if the adolescent were relaxed.

Patient Education   Patient education programs should include:

1. Provider demonstration of insertion and removal techniques: After being shown how to place the diaphragm, the teen should insert and remove it at least once in the office and have her placement checked by the provider.
2. Detailed guidance about use of spermicide

    a. Coat inner surface of diaphragm with spermicidal gel which is then effective for 6 hours.

    b. Add additional spermicide with applicator if intercourse is anticipated later.

    c. Apply extra dose immediately if diaphragm is dislodged during intercourse and consider using emergency contraception.

3. Removal instructions

    a. Wait at least 6 hours after coitus to remove device.

    b. Remove before 24 hours of use to reduce risk of toxic shock syndrome.

4. Concrete instructions about cleaning and storage of device: Recommend washing device in soap and water then soaking in alcohol solution (70% isopropanol or 80% ethanol) for at least 20 minutes after each application. Store in a dry container. Coat with cornstarch or other agents to prevent contamination or cracking.

5. Return for refitting of diaphragm every 1–2 years, after every pregnancy, and after any 10–20% change in body weight.

Advantages

The diaphragm is the most effective of the female barrier methods available today, offers some reduction in risk of cervical and vaginal STDs, and may be placed in anticipation of coitus.

Disadvantages

The diaphragm requires professional sizing and is available only by prescription. It requires motivation and extensive education for proper use. It also requires preparation and access to supplies, may limit spontaneity, and not meet the impulsive needs of the adolescent. It may also be considered messy, especially for multiple acts of intercourse. If either partner is allergic to spermicide, this is not an acceptable method. There is also a small risk of toxic shock syndrome associated with poorly timed or prolonged use. All female barrier methods also increase the risk of cystitis by increasing the counts of enteric organisms within the vagina.

CERVICAL CAP

The cervical cap is a thimble-shaped rubber device with a firm round rim. A small amount of spermicide is placed in the dome of the device. A groove on the inner aspect of the rim helps create and maintain a vacuum seal over the cervix and holds the spermicide in place. The cervical cap provides contraceptive protection for multiple acts of intercourse for up to 48 hours without device removal or additional spermicide. It can be placed hours prior to coitus but must be removed 48 hours after placement to reduce problems with odor and the possibility of toxic shock syndrome. The cervical cap comes in four different sizes measured by internal rim diameters (22 mm, 25 mm, 38 mm, and 31 mm); approximately 80% of women can be fitted.

    Contraindications for the cervical cap include all those mentioned for the diaphragm but also include current problems with known or suspected cervical or uterine malignancies, an abnormal result from a Pap smear, or vaginal or cervical infections. It is not intended for use during menses.

Efficacy

Typical first-year failure rates for the cervical cap are 18%, virtually the same as the diaphragm. Perfect use failure rates in nulliparous women are calculated to be 6%. Younger cervical cap users have lower failure rates than more mature women. Part of this difference may be explained by parity. A parous cervix covered with nabothian cysts and superficial irregularities is more challenging to correctly fit. Pregnancy prevention is enhanced by combining the cap's use with male condoms or emergency contraception.

Fitting the Cervical Cap

Formal training is necessary to obtain proficiency with the fitting procedure for cervical caps. In general the position and size of the cervix are gauged by bimanual examination. Size and contour are evaluated by speculum examination. A fitting cap is placed, a seal created, and the position of the rim to the cervix is verified by palpating the circumference of the cap to confirm that there are no gaps between the cap and the cervix. Stability is tested by attempting to dislodge the cap by thrusting against the cap with the examining finger. After the cap has been in place for 1–2 minutes, the suction should be tested. When traction is placed on the dome, it should remain collapsed and maintain its position. The final test is to rotate the cap. If the cap resists rotation, it is too tight. If it rotates too easily or falls off, it is too loose.

Advantages

1. A single application is effective up to 48 hours: The cap may be used for multiple acts of intercourse at a low cost for spermicide.
2. The cap may be placed early and is usually not detected by partner.
3. The cap offers some reduction of STD risk, especially those causing cervical and upper genitourinary tract infections.

Disadvantages

1. Must be professionally fitted and requires prescription
2. Requires training in placement, removal, cleansing, and storage
3. Requires application with each series of acts of intercourse
4. Requires a second Pap smear in 3 months after initiation of use: In clinical trials, an increase of dysplasia was noted at 3 months when compared to diaphragm users; the risk of dysplasia at 12 months was the same for both groups.
5. Replacement necessary every 2–3 years and refitting needed after each pregnancy
6. Increases enteric organisms in vaginal flora and may cause cystitis

Vaginal Spermicides

Vaginal spermicides (Fig. 46.4) are available in a wide array of delivery systems of the agents nonoxynol 9 (N = 9) or octoxynol 9. Both of these agents are surfactants that destroy the sperm cell membranes. They can be used alone or in combination with barrier methods. Spermicides have shown in vitro activity against many organisms that cause STDs, including HIV. They can play an important role in contraception for the adolescent, as they require neither a prescription nor a pelvic examination and are free from systemic side effects.

Types of Spermicides

The various spermicidal preparations differ in their onset and duration of action and mode of application. Table 46.1 displays the more commonly used spermicidal agents. In general, each agent is active for approximately 1 hour unless used with a diaphragm or cap. Foam is

CONTRACEPTIVE SPERMICIDES

Contraceptive spermicides contain a chemical that immobilizes and kills sperm. Spermicides can come as a foam, a jelly, a cream, a suppository, or a thin piece of film. The spermicide itself, when inserted into the vagina, may also act as a physical barrier between the sperm and the uterus (womb). When a spermicide is used correctly, it is about 90–95% effective as a method of birth control. By combining the use of a spermicide with the use of condoms, the effectiveness rate is increased to almost 100%.

INSTRUCTIONS TO PATIENTS

1. Use the spermicide every time you have intercourse. It should be in place before the penis is put into the vagina.
2. Be sure you have everything you need before you have intercourse. That includes a plastic applicator if you are using foam or jelly.
3. Be sure you understand the instructions on how to use the type of spermicide you are using.

FOAM

1. Foam is effective immediately after insertion. Foam may come preloaded in an applicator or in a separate container with an applicator included.
2. Shake the foam container at least 20 times. This will create plenty of bubbles for the barrier and will mix the sperm-killing chemical with the foam.
3. Fill the applicator with the foam. Insert the applicator 3–4 inches into the vagina and then withdraw the applicator about $1/2$ inch. Press the plunger slowly to deposit the foam. Remove the applicator without pulling out the plunger or you might suck some foam back into the applicator.
4. The bubbles start to go flat within $1/2$ hour, so try to insert the foam just before intercourse. If $1/2$ hour has passed and intercourse has not occurred, more foam must be inserted.
5. A fresh applicator of foam must be inserted every time you have intercourse.
6. Douching is not recommended but if you want to douche, wait at least 8 hours after your last intercourse.
7. To keep applicator clean, wash it with soap and lukewarm water.

If your brand of foam is irritating to you or your partner, try another brand.

Do not confuse feminine deodorants with contraceptive foam or suppositories.

JELLY OR CREAM: Fill the applicator by squeezing the spermicide tube. The instructions are similar to foam except that the container does not need to be shaken.

SUPPOSITORY: Remove the wrapping of the suppository and slide it into the vagina. It should be pushed along the back wall of the vagina as far as it can be placed so that it rests on or near the cervix. Instructions for suppositories are also similar to above except that a short waiting period (10–15 minutes) is needed for the suppository to melt and spread inside the vagina before intercourse. The package instructions should explain the exact time required.

FILM: Your fingers should be completely dry before insertion. Place one of the sheets of film on your fingertip and slide it along the back wall of your vagina as far as you can so it rests near or on your cervix. Instructions for film are also similar to foam except that a short waiting period (5 minutes) is needed for the film to melt and spread inside the vagina before intercourse. The package instructions should explain the exact time required.

SIDE EFFECTS

A very few individuals have had an allergic reaction to suppositories. Should this occur, try changing products or brands.

FIGURE 46.4. Sample instruction sheet for spermicides. (Courtesy Teenage Health Center, Childrens Hospital of Los Angeles.) *Figure continued on following page.*

ADVANTAGES

1. Spermicides are safe with no major health risks.
2. When used with condoms, spermicides are highly effective, almost 100%.
3. Spermicides are available at a drugstore without a prescription.
4. Spermicides are quick and easy to use.
5. Spermicides may provide vaginal lubrication.
6. Spermicides may provide some protection against sexually transmitted diseases.

DISADVANTAGES

1. When used alone, spermicides are only 90–95% effective in preventing pregnancy.
2. Spermicides must be inserted near the time of intercourse, which some people feel interrupts lovemaking.
3. Spermicides can be messy.
4. Spermicides may not always be available for unanticipated lovemaking.

Fɪɢᴜʀᴇ **46.4.**   *continued*

Tᴀʙʟᴇ **46.1.**   Spermicidal Preparations Used as Single Agent

Base or Carrier	Onset of Action	Duration of Action	Spermicide	Representative Products (Brand Names)
Foam				
Aerosol container	Immediate	≥60 minutes	Nonoxynol 9	Delfen, Emko, Koromex
Small container	Immediate	≥60 minutes	Nonoxynol 9	Emko, Because, Emko Prefil
Creams and jellies				
Singe-use packets	Immediate	≥60 minutes	Nonoxynol 9	Conceptrol Jel, Milex Shur Seal Jel
Reusable applicator	Immediate	≥60 minutes	Nonoxynol 9	Conceptrol, Delfen, Koromex Jel, Ortho-Gynol II, Ramses
Reusable applicator	Immediate	≥60 minutes	Octoxynol 9	Koromex Cream, Ortho-Gynol
Suppositories and pills	10–15 minutes	<60 minutes	Nonoxynol 9	Encare, Intercept, Koromex Inserts, Prevent, Semicid
Film	15 minutes	<60 minutes	Nonoxynol 9	Vaginal contraceptive film (VCF)

Adapted from Hatcher RA, Trussell J, Stewart F, et al. Contraceptive technology, 17th revised ed. New York: Irvington Publishers, 1994:180.

the most commonly used, instantly effective spermicide. Suppositories and film require 10–15 minutes to melt and distribute over the cervix.

Efficacy

Typical first-year failure rates of spermicidal agents used alone are 18–21%, with a very wide range. Perfect use of spermicidal agents is estimated to reduce the pregnancy rate to 6%. When used in conjunction with other methods, the pregnancy rate also drops.

Mechanism of Action

The components of spermicidal agents include an inert base (such as foam, cream, or jelly), which holds the spermicidal agent and blocks sperm from entering the cervical os, and a spermicidal chemical to immobilize and kill sperm. The most commonly used agent is nonoxynol 9.

Contraindications

1. Allergy or sensitivity to spermicidal agents or to the ingredients in the base
2. Inability to use due to vaginal abnormalities or inability to master insertion technique

Advantages

1. No proven systemic side effects
2. Readily available without prescription
3. A fairly convenient, easy-to-learn method for teenagers
4. May be used by women with or without involvement of partner
5. May provide lubrication
6. May be useful as backup method for other contraceptives

Disadvantages

1. Relatively high failure rate
2. Considered messy by some teenagers (some forms)
3. Must be used only a short time before intercourse is started
4. Requires 10–15 minutes for activation (some formulations)
5. Requires teenagers to be comfortable with touching their genitals
6. Unpleasant taste if oral genital sex is involved
7. May cause local allergic reaction

CONTRACEPTIVE (TODAY) SPONGE

The nonprescription vaginal contraceptive sponge contains nonoxynol 9. The only manufacturer of sponges in the United States discontinued production in early 1995. While there were no problems with the safety of the product, the Food and Drug Administration found unacceptably high bacteria rates in the air and water at the factory, and the manufacturer voluntarily suspended sponge production. At present there is no plan to remanufacture the sponge.

BIBLIOGRAPHY

ACOG Committee Opinion. Condom availability for adolescents. 1995;154.

American Academy of Pediatrics. Condom availability for youth. Pediatrics 1995;95:281.

Anderson FWJ. Condoms: a technical guide. Female Patient 1993;18:21.

Brown LK, Diclemente RJ, Park T. Predictors of condom use in sexually active adolescents. J Adolesc Health 1992;13:651.

d'Oro LC, Parazzini F, Naldi L, et al. Barrier methods of contraception, spermicides, and sexually transmitted diseases: a review. Genitourin Med 1994;70:410.

Donald M, Lucke J, Dunne M, et al. Determinants of condom use by Australian secondary school students. J Adolesc Health 1994;15:503.

Faundes A, Elias C, Coggins C. Spermicides and barrier contraception. Curr Opin Obstet Gynecol 1994;6:552.

Food and Drug Administration. Polyurethane condom carrier "extremely misleading" label. Contraceptive Technology Update 1995;16(2):17.

Hatcher RA, Trussell J, Stewart F, et al. Contraceptive technology, 16th revised ed. New York: Irvington Publishers, 1994.

"How reliable are condoms?" Consumer Reports 1995; 60(5):320.

Hufford D. Adolescents and condom use. Arch Pediatr Adolesc Med 1994;148:879.

Joffe A. Adolescents and condom use. Am J Dis Child 1993;147:746.

Joffe A, Radius SM. Self-efficacy and intent to use condoms among entering college freshmen. J Adolesc Health 1993;14:262.

Jones EF, Forrest JO. Contraceptive failure rates based on the 1988 NSFG. Fam Plann Perspect 1992;24 (1):12.

Ku L, Sonenstein FL, Pleck JH. The dynamics of young men's condom use during and across relationships. Fam Plann Perspect 1994;26:246.

Leland WL, Barton RP. Gender differences in knowledge, intentions, and behaviors concerning pregnancy and sexually transmitted disease prevention among adolescents. J Adolesc Health 1992; 13:589.

O'Donnell L, Doval AS, Duran R, et al. Predictors of condom acquisition after an STD clinic visit. Fam Plann Perspect 1995;27(1):29.

Orr DP, Langefeld CD. Factors associated with condom use by sexually active male adolescents at risk for sexually transmitted disease. Pediatrics 1993; 91(5):873.

Rosenthal SL, Biro FM, Succop PA, et al. Reasons for condom utilization among high-risk adolescent girls. Clin Pediatr 1994;33:706.

Sex and American teenagers. New York: Alan Guttmacher Institute, 1994.

Stiffman AR, Dore P, Cunningham RM. Inner-city youths and condom use: health beliefs, clinic care, welfare, and the HIV epidemic. Adolescence 1994;29:805.

Trussell J. Contraceptive efficacy of barrier contraceptives. In: Mauck C, Cordero M, Gabelnick H, et al., eds. Barrier contraceptives: current status and future prospects—an international workshop. New York: Wiley-Liss, 1994:17–48.

Trussell J, Sturgen K, Strickler J, Dominik R. Comparative contraceptive efficacy of the female condom and other barrier methods. Fam Plann Perspect 1994; 26(2):66–72.

Woods ER. Contraceptive choices for adolescents. Pediatr Ann 1991;20(6):313.

Wood VD, Buckle RA. Condom misuse among adolescents. J Natl Med Assoc 1994;86:39.

CHAPTER 47

Emergency Contraception

Anita Nelson and Lawrence S. Neinstein

Although recent surveys indicate that adolescents are improving their use of contraception, particularly at the first intercourse, a large percentage of adolescents are still at risk for unintended pregnancy. Only 35% of adolescents reported in 1992 that they had used no method of birth control with first intercourse compared to 52% in the 1988 survey. Recent analysis by the Alan Guttmacher Institute (1994) demonstrates that 72% of sexually experienced adolescents aged 15–17 used some form of a contraception and 84% of those aged 18–19 did so. However, even among those teens contraceptive use is not consistent. In the same survey only 80% of those who reported relying on condoms actually used one at last intercourse. Unprotected acts of intercourse are high not only because of risk-taking behaviors of adolescents but also because of date rape, sexual abuse, and other coercive acts. The high rate of unprotected intercourse puts adolescent women at high risk for unplanned pregnancy.

Although experienced unmarried adolescents are slightly more successful at avoiding pregnancy with pill or condom use than the married 20- to 24-year-olds, many other teens still have poor understanding and compliance with contraceptive methods, which leads to higher rates of condom breakage, inappropriate pill usage, and poor withdrawal practices. That many of the resultant pregnancies were highly unwanted is reflected in the abortion statistics. Estimates are that 35% of adolescent pregnancies in the United States are terminated each year, and even higher rates have been noted in those younger than 14 years old. Emergency contraception can prevent unprotected intercourse from translating into adolescent pregnancy or adolescent abortion. It has been estimated that emergency contraception could reduce by 1.7 million the number of unintended pregnancies in the United States each year and reduce the number of abortions by 800,000 annually, but ready access and awareness of this intervention are crucial if these benefits are to be realized.

EMERGENCY CONTRACEPTION USING BIRTH CONTROL PILLS

The Yuzpe regimen is the most frequently used method of emergency contraception. It involves using two doses of birth control pills totaling 200 mg of ethinyl estradiol and 2 mg norgestrel (or 1 mg levonorgestrel) taken 12 hours apart. Original protocols recommended that treatment should be initiated within 72 hours of the exposure to sperm, although more recent articles have speculated that the regimen could be offered even beyond that 3-day limit. Any norgestrel- or levonorgestrel-containing birth control pill can be used, adjusting the number of pills for dosage:

	Tablets within 72 Hours	*Tablets 12 Hours Later*
Ovral	2	2
Lo/Ovral; Nordette; Levlen	4	4
Triphasil or Tri-Levlen (yellow tablets only)	4	4

It is quite possible that other oral contraceptive formulations with adequate amounts of sex steroids might be effective, but research data are available only for the norgestrel or levonorgestrel progestin-containing birth control pills.

Efficacy

The failure rate for single use emergency contraception with birth control pills is 2%. Because that 2% would be repeated each month and annualized to a 24% annual failure rate, emergency contraception is advocated as a backup and not as a primary method of birth control. However, reducing a woman's risk of pregnancy with single episode exposure from 15–26% to 2% (75% reduction) represents an important clinical achievement. There are no data to support a concern about the impact of the use of emergency contraception on the pregnancy that is resistant to treatment. Studies of pregnancies exposed to such treatment do not demonstrate any increased risk of miscarriages, malformation, or other obstetric complications. It should be noted that the failure rates have been low, so extensive data are not available; but all the available data support the safety of this method. For this reason, restricting the use of emergency contraception to patients who would agree to abort the pregnancy is inappropriate.

Side Effects

Nausea occurs in 50–70% of those treated with oral contraceptive pills for emergency contraception; up to 22% of users also experience vomiting. At a minimum, clinicians recommend that an antiemetic be taken 30 minutes prior to the second dose if nausea is experienced with the first dose. Most clinicians provide antiemetics prophylactically. Several choices are available to control the symptoms of nausea, including:

1. Dimenhydrinate (Dramamine) 50 mg one to two tablets by mouth every 4–6 hours
2. Cyclizine hydrochloride (Marzine) 50 mg one tablet by mouth every 4–6 hours
3. Prescription for trimethobenzamide (Tigan), promethazine (Phenergan), or prochlorperazine (Compazine)—prescriptions rarely needed

If the patient vomits within 1–3 hours of either steroidal dose, a second dose should be given. For this reason, patients are often automatically provided three doses. Other hormonally related side effects such as breast tenderness, abdominal pain, headache, and dizziness have been reported, but these resolve within a day or two after treatment. Menstrual changes are also to be expected, and the patient should be counseled. As she experiences withdrawal of the pharmacologically high doses of sex steroids, a withdrawal bleed is anticipated. Her next menses may occur a few days earlier or later than usual, depending where she is in her cycle when she initiates emergency contraception. She also must be instructed to return for a second pregnancy testing if she has no menses in 3 weeks.

Identification of Candidate

Patients who do not have absolute contraindications to oral contraceptive pill use are able to use them for emergency contraception. However, patients who have experienced strokes, breast cancer, deep venous thrombosis, pulmonary embolism, or uncontrolled hypertension must balance the risks and benefits of therapy carefully. Webb et al. (1993) were unable to detect an effect on clotting factors in women using emergency contraceptive doses of estrogen. Fortunately, few adolescents have absolute contraindications. Relative contraindications to birth control pill use are almost invariably related to long-term oral contraceptive use; short-course use, as for emergency contraception, is usually quite acceptable. It should be noted that patients with abnormal vaginal bleeding require careful evaluation prior to administration of emergency contraception. The list of patients at risk for unintended pregnancy is quite extensive and includes any woman who has had unprotected intercourse (either consensual or assault). Specifically eligible is the patient who has missed more than three pills in the 2 weeks prior to intercourse or who has had 7–9 days with no active combined pills; the patient who has missed one or more progestin-only pills; the patient whose barrier method broke, dislodged, slipped, leaked, or was defective; the patient with failed coitus interruptus, or mistimed intercourse with natural family planning (NFP) or fertility awareness (FA); the patient who experienced ejaculation on her external genitalia; and the woman who had intercourse and whose intrauterine device (IUD) was removed midcycle, expelled, or partially expelled.

Adolescents who have had multiple acts of unprotected intercourse during the cycle are still eligible for emergency contraception as long as the last episode occurred within the 72-hour window. It may be prudent under these circumstances to perform a pregnancy test. It is important to remember that if the patient is already pregnant, emergency contraception will not be effective, but it will not harm the pregnancy. If, on the other hand, she is not pregnant, emergency contraception has a good chance to prevent the latest act of coitus from resulting in a pregnancy.

Emergency contraception can be offered to an adolescent woman at any time in her cycle, even if the risk of conception then is minimal. Prediction of ovulation is not a perfect science, especially when it depends on patient recall of last menses. Therefore, to minimize the risk of pregnancy, emergency contraception should not be withheld because coitus occurred at a time of apparent low risk for pregnancy. Patients may decide not to accept the emergency contraception once their pregnancy risk has been quantified for them, but it should still be offered.

Mechanism of Action of Emergency Contraception with Birth Control Pills

The mechanism of action of high-dose birth control pills changes throughout the menstrual cycle. The most important fact is that emergency contraception does *not* work as an abortifacient. It will not terminate a pregnancy that has already been established. Early in the cycle the high-dose pills disrupt ovarian hormone production and may inhibit ovulation. Midcycle they may inhibit fertilization or disrupt tubal transportation. Later in the cycle high steroidal levels may disrupt the luteal phase and result in an out-of-phase endometrial lining that is unsuitable for implantation. At another extreme the withdrawal of the high-dose hormones may cause the endometrium to slough and prohibit nidation. It should be acknowledged that while many of these mechanisms are traditionally categorized as contraception (blocked ovulation or inhibiting fertilization), some may act after conception but prior to implantation (the establishment of pregnancy). Birth control methods in this time frame have been called "interception." Many women who would decline pregnancy termination feel much more comfortable with interception.

OTHER TECHNIQUES OF EMERGENCY CONTRACEPTION

Danazol for Emergency Contraception

Two regimens have been tested for use of danazol for emergency contraception:

1. Two doses of danazol 400 mg orally taken 12 hours apart OR
2. Three doses of danazol 400 mg orally taken 12 hours

The efficacy of these methods has varied, in some studies being equivalent to emergency contraception with the Yuzpe method, in another having very low efficacy. Danazol has been associated with lower gastrointestinal side effects. However, given the strong androgenicity of this medication, its use (if any) should be restricted to women with contraindications to the use of estrogen. Given the lack of consistent efficacy, its use may also be more appropriate for women who would plan to terminate their pregnancy should the method fail.

Mifepristone (RU 486)

Mifepristone (RU 486) is a synthetic steroid with potent antiprogestational and antigluco-corticoid properties. It has been tested and found effective as a medical method of inducing abortion in early pregnancy. Glasier et al. (1992) tested mifepristone versus standard treatment of ethinyl estradiol and norgestrel in 800 women and adolescents for emergency postcoital contraception who had unprotected intercourse within the preceding 72 hours. There was no statistically significant difference between the two groups, with none of the women treated with mifepristone becoming pregnant compared with four of those receiving standard therapy. Other studies have shown mifepristone to have very low pregnancy rates and fewer side effects when compared to standard methods. While mifepristone may someday replace high doses of oral contraceptives as emergency contraception, it is not currently available for use in the United States.

Postcoital Intrauterine Device Insertion

Insertion of a copper intrauterine device (IUD) within 5–7 days after unprotected intercourse has occurred is extremely efficacious in preventing pregnancy (one pregnancy and only possible miscarriage in 879 women). The exact mechanism of action is not understood. For adolescent patients this method is probably of limited application since the patient who would be a candidate for this method of emergency contraception would also have to qualify for long-term IUD use (i.e., be parous in a stable mutually monogamous relationship). However, if a patient who is scheduled for IUD insertion with her next menses has unprotected coitus, early insertion may provide both emergency contraception and long-term contraceptive efficacy.

ACCESS TO EMERGENCY CONTRACEPTION

Recent surveys have shown that there is relatively little use of emergency contraception in this country, especially when contrasted to the number of episodes of unintended pregnancy. In a 1993 survey of 295 reproductive health-care providers, family practitioners, and emergency room physicians, it was found that emergency contraception had been provided on an average of 3.4 times in the preceding 12 months. Almost one-third of the prescriptions were for rape victims. Few providers had ever discussed emergency contraception with patients or had literature available on the topic.

There are at least two approaches to making emergency contraception available to patients in need. One would be to advise all contracepting patients of the availability of emergency contraception and to ensure immediate appointments for treatment. Each adolescent would be encouraged to call for an appointment to be seen as soon as possible within 72 hours. At that time, a complete history of recent menses, unprotected intercourse, and evaluation of pregnancy risk would be obtained. A urine pregnancy test could be performed and emergency contraception and counseling be provided for immediate use. The advantages of this approach include a professional determination of risk, an evaluation of possible ongoing pregnancy, and a reinstruction of method use and side effect management. In addition, the encounter provides a unique opportunity to re-evaluate the effectiveness of the patient's primary method of birth control and its appropriateness for her. This last feature is quite persuasive for the adolescent who may need additional instruction and motivation to make her primary method work for her.

The second alternative is to provide patients with emergency contraception kits composed of a home pregnancy test, three doses of emergency contraception, at least two doses of antiemetic, and detailed instructions. The patients can have these kits available to them at *any* time in *any* setting without the need to interact with the health-care system. This feature is very attractive for adolescents who may have difficulty confidentially accessing care.

The adolescent's understanding, motivation, and other parameters can guide a provider in deciding which approach to take with each individual patient.

Some providers have hesitated to offer emergency contraception because of concerns that adolescents will use it as a primary method of birth control. However, the side effects with emergency contraception are not pleasant and tend to discourage its repeated use. Others have feared that it would encourage sexual activity. This represents a subset of the larger concern that pregnancy prevention removes a disincentive to coitus; statistics demonstrate the fallacy of this argument.

SUMMARY

Emergency contraception is the only method available to prevent pregnancy once accidental exposure to sperm has occurred. Its widespread use could significantly reduce unintended pregnancy and abortion, already significant problems for adolescents. Unfortunately, most providers have not established this as a priority health service, and most adolescents are unaware that the service is available to them.

BIBLIOGRAPHY

Alan Guttmacher Institute. Sex and America's teenagers. New York: Alan Guttmacher Institute, 1994.

Barnhart KT, Sondheimer SJ. Emergency contraception. Curr Opin Obstet Gynecol 1994;6:559.

Contraceptive Technology Update: Postcoital pills could cut unplanned pregnancies by half. Contraceptive Technology 1993;14:33.

Derman SG, Peralta LM. Postcoital contraception: present and future options. J Adolesc Health. 1995; 16:6.

Glasier A, Thong KJ, Dewar M, et al. Mifepristone (RU 486) compared with high-dose estrogen and progestogen for emergency postcoital contraception. N Engl J Med 1992;327:1041.

Grossman RA, Grossman BD. How frequently is emergency contraception prescribed? Fam Plann Perspect 1994;26:271.

Grou F, Rodriguez I. The morning-after pill—How long after? Am J Obstet Gynecol 1994;171:1529.

Haspels AA. Emergency contraception: a review. Contraception 1994;50:101.

Hatcher RA, Trussell J, Stewart F, et al. Contraceptive technology, 16th revised ed. New York: Irvington Publishers, 1994:415.

Ho PC, Kwan MS. A prospective randomized comparison of levonorgestrel with the Yuzpe regimen in post-coital contraception. Hum Reprod 1993;8:389.

Hoffman J. Morning after pill. New York Times Magazine Jan 10 1993;12.

Johnson JH. Contraception—the morning after. Fam Plann Perspect 1984;16:266.

Koval JE. Violence in dating relationships. J Pediatr Health Care 1989;3(6):298.

Porter J, Warren J. Postcoital contraception. Med J Aust 1981;1(68):85.

Smith RP, Ross A. Post-coital contraception using de-norgestrel/ethinyl estradiol combination. Contraception 1978;17(3):247.

Webb A, Taberner D. Clotting factors after emergency contraception. Adv Contracept 1993;9:75.

Young L, McCowan LM, Roberts HE, et al. Emergency contraception—why women don't use it. N Z Med J 1995;108:145.

Yuzpe AA, Lace WJ. Ethinyl estradiol and norgestrel and postcoital contraception. Fertil Steril 1977;9:932.

CHAPTER 48

Long-Acting Progestins

Anita Nelson and Lawrence S. Neinstein

Long-acting progestin contraceptives are available in two forms in the United States: subdermal progestin implants (Norplant System) and the depo-medroxyprogesterone acetate injection (DMPA or Depo-Provera). These progestin-only methods offer the lowest failure rates of any reversible method of birth control, as well as considerable convenience. Each is devoid of estrogen, and therefore, both may be used by women with isolated contraindications to estrogens, such as women with histories of deep venous thrombosis or pulmonary emboli.

SUBDERMAL PROGESTIN IMPLANTS (NORPLANT SYSTEM)

Description of System

The Norplant System, which is effective for 5 years, is composed of a set of six levonorgestrel-filled silastic capsules that are implanted in the superficial adipose tissue below the dermis of the medial aspect of the patient's nondominant arm. The capsules steadily release levonorgestrel into the surrounding adipose tissue, from which it is absorbed into the general circulation. Initially, 85 µg of levonorgestrel per day is released; by 48 months this will drop to 35 µg. Thereafter the amounts remain relatively steady, dropping to a nadir of 30 µg. The changing blood levels alter the system's mechanism of action and the side effect profile over the 5 years of use but does not have a noticeable impact on efficacy. Virtually 100% of the drug is available, since it is not subject to the hepatic first-pass clearance effect.

Using local anesthetic during a short office procedure, the system is implanted through a small incision during the first 7 days of a woman's menstrual cycle. Removal is more challenging than insertion but usually can be achieved rather straightforwardly in uncomplicated cases in less than 15–20 minutes by trained practitioners. Once the implants are removed, full return to fertility is very prompt, and any side effects resolve rapidly because the low circulating hormone levels are cleared from the circulation within days. Several studies have shown that adolescent acceptance of this method and its side effects has been at least as good as its acceptance by older women. Teen continuation rates and satisfaction ratings with Norplant are considerably higher than with oral contraceptives, even though the implants may cause more side effects in the early months after initiation.

Efficacy

The Norplant System is the most effective method of reversible birth control available. Typical first-year failure rates are quoted by the Food and Drug Administration (FDA) to be 0.09%; cumulative 5-year failure rates are 0.9–1.1%.

Mechanism of Action

The implantable progestin-only method has several important contraceptive effects listed in descending order of significance:

1. Thick cervical mucus: The progestin thickens the cervical mucus and is hostile to sperm penetration. This is the single most important mechanism of action throughout all the years of use.
2. Inhibition of ovulation: Ovulation is inhibited in the majority of cycles for the first year or two of use. Ovulation returns for most women in the final years of use.
3. Endometrial atrophy: Progestin causes endometrial atrophy.
4. Suppression of luteal progesterone production: Should ovulation occur, the pharmacologic doses of progestin suppress luteal progesterone production, simulating luteal phase defect patterns.
5. Tubal motility is altered by progestin.

Metabolic Impacts

The dose of levonorgestrel is relatively low, so metabolic impacts are minimal. Glucose tolerance is only marginally affected. In trials of normal subjects tested prior to implant insertion and after 2 years of use, fasting glucose and 2-hour levels were unchanged. One-hour levels were minimally impacted. The studies on lipid metabolism have been mixed but overall also appear minor. Total cholesterol and triglyceride levels fall. High-density lipoprotein (HDL) cholesterol has been reported to remain the same or decrease slightly; no consistent increase in low-density lipoprotein (LDL) cholesterol has been seen.

Contraindications

1. Suspected or confirmed pregnancy
2. Acute liver disease; benign or malignant liver tumors
3. Unexplained vaginal bleeding
4. Known or suspected carcinoma of the breast
5. Active thrombophlebitis or thromboembolic disorder

Relative Contraindications

1. Breast nodules; an abnormal mammogram
2. Diabetes
3. Dyslipidemia
4. Hypertension
5. Cholecystitis, coronary artery disease, or renal failure
6. History of deep venous thrombosis (DVT), pulmonary embolism (PE), myocardial infarction, or stroke

Drug-Drug Interactions

Because circulating levels of levonorgestrel are minimal, any drug that activates the cytochrome P-450 hepatic enzyme system will compromise Norplant's efficacy. In one small series of patients receiving anticonvulsants (carbamazepine, phenytoin, phenobarbital, primidone (Mysoline), and phenylbutazone but not valproic acid) the first-year failure rates soared to 20%. Similarly, use of the implantable progestin system should not be used in patients receiving rifampin.

Not Contraindicated

1. Postpartum women: This is an excellent method, particularly for postpartum adolescent women. The only caveat is that involution of the uterus may be slowed by progestin.
2. Breast-feeding women: Studies of babies exclusively breast-fed by Norplant users have shown no adverse impact on any infant growth parameters.

Advantages

1. Extremely effective method of birth control
2. Decreases risk of ectopic pregnancy
3. Constant low dose of hormone: No swings occur throughout the day.
4. Long lasting: One set may be used for 5 years.
5. Convenient and low maintenance: A single insertion procedure provides continuous contraception for 5 years.
6. Discrete (but not invisible)
7. Rapidly reversible: Return to fertility is rapid.
8. Progestin only and therefore available to women with contraindications to estrogens
9. Cost effective: The set may be returned to the manufacturer for rebate if it must be removed within the first 6 months.
10. Decreases menstrual blood loss, less anemia
11. May be used immediately by postpartum breast-feeding women, even though FDA labeling is not encouraging
12. Thick cervical mucus may protect against pelvic inflammatory disease (PID), should a woman contract cervicitis.

Disadvantages

1. Progestin-only side effects (see below).
2. Must remind patients to practice safer sex and provide barriers to susceptible patients
3. Has relatively large initial cost
4. Requires trained provider for insertion and removal
5. Counseling: Is initially more time consuming than many other methods
6. Removal: May be complicated and associated with return visits and may rarely require operative removal
7. Litigious environment (Woodman, 1994)

Side Effects

1. Menstrual disturbances: Virtually every user of the implantable progestin system experiences some changes in menstrual patterns. These changes include prolonged bleeding (40%), irregular bleeding (38%), intermenstrual spotting (32%), more frequent bleeding (16%), and amenorrhea (12%). However, unlike other progestin-only contraceptives, the Norplant device usually results in normal menses after the first year of use. By the 5th year 62% have regular cycles, 38% have irregular periods, and none has amenorrhea.

a. Decreased flow: About 20% notice a slightly decreased flow but continue to have predictable withdrawal bleeding from the time of insertion.

b. Amenorrhea: About 10–15% of women initially experience amenorrhea or very infrequent menstrual bleeding. If they can be reassured that they are not pregnant and are not expected to have withdrawal bleeding (because the endometrium is so very thin that there is nothing to slough or "cleanse out" at the end of the month), many teens tend to enjoy this change. Certainly there is no justification to attempt to induce menses in these patients.

c. Spotting: The teens most concerned are often the individuals with prolonged or unpredictable spotting. The progestin causes an atrophy of the endometrium resulting in capillary oozing (daily spotting) or abnormal estrogen cycling (intermittent spotting and bleeding).

Medical treatments can be quite helpful if correctly targeted to the cause of abnormal bleeding. The goal is to build up the endometrium until the circulating levels of levonorgestrel fall enough to permit resumption of more normal levels of ovarian estrogen production. Adding more progestin is counter-intuitive and not particularly helpful. The following therapies have demonstrated efficiency:

a. Nonsteroidal anti-inflammatory drugs (NSAIDs) such as ibuprofen 800 mg PO t.i.d. for 5 days starting when the menses stops and the spotting commences: This is taken only during affected cycles. (An alternative dosage is ibuprofen 200 mg PO every 4–6 hours for 5 days).

b. Estrogen supplements
   — Ethinyl estradiol 0.02–0.05 mg PO every night days 8–28 of cycle for 1–3 months
   — Conjugated equine estrogens 0.625–1.25 mg PO every night days 8–28 of cycle for 1–3 months: Other equivalent estrogen replacement preparations are helpful too.
   — Estrogenic oral contraceptive pills with low progestin content 1 tablet PO every night for 1–3 cycles

Pretesting women with other progestin-only products, such as DMPA or the progestin-only "minipill," will predict neither the *type* of bleeding complication a particular patient may develop with the implants nor *how* she will respond to it. It should also be noted that in real use, adolescent Norplant users have tended to tolerate the menstrual disorders with at least as much equanimity as their adult counterparts (Berenson and Wiemann, 1995; Cromer et al., 1994; Cullins et al., 1994; Darney et al., 1990; Shoupe et al., 1993).

2. Weight changes: Slightly over half of Norplant users gain weight, about one-third lose weight, and the rest experience no weight change. Some Norplant users note abdominal bloating and more generalized fluid retention.

3. Breast tenderness: Some women complain of mastalgia, which may lessen as levonorgestrel levels fall over time but occasionally may require capsule removal.

4. Mood changes: Progesterone has been linked to an increased incidence of depression but in clinical trials the implants have not significantly worsened the moods of depressed patients. However, occasionally, mood changes do force the removal of the implants. Fortunately, since the progestin is so rapidly cleared, the attributable mood changes are quickly resolved. Some patients complain of anxiety or nervousness and others of fatigue.

5. Local changes at insertion site: Infection occurs in less than 1% of cases. Cellulitis may be treated with antibiotics; abscess formation requires incision, drainage, and capsule removal. Expulsion occurs in 0.4% of cases. Norplant can be visible especially if implanted very superficially. In addition, hyperpigmentation may occur over the capsules, which is reversible. Some patients describe a temporary internal tugging or pulling sensation with elbow extension, which responds to local massage.

6. Ovarian cysts: Norplant does not suppress physiologic cyst formation on the ovary as effectively as DMPA or oral contraceptives. Levonorgestrel may even slow the involution of those cysts. Patience is prudent in managing the small simple ovarian cysts palpated in implant users unless the patients develop symptoms.

7. Headaches: Migraine headaches are not a contraindication to progestin-only methods, but some women do complain of worsening or more frequent tension headaches when using Norplant. If a woman complains of visual changes or of severe headaches not relieved by over-the-counter medications or rest, she should have a fundoscopic examination to rule out papilledema, which might indicate the development of pseudotumor cerebri (idiopathic intracranial hypertension).

8. Other changes: A wide range of complaints has been reported at low frequency in Norplant users including acne, hair loss, vaginal distress, increased varicosities, changes in libido, and nausea.

Access and Implementation Issues

The introduction of an implantable contraceptive system raised concerns in some communities, especially around the use of Norplant in adolescents. In Baltimore, several important lessons were learned about the need to involve a broad constituency of community leaders before launching a program to offer Norplant to teens (Beilenson et al., 1995). Early in the introduction of the implant system, investigators were worried that teens would have low continuation rates, but experience has shown the opposite. In one study of parous teens comparing oral contraceptives and implants, only 33% of teens were still taking birth control pills after an average follow-up period of 15.5 months compared to a 95% continuation rate among the Norplant users over a similar period (Polaneczky et al., 1994). Another study in Texas showed over a 6-month period no discontinuation of Norplant use but a 43% dropout rate among oral contraceptive users.

Other crucial concerns were that if adolescents were provided long-term contraception, they would not return for routine health screening appointments and would not use barrier methods to reduce their risks for STDs. In comparative trials, appointment compliance was about equal for pill users and implant users (Cromer et al., 1994; Polaneczky et al., 1994). Another study showed that teens were equal to adult users of implants in their failure to comply with follow-up appointments (Cullins et al., 1994). Providers of the implantable levonorgestrel capsules require training and adequate supervised experience with insertion and removals. With adequate training, removals are usually quite straightforward, with complications reported in less than 5% of cases (Dunson et al., 1995). In addition, newer, easier techniques for removal are being developed.

Future Implants

Several alternative contraceptive implants are under study. These include:

1. Norplant 2 implants: These have been studied since the 1980s and contain two larger rods of levonorgestrel. These are easier and less painful to insert and remove; however, they are not yet approved in the United States.

2. Implants releasing desogestrel and other progestins; single implants for 1 year

3. Biodegradable implants: These do not require removal, but if removal is desired, appear to be much easier because fibrous sheaths do not form around the capsules.

4. Biodegradable subdermal norethindrone pellets

Depo-medroxyprogesterone Acetate Injection

The efficacy and ease of DMPA as a once-every-11–13-week injectable contraceptive method was well recognized over three decades ago, but FDA approval of Depo-Provera for contraceptive use was delayed by the development of breast tumors in beagles and endometrial cancer in rhesus monkeys given high doses of DMPA. It was not until 1990, after the World Health Organization (WHO) published data from international studies (Thomas et al., 1995) that demonstrated the risk of breast cancer in women who used DMPA was not increased and that the risk of endometrial cancer was markedly reduced, that the FDA approved DMPA for contraceptive use. In the interim considerable clinical experience had been accumulated abroad among millions of users and locally with off-label use.

Skegg et al. (1995) reviewed the two major case control studies evaluating the relationship between breast cancer and DMPA. There was no increase in the relative risk for women who had ever used DMPA. There was also no increase in risk with increasing duration of use of DMPA. However, there was a slightly elevated risk for women who started using DMPA within the previous 5 years that was thought to possibly be due to either enhanced detection of breast tumors in women using DMPA or to acceleration of the growth of pre-existing tumors.

Description of Method

DMPA is a crystalline suspension in single vial doses of 150 mg/mL. Before drawing up the drug, the vial should be shaken to evenly distribute the crystals. The suspension should be injected intramuscularly with a 21- to 23-gauge needle measuring 2.5–4 mL in length into a large muscle mass (gluteal or deltoid) within the first 5 days of the menstrual cycle. Caution should be exercised to avoid massaging the area directly after injections, since that spreads the drug over a larger surface area. When such an increased surface area occurs, drug uptake is more rapid and the effect more short lived. Each dose is effective for 11–13 weeks. Questions have been raised about the use of the less expensive preparation of DMPA used for cancer therapy with a concentration of 400 mg/mL. There are several problems with this preparation:

1. It is difficult to measure 150/400 or 0.37 mL.
2. This preparation is not FDA approved for contraception.
3. The injection of the more concentrated DMPA is painful.
4. Clinical trials with 1 mL of this preparation tested as a contraceptive had unacceptably high failure rates throughout the treatment period (Hatcher et al., 1994).

Efficacy

Typical first-year failure rate for DMPA is 0.3%. The cumulative 5-year failure rate is 0.9%.

Mechanism of Action

DMPA is a progestin-only method with similar mechanisms of action as Norplant but with different emphasis. DMPA also relies on cervical mucus changes, but it has a more profound impact on midcycle gonadotropin suppression and reliably blocks ovulation.

Contraindications

Contraindications are the same as those for the Norplant System except that the injection is contraindicated in patients with known sensitivity to DMPA sterile aqueous suspension.

Drug-Drug Interactions

Levels of DMPA are sufficient not to be affected by increased cytochrome P-450 activity resulting from anticonvulsant drug use. In fact, because progesterone has antiseizure activity itself, DMPA is an excellent choice for teens with convulsive disorders. Aminoglutethimide depresses the availability of DMPA. Rifampin use probably decreases contraceptive efficacy.

Metabolic Impacts

Because there is no estrogen component, there are no alterations in coagulation factors, angiotensinogen, or hepatic globulin production. Blood pressure measurements are unchanged with DMPA (WHO, 1983). However, the levels of progestin with this method are higher and do have a greater impact on glucose tolerance, insulin levels, and lipid profiles than do the implants. For healthy, normal subjects the changes in glucose tolerance are not clinically significant (Liew et al., 1985). Since glucose and the insulin levels were increased during DMPA use at all time points of the tolerance test, teens with glucose intolerance or overt diabetes must be monitored closely when using the injections. DMPA was seen to lower total cholesterol, triglycerides, and HDL cholesterol but to have a negligible impact on LDL cholesterol. While this might raise concerns about long-term atherosclerotic risks for adolescent women, the same studies found that the changes in HDL were not statistically significant (Deslypere et al., 1985).

Advantages

1. Extremely effective
2. Private method
3. Convenient and low maintenance
4. Cost effective without high initial costs
5. Intermediate-term method with built-in grace period
6. No estrogen contraindications or side effects
7. Ultimate amenorrhea: Helpful for severely retarded women, busy women, athletes, sickle cell patients, patient with coagulopathies, HIV patients
8. Decreases risk of endometrial and epithelial ovarian cancer
9. May be used by breast-feeding women
10. Thick cervical mucus and amenorrhea: Limit the incidence of PID in patients with cervicitis
11. Acceptable continuation rates (60% at 1 year; 41.5% at 2 years)

Disadvantages

1. Side effects (see below)
2. Must remind patients of safer sex practices and provide method to reduce risks of sexually transmitted disease (STD)
3. Requires medical intervention
4. Delays return to fertility: Average delay is 10 months after last injection (not dependent on the number of injections but on patient weight).
5. Immediate anaphylactic reactions (rare)

Side Effects

1. Menstrual changes: Missed menstrual periods and amenorrhea become more common over time with DMPA. After the first year of use about 50% of DMPA users are amenorrheic, and after several years that number rises to 75%. Some women also experience irregular menstrual spotting and heavy bleeding.

   The bleeding changes with DMPA are more challenging to manage during the first few injections. In addition to the treatments outlined for control of abnormal spotting and bleeding for implants, DMPA users may be offered the second dose earlier, at 10 weeks. The practice of giving a 300-mg dose initially is not recommended because the risk of developing side effects is proportionately increased.

2. Weight changes. Uncontrolled studies conducted in the late 1960s–1970s seemed to indicate that DMPA was associated with considerable weight gain (5 pounds first year with an additional 2–3 pounds each year). Subsequently carefully controlled studies have demonstrated that weight gain attributable to DMPA use totals only 1–2 pounds per year. Clinic patients tend to gain more weight than private provider patients. Preuse weight is not predictive of subsequent DMPA gain. Moore et al. (1995) followed women who used oral contraceptives, DMPA, and implants and found no significant weight gain in any group. Ongoing postmarketing studies should help provide even better data.

3. Breast tenderness: Progesterone stimulates ductal activity and fluid retention in the breast. Mastalgia is reported in 15–20% of women but usually decreases over time.

4. Hypoestrogenic effects: Virtually all users of DMPA maintain early follicular phase estradiol levels. However, in a small percentage ovarian hormonal production is even more profoundly suppressed. These women experience lower estradiol levels, a few even in the postmenopausal range. Those rare patients may complain of dry vagina, dyspareunia, and even hot flashes. Once other causes have been excluded, these symptoms respond well to physiologic estrogen replacement.

   This small cohort has also raised the possibility that DMPA might cause decreases in bone mass. The concern was expressed that DMPA use in adolescents would then decrease ultimate peak bone mass. To date this concern has not been validated. Controlled cross-sectional studies of long-term DMPA users have found that the bone mass of DMPA users was statistically significantly lower than premenopausal controls; however, these studies have been criticized because 40% of the DMPA users were smokers, compared to only 10% of women in the control group. In postmenopausal women DMPA has been shown to increase bone mass. Furthermore, it has been suggested that once women stop DMPA, bone mass normalizes. The current understanding is that DMPA may create temporary reversible decreases in bone mass, akin to the changes seen in pregnancy and breast-feeding. As such, there is minimal concern for the use of DMPA in teens. Postmarketing studies will provide more information.

5. Mood disturbances: DMPA has been associated with a wide range of psychological impacts such as nervousness, insomnia, somnolence, fatigue, dizziness, and depression. Many patients with chronic depression tolerate DMPA, but use in those cases must be individualized.

6. Headaches: Progestin may increase headaches by increasing fluid retention. No association has been noticed with pseudotumor cerebri.

7. Other changes: Acne, alopecia, hirsutism, fluid retention, changes in libido, changes in cervical secretions, nausea, cholestatic jaundice, and local skin reaction to injection have been reported but seldom have been serious enough to change method.

Protocols for DMPA Use

There is a lingering effect of DMPA that gives providers and patients some flexibility in the administration of the drug to meet the needs of challenging patients and unusual situations.

1. Standard protocols

Procedure	*Menstrual Status*	*Recommendation*
Initial injection	Regularly cycling	Administer with first 5 days of cycle
	Amenorrhea (e.g., postpartum or breast-feeding)	Pregnancy test today with barrier method for 2 weeks, then repeat pregnancy test; if negative, administer DMPA OR await next menses
	Irregular cycles	Same as amenorrhea but may offer progestin withdrawal to induce menses, then administer DMPA
Reinjection after 12–13 weeks	Any	Review side effects, reinject if no serious complaints
Reinjection after 13 weeks	Regular cycles	Barrier method, reinject at next menses
	Amenorrhea	Same as initial amenorrheic patient

2. Alternative protocols: May consider for poorly compliant patients or those at higher risk for pregnancy

Procedure	*Menstrual Status*	*Recommendation*
Initial Injection	Any	Pregnancy test; if negative, 2 weeks combination oral contraceptives and barrier method; at 2 weeks, repeat pregnancy test; if negative, give DMPA (give earlier if on menses)
Reinjection less than 13 weeks	Any	Reinjection
Reinjection 13–20 weeks	Any	Pregnancy test, if negative, reinject
Reinjection greater than 20 weeks	Any	Same as initial patient

It should be noted that these alternatives can be modified to include emergency contraception (see Chapter 47), if indicated. The patient could be given birth control pills for emergency contraception and barrier method for interim contraception and advised to return when she has her withdrawal bleeding or in 2 weeks, whichever is earlier.

Bibliography

Affandi B, Karmadibrata S, Prihartono J, et al. Effect of Norplant on mothers and infants in the postpartum period. Adv Contracept 1986;2:371.

Beilenson PL, Miola ES, Farmer M. Politics and practice: introducing Norplant into a school-based health center in Baltimore. Am J Public Health 1995;85:309.

Berenson AB, Wiemann CM. Patient satisfaction and side effects with levonorgestrel implant (Norplant) use in adolescents 18 years of age or younger. Pediatrics 1993;92:257.

Berenson AB, Wiemann CM. Use of levonorgestrel implants versus oral contraceptives in adolescence: a case-control study. Am J Obstet Gynecol 1995;172: 1128.

Contraception Report. Overview of DMPA. 1992;3:1.

Cromer BA, Smith RD, McArdle-Blair J, et al. A prospective study of adolescents who choose among levonorgestrel implant (Norplant), medroxyprogesterone acetate (Depo-Provera), or the combined oral contraceptive pill as contraception. Pediatrics 1994; 94:687.

Cullins VF, Remsburg RE, Blumenthal PP, et al. Comparison of adolescent and adult experiences with Norplant levonorgestrel contraceptive implants. Obstet Gynecol 1994;83:1026.

Darney PD. Hormonal implants: contraception for a new century. Am J Obstet Gynecol 1994;170:1536.

Darney PD, Atkinson E, Tanner S, et al. Acceptance and perceptions of Norplant users in San Francisco, USA. Stud Fam Plann 1990;21:152.

Deslypere JP, Thiery M, Vermeulen A. Effect of hormonal contraception on plasma lipids. Contraception 1985;31:633.

Diaz S, Herreros C, Juez G, et al. Fertility regulation in nursing women: VII. Influence of Norplant levonorgestrel implants upon lactation and infant growth. Contraception 1985;32(1):53.

Diaz S, Croxatto HB, Pavez M, et al. Clinical assessment of treatments for prolonged bleeding in users of Norplant implants. Contraception 1990;42:97.

Dunson TR, Amatya RN, Kreuger SL. Complications and risk factors associated with removal of Norplant implants. Obstet Gynecol 1995;85:543.

Earl DT, David DJ. Depo-provera: an injectable contraceptive. Am Fam Physician 1994;49:891.

Gold MA. Contraception update: implantable and injectable methods. Pediatr Ann 1995;24:203.

Hatcher RA, Trussell J, Stewart F, et al. Contraceptive technology, 16th revised ed. New York: Irvington Publishers, 1994.

Haukkamea M. Contraception by Norplant subdermal capsules is not reliable in epileptic patients on anticonvulsant treatment. Contraception 1986;33:559.

Kaunitz AM. Long-acting injectable contraception with depot medroxyprogesterone acetate. Am J Obstet Gynecol 1994;170:1543.

Klavon SL, Grubb G. Insertion site complications during the first year of Norplant use. Contraception 1990;41:27.

Liew DFM, Ng CSA, Yong YM, et al. Long-term effects of Depo-Provera on carbohydrate and lipid metabolism. Contraception 1985;31:51.

Mishell DR Jr, Kharma KM, Thorneycroft IH, et al. Estrogenic activity in women receiving an injectable progesterone for contraception. Am J Obstet Gynecol 1972;113:372.

Moore LL, Valuck R, McDougall C, et al. A comparative study of one-year weight gain among users of medroxyprogesterone acetate, levonorgestrel implants, and oral contraceptives. Contraception 1995;52(4): 215.

Phemister DA, Laurent S, Harrison FNH. Use of Norplant contraceptive implants in the immediate postpartum period: safety and tolerance. Am J Obstet Gynecol 1995;172:175.

Pinkston-Koenigs LM, Miller NH. The contraceptive use of Depo-Provera in U.S. adolescents. J Adolesc Health 1995;16:347.

Polaneczky M, Slap G, Forke C, et al. The use of levonorgestrel implants (Norplant) for contraception in adolescent mothers. N Engl J Med 1994;331: 1201.

Shoupe D, Mishell DP Jr, Bopp B, et al. The significance of bleeding patterns in Norplant implant users. Obstet Gynecol 1993;77:256.

Silva PD, Kay NR. Comparing the new progestin contraceptives. Female Patient 1994;19:17.

Skegg DC, Noonan EA, Paul C, et al. Depo-medroxyprogesterone acetate and breast cancer. A pooled analysis of the World Health Organization and New Zealand studies. JAMA 1995;273:799.

Thomas DB, Ye Z, Ray RM. Cervical carcinoma in situ and use of depo-medroxyprogesterone acetate (DMPA). WHO Collaborative Study of Neoplasia and Steroid Contraceptives. Contraception 1995; 51:25.

Woodman S. The trouble with Norplant. Allure 1994; (October):126.

World Health Organization (WHO) Expanded Programme of Research, Development and Research Training in Human Reproduction Task Force on Long-Acting Systemic Agents for Regulation of Fertility. Multinational comparative clinical evaluation of two long-acting injectable contraceptive steroids: norethisterone enanthate and medroxyprogesterone acetate. Contraception 1983;28:1.

SECTION XII

Adolescent Gynecology

CHAPTER 49

Gynecological Examination of the Adolescent Female

Eric Cohen, Deborah C. Stewart, and Lawrence S. Neinstein

A gynecological examination is an essential component of the health care of adolescent females. Most adolescent females are apprehensive about the examination of their genitalia, especially during a first examination. A lack of sensitivity for the adolescent's concerns and needs can turn a potentially instructive event into a physically and emotionally traumatic experience. The first pelvic examination can influence an adolescent's attitudes about physicians for the rest of her life.

To create a positive atmosphere a health-care provider should:

1. Interview the adolescent privately in a comfortable environment. The first contact should not be with an undressed adolescent lying on a pelvic table. She should be fully clothed seated eye to eye with the examiner.
2. Reassure the adolescent that what she communicates regarding her reproductive health will be held in strict confidence. She should be aware that the results of the examination will not be discussed with her parents and others without her permission.
3. Be aware of the fears the adolescent has regarding the pelvic examination. Often these fears are expressed as a lack of interest or as frank hostility.
4. Explore with the adolescent her feelings about the examination and the concerns she may have regarding her body.
5. Listen to the adolescent rather than lecturing her.
6. Use the examination as a time for health education.
7. The practitioner may need to address the misconceptions and worries the teenager has regarding the first pelvic examination, including anxieties such as the following:
   a. "It will hurt."
   b. "I will no longer be a virgin."
   c. "I look (or smell) bad."
   d. "Needing a pelvic means I'm sick or something is wrong."
   e. "The doctor will discover my secrets."
   f. "The doctor will judge me."
   g. "I will lose control."
   h. "I'm not OK."
8. Examine your own concerns about performing a pelvic examination, including anxieties such as:
   a. "I won't be competent."
   b. "I will hurt her."
   c. "She won't trust or confide in me."

9. Finally, and most importantly, reassure the teen of her normality, as appropriate. The question "Am I normal?" is often an underlying reason for any teen's visit, particularly when the reproductive organs are being examined.

The need for education, information, and reassurance is demonstrated in a study of 1500 Danish adolescents who responded to a survey regarding their pelvic examination experience (Larsen and Kragstrup, 1995). Of the total group 32% gave a negative general evaluation of the examination, and 13% found the examination very painful. The negative evaluation was strongly associated with the experience of pain, embarrassment, perceived lack of control in not being able to interrupt the examination, not knowing what the doctor was doing, learning nothing during the examination, and having the feeling of inadequate knowledge when arriving for the first examination.

INDICATIONS

Indications for a pelvic examination in an adolescent include:

1. Any sexually active adolescent
2. Symptoms of vaginal or uterine infection
3. Menstrual disorders including amenorrhea, dysfunctional uterine bleeding, severe dysmenorrhea, or mild-to-moderate dysmenorrhea unresponsive to therapy
4. Undiagnosed abdominal pain
5. Sexual assault
6. Birth control: Some practitioners are comfortable in prescribing hormonal contraceptives before the first pelvic examination, particularly if the teen is not yet sexually active but is planning to have sexual intercourse in the near future. In this situation the practitioner would, for example, prescribe oral contraceptives for 1–2 months and then complete the pelvic examination after the teen became sexually active. This might make the first pelvic examination easier to perform.
7. Suspected pelvic mass
8. Diethylstilbestrol (DES) exposure: Adolescents are now out of the age group of exposure.
9. Request by the adolescent
10. Other: The exact age that a pelvic examination is indicated without a history of any of the preceding indications is controversial. Some authorities advocate a pelvic examination within 1 year after menarche, and others advocate an examination at age 18. The authors prefer using the latter age as a guideline. A decision about this will depend on the feelings and background of the patient, her family, and the health-care provider.

HISTORY

Some or all of the history should be taken in private with the adolescent.

1. The chief complaint should be dealt with first and may involve concerns about pelvic pain, vaginal discharge, a menstrual disorder, or a possible pregnancy. As pointed out previously in this book, often a presenting complaint, such as irregular periods, will be used to shield the true concern, such as pregnancy. Even if the chief complaint is not related to the teen's reproductive organs, a gynecological history should be taken.
2. Menstrual history: This should include:
   a. Age at menarche
   b. Duration of menses and interval between periods
   c. Amount of flow and any recent changes in amount of flow

    d. Last menstrual period

    e. Dysmenorrhea if present, severity

    f. Any problems or concerns of the adolescent regarding her reproductive function

3. History and type of vaginal discharge

4. Sexual history: This is often a difficult topic for both health-care providers and adolescents. Suggestions for easing discussion include:

    a. Obtaining the sexual history in private

    b. Not taking notes during this part of the history

    c. Trying to use the same manner and tones as during the rest of the examination

    d. Beginning with questions about nonthreatening areas like menses rather than with the sexual history

    e. Using nonjudgmental questions and responses

Feeling comfortable with a sexual history takes practice but is essential to the health care of the adolescent. One should include questions about:

    a. Sexual activity, both heterosexual and homosexual

    b. Contraception

    c. Sexually transmitted diseases

GYNECOLOGICAL EXAMINATION EQUIPMENT

Materials needed for the gynecological examination include:

1. Examination table with ankle supports: Oven mittens placed over the metal supports increase foot comfort.

2. Gowns, sheet

3. Light source

4. Speculum: Metal (Pedersen's or Huffman-Grave's) or plastic (medium and small). The plastic disposable speculums with attachable light source provide an excellent light source.

5. Gonorrhea culture media or other nonculture gonorrhea test

6. *Chlamydia* culture or other *Chlamydia* screening test: Swabs should be rayon or dacron.

7. Wooden spatula and cytobrush for Pap smear

8. Cotton swabs and either tubes or slides for wet mounts

9. Ten percent potassium hydroxide (KOH) and saline

10. Bottles for Pap solution or Pap slide containers

11. Water-soluble lubricating jelly

12. Warm water source

13. Nonsterile gloves

14. Hand-held mirror (use is optional and up to the patient)

15. Kleenex

16. Tampons and sanitary napkins

PHYSICAL EXAMINATION

A pelvic examination should be performed at least once a year in the sexually active adolescent. It should be performed with only the examining professional and a nurse or chaperon present. Younger adolescents may wish to have their mothers present, and this should be respected. The adolescent should be made to feel that she is in control and can stop the examination at any point to ask questions or, if need be, stop the examination entirely. Often a hand-held mirror to permit the adolescent to view her own genitalia is instructive during the examination. During the examination the patient should be continuously reassured about normal findings. Each step should be explained as the examination proceeds. The steps are as follows:

1. Ask the patient to undress completely and put on a gown.
2. Make sure the patient has emptied her bladder prior to the examination.
3. Examine the adolescent's breasts and abdomen.
4. Have the patient lie with her back on the examination table, feet comfortably resting either in or on the ankle supports. Instruct the patient to slide her buttocks to the edge of the table. A hand placed on the table and toward the lateral aspect of the thigh will signal her that she has reached the correct position. Avoid any contact with the vulva at this time. Elevating the head of the table 30 degrees gives the adolescent an increased sense of control and makes sliding down easier. The foot of the examination table should be turned away from a doorway. The drape or sheet should be positioned so that eye contact can be maintained with the patient.
5. Ask the patient to touch her knees to your hands, which are held out to the side. Do not try to pry her legs apart.
6. Inspect the external genitalia.
   a. Note pubic hair distribution and sexual maturity rating.
   b. Note the general condition of the perineum. This includes looking for any inflamed or abnormal areas over the perineum, thighs, mons veneris, and perianal region. After informing the patient that you are about to do so, place the back of one of your hands high on her inner thigh and examine the external structures.
   c. Visualize the clitoris, the urethra, and the Bartholin's glands.
      — Clitoris: Inform the patient of what the clitoris is (its function should be discussed at another time). The normal clitoral gland is 2–5 mm wide; a width of greater than 6 mm in a teen is considered a possible sign of virilization.
      — Skene's glands: These are two small glands located just inside the urethra. They are usually not visible. If there is reason to suspect a gonococcal infection, the glands can be milked to produce an exudate that can be cultured.
      — Bartholin's glands: These are two small mucus-secreting glands located just outside the hymenal ring at 4:30 and 7:30. Though normally not felt, they can be palpated by placing one finger just inside the hymenal ring and the thumb on the perineum.
   d. Examine the hymenal ring to make a decision about a speculum examination. In adolescents with intact hymenal rings, one can use either a Pedersen's speculum, a Kelly cystoscope, or an otoscope with a veterinary horse otoscope attachment. A Huffman-Grave's speculum or medium plastic speculum can be used on most sexually active adolescents or adolescents who have used tampons. In the Teenage Health Center at the Childrens Hospital of Los Angeles, we use a small or medium plastic speculum in most teenagers. Attached to a light source, it provides excellent visualization.
7. Speculum examination: The speculum should be warmed with warm water (not hot). Your patients will be eternally grateful for this simple act of consideration. It should not be lubricated with anything other than water if a Pap smear or culture are to be taken. It is often helpful for the examiner to perform a one-finger examination to determine the size of the introitus and the location of the cervix, as well as the angle of the vagina. A frequent error in examination is the failure to realize that the vagina is not directed in a horizontal plane but is actually directed about 45 degrees below the horizontal. The one-finger examination facilitates the insertion of the speculum and also relaxes the pelvic

muscles by using gentle downward pressure immediately prior to the speculum insertion. The speculum should be inserted at an angle of approximately 45 degrees and in a downward direction toward the hollow of the sacrum. Avoid any contact with the urethra. Maintain downward pressure while inserting the speculum. The examiner should be careful to avoid pinching the labia or trapping pubic hair with the blades. If using a plastic speculum, the patient should be forewarned regarding the clicking sound that is made while opening the speculum; this can be a frightening sound to the adolescent. With the speculum in place, the practitioner should:

a. Observe the vaginal walls for signs of estrogenization, inflammation, or tumors.

b. Inspect the cervix. The stratified squamous epithelium of the external os is usually a dull pink color. However, younger adolescents have a darker, more erythematous area surrounding the cervical os; this is the columnar mucosal lining of the internal os. The junction between the two types of mucosa is called the squamocolumnar junction. While in most adults it is located within the internal os, in adolescents it is frequently located at the external os. This condition is called ectopy or cervical eversion and is completely normal. Abnormalities of the cervix can include a cervicitis that is often due to either *Chlamydia*, gonorrhea, or *Trichomonas* infections. Cervical polyps may also be found. Women exposed to diethylstilbestrol (DES) in utero should be examined carefully for abnormalities of the vagina and cervix. Gross anatomical abnormalities include transverse ridges, circular sulci, and deformities of the cervix ranging from a small protuberance on the anterior lip to a cockscomb formation to complete hypoplasia of the cervix. Women with a history of DES exposure should be referred for colposcopic examination. The incidence of clear cell adenocarcinoma of the vagina in DES-exposed individuals is estimated to be between 1.4 per 1000 and 1.4 per 10,000 through age 24.

c. Obtain a gonorrhea culture from the endocervix. A sterile cotton swab should be inserted into the endocervix and left in place for 10–15 seconds. It should be rotated 180 degrees before being withdrawn and then streaked on a Thayer-Martin plate or held in transport media. (The use of transport media should be discouraged, as a significant percentage of positive cultures may be missed). Nonculture screening tests can also be used.

d. Obtain a specimen for *Chlamydia* testing. Since chlamydia is an intracellular organism, cells are best collected by a nylon, dacron swab or brush. Obtain the sample in the same manner as the gonorrhea culture. Most health-care providers use one of the commercially available rapid screening techniques, such as a direct fluorescent antibody test or an enzyme immunoassay.

e. Obtain swabs for wet mount and KOH preparation. The swabs can be placed in a test tube with saline for later use or directly smeared onto a slide with several drops of either saline (for *Trichomonas*, white cells, or "clue cells") or KOH (for pseudohyphae). Pascoe et al. (1994) compared vaginal versus endocervical swabs during the pelvic examination. The sensitivity was highest for the vaginal specimen in detecting the presence of trichomonads (100% versus 50%), pseudohyphae (76% versus 65%), and clue cells (95% versus 50%).

f. Obtain a Pap smear of the endocervix. This should include at least a 360-degree rotation of the spatula as it remains in contact with the cervix. Nylon cytobrushes are also commonly used in addition to the spatula, thus ensuring the collection of cells from the squamocolumnar junction. The speculum should then be removed while inspecting the vaginal walls. At any point during the examination the patient may contract the vaginal muscles, causing discomfort to herself. If that happens, stop what you are doing and allow the patient to relax. Slow, deep breathing may help.

8. Bimanual examination: The bimanual examination begins with the insertion of the gloved, lubricated, index finger into the vagina. Remind the patient that you will be examining her uterus and ovaries, using one or two fingers in her vagina and the other hand on her stomach. Remind her to communicate any feelings of discomfort she may be experiencing during the examination. After allowing for pelvic muscle relaxation, the insertion of the middle finger should be added. The other hand can then be placed on the abdomen. The examination should include:
   a. Palpation of the cervix: Check for tenderness on cervical motion.
   b. Palpation of the uterus: The examination record should include the size, position of the uterus, and any masses or tenderness. Pushing backward on the cervix causes the uterus to move anteriorly, allowing for its palpation with the abdominal hand.
   c. Gently explore the posterior fornix and the rectouterine pouch (pouch of Douglas) for masses, fullness, fluctuation, and sensitivity.
   d. Palpation of the adnexa: A record should be made of any masses, tenderness, or abnormalities of the ovaries or the adnexal area. To palpate these structures, insert the examining fingers into each lateral fornix, position them slightly posteriorly and high. Sweep the abdominal examining hand downward over the internal fingers, forming a cup between the fingers of both hands. Maintain this cup position of the fingers and sweep downward and medially toward the pubis. The ovary is often very difficult to palpate, especially in obese and nonrelaxed patients. If felt, the ovary will usually be palpated with the vaginal fingers and in the region of the top of the pubic hair line. It is normally slightly tender, as distinguished from other adnexal masses such as bowel. To improve the practitioners accuracy the patient may be asked to inform the examiner when she feels her ovary being palpated. This is usually experienced as a slight cramp or pinching sensation. Any thickening of the fallopian tubes should be noted.

   A rectovaginal examination may be necessary to complete the evaluation of the adnexa or uterus as well as the rectum, anus, and the posterior cul-de-sac. However, especially in younger adolescents, if the rest of the examination has yielded the needed information, the rectovaginal examination can be deferred. To perform the examination, put on a clean glove and while applying gentle pressure to the external anus, have the patient bear down slightly relaxing the anal sphincter. Insert the lubricated middle finger into the anal canal and toward the umbilicus for the initial 2–3 cm. Insert the lubricated forefinger into the vaginal canal. Then change the angle of insertion so that both fingers are heading downward toward the hollow of the sacrum. It is important to inform the patient that she may experience an urge to defecate and to reassure her that she will not. Reach with the tips of both the vaginal and rectal fingers as high as possible and note any masses or tenderness. The rectovaginal septum should be thin and pliable and the pelvic floor should be free of masses and tenderness. On indication, stool retrieved should be tested for occult blood.

9. At the completion of the examination, offer the patient tissue to be used to remove the lubrication from her perineum after you leave the room. Some patients may require assistance in sliding up the table before taking their feet out of the ankle supports. Instruct her to fully dress and return to the office for a discussion of your findings and plan. Before the practitioner leaves the room, the patient should be in a sitting position and draped.

   During the postexamination discussion, the findings of the examination should be discussed, questions should be answered, and any therapy should be outlined. This is an important time for discussion of the adolescent's concerns about normal anatomy and physiology, contraception, and sexuality. During this discussion with the adolescent, it is important for the examiner to listen "between the lines," remembering that teenagers will frequently not directly communicate their concerns. At the conclusion of the discussion, at the discretion of the teenager, the parent or partner can be invited to join the health practitioner and the teenager. The parent can be asked any further historical questions and informed of the results of the examination, as well as of any treatment plan. Any confidential information that is revealed to the parent should have been previously agreed on with the teenager, so as to maintain trust. (In this connection, practitioners should be aware of their state's laws regarding limits of confidentiality.) Parents should be encouraged to ask questions and to voice concerns.

Obtaining a complete gynecological history and conducting a thorough pelvic examination can be a rewarding and educational experience for the teenager if it is performed sensitively, if confidentiality is maintained to the extent allowable by state law, and if the health provider exhibits a clear understanding of the special needs of the adolescent. The examination also provides the physician an opportunity to impart to the teenager a positive attitude toward her body and the maintenance of her health.

BIBLIOGRAPHY

Bibbo M, Gill WB. Screening of adolescents exposed to diethylstilbestrol in utero. Pediatr Clin North Am 1981;28:379.

Capraro VJ, Kinch MR. Examination of the female genitalia. In: Adolescent gynecology. Report of the Seventh Ross Roundtable on Critical Approaches in Common Pediatric Problems, 11–15. Columbus, Ohio: Ross Laboratories, 1977.

Cavanaugh RM Jr. Pelvic examination of adolescent girls. Am Fam Pract 1982;26:105.

Donovan P. Delaying pelvic exams to encourage contraceptive use. Fam Plann Perspect 1992;24:136.

Emans SJ. Pelvic examination of the adolescent patient. Pediatr Rev 1983;4:307.

Frye CA, Weisberg RB. Increasing the incidence of routine pelvic examinations: behavioral medicine's contribution. Women and Health 1994;21:33.

Koadlow F. The pelvic examination. The first vaginal examination for a healthy young woman. Aust Fam Physician 1990;19:665.

Larsen SB, Kragstrup J. Experiences of the first pelvic examination in a random sample of Danish teenagers. Acta Obstet Gynecol Scand 1995;74:137.

Leppert PC. Adolescent anxiety at first pelvic examination. Medical Aspects of Human Sexuality 1985; 19:24.

Magee J. The pelvic examination: a view from the other end of the table. Ann Intern Med 1975;83:563.

Neinstein LS. Pelvic examination of the adolescent. Phys Assist 1988;(March):87.

Pascoe RS, Neinstein LS, Pennbridge J. Comparison between vaginal swab and endocervical swab during pelvic examination. J Adolesc Health 1994;15:245.

Patton DD, Bodtke S, Horner RD. Patient perceptions of the need for chaperones during pelvic exams. Fam Med 1990;22:215.

Talbot CW. The gynecologic examination of the pediatric patient. Pediatr Ann 1986;15:501.

Tolmas HC. Adolescent pelvic examination. An effective practical approach. Am J Dis Child 1991;145: 1269.

Tolmas HC. The adolescent pelvic examination: an update of a successful program [letter]. Arch Pediatr Adolesc Med 1994;148:435.

Wilson MD, Joffe A. Step-by-step through the pelvic exam. Contemp Pediatr 1988;(March):92.

CHAPTER 50

Normal Menstrual Physiology

This chapter will review normal menstrual physiology, with the following several chapters discussing common abnormalities to menstrual function in adolescents.

MENARCHE

While the exact trigger for puberty is unknown, hypothesized mechanisms for the onset of menarche and puberty include:

1. A progressive decrease in the sensitivity of the hypothalamus to gonadal steroids
2. A critical body composition or percent body fat
3. An increase in the pulsatile secretion of gonadotropin-releasing hormone (GnRH) both in amplitude and frequency, leading to an increase in sex steroids

Menarche has been reported to occur at about 17% body fat, with 22% body fat reported to be required to maintain or restore menstruation. In the United States, menarche occurs in girls at an average of about 12.7 years with a 2 standard deviation range of between 11 and 15. In most teens menarche occurs at sexual maturity rating (SMR) 4 (about two-thirds). Menarche occurs in SMR 2 in 5% of girls, SMR 3 in 25%, and not until SMR 5 in 10%. Menarche occurs about 3.3 years after the start of the growth spurt, about 2 years after thelarche, and about 1.1 years after the peak height velocity. The development of the menstrual cycle is dependent on several hypothalamic changes that occur during puberty. These include:

1. A rise in luteinizing hormone (LH) secretion: During early puberty these spikes occur at night, in a pulsatile fashion. In late puberty and adulthood, pulsatile LH secretion occurs throughout the day and night.
2. A decrease in the negative feedback settings of the hypothalamus to estradiol and testosterone, resulting in higher levels of LH and follicle-stimulating hormone (FSH): The rise in LH and FSH may be secondary to changes in GnRH based on a central biological clock and unrelated to feedback sensitivity to gonadal steroid secretion.
3. The development of a positive feedback system, allowing critical levels of estradiol to trigger a burst of GnRH and thus LH

DEFINITION OF MENSTRUAL CYCLE

A menstrual cycle is defined as that period of time from the beginning of one menstrual flow to the beginning of the next menstrual flow. Based on current understanding, the menstrual cycle may be defined at the levels of the endometrial response (proliferative and secretory phases), the ovarian response (follicular, ovulatory, and luteal phases), and the pituitary response (FSH and LH levels; (Fig. 50.1). The most pivotal level of the menstrual cycle, and the level that is most useful clinically, is the ovarian cycle.

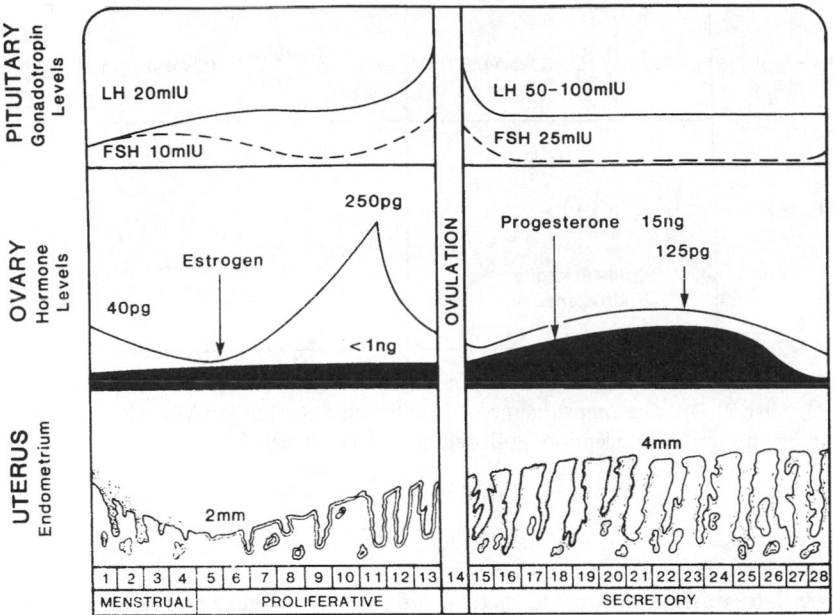

FIGURE 50.1.   Normal menstrual cycle. (From Neinstein LS. Menstrual disorders. Semin Fam Med 1981;2:184.)

Follicular Phase

The duration of the follicular phase is usually 14 days, but the length is highly variable with a range of from 7 to 22 days, ending with ovulation.

1. During the end of the prior menstrual cycle, corpus luteum involution occurs, with resulting low levels of estradiol and progesterone. Low levels of these hormones stimulate the hypothalamic release of GnRH, which, in turn, increases the pituitary's release of FSH and LH.
2. FSH stimulates the maturation of ovarian follicles, with usually one follicle predominating.
3. At present, it is believed that LH stimulates theca cells of the ovary to produce androgens, which are then converted to estrogens in the granulosa cells of the ovary under the influence of FSH (Fig. 50.2). Estradiol increases FSH binding to granulosa cell receptors, leading to amplification of the FSH effect.
4. Under the influence of estrogen, the proliferative phase of the endometrium occurs. The binding of estradiol to its receptor sites on the endometrium results in the production of growth factors that stimulate marked proliferation within the glandular and stromal compartments of the endometrium. This results in the increase in height of the endometrium from about 1 mm at the time of menstruation to 5 mm at the time of ovulation. The major effect of estrogen on the endometrium is that of growth. Estrogen also increases the number of estrogen and progesterone receptors on endometrial cells.
5. Estrogen causes maturation of vaginal basal cells into superficial squamous epithelial cells and the formation of watery vaginal mucus, which can be strung out (spinnbarkeit) or dried into a ferning pattern.
6. In response to rising estradiol levels in the mid- and late-follicular phase, FSH release begins to fall.

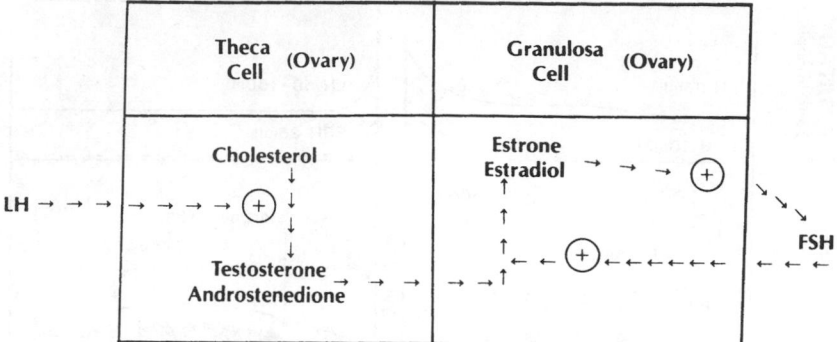

FIGURE 50.2.   Two-cell two-gonadotropin hypothesis of gonadal steroid synthesis. (Adapted from Gobelsmann U, Mishell DR. The menstrual cycle. In: Mishell DR, Davajan VC, eds. Reproductive endocrinology, infertility, and contraception. Philadelphia: FA Davis, 1979.)

Ovulation

1. A preovulatory estradiol surge leads to a midcycle LH surge, which initiates ovulation approximately 10–16 hours after the LH surge. An estradiol level of approximately 200 pg/mL or higher for at least 2 days is needed to induce ovulation. A small preovulatory rise in progesterone is required to induce the FSH surge.
2. A mature follicle releases an oocyte and becomes a functioning corpus luteum.
3. At this stage there are copious, clear vaginal secretions, with maximum spinnbarkeit and a positive ferning test result.

Luteal Phase

The luteal phase begins with ovulation and ends with the menstrual flow. This phase is more constant, lasting about 14 ± 2 days, reflecting the life of the corpus luteum.

1. The corpus luteum produces large amounts of progesterone, as well as increased levels of estrogen. This results from an invasion of blood vessels into the collapsed follicle, exposing granulosa cells to low-density lipoprotein cholesterol, which acts as a substrate for progesterone synthesis. A progesterone serum level of greater than 3 ng/mL is presumptive evidence of ovulation. Rising levels of estrogen and progesterone lead to falling levels of FSH and LH.
2. Progesterone antagonizes the action of estrogen by reducing estrogen receptor sites and increasing conversion of estradiol to estrone, a less potent estrogen. Progesterone halts the growth of the endometrium and stimulates differentiation into a secretory endometrium. The secretory phase is characterized histologically by increased tortuosity of glands and spiraling of blood vessels. Secretory activity is maximal and stromal edema occurs. The secretory endometrium is prepared for implantation.
3. Local progesterone produced by the corpus luteum suppresses follicular development in the ipsilateral ovary so that ovulation the following month usually occurs in the contralateral ovary.
4. The cervical mucus becomes thick during the luteal phase, owing to the influence of progesterone, and no ferning or spinnbarkeit occurs.
5. Unless there is fertilization with subsequent human chorionic gonadotropin production, the corpus luteum involutes after about 10–12 days. This leads to sloughing of the en-

dometrium, secondary to a loss both of estrogen and of supporting progesterone. Local prostaglandins lead to vasoconstriction and uterine contractions.

6. The decreased levels of estrogen and progesterone lead to increased levels of LH and FSH, with a repetition of the menstrual cycle.

For normal ovulation to occur, both the positive and negative feedback systems must be functioning.

1. Negative feedback: Estradiol and progesterone suppress LH and FSH. Estradiol predominantly suppresses FSH, while estradiol and progesterone together suppress LH. With low levels of estradiol, LH and FSH are stimulated.

2. Positive feedback: Rising estradiol above 200 pg/mL during preovulation leads to a positive feedback surge of LH, causing ovulation. This positive feedback only occurs after puberty has begun and ovulation occurs.

LH and FSH are secreted in a pulsatile fashion about every 60 minutes during the follicular phase and every 90 minutes during the luteal phase. The pulsatile spikes are higher during the luteal phase. The pulsatile secretions of LH and FSH are secondary to the pulsatile secretion of GnRH from the hypothalamus. The pulsatile secretion of GnRH can be modulated by estradiol and progesterone feedback but also from other neurotransmitters (i.e., dopamine and norepinephrine). Endorphins also seem to play a role in modulating GnRH secretion. It is possible that these other compounds, in centers above the hypothalamus, lead to the effects of weight loss, stress, exercise, and drugs on the menstrual cycle.

BIBLIOGRAPHY

Blythe M, Orr D. Common menstrual problems: part 1, adolescent health update, Elk Grove Village, Illinois: American Academy of Pediatrics, 1993.

Emans JH, Goldstein DP. Pediatric and adolescent gynecology, 3rd ed. Boston: Little, Brown & Co, 1990.

Filicori M, Santoro N, Merriam GR, et al. Characteristics of the physiological pattern of episodic gonadotropin secretion throughout the human menstrual cycle. J Clin Endocrinol Metab 1986;6:1136.

Fritz MA, Speroff L. The endocrinology of the menstrual cycle: the interaction of the folliculogenesis and neuroendocrine mechanisms. Fertil Steril 1982;38:509.

Gobelsmann U. The menstrual cycle. In: Mishell DR Jr, Davajan V, eds. Infertility, contraception, and reproductive endocrinology. Oradell, New Jersey: Medical Economics Books, 1986.

Gobelsmann U, Mishell DR. The menstrual cycle. In: Mishell DR Jr, Davajan V, Lobo A, eds. Infertility, contraception, and reproductive endocrinology, 3rd ed. Boston: Blackwell Scientific, 1991.

McDonough PG, Ganett P. Dysfunctional uterine bleeding in the adolescent In: Barron BN, Belisle BS, eds. Adolescent gynecology and sexuality. New York: Masson Publishing, 1982.

Neinstein LS. Menstrual disorders. Semin Fam Med 1981;2:184.

Neinstein LS. Menstrual problems in adolescents. Med Clin North Am 1990;74;1181.

Rosenfield RL, Barnes RB. Menstrual disorders in adolescence. Endocrinol Metab Clin North Am 1993;22:491.

Shaw R. Neuroendocrinology of the menstrual cycle in humans. Clin Endocrinol Metab 1978;7:531.

Speroff L, Glass RH, Kase NG, eds. Clinical gynecologic endocrinology and infertility, 5th ed. Baltimore: Williams & Wilkins, 1994.

Vuorento T, Huhtaniemi I. Daily levels of salivary progesterone during menstrual cycle in adolescent girls. Fertil Steril 1992;58:685.

Yen SSC, Jaffe RB. The endometrium. In: Yen SSC, ed. Reproductive endocrinology physiology, pathophysiology, and clinical management. Philadelphia: WB Saunders, 1978.

CHAPTER 51

Dysmenorrhea and Premenstrual Syndrome

About 50% of adolescent females experience some menstrual dysfunction, including dysfunctional uterine bleeding, amenorrhea, dysmenorrhea, and premenstrual syndrome. Many of the problems are minor, including mild dysmenorrhea and minor variations in cycle length or amount of flow. However, the dysfunction can become more severe when amenorrhea, debilitating dysmenorrhea, or severe dysfunctional bleeding occurs.

Most adolescent females regard menarche as an important event in their development. Depending on the female's knowledge of sexual development and her attitudes toward her own body, the onset of menstruation may invoke feelings of excitement, fear, or curiosity. The physician can do much to correct myths and misinformation that the teenager may have concerning her menstrual cycles, in addition to providing reassurance. Discussion of problems regarding menses is often embarrassing and difficult for teenagers. Physicians should be sensitive to this and should endeavor to convey to teenagers that they care about and understand their feelings and desire for confidentiality.

The goals of the practitioner dealing with adolescents with menstrual problems include:

1. Preventing significant menstrual abnormalities such as dysmenorrhea or heavy prolonged bleeding
2. Evaluating for any underlying potentially harmful pathologic state or psychosocial problem that could present as a menstrual problem
3. Preventing problems that could disfigure the teen, such as hirsutism or acne, that may be part of a problem associated with a menstrual abnormality
4. Preventing the possible long-term sequelae of these problems

This and the next several chapters deal with the evaluation of common adolescent menstrual dysfunctions. Dysmenorrhea, the most prevalent of these, is considered first.

DYSMENORRHEA

Primary dysmenorrhea refers to pain associated with the menstrual flow, with no evidence of organic pelvic disease. Secondary dysmenorrhea refers to pain associated with menses secondary to organic disease such as endometriosis, ovarian cysts, adhesions, pelvic inflammatory disease, and so forth.

Etiology

Psychological Factors Probably a small association exists between dysmenorrhea and the power of suggestion and imitation of mother or peers. Table 51.1 summarizes the results of a study by Widholm and Kantero (1971) on the role of mothers' influence.

Table **51.1.** Role of Mothers' Influence in Dysmenorrhea

Incidence of Dysmenorrhea in Daughters	Daughters of Mothers with No Dysmenorrhea (%)	Daughters of Mothers with Dysmenorrhea (%)
None	67	30
Occasional	27	40
Regular	7	30

Adapted from Widholm O, Kantero RL. Correlation of menstrual traits between adolescent girls and their mothers. Acta Obstet Gynecol Scand 1971;50(14, suppl):30.

Myometrial Factors

1. Follicular phase: Uterine contractions occur 1–3 times per minute and at 10–30 mm Hg, with a basal pressure of 0–10 mm Hg.
2. Ovulation: Basal pressure is 40–60 mm Hg, with low-intensity contractions of 5–10 mm Hg every 3–5 minutes.
3. Luteal phase: During this phase basal pressure is 10–20 mm Hg, with infrequent (less than one per minute) contractions of 40–60 mm Hg.
4. Menses: Basal pressure is 0–10 mm Hg, with infrequent laborlike contractions of 100–120 mm Hg.
5. Anovulatory cycles: Contractions occur similar to those in the follicular phase, with no strong contractions or pain.
6. Dysmenorrhea: Four changes occur that contribute to pain. These include an elevation of myometrial resting tone to above 10 mm Hg, an elevation of contractile myometrial pressure to above 120 mm Hg, an increase in the frequency of contractions, and a dysrhythmia of uterine contractions.

Prostaglandins   Prostaglandins seem to be the cause of the changes noted above that lead to dysmenorrhea. Prostaglandins are 10-carbon-hydroxy unsaturated fatty acids with a cyclopentane ring and two side chains. Prostaglandin $F_{2\alpha}$ causes myometrial contractions, vasoconstriction, and ischemia, while prostaglandin E_2 causes vasodilation and hypersensitivity of pain nerve terminals in the myometrium. Prostaglandins are synthesized locally in endometrial tissue. Their production seems to be enhanced by progesterone and the presence of a secretory endometrium. It has been noted that:

1. Exogenous injection of prostaglandin E_2 and $F_{2\alpha}$ produce myometrial contractions and pain similar to dysmenorrhea.
2. Anovulatory cycles are associated with lower prostaglandin levels and usually no dysmenorrhea.
3. Patients with dysmenorrhea have higher levels of prostaglandins in the endometrium.
4. Prostaglandin inhibitors decrease dysmenorrhea.

From this evidence it has been presumed that primary dysmenorrhea is related to prostaglandins released during menses, which seem to be increased during ovulatory cycles under the influence of progesterone. Prostaglandins have also been shown to be locally elevated in cases of secondary dysmenorrhea such as fibroids, intrauterine devices, and endometriosis.

Epidemiology

Prevalence   About 45–60% of all postpubescent females have some degree of dysmenorrhea, with 10% of these females being incapacitated for 1–3 days per month. Dysmenorrhea is the greatest single cause of lost work and school hours in females, with more than 140 million hours lost per year. Robinson et al. (1992) found a prevalence of 79.6% in a group of 308 adolescent females. The prevalence rises from 39% of 12-year-old girls to 72% of 17-year-old girls. The prevalence of dysmenorrhea also increases from 38% at sexual maturity rating of 3 (SMR 3) to 66% at SMR 5.

Clinical Manifestations

1. Primary dysmenorrhea usually begins 6–12 months after menarche and usually before the age of 20.
2. Local symptoms: Pain is spasmodic in nature and is strongest in the lower abdomen, with radiation to the back and the anterior aspects of the thighs.
3. Systemic symptoms: About 50% of females have associated systemic symptoms including:

Nausea or vomiting	89%
Fatigue	85%
Nervousness	67%
Dizziness	60%
Diarrhea	60%
Backache	60%
Headache	45%

4. Grades: It is useful to grade dysmenorrhea from I to III.
   a. Grade I: Mild dysmenorrhea that does not interfere with the adolescent's participation in everyday activity
   b. Grade II: Moderate dysmenorrhea that may interfere in the adolescent's participation in some activities; minimal, if any, systemic symptoms
   c. Grade III: Severe discomfort; adolescent restricted from activities for several days; often associated with systemic symptoms

Differential Diagnosis

1. Endometriosis: Endometriosis involves endometrial implants in various locations throughout the pelvis. Although not common in adolescents, this condition is probably not so rare in adolescents as previously thought. Goldstein et al. (1980) found endometriosis in 66 of 140 adolescents undergoing laparoscopy for chronic pelvic pain. Strickland et al. (1989) found 12 of 100 adolescents with endometriosis in a study evaluating chronic pelvic pain in adolescent females. The typical symptoms of endometriosis in adolescents may include chronic pelvic pain, which may precede menses and continue after menses; abnormal uterine bleeding; pain on defecation; and dyspareunia. On examination a tender or nodular cul-de-sac or tender uterosacral ligaments may be found. Goldstein et al. (1980) found pelvic tenderness in 76% of adolescents with endometriosis. Often a combination of antiprostaglandins and oral contraceptive pills will relieve the symptoms. Adolescents with endometriosis may not have the classic presentation with thickened nodular sacrouterine ligaments. The more common presentation is cyclic pain with localized pelvic cul-de-sac tenderness just before menses.
2. Pelvic inflammatory disease
3. Benign uterine tumors: Polyps, fibroids
4. Intrauterine device
5. Anatomic abnormalities: Uterus with blind horn

Diagnosis

1. History
   a. Menstrual history: Primary dysmenorrhea usually starts 6–12 months after menarche, most commonly begins between the ages of 14–16, and peaks around 17–18. It usually decreases during the twenties and thirties. Secondary dysmenorrhea is especially a concern if the pain starts with the onset of menarche or after the age of 20.
   b. Prior sexually transmitted diseases and sexual history: Helps to eliminate infection as a cause
   c. Gastrointestinal and genitourinary systems history: Helps to eliminate gastrointestinal or genitourinary problems, such as cystitis or irritable bowel syndrome as a cause of pain
2. Physical examination: Examine pelvis for evidence of endometriosis, endometritis, polyps, fibroids, or uterine or cervical abnormalities. However, if the teen is not sexually active and the history is typical for dysmenorrhea, a pelvic examination is only indicated if symptoms do not respond to standard medical therapy.
3. Laboratory tests: A complete blood count and an erythrocyte sedimentation rate should be taken if pelvic inflammatory disease is suspected. If evaluation of the genitourinary and gastrointestinal tracts fails to find a cause and the pain is severe and intractable despite treatment with antiprostaglandins and oral contraceptives, then consideration should be made for diagnostic laparoscopy.

Therapy

The two most effective treatments for primary dysmenorrhea are nonsteroidal anti-inflammatory drugs (NSAIDs) and oral contraceptives.

1. Education of patient and reassurance that problem is physiological and can be helped.
2. NSAIDs: These are the primary modality of therapy. Because much of primary dysmenorrhea is secondary to prostaglandin-mediated uterine hyperactivity, prostaglandin inhibitors can alleviate menstrual cramps and associated systemic symptoms. Many NSAIDs have been found effective in alleviating menstrual cramps. The two most useful classes of NSAIDs include the propionic acids such as ibuprofen (Motrin), naproxen (Naprosyn), and naproxen sodium (Anaprox) and the fenamates such as mefenamic acid (Ponstel). These drugs and doses include:

Drug (Trade Name)	Initial Dose (mg)	Following Dose (mg)
Propionic acids		
Ibuprofen (Motrin)	400	400, 3–4 times/day
Naproxen (Naprosyn)	500	250, q6–8h
Naproxen sodium (Anaprox)	550	275, q6–8h
Fenamates		
Mefenamic acid (Ponstel)[a]	500	250, q4–6h

[a]Mefenamic acid has been undergoing recertification in the United States in recent years. It is available in Canada and elsewhere and will become available in the United States in the near future.

Over-the-counter ibuprofen is also available in preparations such as Advil and Nuprin. Since these medications come as 200-mg tablets, a larger number of tablets may be needed for effectiveness. The medications should be started as soon as possible when dysmenorrheic symptoms occur and usually are only needed for 1–3 days. After starting to use one of the NSAIDs, the drug should be tried for 3–4 menstrual cycles before judged ineffective. At that time a trial of a different prostaglandin inhibitor should be performed. With these doses used for short periods of time, side effects are usually minimal but include:

  a. Greater than 1%
- Gastrointestinal: Nausea, epigastric pain, vomiting, constipation
- Central nervous system (CNS): Dizziness, headache
- Skin: Rash
- Cardiovascular: Edema, fluid retention
- Other: Tinnitus

  b. Less than 1%
- Gastrointestinal: Ulcer, hepatitis
- CNS: Depression, confusion
- Skin: Stevens-Johnson syndrome, alopecia
- Hematological: Pancytopenia, hemolysis
- Other: Hearing loss, scotoma, dry eyes

3. Hormonal: If patient wishes contraception or the pain is severe and not responsive to NSAIDs, oral contraceptives can be tried. As combined oral contraceptives inhibit ovulation and prostaglandin release, they decrease symptoms in more than 90% of patients with primary dysmenorrhea. Oral contraceptives are also useful to treat endometriosis, as they decrease endometrial proliferation and thus decrease total local prostaglandin production. The maximal effect may not become apparent for several months.

4. Other modalities: Earl and Mercola (1992) reported on the use of the calcium channel blocker, nicardipine, to successfully treat one teen with severe dysmenorrhea refractory to other modalities.

PREMENSTRUAL SYNDROME

The premenstrual syndrome (PMS) is a nebulous condition characterized by a broad spectrum of symptoms. PMS is surrounded by confusing definitions, which has resulted in some women seeking treatment being excluded from the diagnosis. Evidence is accumulating that PMS is not a single condition but a set of interrelated symptom complexes, each with its own pathophysiological mechanism. The exact prevalence is unknown, but estimates are that 20–40% of women have some degree of symptoms before menses and that 5–10% are so severely afflicted that daily activities are hindered (Chakmakjian, 1983). In one longitudinal study of 384 15-year-old adolescent girls, Raja et al. (1992) found a 14% prevalence of PMS symptoms. In another survey study of 207 adolescents, 89% reported at least one PMS symptom that the teens considered moderately severe, 59% reported at least one symptom considered severe, and 43% at least one symptom considered extreme (Fisher et al., 1989).

Definition

PMS is used to describe an array of physical, cognitive, affective, and behavioral symptoms occurring cyclically during the luteal phase of the menstrual cycle and resolving quickly at or near the onset of menstruation.

Pathophysiology

The exact mechanism is unknown, but theories include:

1. Estrogen excess or progesterone deficiency

2. Alterations in hormones including prolactin, growth hormone, thyroid hormone, luteinizing hormone (LH), follicle-stimulating hormone (FSH), antidiuretic hormone, insulin and cortisol: None of these has been proven.
3. Pyridoxine (vitamin B_6 deficiency): Has been implicated but not documented
4. Alteration in glucose metabolism
5. Alterations in neurotransmitters: Endorphins, monoamines, and serotonin have been implicated.

Clinical Manifestations

More than 150 symptoms have been described in literature on PMS ranging from mild to severe enough to interfere with normal activities.

1. Emotional symptoms
   a. Irritability
   b. Depression
   c. Fatigue or lethargy
   d. Altered libido
   e. Anger
   f. Insomnia
   g. Mood lability
   h. Panic attacks
   i. Poor concentration
   j. Tearfulness
2. Physical symptoms
   a. Headaches
   b. Edema: Legs, abdomen, or breasts
   c. Increased appetite
   d. Food cravings
   e. Weight gain
   f. Increased acne
   g. Constipation
   h. Dizziness
   i. Fatigue
   j. Muscle aches and pains
   k. Palpitations

Diagnosis

The diagnosis relies on the history of cyclic symptoms. No specific physical findings or laboratory tests have proven useful. Three important findings are usually needed to diagnosis PMS:

1. Symptoms must occur in the luteal phase and resolve within 1–2 days after onset of menstruation. Symptoms should not be present in the follicular phase.
2. The symptoms must be documented over several menstrual cycles and not caused by other physical or psychological problems.
3. Symptoms must be recurrent and severe enough to disrupt normal activities.

A calendar as in Figure 51.1 can be helpful in the diagnosis and in following teens after the start of any therapy. Other assessment tools include the Self-Assessment Disk (Magos and

Premenstrual Changes

Name: _____

Rate each of the following words or phrases according to how you feel today. Each item should be rated on a 5-point scale. The numbers refer to the following: 0 = not at all; 1 = a little; 2 = moderately; 3 = quite a bit; 4 = extremely. For each item, write the number in the box for the response that best describes your feeling or behavior today. The best time of day to complete this questionnaire is early evening. Grading of menses: 0 = none; 1 = slight spotting; 2 = moderate; 3 = heavy; 4 = heavy and clots.

DAY OF CYCLE	1	2	3	4	5	6	7	8	9	10	11	12	13	14	15	16	17	18	19	20	21	22	23	24	25	26	27	28	29	30
Menstruation																														
Angry																														
Unable to concentrate																														
Fatigue																														
Anxious, tense																														
Constipation																														
Confused																														
Nervous																														
Avoiding social activities																														
Tender or painful breasts																														
Bad temper																														
Headaches																														
Craving for foods																														
Swelling of breasts, ankles, or abdomen																														

FIGURE 51.1.   Premenstrual symptom calendar.

Studd, 1988), the Premenstrual Assessment Form (Halbreich et al., 1982), and the Prospective Record of the Impact and Severity of Menstrual Symptoms (PRISM) (Reid, 1987).

Therapy

No single treatment is universally acceptable as effective. Studies have yielded conflicting results with all therapies and most trials have not been well controlled. Treatments include:

1. Education: Teen should be educated regarding menstrual physiology and the relationship of changing hormones to symptoms.
2. Stress management: Teen can be taught or referred for techniques to manage stress such as biofeedback, self-hypnosis, and relaxation exercises.
3. Exercise: Regular exercise has been reported to help some individuals with PMS.
4. Vitamin and mineral supplementations
   a. Pyridoxine (vitamin B_6): Pyridoxine has been used extensively, particularly in treating the emotional symptomatology of PMS. This should be a first-line drug, as it seems to be effective in some patients and is usually well tolerated. Pyridoxine is used in doses of 50–100 mg/day throughout the cycle. Some controlled studies have shown positive results, while others show no benefit (Kendall and Schnurr, 1987). Side effects are rare, but a sensory neuropathy has been reported in individuals taking doses as low as 50–200 mg/day for several months. Therapy should be discontinued if neurologic sequelae develop or no improvement in symptoms occurs.
   b. Calcium: Calcium 1 g/day has been reported to reduce physical and emotional symptoms. Mechanism of action is unclear, and usage is not well studied.
   c. Magnesium: Magnesium 360 mg/day has been noted to reduce negative mood and reduce water retention. Mechanism of action is not known, and usage is not well studied.
5. Suppression of ovulation: Since PMS appears to be a cyclic disorder of menses occurring in the luteal phase, suppression of ovulation has been used as a therapy.
   a. Combination oral contraceptives: These have been tried, and some authorities consider them as first-line medications. However, symptoms in some individuals with PMS worsen with use of oral contraceptives, especially triphasic preparations.
   b. Medroxyprogesterone acetate (Depo-Provera): Depo-Provera is an alternative contraceptive to suppress ovulation.
6. Natural progesterones: Progesterone suppositories have been reported to help in doses of 200–400 mg/day used from midcycle to menses (days 17–28 of cycle). However, double-blind crossover placebo-controlled trials of vaginal or rectal suppositories have failed to show any benefit.
7. Gamma-linolenic acid: This has been tried in the form of Evening Primrose Oil, 1.5 g twice daily from day 15 of the cycle until menses.
8. Medications to suppress symptoms
   a. Naproxen and mefenamic acid: NSAIDs have been used to treat PMS including naproxen sodium 550 mg or naproxen 500 mg twice daily on days 17–28 of the menstrual cycles and mefenamic acid 250 mg three times daily on days 24–28 for fluid retention and 500 mg three times daily on days 19–28 for pain. Therapy is stopped after menses begins.
   b. Other therapies: Other therapies prescribed for some adults include use of danazol, bromocriptine, spironolactone, and tamoxifen. The adverse effects of these medications may well outweigh their benefits and at present cannot be recommended for routine use in adolescents.

9. Medications to suppress psychologic symptoms: Suggested therapies have included use of the benzodiazepines (especially alprazolam), selective serotonin reuptake inhibitors (especially fluoxetine), β-blockers including atenolol and propranolol, and calcium channel blockers including verapamil. None of these would be recommended for routine use in adolescents but only for use in selected adolescents with severe symptoms unresponsive to other modalities.

BIBLIOGRAPHY

Altchek A. Dysmenorrhea in the young patient. Female Patient 1984;9:61.

Altchek A. Pediatric and adolescent gynecology. Compr Ther 1995;21:235.

Bancroft J. The premenstrual syndrome: a reappraisal of the concept and the evidence. Psychol Med [Monogr Suppl] 1993;24:1.

Bancroft J, Williamson L, Warner P, et al. Premenstrual complaints in women complaining of PMS, menorrhagia, and dysmenorrhea: toward a dismantling of the premenstrual syndrome. Psychosom Med 1993; 55:133.

Barber HRK. A modern enigma: premenstrual syndrome or syndromes. Female Patient 1986;11:9.

Blythe M, Orr D. Common menstrual problems: part 1, adolescent health update. Elk Grove Village, Illinois: American Academy of Pediatrics, 1993.

Budeiri DJ, Li-Wan A, Dornan JC. Clinical trials of treatments of premenstrual syndrome: entry criteria and scales for measuring treatment outcomes. Br J Obstet Gynaecol 1994;101:689.

Carter J, Verhoef MJ. Efficacy of self-help and alternative treatments of premenstrual syndrome. Womens Health Issues 1994;4:130.

Chakmakjian ZH. A critical assessment of therapy for the premenstrual tension syndrome. J Reprod Med 1983;28:532.

Coupey SM. Common menstrual disorders. Pediatr Clin North Am. 1989;36:551.

DeMonico SO, Brown CS, Ling FW. Premenstrual syndrome. Curr Opin Obstet Gynecol 1994;6:499.

Earl DT, Mercola JM. Calcium channel blockers and dysmenorrhea. J Adolesc Health 1992;13;107.

Emans JH, Goldstein DP. Pediatric and adolescent gynecology, 3rd ed. Boston: Little, Brown & Co, 1990.

Facchinetti F, Borella P, Sances G, et al. Oral magnesium successfully relieves premenstrual mood changes. Obstet Gynecol 1991;78:177.

Facchinetti F, Genazzani AD, Martignoni E, et al. Neuroendocrine changes in luteal function in patients with premenstrual syndrome. J Clin Endocrinol Metab 1993;76:1123.

Fisher M, Trieller K, Napolitano B. Premenstrual syndrome in adolescents. J Adolesc Health Care 1989; 10:369.

Freeman EW, Rickels K, Sondheimer SJ. Premenstrual symptoms and dysmenorrhea in relation to emotional distress factors in adolescents. J Psychosom Obstet Gynaecol 1993;14:41.

Freeman EW, Rickels K, Sondheimer SJ, et al. A double-blind trial of oral progesterone, alprazolam, and placebo in treatment of severe premenstrual syndrome. JAMA 1995;274:51.

Gantt PA, McDonough PG. Adolescent dysmenorrhea. Pediatr Clin North Am 1981;28:389.

Gidwani GP. Endometriosis: more common than you think. Contemp Pediatr 1989;(October):99.

Goldstein DP, Cholnoky C, Emans SJ. Adolescent endometriosis. J Adolesc Health Care 1980;1:37.

Halbreich U, Endicott J, Schact S, et al. The diversity of premenstrual changes as reflected in the Premenstrual Assessment Form. Acta Psychiatr Scand 1982; 65:46.

Harrison WM, Endicott J, Nee J. Treatment of premenstrual dysphoria with alprazolam. Arch Gen Psychiatry 1990;47:270.

Henzl MR, Ortega-Herrera E, Rodriguez C, et al. Anaprox in dysmenorrhea: reduction of pain and intrauterine pressure. Am J Obstet Gynecol 1979;135:455.

Kendall KE, Schnurr PP. The effects of vitamin B_6 supplementation on premenstrual symptoms. Obstet Gynecol 1987;70:145.

Klein JR, Litt IF. Epidemiology of adolescent dysmenorrhea. Pediatrics 1981;68:661.

Lewis LL. One year in the life of a woman with premenstrual syndrome: a case study. Nurs Res 1995;44:111.

Magos JAL, Studd JWW. A simple method for the diagnosis of premenstrual syndrome by use of a self-assessment disk. Am J Obstet Gynecol 1988;158:1024.

Massil H, O'Brien PM. Premenstrual syndrome. Br Med J 1986;293:1289.

Mortola JF. A risk-benefit appraisal of drugs used in the management of premenstrual syndrome. Drug Safety 1994;10:160.

Neinstein LS. Menstrual problems in adolescents. Med Clin North Am 1990;74:1181.

O'Brien PM. Helping women with premenstrual syndrome. BMJ 1993;307:1471.

Owen PR. Prostaglandin synthetase inhibitors in the treatment of primary dysmenorrhea: outcome trials reviewed. Am J Obstet Gynecol 1984;148:96.

Parker PD. Premenstrual syndrome. Am Fam Physician 1994;50:1309.

Pearlstein TB. Hormones and depression: what are the facts about premenstrual syndrome, menopause, and hormone replacement therapy? Am J Obstet Gynecol 1995;173:646.

Plouffe L Jr, Stewart K, Craft KS, et al. Diagnostic and treatment results from a southeastern academic center-based premenstrual syndrome clinic: the first year. Am J Obstet Gynecol 1993;169:295.

Polaneczky MM, Slap GB. Menstrual disorders in the adolescent: dysmenorrhea and dysfunctional uterine bleeding. Pediatr Rev 1992;13;83.

Raja SN, Feehan M, Stanton WR, McGee R. Prevalence and correlates of the premenstrual syndrome in adolescence. J Am Acad Child Adolesc Psychiatry 1992; 31:783.

Reid RL. Premenstrual syndrome. Am Assoc Clin Chem 1987;5:1.

Robinson GE. Premenstrual syndrome: current knowledge and management. Can Med Assoc J 1989;140: 605.

Robinson JC, Plichta S, Weisman CS, et al. Dysmenorrhea and use of oral contraceptives in adolescent women attending a family planning clinic. Am J Obstet Gynecol 1992;166:578.

Rosenfield RL, Barnes RB. Menstrual disorders in adolescence. Endocrinol Metab Clin North Am 1993; 22:491.

Severino SK, Moline ML. Premenstrual syndrome. Identification and management. Drugs 1995;49:71.

Smith RP. Primary dysmenorrhea and the adolescent patient. Adolesc Pediatr Gynecol 1988;1:23.

Smith RP. Cyclic pelvic pain and dysmenorrhea. Obstet Gynecol Clin North Am 1993;20:753.

Steinberg SK, Sylvester WH, Dean C. Pharmacologic management of premenstrual syndrome. Mod Med 1986;54:149.

Steiner M, Steinberg S, Stewart D, et al. Fluoxetine in the treatment of premenstrual dysphoria. N Engl J Med 1995;332:1529.

Strickland DM, Hauth JC, Strickland KM. Laparoscopy for chronic pelvic pain in adolescent women. Adolesc Pediatr Gynecol 1989;1:31.

Svanberg L, Ulmsten U. The incidence of primary dysmenorrhea in teenagers. Arch Gynecol 1981;230: 173.

Taghavi E, Menkes DB, Howard RC, et al. Premenstrual syndrome: a double-blind controlled trial of desipramine and methylscopolamine. Int Clin Psychopharmacol 1995;10:119.

Thys-Jacobs S, Ceccarelli S, Bierman A, et al. Calcium supplementation in premenstrual syndrome: a randomized crossover trial. J Gen Intern Med 1989;4: 183.

Widholm O, Kantero RL. Correlation of menstrual traits between adolescent girls and their mothers. Acta Obstet Gynecol Scand 1971;50(14, suppl):30.

Ylikorkala O, Dawood MY. New concepts in dysmenorrhea. Am J Obstet Gynecol 1978;130:833.

CHAPTER 52
Dysfunctional Uterine Bleeding

Dysfunctional uterine bleeding, another common menstrual problem in adolescents, is an important concern, as it can present as a gynecological emergency. Even if mild, it can be of serious concern to the adolescent and her parents. While most abnormal bleeding is the result of anovulatory menstrual cycles, the problem must be differentiated from possible organic lesions. Organic lesions account for only about 9% of abnormal uterine bleeding in the 10- to 20-year-old age group.

DEFINITIONS

1. Normal menstrual bleeding
   a. Duration of flow: 2–8 days
   b. Cycle length: 21–40 days with normal up to 45-day intervals in adolescents
   c. Blood loss: Average blood loss is 35–40 mL ranging from between 25 and 69 mL. 80 mL is considered excessive.
2. Abnormal uterine bleeding: Menstrual cycles less than 20 days apart, lasting over 8 days or with a blood loss over 80 mL.
3. Dysfunctional uterine bleeding: Abnormal uterine bleeding with no demonstrable organic lesion; usually a result of an anovulatory cycle
4. Polymenorrhea: Uterine bleeding that occurs at regular intervals of less than 21 days
5. Hypermenorrhea or menorrhagia: Prolonged or excessive uterine bleeding that occurs at regular intervals
6. Metrorrhagia: Uterine bleeding occurring at irregular intervals
7. Menometrorrhagia: Prolonged or excessive uterine bleeding that occurs at irregular intervals

ETIOLOGY

The vast majority of cases of dysfunctional uterine bleeding in adolescents are due to anovulatory cycles resulting from an immature hypothalamic-pituitary-ovarian axis. Approximately 55–82% of cycles are anovulatory from menarche to 2 years after menarche, 30–55% are anovulatory from 2–4 years after menarche, and up to 20% are anovulatory after 4–5 years after menarche (Hertweck, 1992). In general, the later menarche occurs during adolescence, the longer the period of anovulation, such that for adolescents whose menarche is prior to age 12 about 50% of cycles are ovulatory by 1 year after menarche. The time interval until 50% of cycles are ovulatory lengthens to 3 years for those whose menarche is between 12 and 13 and to between 4 and 5 years for those whose first menstrual cycle is after age 13.

Rising levels of follicle-stimulating hormone (FSH) at menarche cause follicular maturation in the ovaries, with resultant elevations in estrogen levels. These rising estrogen levels cause a proliferative endometrium to form in the uterus, with the replication and growth of endometrial glands. Progesterone produced during ovulatory cycles halts endometrial growth, stabilizes the endometrium, and decreases estrogen and progesterone receptors in the endometrium. With anovulation and no resultant corpus luteum or progesterone production, a secretory endometrium does not develop. This unopposed estrogen production during an anovulatory cycle can result in the following:

1. Estrogen withdrawal or estrogen breakthrough bleeding, when the estrogen level falls or is too low to support an increasingly thick proliferative endometrium: The unopposed estrogen also leads to asynchronous development of stroma, glands, and blood vessels, which contribute to the irregular endometrial shedding. Breakthrough bleeding can occur at frequent or irregular intervals.
2. Heavy and prolonged menstrual flow: The lack of progesterone and consequent low levels of local uterine prostaglandins result in lower-than-normal myometrial and vascular contractions to aid in stopping menstrual blood flow.

Surprisingly, most anovulatory menstrual cycles are not associated with bleeding or cycle lengths significantly different from ovulatory cycles. This is because in most adolescent females the negative feedback system of estrogen on luteinizing hormone (LH) or FSH allows for some cyclicity. When estrogen levels rise, gonadotropin levels are suppressed with resultant lower levels of estrogen. The falling levels of estrogen lead to endometrial shedding usually before the endometrium is excessively thickened.

Occasionally, dysfunctional uterine bleeding can occur in an ovulatory cycle. This is the result of a defect in the corpus luteum, leading to a shortened corpus luteum life span and inadequate progesterone production. Patients with dysfunctional uterine bleeding may also have higher levels of prostaglandin E_2 receptors. Prostaglandin E_2 is a vasodilator, and this may lead to heavier bleeding. Other causes of abnormal uterine bleeding are listed in the next section under "Differential Diagnosis."

In a study by Claessens and Cowell (1981) 26% of hospitalized adolescents were found to have an underlying organic cause for their abnormal uterine bleeding. This is higher than found in an outpatient population. In this study of hospitalized adolescents, risks for underlying organic disorders included:

1. Hospitalization: One in five risk of organic cause
2. Hospitalization and hemoglobin less than 10 g/dL: One in four risk
3. Transfusion required: One in three risk
4. Hospitalization required and hemoglobin less than 10 g/dL occurring at menarche: One in two risk

Falcone et al. (1994) also conducted a retrospective inpatient study involving all adolescents admitted to three pediatric hospitals in Montreal over a 10-year period (1981–1991) with a primary diagnosis of dysfunctional uterine bleeding. Of the 61 teens with dysfunctional uterine bleeding, two had a newly diagnosed hematologic abnormality (one with immune thrombocytopenic purpura and one with acute promyelocytic leukemia). Twenty-nine percent of the patients had a past history of a significant medical problem. All patients who were evaluated had normal factor VIII levels, partial thromboplastin times, and prothrombin times.

DIFFERENTIAL DIAGNOSIS

The most common organic causes of abnormal uterine bleeding in the adolescent include ectopic pregnancy, threatened abortion, endometritis, the intrauterine device, and hormonal contraceptives. The differential diagnosis of abnormal uterine bleeding in adolescents includes:

1. Dysfunctional uterine bleeding (anovulation): The cause of about 90% of abnormal uterine bleeding in adolescents
2. Complications of pregnancy
   a. Ectopic pregnancy
   b. Threatened or incomplete abortion
   c. Spontaneous abortion
   d. Placental polyp: Hydatidiform mole
3. Local pathology
   a. Endometritis or cervicitis
   b. Vaginal or intrauterine polyp
   c. Uterine myoma
   d. Trauma
   e. Foreign body
   f. Malignancy: Clear cell adenocarcinomas of the vagina or cervix in the diethylstilbestrol (DES)-exposed woman have been reported. However, DES exposure would be unusual in the adolescent age group, as DES was discontinued from common use in 1960 and from all use during pregnancy in 1971. Endometrial adenocarcinomas are extremely rare in adolescents. Stovall et al. (1989) reported two adolescents with this problem, both with a history of prolonged periods of anovulation.
   g. Ovarian pathology: Polycystic ovarian syndrome, tumors, corpus luteum failure
4. Systemic illnesses
   a. Blood dyscrasias: Von Willebrand's disease, idiopathic thrombocytopenic purpura, platelet disorders
   b. Systemic lupus erythematosus
   c. Chronic renal failure
   d. Leukemia and other malignancies
   e. Severe liver disease
   f. Hypothyroidism
   g. Hyperdysfunction and hypodysfunction of the adrenal gland
5. Medications
   a. Tranquilizers
   b. Hormonal contraceptives
   c. IUD
   d. Seizure medications
   e. Anticoagulation
   f. Antineoplastic agents

EVALUATION

Evaluation of the adolescent with abnormal vaginal bleeding includes a thorough history, physical examination, and laboratory tests. This evaluation should assess the degree of blood loss and the need for fluid or blood replacement, hospitalization, and hormonal intervention.

History

The history should contain a menstrual history including dates of the adolescent's last three cycles, presence or absence of pain, number of pads or tampons used and amount of saturation, age of menarche, and prior menstrual history. Statements about the degree of blood loss and the number of pads used may not be reliable indicators of blood loss. Subjective assessment of bleeding can vary widely, and there is marked individual variability of pad use between teens. Better indicators include a change in the daily use of pads, the use of two pads at once, a change to super pads and accidental breakthroughs. Other historical data should include any medications, trauma, masturbation with foreign objects, marked weight changes, diets or binge-purging behavior, heavy physical activity, sexual activity, contraception, symptoms of pregnancy, systemic diseases, and evidence of any other bleeding problems. The color of the blood may help in the diagnosis. Most etiological factors cause red or pink blood. Brown or prune-colored blood (degraded hemoglobin) is suggestive of endometriosis or an obstructed genital tract. Dysfunctional uterine bleeding should be painless bleeding. If pain is present, a uterine infection or complication of pregnancy should be considered.

The timing of the abnormal bleeding can help in the diagnosis. Abnormal bleeding at the usual time of cyclic menses suggests a possible blood dyscrasia or uterine abnormality. Cyclic bleeding with abnormal interval bleeding suggests possible trauma, a uterine polyp, a cervical lesion, infection, or endometriosis. Abnormal bleeding in adolescents occurring outside the 21- to 40-day interval suggests an immature or disrupted hypothalamic-pituitary axis. This may include normal puberty, polycystic ovary syndrome, stress, anorexia nervosa, exercise, or thyroid dysfunction. In teens with heavy bleeding after pregnancy, consider a possible choriocarcinoma.

Physical Examination

1. A general physical examination is necessary to rule out thyroid disease, liver disease, and bleeding dyscrasia. This should include blood pressure and pulse recordings in both supine and upright positions to detect orthostatic changes. Height and weight and any significant changes from last visit should be noted. In addition, the practitioner should check for signs of excessive hair, suggesting polycystic ovary syndrome (PCOS) or another hyperandrogenic state.
2. Breast examination: Check for galactorrhea.
3. Pelvic examination: This helps to eliminate vaginal, cervical, or uterine pathology; endometritis; and any evidence of trauma. A pelvic examination is certainly indicated in the teen who either has a history of sexual activity or painful bleeding. In the teen with painless, mild dysfunctional uterine bleeding (hemoglobin >11 g/dL) who is within the first 1–2 years of menarche and has never been sexually active, a pelvic examination could be deferred. The practitioner must be very careful determining if the teen is sexually active. A pregnancy test would always be a valuable additional check to rule out a complication of pregnancy.

Laboratory Tests

Laboratory tests should include:

1. Gonorrhea and *Chlamydia* tests from endocervix in sexually active teens
2. A complete blood count to establish degree of bleeding: The mean corpuscular volume (MCV) may help in determining if there is an underlying iron deficiency anemia, suggesting long-term blood loss.
3. Pregnancy test: The test should be sensitive enough to measure 50 mIU of β-human chorionic gonadotropin (β-hCG) so as not to miss ectopic pregnancies or miscarriages.
4. If necessary as indicated:
   a. Liver function tests
   b. Thyroid function
   c. Prothrombin time, partial thromboplastin time (PTT), bleeding time, and platelet count

  d. If chronic anovulation is present, LH and FSH, thyroid studies, and a serum prolactin should be considered.
  e. If there is clinical evidence of hyperandrogenism, an appropriate evaluation is in order, see Chapter 58.

Endometrial biopsy is not indicated in adolescents. An endometrial biopsy is indicated in women over age 35 or younger if they have a risk factor for endometrial cancer such as chronic anovulation or obesity.

THERAPY

The objectives of management of abnormal uterine bleeding in adolescents are to control bleeding if necessary, prevent recurrences, and correct any organic pathology. The adolescent with dysfunctional uterine bleeding secondary to anovulatory cycles also requires education and reassurance regarding her menses and reproductive function.

In managing abnormal menstrual bleeding it is essential for the patient to keep a careful menstrual calendar. Treatment of dysfunctional uterine bleeding depends on the severity.

1. First episode, hematocrit stable: This patient should be treated with reassurance, education, and observation. The teen should be given a menstrual calendar to record her menstrual pattern. Also consider iron supplementation.
2. Multiple episodes, hematocrit stable, not actively bleeding: This patient should be treated with cyclic medroxyprogesterone acetate 10 mg daily for 10 days per month for 3–6 months or cyclic oral contraceptives.
3. Acute bleeding and anemia, not requiring hospitalization: Several hormonal approaches are acceptable and include:
  a. Medroxyprogesterone acetate (Provera) 10 mg/day for 10–14 days: Patient must be told she will bleed again after medication is stopped. Minimal effective duration of medroxyprogesterone acetate is not known but endometrial maturation requires no less than 6 days and is maximal after 12 days.
  b. Cyclic oral contraceptives for 1–3 months: With heavy or more prolonged bleeding, one should start with two to four pills for several days until bleeding stops and decrease to 1 pill per day for the rest of the cycle. One regimen would include one pill q.i.d. until bleeding stops and then one pill t.i.d. for 4 days, one pill b.i.d. for 4 days and then one pill every day for the rest of a 21-day cycle. The teen should then be cycled for several months. These teens can use a 1/35 oral contraceptive pill.
  c. Conjugated estrogen (Premarin) 2.5 mg four times a day for 21 days, plus medroxyprogesterone acetate 10 mg/day on days 17–21.
  In addition, all these patients should receive iron therapy to compensate for decreased iron stores. All the preceding regimens have their advocates. Regimens *a* and *b* are the easiest in terms of compliance. Medroxyprogesterone (Provera) alone probably has the lowest success rate, while the combination of estrogen and progesterone probably has the lowest rate of subsequent recurrent dysfunctional uterine bleeding, as indicated by a study by March et al. (1991) at the University of Southern California Women's Hospital. Whether the newer lower dose combination oral contraceptives are as effective as older higher dose pills has not been studied.
4. Heavy bleeding with significant drop in hematocrit requiring hospitalization: Hospitalization is indicated in those adolescents with a hemoglobin less than 7 g/dL or with a hemoglobin more than 10 g/dL but with either significant postural changes or excessive heavy bleeding. Hormonal therapy usually stops even the most severe bleeding. These patients will require Premarin 20–40 mg every 4 hours up to 24 hours given intra-

venously. At the same time a combination contraception pill should be given as 4 pills per day. Preferably use a combination pill with either 50 μg of ethinyl estradiol or a potent progestational pill such as Ovral. Alternatively, a progestational agent, such as norethindrone 5 mg orally four times a day or medroxyprogesterone acetate 5–10 mg four times a day, could be used with conjugated estrogen. While these initial doses of estrogens are extremely high, reports of complications associated with the short-term use in such cases has not been reported.

Estrogen seems to have a direct effect on clotting, including increased platelet aggregation, increased fibrinogen levels, increased factors V and IX, and decreased effectiveness of bradykinin causing capillary hemostasis. In the longer term there is stabilization of the endometrium by growth and healing effects.

Therapy usually stops bleeding within 24 hours. If this does not occur, the adolescent should be reevaluated for a bleeding problem or another organic problem. If hormonal therapy cannot control the bleeding, an unusual occurrence, a dilation and curettage is advisable for both diagnostic and therapeutic purposes.

When bleeding stops, one should:

a. Continue the oral contraceptive or progestational agent q.i.d. for 4 days, t.i.d. for 4 days, then b.i.d. for 2 weeks. Afterward, the adolescent should be cycled on birth control pills for several months. In a teen with a low hemoglobin level, the practitioner may wish to continue oral contraceptives daily without withdrawal bleeding during the first cycles until the hemoglobin level increases.

b. The patients should receive iron therapy.

5. Adolescents with dysfunctional uterine bleeding while using long-standing oral contraceptives or medroxyprogesterone (Depo-Provera): These teens may benefit from Premarin 2.5 mg for 7 days.

Other drugs used in the treatment of dysfunctional uterine bleeding have included nonsteroidal anti-inflammatory drugs (NSAIDs), which can decrease menstrual loss by about 50% in women with heavy bleeding.

If the adolescent continues to have recurring anovulatory bleeding despite the preceding hormonal therapy, one should again rule out organic pathology and treat with Provera 10 mg for 7–10 days every 1–2 months to convert a proliferative endometrium to the secretory phase and thus prevent unopposed estrogen stimulation.

A dilation and curettage should rarely be used in an adolescent and should be reserved for cases of extreme profuse bleeding or for patients who fail medical therapy.

The adolescent who continues to have dysfunctional uterine bleeding or oligomenorrhea 2–4 years after menarche is at a greater risk of continued menstrual irregularities and infertility. Such patients may require clomiphene citrate to conceive.

A long-term risk (three times risk) of anovulatory cycles is the development of endometrial cancer from chronic unopposed estrogen stimulation. The majority of women under 40 with endometrial cancer have chronic anovulation. Endometrial cancer is extremely rare in adolescents.

BIBLIOGRAPHY

Altchek A. Dysfunctional uterine bleeding in the adolescent. Female Patient 1991;16:53.

Anderson NM, Irwin CE, Snyder DL. Abnormal vaginal bleeding in adolescents. Pediatr Ann 1986;15:697.

Bayer SR, DeCherney AH. Clinical manifestations and treatment of dysfunctional uterine bleeding. JAMA 1993;14:1823.

Bulletti C, Flamigni C, Prefetto RA, et al. Dysfunctional uterine bleeding (DUB). Ann NY Acad Sci 1994; 734:80.

Claessens EA, Cowell CA. Acute adolescent menorrhagia. Am J Obstet Gynecol 1981;139:277.

Claessens EA, Cowell CA. Dysfunctional uterine bleeding in the adolescent. Pediatr Clin North Am 1981;28:369.

Coupey SM. Common menstrual disorders. Pediatr Clin North Am 1989;36:551.

Cowan BD, Morrison JC. Management of abnormal genital bleeding in girls and women. N Engl J Med 1991;324:1710.

Emans SJ. Adolescent gynecology, part II. DUB and contraceptive counseling. Female Patient 1988;13:15.

Emans SJ, Goldstein DP. Delayed puberty and menstrual irregularities. In: Pediatric and adolescent gynecology, 3rd ed. Boston: Little, Brown & Co, 1990.

Falcone T, Desjardins C, Bourque J, et al. Dysfunctional uterine bleeding in adolescents. J Reprod Med 1994; 39:761.

Fraser IS. Menorrhagia—a pragmatic approach to the understanding of causes and the need for investigations. Br J Obstet Gynaecol 1994;101(suppl 11):3.

Galle PC, McRae MA. Abnormal uterine bleeding: finding and treating the cause. Postgrad Med 1993;93:73.

Gidwani GP. Vaginal bleeding in adolescents. J Reprod Med 1984;29:417.

Hertweck SP. Dysfunctional uterine bleeding. Obstet Gynecol Clin North Am 1992;19:129.

Khoiny FE. Dysfunctional uterine bleeding. J Am Acad Nurse Pract 1993;5:159.

March CM, Hoffman DI, Lobo RA. Dysfunctional uterine bleeding. In: Mishell DR Jr, Davajan V, Lobo A, eds. Infertility, contraception, and reproductive endocrinology, 3rd ed. Boston: Blackwell Scientific, 1991.

Mishell DM, Fisher HW, Haynes PJ. Menorrhagia: a symposium. J Reprod Med 1984;29:763.

Neinstein LS. Menstrual problems in adolescents. Med Clin North Am 1990;74:1181.

Nygren KG, Rybo G. Prostaglandins and menorrhagia. ACTA Obstet Gynecol Scand 1983;113(suppl):101.

Polaneczky MM, Slap GB. Menstrual disorders in the adolescent: dysmenorrhea and dysfunctional uterine bleeding. Pediatr Rev 1992;13:83.

Rosenfield RL, Barnes RB. Menstrual disorders in adolescence. Endocrinol Metab Clin North Am 1993;22: 491.

Shaw RW. Assessment of medical treatments for menorrhagia. Br J Obstet Gynaecol 1994;101(suppl 11):15.

Southam LA, Richart RM. The prognosis for adolescents with menstrual abnormalities. Am J Obstet Gynecol 1966;94:637.

Speroff L, Glass RH, Kase NG. Dysfunctional uterine bleeding. In: Clinical gynecological endocrinology and infertility, 4th ed. Baltimore: Williams & Wilkins, 1989.

Stovall DW, Anderson RJ, DeLeon FD. Endometrial adenocarcinoma in teenagers. Adolesc Pediatr Gynecol 1989;2:157.

Wathen PI, Henderson MC, Witz CA. Abnormal uterine bleeding. Med Clin North Am 1995;79:329.

Worley RJ. Dysfunctional uterine bleeding. Postgrad Med 1986;79:101.

CHAPTER 53

Amenorrhea

DEFINITION

There are many reported definitions of amenorrhea. However, strict adherence to these criteria results in improper management in some cases. Chronological age and developmental age, plus clinical data, must be integrated into the criteria to establish more useful evaluation guidelines. Such guidelines are included below (the more criteria present, the stronger the case for evaluation). First, a review of normal development: Ninety-five to 97% of females reach menarche by 16 years of age and 98% by 18 years of age. There is an average of 2 years between the start of thelarche and the onset of menarche. The onset of menarche is fairly constant in adolescent development, with about two-thirds of females becoming menarchal at a sexual maturity rating of 4 (SMR 4). Menarche occurs at SMR 2 in 5% of girls, SMR 3 in 25%, and not until SMR 5 in 10%. Ninety-five percent have attained their menarche 1 year after attaining SMR 5. The average age of the American adolescent's menarche is 12.7 years of age, with a two standard deviation range of 11–15.

1. Primary amenorrhea
   a. No episodes of spontaneous uterine bleeding by the age of 14–15 with secondary sex characteristics absent or by age 16–16.5 regardless of normal secondary sex characteristics (chronological age)
   b. No episodes of spontaneous uterine bleeding, despite having attained SMR 5 for at least 1 year or despite the onset of breast development 4 years previously (developmental age): Most teens have menarche within 2–2.5 years after thelarche.
   c. No episodes of spontaneous uterine bleeding in any individual with clinical stigmata of Turner syndrome (clinical correlation)
2. Secondary amenorrhea: After previous uterine bleeding, no subsequent menses for 6 months or a length of time equal to three previous cycles

ETIOLOGY

1. Primary amenorrhea without secondary sex characteristics (absent breast development) but with normal genitalia (uterus and vagina)
   a. Genetic or enzymatic defects (hypergonadotropic hypogonadism): About 30% of primary amenorrhea is secondary to a genetic cause. The most common disorders are:
      — Turner syndrome (45,X): Stigmata include short stature (height usually less than 60 inches); streak gonads; sexual infantilism; and somatic anomalies (web neck, short fourth metacarpal, cubitus valgus, coarctation of the aorta).
      — Structurally abnormal X chromosome: Short- or long-arm deletion. Phenotype varies. Long-arm deletion commonly causes normal stature, no somatic abnormalities, streak gonads, and sexual infantilism. Short-arm deletion defects lead to a phenotype similar to Turner syndrome.

— Mosaicism: X/XX. Eighty percent of such individuals are short, 66% have some somatic anomaly, and 20% have spontaneous menses. The characteristics for X/XXX and X/XX/XXX individuals are similar to X/XX.

— Pure gonadal dysgenesis (46,XX with streak gonads): Stigmata include normal stature; streak gonads; sexual infantilism; and usually no somatic abnormalities.

— 17α-Hydroxylase deficiency with 46 XX karyotype: These individuals have normal stature, sexual infantilism, hypertension, and hypokalemia. Their laboratory tests show an elevated progesterone (>3 ng/mL), low 17α-hydroxyprogesterone (<0.2 ng/mL), and elevated serum deoxycorticosterone.

   b. Isolated pituitary gonadotropin insufficiency: Very rare
   c. Hypothalamic failure secondary to inadequate gonadotropin-releasing hormone (GnRH) release

2. Primary amenorrhea with normal breast development but absent uterus:
   a. Testicular feminization (complete form): In these individuals the wolffian ducts fail to develop and the external genitalia develop as female in absence of a response to testosterone stimulation. Since müllerian inhibitory factor (MIF) is still made by the male gonads, müllerian ducts regress, and the teen does not form internal female genitalia. Internally, the teens have normal male gonads and fibrous müllerian remnants. The low levels of endogenous gonadal and adrenal estrogens, unopposed by androgens, result in breast development. Because of the end-organ insensitivity to androgens, the teens develop sparse or absent pubic and axillary hair. In summary, manifestations include:
      — 46 XY karyotype
      — Female phenotype
      — Testes present
      — Lack of axillary and pubic hair
      — Normal breast development
      — Blind vaginal pouch with absence of ovaries, uterus, and fallopian tubes
      — Normal male levels of testosterone
   b. Congenital absence of uterus: Characteristics include:
      — 46 XX karyotype
      — Ovaries are present: These adolescents may experience cyclic breast and mood changes.
      — Normal secondary sexual characteristics
      — Uterus absent or rudimentary cords
      — Absent or blind vaginal pouch
      — Normal female levels of testosterone
      — May have associated renal, skeletal, and other congenital anomalies

3. Primary amenorrhea with no breast development and no uterus: This condition is extremely rare. The individual usually has a male karyotype, elevated gonadotropins, and testosterone values that are either equal to or less than a normal female level. These individuals produce enough müllerian inhibitory factor to inhibit development of female internal genital structures but not enough testosterone to develop male internal and external genitalia. The causes include:
   a. 17,20 desmolase deficiency
   b. Agonadism, including no internal sex organs
   c. 17α-hydroxylase deficiency with 46 XY karyotype: Manifestations include sexual infantilism, absent uterus, and hypertension.

4. Primary and secondary amenorrhea with normal secondary sex characteristics (breast development) and normal genitalia (uterus and vagina):

a. Hypothalamic causes
   — Idiopathic: Usually associated with a normal response of luteinizing hormone (LH) and follicle-stimulating hormone (FSH) to GnRH. The disorder is probably secondary to a subtle defect in GnRH secretion.
   — Medications and drugs: Especially phenothiazines, contraceptive steroids, and heroin.
   — Stress: Common in adolescents and may relate to family, school, or peer problems or to the fear of pregnancy.
   — Exercise: Athletes, particularly runners, gymnasts, and ballet dancers have higher rates of amenorrhea. As many as 18% of women recreational runners, 50% of competitive runners training 80 miles per week, and 47–79% of ballet dancers may be amenorrheic (Calabrese et al., 1983; Cumming and Rebar, 1983). While the cause is unknown, exercise-induced menstrual dysfunction may relate to elevated dopamines or endorphins altering GnRH secretion. Alterations of the hypothalamic-pituitary-ovarian-adrenal axes appear more severe in those athletes who are amenorrheic as compared to those with normal cycles. Constantini et al. (1995) report on amenorrhea in swimmers. The results of their study seem to indicate that female competitive swimmers are vulnerable to delayed puberty and menstrual irregularities, but the associated hormonal profile is very different from the hypothalamic amenorrhea described in dancers and runners. The study suggested a different mechanism for reproductive dysfunction in swimmers that is associated not with hypoestrogenism but rather with mild hyperandrogenism. Predisposing factors to exercise-induced amenorrhea include:
     (1) Training intensity
     (2) Weight loss
     (3) Changes in percentage of body fat
     (4) Nulliparity
     (5) Prior menstrual dysfunction before exercise
     (6) Years before menarche of the onset of intense training
      Low levels of estradiol may be present, which has been implicated as a source of loss of bone mineralization and increased risk of stress fractures. The condition is usually reversible with weight gain or with lessening of the intensity of exercise. There are many questions about exercise-induced amenorrhea that remained unanswered:
     (1) What effect does delayed menarche secondary to athletics have on eventual bone density?
     (2) Which athletes with amenorrhea need estrogen replacement?
     (3) How effective is estrogen replacement in reducing the risk for decreased bone density?
   — Weight loss: This group includes adolescents with simple weight loss and those with anorexia nervosa (see Chapter 33). In both anorexia nervosa and simple weight loss the mechanism of amenorrhea appears to be hypothalamic derangement. This derangement appears to be more severe in adolescents with anorexia nervosa. The estradiol levels in patients with weight loss and anorexia nervosa can vary from low to normal; consequently, such individuals may or may not respond to progesterone withdrawal with uterine bleeding. The teens with amenorrhea and severe weight loss also are at risk for decreased bone density. Many of the same questions as listed under athletic-induced amenorrhea are unanswered for this group also.
   — Chronic illnesses: Certain chronic illnesses can affect the hypothalamic-pituitary axis. Examples include cystic fibrosis (Moshang and Holsclaw, 1980; Neinstein et

al., 1983b) and chronic renal disease (Lim et al., 1977; Mooradian and Morley, 1984).

— Hypothalamic failure
(1) Idiopathic
(2) Lesions: Rare but can be secondary to craniopharyngioma, tuberculous granuloma, or meningoencephalitis.

— Polycystic ovary syndrome (PCOS): Many researchers believe PCOS to be a primary hypothalamic disorder. Many affected individuals have an LH-FSH ratio of more than 3, with an LH of more than 10 mIU and often more than 25 mIU.

b. Pituitary causes
— Nonneoplastic lesions: Sheehan's syndrome (pregnancy related), Simmonds' disease (nonpregnancy related), aneurysm, or empty sella
— Tumors: Adenoma or carcinoma
— Idiopathic
— Infiltrative: Hemochromatosis

c. Ovarian causes
Premature ovarian failure: Menopause earlier than age 35. This is often associated with autoantibodies directed against ovarian tissue and is often found also in association with thyroid and adrenal antibodies. This can also occur in some individuals receiving chemotherapy or radiation therapy for cancer as children or adolescents (Byrne, 1987, 1992; Shalet, 1980; Stillman et al., 1981; Waxman, 1983).

d. Uterine causes: Uterine synechiae (Asherman's syndrome)

e. Pregnancy

5. Causes of amenorrhea in a study of 138 adolescent patients 13–20 years of age (Behrman, 1967):

a. Primary amenorrhea, 30 patients
— Personality disorders, 3
— Streak ovaries, 3
— Pituitary selective deficiency, 1
— Turner syndrome, 1
— Polycystic ovaries, 1
— Cushing's disease, 2
— Hypothyroid, 1
— Vaginal agenesis, 2
— Stenotic cervix, 1
— Uterine absence, 3
— Pregnant, 1
— Delayed menses, 2
— Systemic disease, 1
— Unknown, 7
— Pituitary tumor, 1

b. Secondary amenorrhea, 108 patients
— Personality disorders, 23
— Pituitary failure, 15
— Pituitary tumor, 1
— Polycystic ovaries, 11
— Ovarian tumor, 2
— Thyroid disturbance, 4
— Ovarian failure, 5

      — Systemic disease, 12
      — Adrenal disturbance, 3
      — Unclassified, 24
      — Obesity, 8

6. Another study of 62 patients with primary amenorrhea showed the following distribution of etiologies (Mashchak et al., 1981):
   a. Absent breasts, uterus present
      — Gonadal dysgenesis, 17
      — Hypogonadotropic hypogonadism, 12
   b. Absent uterus, breasts present
      — Congenital absence of uterus, 6
      — Testicular feminization, 3
   c. Absent uterus, breasts absent
      — Enzyme deficiency, 1
      — Agonadism, 1
   d. Uterus present, breasts present
      — Hypothalamic pituitary failure, 6
      — Hypothalamic dysfunction, 5
      — Ovarian failure, 4
      — PCOS, 2

DIAGNOSIS

The evaluation of amenorrhea can be done easily with a thorough history, physical examination, and performance of several laboratory tests in a logical sequence. Too often, adolescents are subjected to an expensive shotgun approach to evaluation. It is essential to rule out the diagnosis of pregnancy before an extensive evaluation is made.

History

History should include:

1. Systemic diseases: History of diseases associated with secondary amenorrhea should include anorexia nervosa, inflammatory bowel disease, diabetes mellitus, and pituitary adenoma. A history of thyroid dysfunction is of particular importance, as even mild thyroid dysfunction can lead to menstrual dysfunction.
2. Family history, including ages of parental growth and development, as well as mother's and sister's ages of menarche: In addition, a family history of any thyroid disease, diabetes mellitus, eating disorders or menstrual problems
3. Past medical history including childhood development
4. Pubertal growth and development, including breast and pubic hair development, and the presence of a growth spurt
5. Emotional status
6. Medications: This would include illicit drugs (heroin and methadone are strongly correlated with menstrual dysfunction).
7. Nutritional status and recent weight changes
8. Exercise history
9. Sexual history, contraception, and symptoms of pregnancy
10. Past menstrual history
11. History of androgen excess suggesting PCOS or another ovarian or adrenal abnormality

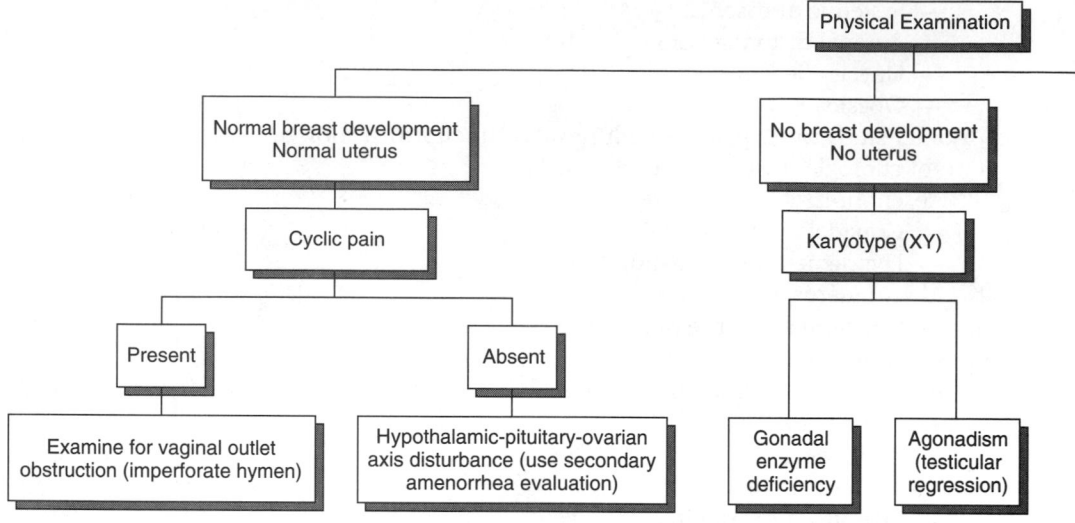

FIGURE 53.1.   The evaluation of primary amenorrhea.

Physical Examination

The physical examination should include:

1. Check for signs of systemic disease or malnutrition.
2. Evaluate for sexual maturity rating: This is important for evaluating progress in secondary sex characteristics, since most adolescents are not menarchal until SMR 4, and 95% are menarchal by 1 year after SMR 5.
3. Check height and weight.
4. Check for signs of androgen excess.
5. Check for signs of thyroid dysfunction.
6. Check for signs of gonadal dysgenesis: Webbed neck, low setting of ears, broad shield-like chest, short fourth metacarpal, and increased carrying angle of the arms
7. Test for anosmia in the female with primary amenorrhea to evaluate for Kallmann's syndrome.
8. Breast examination: Check for galactorrhea.
9. Pelvic examination: Search especially for a stenotic cervix, vaginal agenesis, imperforate hymen, transverse vaginal septum, absent uterus, or pregnancy. A pelvic examination may not be necessary if the teen is not sexually active and the history or physical examination has detected the cause of amenorrhea.

Laboratory Evaluation

The laboratory evaluation can be divided into those adolescents with:

1. Primary and secondary amenorrhea with normal secondary sexual characteristics and normal genitalia
2. Primary amenorrhea and absent secondary sexual characteristics or absent uterus or vagina

Figures 53.1 and 53.2 review the evaluation of primary and secondary amenorrhea.

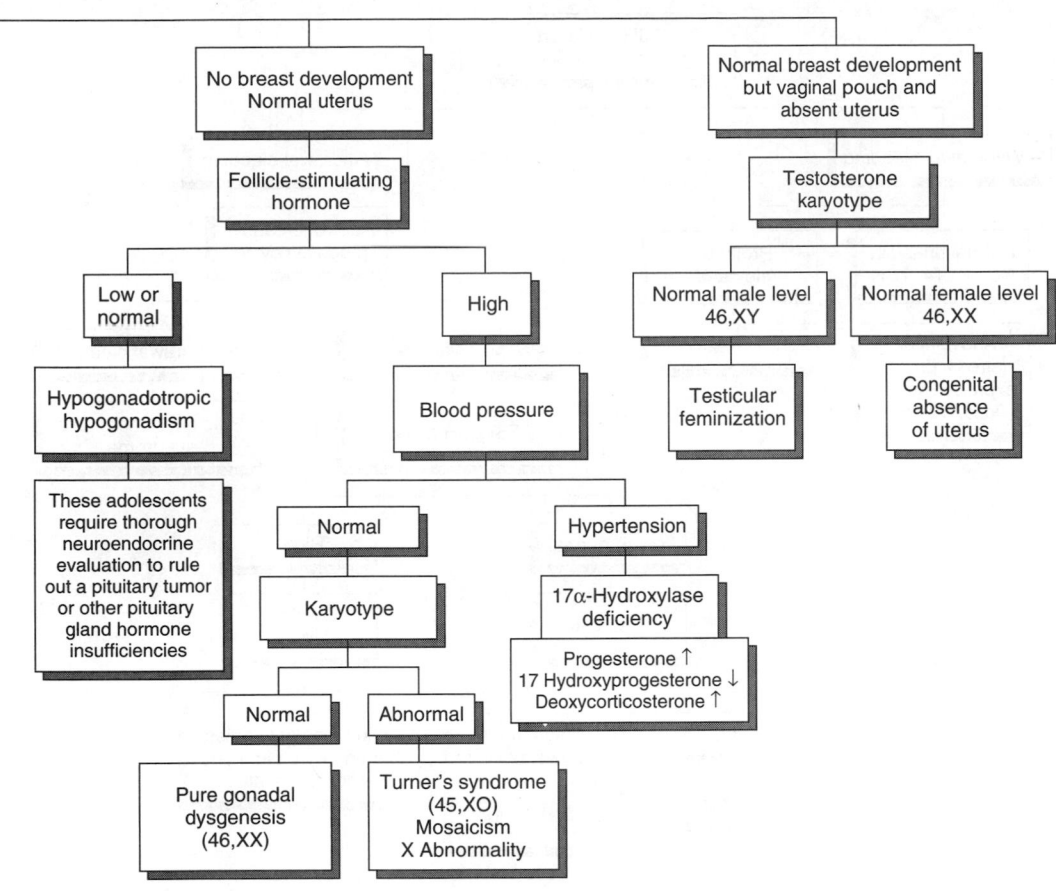

1. For primary and secondary amenorrhea with normal secondary sexual characteristics:
    a. If evidence of androgen excess or galactorrhea is present, the adolescent should be evaluated as described in Chapters 57 and 58.
    b. Pregnancy should always be considered and ruled out.
    c. Diabetes mellitus and hypothyroidism should be considered and, if clinically indicated, ruled out with fasting blood sugar or thyroid function tests.
    d. Uterine synechiae, or Asherman's syndrome, should be considered if there is a history of dilation and curettage or endometritis. This condition may cause partial or total obliteration of the uterine cavity. If this problem is suggested by the history, a gynecological referral for evaluation by hysteroscopy or hysterosalpingography is indicated.

    If the above evaluation result is negative, the workup should proceed as follows (Fig. 53.2):
    — Administer progesterone withdrawal test: A positive response correlates with circulating estradiol levels adequate to prime the endometrium. A positive response (ranges from minimal brown staining to normal menstrual flow) indicates a serum estradiol level greater than 40 pg/mL.
    — A positive response to progesterone indicates either hypothalamic-pituitary dysfunction or PCOS. A prolactin level should be measured, as this is the most sensitive test for pituitary microadenomas. Rarely, a patient who withdraws to proges-

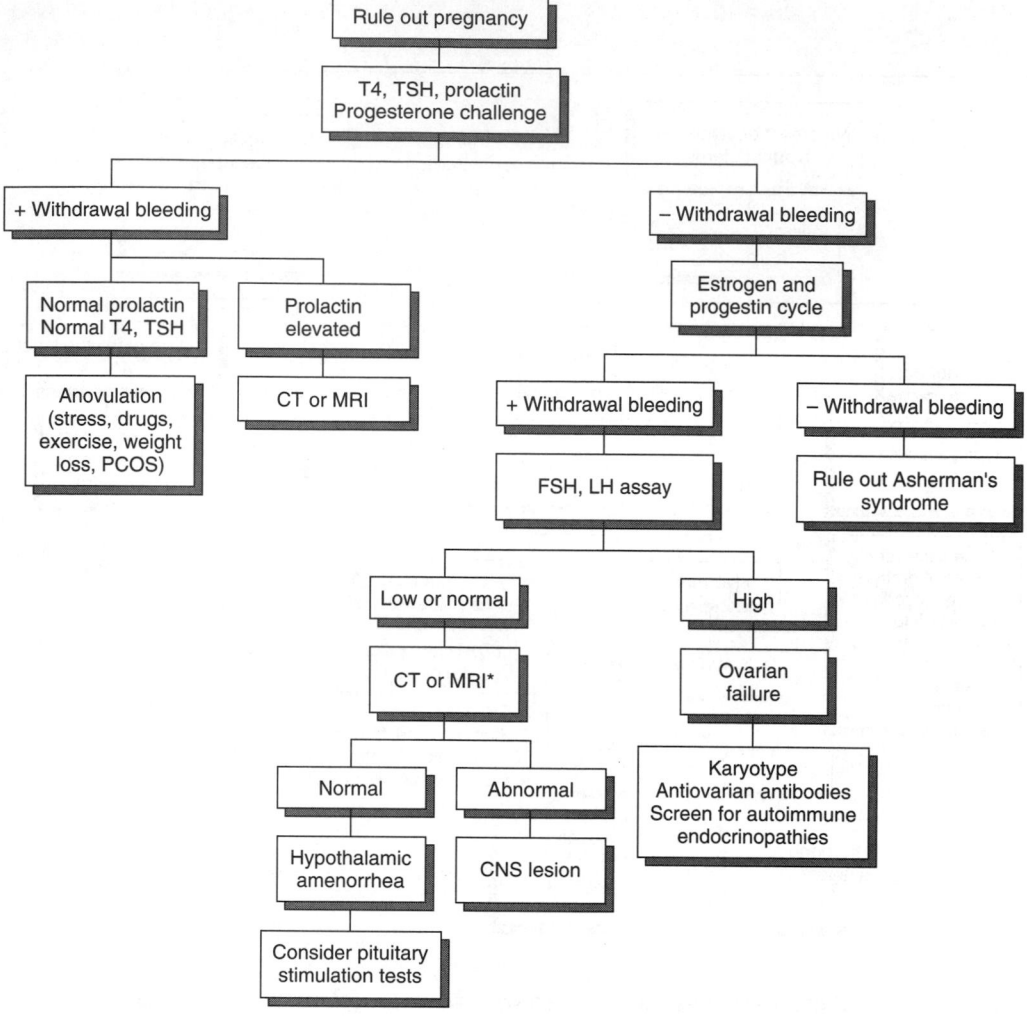

*Except in the presence of heavy exercise, weight loss, or drug abuse with a normal prolactin

FIGURE 53.2.   The evaluation of secondary amenorrhea. *CNS,* central nervous system; *CT,* computed tomography; *FSH,* follicle-stimulating hormone; *LH,* luteinizing hormone; *MRI,* magnetic resonance imaging; *PCOS,* polycystic ovary syndrome; *T4,* thyroxine; *TSH,* thyroid-stimulating hormone.

terone can have a microadenoma. In addition, thyroid-stimulating hormone (TSH) with or without thyroxine (T4) should be measured to eliminate the possibility of subtle thyroid dysfunction. LH or LH-FSH ratios have been used in the past to evaluate for PCOS; however, these values are not very sensitive nor specific.
— If there is no response to progesterone, then either hypothalamic-pituitary failure or ovarian failure is likely. A high FSH level indicates ovarian failure, whereas a normal or low FSH suggests hypothalamic-pituitary failure. If ovarian failure is suspected then a karyotype, antiovarian antibodies, and screening for autoimmune endocrinopathies should be considered. If hypothalamic pituitary failure is suspected, a magnetic resonance imaging (MRI) scan, visual fields, and pituitary stimulation tests should be considered.

— Individuals with weight loss, anorexia nervosa, heavy substance abuse, or heavy exercise may or may not withdraw to progesterone. If they do not withdraw to progesterone, it is an indication of low estradiol levels. If the teen has a normal prolactin level, she would not require an MRI scan unless otherwise indicated on the history and physical examination. However, a prolactin test would be indicated every 6–12 months if there are no spontaneous menses.

2. For primary amenorrhea with either absent uterus or absent secondary sexual characteristics (Fig. 53.1):

a. A physical examination will divide the teens into three groups:

— Absent uterus, normal breasts; absent breasts, normal uterus; and absent breasts, absent uterus: In general, breast development should be at least an SMR 4 to be considered indicative of full normal gonadal function. A breast stage of SMR 2 or SMR 3 may indicate adrenal function alone without gonadal function.

b. If the examination reveals normal breast development but an absent uterus and blind vaginal pouch, a karyotype and a test for testosterone level are indicated.

— XX karyotype plus female level of testosterone: Congenital absence of uterus

— XY karyotype plus male level of testosterone: Testicular feminization

c. If the examination reveals absent secondary sexual characteristics but a normal uterus, an FSH test is ordered.

— A low or normal FSH suggests a hypothalamic or pituitary abnormality, and a careful neuroendocrine evaluation is in order.

— A high FSH and normal blood pressure suggest a genetic disorder or gonadal dysgenesis. A karyotype should be ordered.

— A high FSH and hypertension suggest a 17α-hydroxylase deficiency. This is confirmed by an elevated progesterone (>3 ng/mL), low 17α-hydroxyprogesterone (<0.2 ng/mL), and an elevated serum deoxycorticosterone.

d. The absence of both breast development and uterus or vagina is very rare. These findings suggest gonadal failure and the presence of MIF secretion from a testis. This could arise from anorchia occurring after MIF activity was present or an enzyme block, such as a 17,20-desmolase defect. The evaluation should include LH, FSH, progesterone, and 17-hydroxyprogesterone measurements and a karyotype.

TREATMENT

Primary Amenorrhea

Hypothalamic Hypogonadotropic Hypogonadism (Hypothalamic Failure)   Therapy should begin with estrogen therapy 0.3 mg/day, or less if the adolescent is short, to avoid premature epiphyseal closure. Patients with normal height can receive 0.625 mg/day of conjugated estrogen (Premarin). High doses of estrogen should be avoided early to avoid abnormal breast development manifested by increased subareolar breast development and abnormal contours.

A maintenance schedule would be 0.625–2.5 mg/day of conjugated estrogens on days 1–25 of each month, with 10 mg of medroxyprogesterone acetate (Provera) on days 12–25. The progestin is added to induce withdrawal bleeding and thus avoid endometrial hyperplasia. This schedule can be repeated beginning the first of each month. The dosage of estrogen may range from 0.625–2.5 mg/day, depending on the individual and the estrogen response. In the future GnRH will probably be used for these conditions when a more easily tolerated delivery system is available. If pregnancy is desired, pulsatile GnRH can be used.

Pituitary Defect   Hormonal therapy as outlined above.

Genetic Abnormalities Leading to Gonadal Defects   Hormonal therapy as already outlined. If a Y chromosome is present, gonadal removal is necessary. If a 46,XX karyotype is present, then the gonadal tissue should be visualized to see if more than a streak gonad is present. Hormonal replacement is important to start early in adolescence. These individuals are universally sterile. However, with an intact uterus, the individual could be able to bear children after donor oocyte implantation and hormonal support.

Enzyme Defects   For 17α-hydroxylase deficiency use Cortisone plus estrogen-progesterone replacement; remove gonads if Y chromosome is present. For 17,20-desmolase deficiency prescribe estrogen-progesterone replacement; remove gonads if Y chromosome is present.

Testicular Feminization

1. Gonadal removal: All intra-abdominal gonads associated with a Y chromosome have a relatively high potential for malignancy. Tumors in testicular feminization patients are rare before the age of 25. Since the gonadal secretion contributes to secondary sexual characteristics, gonad removal should be delayed until the age of 20 in testicular feminization patients.
2. After the testes are removed, maintenance estrogen therapy is needed.
3. The adolescent should be informed that she may require vaginoplasty to have normal sexual function.
4. The adolescent should be informed that she cannot become pregnant.
5. Counseling: The adolescent should be informed that she has an abnormal sex chromosome, not that she has male chromosomes. She may require extra reassurance and counseling regarding her identity and concerns about infertility and sexual function.

Congenital Absence of the Uterus   Since these adolescents have normal-functioning ovaries, they do not require hormonal replacement. They may require a vaginoplasty for normal sexual function and an intravenous pyelogram to rule out renal anomalies. These adolescents must be informed that they cannot become pregnant; they may require additional support and counseling regarding their identity and body image.

Primary and Secondary Amenorrhea with Normal Secondary Sex Characteristics

1. PCOS
   a. Medroxyprogesterone acetate (Provera) 10 mg should be given for 10–12 days every 1–2 months to induce withdrawal bleeding or oral contraceptives with or without spironolactone, if androgens are elevated.
   b. When pregnancy is desired, referral for use of clomiphene citrate can be recommended.
2. Hypothalamic-pituitary dysfunction
   a. Alleviate the precipitating cause if known.
   b. Hormonal therapy with progestins to induce uterine bleeding every 1–2 months is recommended.
3. Hypothalamic-pituitary failure
   a. The cause must be evaluated and corrected if possible.
   b. Replacement therapy with cyclic conjugated estrogens and progestins as outlined earlier in hypothalamic failure is recommended.
   c. If the adolescent or young adult desires pregnancy, refer her to an infertility clinic.

4. Ovarian failure
   a. These adolescents also require cyclic estrogen and progestin therapy.
   b. These adolescents are generally sterile and should be counseled regarding this aspect of their problem.
5. Uterine synechiae: This problem requires referral to a gynecologist for possible transhysteroscopic lysis of the adhesions.

Amenorrhea Associated with Weight Loss

In young women with amenorrhea associated with weight loss, bone mineral density (BMD) loss can occur soon after amenorrhea develops. Treatment to prevent BMD loss or promote BMD accretion should start probably within 6 months after amenorrhea occurs (Hergenroeder, 1995). Most adolescents who recover from anorexia nervosa at a young age (<15 years of age) can have normal total body BMD, but regional (lumbar spine and femoral neck) BMD may remain low (Hergenroeder, 1995). The longer the weight loss, the less likely the BMD will return to normal.

Sports Amenorrhea

Athletes, particularly runners, gymnasts, and dancers, with secondary amenorrhea may fall into either the hypothalamic-pituitary dysfunction or failure category. There is evidence to suggest that athletes with amenorrhea have low levels of estrogen and may be at risk for osteoporosis and stress fractures (Cann et al., 1984; Drinkwater et al., 1986; Marcus et al., 1985). Some studies suggest that when amenorrhea persists for 6 months with bone loss, the bone loss may never be regained, while other studies indicate a 20% increase in bone mass when weight is gained. Baer (1993) compared reproductive function in ten amenorrheic (AR) and eumenorrheic (ER) adolescent female runners and seven untrained controls (SE). AR were found to run more miles per day and consume fewer calories per day compared to ER. Mean levels of fasting plasma estradiol, LH, FSH, free thyroxine, and triiodothyronine were significantly lower in AR compared to ER and SE. In addition, AR indicated that they were very concerned about their weight and fearful of gaining fat mass. Other studies have indicated that the change in bone density may also relate to the type of athletics performed, with gymnastic exercises, for example, yielding better bone mass. One recent Scandinavian study has demonstrated that most women who exercise regularly at moderate levels are not at significant risk for athletic amenorrhea and a decrease in bone mineral density. Summary considerations for athletes with amenorrhea include (Hergenroeder, 1995):

1. The vast majority of bone mineralization in adolescent females occurs by the middle of the second decade.
2. Premature bone demineralization occurs in women with hypothalamic dysfunction manifest as amenorrhea and oligomenorrhea, associated with athletics, dancing, and eating disorders.
3. Regular menses and fertility should return with a decrease in the intensity of activity.
4. Calcium intake should be increased to 1500 mg/day.
5. Hormonal therapy: If the teen does not withdraw to progesterone or has a documented low circulating estradiol level, estrogen and progesterone replacement should be considered, particularly in amenorrheic athletes who show no signs of gaining weight or reducing activity after 6 months. These individuals may require higher doses of estrogen than replacement doses (1.25 mg/day of conjugated estrogen [Premarin] rather than 0.625 mg/day). However, controversy still exists regarding the beneficial effects on BMD in amenorrheic athletes, particularly those who are underweight. Conjugated estrogen, in

doses that improve BMD in postmenopausal women and in combination with medroxyprogesterone, has not been shown to improve BMD in young women with hypothalamic amenorrhea. The role of oral medroxyprogesterone (10 mg/day, 10 days/month) in improving BMD in teenage girls with hypothalamic amenorrhea or oligomenorrhea also remains to be established. Some authorities have advocated the use of combination oral contraceptive pills in young women with hypothalamic amenorrhea. The benefits of this approach have also not been established in a randomized, controlled trial.

6. The practitioner should evaluate these individuals, as outlined in this chapter, to eliminate the possibility of pregnancy, thyroid dysfunction, prolactinoma, or a disorder of androgen excess. It should not just be assumed that amenorrhea is secondary to exercise.

BIBLIOGRAPHY

Alper MM, Garner PR. Premature ovarian failure: its relationship to autoimmune disease. Obstet Gynecol 1985;66:27.

Bachmann GA, Kemmann E. Prevalence of oligomenorrhea and amenorrhea in a college population. Am J Obstet Gynecol 1982;144:98.

Bachrach LK, Katzman DK, Litt IF, et al. Recovery from osteopenia in adolescent girls with anorexia nervosa. J Clin Endocrinol Metab 1991;72:602.

Baer JT. Endocrine parameters in amenorrheic and eumenorrheic adolescent female runners. Int J Sports Med 1993;14:191.

Baer JT, Taper LJ, Gwazdauskas FG, et al. Hormonal and metabolic factors affecting bone mineral density in adolescent amenorrheic and eumenorrheic female runners. J Sports Med Phys Fitness 1992;32:51.

Baker ER. Menstrual dysfunction and hormonal status in athletic women: a review. Fertil Steril 1981;36:691.

Bar-Or O, Lombardo JA, Rowland TW. Prepubertal exercise: how much, when? Patient Care 1988;22:59.

Barrow GW, Sama S. Menstrual irregularity and stress fractures in collegiate female distance runners. Am J Sports Med 1988;16:209.

Behrman SJ. Adolescent amenorrhea. Ann NY Acad Sci 1967;142:807.

Blythe M. Common menstrual problems, amenorrhea and oligomenorrhea. In: Adolescent Health Update. Elk Grove Village, Illinois: American Academy of Pediatrics, 1991.

Brooks-Gunn J, Warren MP, Hamilton LH. The relation of eating problems and amenorrhea in ballet dancers. Med Sci Sports Exerc 1987;19:41.

Bullen BA, Skrinar GS, Beitins IZ, et al. Induction of menstrual disorders by strenuous exercise in untrained women. N Engl J Med 1985;312:1349.

Byrne J, Fears TR, Gail MH, et al. Early menopause in long-term survivors of cancer during adolescence. Am J Obstet Gynecol 1992;1666:788.

Byrne J, Mulvihill JJ, Myers MH, et al. Effects of treatment on fertility in long-term survivors of childhood and adolescent cancer. N Engl J Med 1987;317:1315.

Calabrese LH, Kirkendall DT, Floyd M, et al. Menstrual abnormalities, nutritional and body composition patterns in female ballet dancers. Phys Sportsmed 1983;2:86.

Cann CE, Martin MC, Genant HK, et al. Decreased spinal mineral content in amenorrheic women. JAMA 1984;251:626.

Carpenter SE. Psychosocial menstrual disorders: stress, exercise and diet's effect on the menstrual cycle. Curr Opin Obstet Gynecol 1994;6:536.

Cohen JL, Kim CS, May PB, et al. Exercise, body weight, and professional ballet dancers. Phys Sportsmed 1982;4:92.

Constantini NW, Warren MP. Menstrual dysfunction in swimmers: a distinct entity. J Clin Endocrinol Metab 1995;80:2740.

Copeland PM, Sacks NR, Herzog DB. Longitudinal follow-up of amenorrhea in eating disorders. Psychosom Med 1995;57:121.

Coupey SM. Common menstrual disorders. Pediatr Clin North Am 1989;36:551.

Cumming DC, Rebar JRW. Exercise and reproductive function in women. Am J Indust Med 1983;4:113.

Cumming DC, Strich G, Brunsting L. Amenorrheic joggers differ in hormone profile. Obstet Gynecol News 1982;17:12.

Dale E, Gerlach DH, Wilhite AL. Menstrual dysfunction in distance runners. Obstet Gynecol 1979;54:47.

Davajan V. Primary amenorrhea. In: Mishell DR Jr, Davagan V, Lobo A, eds. Infertility, contraception, and reproductive endocrinology, 3rd ed. Boston: Blackwell Scientific, 1991a.

Davajan V. Secondary amenorrhea. In: Mishell DR Jr, Davagan V, Lobo A, eds. Infertility, contraception, and reproductive endocrinology, 3rd ed. Boston: Blackwell Scientific, 1991b.

Dawood MY, Ravnikar VA, Schneider GT, et al. A practical approach to amenorrhea. Patient Care Supplement, 1992;(May 15):12–21.

Devereaux MD, Parr GR, Lachmann SM, et al. The diagnosis of stress fractures in athletes. JAMA 1984;252:531.

Diddle AW. Athletic activity and menstruation: review articles. South Med J 1983;76:619.

Drinkwater BL, Nilson K, Chesnut CH III, et al. Bone mineral content of amenorrheic and eumenorrheic athletes. N Engl J Med 1984;311:277.

Drinkwater BL, Nilson K, Ott S, et al. Bone mineral density after resumption of menses in amenorrheic athletes. JAMA 1986;256:380.

Emans SJ. The athletic adolescent with amenorrhea. Pediatr Ann 1984;13:605.

Frisch RE, Wyshak G, Vincent L. Delayed menarche and amenorrhea in ballet dancers. N Engl J Med 1980; 303:17.

Greene JW. Exercise-induced menstrual irregularities. Compr Ther 1993;19:116.

Griffin JE, Edwards C, Madden JD, et al. Congenital absence of the vagina: clinical review. Ann Intern Med 1976;85:224.

Hergenroeder AC. Bone mineralization, hypothalamic amenorrhea, and sex steroid therapy in female adolescents and young adults. J Pediatr 1995;126:683.

Hintz RL. New approaches to growth failure in Turner syndrome. Adolesc Pediatr Gynecol 1989;2:172.

Jonnavithula S, Warren MP, Fox RP, et al. Bone density is compromised in amenorrheic women despite return of menses: a 2-year study. Obstet Gynecol 1993; 81:669.

Lim VS, Auletta F, Kathpalia S. Gonadal function in women with chronic renal failure: a study of the hypothalamo-pituitary axis. Proceedings of the Clinical Dialysis and Transplant Forum (Washington) 1977; 7:39.

Lindberg JS, Fears WB, Hunt MM, et al. Exercise-induced amenorrhea and bone density. Ann Intern Med 1984;101:647.

Lindberg JS, Powell MR, Hunt MM, et al. Increased vertebral bone mineral in response to reduced exercise in amenorrheic runners. West J Med 1987;146:39.

Lutter JM, Cushman S. Menstrual patterns in female runners. Phys Sportsmed 1982;10:60.

Marcus R, Cann C, Madvig P, et al. Menstrual function and bone mass in elite women distance runners. Ann Intern Med 1985;102:158.

Marshall LA. Clinical evaluation of amenorrhea in active and athletic women. Clin Sports Med 1994;13:371.

Mashchak CA, Kletzky OA, Davajan V, et al. Clinical and laboratory evaluation of patients with primary amenorrhea. Obstet Gynecol 1981;57:715.

Micklesfield LK, Lambert EV, Fataar AB. Bone mineral density in mature, premenopausal ultramarathon runners. Med Sci Sports Exerc 1995;27:688.

Mooradian AD, Morley JE. Endocrine dysfunction in chronic renal failure. Arch Intern Med 1984;144:351.

Moshang T, Holsclaw DS. Menarchal determinants in cystic fibrosis. Am J Dis Child 1980;134:1139.

Neinstein LS. Menstrual dysfunction in pathophysiologic states. West J Med 1985;143:476.

Neinstein LS. Menstrual problems in adolescents. Med Clin North Am 1990;74:1181.

Neinstein LS, Castle GF. Congenital absence of the vagina. Am J Dis Child 1983a;137:669.

Neinstein LS, Stewart D, Wang CI, et al. Menstrual dysfunction in cystic fibrosis. J Adolesc Health Care 1983b;4:153.

Okano H, Mizunuma H, Soda M. Effects of exercise and amenorrhea on bone mineral density in teenage runners. Endocrinol JPN 1995;42:271.

Olson BR. Exercise-induced amenorrhea. Am Fam Physician 1989;39:213.

Pasloff ES, Slap GB, Pertschuk MJ, et al. A longitudinal study of metacarpal bone morphometry in anorexia nervosa. Clin Orthop 1992;278:217.

Patterson DF. Menstrual dysfunction in athletes: assessment and treatment. Pediatr Nurs 1995;21:310.

Polaneczky MM, Slap GB. Menstrual disorders in the adolescent: amenorrhea. Pediatr Rev 1992;13:43.

Puffer JC. Athletic amenorrhea and its influence on skeletal integrity. Bull Rheum Dis 1994;43:5.

Russell JB, Mitchell D, Musey PI, et al. The relationship of exercise to anovulatory cycles in female athletes: hormonal and physical characteristics. Obstet Gynecol 1984a;63:452.

Russell JB, Mitchell DE, Musey PI, et al. The role of α-endorphins and catechol estrogens on the hypothalamic-pituitary axis in female athletes. Fertil Steril 1984b;42:690.

Schwartz B, Rebar RW, Yen SSC. Amenorrhea and long distance running. Fertil Steril 1980;34:306.

Shalet SM. Effects of cancer chemotherapy on gonadal function of patients. Cancer Treat Rev 1980; 7:141.

Shangold MM. How I manage exercise-related menstrual disturbances. Phys Sportsmed 1986;14:113.

Singh KB. Menstrual disorders in college students. Am J Obstet Gynecol 1981;140:299.

Speroff L, Glass RH, Kase NG. Amenorrhea. In: Clinical gynecologic endocrinology and infertility, 4th ed. Baltimore: Williams & Wilkins, 1989.

Speroff L, Shangold MM, Dale E. Impact of exercise on menstruation and reproduction. Contrib Gynecol Obstet 1982;19:54.

Stager JM, Ritchie-Flanagan B, Robertshaw D. Reversibility of amenorrhea in athletes. N Engl J Med 1984;310:51.

Stillman RJ, Schinfeld JS, Schiff I. Ovarian failure in long term survivors of childhood malignancy. Am J Obstet Gynecol 1981;139:62.

Vigersky RM, Andersen AE, Thompson RN, et al. Hypothalamic dysfunction in secondary amenorrhea associated with simple weight loss. N Engl J Med 1977; 297:1141.

Warren MP. The effects of exercise on pubertal progression and reproductive function in girls. J Clin Endocrinol Metab 1980;51:1150.

Warren MP, Jewelewicz R, Dyrenfurth I, et al. The significance of weight loss in the evaluation of pituitary response to LH-RH in women with secondary amenorrhea. J Clin Endocrinol Metab 1975;40: 601.

Waxman J. Chemotherapy and the adult gonad: a review. J R Soc Med 1983;76:144–148.

Yurth EF. Female athlete triad. West J Med 1995;162: 149.

CHAPTER 54

Polycystic Ovary Syndrome and Ovarian Cysts and Tumors

Lawrence S. Neinstein and Karen S. Himebaugh

POLYCYSTIC OVARY SYNDROME

Definition

Polycystic ovary syndrome (PCOS) is a disorder of the hypothalamic-pituitary-ovarian system, giving rise to temporary or persistent anovulation and usually androgen excess. The syndrome was originally described in 1935 by Stein and Leventhal as amenorrhea, hirsutism, and obesity associated with enlarged polycystic ovaries. For many years there was an emphasis on the morphologic changes in the ovary. However, enlarged polycystic ovaries may occur with other conditions such as Cushing's syndrome and congenital adrenal hyperplasia, and women with other classic features of PCOS may have ovaries of normal size. The features stressed in recent years for PCOS include clinical evidence of hyperandrogenism such as facial hair and acne, anovulation, and laboratory evidence of elevated androgens. PCOS affects approximately 5–7% of women of reproductive age.

Etiology

Endocrine Findings   PCOS is characterized by menstrual irregularities ranging from amenorrhea to oligomenorrhea to dysfunctional uterine bleeding. An androgen excess state is often present, leading to hirsutism and rarely virilization. The changes in gonadotropins and steroid hormones that cause these manifestations are listed below:

1. Inappropriate gonadotropin secretion (IGS) characterized by:
   a. Elevated serum luteinizing hormone (LH) level (>21 mIU/mL)
   b. Normal or low follicle-stimulating hormone (FSH) level
   c. Exaggerated response of LH, not FSH, to gonadotropin-releasing hormone (GnRH)
   d. LH-FSH ratio often greater than 3
   e. Elevated bioactive LH (generally a research tool, but even more sensitive for PCOS than an elevated immunoreactive LH)
2. Steroid hormones
   a. Estrone (E_1): Significantly elevated serum levels
   b. Estradiol (E_2): Normal total estradiol, but elevated unbound or free estradiol
   c. Androstenedione and dehydroepiandrosterone-sulfate: Elevated serum levels
   d. Testosterone: Occasionally minimally elevated serum levels
3. Source of excess androgens: The source may be secretion from the ovaries, the adrenal gland, or both. Two other sources contribute to androgen excess:

a. Androstenedione is converted peripherally in adipose tissue to testosterone.
b. There is a decrease in binding of testosterone to sex hormone–binding globulin (SHBG). Normal females have approximately 96% of their testosterone bound to SHBG, where it is inactive, while PCOS patients have only 92% of their testosterone bound; thus, there is a larger percentage of free and active testosterone in PCOS patients.

Pathophysiology   The exact initiating cause of PCOS is not known but may be related to:

1. Abnormal hypothalamic-pituitary function
2. Abnormal ovarian function
3. Abnormal adrenal androgen metabolism
4. Insulin resistance: Insulin resistance may exist in women with PCOS in obese as well as lean individuals. Some individuals may develop HAIRAN syndrome, a combination of hyperandrogenism, insulin resistance, and acanthosis nigricans.

Factors leading to the development of PCOS include the following factors:

1. Insulin increases at the time of puberty, since insulin resistance selectively affects peripheral glucose metabolism.
2. Insulin and insulin-like growth factor I (IGF-I) have mitogenic effects on the ovaries, causing theca cell hyperplasia, which leads to excessive androgen production.
3. The increased ovarian androgen levels cause follicular atresia, impairing estradiol production.
4. The estrone levels are elevated due to increased conversion of androstenedione to estrone in adipose cells, which leads to suppression of FSH and tonic stimulation of LH, which further aggravates theca cell stimulation.
5. The combination of theca cell hyperplasia and arrested follicular maturation constitutes the typical histological features of PCOS.
6. Since not all adolescents ultimately develop PCOS, it is thought there is a genetic factor involved. Genetic studies of family clusters have shown a high incidence of affected relatives (Legro, 1995). A dominant mode of inheritance seems most likely, but the type and degree of expression may vary within the same family. The syndrome may be transmitted through paternal or maternal sides of a family. It is of interest that both the insulin receptor genes and the LH-β-subunit gene have been mapped to chromosome 19. However, chromosomal studies of patients with PCOS have shown no consistent abnormality.

Gulekli et al. (1993) compared adolescent and adult women with PCOS and found that clinical manifestations and hormonal changes were similar.

Valproate can also induce menstrual disturbances, polycystic ovaries, and hyperandrogenism (Isojarvi et al., 1993). In a study of 238 women with epilepsy, Isojarvi et al. (1993) found 43% of the women using valproate had polycystic ovaries. In those women using valproate before the age of 20 years 80% had polycystic ovaries or hyperandrogenism.

Clinical Consequences

PCOS can present with many symptoms. Table 54.1 indicates the prevalence of various signs and symptoms associated with PCOS.

1. Anovulation is the key feature: The ovaries in PCOS patients are usually enlarged, pearly white, sclerotic with multiple (20–100) cystic follicles. Normally, follicles develop to about 19–20 mm and then ovulation occurs. In women with PCOS, multiple

TABLE 54.1.   Signs and Symptoms of Polycystic Ovary Syndrome

Symptom	Mean (%)	Range (%)
Infertility	74	35–95
Hirsutism	69	17–83
Amenorrhea	51	15–77
Obesity	41	16–49
Functional bleeding	29	6–65
Dysmenorrhea	23	NA[a]
Corpus luteum at surgery	22	0–71
Virilization	21	0–28
Biphasic basal body temperature	15	12–40
Cyclic menses	12	7–28

Adapted from Lobo RA. Polycystic ovary syndrome. In: Mishell DR Jr, Davajan V, eds. Infertility contraception, and reproductive endocrinology. Oradell, New Jersey: Medical Economics Books, 1986.
[a]NA, not available.

follicles develop but only to about 9–10 mm in size. Histologically, the ovaries have the same number of primordial follicles, but the number of atretic follicles is doubled. Also there is an absence of corpora lutea. The polycystic ovary is a sign, not a disease entity on its own. The typical histological changes of the polycystic ovary can be seen with any size ovary.

2. Hirsutism: The development of hirsutism depends not only on the concentration of androgens in the blood but also on the genetic sensitivity of the hair follicles to androgens. Clinical hirsutism may not occur in all women with PCOS, but nearly all women with PCOS have elevated blood androgen levels.

3. Obesity: Originally, obesity was regarded as a classic feature, but its presence is extremely variable and not mandatory for diagnosis.

4. Infertility: Infertility is usually not of concern to the adolescent patient.

5. Increased risk for cancer of the endometrium due to prolonged unopposed estrogen stimulation of the endometrial lining: Also there is an increased risk of breast cancer associated with chronic anovulation during the reproductive years. The risk of endometrial cancer is increased threefold, while the risk of developing breast cancer is increased three to four times.

6. Elevated lipoprotein profile: The lipid profile in androgenized women with PCOS is similar to the male pattern, which may increase the risk of cardiovascular disease in this group of patients. The long-term impact is not known and remains to be studied.

7. Insulin resistance and hyperinsulinemia: Both are well-recognized features of PCOS. Approximately 50% of women with PCOS are insulin resistant. The insulin resistance in PCOS patients is unrelated to body weight or composition. The cause-and-effect relationships between insulin and androgens in PCOS is still controversial and is under investigation.

Differential Diagnosis

1. Familial hirsutism
2. Androgen-producing ovarian and adrenal tumors: For further discussion, see Chapter 58 on hirsutism and virilism.
3. Cushing's syndrome: Potential influence of Cushing's syndrome is usually excluded by history and physical examination and, if needed, an overnight dexamethasone suppression test.

4. Congenital adrenal hyperplasia (CAH): An incomplete 21-hydroxylase deficiency can mimic PCOS. The diagnosis of CAH is based on elevated serum 17-hydroxyprogesterone, especially after a 0.25-mg single-dose injection of adrenocorticotropic hormone (ACTH).
5. Stromal hyperthecosis: Stromal hyperthecosis probably represents a disorder related to PCOS. However, in this disorder the testosterone levels are higher and may be as high as in patients with androgen-producing tumors. These patients may be not only hirsute but virilized. The history is one of slow onset and progression of symptoms and signs. Ovarian vein catheterization shows increased but equal amounts of testosterone from each ovary.

Diagnosis

Criteria for the diagnosis of PCOS include:

1. Chronic anovulation with a perimenarchal onset of menstrual irregularities
2. Hormonal evidence of androgen excess
   The following are not needed for diagnosis:
3. Increased body weight (ponderal index: height [inches] divided by the cube root of weight [pounds] is less than 12): Obesity is not absolutely necessary for the diagnosis if the other criteria are present. However, while all patients may not appear obese, most should have a ponderal index below 12.
4. Inappropriate gonadotropin secretion (LH or FSH = >3, provided LH level is not below 8 mIU/mL): While LH and FSH have been widely used, the sensitivity and specificity of these hormones are not particularly high.
5. Euprolactinemia: Most individuals with PCOS have normal levels of prolactin. Some patients with PCOS have mildly elevated prolactin levels. It is unclear whether this is a special group of PCOS patients.

Therapy

Infertility   Infertility is usually not a concern in the adolescent patient. However, when fertility is desired, clomiphene citrate is used to stimulate ovulation.

Hirsutism

1. Cosmetic methods including shaving wax or electrolysis
2. Oral contraceptives work in 60–100% of women but require 6–12 months. Combination pills should be used that contain low androgenic progestins such as norethindrone, norgestimate, or desogestrel. Oral contraceptives work by:
   a. Suppressing LH production and thus reducing ovarian androgen production
   b. Increasing the binding capacity of SHBG and thus decreasing free testosterone
   c. Decreasing adrenal androgen production
   d. Decreasing 5α-reductase activity

In addition to oral contraceptives, antiandrogens such as spironolactone can be used (see Chapter 58). The combination of low-dose oral contraceptives and spironolactone is very effective.

Menstrual Irregularities   The patient with amenorrhea or oligomenorrhea should receive medroxyprogesterone acetate (Provera) (10 mg a day for 10–12 days) every 1–2 months for withdrawal bleeding. The monthly use of medroxyprogesterone acetate has no significant effect on androgen production by the ovaries, so it is not helpful if hirsutism is present. Combination oral contraceptives can also be used.

OVARIAN CYSTS AND TUMORS

The finding of an enlarged ovary may represent either the development of a functional ovarian cyst or may indicate the presence of a benign or malignant, cystic or solid, neoplasm of the ovary. Although physiologic cysts of the ovary are common during adolescence, ovarian neoplasms, particularly malignant ovarian tumors, are uncommon. However, ovarian tumors are the most frequent genital neoplasm in childhood and adolescence. This section describes various types of ovarian cysts and neoplasms and management of the adolescent with an ovarian mass.

Classification of Ovarian Masses

1. Physiological cysts
   a. Follicular cyst
   b. Corpus luteum cysts
   c. Theca lutein cysts
   d. Luteal cyst of pregnancy
   e. Endometrioma
2. Germinal epithelium
   a. Teratomas
      — Immature
      — Mature: Solid or cystic, benign or with malignant transformation
   b. Embryonal carcinoma
   c. Dysgerminoma
   d. Endodermal sinus tumor
   e. Choriocarcinoma
3. Epithelial cell tumors
   a. Serous cystadenomas and cystadenocarcinomas
   b. Mucinous cystadenomas and cystadenocarcinomas
   c. Undifferentiated carcinoma
4. Connective tissue tumors
   a. Fibromas
   b. Sarcomas
   c. Granulosa cell and theca cell tumors
   d. Arrhenoblastomas
5. Metastatic lesions
6. Tumors deriving from mesenchymal tissue from the kidney or adrenal gland
   a. Brenner tumors, derived from tissue similar to renal, pelvis, or ureter
   b. Adrenal cell rest tumors
   c. Parovarian cysts derived from wolffian duct remnants

Physiological Cysts

Follicular Cysts   Follicular cysts may result from failure of the dominant follicle to ovulate or from the failure of other follicles to undergo atresia. Follicular cysts are usually an incidental finding on physical examination or ultrasound, but they may become as large as 6–8 cm in diameter. These cysts may produce estrogen, leading to menstrual irregularity. There are usually no symptoms unless rupture or torsion of the ovary occurs, both of which can cause peritoneal signs. With rupture of cysts peritoneal signs usually resolve within 24 hours. Follicular cysts usually resolve spontaneously within 4–8 weeks.

Corpus Luteum Cysts   Corpus luteum cysts result from a persistent corpus luteum often associated with hemorrhage into the cysts. They are usually larger than follicular cysts (5–10 cm in diameter). Corpus luteum cysts are more likely than follicular cysts to produce menstrual irregularities, including delayed menses or heavy menses. These cysts may contain significant amounts of progesterone. They are more likely, because of their size, to cause pelvic and lower abdominal, usually unilateral, pain. Adolescents with a corpus luteum cyst may present as a surgical emergency because of rupture with significant hemorrhage. Smaller luteal cysts will often resolve spontaneously. Larger cysts may require surgical intervention.

Ovarian Tumors

Germ cell tumors are the most common ovarian tumors found in adolescent females with a frequency of 67–89% (Ehren et al., 1984). The most common germ cell tumors are the teratomas. They are derived from the germ cell layer of the ovary and contain endoderm, mesoderm, and ectoderm elements. They may contain hair and teeth, as well as evidence of embryonic gastrointestinal, genitourinary, and muscle tissue. Although the majority of the teratomas are benign, malignant teratomas do occur. These are often diagnosed late after abdominal swelling, cachexia, and metastases have occurred. Dysgerminomas, another germ cell tumor, are an uncommon tumor. However, they are the most common ovarian malignancy in adolescent females.

In adults two-thirds of primary ovarian tumors and 90% of ovarian cancers are of epithelial origin. In children and adolescents epithelium-derived ovarian tumors are much less common, representing about 5–19% of ovarian tumors. In a series from Childrens Hospital of Los Angeles (Ehren et al., 1984) the following distribution of ovarian tumors was found:

Tumor Type	Patients	Tumors	Bilateral
Germ cell tumors	56		
Teratomas		47	
Benign		41	2
Embryonic		3	
Malignant		3	
Germinomas		6	2
Endodermal sinus tumors		1	
Mixed germ cell tumors		2	
Epithelial tumors	7		
Cystadenoma		6	
Cystadenocarcinoma		1	

None of the epithelial tumors occurred in patients younger than 12 years of age.

Tumors derived from stromal elements account for about 12–20% of ovarian tumors in adolescents. Stromal element tumors are often hormonally active. The granulosa or theca cell tumors produce high amounts of estradiol, and thus produce precocious puberty in young children and menstrual abnormalities in adolescents. The arrhenoblastoma produces testosterone and androstenedione, and thus produces virilization and amenorrhea. Struma ovarii is a form of benign ovarian tumor composed primarily of ectopic thyroid tissue, rarely producing sufficient amounts of thyroxine to cause hyperthyroidism.

The diagnosis of ovarian tumors is hindered by their locations and relatively asymptomatic courses. Many adolescents with ovarian tumors are asymptomatic, with the mass being discovered on routine examination. At presentation, the most common complaint of adolescents with these tumors is abdominal pain. In the above series of patients 76% had abdominal pain when first seen. Other presenting symptoms include increased abdominal girth, weight gain or weight loss, lethargy, dysuria, constipation, and in children, precocious puberty. Another presentation is Meigs' syndrome, which includes ascites and pleural effusion secondary to a benign fibroma of the ovary (fibroma), with symptom resolution after tumor removal. Occasionally, an adolescent with an ovarian mass will present with acute abdominal symptoms secondary to gonadal torsion or rupture of a cyst.

Differential Diagnosis

1. Gastrointestinal masses: Retained stools, appendiceal abscess
2. Genitourinary masses: Distended bladder, ectopic kidney, and polycystic kidneys
3. Pelvic masses: Intrauterine pregnancy, ectopic pregnancy, and tubo-ovarian abscess
4. Traumatic hematoma

Management of Enlarged Ovary

The prepubertal ovary is about 1.5–2.0 cm in length and 0.5 cm in width. After menarche, the ovary is about 3.0–3.5 cm in length, 1.5–2.0 cm in width, and 1.0–1.5-cm thick. The practitioner is reminded that small ovarian cysts during adolescence are common and are not an unusual finding on ultrasound. Winer-Muram et al. (1989) found that 59 of 83 adolescents had 1.0- to 1.5-cm ovarian cysts found on ultrasound. These small cysts should not be associated with abdominal pain. If a cystic ovarian mass is found that is less than 6–8 cm, observation for a 6-week period with hormonal suppression can be helpful in the differential diagnosis.

In the classic article by Spanos (1973), 285 females were treated with a combination of oral contraceptive pills. After 6 weeks 81 patients still had masses and underwent exploratory laparotomy. Of these 81 patients none had functional cysts.

With contemporary low-dose oral contraceptive pills, suppression of follicular development may be incomplete as suggested by several recent studies. Triphasic oral contraceptive pills appear to offer no protection against ovarian cysts. Although both high- and low-dose monophasic contraceptive pills decrease the incidence of ovarian cysts, the effect is greater with higher dose monophasic pills. Also follicular development may continue with the progestin-only pill and with the levonorgestrel implants. Therefore, patients who develop a simple cystic mass while taking oral contraceptive pills should be followed for 6–8 weeks. If the cystic mass is still present, surgical evaluation is recommended.

Other indications for surgical evaluation of an adnexal mass include:

1. Any solid or fixed tumor
2. Any adnexal mass in a prepubertal female that measures greater than 9 mm
3. Any adnexal mass greater than 6–8 cm
4. Any adnexal mass greater than 5 cm not responding to 6 weeks of hormonal suppression
5. Signs or symptoms of adnexal torsion or ovarian rupture
6. Unexplained ascites with malignant cells in the peritoneal fluid

Those adolescents with tumors over 5–6 cm deserve an ultrasound before suppressive therapy. If a solid tumor is found, it should be removed. The practitioner should also consider the other diagnoses as listed previously. A pelvic examination with cultures, a pregnancy test, and a pelvic ultrasound usually help to sort out the diagnosis.

Bibliography

Adashi EY, Resnick CE, Ricciarella E, et al. Granulosa cell–derived insulin-like growth factor (IGF) binding proteins are inhibitory to IGF-I hormonal action: evidence derived from the use of a truncated IGF-I analog. J Clin Invest 1992;90:1593.

Carmina E, Gonzalez F, Chang L, et al. Reassessment of adrenal androgen secretion in women with polycystic ovary syndrome. Obstet Gynecol 1995;85:971.

Dale PO, Tomb T, Voalir S, et al. Body weight, hyperinsulinemia, and gonadotropin levels in the polycystic ovary syndrome: evidence of two distinct populations. Fertil Steril 1992;58:487.

Ditkoff EC, Fruzzetti F, Chang L, et al. The impact of estrogen on adrenal androgen sensitivity and secretion in polycystic ovary syndrome. J Clin Endocrinol Metab 1995;80:603.

Dunaif A. Insulin resistance and ovarian dysfunction. In: Moller DE, ed. Insulin resistance. Boston: Wiley & Sons, 1993:301.

Dunaif A, Seqal KR, Shelley DR, et al. Evidence for distinctive and intrinsic defects in insulin action in polycystic ovary syndrome. Diabetes 1992;41:1257.

Ehren EM, Mahour GH, Isaacs H Jr. Benign and malignant ovarian tumors in children and adolescents: a review of 63 cases. Am J Surg 1984;147:339.

Franks S. Polycystic ovary syndrome. N Engl J Med 1995;333:853.

Functional ovarian cysts in relation to the use of monophasic and triphasic oral contraceptives. Obstet Gynecol 1992;79:529.

Gibson M. Reproductive health and polycystic ovary syndrome. Am J Med 1995;98(1A):67S.

Goldzieher JW. Polycystic ovarian disease. Fertil Steril 1981;35:371.

Grimes DA, Godwin AJ, Rubin A, et al. Ovulation and follicular development associated with three low-dose oral contraceptives: a randomized controlled trial. Obstet Gynecol 1994;83(1):29.

Gulekli B, Turhan NO, Senoz S, et al. Endocrinological, ultrasonographic and clinical findings in adolescent and adult polycystic ovary patients: a comparative study. Gynecol Endocrinol 1993;7:273.

Huffman JW, Dewhurst CJ, Capraro UJ, eds. Ovarian tumors in children and adolescents. In: The gynecology of children and adolescence. 2nd ed. Philadelphia: WB Saunders, 1981.

Imai A, Furui T, Tamaya T. Gynecologic tumors and symptoms in childhood and adolescence: 10-years' experience. Int J Gynaecol Obstet 1994;5:227.

Isojarvi JIT, Laatikainen TJ, Pakarinen AJ, et al. Polycystic ovaries and hyperandrogenism in women taking valproate for epilepsy. N Engl J Med 1993;329:1383.

Jacobs HS. Polycystic ovary syndrome: etiology and management. Curr Opin Obstet Gynecol 1995;7:203.

Jansen RP. Ovulation and the polycystic ovary syndrome. Aust N Z J Obstet Gynaecol 1994;34:277.

Lanes SF, Birmann B, Walker AM, et al. Oral contraceptive type and functional ovarian cysts. Am J Obstet Gynecol 1992;166:95.

Lauritzen C. Tumors of the ovary in childhood and adolescence. Pediatr Adolesc Gynecol 1984;2:111.

Legro RS. The genetics of polycystic ovary syndrome. Am J Med 1995;98:9S.

Lobo, RA. Polycystic ovary syndrome. In: Mishell DR Jr, Davajan V, eds. Infertility, contraception, and reproductive endocrinology. Oradell, New Jersey: Medical Economics Books, 1986.

McGowan L. Adnexal masses: a visual guide. Female Patient 1989;14:48.

McKenna TJ. Pathogenesis and treatment of polycystic ovary syndrome. N Engl J Med 1988;318:558.

Nader S. Polycystic ovary syndrome and the androgen-insulin connection. Am J Obstet Gynecol 1991;165:346.

Porcu E, Venturoli S, Prato LD, et al. Frequency and treatment of ovarian cysts in adolescence. Arch Gynecol Obstet 1994;255:69.

Poretsky L, Piper B. Insulin resistance, hypersecretion of LH, and a dual-defect hypothesis for the pathogenesis of polycystic ovarian syndrome. Obstet Gynecol 1994;84(4):613.

Rajkhowa M, Bicknell J, Jones M, Clayton RN. Insulin sensitivity in women with polycystic ovary syndrome: relationship to hyperandrogenemia. Fertil Steril 1994;61(4):605.

Richardson GS, Scully RE, Nikrui N, Nelson JH Jr. Common epithelial cancers of the ovary (two parts). N Engl J Med 1985;312:415 & 474.

Rodin A, Thakkar H, Taylor N, et al. Hyperandrogenism in polycystic ovary syndrome. N Engl J Med 1994;330:460.

Seino S, Seino M, Bell GI. Human insulin—receptor gene. Diabetes 1990;39:129.

Siegel MJ, Surratt JT. Pediatric gynecologic imaging. Obstet Gynecol Clin North Am 1992;19:103.

Spanos WJ. Preoperative hormonal therapy of cystic adnexal masses. Am J Obstet Gynecol 1973;116:551.

Watson RE, Bouknight R, Alguire PC. Hirsutism: evaluation and management. J Gen Intern Med 1995;10:283.

Westfall CT, Andrassy RJ. Giant ovarian cyst. Clin Pediatr (Phila) 1982;9:228.

Winer-Muram MT, Emerson DE, Muram D, et al. The sonographic features of the peripubertal ovaries. Adolesc Pediatr Gynecol 1989;2:160.

CHAPTER 55
Vaginitis and Cervicitis

VAGINITIS

Vagina: Normal State

The vagina is a potential space approximately $3\frac{1}{2}$ inches long by $1\frac{1}{2}$ inches in diameter, extending from the vulva to the cervix uteri. Embryologically the upper four-fifths of the vagina is derived from the müllerian ducts and the lower one-fifth from the urogenital sinus. The vagina is lined with epithelial cells that are estrogen dependent. Before puberty and after menopause the cells are thin, leading to heightened susceptibility to infection. During adolescence increased sexual contact may result in a greater number and variety of infections.

Vaginal Flora   The normal flora, composed of over 95% lactobacilli, appears to protect the individual from colonization by more pathogenic organisms. These organisms are normally associated with the vaginal epithelium in a stable relationship. A change in the environmental conditions provided by the vaginal epithelium can cause a significant change in the bacterial flora of the vagina.

Vaginal Secretions   Vaginal secretions are a normal result of the changing hormonal milieu of the menstrual cycle. Six to 12 months prior to menarche there may be a physiological increase in vaginal secretions. This may be copious but is not associated with an odor or with pruritus.
Changes during the menstrual cycles:

1. After menses there is little secretion, but with increasing estrogen levels a cloudy, sticky, whitish secretion develops.
2. Just before ovulation the secretions become profuse and clear.
3. After ovulation, progesterone stimulates a thick and sticky secretion.
4. Before menses a watery secretion develops again.

These normal secretions, which are odorless and nonirritating, are composed of mucus, with occasional squamous cells from the vaginal wall.

Defense Mechanisms of the Vagina   Normal defense mechanisms in the postpubertal teen include:

1. Acid pH of 3.8–4.4: This is a result of lactic acid production from the breakdown of glycogen laid down in vaginal epithelial cells. The low pH fosters growth of acidophilic lactobacilli. The epithelial cell glycogen is dependent on estrogen secretion. The lack of estrogen-stimulated glycogen production is the major reason for the relatively alkaline vaginal pH in prepubertal girls and postmenopausal women.
2. Protective thick epithelium

3. Estrogen support
4. Commensal bacterial flora, leading to low pH
5. Physiological mucous secretion

Factors Predisposing to Infection

Factors predisposing to infection include:

1. Low estrogen levels, especially in girls before puberty and in postmenopausal women
2. Pregnancy
3. Menstruation, due to menstrual blood acting as a culture media and the loss of a protective mucous plug
4. Multiple sexual partners
5. Diabetes mellitus
6. Broad-spectrum antibiotics
7. Immunosuppression
8. Tight clothing
9. Poor hygiene

Vulvovaginitis in Prepubertal Females

Vulvar skin in prepubertal girls is more susceptible to irritation because of the lack of estrogenization and the absence of protective labial hair and fat. Most vulvovaginitis in this group is related to either poor hygiene, obesity, tight clothing, or nonabsorbent underpants. Usually the organisms involved are normal floral including lactobacilli, diphtheroids, α-streptococci, and *Staphylococcus epidermidis* or Gram-negative enteric organisms, usually *Escherichia coli*. The respiratory and enteric pathogens can also play a role in causing vaginal infections in these individuals. Other organisms to be concerned about in prepubertal females are the sexually transmitted organisms. All sexually transmitted organisms can be associated with a vaginitis in prepubertal females. The finding of *Neisseria gonorrhoeae* or *Chlamydia trachomatis* should be regarded as evidence of sexual contact and lead to an investigation of sexual abuse. Vaginal rather than cervical cultures for these organisms are sufficient, as *N. gonorrhoeae* or *C. trachomatis* infect the vagina and not the cervix in prepubertal females.

Vulvovaginitis in Pubertal Females

Prevalence Approximately one-third of women have vaginitis during their lifetime, with the majority of first episodes occurring during adolescence. In most cases vaginitis results in a vaginal discharge or vulvar irritation and itching. In addition, a vaginal odor may be present. Trichomoniasis (caused by *Trichomonas vaginalis*), bacterial vaginosis (BV, caused by a replacement of normal vaginal flora with anaerobic bacteria and *Gardnerella vaginalis*), and candidiasis (usually caused by *Candida albicans*) cause about 97% of nongonococcal infectious vaginitis. Other causes of discharge include birth control pills (estrogen effect), stress (psychophysiological), chemical irritants, tampons left in place, trauma, allergies, and poor hygiene. A vaginal discharge secondary to a cervicitis from *N. gonorrhoeae* or *C. trachomatis* can be indistinguishable to the teen from a discharge secondary to a vaginitis.

Evaluation

History The history in an adolescent female with vaginitis should include questions regarding:

1. Sexual activity including changes in sexual partners
2. Type, duration, and extent of symptoms
3. Contraceptive method and any recent changes in method
4. Changes in diet, exercise, and medications including antibiotics, steroids, use of spray deodorants, soaps, or douches
5. History of prior sexually transmitted diseases (STDs)
6. Family history of diabetes mellitus
7. Location of the pain: The location of any associated pain may help to differentiate urinary tract infection from vaginitis (Demetriou et al., 1982). External pain with urination is usually associated with a vaginitis, while internal pain may occur with either condition.

Examination   The physical examination in a teen with a vaginitis includes checking:

1. The perineum, vulva, vagina, and cervix for erythema, swelling, or lesions
2. The introitus for tenderness
3. The color, texture, and odor of the vaginal discharge
4. The uterus and adnexa for tenderness or masses
5. For other infections such as a cervicitis, herpes, or syphilis

Laboratory   The office evaluation should include:

1. pH of vaginal secretions: The normal pH of the vagina is less than 4.5 (3.8–4.4). A pH greater than 5 is commonly found with *T. vaginalis* and *G. vaginalis* infections. *Candida* is usually associated with a pH in the normal range. The pH should be sampled from the anterior vaginal fornix or lateral side wall; cervical mucus should not be used, since it has a pH of about 7.
2. Amine or "whiff test": Fishy, amine odor after addition of potassium hydroxide (KOH) to vaginal discharge
3. Saline wet mount preparation for microscopic evaluation looking for:
   a. Presence of white blood cells (WBCs): The normal wet mount should have less than 5–10 WBCs per high-power field or less than or 1 WBC per epithelial cell.
   b. Motile trichomonads
   c. Type of background bacterial flora: Normal long lactobacillus versus pleomorphic coccobacilli
   d. "Clue cells": Epithelial cells covered with bacteria and indistinct borders
4. KOH preparation for microscopic evaluation: Checking for the presence of pseudohyphae or budding yeast forms
5. A *Chlamydia* and gonorrhea screening test: To rule out a cervicitis

Other laboratory tests as needed include:

Gram stain of vaginal or cervical secretions
Urinalysis
Pregnancy test

Vulvovaginal Candidiasis

Vulvovaginal candidiasis is a common form of vaginitis in females. A major problem in diagnosis is that of determining true infection from nonpathogenic colonization.

Etiology   Vulvovaginal candidiasis is usually caused by *C. albicans* in about 85% of clinical cases and occasionally by other *Candida* sp., *Torulopsis* sp., or other yeasts.

Epidemiology

1. Prevalence: The overall prevalence of *Candida* vulvovaginitis is unknown. *Candida* is present in the vagina of 25–50% of healthy females, with an increased prevalence in oral contraceptive users. An estimated 75% of women have at least one episode of *Candida* vulvovaginitis.
2. Transmission: While *Candida* vulvovaginitis is usually not sexually acquired or transmitted, evidence exists that sexual contact plays a role in transmitting *Candida* infections in some patients. About 20% of male partners have asymptomatic penile colonization.
3. Predisposing factors: Strong evidence exists that infection and particularly recurrent infections are a result of certain predisposing factors including:
   a. Diabetes mellitus
   b. Pregnancy
   c. Oral contraceptive use
   d. Steroids
   e. Antibiotic therapy: Especially, broad-spectrum antibiotics such as tetracycline
   f. Immunosuppressive therapy
   g. Human immunodeficiency virus (HIV) infection
   h. Some evidence suggests a selective macrophage defect (Witkin et al., 1986) or an acquired *Candida* antigen-specific immunological deficiency (Sobel, 1992a) in women with recurrent candidiasis.
   For adolescents, antibiotics and oral contraceptives are the most frequent predisposing factors.
4. Age: The highest prevalence of infections occurs between the ages of 16 and 30 years.

Clinical Manifestations

1. Usually accompanied by intense burning, pruritus, vulvar pruritus, and erythema
2. Milky-white discharge: May have a cottage cheese appearance
3. Usually no odor
4. Occasional dysuria or dyspareunia
5. May affect the thighs and skin folds, especially in obese females
6. Often accompanied by a history of risk factors such as pregnancy, antibiotic use, or oral contraceptive use
7. The examination reveals:
   a. Normal or erythematous vulva
   b. Vulvar edema
   c. Thick, white, cheesy, adherent discharge

Diagnosis

1. A wet mount with saline or KOH shows budding yeast with pseudohyphae. The use of KOH lyses epithelial cells, allowing better visualization of yeast. A KOH preparation has a sensitivity of 40–80%.
2. The pH range is usually less than 4.5.
3. Yeast cells appear as Gram-positive oval masses, and pseudohyphae appear as long Gram-positive tubes. The sensitivity of the Gram stain is about 70% to almost 100%.
4. Rapid in-office tests for *Candida* antigens in vaginal discharge are commercially available and appear to be more sensitive than the KOH preparation. Their use in the clinical setting has not been well studied.
5. Culture is expensive and time consuming. The culture may be useful in the individual with symptoms consistent with *Candida* vulvovaginitis and negative results from KOH preparation.

6. The diagnosis is suggested by vulvar pruritus and erythema. The diagnosis can be made in the presence of signs and symptoms of vaginitis with positive results from wet mount or KOH smear demonstrating yeasts or pseudohyphae. Colonization can be difficult to differentiate from infection. Women who have the presence of *Candida* but are asymptomatic should not be treated.

Therapy

1. Topical agents: Three-day and 7-day regimens are probably superior to single-dose therapy, particularly for more severe infections. Nystatin is also less effective than the regimens included here. Effective regimens include the following. An asterisk (*) indicates agents that are oil based and may weaken a latex condom or diaphragm. OTC indicates over-the-counter preparations.
   a. Butoconazole 2% cream (Femstat) 5 g intravaginally for 3 days*; or
   b. Clotrimazole 1% cream (Gyne-Lotrimin, Mycelex-G) 5 g intravaginally for 7–14 days[OTC]; or
   c. Clotrimazole 100 mg vaginal tablet (Gyne-Lotrimin, Mycelex-G) for 7 days[OTC]; or
   d. Clotrimazole 100 mg vaginal tablet (Gyne-Lotrimin, Mycelex-G), two tablets for 3 days; or
   e. Clotrimazole 500 mg vaginal tablet (Mycelex), one tablet single application; or
   f. Miconazole 2% cream (Monistat-7) 5 g intravaginally for 7 days*[OTC]; or
   g. Miconazole 200 mg vaginal suppository (Monistat-3), one suppository for 3 days*; or
   h. Miconazole 100 mg vaginal suppository (Monistat), one suppository for 7 days*[OTC]; or
   i. Tioconazole 6.5% ointment (Vagistat) 5 g intravaginally in a single application*; or
   j. Terconazole 0.4% cream (Terazol 7) 5 g intravaginally for 7 days; or
   k. Terconazole 0.8% cream (Terazol 3) 5 g intravaginally for 3 days; or
   l. Terconazole 80 mg suppository (Terazol 3), one suppository for 3 days.*
2. Alternative regimens: Oral azole agents including fluconazole, ketoconazole, and itraconazole have been shown to be as effective in some clinical trials as topical azole agents. Most of the studies have used 1–5 days of therapy. The optimal dose and duration of these drugs is still being studied. One advantage of the oral medications is their ease of use. In most studies women prefer oral therapy over intravaginal therapy. However, because of the potential toxicity, there is still concern about using oral agents as first-line agents. Oral ketoconazole has a risk of mild reversible hepatitis of 5–10% and a risk of serious, potentially life-threatening hepatitis of one in 15,000. Ketoconazole should therefore be reserved for only resistant, recurrent cases of *Candida* vulvovaginitis. Fluconazole in a single 150-mg dose will play an increasingly larger role in treatment, particularly for those women who prefer oral therapy. Sobel et al. (1995) conducted a multicenter, randomized, prospective, single-blinded study of 429 patients with acute *Candida* vaginitis, comparing the efficacy and safety of a single oral 150-mg dose of fluconazole with 7-day clotrimazole 100 mg vaginal treatment. There were no statistically significant differences between fluconazole and clotrimazole in the clinical, mycological, or therapeutic responses. After 14 days clinical cure or improvement was seen in 94% of fluconazole-treated patients and 97% of clotrimazole-treated patients. Mycological and therapeutic cures were seen in 77% and 76% of the fluconazole and 72% of the clotrimazole groups, respectively. At the 35-day evaluation 75% of both groups remained clinically cured, while 56% of the fluconazole and 52% of the clotrimazole group were considered therapeutic cures. Both treatments were less effective in those women with a history of recurrent vaginitis. Mild side effects were reported in 27% of the fluconazole-treated patients and 17% of the clotrimazole-treated patients. The treatment of *Candida*

vaginitis should take into account the severity of disease, the history of recurrent vaginitis, and patient preference.

3. Treatment of sexual partners: Treatment of the adolescent's sex partner is not recommended in most cases. Treatment has not been demonstrated to reduce recurrence rates. If a male partner has a candidal balanitis, he should be treated with topical antifungal agents.

4. Follow-up: Follow-up is not necessary for individuals who become asymptomatic after treatment. If symptoms occur three or more times in a year, an evaluation should be performed for the predisposing conditions listed above.

5. Pregnancy: Topical azole medications can be used during pregnancy, but oral agents should be avoided. Seven-day therapy is preferred during pregnancy.

6. Allergies and side effects to therapy: Topical azole medications do not usually cause systemic side effects. Occasionally, individuals will complain of local irritation or burning. Oral azole agents can cause nausea, abdominal pain, headaches, and an elevation in liver enzymes. Ketoconazole can be associated rarely with severe hepatotoxicity.

7. HIV infection: Adolescents with HIV infection should usually be treated for *Candida* vulvovaginitis in a similar fashion to those without HIV infection. However, *Candida* vulvovaginitis may be more severe in these women, and some experts have employed oral agents more frequently.

8. Recurrent vulvovaginal candidiasis (three or more episodes per year):
   a. Eliminate or reduce risk factors
      — Switch to a lower estrogen oral contraceptive agent
      — Discontinue broad-spectrum antibiotics
      — Discontinue or reduce steroids
      — Review control of diabetes
      — Avoid constricting clothing and vaginal sprays
      — Wear cotton underwear
      — Ingest yogurt with live lactobacillus to recolonize the intestines
   b. Eliminate any sources of reinfection
      — Dry clean or wash all underwear in hot water
      — Dispose of all diaphragms and obtain new ones
      — Discontinue oral-genital contact
      — Oral nystatin 500,000 units, two to three times a day for 10 days. The intestines may serve as a source for reinfection. However, Spinillo et al. (1992) could not demonstrate a lower recurrence rate after treatment of *Candida* colonization in the female intestinal tract in women with recurrent vaginal candidiasis.
      — Examine and treat partner if candidal balanitis is present. Spinillo et al. (1992) found that identification and treatment of male sexual partners' Candida colonization led to lower recurrence rates in women with recurrent candidal vaginitis.
   c. Treatment with longer course of topical agents or use of oral agents. Recommendations have included:
      — Topical azole for 14–21 days intravaginally
      — Fluconazole (Diflucan) 100–150 mg orally one time
      — Ketoconazole (Nizoral) 200 mg orally twice daily for 5–14 days
      — Itraconazole (Sporanox) 200 mg orally once daily for 3 days
      — Boric acid, 600-mg capsule twice daily intravaginally for 14 days (requires special formulation by pharmacist)
   d. Long-term prophylaxis: Several studies have shown decreased recurrences with long-term prophylaxis. Regimens have included:
      — Clotrimazole, one 500-mg vaginal tablet each month
      — Miconazole, 100-mg vaginal tablet two times weekly

— Fluconazole 150 mg orally once each month
— Ketoconazole 200 mg orally twice daily for 5 days each month or 100 mg orally, once daily for up to 6–12 months (less preferred to fluconazole because of higher toxicity of ketoconazole)
— Vaginal suppositories with 600 mg boric acid powder in gelatin capsules, one every day for 14 days, then three per week for up to 12 months or longer: There is little systemic absorption, so these are well tolerated. However, the capsules appear similar to vanilla jelly beans and should be kept out of the way of small children. The oral regimens, especially ketoconazole, can be associated with systemic toxicity and are expensive for long-term therapy. The doses and relative effectiveness and toxicity of these regimens still require further study.

Trichomoniasis

Etiology   *T. vaginalis* infection is caused by a flagellated protozoa with three to five anterior flagella and one posterior flagellum.

Epidemiology

1. Prevalence: *T. vaginalis* is one of the most frequently acquired STDs, with an estimated $2\frac{1}{2}$–3 million cases annually in the United States and as many as 180 million cases worldwide. The organism is found in 28% of adolescent females in juvenile detention centers.
2. Transmission: The organism is almost always sexually transmitted. Since the organism can survive for about $1\frac{1}{2}$ hours on a wet sponge, transmission can possibly occur through sharing of wash cloths, communal bathing, or during routine child care.
3. Age: The peak prevalence rates are between the ages of 16 and 35.
4. Incubation period: 4–28 days
5. Sites of colonization: Trichomonads, when present, usually occur at other sites in addition to the vagina, the most common extravaginal sites being the urethra (82.5% of cases) and the periurethral glands (98% of cases).

Clinical Manifestations

1. Up to 25–50% of females may be asymptomatic. The majority (90%) of men are symptomatic.
2. Symptoms
   a. Pruritus: 60–75% of cases
   b. Discharge: Fifty percent of cases. The discharge is usually diffuse, bubbly, or frothy. The color is cream-colored or greenish. Only about 10% of females complain of an odorous discharge.
   c. Dysuria: Twenty percent of cases
   d. Dyspareunia
   e. Lower abdominal pain: Approximately 5% of cases
3. Signs
   a. Edema and excoriation of the external genitalia
   b. Frothy, foul-smelling vaginal discharge
   c. Erythematous, edematous, and granular vaginal walls
   d. Cervicitis: May have erosions or petechiae of the cervix (colpitis macularis, "strawberry spots")
   e. Bartholinitis

  f. Urethritis

  g. Rarely, abdominal tenderness

 4. Complications: Trichomoniasis does not cause disseminated disease; however, it has been associated with a higher incidence of postpartum endometritis.

Diagnosis

 1. Wet mount: This is the simplest and most frequently used method for demonstrating the presence of trichomonads. The sensitivity is around 60–80%.

  a. Collection: The specimen should be obtained from the pool of discharge in the posterior vaginal fornix.

  b. Processing: Two common, simple methods are used.

   — Direct-slide technique: A drop of saline is placed on a slide and then a drop of the discharge is introduced into the saline and mixed. A cover slip is applied.

   — Test tube technique: Saline in the amount of 0.5–1 mL is placed into a small test tube. A drop of the discharge is collected and mixed into the test tube. Then a drop of suspension is transferred to a slide with a dropper, and a cover slip is applied. It is essential to view the slide as soon as possible because the trichomonads are more motile if warm and fresh. It is also important to examine at least 10 microscopic fields and to search for trichomonads in the center of WBC clumps where they often tend to accumulate.

  c. Appearance: Positive wet mount results reveal a few to a multitude of pear-shaped motile organisms about the size of a polymorphonuclear leukocyte with anterior flagella and an undulating membrane.

 2. ph: The pH is usually higher than 4.5.

 3. Stained smears: Smears are more difficult and time consuming to perform than are wet mounts.

 4. Cultures: Cultures are more time consuming and expensive than are wet mounts. However, these can be used in cases of treatment failure or recurrence of symptoms, if the diagnosis is in question.

 5. Pap smear: Pap smears are unreliable for the diagnosis of *Trichomonas* infection. Up to 42% of reports will be false positives or false negatives.

 6. Urine sediment: Trichomonads are occasionally seen in the urinary sediment. The sensitivity is 60% in infected females. However, this can be a useful technique in the diagnosis of infections in males (80% sensitivity).

 7. Immunological testing: This includes the direct monoclonal antibody test, a rapid test with similar sensitivity as a culture. These tests require further evaluation before their use in the primary care setting can be recommended.

Therapy

 1. Regimen

  a. Recommended: Metronidazole 2 g orally in a single dose can be used.

  b. Alternative: Metronidazole 500 mg twice daily for 7 days can be used.

  c. Both these regimens have a cure rate of about 95%. The single-dose regimen is preferred in adolescents to increase compliance. Systemic therapy with metronidazole is the only therapy well documented to be effective. Treatment of asymptomatic females is advisable.

 2. Side effects of therapy: Nausea and vomiting, a metallic taste, and effects similar to those caused by disulfiram (Antabuse) occur if alcohol is ingested. No alcohol should be used the same day and for 24 hours after the medication is taken.

3. Treatment of sexual partners: Treatment of the adolescent's sex partner is essential. Patients should avoid sex until both patient and partner(s) are cured. Since test of cures are not recommended, "cure" means that both partners have taken the medication and are asymptomatic.

4. Follow-up: Follow-up is not necessary for individuals who become asymptomatic after treatment. If failure occurs with either regimen, the adolescent should be retreated with metronidazole 500 mg twice daily for 7 days. For repeated failures the teen can be treated with a single 2-g dose of metronidazole daily for 3–5 days. A small but increasing number of individuals are infected with trichomonal strains with varying resistance to metronidazole. Grossman et al. (1990) reported some success in women with resistant infection by using metronidazole 500 mg orally three times daily for 14 days, intravaginal metronidazole for 14 days and twice weekly swabbing of the vagina with 3% acetic acid. This regimen has not been studied in any controlled study.

5. Pregnancy: While metronidazole is still contraindicated during the first trimester of pregnancy and lactation, evidence for its safety does exist. Burtin et al. (1995) performed a meta-analysis on the use of metronidazole in the first trimester of pregnancy and were unable to find any evidence of an increased teratogenic risk for its use during the first trimester of pregnancy. At present no other adequate therapy exists. Women may be treated after the first trimester with 2 g of metronidazole in a single dose. Symptomatic relief during the first trimester may be obtained with clotrimazole vaginal cream. Lactating women may be treated with a single 2-g oral dose of metronidazole, but breast-feeding should be discontinued for 24 hours after treatment.

6. Allergies to metronidazole: Effective therapies as alternatives to metronidazole are not currently available.

7. HIV infection: Adolescents with HIV infection should be treated for trichomoniasis in a similar fashion to those without HIV infection.

Complications

1. Usually there is no significant morbidity beyond an uncomfortable vaginitis.
2. There may be an increased risk for adverse pregnancy outcomes including premature rupture of the membranes and preterm delivery. There also may be a higher rate of postpartum infections.
3. There is an increased prevalence of cellular atypia on Pap smear. No association with cervical cancer has been demonstrated.

Bacterial Vaginosis (Gardnerella *Vaginitis*)

Bacterial vaginosis (BV) has also been known as *Gardnerella* vaginitis, "clue cell" vaginitis, *Haemophilus vaginalis* vaginitis, or *Corynebacterium vaginale* vaginitis. The term *bacterial vaginosis* has recently been adopted for this syndrome because many diverse bacteria are found in the vagina of individuals with this syndrome and the clinical signs of inflammation are absent.

Etiology   The syndrome results from the replacement of normal *Lactobacillus* in the vagina with anaerobic bacteria (*Bacteroides* sp., *Mobiluncus* sp.), *G. vaginalis,* and *Mycoplasma hominis.* In most females without bacterial vaginosis the dominant organism is *Lactobacillus* species (>95% of all vaginal organisms), while in infected females *Lactobacillus* is often not found or found in much lower bacterial counts (100- to 1000-fold decrease) (Sobel, 1989). In addition, the hydrogen peroxide (H_2O_2)–producing strains of lactobacilli are found in only 11% of women with BV. It is not known whether the initial problem is a fall in *Lactobacillus* species or a rise in these other bacteria.

The normal lactobacilli help maintain an acid pH by converting glucose into lactic acid. The normally lower pH helps to prevent the growth of *G. vaginalis* and anaerobes such as *Mobiluncus* sp. With an elevated pH there is a loss of lactobacilli and an overgrowth in high concentrations of *G. vaginalis;* anaerobes such as *Bacteroides, Peptostreptococcus,* and *Mobiluncus* sp.; and genital mycoplasmas.

G. vaginalis is present in about 40% of sexually active unmarried females without signs or symptoms of vaginitis. So while this organism is a common commensal in many females, it appears that in combination with other vaginal bacteria, particularly anaerobes, it can be a pathogenic organism. Even in women who meet the clinical criteria for bacterial vaginosis, as many as 50% have no symptoms. In only a minority of asymptomatic females with clue cells or positive cultures for *G. vaginalis* do these laboratory findings persist without treatment.

Epidemiology

1. Transmission: The transmission of bacterial vaginosis is unresolved. Sexual transmission is suggested by the age of the patients involved, the previous sexual experience of the patients involved, and the fact that 70–90% of male partners can have the organism isolated from their urethra. BV only rarely affects individuals who have not been sexually active, but it is not an exclusively sexually transmitted disease. *G. vaginalis, Mobiluncus* spp., and *M. hominis* have been isolated from the rectum of women with BV and indicate a potential source of autoinfection (Catlin, 1992).
2. Prevalence: Bacterial vaginosis is one of the most common infections in females. Since the condition is not required to be reported to local health departments, the exact prevalence is unknown. However, bacterial vaginosis has been reported in 15% of women at a university student gynecology clinic, 12–25% in family practice settings, 10–26% of pregnant women, and 32–64% of women being seen at an STD clinic (McGregor, 1993; Sobel, 1989).

Clinical Manifestations

1. Vaginal discharge
   a. Onset: Unrelated to menses
   b. Amount: Slight in 85% of cases and moderate in about 15% of cases
   c. Color: Grayish white
   d. Odor: Often a fishy smell, especially in the presence of either semen or KOH. The combination of *G. vaginalis* and anaerobes produces organic acids and several amines that in the presence of an elevated vaginal pH volatilize to the malodorous compounds of putrescine and cadaverine. Trimethylamine may also be a cause of the fishy odor associated with BV.
2. Pruritus or burning is either absent or mild.
3. Up to 50% of patients with bacterial vaginosis are asymptomatic.
4. Physical examination
   a. Thin, frothy, grayish-white discharge, adhering to the vaginal walls
   b. Usually no vulvar or vaginal-wall changes
   c. Possibly a pungent "fishy" odor

Diagnosis

1. Wet mount: On wet mount one looks for:
   a. Few polymorphonuclear leukocytes
   b. "Clue cells": Granular, stippled appearing epithelial cells. The cells also have indistinct cell borders due to the adherence of *G. vaginalis.* In women with BV, clue cells should comprise at least 20% of the cells examined.

c. Replacement of the normal *Lactobacillus* (large rods), with small, pleomorphic, coccobacilli as the predominant flora
2. The pH is higher than 4.5.
3. "Whiff test": The addition of KOH to a drop of the vaginal discharge releases a fishy, amine odor in 90% of women with BV. This may also occur in *Trichomonas* infections.
4. Gram stain: The relative concentration of the bacterial morphotypes (nonlactobacilli morphotypes exceed lactobacilli morphotypes) can be used to diagnose BV.
5. Culture: This is not recommended as a diagnostic test because of its questionable specificity.
6. Under current investigation are newer commercial probe tests that detect vaginal pathogens including *G. vaginalis.*
7. Diagnostic criteria: Should have three out of four of the following criteria:
    a. Homogeneous, white noninflammatory vaginal discharge
    b. pH of vaginal fluid higher than 4.5
    c. Positive amine or "whiff test"
    d. Presence of clue cells on wet mount microscopic examination

Complications   There is growing concern that BV has an important role in the development of clinical chorioamnionitis, postpartum endometritis, posthysterectomy vaginal cuff cellulitis, postabortion pelvic inflammatory disease (PID), and upper genital tract infections such as amniotic fluid infection and chorioamnionic infection associated with premature delivery (Eschenbach, 1993a,b; Gibbs, 1993).

Therapy

1. In most instances only women with vaginal signs or symptoms should be treated. Prevention of transmission to males is not a goal of therapy as males are asymptomatic and the treatment of partners has not altered the course in women in regard to relapse or reinfection rates. Because of the possible risk of invasion of these organisms into the genital tract with invasive procedures including uterine curettage and intrauterine device (IUD) placement, it may be reasonable to treat symptomatic or asymptomatic BV before a surgical abortion procedure. Treatment of BV with metronidazole has been shown to reduce postabortion PID rates.
2. Regimen:
    a. Recommended: Metronidazole 500 mg orally 2 times a day for 7 days
    b. Alternative: Metronidazole 2 g orally in a single dose
    c. Other alternatives that have been shown to be effective but have less clinical experience include:
        — Clindamycin cream, 2%, one full applicator (5 g) intravaginally at bedtime for 7 days
        — Metronidazole gel, 0.75%, one full applicator (5 g) intravaginally, two times a day for 5 days
        — Clindamycin 300 mg orally two times a day for 7 days
        Several other antibiotics may turn out to be effective including ciprofloxacin, amoxicillin plus clavulanic acid, and cephalexin.
        The single-dose metronidazole regimen has the advantage in adolescents of having a higher compliance rate. Minkowski et al. (1983) demonstrated a 95% cure rate in 882 symptomatic adolescents using a single 2-g oral dose of metronidazole. In their reviews of treatments of BV, Sweet (1993) and Lugo-Miro et al. (1992) found that single-dose metronidazole was as effective as 5- to 7-day courses of oral metronidazole. Sweet (1993)

also found that intravaginal clindamycin cream 2% and intravaginal metronidazole gel 0.75% were associated with clinical cure rates similar to those obtained with oral metronidazole. The Centers for Disease Control (CDC) in their 1993 STD guidelines list a 95% cure rate for the 7-day regimen and 84% for the 2-g single-dose regimen. Individuals should be warned not to use alcohol during treatment and for 24 hours after completion to avoid nausea and vomiting secondary to a disulfiram-like reaction.

The serum levels associated with intravaginal metronidazole are 2% those of 500-mg oral doses, and intravaginal clindamycin has about 4% of the serum level of oral clindamycin. The mineral oil base in the clindamycin cream may weaken latex; therefore teens should avoid the use of condoms and contraceptive diaphragms for 72 hours after using the cream. Standard therapy with oral metronidazole is about one-sixth the cost of either metronidazole gel or oral or topical clindamycin.

3. Treatment of sex partners: Treatment of contacts is not routinely recommended because it does not alter the response rate or the rate of relapse or recurrences.

4. Follow-up: Follow-up is not necessary if the teen becomes asymptomatic. Adolescents with recurrent or persistent infections should be reevaluated for other infections. Several approaches can be tried in individuals with recurrent infections, including:
   a. Treatment of partner(s) in individuals with recurrent infections who have a stable partner
   b. Having the partner(s) use condoms for several months after therapy is complete
   c. Trial of alternative therapy such as oral clindamycin

5. Pregnancy
   a. First trimester: Clindamycin cream is the preferred treatment.
   b. Second and third trimester: Oral metronidazole can be used, but vaginal metronidazole cream or clindamycin cream may be preferred to limit the fetal exposure to medications. Neri et al. (1993) found favorable results in 32 pregnant women using commercial yogurt intravaginally.
   c. In one large collaborative study of women with BV during pregnancy, the prematurity rate was approximately 11% without treatment and 5% with metronidazole therapy. However, the treatment of BV among pregnant women require further confirmatory studies before routine screening and treatment during pregnancy is recommended.

6. HIV infection: HIV-infected teens can be treated for BV with the same regimens as those individuals without HIV.

Other Causes of Vaginal Discharge

1. Pubertal physiological discharge: A normal increase in vaginal secretions occurs 6–12 months before menarche.

2. Extravaginal disease: Extravaginal lesions may cause staining of the underwear, suggesting a vaginal discharge to the adolescent. These lesions include:
   a. Perineal lesions: Herpes, syphilis, intertrigo
   b. Bartholin's gland abscess
   c. Proctitis

3. Physiological discharge: Vaginal and cervical secretions change depending on the hormonal state. High-estrogen levels induce a more profuse discharge. At the time of ovulation or just before menses vaginal secretions are more likely to increase. Progesterone induces a thicker discharge. Physiological discharge is characterized by:
   a. Lack of offensive odor
   b. Lack of pruritus or burning

TABLE 55.1.   Vaginal Discharge in the Adolescent

Condition	Signs and Symptoms	Diagnosis	Treatment
Physiological discharge	Clear gray discharge No offensive odor No burning or itching	Wet mount: Epithelial cells with no or few polymorphonuclear cells; no pathogens	Reassurance and explanation
Moniliasis (candidiasis)	Curdlike discharge Intense burning and pruritus Usually no odor Often associated vulvitis	KOH: Budding yeast and pseudohyphae	Miconazole or clotrimazole suppositories, 200 mg at bedtime for 3 days or 100 mg suppositories or cream daily for 7 days
Trichomoniasis	Pruritus Malodorous, frothy, cream-colored discharge Dysuria Rarely, abdominal pain Granular vaginitis and cervicitis	Wet mount: Pear-shaped organism with motile flagella	Metronidazole (Flagyl): 2 g (eight 250-mg tablets) at one time Avoid if pregnant Treat partner
Gardnerella vaginitis	Mild, gray-white discharge Discharge may have an odor Usually mild or no pruritus or burning	Wet mount: Epithelial cells covered with Gram-negative rods Few polymorphonuclear leukocytes pH >4.5	Metronidazole: 500 mg twice daily for 7 days, or single oral 2-g dose Treat partner if recurrent infection Treat partner with metronidazole or ampicillin
Gonorrhea	Majority asymptomatic Gray-white cervical discharge	Culture Gram stain can be used, but a negative smear must be confirmed by culture	Ceftriaxone 250 mg IM once plus doxycycline 100 mg orally two times a day for 7 days
Chlamydia infection	Asymptomatic Yellowish vaginal discharge Cervicitis	Culture Exclusion of other organisms in a female with cervicitis	Doxycycline 100 mg orally two times a day for 7 days OR Tetracycline 500 mg four times daily for 7 days
Retained tampon	Malodorous discharge	History and physical examination	Removal of tampon
Allergic vaginitis	Local pain Vaginal erythema	History of exposure to deodorant spray or scented tampons	Cessation of sensitizing spray

    c. Lack of vulvar, vaginal, or cervical erythema

    d. May leave a brown stain on the underwear

    e. Lack of polymorphonuclear leukocytes on wet mount

  4. *Enterobius vermicularis* (pinworms)

  5. Irritant vaginitis: Irritations can occur with chemical douches, vaginal deodorants, vaginal sprays, tampons or pads, colored or perfumed toilet paper, bubble bath, laundry detergents, fabric softeners, swimming pools or hot tubs, powders, soaps, spermicides, or medications used by the male that remain on the penis.

  6. Foreign bodies: Foreign bodies causing a vaginal discharge include forgotten tampons, intrauterine devices (uterine discharge), and objects for masturbation.

  7. Vulvodynia or vulvar vestibulitis: Clinical manifestations include pain with penetration during intercourse and small inflamed areas at 5 and 7 o'clock on the perineum that are exquisitely tender to touch. The vaginal examination results, including pH, flora, and wet mount, are normal. A course of topical steroids may be of benefit.

  8. Gonorrhea: See Chapter 61. Gonorrhea generally infects the endocervix and not the vaginal walls. The majority of females are asymptomatic, while approximately 25% experience a foul-smelling discharge.

9. *C. trachomatis* cervical infections are common; because of the cervical discharge patients may complain of vaginal discharge (see Chapter 62).

Table 55.1 outlines treatment of vaginitis in adolescents.

CERVICITIS

Cervicitis is common in sexually active women. The condition is usually caused by STDs and is a significant problem because it often produces very few, if any, symptoms. Infections of the cervix are a source for transmission of STDs to males and newborns. Cervical infections also precede PID.

Cervicitis represents an infection of the cervix and should not be confused with cervical ectopy. During adolescence and young adulthood, the junction of columnar and squamous epithelium is on the ectocervix. This condition has unfortunately often been mislabeled as cervicitis. With increasing age and after a pregnancy, the squamocolumnar junction recedes into the endocervical canal.

Cervicitis may produce a significant enough discharge to be confused with a vaginal infection.

Etiology

Common causative microorganisms include:

1. *C. trachomatis*
2. *N. gonorrhoeae*
3. *T. vaginalis*
4. *C. albicans*
5. Herpes simplex

Symptoms

1. Vaginal discharge
2. Dyspareunia
3. Postcoital spotting

Signs

Cervicitis is presumed if all the following are found on pelvic examination:

1. Mucopurulent endocervical discharge visible on a white swab
2. Ten or more white blood cells per high-power field on Gram-stained specimen from the endocervix that is not contaminated with vaginal secretions
3. Endocervical friability: Easy bleeding from endocervical tissue after contact with first swab

Diagnostic Tests

1. Wet mount: Examine for evidence of trichomonads
2. Gram stain of endocervical specimen
3. Gonorrhea culture or other screening test
4. Chlamydia culture or screening test
5. KOH

Treatment should cover both gonorrhea and *Chlamydia,* unless the cervicitis is known to be caused by *Trichomonas* or herpes.

For a further discussion of gonococcal and chlamydial cervicitis, see Chapters 61 and 62.

BIBLIOGRAPHY

Amsel R, Totten PA, Spiegel CA, et al. Non-specific vaginitis: diagnostic criteria and microbial and epidemiologic associations. Am J Med 1983;74:14.

Andrews H, Acheson N, Huengsberg M. The role of microscopy in the diagnosis of sexually transmitted infections in women. Genitourin Med 1994;70:118.

Baldson HJ, Pead L, Taylor GE, et al. *Corynebacterium vaginale* and vaginitis: a controlled trial of treatment. Obstet Gynecol 1981;57:711.

Bertholf ME, Stafford MJ. An office laboratory panel to assess vaginal problems. Am Fam Physician 1985; 32:113.

Biswas MK. Bacterial vaginosis. Clin Obstet Gynecol 1993;36:166.

Blackwell AL, Fox AR, Phillips I, et al. Anaerobic vaginosis (non-specific vaginitis): clinical, microbiological, and therapeutic findings. Lancet 1983;2:1379.

Boeke AJ, Dekker JH, Peerbooms PG. A comparison of yield from cervix versus vagina for culturing *Candida albicans* and *Trichomonas vaginalis.* Genitourin Med 1993;69:41.

Briselden AM, Hillier SL. Evaluation of affirm VP microbial identification test for *Gardnerella vaginalis* and *Trichomonas vaginalis.* J Clin Microbiol 1994;32: 148.

Bump RC, Zuspan FP, Buesching WJ III, et al. The prevalence, six month persistence, and predictive values of laboratory indicators of bacterial vaginosis (non-specific vaginitis) in asymptomatic women. Am J Obstet Gynecol 1984;150:917.

Burns FM, Gould IM, Patterson A, et al. Diagnosis of bacterial vaginosis in a routine diagnostic laboratory. Med Lab Sci 1992;49:8.

Burtin P, Taddio A, Ariburnu O, et al. Safety of metronidazole in pregnancy: a meta-analysis. Am J Obstet Gynecol 1995;172:525.

Catlin BW. *Gardnerella vaginalis:* characteristics, clinical considerations, and controversies. Clin Microbiol Rev 1992;5:213.

Centers for Disease Control. 1993 Sexually transmitted diseases treatment guidelines. MMWR 1993;42 (RR–14).

Chapin-Robertson K. Use of molecular diagnostics in sexually transmitted diseases. Critical assessment. Diagn Microbiol Infect Dis 1993;16:173.

Combined therapy helps cure resistant trichomoniasis. Contraceptive technology update 1992;(February):27.

Communicable disease report: drug-resistant *Trichomonas vaginalis.* Commun Dis Rep CDR Wkly 1993;3:141.

Cook RL, Redondo-Lopez V, Schmitt C, et al. Clinical, microbiological, and biochemical factors in recurrent bacterial vaginosis. J Clin Microbiol 1992;30:870.

Demetriou E, Emans SJ, Masland RP. Dysuria in adolescent girls: urinary tract infection or vaginitis. Pediatrics 1982;70:299.

Deutchman ME, Leaman D, Thomason JL. Vaginitis: diagnosis is the key. Patient Care 1994;(September 15):39.

Easmon CS, Hay PE, Ison CA. Bacterial vaginosis: a diagnostic approach. Genitourin Med 1992;68:134.

Eschenbach DA. Bacterial vaginosis and anaerobes in obstetric-gynecologic infections. Clin Infect Dis 1993a;16:S282.

Eschenbach DA. History and review of bacterial vaginosis. Am J Obstet Gynecol 1993b;169:441.

Eschenbach DA, Mead PB. Managing problem vaginitis. Patient Care 1992;(September 15):137.

Fischbach F, Petersen EE, Weissenbacher ER, et al. Efficacy of clindamycin vaginal cream versus oral metronidazole in the treatment of bacterial vaginosis. Obstet Gynecol 1993;82:405.

Foster DC. Vulvitis and vaginitis. Curr Opin Obstet Gynecol 1993;5:726.

Friedrich EG Jr. Vaginitis. Am J Obstet Gynecol 1985; 152:247.

Gardner HL. *Haemophilus vaginalis* after twenty-five years. Am J Obstet Gynecol 1980;137:385.

Gibbs RS. Chorioamnionitis and bacterial vaginosis. Am J Obstet Gynecol 1993;169:460.

Graves A, Gardner WA Jr. Pathogenicity of *Trichomonas vaginalis.* Clin Obstet Gynecol 1993;36:145.

Gravett MG, Nelson HP, DeRouen T, et al. Independent associations of bacterial vaginosis and *Chlamydia trachomatis* infection with adverse pregnancy outcome. JAMA 1986;256:1899.

Grossman JH III, Galask RP. Persistent vaginitis caused by metronidazole-resistant trichomonas. Obstet Gynecol 1990;76:521.

Hager WD, Rapp RP. Metronidazole. Obstet Gynecol Clin North Am. 1992;19:497.

Hallen A, Jarstrand C, Pahlson C. Treatment of bacterial vaginosis with lactobacilli. Sex Transm Dis. 1992; 19:146.

Hay PE, Taylor-Robinson D, Lamont RF. Diagnosis of bacterial vaginosis in a gynaecology clinic. Br J Obstet Gynaecol 1992;99:63.

Heine P, McGregor JA. *Trichomonas vaginalis:* a reemerging pathogen. Clin Obstet Gynecol 1993;36:137.

Hillier SL. Diagnostic microbiology of bacterial vaginosis. Am J Obstet Gynecol 1993;169:455.

Hillier S, Holmes KK. Bacterial vaginosis. In: Holmes KK, Mardh PA, Sparling PF, Wiesner PJ, eds. Sexually transmitted diseases. 2nd ed. New York: McGraw-Hill Information Services, 1990.

Hillier SL, Lipinski C, Briselden AM, et al. Efficacy of intravaginal 0.75% metronidazole gel for the treatment of bacterial vaginosis. Obstet Gynecol 1993; 81:963.

Hilton E, Isenberg HD, Alperstein P, et al. Ingestion of yogurt containing *Lactobacillus acidophilus* as prophylaxis for candidal vaginitis. Ann Intern Med 1992; 116:353.

Holmes KK. Lower genital tract infections in women: cystitis, urethritis, vulvovaginitis, and cervicitis. In: Holmes KK, Mardh PA, Sparling PF, Wiesner PJ, eds. Sexually transmitted diseases. 2nd ed. New York: McGraw-Hill Information Services, 1990.

Larsen B. Vaginal flora in health and disease. Clin Obstet Gynecol 1993;36:107.

Livengood CH III, McGregor JA, Soper DE, et al. Bacterial vaginosis: efficacy and safety of intravaginal metronidazole treatment. Am J Obstet Gynecol 1994;170:759.

Lugo-Miro VI, Green M, Mazur L. Comparison of different metronidazole therapeutic regimens for bacterial vaginosis. A meta-analysis. JAMA 1992;268:92.

MacDermott RI. Bacterial vaginosis. Br J Obstet Gynaecol 1995;102:92.

Mardh PA. The vaginal ecosystem. Am J Obstet Gynecol 1991;165:1163.

McCue JD. Evaluation and management of vaginitis: an update for primary care practitioners. Arch Intern Med 1989;149:565.

McGregor JA. Bacterial vaginosis: screening and treatment. Female Patient 1993;18:81.

Mead PB. Epidemiology of bacterial vaginosis. Am J Obstet Gynecol 1993;169:446.

Minkowski WL, Baker CJ, Alleyne D, et al. Single oral dose metronidazole therapy for *Gardnerella vaginalis* vaginitis in adolescent females. J Adolesc Health Care 1983;4:113.

Neri A, Sabah G, Samra Z. Bacterial vaginosis in pregnancy treated with yoghurt. Acta Obstet Gynecol Scand 1993;72:17.

Reed BD, Eyler A. Vaginal infections: diagnosis and management. Am Fam Physician 1993;47:1805.

Rein MF. How to treat the three most common vaginal infections. Mod Med 1986;54:126.

Rein MF, Muller M. *Trichomonas vaginalis* and trichomoniasis. In: Holmes KK, Mardh PA, Sparling PF, Wiesner PJ, eds. Sexually transmitted diseases. 2nd ed. New York: McGraw-Hill Information Services, 1990.

Sanfilippo JS. Adolescent girls with vaginal discharge. Pediatr Ann 1986;15:509.

Schaaf VM, Perez-Stable EJ, Borchardt K. The limited value of symptoms and signs in the diagnosis of vaginal infections. Arch Intern Med 1990;150:1929.

Schydlower M, Shafer MA. *Chlamydia trachomatis* infections in adolescents. Adolesc Med 1990;1:615.

Slavin MB, Benrubi GI, Parker R, et al. Single dose oral fluconazole vs intravaginal terconazole in treatment of candida vaginitis. Comparison and pilot study. J Fla Med Assoc 1992;79:693.

Sobel JD. Recurrent *Candida* vaginitis. Drug Ther Bull 1982;12:41.

Sobel JD. Vulvovaginal candidiasis: what we do and do not know. Ann Intern Med 1984;101:390.

Sobel JD. Recurrent vulvovaginal candidiasis: a prospective study of the efficacy of maintenance ketoconazole therapy. N Engl J Med 1986;315:1455.

Sobel JD. Bacterial vaginosis: An ecologic mystery. Ann Intern Med 1989;111:551.

Sobel JD. Vulvovaginal candidiasis. In: Holmes KK, Mardh PA, Sparling PF, Wiesner, eds. Sexually transmitted diseases, 2nd ed. New York: McGraw-Hill Information Services, 1990.

Sobel JD. Pathogenesis and treatment of recurrent vulvovaginal candidiasis. Clin Infect Dis 1992a;14:S148.

Sobel JD. Vulvovaginitis. Dermatol Clin 1992b;10:339.

Sobel JD, Brooker D, Stein GE, et al. Single oral dose fluconazole compared with conventional clotrimazole topical therapy of *Candida* vaginitis. Fluconazole Vaginitis Study Group. Am J Obstet Gynecol 1995;172:1263.

Spinillo A, Carratta L, Pizzoli G, et al. Recurrent vaginal candidiasis. Results of a cohort study of sexual transmission and intestinal reservoir. J Reprod Med 1992; 37:343.

Stein GE, Christensen SL, Mummaw NL, et al. Placebo-controlled trial of intravaginal clindamycin 2% cream for the treatment of bacterial vaginosis. Ann Pharmacother 1993;27:1343.

Swedberg J, Steiner JF, Deiss F, et al. Comparison of single-dose vs. one-week course of metronidazole for symptomatic bacterial vaginosis. JAMA 1985;254: 1046.

Sweet RL. New approaches for the treatment of bacterial vaginosis. Am J Obstet Gynecol 1993;169:479.

Thomason JL, Anderson RJ, Gelbart SM, et al. Simplified gram stain interpretive method for diagnosis of bacterial vaginosis. Am J Obstet Gynecol 1992; 167:16.

Tidwell BH, Lushbaugh WB, Laughlin MD, et al. A double-blind placebo-controlled trial of single-dose intravaginal versus single-dose oral metronidazole in the treatment of trichomonal vaginitis. J Infect Dis 1994;170:242.

Vandeven AM, Emans SJ. Vulvovaginitis in the child and adolescent. Pediatr Rev 1993;14:141.

Witkin SS, Hirsch J, Ledger WJ. A macrophage defect in women with recurrent Candida vaginitis and its reversal in vitro by prostaglandin inhibitors. Am J Obstet Gynecol 1986;155:790.

Wolner-Hanssen PA, Krieger JN, Stevens CE, et al. Clinical manifestations of vaginal trichomoniasis. JAMA 1989;261:571.

CHAPTER 56

Ectopic Pregnancy

Lawrence S. Neinstein and Karen S. Himebaugh

Ectopic pregnancies must be considered in the differential diagnosis of the adolescent with pelvic pain, especially if such pain is associated with abnormal uterine bleeding or amenorrhea. The number of ectopic pregnancies has increased from 17,800 (4.8 per 1000 live births) in 1970 to 108,800 (19.7 per 1000) in 1992. In 1992 ectopic pregnancies accounted for 2% of reported pregnancies and 9% of all pregnancy-related deaths. Ectopic pregnancies are now the second leading cause of maternal mortality in the United States and the leading cause of death during the first trimester. Washington and Katz (1993) estimated the total cost of ectopic pregnancies in the United States in 1990 at $1.1 billion, with hospitalization and other medical treatments contributing to 77% of the total costs. About 50% of ectopic pregnancies in 1992 did not require hospitalization, as management has progressively emphasized less invasive procedures (laparotomy and medical therapy).

EPIDEMIOLOGY: RISK FACTORS

1. Tubal abnormalities: The most common cause of tubal abnormalities is secondary to acute salpingitis. Other tubal problems include previous tubal surgery from a prior ectopic pregnancy or prior pelvic surgery with tubal adhesions.
2. Altered tubal motility: The progestin-only contraceptive pill ("minipill") may decrease tubal motility and alter tubal microanatomy.
3. Intrauterine device (IUD): Use of an IUD may increase the risk of tubal infection. The progesterone-containing IUD can alter tubal motility. The risk of ectopic pregnancy is six times higher among women using progesterone IUDs versus copper systems.
4. Age: The rate is highest among the 35- to 44-year-old age group. The rate is lowest among the 15- to 24-year-old age group, but this group has the highest reported death rate.

CLINICAL MANIFESTATIONS

History

The classic presentation of an ectopic pregnancy includes the sudden onset of unilateral pain 6–8 weeks after the last menstrual period with a 1-week history of abnormal uterine bleeding. However, most patients with ectopic pregnancies do not follow a classic course. Common signs and symptoms are:

Symptoms

1. Abdominal pain, 95–100% of cases
   a. Generalized, 44%

    b. Unilateral, 33%

    c. Radiating, 23%

2. Amenorrhea, 75–95%
3. Vaginal bleeding or spotting, 50–80%
4. Other symptoms: Syncope and shoulder or back pain

Signs

1. Vital signs: Variable, fever, 5–10%
2. Adnexal tenderness, 80–95% of cases, unilateral more common than bilateral
3. Adnexal mass, 40–60%
4. Uterine enlargement, 25–70%
5. Clinical shock, 10–17%

Laboratory Tests

1. White blood cell count: Of little diagnostic value; usually normal or slightly elevated
2. Sedimentation rate: Usually no change
3. Hematocrit: Usually over 30%, occasionally under 30% or with rupture under 20%
4. Pregnancy tests: The pregnancy test is essential in an adolescent with a suspected ectopic pregnancy. Currently available serum human chorionic gonadotropin (hCG) radioimmunoassays offer higher than a 99% sensitivity in detecting the presence of a pregnancy compared to the 50% sensitivity in detecting ectopic pregnancies offered by the urinary pregnancy tests from 20 years ago.

    Produced by the placenta, hCG is first measurable in the serum 8–12 days after conception. On the basis of production rates hCG has a normal doubling time of 1.9–2.0 days within the first 30 days of a normal gestation. Abnormal pregnancies are associated with an abnormal production of hCG, and so the doubling time may be longer. In general, a doubling time of less than 66% in 48 hours is predictive of an ectopic pregnancy or an intrauterine pregnancy that is destined to abort. Ninety percent of ectopic pregnancies have a β-hCG level of less than 6500 mIU.

    In the office or emergency care setting, urine pregnancy tests can be performed with immediate results. If the patient is to be followed, a serum test should be drawn simultaneously to verify and quantify β-hCG. The urine specific gravity should be higher than 1.015 for increased accuracy.

    Stewart et al. (1995) examined the rate of change of hCG levels and progesterone concentration to distinguish ectopic from normal intrauterine pregnancies. They found that by following these two markers, one could distinguish between abnormal pregnancies, including ectopic pregnancies and inevitable abortions, and normal intrauterine pregnancies. However, the rate of changes overlapped between the ectopic pregnancies and the inevitable abortions.
5. Serum progesterone: Low serum progesterone levels have been associated with ectopic pregnancies and impending abortions. During the first 8–10 weeks of gestation, serum progesterone concentrations change little. Levels of 25 ng/mL or more are 97.5% sensitive in excluding ectopic pregnancy. Conversely, levels of 5 ng/mL or less are 100% sensitive in identifying nonviable pregnancies. Levels between these values can represent a normal or abnormal pregnancy and require a transvaginal ultrasound for further diagnosis.
6. Ultrasound: An ultrasound can be helpful in diagnosing ectopic pregnancy by confirming either an intrauterine pregnancy or the presence of a tubal mass. A normal intrauterine pregnancy can be detected at 21 days postconception or by 5 menstrual

weeks. By 7 menstrual weeks the embryo can be seen and cardiac activity noted in an intrauterine pregnancy. During the period of 5–6.5 weeks an ectopic pregnancy may be confused with an intrauterine pregnancy due to a pseudogestational sac. This occurs in 10–20% of ectopic pregnancies. Another ultrasound finding that suggests an ectopic pregnancy is the presence of a mass or fluid in the cul-de-sac. An intrauterine pregnancy can usually be visualized with a quantitative hCG level of 6500 mIU on transabdominal ultrasound scanning. The use of a vaginal probe for ultrasound aids in earlier diagnosis and can detect an intrauterine pregnancy at levels of 1200–1500 IU/L of hCG. The discriminatory zone of minimal hCG in detecting normal versus abnormal pregnancies is influenced by the type, resolution, and quality of the ultrasound, as well as the particular hCG assay used.

7. Culdocentesis: Culdocentesis is a helpful test if the result is positive for nonclotting blood with a hematocrit higher than 15%. A negative test result does not eliminate the presence of a nonruptured ectopic pregnancy. Compared to the combination of a serum pregnancy test and ultrasound, culdocentesis is less sensitive, less specific, and more invasive. This test is rarely used now, since currently available pregnancy tests and ultrasounds are more sensitive.

8. Dilation and curettage: A D & C may distinguish between an ectopic pregnancy or an incomplete or threatened abortion due to the presence of products of conception with the latter.

9. Laparoscopy: In difficult diagnostic cases laparoscopy can not only eliminate the diagnosis of ectopic pregnancy but can establish the correct diagnosis. If an ectopic pregnancy is diagnosed, it can often be treated through laparoscopic surgery, thus avoiding a laparotomy.

DIAGNOSIS

The diagnosis of ectopic pregnancy can be difficult, as evidenced by the number of prior visits women with ectopic pregnancy have made to emergency rooms before a diagnosis is made. A thorough history eliciting risk factors, a sexual history, symptoms of pregnancy, menstrual history, and history of pain is essential in diagnosing an ectopic pregnancy. The physical examination is important in looking for signs of shock, unilateral pelvic tenderness, or mass. Fever is usually absent. The pregnancy test can be helpful, especially if results are positive. The combination of a sensitive serum pregnancy test and ultrasound can correctly predict an ectopic pregnancy in 93% or more of patients. A quantitative serum β-hCG test can also be of value in the diagnosis. A β-hCG level of 6500 mIU/mL or approximately 6 weeks past the last menstrual period has been correlated to the time at which a gestational sac should be present on an abdominal pelvic ultrasound. A level of 6500 mIU/mL and the absence of gestational sac is 100% sensitive and 96% specific for an ectopic pregnancy. In fact, 96% of intrauterine pregnancies have a gestational sac at a β-hCG level of 6500 mIU/mL. The presence or absence of a gestational sac on ultrasound at β-hCG levels less than 6500 mIU/mL is nonspecific and can indicate either a normal pregnancy, an ectopic pregnancy, or a spontaneous abortion. If the teen is less than 6 weeks' pregnant or the β-hCG level is less than 6500 mIU/mL, a second quantitative β-hCG test is valuable. As indicated previously, between 1 and 2 months after the last menstrual period, a β-hCG level doubles every 2 days. An increase of less than 66% after 48 hours suggests an abnormal pregnancy (ectopic pregnancy or spontaneous abortion). If the teen is acutely ill, however, a laparoscopy is indicated. The β-hCG cutoff level of 6500 mIU/mL should be changed to 1500 mIU/mL if a pelvic ultrasound is performed with a vaginal transducer.

TABLE 56.1. Differential Diagnosis of Ectopic Pregnancy

	Ectopic	Abortion	Corpus Luteum Cyst	Salpingitis	Appendicitis
Pain	Crampy, dull lower abdominal pain may be unilateral or bilateral, may radiate to shoulder	Crampy, dull, suprapubic	Unilateral unless rupture	Usually bilateral	Epigastric, moving to right upper quadrant
History	Prior tubal surgery, IUD, PID, or ectopic pregnancy	Prior fetal abnormalities, maternal systemic problems		IUD, age 12–25, history of prior PID, or gonorrhea, or *Chlamydia* culture	
Associated symptoms	Pregnancy symptoms	Symptoms of pregnancy that disappear		Fever, dysuria	Anorexia, nausea, vomiting, constipation
Menses	Missed period followed by abnormal period	Amenorrhea followed by abnormal bleeding	Amenorrhea followed by irregular bleeding	Hypermenorrhea	Unaffected
Temperature	Normal	Normal	Normal	May be elevated	May be elevated
Examination	Fullness in cul-de-sac; cervical and adnexal tenderness; may have adnexal mass	Uterus soft and enlarged; cervix may be open with protruding tissue	Enlarged ovary	Bilateral adnexal tenderness, cervical motion tenderness, vaginal discharge	Rebound abdominal tenderness, rectal tenderness on right side
Laboratory	Positive β-hCG; ultrasound usually shows no gestational sac; hemoglobin low if ruptured ectopic	Falling level of β-hCG	Negative β-hCG; normal white count; hemoglobin low if ruptured cyst	Negative β-hCG; may have elevated white count and sedimentation rate; positive gonorrhea or Chlamydia culture	Negative β-hCG, elevated white count

DIFFERENTIAL DIAGNOSIS

The differential diagnosis includes (see also Table 56.1):

1. Pelvic inflammatory disease (PID)
2. Threatened or spontaneous abortion
3. Appendicitis
4. Corpus luteum cyst
5. Torsion of the adnexa
6. Ruptured ovarian cyst
7. Acute gastroenteritis

THERAPY

Ectopic pregnancy is a gynecologic emergency and requires referral to a gynecologist. In the past ectopic pregnancy was considered a surgical emergency requiring laparotomy. This is still true for the ruptured ectopic pregnancy. Alternative treatments now include laproscopic surgery and parenteral methotrexate. Single-dose parenteral methotrexate is safe and effective, particularly in those with an unruptured ectopic pregnancy with evidence of an adnexal mass less than 3.5 cm in size and absence of any fetal cardiac activity on ultrasound. Slaughter and Grimes (1995) reviewed 17 studies reporting on 400 patients treated with methotrexate for ectopic pregnancies. The overall success rate was 92%. A prospective, randomized clinical trial comparing medical and surgical management of ectopic pregnancy is needed to assess the risks, benefits, and costs of these two approaches.

Gray et al. (1995) evaluated the cost-effectiveness of therapeutic laparoscopy and open laparotomy for treatment of laparoscopically diagnosed ectopic pregnancy. By specified criteria the initial procedure eliminated trophoblastic activity without major complications in 81% of 52 laparoscopy patients versus 95% of 57 laparotomy patients. Residual trophoblasts or complications were successfully treated in all. Laparoscopy produced final outcomes equivalent to those of laparotomy at lower costs.

COMPLICATIONS

Following one ectopic pregnancy 66% of females fail to have a subsequent pregnancy, and of the one-third who conceive, only 64% deliver a term baby. The incidence of further ectopic pregnancies is increased.

BIBLIOGRAPHY

Ammerman S, Shafer MA, Snyder D. Ectopic pregnancy in adolescents: a clinical review for pediatricians. J Pediatr 1990;117(5):677.

Asseryanis E, Frigo P, Schurz B, et al. A new diagnostic method to detect ectopic pregnancy at a very early stage. Am J Obstet Gynecol 1995;173:236.

Atrash HK, Freide A, Hogue CJ. Ectopic pregnancy mortality in the United States 1970–1983. Obstet Gynecol 1987;70:817.

Barnhart K, Mennuti MT, Benjamin I. Prompt diagnosis of ectopic pregnancy in an emergency department setting. Obstet Gynecol 1994;84:1010.

Behrman SJ, Burchell RC, Goebelsmann UT, et al. When to think ectopic pregnancy. Patient Care 1984; 18:63.

Brenner PF, Roy S, Mishell DR. Ectopic pregnancy: a study of 300 consecutive surgically treated cases. JAMA 1980;243:673.

Bryson SCP. β-subunit of human chorionic gonadotropin, ultrasound, and ectopic pregnancy: a prospective study. Am J Obstet Gynecol 1983;146:163.

Carson SA, Buster JE. Ectopic pregnancy. N Engl J Med 1993;329:1174.

Centers for Disease Control. Ectopic pregnancy. United States, 1981. MMWR 1986;35:298.

Centers for Disease Control and Prevention. Ectopic pregnancy—United States, 1990–1992. JAMA 1995; 273:533.

Churgay CA, Apgar BS. Ectopic pregnancy: an update on technologic advances in diagnosis and treatment. Prim Care 1993;20:629.

Corson SL, Batzer FR. Ectopic pregnancy: a review of the etiologic factors. J Reprod Med 1986;31:78.

Decherney AH. Ectopic pregnancy. American College of Obstetrics and Gynecology Technical Bulletin 1989; 126:3.

Decherney AH, Diamond MP. Laparoscopic salpingostomy for ectopic pregnancy. Obstet Gynecol 1987; 70:948.

Easly HA, Olive DL, Holman JF. Contemporary evaluation of suspected ectopic pregnancy. J Reprod Med 1987;32:901.

Filly RA. Ectopic pregnancy: the role of sonography. Radiology 1987;162:661.

Frates MC, Laing FC. Sonographic evaluation of ectopic pregnancy: an update. Am J Roentgenol 1995;165:251.

Gale CL, Stovall TG, Muram D. Tubal pregnancy in adolescence. J Adolesc Health Care 1990;11(4):304.

Gray DT, Thorbum J, Lundorff P, et al. A cost-effectiveness study of a randomised trial of laparoscopy versus laparotomy for ectopic pregnancy. Lancet 1995; 345:1139.

Henry MA, Gentry WL. Single injection of methotrexate for treatment of ectopic pregnancies. Am J Obstet Gynecol 1994;171:1584.

Kim DS, Chung SR, Park MI. Comparative review of diagnostic accuracy in tubal pregnancy: a 14 year survey of 1040 cases. Obstet Gynecol 1982;70:547.

Marchbanks PA, Annegers JF, Coulam CB, et al. Risk factors for ectopic pregnancy: a population-based study. JAMA 1988;259:1823.

Nyberg DA, Filly RA, Mahony BS. Early gestation: correlation of HCG levels and sonographic identification. AJR 1985;144:951.

Nyberg DA, Mack LA, Laing FC, et al. Early pregnancy complications: endo-vaginal sonographic findings correlated with human chorionic gonadotropin levels. Radiology 1988;167:619.

Ory SJ. New options for diagnosis and treatment of ectopic pregnancy. JAMA 1992;267:534.

Romero R, Kader N, Jeanty P, et al. Diagnosis of ectopic pregnancy: value of the discriminatory human chorionic gonadotropin zone. Obstet Gynecol 1985;66:357.

Slaughter JL, Grimes DA. Methotrexate therapy. Nonsurgical management of ectopic pregnancy. West J Med 1995;162:225.

Stewart BK, Nazar-Stewart V, Toivola B, et al. Biochemical discrimination of pathologic pregnancy from early, normal intrauterine gestation in symptomatic patients. Am J Clin Pathol 1995;103:386.

Stovall TG, Ling FW, Carson SA, et al. Nonsurgical diagnosis and treatment of tubal pregnancy. Fertil Steril 1990;54:537–538.

Washington AE, Katz P. Ectopic pregnancy in the United States: economic consequences and payment source trends. Obstet Gynecol 1993;81:287.

Weckstein LN, Boucher AR, Tucker N, et al. Accurate diagnosis of early ectopic pregnancy. Obstet Gynecol 1985;65:393.

Ziederman AM, Wiles PJ, Espino DV. Ectopic pregnancy: six atypical cases. Postgrad Med 1988;83:297.

CHAPTER 57

Galactorrhea

Lawrence S. Neinstein and Karen S. Himebaugh

Galactorrhea refers to the secretion of a milky fluid, from one or both breasts, which is non-physiological and is considered to be inappropriate (i.e., not related to pregnancy or breast-feeding). This fluid is usually white or clear, but it may be yellow or even a greenish color. With a yellow or greenish discharge, local breast disease may also need to be considered. A bloody discharge is also suggestive of local breast disease. Galactorrhea demands evaluation in a nulliparous woman and if at least 1 year has elapsed since the last pregnancy or weaning in a parous woman. Amenorrhea often accompanies galactorrhea but may not.

ETIOLOGY

Prolactin is secreted by the anterior pituitary gland under the control of the hypothalamus. The basal hypothalamus secretes prolactin-inhibiting factor (PIF), or dopamine, into the portal system. Dopamine then binds to the lactotroph cells and suppresses the release of prolactin. Prolactin secretion may also be stimulated by thyroid-releasing hormone (TRH) from the hypothalamus, which would explain the occurrence of galactorrhea with hypothyroidism. A schema of prolactin control is shown in Figure 57.1.

A large collection of peptides has been reported to stimulate the release of prolactin in vitro. This includes gonadotropin-releasing hormones (GnRH), vasopressin, angiotensin II, and growth factors. Galactorrhea is usually a result of drug use, hypothalamic-pituitary lesions, thyroid dysfunction, chronic renal disease, or unknown factors affecting the normal physiological feedback on prolactin. Normal prolactin and lactation physiology include:

1. Pregnancy: Breast glandular tissue increases under the influence of increased levels of estrogen, progesterone, and prolactin.
2. Postpartum: Secondary to falling levels of estrogen and progesterone and continued stimulation of prolactin, lactation occurs. Prolactin is further stimulated by infant sucking of breasts.
3. Prolactin control
   a. Prolactin is secreted by the pituitary gland, under the control of the hypothalamus. The predominant action of the hypothalamus is inhibitory, via dopamine. Elevated prolactin levels may lower GnRH, luteinizing hormone (LH), and follicle-stimulating hormone (FSH). Elevated levels are frequently associated with oligomenorrhea and amenorrhea.
   b. Stimulation of prolactin
      — TRH: Direct pituitary stimulation
      — Insulin-induced hypoglycemia: Leads to increased serotonin
      — Phenothiazines, reserpine, methyldopa (Aldomet): Leads to decreased dopamine secretion

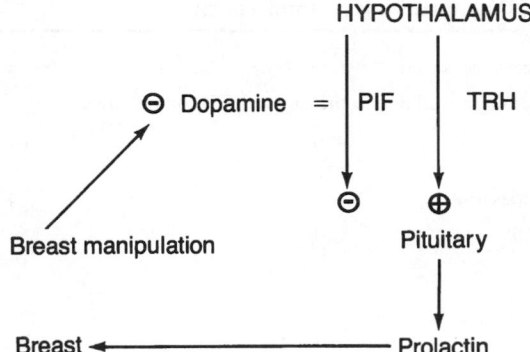

FIGURE 57.1.   Schema of prolactin control. *PIF,* prolactin-inhibiting factor; *TRH,* thyrotropin-releasing hormone.

    c. Inhibition of prolactin
- Levodopa
- Ergot alkaloids (e.g., bromocriptine, a dopaminergic agonist)
- Serotonin antagonists

DIFFERENTIAL DIAGNOSIS

The differential diagnosis for hyperprolactinemia is listed in Table 57.1. The differential diagnosis of galactorrhea may be very complex due to the many factors that control prolactin secretion. Normal prolactin secretion and lactation occur in pregnancy and in the postpartum period.

Excessive estrogen (e.g., birth control pills) has been noted to cause galactorrhea secondary to hypothalamic suppression, leading to a reduction of PIF and increased release of prolactin. Galactorrhea may be most noticeable during days when the medication is not taken and usually disappears by 3–6 months after discontinuing use of oral contraceptives. Newer, low-dose pills have a lower prevalence of galactorrhea. Galactorrhea related to phenothiazines and other medications usually does not persist beyond 3–6 months after drug discontinuation.

DIAGNOSIS

Multiple factors must be considered in the evaluation and treatment of serum prolactin elevation. In the presence of hyperprolactinemia and in the absence of pregnancy, renal failure, hypothyroidism, or the use of a medication known to induce hyperprolactinemia, a neuroradiologic investigation must be carried out to evaluate the pituitary gland. Magnetic resonance imaging (MRI) represents an improvement over computed tomography (CT) in the visualization of the structures adjacent to the pituitary, especially the lateral margins and in the diagnosis of "empty sella." The practitioner should first have the adolescent discontinue any drugs associated with elevated prolactin or galactorrhea. If galactorrhea persists, proceed as outlined in Figure 57.2.

Symptoms in women tend to be proportional to circulating levels of prolactin. Men may experience infertility or impotence, or they may present later in the course of the disease when a mass effect from a growing tumor produces changes in visual fields or headaches. Absence or delay of pubertal development may occur in either sex.

TABLE 57.1.   Differential Diagnosis for Hyperprolactinemia

1. Idiopathic
2. Physiological causes
   a. Excessive stimulation of chest wall due to breast manipulation or surgery
   b. Stress
   c. Exercise
3. Pharmacological causes
   a. Depleted storage of dopamine
      — Reserpine
   b. Blocked dopamine receptor
      — Phenothiazines
      — Thioxanthenes
      — Butyrophenones
      — Benzamines
   c. Inhibition of dopamine release
      — Chronic opioid use
   d. Blocked histamine receptor
      — Cimetidine
   e. Estrogen-containing oral contraceptives: Galactorrhea can occur during use of birth control pills or after stopping.
   f. Calcium channel blockers
   g. General anesthesia
4. Pathological causes
   a. Hypothyroidism: Secondary to elevated thyrotropin-releasing hormone (TRH) with resultant increased prolactin secretion
   b. Hypothalamic disorders: Tumors such as craniopharyngioma, infections, or infiltrative diseases such as sarcoid and histiocytosis
   c. Pituitary disorders
      — Adenomas: Micro (<10 mm diameter), macro (>10 mm diameter)
      — Acromegaly
      — Cushing's disease
      — Empty-sella syndrome
5. Ectopic production of prolactin
   a. Breast carcinoma
   b. Bronchogenic carcinoma
   c. Hypernephroma
6. Chest wall lesions
   a. Surgical scar
   b. Herpes zoster
   c. Burns
7. Others
   a. Renal failure: Related to delayed clearance of prolactin
   b. Hepatic cirrhosis
   c. Acute intermittent porphyria
   d. Spinal cord injury: Has been reported to be associated with both amenorrhea and hyperprolactinemia

The level of serum prolactin is somewhat useful for predicting diagnosis in that:

1. Levels less than 100 ng/mL are often unassociated with a discrete tumor. Women with normal prolactin levels and normal menses are in particular at low risk for a prolactinoma.
2. Levels 100–250 ng/mL are often associated with a microadenoma.
3. Levels greater than 250 ng/mL usually are secondary to macroadenomas.

Kane et al. (1994) evaluated the signs, symptoms, and outcomes of 56 children and adolescents with pituitary adenomas.

1. Types of adenoma: Macroadenomas were more common than microadenomas (1.4:1).
   a. Prolactin alone, 41
   b. Prolactin and GH, 8
   c. Multiple hormones, 6
   d. Glycoproteins, 1

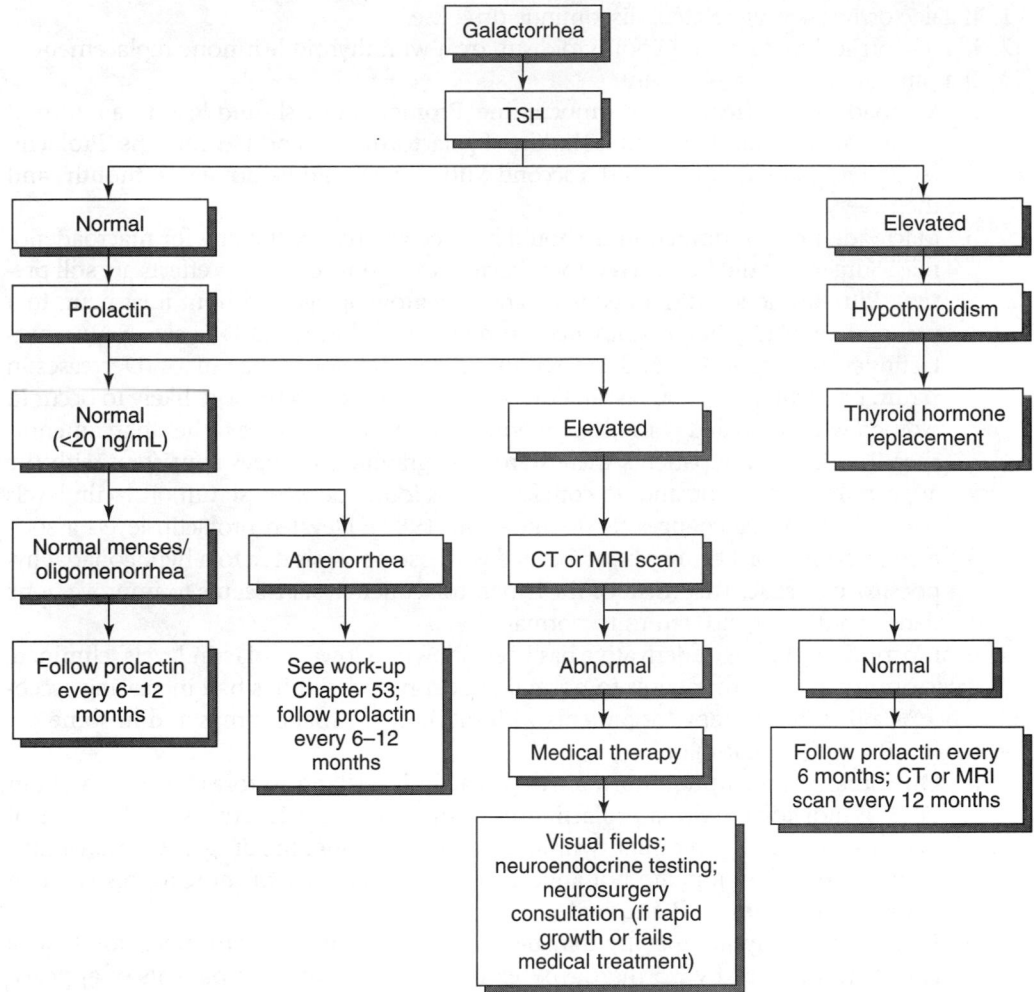

FIGURE 57.2.   Flow chart of evaluation for galactorrhea. MRI represents an improvement over CT in the visualization of the structures adjacent to the pituitary, especially the lateral margins and in the diagnosis of "empty sella". However, CT scanning still remains most useful in the diagnosis of the small tumors that do not distort or alter the size of the gland. *TSH,* thyroid-stimulating hormone.

2. Prevalence by sex
    a. No males had microadenomas.
    b. Females outnumbered males (3.3:1).
3. Symptoms: Patients presented most frequently with headache, menstrual dysfunction (in females), galactorrhea, and hypopituitarism. All but one of the patients with hypopituitarism at presentation had macroadenomas.

THERAPY

Forty percent of patients using oral contraceptives have mildly elevated basal prolactin levels (20–40 ng/mL). Most do not have galactorrhea. If galactorrhea occurs, the oral contraceptive should be stopped for 1 month and prolactin levels tested.

1. If galactorrhea is drug related, discontinue drug use.
2. If galactorrhea is related to hypothyroidism, treat with thyroid hormone replacement.
3. If a pituitary adenoma is present:
    a. Microadenoma: Treat with bromocriptine. Bromocriptine should lead to a return of menses in 2–3 months and resolution of galactorrhea in about 3 months. Prolactin levels should be followed, and a second MRI scan should be done in 6 months and then every 2–3 years.
    b. Macroadenoma: Bromocriptine should be used as primary therapy for macroadenomas. Surgery should be reserved for refractory cases only or if mass effects are still present. Pituitary adenomas, in general, are slow growing even without treatment. In a prospective evaluation, 30 untreated women were followed for 3–7 years. Serum prolactin levels increased in 6, decreased in 10, and did not change in 14. Decreases in serum prolactin levels and restoration of normal menses were more likely to occur in women who presented with oligomenorrhea or normal menses rather than amenorrhea. In 22% of the patients there were radiographical changes consistent with the appearance of a tumor, and no correlation was found between serum prolactin levels and radiographical changes (Schlechte et al., 1989). Elevated prolactin levels associated with amenorrhea may be associated with osteoporosis due to a hypogonadal hypoestrogenic state. Treatment of the hyperprolactinemia state seems to improve bone density but it may not return to normal.
4. Bromocriptine: This ergot derivative has been shown to lower prolactin levels, eliminate galactorrhea, and return menses to normal ovulatory cycles. It has had increasing acceptance as a first-line therapy for patients with pituitary microadenomas and in some patients with macroadenomas.
    a. Outcome: Bromocriptine normalizes prolactin levels and restores fertility in about 90% of individuals with a prolactinoma. Tumor diameter is reduced in 60–79% of patients within 3–12 months. Symptoms may return after the drug is withdrawn. Pediatric pituitary tumors did not appear to be more invasive or more aggressive than adult pituitary tumors (Kane et al., 1994).
    b. Doses: Bromocriptine therapy may be started at 2.5 mg/day with meals for 1 week and then increased by 2.5 mg/day/week until a dosage in most patients of approximately 2.5 mg t.i.d. is reached.
    c. Side effects: The side effects include hypotension, nausea, vomiting, lethargy, dizziness, syncope, tachyarrhythmias, and psychosis.
5. Alternative treatments: Pergolide mesylate is an ergot-derived dopamine receptor agonist. The drug is active in treating prolactin elevation in the 25- to 100-µg dose range. The major advantage is once-a-day dosing, which may improve compliance as well as decrease side effects.
6. Surgery: Neurosurgical intervention is required for rapidly growing prolactinomas or those tumors failing response to medical therapy.

BIBLIOGRAPHY

Abdel-Gadir A, Khatim MS, Muharib NS, et al. The etiology of galactorrhoea in women with regular menstruation and normal prolactin levels. Hum Reprod 1992;7:912.

Aron DC, Tyrrell JB, Wilson CB. Pituitary tumors. Current concepts in diagnosis and management. West J Med 1995;162:340.

Benjamin F. Normal lactation and galactorrhea. Clin Obstet Gynecol 1994;37:887.

Caputy GG, Flowers RS. Copious lactation following augmentation mammaplasty: an uncommon but not rare condition. Anesth Plast Surg 1994;18:393.

Cunnah D, Besser M. Management of prolactinomas. Clin Endocrinol 1991;34:231.

Divers WA, Yen SSC. Prolactin-producing microadenomas in pregnancy. Am J Obstet Gynecol 1983;61:425.

Gold EB, Bush T, Chee E. Risk factors for secondary amenorrhea and galactorrhea. Int J Fertil Menopausal Stud 1994;39:177.

Gonzales GF, Carrillo CF. Low serum prolactin levels in native women at high altitude. Int J Gynaecol Obstet 1993;43:169.

Greenspan SL, Klibanski A. Increase in bone mass after treatment of hyperprolactinemic amenorrhea. N Engl J Med 1986;315:542.

Howlett TA, Wass JAH, Grossman A, et al. Prolactinomas presenting as primary amenorrhea and delayed or arrested puberty: response to medical therapy. Clin Endocrinol 1989;30:131.

Jaquet P. Medical therapy of prolactinomas. Acta Endocrinol 1993;129(suppl 1):31.

Kane LA, Leinung MC, Scheithauer BW, et al. Pituitary adenomas in childhood and adolescence. J Clin Endocrinol Metab 1994;79:1135.

Katz E, Adashi EY. Hyperprolactinemia disorders. Clin Obstet Gynecol 1990;33:622.

Kletzky OA, Davajan V. Hyperprolactinemia. In: Mishell JR Jr, Davajan V, eds. Infertility, contraception, and reproductive endocrinology. Oradell, New Jersey: Medical Economics Books, 1986.

Klibanski A, Biller BMK, Rosenthal DI, et al. Effects of prolactin and estrogen deficiency in amenorrhea bone loss. J Clin Endocrinol Metab 1988;67:124.

Klibanski A, Greenspan SL. Increase in bone mass after treatment of hyperprolactinemic amenorrhea. N Engl J Med 1986;315:542.

Klibanski A, Neer RM, Beitins IZ, et al. Decreased bone density in hyperprolactinemic women. N Engl J Med 1980;303:1511.

Klibanski A, Zervas NT. Diagnosis and management of hormone-secreting pituitary adenomas. N Engl J Med 1991;324:822.

Kohler PO. Treatment of pituitary adenomas. N Engl J Med 1987;317:44.

McCutcheon IE. Management of individual tumor syndromes. Pituitary neoplasia. Endocrinol Metab Clin North Am 1994;23:37.

Melmed S, Braunstein GD, Chang RJ. Pituitary tumors secreting growth hormone and prolactin. Ann Intern Med 1986;105:238.

Molitch ME. Endocrine problems of adolescent pregnancy. Endocrinol Metab Clin North Am 1993;22:649.

Nalbach DA, Carson MA. Prolactinoma: a review and case study. Crit Care Nurse 1991;11:48.

Neal JH, Weiss MH. Management of prolactin-secreting pituitary adenomas. West J Med 1990;153:546.

Nunes MCP, Sobrinho LG, Calhaz-Jorge C, et al. Psychosomatic factors in patients with hyperprolactinemia and/or galactorrhea. Obstet Gynecol 1980;55:591.

Scamoni C, Balzarini C, Crivelli G, et al. Treatment and long-term follow-up results of prolactin secreting pituitary adenomas. J Neurosurg Sci 1991;35:9.

Schlechte J, Dolan K, Sherman B, et al. The natural history of untreated hyperprolactinemia: a prospective analysis. J Clin Endocrinol Metab 1989;64:412.

Schlechte J, Walkner L, Kathol M. A longitudinal analysis of premenopausal bone loss in healthy women and women with hyperprolactinemia. J Clin Endocrinol Metab 1992;75:698.

Sheeler LR. Medical treatment of pituitary tumors. Cleve Clin J Med 1994;61:99.

State D. Nipple discharge in women. Is it cause for concern? Postgrad Med 1991;89:65.

Stein AL, Levenick MN, Kletzky DA. Computed tomography versus magnetic resonance imaging for the evaluation of suspected pituitary adenomas. Obstet Gynecol 1989;73:996.

Taler SJ, Coulam CB, Annegers JF, et al. Case-control study of galactorrhea and its relationship to the use of oral contraceptives. Obstet Gynecol 1985;65:665.

Tonner D, Schlechte J. Contemporary therapy of prolactin secreting adenomas. Am J Med Sci 1993;306:395.

Tyson D, Reggiardo D, Sklar C, et al. Prolactin secreting macroadenomas in adolescents. Response to bromocriptine therapy. Am J Dis Child 1993;147:1057.

Yarkony GM, Novick AK, Roth EJ, et al. Galactorrhea: a complication of spinal cord injury. Arch Phys Med Rehabil 1992;73:878.

CHAPTER 58

Hirsutism and Virilism

Lawrence S. Neinstein and Francine Ratner Kaufman

Hirsutism is defined as increased growth of terminal (long, coarse, and pigmented) hair in the female, in an amount greater than is cosmetically acceptable in a certain culture. The condition commonly refers to an increase in length and coarseness of the hair, in a male pattern, including predominantly midline hair of the upper lip, chin, cheeks, inner thighs, lower back, and intermammary, abdominal, and intergluteal regions. Virilism implies the development of male secondary sex characteristics in the female. This may include:

1. Defeminizing symptoms: Vaginal wall atrophy, decreased vaginal secretions, decreased breast tissue, oligomenorrhea, and amenorrhea.
2. Masculinizing symptoms: Hirsutism, deepened voice, increased libido, increased muscle mass, clitoromegaly (greater than 1 cm in diameter), temporal balding, and acne.

Hypertrichosis implies the predominance of excessive vellus hair on the body, particularly the forehead, forearms, or lower legs.

Androgen excess causes changes in appearance of the female and can be associated with abnormal menstrual patterns, infertility, and metabolic disturbances that include decreased high-density lipoprotein (HDL) cholesterol, increased insulin resistance, decreased sex hormone–binding globulin (SHBG), and alterations of the balance between thromboxane and α_2-prostacyclin (Haseltine et al., 1994).

Androgen disorders should be evaluated, particularly in adolescent females, since appropriate interventions are now available; the evaluation does not require complicated, expensive procedures; and if untreated, the hyperandrogenism will persist and lead to excess morbidity and psychosocial dysfunction.

HAIR PHYSIOLOGY

Hair grows from hair follicles that develop at 8 weeks of gestation. All hair follicles are developed in utero, and no new follicles develop during life. The concentration of hair follicles per unit area of skin is similar in males and females but differs between races and ethnic groups. Caucasians have a greater concentration than Asians, and Mediterraneans have a greater concentration than Nordic persons. Hair grows in cycles according to the following phases:

1. Anagen phase: Growing phase
2. Catagen phase: Rapid involution phase
3. Telogen phase: Resting phase

Hair length is determined by the duration of the growing phase. Factors influencing hair growth include:

1. Androgens: Androgens initiate hair growth and increase hair diameter and pigmentation. These changes occur secondary to dihydrotestosterone's effect on altering vellus hair to terminal hair. Once hair growth is established, the pattern may continue despite androgen withdrawal, albeit at a slower rate. Once the androgen level is reduced, there may be a lag time of 6–9 months before a significant change is noticed, as old terminal hairs fall out and new vellus hairs take their place.
2. Estrogens: Estrogens retard initiation and the rate of hair growth and may prolong the anagen phase.

ANDROGEN PHYSIOLOGY

Androgens are synthesized during the metabolic pathways of progesterone, cortisol, and estrogen (Figure 58.1).

1. Circulating androgenic steroids in females
   a. 17-Ketosteroids
      — Dehydroepiandrosterone sulfate (DHAS)
      — Dehydroepiandrosterone (DHA)
      — Androstenedione
      — Androsterone
   b. 17β-Hydroxysteroids
      — Testosterone

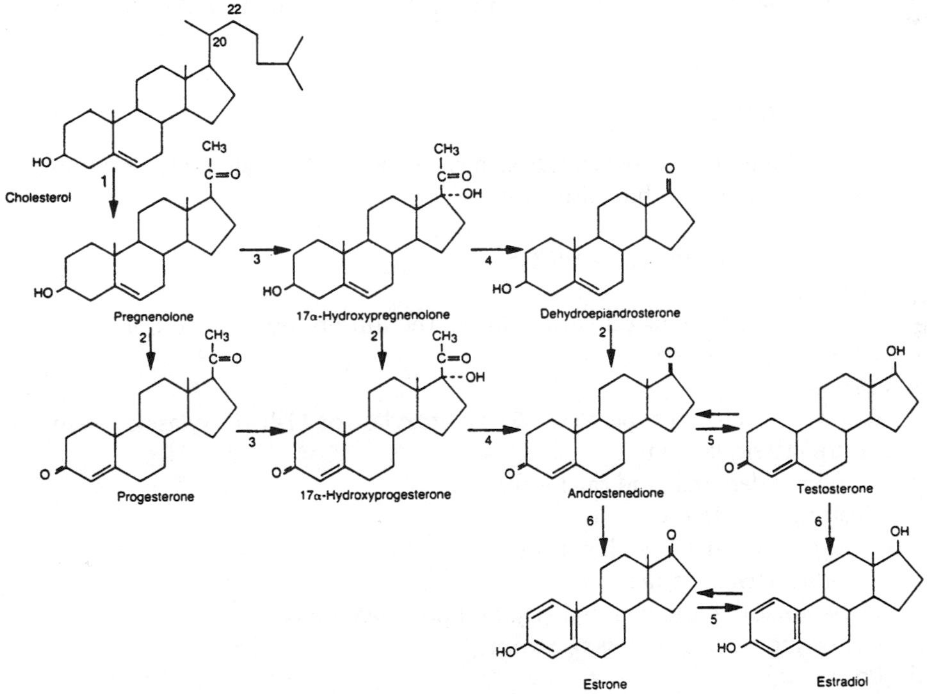

FIGURE 58.1. Ovarian steroid biosynthetic pathways. The following enzymes are required where indicated: (*1*) 20-hydroxylase, 22-hydroxylase, and 20,22-desmolase; (*2*) 3β-hydroxysteroid dehydrogenase and $\Delta^5 \rightarrow \Delta^4$-isomerase; (*3*) 17α-hydroxylase; (*4*) 17,20-desmolase; (*5*) 17β-hydroxysteroid dehydrogenase; and (*6*) aromatizing enzyme system. (Reprinted by permission of Blackwell Science, Inc. From Goebelsmann U. Steroid hormones. In: Mishell DR Jr, Davajan V, eds. Infertility, contraception and reproductive endocrinology. Oradell, New Jersey: Medical Economics, 1986.)

— Dihydrotestosterone
— Androstenediol
— 3β-Androstenediol

2. Metabolism: Androgens originate in the adrenal gland and ovaries, either via direct secretion or peripheral conversion of precursors. DHAS, DHA, and androstenedione, which are mainly produced in the adrenal gland, exert their androgenic activity after peripheral conversion to testosterone or its metabolites.

   a. Adrenal secretion: Androgens are by-products of cortisol synthesis.

      — 17-Ketosteroids: The majority of 17-ketosteroids are generated from adrenal sources. This includes a daily secretion of 7 mg of DHAS (90% of total daily secretion), 5.5 mg of DHA, and 1.8 mg of androstenedione (50% of total daily secretion). All these compounds have low androgenic activity.

      — Testosterone: Twenty-five percent is derived from adrenal secretions, or a total of 0.06 mg/day is secreted from the adrenal gland. Testosterone is a potent androgen.

   b. Ovarian secretions: Androgens from the ovary are metabolized as intermediates in the production of estrogen and progesterone. Major ovarian androgenic secretions include:

      — Testosterone: About 25% of total daily secretion (0.06 mg/day)
      — Androstenedione: About 50% of total daily secretion (1.7 mg/day)

   c. Peripheral conversion: About 50% of testosterone is derived from peripheral conversion of androstenedione in liver, fat, and skin cells.

   d. Testosterone is 95.5% bound to SHBG in females; only the free portion is active. During pregnancy about 99% is bound. In the normal male 92.8% of testosterone is bound.

DIFFERENTIAL DIAGNOSIS

1. Idiopathic hirsutism: As hyperandrogenism is better delineated, the percent of hirsute women with idiopathic hirsutism continues to fall.

2. Ovarian causes
   a. Polycystic ovary syndrome (PCOS)
   b. Hyperthecosis
   c. Tumor: Sertoli-Leydig cell tumor, lipoid cell tumors, hilar cell tumor
   d. Pregnancy: Luteoma

3. Adrenal causes
   a. Congenital adrenal hyperplasia: 21-Hydroxylase or 11-hydroxylase deficiency, classic or nonclassic, late onset
   b. Tumors: Adenomas and carcinomas
   c. Cushing's syndrome

4. Nonandrogenic dependent hirsutism
   a. Genetic: Racial, familial
   b. Physiological: Pregnancy, puberty, and postmenopausal
   c. Endocrine: Hypothyroidism, acromegaly
   d. Porphyria
   e. Hamartomas
   f. Drug-induced: Phenytoin, diazoxide, steroids, adrenocorticotropic hormone (ACTH), Geritol, minoxidil, cyclosporine; valproate is associated with menstrual disturbances and hyperandrogenism (Isojarvi et al., 1993).
   g. Central nervous system lesions: Multiple sclerosis, encephalitis
   h. Congenital lesions: Hurler's syndrome, De Lange syndrome

Ehrmann et al. (1992) examined 40 women with hyperandrogenism and found that 25% had ovarian dysfunction, 33% combined ovarian and adrenal dysfunction, and 25% adrenal dysfunction alone. Only one patient had adult-onset adrenal 21-hydroxylase deficiency. Overall, most diagnostic tests including LH and FSH and stimulation tests were not highly specific.

DIAGNOSIS

Indications for Evaluation

1. Rapid onset of signs and symptoms
2. Virilization
3. Onset of hirsutism or virilism that is not peripubertal
4. Symptoms suggesting Cushing's syndrome (i.e., weight gain, weakness, or hypertension)

Consider hyperandrogenism in any female with either premature pubarche, unusual acne, hirsutism, or androgenetic alopecia.

History

1. Menstrual history, evaluating for amenorrhea or oligomenorrhea
2. Drug history
3. Ethnic background and family history of hirsutism
4. Rapidity of androgenizing or virilizing symptoms and signs: Most women with an androgen-producing ovarian or adrenal tumor have rapid onset of virilization.

Physical Examination

1. Extent of hirsutism: A grading system for hirsutism is illustrated and discussed in Hatch et al. (1981), based on grading nine areas of the body from 1 to 4. Some terminal hair on lower abdomen, face, and around the areola is normal, but hair on the upper back, shoulders, sternum, and upper abdomen suggests more marked androgen activity.
2. Stigmata of Cushing's syndrome
3. Signs of virilism: Check clitoral diameter or index. Clitoral diameter should be less than 1 cm. The clitoral index is the product of the vertical and horizontal dimensions of the glans. The normal range is 9–35 mm^2; a clitoral index greater than 100 mm^2 suggests a serious underlying disorder.
4. Presence of ovarian or adrenal masses

Laboratory Evaluation

The goals of the laboratory evaluation include demonstrating androgen excess and locating the source of the excess.

1. Measuring androgen excess
   a. Plasma testosterone is the most important measurement. Levels above 200 ng/dL suggest a serious disease.
   b. Other important indicators include:
      — DHAS
      — 17-Hydroxyprogesterone: This is often elevated in patients with congenital adrenal hyperplasia due to 21-hydroxylase deficiency. 17-Hydroxyprogesterene should be

measured between 7 AM and 9 AM. Can also measure 11-desoxycortisol to rule out 11-hydroxylase deficiency.
  — Free testosterone: Free testosterone may be elevated in the presence of normal total testosterone. However, free testosterone will be elevated in the presence of hirsutism, so it is not a very specific test. Total testosterone is less expensive and may be enough to point the diagnosis toward an ovarian cause.
  c. 17-Ketosteroids: This is not a particularly specific test, as some 17-ketosteroids are nonandrogenic and the potent 17β-hydroxysteroids are not measured.
  d. If the teen is oligomenorrheic, prolactin and thyroid-stimulating hormone (TSH) should be measured and a pregnancy test performed.
Overall, in most individuals a minimum of laboratory testing is necessary because of the complete response to combination oral contraceptives with or without spironolactone. This includes a total testosterone determination to eliminate the rare individual with a testosterone-secreting tumor. A baseline early morning level of 17-hydroxyprogesterone is useful. DHAS is usually also measured, but in many instances a moderate increase is found in women with anovulation who have no adrenal disease.
2. Locating the source of androgen excess
  a. If male levels of testosterone are obtained or a mass is felt on examination, perform an ultrasound or computed tomography (CT) scan of adrenal glands and of ovaries. Markedly elevated serum testosterone and DHAS suggest an adrenal tumor and the need for a CT scan, while markedly elevated serum testosterone and normal DHAS suggest an ovarian source and the need for ultrasound of the ovaries.
  b. If any of the androgens are elevated or signs suggest hypercortisolism, perform a dexamethasone suppression test.
    — An ovarian source is suggested by cortisol suppression but a lack of androgen suppression. An ultrasound of the ovaries is helpful in this instance.
    — Both adrenogenital syndrome and idiopathic hirsutism are suggested by suppression of cortisol and androgens after dexamethasone.
    — Cushing's syndrome or an adrenal tumor is suggested by lack of cortisol suppression. Indicators of suppression after dexamethasone (0.5 mg four times daily for 7 days) include:
    — Free testosterone less than 8 pg/mL
    — Total testosterone less than 58 ng/dL
    — Free plasma 17β-hydroxysteroid level less than 42 pg/mL
    — Fall in DHAS of at least 50%
  c. If 17-hydroxyprogesterone is elevated, perform an ACTH stimulation test. This is helpful in differentiating normal and idiopathic hirsute females from those with late-onset congenital adrenal hyperplasia due to incomplete 21-hydroxylase deficiency.
    — To perform the test: Measure a baseline 17-hydroxyprogesterone and repeat a serum level 60 minutes after 0.25 mg of ACTH is administered intravenously. In a positive result, there is an increase in the serum level to greater than 30 ng/mL, whereas in normal or idiopathic hirsute females the levels are usually less than 5 ng/mL. This test can also be used to rule out late-onset congenital adrenal hyperplasia due to 11-hydroxylase or 3β-hydroxysteroid dehydrogenase deficiency.
3. Specific diagnoses
  a. Idiopathic hirsutism: These women generally ovulate regularly and have normal levels of androgens. As hyperandrogenism is better understood, the number of women with a hyperandrogenic state ascribed to idiopathic hirsutism will decline. The underlying mechanism remains to be identified, with the following possible causes of androgen excess:

— Altered gonadotropin secretory patterns
— Exaggerated adrenal androgen secretion
— Increased prolactin levels altering adrenal androgen secretion
— Alteration of SHBG
— Obesity
— Hyperinsulinism
— Altered skin metabolism of androgens

b. Ovarian tumors
— Palpable adnexal mass
— Testosterone level greater than 200 ng/mL
— Nonsuppression of androgens with dexamethasone

c. PCOS or hyperthecosis of the ovaries
— Hirsutism, infertility, menstrual irregularities, obesity
— Slight elevations in androgen levels
— Increase in LH level and LH-FSH ratio: LH and FSH have been suggested as markers for PCOS with a high LH and low-normal FSH (ratio > 3:1), but this test is neither sensitive nor specific.
— Young women with severe acne: High incidence of PCOS

d. Congenital adrenal hyperplasia: Elevated 17- hydroxyprogesterone, with large increase after ACTH is diagnostic of incomplete 21-hydroxylase deficiency. This condition is often recognized during adolescence with presentation similar to PCOS syndrome. An elevated 11-desoxycortisol or DHAS and 17-hydroxypregnenolone is found in 11-hydroxylase and 3β-hydroxysteroid dehydrogenase deficiencies.

e. Adrenal tumors
— Adrenal androgenizing tumors: Rare and associated with rapid defeminization
— Adrenal mass: Palpable in many individuals
— Elevated 17-ketosteroids, DHAS, and DHA
— Subnormal suppression with dexamethasone
— Mass on ultrasound, intravenous pyelogram, or CT scan

f. Drug-induced hirsutism: The cause of nonandrogen drug-induced hirsutism is not well understood. The pattern is not restricted to androgen-dependent areas, and the hair is usually vellus in nature.

g. Anabolic androgen abuse

h. HAIRAN syndrome: This includes a combination of *h*yperandrogenism, *i*nsulin *r*esistance, and *a*canthosis *n*igricans. The syndrome is also associated with PCOS and myocardial hypertrophy. Insulin receptor blockade leads to more insulin acting on the insulin-like growth factor (IGF-I) receptor. This is associated with growth promotion, including acanthosis nigricans and potential myometrial hypertrophy. These individuals have fasting basal insulin levels of over 80 μU/mL compared to normal levels of about 7–8 μU/mL, and peaks of over 1000 μU/mL compared to about 60 μU/mL in normal individuals.

THERAPY

1. Tumor: Remove the androgen source.
2. Drug-induced: Stop medication.
3. Congenital adrenal hyperplasia: Replace cortisol with oral hydrocortisone or cortisone acetate. In rare instances, use low-dose dexamethasone (0.25 mg every day).
4. Functional ovarian hyperandrogenemia (e.g., PCOS)
   a. Hirsutism

— Cosmetic: Temporary methods such as shaving, waxing, and bleaches; or permanent methods such as electrolysis (Richards, 1995)

— Estrogen-progestins: Oral contraceptives work in 60–100% of women. Medical therapy is slow and requires 6–12 months to judge effectiveness. Lag time occurs because of the delay before terminal hair falls out and is replaced by thinner less pigmented hair. Combination pills that contain low androgenic progestins such as norethindrone, norgestimate, or desogestrel should be used. Oral contraceptives decrease androgen production by:
   (1) Lowering LH and thus decreasing androgen production
   (2) Increasing SHBG and thus lowering free androgens
   (3) Decreasing adrenal androgen production
   (4) Decreasing 5α-reductase activity

— Antiandrogens: Spironolactone and cyproterone acetate (investigational) have been used. Spironolactone competes with androgen receptors peripherally and inhibits 5α-reductase. The starting dosage is usually 50 mg/day and is usually effective between about 75–200 mg/day. The medication can be increased by 25 mg every 1–2 weeks. However, the maximal response is not seen for 6 months to 1 year. Side effects are minimal but can include dry mouth, diuresis, fatigue, and menstrual spotting. The drug is contraindicated during pregnancy, as it can lead to feminization of the male fetus. Also in use are flutamide (a nonsteroidal antiandrogen) and 5α-reductase inhibitors (such as finasteride).

— Combination therapy: The combination of low-dose oral contraceptives and spironolactone is very effective.

— Future directions: Future therapies will probably include topical antiandrogens, inhibitors of the enzyme 5α-reductase and long-acting GnRH agonists. GnRH agonists are best reserved for very severe hyperandrogen states such as those individuals with HAIRAN. Carr et al. (1995) compared the use of oral contraceptives alone, GnRH agonists alone, or the two in combination and found that by 6 months measurements of hirsutism were not different between the groups. GnRH agonists alone had a negative impact on bone density. If GnRH agonists are used, it is best to use in conjunction with oral contraceptives to avoid the hypoestrogenic state that GnRH agonists can induce when used alone.

b. Menstrual abnormality
   — Cyclic progestin
   — Combined oral contraceptives

c. Infertility (referral to infertility specialist)
   — Clomiphene citrate
   — Dexamethasone
   — Human chorionic gonadotropin

Bibliography

ACOG technical bulletin. Hyperandrogenic chronic anovulation. Number 202—February 1995. Committee on Technical Bulletins of the American College of Obstetricians and Gynecologists. Int J Gynaecol Obstet 1995;49:201.

Burkman RT Jr. The role of oral contraceptives in the treatment of hyperandrogenic disorders. Am J Med 1995;98:130S.

Carr BR. Disorders of the ovary and female reproductive tract. In: Wilson JD, Foster DW, eds. Williams textbook of endocrinology. 8th ed. Philadelphia: WB Saunders, 1992.

Carr BR, Breslau NA, Givens C, et al. Oral contraceptive pills, gonadotropin-releasing hormone agonists, or use in combination for treatment of hirsutism: a clinical research center study. J Clin Endocrinol Metab 1995;80:1169.

Chetkowski RJ, DeFrazid J, Shamonki I, et al. The incidence of late-onset congenital adrenal hyperplasia due to 21-hydroxylase deficiency among hirsute women. J Clin Endocrinol Metab 1984;58:595.

Ehrmann DA, Rosenfield RL, Barnes RB, et al. Detection of functional ovarian hyperandrogenism in women with androgen excess. N Engl J Med 1992; 327:157.

Goebelsmann U, Lobo RA. Androgen excess. In: Mishell DR Jr, Davajan V, Lobo A, eds. Infertility, contraception, and reproductive endocrinology. 3rd ed. Boston: Blackwell Scientific, 1991.

Hammond MG, Talbert LM, Groff TR. Hyperandrogenism. Postgrad Med 1986;79:107.

Haseltine F, Wentz AC, Redmond GP, et al. Androgens and women's health: NICHD Conference. Clinician 1994;12:3.

Hatch R, Rosenfield RL, Kim MH, et al. Hirsutism: implications, etiology, and management. Am J Obstet Gynecol 1981;140:815.

Herter LD, Magalhaes JA, Spritzer PM. Association of ovarian volume and serum LH levels in adolescent patients with menstrual disorders and/or hirsutism. Braz J Med Biol Res 1993;26:1041.

Isojarvi JI, Laatikainen TJ, Pakarinen AJ. Polycystic ovaries and hyperandrogenism in women taking valproate for epilepsy. N Engl J Med 1993;329:1383.

Jahanfar S, Eden JA. Idiopathic hirsutism or polycystic ovary syndrome? Aust N Z J Obstet Gynaecol 1993; 33:414.

Kustin J, Rebar RW. Hirsutism in young adolescent girls. Pediatr Ann 1986;15:522.

Lobo RA, Goebelsman V. Adult manifestation of congenital adrenal hyperplasia due to incomplete 21-hydroxylase deficiency mimicking polycystic ovarian disease. Am J Obstet Gynecol 1980;138:720.

Lucky AW. Hormonal correlates of acne and hirsutism. Am J Med 1995;98(1A):89S.

Marshburn PB, Carr BR. Hirsutism and virilization. A systematic approach to benign and potentially serious causes. Postgrad Med 1995;97:99.

Morris DV. Hirsutism. Clin Obstet Gynecol 1985;12:649.

Pittaway DE, Wentz AC. Therapeutic alternatives for the hirsute patient. Drug Ther Bull 1982;(April):97.

Redmond GP. Androgenic disorders of women: diagnostic and therapeutic decision making. Am J Med 1995;98:120S.

Richards RN, Meharg GE. Electrolysis: observations from 13 years and 140,000 hours of experience. J Am Acad Dermatol 1995;33:662.

Rittmaster RS. Clinical relevance of testosterone and dihydrotestosterone metabolism in women. Am J Med 1995;98:17S.

Rittmaster RS. Clinical review 73: medical treatment of androgen-dependent hirsutism. J Clin Endocrinol Metab 1995;80:2559.

Rittmaster RS, Loriaux DL. Hirsutism. Ann Intern Med 1987;109:95.

Rosenfield RL, Lucky AW. Acne, hirsutism, and alopecia in adolescent girls. Clinical expressions of androgen excess. Endocrinol Metab Clin North Am 1993;22: 507.

Sane K, Pescovitz OH. The clitoral index: a determination of clitoral size in normal girls and girls with abnormal sexual development. J Pediatr 1992;120:265.

Schwartz FL, Flink EB. Hirsutism: pathophysiology, clinical evaluation, treatment. Postgrad Med 1985; 77:81.

Vetr M, Sobek A. Low dose spironolactone in the treatment of female hyperandrogenemia and hirsutism. Acta Univ Palacki Olomuc Fac Med 1993;135:55.

Wild RA. Obesity, lipids, cardiovascular risk, and androgen excess. Am J Med 1995;98:27S.

Wild RA, Demers LM, Applebaum-Bowden D, et al. Hirsutism: metabolic effects of two commonly used oral contraceptives and spironolactone. Contraception 1991;44:113.

CHAPTER 59

Breast Disorders

This chapter discusses breast disorders that can occur in female adolescents: asymmetrical breast development, accessory breast tissue, benign breast tumors, and virginal hypertrophy of the breast. Galactorrhea (abnormal lactation) is discussed in Chapter 57.

DEVELOPMENTAL ANOMALIES

Asymmetrical Breast Development

For unknown reasons, one breast may develop faster during puberty than the other. Usually the breasts equalize by adulthood. Occasionally, when notable asymmetry is present, corrective surgery can be performed with augmentation of one breast. This can be done in stages with an implant placed in one side that allows for increasing amounts of saline to match growth on the other side. After puberty, this implant is replaced with a permanent implant. One can monitor differences in breast sizes by measuring breast units, which equal vertical distance multiplied by horizontal distance.

Absence of Breast Tissue

Amastia is the total absence of one breast. The condition is usually associated with an anomaly in the chest wall, consisting of the absence of the pectoralis major or other muscles. The condition may also be associated with Poland's syndrome, which includes a rib deformity, webbed fingers, and radial nerve palsy. Atelia is the absence of the nipple on one or both sides.

Accessory Breast Tissue

Accessory breast tissue is the most common breast anomaly, found in 1–2% of females. Polythelia refers to supernumerary nipples and polymastia to any accessory breast elements. The accessory tissue is usually located along the embryonic milk line anywhere from the midclavicular or axillary area to the middle of the inguinal ligament in the groin. This condition has been occasionally associated with cardiovascular and genitourinary anomalies. While the problem is usually of no significance, the extra nipples may become engorged postpartum and create painful swellings. The extra nipples can be excised for cosmetic reasons.

BREAST TUMORS

Types of Tumors

In reviewing 15 retrospective studies involving breast lesions in adolescents and young adults, the following prevalences were found (studies include Bauer et al., 1987; Bower et al.,

840

1976; Daniel and Mathews, 1968; Farrow and Ashikari, 1969; Gogas et al., 1979; Goldstein and Miler, 1982; Neinstein et al., 1993; Raju, 1985; Sandison and Walker, 1968; Seashore, 1975; Simmons and Wold, 1989; Simpson and Barson, 1969; Skiles and Seltzer, 1980; Stone et al., 1977; Turbery et al., 1975):

Fibroadenoma	68.3%
Fibrocystic changes	18.5%
Abscess or mastitis	3.7%
Other benign lesions or tumors	2.6%
Virginal or juvenile hypertrophy	1.9%
Intraductal papilloma	1.2%
Cyst	1.2%
Giant fibroadenoma	1.1%
Cancer	0.9%
Cystosarcoma phyllodes	0.4%

Of the 12 malignant lesions reported in the above studies, five were primary breast cancer while the others consisted of Hodgkin's lymphoma, lymphosarcoma, angiosarcoma, and other metastatic tumors.

The prevalence of breast cancer in adolescents is extremely low. The practitioner should remember that these prevalences reflect surgically excised lesions. Fibrocystic disease or proliferative breast changes are probably more common than represented here.

Benign Breast Disease

Love (1990) suggests classifying benign breast lesions into the categories of physiological swelling and tenderness, mastalgia, nodularity, breast lumps or masses, and breast infections. These conditions, as well as malignant breast diseases in adolescents, are discussed in the remainder of this chapter.

Physiological Swelling and Tenderness   The breasts of most women of reproductive age have a nodular texture representing the glandular units or lobules of the breast. Under hormonal stimulation during each menstrual cycle, these lobules undergo proliferative changes. This results in changes varying from a feeling of fullness in the breast to distinct masses suggestive of a pathological process. Such physiological changes account for as many as 50% of breast complaints in adolescent females. If treatment is needed, analgesics or the use of a well-fitting brassiere worn both day and night can be tried.

Mastalgia (Severe Pain, Either Cyclic or Noncyclic)   Moderate-to-severe breast pain is another relatively common and occasionally distressing breast symptom. These symptoms have not been correlated to any histological changes. While the prevalence in adult females has been reported to be has high as 66% (Maddox and Mansel, 1989), the prevalence of mastalgia in adolescents is unknown. With noncyclic mastalgia the affected female can often point to a spot that hurts all the time, commonly located bilaterally in the upper outer quadrant of the breasts.

Modalities used to treat mastalgia have included heat, firm support, analgesics, hormonal therapy, evening primrose oil, diuretics, and in adults, danazol, bromocriptine, and tamoxifen. These latter drugs are not recommended for adolescents. Most adolescents only require reassurance and analgesics, such as the nonsteroidal antiinflammatory agents. Evening primrose oil, a compound primarily used in Europe, has been shown to be of benefit to some females with mastalgia (Pye et al., 1985). The overall response rate is 44% to a regimen consisting of two 500-mg capsules three times a day. The drug is usually tried for 3 months, and if the response is good, continued for 2 more months before withdrawal.

Proliferative Breast Changes (Nodularity, Fibrocystic Changes)

Most nodularity in adolescents and young adults is associated with proliferative breast changes or fibrocystic changes. Some authorities consider this condition a nondisease (Love et al., 1982) and recommend elimination of the term *fibrocystic disease.*

1. Prevalence: The prevalence in adolescents is unknown. If examined carefully, probably over 50% of women in the reproductive age group have some degree of fibrocystic changes. The prevalence increases during the third and fourth decade. At autopsy, 58–90% of women of virtually all ages have histologic changes associated with the name *fibrocystic disease.*
2. Pathophysiology: The exact cause of breast nodularity or fibrocystic changes is unknown. However, an imbalance between estrogen and progesterone has been implicated (Vorherr, 1986). With relatively higher estradiol-to-progesterone levels, connective and epithelial tissue proliferation occurs. Women with fibrocystic changes also have obstruction and persistent secretory material in alveoli and terminal ducts causing alveolar enlargement and cyst formation. In some studies methylxanthines (caffeine) have been implicated to worsen the condition.

   Fibrocystic changes usually occur in stages that correlate to the individual's age. Adolescents and women in their twenties have minimally symptomatic fibrotic tissue changes, particularly in the upper outer quadrants of the breasts. Changes in women in their thirties and forties usually include multiple small cysts with a diffuse increase in glandular tissue and increasing complaints of pain. Single large cysts are more common in women 35 years of age or older.
3. Clinical manifestations
   a. Fibrocystic changes are usually found either as painless lumps on examination or because of pain or discomfort.
   b. Symptoms, including tenderness, are most common about 1 week prior to menstruation and are often relieved by menstruation.
   c. Characteristic nodularity consists of hard and tender areas of a few millimeters to 1 cm in diameter.
4. Risk of breast cancer: In most instances there is no additional risk of breast cancer. In those unusual females with proliferative lesions with atypia, usually adult females, there is a five times increased risk of breast cancer.
5. Treatment: Many modalities have been suggested for treating fibrocystic changes. In most adolescents the symptoms are not severe enough to warrant aggressive measures.
   a. Supportive measures include well-padded brassieres in addition to mild analgesics.
   b. Hormonal modalities: Oral contraceptives can help in up to 70–90% of individuals, while medroxyprogesterone acetate (Provera) 10 mg on days 15–25 of the menstrual cycle has had success in up to 85% of women (Cox, 1986).
   c. Caffeine: A decrease in caffeine intake is advocated by some; however because of its very questionable effects, heavy restriction of diet should not be encouraged.
   d. Vitamin therapy, including vitamins B_1, A, and E, has been used, but a beneficial effect has not been proven.
   e. Danazol: While danazol has been used in adult women for severe fibrocystic breast changes, there is little experience with its use in adolescent females.

Fibroadenomas (Breast Lumps or Masses)

1. Definition: A fibroadenoma is a benign neoplasm of mammary gland that microscopically has stromal proliferation surrounding aggregates of compressed or uncompressed, elongated and distorted ducts.
2. Prevalence: Fibroadenomas are the most common breast tumor found in adolescents in surgical reports, comprising 60–90% of benign breast lesions. Most adolescents with this condition are over 14 with a large increase in prevalence in 15- and 16-year-olds. The condition has been reported to be twice as common in African-Americans. There is no evidence of progression to cancer.
3. Clinical manifestations
    a. Fibroadenomas are frequently discovered by the adolescent, often while bathing.
    b. Associated symptoms, other than the presence of a breast mass, are unusual. However, some adolescents will complain of breast discomfort during menstruation or pregnancy.
    c. The average duration of symptoms is about 5 months.
    d. On examination, the mass is usually a rubbery, firm, mobile, well demarcated, and nontender lesion. It is usually easy to distinguish the mass from surrounding breast tissue.
    e. Most commonly, there is only one fibroadenoma, with the largest prevalence in the upper outer quadrant of the breast. Sixty-three percent are in the lateral quadrants. Fibroadenomas are multiple in 10–25% of cases and bilateral in about 10%.
    f. Fibroadenomas range in size from less than 1 cm to more than 10 cm, with an average size of 2–3 cm.
4. Treatment: Treatment for fibroadenomas may involve either careful follow-up, especially if diagnosis has been confirmed by fine-needle aspiration cytology or elective surgical excision. These operations can often be performed under local anesthesia and sedation on an outpatient basis sparing teens the risk of general anesthesia. However, general anesthesia is recommended in adolescents with undue anxiety, with large pendulous breasts, or with deep lesions.

Cysts

Large cysts are another cause of benign breast masses. Cysts larger than 1 cm usually occur in women in their forties. Cysts are associated with few symptoms and on examination feel like a well-circumscribed, small, freely movable mass. These can usually be diagnosed and treated by fine-needle aspiration.

Giant Fibroadenoma

Some fibroadenomas, labeled juvenile or giant fibroadenomas, have much more rapid growth with a greater degree of stromal cellularity and the potential to grow to a large size, usually larger than 5 cm in diameter. Giant fibroadenomas, while uncommon, are found most commonly in young adolescents, with a greater prevalence in African-American teens. The mass has a rapid and asymmetric growth pattern, which may cause compression of adjacent breast tissue. The area may feel warmer due to the increased blood supply of the tumor. While encapsulated, the tumor may have a consistency similar to normal breast tissue, which may make it difficult to differentiate from normal tissue or unilateral virginal hypertrophy. Treatment of giant fibroadenomas is by simple excision sparing as much mammary tissue as possible. A simple mastectomy for this lesion is not warranted.

Phyllodes Tumors (Cystosarcoma Phyllodes)

Cystosarcoma phyllodes tumors usually present as a bulky mass in the breast. The lesions tend to be large, up to 20 cm, and sharply circumscribed. The mass is firm, mobile, and smooth or irregular. Overlaying skin may be stretched and shiny, with distended veins from the rapid growth of the tumor. Compared to juvenile giant fibroadenoma this lesion is more firm and more discrete. The lesion is almost always benign, but malignant lesions have been reported in adolescents. Microscopically, benign phyllodes tumors are similar to fibroadenomas containing both epithelial and connective tissue elements, but with a more cellular hyperplastic stroma. Phyllodes tumors lack complete encapsulation and extend into surrounding tissue in multiple projections of varying size.

Treatment recommendations range from simple excision to radical mastectomy, but little evidence exists to support the use of mastectomy as initial therapy (Mollit et al., 1987). Most adolescents and adults are cured by excision alone. The lesion should be excised completely with a surrounding rim of normal breast tissue. There is no need for a mastectomy unless the tumor is found to be malignant. There is also no reason for adjuvant chemotherapy or radiation in absence of metastatic disease.

Virginal or Juvenile Hypertrophy

Virginal or juvenile hypertrophy implies diffuse enlargement of the breast that is usually symmetrical occurring near the time of menarche.

1. Etiology: The cause of juvenile hypertrophy is not well understood but may represent an abnormal response of the breast to normal serum estrogen levels. Results from hormonal studies are normal in these individuals.
2. Clinical manifestations
   a. Pendulous and diffusely firm breasts without any discrete mass lesions: The breasts can get as large as 30–50 pounds.
   b. The breast tissue may be soft but sometimes has diffuse ropelike thickenings.
   c. Neck and back strain may be associated problems.
   d. The hypertrophy may cause significant psychologic problems and embarrassment.
   e. In contrast to the giant fibroadenoma, there is less thinning of the skin, less prevalence of enlarged veins, and less displacement of the nipple or areola.
3. Treatment: No definite therapeutic guidelines have been developed. While it is preferable to delay any surgery until the breasts have matured, this may not be practical in some adolescents if breast size or weight is unbearable. Four modalities of treatment have been recommended (Bauer et al., 1987).
   a. Reduction mammoplasty: This is the most common therapy but many adolescents may continue to have breast enlargement after this procedure.
   b. Subcutaneous mastectomy with implantation of a prosthesis: This may be the surgical procedure of choice in individuals with massive recurrent enlargement.
   c. Hormonal manipulation: This includes treatment with either medroxyprogesterone, dydrogesterone, or danazol (Danocrine). Dydrogesterone may suppress the secretion of growth hormone and also could interfere with development of secondary sexual characteristics. Teratogenic and carcinogenic effects have also been a concern with these medications.
   d. A combination of medications and surgery: This includes surgery plus the postoperative use of the dydrogesterone to prevent recurrences.

Intraductal Papilloma

An intraductal papilloma arises from an abnormal proliferation of cells in mammary ducts. The lesion is usually small and most frequently microscopic, consisting of simple proliferations of duct epithelium projecting into a dilated lumen. Because the proliferated epithelium is supported by a vascular stalk, slight local trauma may rupture this stalk, leading to a bloody discharge. The proliferation of cells may grow large enough so that a mass may be palpable.

1. Infrequent finding in the adolescent: The lesion is most frequent in women in their twenties through forties.
2. Often present with a bloody nipple discharge
3. Examination: Many individuals with this condition have well-defined nodules or thickenings near the areola.
4. Treatment: These lesions are uniformly benign and amenable to local excision.

Infections and Inflammations

Infections and inflammations include subareolar abscess, lactational mastitis, duct ectasia, and breast abscess.

A breast abscess or cellulitis can occur secondary to bacteria introduced from the skin into the ductal system or from cutaneous infections, foreign bodies, epidermal cysts, and trauma, such as shaving periareolar hair or trauma related to sexual play.

1. Breast abscesses are not common in adolescents, with the majority being related to lactation.
2. Abscesses are usually present similarly to an abscess elsewhere on the body, leading to the sudden onset of a tender or fluctuant mass with skin erythema.
3. Organisms: *Staphylococcus aureus* is the most common organism, followed by *Escherichia coli* and pseudomonas. Other organisms include group B β-hemolytic streptococcus and anaerobes.
4. Risk factors: Preceding factors may include trauma, ductal obstruction, or a preexisting cyst.
5. Treatment: Treatment involves the use of warm compresses and antibiotics.

Mastitis

1. Common occurrence in breast-feeding females
2. Etiology: Mastitis results from abrasions on the nipple that allow for infection and the clogging of lactiferous ducts, allowing for the stasis of milk.
3. Clinical manifestations: Pain, tenderness, induration, and fever. The abscess may be subcutaneous, subareolar, intramammary, or retromammary.
4. Organisms: The most common bacteria involved is *S. aureus*. However other organisms include streptococcus, *Micrococcus dyogenes*, *E. coli*, *Pseudomonas* sp., and others.
5. Diagnosis: An infection is likely with a leukocyte count from breast milk of over 10^6 per mL plus more than 10^3 bacteria per mL on culture. Culture and sensitivity of breast milk of the affected breast is helpful in identifying the organism and choosing an appropriate antibiotic.
6. Treatment: Heat and antibiotics are used in the treatment. Nursing or breast pumping can be continued using the unaffected breast. Nursing on the affected side can be quite painful.

Cancer of the Breast

1. Prevalence: During the past 70 years there have only been sporadic reports of breast cancer in females under the age of 20 (Hammar, 1981; Oberman and Stephens, 1971; Seltzer and Skiles, 1980). Less than 1% of all breast tumors in adolescents are cancerous, and 98% of breast cancer occurs in women older than 25 years. Of breast cancer cases in adolescents about one-third are primary tumors of breast tissue and the rest are either a tumor of nonbreast tissue or some form of metastatic cancer. In tabulation of English mortality data including over 70,000 deaths from breast cancer, there was one case of a child under the age of 5, one between 10–14, five between 15–19, and 27 between 20 and 24 (Close and Maximov, 1965).

2. Clinical manifestations: Schydlower, 1982 found that 90% of children and adolescents with breast cancer present with a breast mass. The mass is usually hard, is most commonly subareolar, and is frequently fixed to the deep tissues. Symptoms are uncommon with axillary lymphadenopathy present in only a few cases. Up to 30% of affected teens have a family history of breast cancer, and the tumor tends to occur earlier in the daughter than in the mother. The size varies from 1 to 2.5 cm in diameter, with the right and left breast equally affected.

3. Prognosis: Among teenagers survival is similar to adults, while the prognosis of carcinoma of the breast in prepubertal children seems better than in adults.

Diagnosis of Breast Masses in Adolescents

1. History
   a. Family history of breast tumors (both benign and malignant): The most significant risk factor is a history of breast cancer in several members of the teen's mother's family. Breast cancer in two or more of following add significantly to the risk profile: the teen's mother, maternal aunts, maternal grandmother, sister, and daughter.
   b. A history of trauma to the breast
   c. Menstrual and reproductive histories and a review of the use of contraceptives and other hormones
2. Breast examination
   a. Inspection: This consists of inspection of both breasts to observe for asymmetry or skin retraction. Traditionally this has been performed with the individual seated and in three different positions: leaning forward, extending her arms over her head, and pressing her hands against her hips (Sapira, 1990). However, these three positions are seldom helpful in the screening examination unless a mass is palpated. Because of this reason and the potential discomfort for the adolescent, the author would recommend skipping this maneuver for the screening examination.
   b. Palpation: The examiner should next palpate the breast for a mass or discharge. Palpation is performed while the teen is in the supine position. First, the teen's arm on the side to be examined should be placed behind her head. The examiner can also place a pillow or folded sheet under the posterior ribs. The breast should be palpated in an orderly fashion. The examiner can examine the breast in one of several ways.
      — In the first method the examiner uses a pattern similar to the spokes of a wheel. Starting with the tail of the breast in the axilla, the examiner moves in a straight line to the nipple. Using straight lines from the outer boundary of the breast to the nipple, the examiner can work around the whole breast.
      — A second method involves covering the breast in either concentric circles or a spiral pattern around the breast.

— A third method involves covering the breast by examining vertical strips.

Whichever method is used, the entire anterior chest wall should be palpated applying varying degrees of pressure with the pads of the second, third, and fourth fingers and rotating in small dime-sized circles. Particular attention should be given to the nipple and areolar areas, as 15% of breast cancers are located here. The areola should be compressed to elicit nipple discharge. The examiner should also palpate for supraclavicular, infraclavicular, and axillary nodes.

Throughout the examination, it is helpful to explain to the teen what is being done, using the examination time to discuss self-examination skills. Explain to the teen that she may be the best individual to notice if something has changed with her breasts. Combining this educational maneuver with the physical examination can be a useful method in alleviating fear and tension during the breast examination. In addition, reassure the teen that the breast has many lumps and bumps that may change, particularly with menstrual cycles.

3. Management of breast masses: The management of breast masses in adolescents still involves some controversy. If a mass were easy to diagnose by palpation, a biopsy would not be required, but palpation cannot exclude a malignant tumor. However, because of the rarity of malignant breast tumors, excisional biopsies should not be an urgent procedure. It is recommended to observe a breast mass in an adolescent through at least one complete menstrual cycle (Emans and Goldstein, 1990). Furnival (1983) reports that 77% of women have some resolution of fibrocystic changes. An excisional biopsy may be necessary if a mass persists over 3–6 months or continues to increase in size. An alternative approach would be to obtain a fine-needle aspiration with cytologic studies in these individuals. The role of fine needle aspiration has not been evaluated in the adolescent population. However, this procedure may be a good diagnostic test for breast masses in adolescents, as the surgical risks and scars of excisional biopsies are avoided. An excisional biopsy is also recommended for a hard mass, a fixed mass, or if there is skin dimpling, edema, ulceration or fixation to the chest wall, patient or parental anxiety about the mass, or a strong positive family history. Multiple or recurrent lesions that are stable in size should not be excised. If feasible, cysts can be aspirated and the fluid, if bloody, sent for cytological examination.

4. Other diagnostic modalities
   a. Mammography: Mammography is not generally helpful in the adolescent because breast tissue is very dense, and the prevalence rate of malignancy is low. In women less than 30 years there is poor correlation between mammographic diagnosis, and tissue diagnosis, as masses may be hidden in dense breast parenchyma.
   b. Ultrasound: An ultrasound is helpful in differentiating a solid mass from a cystic mass. However, the ultrasound cannot differentiate a benign from a malignant solid mass. An ultrasound can also help in guiding a needle into an abscess or cyst. In women aged 30 or less, the ultrasound can be helpful as a primary imaging examination to evaluate a breast mass. If a cyst is found, an aspiration can be done without need for further studies.

      There is no evidence to suggest a role for the ultrasound as a sole imaging technique for breast cancer screening.
   c. Fine-needle aspiration: In some centers a fine-needle aspiration is done as the primary technique without an ultrasound. If nonbloody fluid is found it is considered benign and not sent for cytology. The teen should be checked for a reoccurrence in 4 to 6 weeks. If a solid mass is encountered, an aspiration is performed with a cytologic smear made up for evaluation.

BIBLIOGRAPHY

Ackerman BL, Otis C, Stueber K. Lobular carcinoma in situ in a 15-year-old girl: a case report and review of the literature. Plast Reconstr Surg 1994;94:714.

Adler DD. Ultrasound of benign breast conditions. Semin Ultrasound CT MR 1989;10:106.

Atkins E, Solomon LJ, Worden JK, Foster RS Jr. Relative effectiveness of methods of breast self-examination. J Behav Med 1991;14:357.

Bachman JW. Breast problems. Prim Care 1988;15: 643–664.

Bauer BS, Jones KM, Talbot CW. Mammary masses in the adolescent female. Surg Gynecol Obstet 1987; 165:63.

Bower R, Bell M, Ternberg J. Management of breast lesions in children and adolescents. J Pediatr Surg 1976;3:337.

Cancer Committee, College of American Pathologists. Is fibrocystic disease of the breast precancerous? Report of a consensus meeting [October 3–5, New York]. Arch Pathol Lab Med 1986;110:171.

Close MB, Maximov NG. Carcinoma of breast in young girls. Arch Surg 1965;91:386–389.

Corriveau S, Jacobs JS. Macromastia in adolescence. Clin Plast Surg 1990;17:151.

Cox EB. Benign breast lesions and breast cancer: is there a relation? Female Patient 1986;11:52.

Daniel WA, Mathews MD. Tumors of the breast in adolescent females. Pediatrics 1968;41:743.

Dewhurst J. Breast disorders in children and adolescents. Pediatr Clin North Am 1981;28:287.

Diehl T, Kaplan DW. Breast masses in adolescent females. J Adolesc Health Care 1985;6:353.

Dixon JM. Periductal mastitis/duct ectasia. World J Surg 1989;13:715.

Dodd GD, Goodson WH III, Marchant DJ. Fibrocystic breasts: long-term care. Patient Care 1987;21:41.

Dudgeon DL. Pediatric breast lesions: take the conservative approach. Contemp Pediatr 1985;(January): 61–73.

Emans SJH, Goldstein DP. The breast: examination and lesions. In: Pediatric and adolescent gynecology. 3rd ed. Boston: Little, Brown & Co, 1990:437–450.

Ernster VL, Goodson WH, Hunt TK, et al. Vitamin E and benign breast "disease": a double-blind, randomized, clinical trial. Surgery 1985;4:490.

Ernster VL, Mason L, Goodson WH. Effects of caffeine-free diet on benign breast disease: a randomized trial. Surgery 1982;91:263.

Ernster VL, Mason L, Goodson WH III, et al. Effects of caffeine-free diet on benign breast disease: a randomized trial. Surgery 1982;91:263.

Farrow JH, Ashikari H. Breast lesions in young girls. 1969;49:261.

Furnival CM, Irwin JR, Gray GM. Breast disease in young women: when is biopsy indicated? Med J Aust 1983;2:167.

Gogas J, Sechas M, Skalkeas GR. Surgical management of disease of the adolescent female breast. Am J Surg 1979;137:634.

Goldstein DP, Miler V. Breast masses in adolescent females. Clin Pediatr 1982;21:17.

Greydanus DE, Parks DS, Farrell EG. Breast disorders in children and adolescents. Pediatr Clin North Am 1989;36:601.

Halverson JD, Hori-Fubaina JM. Cystosarcoma phyllodes of the breast. Am Surg 1974;40:295.

Hammar B: Childhood breast carcinoma: report of a case. J Pediatr Surg 1981;16:77.

Hein K, Dell R, Cohen MI. Self detection of a breast mass in adolescent females. J Adolesc Health Care 1982;3:15.

Hindle WH. Changing concepts in the evaluation of dominant breast masses. Female Patient 1990;15:40.

Hindle WH. Examination for breast cancer: assuring against a missed diagnosis. Mod Med 1991;59:34.

Jimerson GK. The adolescent breast: disorders and evaluation. Medical Aspects of Human Sexuality 1985; 19:66.

Ligon RE, Stevenson DR, Diner W, et al. Breast masses in young women. Am J Surg 1980;140:779.

Love SM. Fibrocystic disease: what's in a name? Patient Care 1990;24:65.

Love SM, Gelman RS, Silen W. Fibrocystic disease of the breast: a nondisease? N Engl J Med 1982;307:1010.

Love SM, Schnitt SJ, Connolly JL. Benign breast disorders. In: Harris JR, Hellman S, Henderson IC, eds. Breast diseases. Philadelphia: JB Lippincott, 1987.

Lubin F, Ron E, Wax Y, et al. A case-control study of caffeine and methylxanthines in benign breast disease. JAMA 1985;253:2388.

Maddox PR, Mansel RE. Management of breast pain and nodularity. World J Surg 1989;13:699.

Marchant DJ. Evaluation, diagnosis, and treatment of the fibrocystic breast. Mod Med 1987;55:42.

McGregor GI, Knowling MA, Este FA. Sarcoma and cystosarcoma phyllodes tumors of the breast—a retrospective review of 58 cases. Am J Surg 1994;167: 477.

Mollit DL, Golladay ES, Gloster ES, et al. Cystosarcoma phyllodes in the adolescent female. J Pediatr Surg 1987;22:907.

Neinstein LS, Atkinson J, Diament M. Prevalence and longitudinal study of breast masses in adolescents. J Adolesc Health 1993;14:277.

Oberman HA, Stephens PJ. Carcinoma of the breast in childhood. Cancer 1971;30:470.

Organ CH, Organ BC. Fibroadenoma of the female breast: a critical clinical assessment. J Natl Med Assoc 1983;75:701.

Pye JK, Mansel RE, Hughes LE. Clinical experience of drug treatments for mastalgia. Lancet 1985;2:373.

Raju CG. Breast masses in adolescent patients in Trinidad. Am J Surg 1985;149:219.

Sandison AT, Walker JC. Diseases of the adolescent female breast. Br J Surg 1968;55:443.

Sapira JD. The breast. In: Art and science of bedside diagnosis. Baltimore: Urban & Schwarzenberg, 1990: 239–244.

Schydlower M. Breast masses in adolescents. Am Fam Physician 1982;25:141.

Scott EB. Fibrocystic breast disease. Am Fam Physician 1986;36:119.

Seashore JH. Breast enlargements in infants and children. Pediatr Ann 1975;4:542.

Seltzer MH, Skiles MS. Diseases of the breast in young women. Surg Gynecol Obstet 1980;150:360.

Skiles MS, Seltzer MH. Adolescent breast disease. Nat Med Soc N J 1980;77:891.

Simmons PS, Wold LE. Surgically treated breast disease in adolescent females: a retrospective review of 185 cases. Adolesc Pediatr Gynecol 1989;2:95.

Simpson JS, Barson AJ. Breast tumors in infants and children: a 40-year review of cases at a children's hospital. Can Med Assoc J 1969;101:100.

Stone AM, Shenker IR, McCarthy K. Adolescent breast masses. Am J Surg 1977;134:275.

Turbery WJ, Buntain WL, Dudgeon DL. The surgical management of pediatric breast masses. Pediatrics 1975;56:736.

Vorherr H. Fibrocystic breast disease: pathophysiology, pathomorphology, clinical picture, and management. Am J Obstet Gynecol 1986;154:161.

Watkins F, Giacomantonio M, Salisbury S. Nipple discharge and breast lump related to Montgomery's tubercles in adolescent females. J Pediatr Surg 1988; 23:718.

Sexually Transmitted Diseases

CHAPTER 60

Overview of Sexually Transmitted Diseases

The formerly used term *morbus venereus*, or venereal disease, denoting any of several diseases acquired through sexual intercourse or other genital contact, has been supplanted by the term *sexually transmitted disease* (STD). STDs are an overwhelming problem; the original five classic venereal diseases have now expanded to a list of over 20 diseases. The annual incidence of gonorrhea, nongonococcal urethritis, and trichomoniasis is an estimated 2.5 million cases for each disease. Herpes simplex has an estimated annual incidence of 400,000–600,000 new cases each year; however, as many as 5–25 million Americans may be actively infected. The prevalence rates from studies in sexually active adolescent females include:

1. *Chlamydia trachomatis*, 8–25%
2. *Neisseria gonorrhoeae*, 3–18%
3. *Trichomonas vaginalis*, 0–48%
4. Human papilloma virus infections, 3–33%

The rates in adolescent males have not been so well studied, but the few studies available indicate rates in asymptomatic males of 3–14% for *C. trachomatis* and 1–3% for *N. gonorrhoeae*.

Although the actual numbers of many STDs are highest in the 20- to 24-year-old age group, adolescents still have the highest risk if these rates are corrected to include only those who are sexually active. While most individuals over 20 years of age are sexually active, many adolescents between 12 and 19 years of age are not.

The reasons for this elevated risk are not entirely known but include:

1. Cervical ectopy: *N. gonorrhoeae* and *C. trachomatis* have a predilection for columnar epithelium, and adolescents usually have significant cervical ectopy with much columnar epithelium present on the ectocervix.
2. Immature immune system: Adolescents have had less prior exposure to STDs and thus may be less protected against infections.
3. Contraceptive techniques: Adolescents do not use barrier methods consistently.

There has been a change in the ratio of males to females who have an STD. In prior years, STDs were more common in males, whereas currently in most instances females have higher rates. This may be secondary to greater use by females of STD clinics and also to the fact that adolescent females are becoming sexually active earlier than in prior years, with rates approaching those of adolescent males.

Other groups besides adolescents at increased risk for STDs include:

1. Individuals with multiple sexual partners in the past 6 months
2. Individuals with a past history of STDs
3. Women not using contraception

4. Prostitutes and their contacts
5. Users of illicit drugs
6. Inmates of detention centers

The practitioner should remember that adolescents with one STD may be infected with other STDs. The teen with an STD should thus be screened for other STDs, including gonor-

Tᴀʙʟᴇ 60.1.   Etiological Classification of Sexually Transmitted Diseases

Bacteria	Viruses
Neisseria gonorrhoeae	Herpes simplex
Chlamydia trachomatis	Hepatitis A
Treponema pallidum	Hepatitis B
Ureaplasma urealyticum	Cytomegalovirus (CMV)
Mycoplasma hominis	Genital wart
Haemophilus ducreyi	Molluscum contagiosum
Calymmatobacterium granulomatis	Human immunodeficiency virus (HIV)
Shigella species	Protozoa
Campylobacter fetus	*Trichomonas vaginalis*
Gardnerella vaginalis	*Entamoeba histolytica*
Streptococcus, group B (?)	*Giardia lamblia*
	Ectoparasites
	Pthirus pubis (crab louse)
	Sarcoptes scabiei (scabies mite)

Tᴀʙʟᴇ 60.2.   Sexually Transmitted Diseases by Presenting Symptom

1. Urethritis or dysuria
   a. Gonorrhea
   b. *Chlamydia trachomatis*
   c. *Ureaplasma urealyticum*
   d. Herpes simplex
   e. *Trichomonas vaginalis* (primarily females)
   f. Possibly: *Candida, Mycoplasma hominis*
2. Vaginitis or cervicitis
   a. *Candida:* Vulva and vagina
   b. *Trichimonas:* Vagina and cervix
   c. *Neisseria gonorrhoeae:* Cervix
   d. *Chlamydia trachomatis:* Cervix
   e. *Gardnerella vaginalis:* Vagina
   f. Herpes simplex virus
3. Genital ulcers
   a. Herpes simplex
   b. Syphilis: *Treponema pallidum*
   c. Chancroid: *Haemophilus ducreyi*
   d. Lymphogranuloma venereum: *Chlamydia trachomatis*
   e. Granuloma inguinale: *Calymmatobacterium granulomatis*
4. Genital growths
   a. Genital warts
   b. Molluscum contagiosum
   c. Condylomata lata: Syphilis
5. Abdominal pain
   a. Pelvic inflammatory disease
      — *Neisseria gonorrhoeae*
      — Mixed bacterial infections
      — Aerobes and anaerobes
      — *Chlamydia trachomatis*
   b. *Trichomonas vaginalis:* Rare
6. Enteritis and proctitis: Gay bowel syndrome
   a. *Neisseria gonorrhoeae*
   b. *Shigella*
   c. *Campylobacter fetus*
   d. *Entamoeba histolytica*
   e. *Giardia lamblia*
7. Epididymitis
   a. *Chlamydia trachomatis*
   b. *Neisseria gonorrhoeae*
   c. *Trichonomas vaginalis:* Rare
8. Hepatitis
   a. Hepatitis A and B
   b. Cytomegalovirus (CMV)
9. Arthritis
   a. *Neisseria gonorrhoeae*
   b. Hepatitis B virus
10. Pruritus: Body
   a. Crab louse: *Pthirus pubis*
   b. Scabies mite: *Sarcoptes scabiei*
11. Mononucleosis syndrome
   a. Cytomegalovirus (CMV)
   b. Hepatitis A and B virus
   c. *Chlamydia trachomatis:* Lymphogranuloma venereum (fever and adenopathy)
   d. Human immunodeficiency virus (HIV)
12. Fetal and perinatal infections
   a. Syphilis
   b. *Neisseria gonorrhoeae*
   c. *Chylamydia trachomatis*
   d. Herpes simplex
   e. Hepatitis B
   f. Human immunodeficiency virus (HIV)
   g. Human papilloma virus (HPV)
   h. Cytomegalovirus (CMV)
   i. Bacterial vaginosis

rhea, *Chlamydia,* and syphilis. The practitioner should also consider a serologic test for HIV. For adolescents seeking evaluation or treatment for an STD, the practitioner should use the opportunity to discuss contraception and the importance of condom use.

The adolescent with an STD should receive counseling regarding lowering his or her exposure to future STDs, including abstinence, condom use, spermicide use, periodic examinations, STD screening, and selection of partners.

Table 60.1 provides an etiological classification of STDs. In view of the fact that most adolescents complain of a particular set of symptoms and not a specific organism, a list of presenting symptoms for the STDs is also included (Table 60.2). As a broad overview, the appendix to this chapter summarizes the clinical features and treatment of many of the well-known STDs. The remaining chapters in Section XIII focus on individual STDs in more detail.

APPENDIX:
SEXUALLY TRANSMITTED DISEASES SUMMARY[a]

NOTE: For a full review of information contained in the "Therapy" section for each disease, see Morbidity and Mortality Weekly Report, volume 42, number RR–14. For a copy of this publication, write Centers for Disease Control, Technical Information Services, Atlanta, GA 30333.

---

[a]Adapted from U.S. Department of Health and Human Services, Centers for Disease Control, Center for Prevention Services. Sexually transmitted diseases summary. 1986;35(55):1–57, and Centers for Disease Control, Sexually transmitted diseases treatment guidelines, 1989 and 1993. MMWR 1989;37(54, suppl):1–57 and 1993;42(RR–14).

Nᴏɴɢᴏɴᴏᴄᴏᴄᴄᴀʟ Uʀᴇᴛʜʀɪᴛɪs

Etiologic Agents

Chlamydia trachomatis (23–55%)
Ureaplasma urealyticum (20–40%)
Trichomonas vaginalis (2–5%)
Herpes simplex virus on occasion

TYPICAL CLINICAL PRESENTATION

Men usually have dysuria, frequency, and mucoid-to-purulent urethral discharge. Some men have asymptomatic infections.

Steady female sexual partners of men with chlamydial nongonococcal urethritis (NGU) are likely to have chlamydial endocervicitis.

PRESUMPTIVE DIAGNOSIS

(Warrants full treatment and follow-up)

Men with typical clinical symptoms are presumed to have NGU when gonorrhea test results are negative and they have either >5 polymorphonuclear (PMN) leukocytes per oil immersion field on a smear of an intraurethral swab specimen or sexual exposure to an agent known to cause NGU.

Asymptomatic men with negative gonorrhea test results are also presumed to have NGU if they have at least 5 white blood cells (WBCs) per oil immersion field on an intraurethral smear. Increasingly a leukocyte esterase test (LET) is used to screen asymptomatic males for urethritis. Positive LET results should be confirmed with a Gram-stained smear of a urethral swab specimen or gonorrhea and chlamydia testing.

DEFINITIVE DIAGNOSIS

An agent etiologically associated with NGU is recovered from the male urethra.

NOTE: Gonococcal and nongonococcal urethritis may coexist in the same patient.

THERAPY

Recommended Regimen

Doxycycline 100 mg orally 2 times daily for 7 days; OR

Azithromycin 1 g orally in a single dose.

Alternative Regimens

Erythromycin base 500 mg orally 4 times daily for 7 days; OR

Erythromycin ethylsuccinate 800 mg orally 4 times daily for 7 days.

If patient cannot tolerate high-dose erythromycin schedules, one of the following regimens can be used:

Erythromycin base 250 mg orally 4 times a day for 14 days; OR

Erythromycin ethylsuccinate 400 mg orally 4 times a day for 14 days.

NOTE: Patients with persistent or recurrent objective signs of urethritis after adequate treatment of themselves and their partners warrant further evaluation for less common causes of urethritis.

COMPLICATIONS AND SEQUELAE

Urethral strictures

Prostatitis

Epididymitis

Reiter's syndrome

Chlamydial NGU may be transmitted to female sexual partners, resulting in mucopurulent endocervicitis, pelvic inflammatory disease (PID), and other adverse outcomes. (See entries related to these conditions in the succeeding pages.)

OTHER CONSIDERATIONS

Pregnant Women: Doxycycline is contraindicated for pregnant women. The safety of azithromycin among pregnant and lactating women is not known.

Follow-Up: Patients should return for follow-up if symptoms persist or recur after therapy. If treatment is not completed or patient is re-exposed to an untreated sex partner, patient should be retreated with initial regimen. Otherwise, the patient should have wet mount and culture for *T. vaginalis;* if the results are negative, the patient should be retreated with an alternative regimen extended to 14 days.

Management of Sex Partners: Sex partners should be referred for evaluation and treatment.

HIV Infection: Patients with human immunodeficiency virus (HIV) infection should receive the same treatment as patients without HIV.

Mucopurulent Cervicitis

Etiologic Agents

Chlamydia trachomatis
Neisseria gonorrhoeae

(In most cases neither of these organisms can be isolated.)

TYPICAL CLINICAL PRESENTATION

The patient may be symptomatic or asymptomatic, and a yellow mucopurulent endocervical exudate may be present.

PRESUMPTIVE DIAGNOSIS

(Warrants full treatment and follow-up)

The presence of yellow mucopurulent endocervical exudate or the finding of this exudate on a white cotton-tipped swab of endocervical secretions suggests infection. In women without visible mucopus, the presence of ≥10 PMN leukocytes per X 1000 field on a Gram-stained specimen of endocervical mucus (without contamination by vaginal cells) also allows a presumptive diagnosis.

DEFINITIVE DIAGNOSIS

Definitive diagnosis is made by a positive Chlamydia test result (culture, direct immunofluorescence assay [DFA], or DNA probe) or a positive gonorrhea test result (culture or DNA probe).

THERAPY

Treatment is based on the results of Chlamydia and gonorrhea testing. If the patient is unreliable or in an area of high likelihood of gonorrhea or Chlamydia infection, treat presumptively with coverage for both gonorrhea and Chlamydia.

COMPLICATIONS AND SEQUELAE

Ascending infections may lead to symptomatic or asymptomatic endometritis and salpingitis and subsequent infertility. Ascending infection during pregnancy may lead to adverse obstetric outcomes, conjunctivitis, or pneumonia in the infant, and to puerperal infection.

OTHER CONSIDERATIONS

Follow-Up: Follow-up should be similar to that recommended for the type of STD diagnosed.

Management of Sex Partners: Sex partners should be managed as appropriate for the underlying STD identified. Partners of patients treated presumptively should receive same treatment as patient.

HIV Infection: Patients with HIV infection should receive the same treatment as patients without HIV infection.

Gonorrhea

Etiologic Agent

Neisseria gonorrhoeae
(A Gram-negative diplococcus.)

TYPICAL CLINICAL PRESENTATION	**THERAPY**
When symptomatic, men usually have dysuria, frequency, and purulent urethral discharge. Women may have abnormal vaginal discharge, abnormal menses, or dysuria or be asymptomatic. Women may not have symptoms until complications like PID have occurred. Anorectal and pharyngeal infections are common. These may be symptomatic or asymptomatic.	**Recommended Regimen for Uncomplicated Gonococcal Infections** Ceftriaxone 125 mg IM at one time; OR Cefixime 400 mg orally in a single dose; OR Ciprofloxacin 500 mg orally in a single dose; OR Ofloxacin 400 mg orally in a single dose. – In addition to one of the above regimens, a regimen effective against possible coinfection with *C. trachomatis* such as doxycycline should be added. – These recommended regimens cured >95% of anal and genital infections. Ceftriaxone and ciprofloxacin regimens can cure >90% of pharyngeal infections and should be used if the pharynx is a suspected site of infection. – Cefixime has the advantage of being given orally, but it is not known if it can cure incubating syphilis. – Quinolones are contraindicated for pregnant or nursing women and for persons ≤17 years of age.
PRESUMPTIVE DIAGNOSIS (Warrants full treatment and follow-up) Microscopic identification of typical Gram-negative intracellular diplococci on smear of urethral exudate (men) or endocervical material (women): Cervical specimens that are Gram-stain tested should also be cultured for *N. gonorrhoeae;* OR Growth on selective medium demonstrating typical colonial morphology, positive oxidase reaction, and typical Gram-stain morphology: Alternatively, a positive DNA probe test result.	**Alternative Regimens** Spectinomycin 2 g IM, a single dose. Injectable cephalosporin regimens other than ceftriaxone 125 mg such as ceftizoxime 500 mg IM in a single dose; cefotaxime 500 mg IM in a single dose; cefotetan 1 g IM in a single dose; and cefoxitin 2 g IM in a single dose. Oral cephalosporin regimens other than cefixime such as cefuroxime axetil 1 g orally in a single dose and cefpodoxime proxetil 200 mg orally in a single dose. Quinolone regimens other than ciprofloxacin and ofloxacin such as enoxacin 400 mg orally in a single dose; lomefloxacin 400 mg orally in a single dose; and norfloxacin 800 mg orally in a single dose.
DEFINITIVE DIAGNOSIS Growth on selective medium demonstrating typical colonial morphology, positive oxidase reaction, typical Gram-stain morphology, and confirmed by sugar utilization, coagglutination, or antigonococcal fluorescent antibody (FA) testing. A definitive diagnosis is required if specimen is extragenital, from a child, or medicolegally significant.	**COMPLICATIONS AND SEQUELAE** Ten percent to 20% of women develop PID and are at risk for its sequelae (see entry following). Men are at risk for epididymitis, sterility, urethral stricture, and infertility. Newborns are at risk for ophthalmia neonatorum, scalp abscess at the site of fetal monitors, rhinitis, pneumonia, or anorectal infections. All infected, untreated persons are at risk for disseminated gonococcal infection (includes septicemia, arthritis, dermatitis, meningitis, and endocarditis).
	OTHER CONSIDERATIONS Patients treated for gonorrhea should be screened for syphilis by serologic testing. **Pregnant Women:** Should not be treated with tetracycline or quinolones. **Follow-Up:** No test-of-cure needed for patients with uncomplicated gonorrhea treated with one of the regimens in these guidelines. Treatment failures are most likely due to reinfection. **Management of Sex Partners:** Sex partners should be referred for evaluation and treatment. Treatment should include coverage for both *N. gonorrhoeae* and *C. trachomatis* infections. Sexual intercourse should be avoided until patient and partners are cured. **HIV Infection:** Patients with HIV infection should receive the same treatment as patients without HIV infection.

CHLAMYDIA

Etiologic Agents

Chlamydia trachomatis

TYPICAL CLINICAL PRESENTATION

The patient may be symptomatic or asymptomatic. In females, dysuria and a yellow mucopurulent endocervical exudate may be present. Women may not have symptoms until complications like PID have occurred. When symptomatic, men usually have dysuria, frequency, and a purulent urethral discharge.

PRESUMPTIVE DIAGNOSIS

(Warrants full treatment and follow-up)

Women: The presence of yellow mucopurulent endocervical exudate or the finding of this exudate on a white cotton-tipped swab of endocervical secretions suggests infection. The presence of ≥10 PMN leukocytes per X 1000 field on a Gram-stained specimen of endocervical mucus (without contamination by vaginal cells) also allows a presumptive diagnosis.

Men: Men with typical clinical symptoms are presumed to have *Chlamydia* when gonorrhea test results are negative and they have either >5 PMN leukocytes per oil immersion field on a smear of an intraurethral swab specimen or sexual exposure to *Chlamydia*. Increasingly, a leukocyte esterase test (LET) is used to screen asymptomatic males for Chlamydia urethritis. Positive LET results should be confirmed with a Gram-stained smear of a urethral swab specimen or gonorrhea and Chlamydia testing.

DEFINITIVE DIAGNOSIS

Definitive diagnosis is made with a positive Chlamydia test (culture, DFA, or DNA probe).

THERAPY

Recommended Regimens

Doxycycline 100 mg, orally, 2 times daily for 7 days; OR Azithromycin 1 g, orally, in a single dose.

Alternative Regimens

Ofloxacin 300 mg orally 2 times a day for 7 days; OR
Erythromycin base 500 mg orally 4 times a day for 7 days; OR
Erythromycin ethylsuccinate 800 mg orally 4 times a day for 7 days; OR
Sulfisoxazole 500 mg orally 4 times a day for 10 days (inferior efficacy to other regimens).

Safety of azithromycin for persons 15 years or younger has not been established. Ofloxacin has similar efficacy to doxycycline and azithromycin but is more expensive and cannot be used during pregnancy or with persons 17 years or younger.

COMPLICATIONS AND SEQUELAE

Ascending infections may lead to symptomatic or asymptomatic endometritis and salpingitis and subsequent infertility. Ascending infection during pregnancy may lead to adverse obstetric outcomes, conjunctivitis, or pneumonia in the infant, and to puerperal infection.

OTHER CONSIDERATIONS

Pregnant Women: Doxycycline and ofloxacin are contraindicated for pregnant women, and sulfisoxazole is contraindicated for women during pregnancy near-term and for women who are nursing. The safety of azithromycin among pregnant and lactating women is not known.

Recommended Regimen

Erythromycin base 500 mg orally 4 times a day for 7 days.

Alternative Regimens

Erythromycin base 250 mg orally 4 times a day for 14 days; OR
Erythromycin ethylsuccinate 800 mg orally 4 times a day for 7 days; OR
Erythromycin ethylsuccinate 400 mg orally 4 times a day for 14 days.

Follow-Up: No need for retesting after completing treatment with doxycycline or azithromycin unless symptoms persist or reinfection is suspected. If done, *Chlamydia* retesting at <3 weeks after completion of therapy may be associated with false-positive and false-negative results.

Management of Sex Partners: Sex partners should be referred for evaluation and treatment. Sex partners of symptomatic patients with *C. trachomatis* should be evaluated and treated if their last sexual contact with the index patient was within 30 days of onset of the index patient's symptoms. If the index patient is asymptomatic, referral of sex partners within the last 60 days is recommended.

HIV Infection: Patients with HIV infection should receive the same treatment as patients without HIV infection.

Pᴇʟᴠɪᴄ Iɴꜰʟᴀᴍᴍᴀᴛᴏʀʏ Dɪsᴇᴀsᴇ

Etiologic Agents

In the majority of cases, sexually transmitted organisms, especially *N. gonorrhoeae* and *C. trachomatis*, are implicated. However, other microorganims that can be part of vaginal flora, such as anaerobes, *G. vaginalis, H. influenzae,* enteric Gram-negative rods, and *Streptococcus agalactiae* can cause pelvic inflammatory disease (PID). *M. hominis* and *U. urealyticum* may also play a role.

TYPICAL CLINICAL PRESENTATION

The spectrum of PID includes any combination of endometritis, salpingitis, tubo-ovarian abscess, and pelvic peritonitis. The patient may present with pain and tenderness involving the lower abdomen, cervix, uterus, and adnexae, possibly combined with fever, chills, and elevated WBC count and erythrocyte sedimentation rate (ESR).

PRESUMPTIVE DIAGNOSIS

The clinical diagnosis of PID can be difficult and imprecise because of the wide variation of symptoms and signs. No combination of symptoms, signs, or laboratory findings is both sensitive and specific for diagnosing PID. Because of the difficulty of diagnosis and the potential for damage to the reproductive health of the woman with PID, the provider should maintain a low threshold for the diagnosis of PID.

Minimum Criteria: Empiric treatment of PID should be started in the presence of all the three minimum clinical criteria and in the absence of an established cause of abdominal pain other than PID:

- Lower abdominal tenderness
- Adnexal tenderness
- Cervical motion tenderness

Additional Criteria: These additional criteria may increase the specificity of the diagnosis:

Routine Criteria

- Oral temperature >38.3°C
- Abnormal cervical or vaginal discharge
- Elevated ESR
- Elevated C-reactive protein
- Laboratory documentation of cervical infection with *N. gonorrhoeae* or *C. trachomatis*

Elaborate Criteria

- Histopathologic evidence of endometritis on endometrial biopsy
- Tubo-ovarian abscess on sonography
- Laparoscopic abnormalities consistent with PID

THERAPY

Many experts recommend that all patients with PID be hospitalized to initiate parenteral antibiotics. Hospitalization of patients with PID is especially recommended in the following circumstances:

1. The diagnosis is uncertain; and surgical emergencies such as appendicitis and ectopic pregnancy cannot be excluded.
2. A pelvic abscess is suspected.
3. The patient is pregnant.
4. The patient is an adolescent.
5. The patient has HIV infection.
6. Severe illness or nausea and vomiting preclude outpatient management.
7. The patient is unable to follow or tolerate an outpatient regimen.
8. The patient has failed to respond to outpatient therapy.
9. Clinical follow-up within 72 hours of starting antibiotic treatment cannot be arranged.

INPATIENT TREATMENT

Regimen A

Cefoxitin 2 g IV every 6 hours or cefotetan 2 g IV every 12 hours; PLUS
Doxycycline 100 mg IV or orally every 12 hours.

Regimen B

Clindamycin 900 mg IV every 8 hours; PLUS
Gentamicin loading dose IV or IM (2 mg/kg of body weight) followed by a maintenance dose (1.5 mg/kg) every 8 hours.

These regimens should be continued for at least 48 hours after the patient demonstrates improvement. Thereafter, doxycycline 100 mg orally 2 times a day or clindamycin 450 mg orally 4 times a day should be continued for a total of 14 days.

Pelvic Inflammatory Disease
(Continued)

DEFINITIVE DIAGNOSIS

Direct visualization of inflamed (edema, hyperemia, or tubal exudate) fallopian tube(s) at laparoscopy or laparatomy makes the diagnosis of PID definitive. A culture of tubal exudate establishes the etiology.

OUTPATIENT TREATMENT

Little information is available from clinical trials on intermediate and long- term outcomes using outpatient regimens. If patients do not respond within 72 hours to outpatient regimens, they should be hospitalized to confirm diagnosis and receive parenteral treatment.

Regimen A

Cefoxitin 2 g IM plus probenecid, 1 g orally in a single dose concurrently, or ceftriaxone 250 mg IM or other parenteral third-generation cephalosporin (e.g., ceftizoxime or cefotaxime); PLUS
Doxycycline 100 mg orally 2 times a day for 14 days.

Regimen B

Ofloxacin 400 mg orally 2 times a day for 14 days; PLUS
Either clindamycin 450 mg orally 4 times a day or metronidazole 500 mg orally 2 times a day for 14 days.

COMPLICATIONS AND SEQUELAE

Potentially life-threatening complications include ectopic pregnancy and pelvic abscess. Other complications are involuntary infertility, recurrent PID, chronic PID, chronic abdominal pain, pelvic adhesions, premature hysterectomy, and depression.

OTHER CONSIDERATIONS

Pregnant Women: Should be treated as inpatients.

Follow-Up: Hospitalized patients should show substantial clinical improvement within 3–5 days or require further diagnostic workup. Patients treated as outpatients should be followed up within 72 hours and after significant clinical improvement. Patients should be tested for *N. gonorrhoeae* and *C. trachomatis* 7–10 days after completing therapy.

Management of Sex Partners: Sex partners should be referred for evaluation and treatment. Treatment should include coverage for both *N. gonorrhoeae* and *C. trachomatis* infections. Sexual intercourse should be avoided until patient and partners are cured.

HIV Infection: Patients with HIV infection should be managed aggressively including hospitalization.

VAGINITIS

Etiologic Agent

Trichomonas vaginalis vaginitis
(A motile protozoan with an undulating membrane and four flagella.)

Bacterial vaginosis (also called nonspecific vaginitis or *Gardnerella vaginalis*–associated vaginitis). Clinical syndrome resulting from replacement of normal vaginal flora with anaerobic bacteria, *G. vaginalis*, and *Mycoplasma hominis*.

Fungal vaginitis (predominantly *Candida albicans* or occasionally by other *Candida* sp., *Torulopsis* sp., or other yeasts).

Other vaginitides (vaginitis caused by other infectious, chemical, allergenic, and physical agents).

TYPICAL CLINICAL PRESENTATION

Presentations vary from no signs or symptoms to erythema, edema, and pruritus of the external genitalia. Excessive or malodorous discharge is a common finding.

Male sexual partners may develop urethritis, balanitis, or cutaneous lesions on penis.

PRESUMPTIVE DIAGNOSIS

(Warrants full treatment and follow-up)

The diagnosis of vaginitis is made by pH and microscopic examination of fresh samples of the discharge.

Trichomonas vaginalis Vaginitis

There are no presumptive criteria for this diagnosis.

Bacterial Vaginosis

The clinical criteria include three of the following:

- A homogenous gray or white noninflammatory discharge that adheres to vaginal walls
- Vaginal pH greater than 4.5
- A fishy odor from vaginal fluid before or after addition of 10% potassium hydroxide (KOH)
- Presence of clue cells on microscopic examination

Vulvovaginal Candidiasis (VVC)

The presumptive criteria are the typical symptoms of vaginitis or vulvitis and microscopic identification of yeast forms (budding cells or hyphae) in Gram's stain or KOH wet mount preparation of vaginal discharge.

THERAPY

Trichomonas vaginalis Vaginitis

Recommended Regimen: Metronidazole 2 g orally in a single dose.

Alternative Regimen: Metronidazole 500 mg twice daily for 7 days.

- Both regimens have cure rates of approximately 95%. Metronidazole gel has not been studied for treatment of trichomoniasis.

Bacterial Vaginosis

Recommended Regimen: Metronidazole 500 mg orally 2 times a day for 7 days (95% cure rate).

Alternative Regimen: Metronidazole 2 g in a single oral dose (84% cure rate).

Regimens with Limited Clinical Experience: Clindamycin cream 2%, one full applicator (5 g) intravaginally at bedtime for 7 days; OR

Metronidazole gel 0.75%, one full applicator (5 g) intravaginally, 2 times a day for 5 days; OR

Clindamycin 300 mg orally 2 times a day for 7 days.

Fungal Vaginitis

Clotrimazole, miconazole nitrate, terconazole, or butoconazole creams or vaginal tablets are recommended. Regimens range from 3 to 14 days of treatment. Oral regimens of fluconazole and other agents are being investigated (see Chapter 55).

COMPLICATIONS AND SEQUELAE

Secondary excoriations are common.

Recurrent infections are common.

Bacterial vaginosis may be associated with infectious complications of pregnancy, such as chorioamnionitis and puerperal infection, and with polymicrobial upper genital tract infections in nonpregnant women, such as endometritis and salpingitis.

Fungal vaginitis in pregnancy increases the risk of neonatal oral thrush.

Vaginitis
(Continued)

DEFINITIVE DIAGNOSIS	OTHER CONSIDERATIONS

DEFINITIVE DIAGNOSIS

Trichomonas vaginalis Vaginitis

A vaginal culture is positive for *T. vaginalis;* OR

Typical motile trichomonads are identified in a saline wet mount of vaginal discharge.

Bacterial Vaginosis

The most practical confirmatory microbiological test is the demonstration of characteristic changes in vaginal flora by Gram's stain of vaginal fluid; few or no lactobacilli, with a predominance of *G. vaginalis* plus other organisms resembling Gram-negative *Bacteroides* sp., anaerobic Gram-positive cocci, or curved rods.

Fungal Vaginitis

Culture may be useful when signs and symptoms are suggestive but when the fungus cannot be identified by direct microscopy.

OTHER CONSIDERATIONS

Pregnant Women: Use of metronidazole is contraindicated in first trimester of pregnancy. Metronidazole can be used after the first trimester with a single dose of 2 g. Clindamycin vaginal cream can be used to treat bacterial vaginosis during the first trimester of pregnancy. For treating vulvovaginal candidiasis only topical azole therapies should be used.

Follow-Up

Bacterial Vaginosis: No follow-up visits are necessary.

Trichomoniasis: Follow-up is unnecessary for patients who become asymptomatic after treatment.

Vulvovaginal Candidiasis: Follow-up is unnecessary for patients who respond to therapy.

Management of Sex Partners

Bacterial Vaginosis: Treatment of partners is not recommended.

Trichomoniasis: Sex partners should be treated and sexual contact should be avoided until both patient and partners are cured.

Vulvovaginal Candidiasis: Treatment of sex partners is not routinely warranted unless male sexual partner has balanitis.

HIV Infection

Bacterial Vaginosis, Triconomiasis, and Vulvovaginal Candidiasis: Patients with HIV infection should be managed in the same manner as patients without HIV infection.

Condylomata Acuminata (Genital Warts)
Etiologic Agent
Human papilloma virus (HPV)

(Certain types [usually 6 and 11] cause exophytic benign genital and anal warts. Other types present in the anogenital region [16, 18, 31, 33, and 35] and have been found to be strongly associated with genital dysplasia and carcinoma.)

TYPICAL CLINICAL PRESENTATION

Condylomata acuminata present as single or multiple soft, fleshy, papillary or sessile, painless growths around the anus, vulvovaginal area, penis, urethra, or perineum.

PRESUMPTIVE DIAGNOSIS

(Warrants full treatment and follow-up)

A diagnosis may be made on the basis of the typical clinical presentation.

Colposcopy may also aid in the diagnosis of certain cervical lesions.

The possibility of condylomata lata can be excluded by obtaining a dark-field or serologic test for syphilis.

DEFINITIVE DIAGNOSIS

A biopsy, although usually unnecessary, can make a definitive diagnosis. Very atypical lesions, where neoplasia is a consideration, should be biopsied before initiating therapy.

A Pap smear of cervical lesions shows typical cytologic changes. Direct DNA immunofluorescent staining techniques can diagnose certain types of HPV.

THERAPY

The goal of therapy is removal of exophytic warts and alleviating signs and symptoms, not the eradication of HPV.

External Genital or Perianal and Vaginal Condylomata Acuminata

Cryotherapy with liquid nitrogen or cryoprobe: For vaginal warts do not use cryoprobe (to avoid perforations); OR

Podofilox 0.5% solution for self-treatment (genital warts only): Applied in cycles of twice daily for 3 days followed by 4 days of no therapy. May be repeated for 4 cycles; OR

Podophyllin 10–25% in compound tincture of benzoin: Wash off in 1–4 hours; OR

Trichlorocetic acid (TCA) 80–90%: Weekly for maximum of 6 weeks; OR

Electrodesiccation or electrocautery.

Cervical Condylomata Acuminata

Dysplasia must be excluded before treatment is begun. Management is complicated and should be carried out in consultation with an expert.

Vaginal Warts: Cryotherapy with liquid nitrogen or TCA or podophyllin.

Anal or Oral Warts: Cryotherapy with liquid nitrogen or TCA or surgical removal.

COMPLICATIONS AND SEQUELAE

Lesions may enlarge and produce tissue destruction. Giant condyloma, while histologically benign, may stimulate carcinoma. Cervical lesions have been associated with neoplasia.

In pregnancy, warts enlarge, are extremely vascular, and may obstruct the birth canal, necessitating cesarean section.

OTHER CONSIDERATIONS

Pregnant Women: Use of podophyllin and podofilox are contraindicated.

Follow-Up: Not necessary after warts have responded to therapy. Annual cytologic screening recommended for women with or without genital warts.

Management of Sex Partners: Partners may wish to be examined and treated for clinical lesions. Reinfection from a partner is unusual. Use of condoms may reduce transmission to partners who are uninfected.

HIV Infection: Patients with HIV may not respond to therapy for HPV as well as persons without HIV.

HERPES GENITALIS
Etiologic Agents
Herpes simplex virus (HSV) types 1 and 2

TYPICAL CLINICAL PRESENTATION

Single or multiple vesicles appear anywhere on the genitalia. Vesicles spontaneously rupture to form shallow ulcers that may be very painful. Lesions resolve spontaneously without scarring. The first occurrence is termed initial infection (mean duration 12 days). Subsequent, usually milder, occurrences are termed recurrent infections (mean duration 4–5 days). The interval between clinical episodes is termed latency. Viral shedding occurs intermittently during latency.

PRESUMPTIVE DIAGNOSIS

(Warrants full treatment and follow-up)

When typical genital lesions are present or a pattern of recurrence has developed, herpes infection is likely. A presumptive diagnosis is further supported by direct identification of multinucleated giant cells with intranuclear inclusions in a clinical specimen prepared by Papanicolaou or other histochemical stain; OR typical HSV morphology by electron microscopy; OR detection of HSV antigens by monoclonal or polyclonal antibody detection systems. Primary HSV infection is presumed if an initially negative serologic titer becomes significantly detectable in convalescent serum.

DEFINITIVE DIAGNOSIS

An HSV virus tissue culture demonstrates the characteristic cytopathic effect (CPE) following inoculation of a specimen from the cervix, the urethra, or the base of a genital lesion. The isolates can be identified as type 1 or type 2 by fluorescent antibody, neutralization, or other serological techniques.

THERAPY

There is no known cure.

First Clinical Episode of Genital Herpes

Recommended Regimen: Acyclovir 200 mg orally 5 times a day for 7–10 days or until clinical resolution is attained.

First Clinical Episode of Herpes Proctitis

Recommended Regimen: Acyclovir 400 mg orally 5 times a day for 10 days or until clinical resolution is attained.

Recurrent Episodes of Genital Herpes and Herpes Proctitis:

When treatment is started during prodrome or within 2 days of onset of lesions, some patients experience limited benefit. However, most immunocompetent patients with recurrent disease do not benefit from acyclovir treatment.

Recommended Regimen if Used:

Acyclovir 200 mg orally 5 times a day for 5 days; OR
Acyclovir 400 mg orally 3 times a day for 5 days; OR
Acyclovir 800 mg orally 2 times a day for 5 days.

Daily Suppressive Therapy of Genital Herpes and Herpes Proctitis

Daily suppressive therapy can reduce frequency of HSV recurrences by at least 75% with patients with six or more recurrences per year.

Recommended Regimen: Acyclovir 400 mg orally 2 times a day.

Alternative Regimen: Acyclovir 200 mg orally 3–5 times a day.

COMPLICATIONS AND SEQUELAE

Males and Females: Neuralgia, meningitis, ascending myelitis, urethral strictures, and lymphatic suppuration may occur.

Females: There is possibly an increased risk for cervical cancer and fetal wastage.

Neonates: Virus from an active genital infection may be transmitted during vaginal delivery, causing neonatal herpes infection, which has a high case fatality rate, and many survivors have ocular or neurologic sequelae.

OTHER CONSIDERATIONS

Pregnant Women: The safety of systemic acyclovir during pregnancy has not been established. Women who receive acyclovir during pregnancy should be reported to a Burroughs Wellcome Company registry at 800-722-9292, ext. 58465.

Management of Sex Partners: Patients should abstain from sexual activity while lesions are present. Sexual transmission of HSV can occur during periods without evidence of lesions. The use of condoms should be encouraged during all sexual contact. Sex partners may require evaluation and counseling.

HIV Infection: HSV lesions are common among HIV-infected patients. Intermittent or suppressive therapy with oral acyclovir may be required.

SYPHILIS

Etiologic Agent

Treponema pallidum
(A spirochete with 6–14 spirals and characteristic motility.)

TYPICAL CLINICAL PRESENTATION

Primary: The classic chancre is painless, indurated, and located at the site of exposure. All genital lesions should be suspected to be syphilitic.

Secondary: Patients may have a highly variable skin rash, mucous patches, condylomata lata, lymphadenopathy, or other signs.

Tertiary: Patients have cardiac, neurologic, ophthalmic, auditory, or gummatous lesions.

Latent: Patients are without clinical signs.

PRESUMPTIVE DIAGNOSIS

(Warrants full treatment and follow-up)

Presumptive diagnosis relies on using both nontreponemal tests (VDRL or RPR) and treponemal tests (fluorescent treponemal antibody absorption [FTA-ABS] or microhemagglutination-*Treponema pallidum* [MHA-TP]). Nontreponemal test antibody titers usually correlate with disease activity.

Primary: Patients have typical lesion(s) and either a newly positive serologic test for syphilis (STS) or their present STS titer is at least fourfold greater than the last or there has been syphilis exposure within 90 days of lesion onset.

Secondary: Patients have the typical clinical presentation and a strongly reactive STS.

Latent: Patients have serologic evidence of untreated syphilis without clinical signs.

HIV-Infected Patients: When clinical findings suggest syphilis is present, but serological tests are negative, alternative tests, such as biopsy, dark-field examination, and direct fluorescent antibody (FA) staining of lesion material should be employed.

DEFINITIVE DIAGNOSIS

Primary and secondary syphilis are definitively diagnosed by demonstrating *T. pallidum* with dark-field microcopy of FA techniques in material from a chancre, regional lymph node, or other lesion.

THERAPY

Primary and Secondary Syphilis

Benzathine penicillin G, 2.4 million units IM in a single dose.

Penicillin-Allergic Patients

Doxycycline 100 mg orally 2 times a day for 2 weeks; OR Tetracycline 500 mg orally 4 times a day for 2 weeks.

Latent Syphilis

Early latent (<1 year) Syphilis: Benzathine penicillin G, 2.4 million units IM in a single dose.

Late latent (>1 year) Syphilis or Latent Syphilis of Unknown Duration: Benzathine penicillin G, 7.2 million units total, administered as 3 doses of 2.4 million units IM each at 1-week intervals.

Late Syphilis (Patients with gumma or cardiovascular syphilis but not neurosyphilis): Benzathine penicillin G, 7.2 million units total, administered as 3 doses of 2.4 million units IM at 1-week intervals.

Neurosyphilis

Recommended Regimen: Aqueous crystalline penicillin G, 12–24 million units daily, administered as 2–4 million units IV every 4 hours for 10–14 days.

Alternative Regimen: 2.4 million units procaine penicillin IM daily, plus probenecid 500 mg orally 4 times a day, both for 10–14 days.

COMPLICATIONS AND SEQUELAE

Both late syphilis and congenital syphilis are complications, since they are preventable with prompt diagnosis and treatment of early syphilis. Sequelae of late syphilis include neurologic (general paresis, tabes dorsalis, and focal neurologic signs), cardiovascular syphilis (thoracic aortic aneurism, aortic insufficiency), and localized gumma formation.

OTHER CONSIDERATIONS

Pregnant Women: Pregnant women should receive the same therapy as listed above, except that tetracycline, doxycycline, or erythromycin should not be used. Pregnant women with a history of penicillin allergy should be skin tested and then treated with penicillin or desensitized.

Follow-Up: Patients should be re-examined clinically and serologically at 3 and 6 months for primary and secondary syphilis and 6 and 12 months for latent syphilis.

Management of Sex Partners: Persons exposed to a patient with primary, secondary, or latent (<1 year) syphilis within 90 days should be treated presumptively. Those exposed >90 days should be treated presumptively if serologic tests are not available immediately or follow-up is uncertain. Partners considered at risk are those exposed within 3 months plus duration of symptoms for primary syphilis, 6 months plus duration of symptoms for secondary syphilis, and 1 year for early latent syphilis.

HIV Infection: Unusual serologic response may occur in HIV-infected persons. Penicillin regimens should be used whenever possible. Some authorities recommend cerebrospinal fluid (CSF) examination or treatment with a regimen appropriate for neurosyphilis for all patients coinfected with syphilis and HIV. Patients should be followed clinically and serologically at 1, 2, 3, 6, 9, and 12 months after therapy.

Chancroid

Etiologic Agent

Haemophilus ducreyi

(A Gram-negative bacillus with rounded ends, commonly observed in small clusters along strands of mucus. On culture, the organism tends to form straight or tangled chains.)

TYPICAL CLINICAL PRESENTATION

Usually a single (but sometimes multiple), superficial, painful ulcer appears and is surrounded by an erythematous halo. Ulcers may also be necrotic or severely erosive with ragged serpiginous borders. Accompanying adenopathy is usually unilateral. A characteristic inguinal bubo occurs in 25–60% of cases.

PRESUMPTIVE DIAGNOSIS

(Warrants full treatment and follow-up)

The clinical presentation is consistent with chancroid involving the genitalia. Since many STDs cause genital ulcers, it is crucial to differentiate them. All should be examined with dark-field microscopy. Gram-stained smears of ulcer exudate are unreliable.

DEFINITIVE DIAGNOSIS

The diagnosis is definitive when *H. ducreyi* is recovered by culture.

THERAPY

Recommended Regimens

Azithromycin 1 g orally in a single dose; OR
Ceftriaxone 250 mg IM in a single dose; OR
Erythromycin base 500 mg orally 4 times a day for 7 days.

Alternative Regimens

Amoxicillin 500 mg plus clavulanic acid 125 mg orally 3 times a day for 7 days; OR
Ciprofloxacin 500 mg orally 2 times a day for 3 days.

COMPLICATIONS AND SEQUELAE

Systemic spread is not known to occur.

Lesions may become secondarily infected and necrotic.

Buboes may rupture and suppurate, resulting in fistulae.

Ulcers on the prepuce may cause paraphimosis or phimosis.

OTHER CONSIDERATIONS

Pregnant Women: Safety of azithromycin during pregnancy has not been established. Ciprofloxacin is contradindicated during pregnancy.

Follow-Up: Successfully treated ulcers are almost invariably clinically improved by 7 days after institution of therapy. If the condition does not improve, the clinician should consider whether antimicrobials were taken as prescribed; the *H. ducreyi* is resistant to the prescribed antimicrobial; the diagnosis is correct; there is a coinfestation with another STD; or the patient is infected with HIV.

Management of Sex Partners: Partners who had contact within 10 days prior to the onset of symptoms should be examined and treated.

HIV Infection: Patients with HIV infections should be closely monitored and may require longer courses of therapy.

Lymphogranuloma Venereum

Etiologic Agent

Chlamydia trachomatis
(An obligate intracellular organism of immunotypes L1, L2, or L3.)

TYPICAL CLINICAL PRESENTATION

The primary lesion of lymphogranuloma venereum (LGV) is a 2–3 mm painless vesicle or nonindurated ulcer at the site of inoculation. Patients commonly fail to notice this primary lesion. Regional adenopathy follows a week to a month later and is the most common clinical presentation.

Sensation of stiffness and aching in the groin, followed by swelling of the inguinal region, may be the first indications of infection for most patients. Adenopathy may subside spontaneously or proceed to the formation of abscesses that rupture to produce draining sinuses or fistulae.

PRESUMPTIVE DIAGNOSIS

(Warrants full treatment and follow-up)

The LGV complement fixation test is sensitive; 80% of cases have a titer of 1:16 or higher. Since the sequelae of LGV are serious and preventable, treatment should not be withheld pending laboratory confirmation.

DEFINITIVE DIAGNOSIS

A definitive diagnosis requires isolation of *C. trachomatis* from an appropriate specimen and confirmation of the isolate as an LGV immunotype. However, such laboratory diagnostic capabilities are not widely available.

THERAPY

Recommended Regimen: Doxycycline 100 mg orally 2 times a day for 21 days.

Alternative Regimens: Erythromycin 500 mg orally 4 times a day for 21 days; OR
Sulfisoxazole 500 mg orally 4 times a day for 21 days or equivalent sulfonamide course.

Fluctuant lymph nodes should be aspirated as needed. Incision and drainage or excision of nodes will delay healing and are contraindicated.

Late sequelae such as strictures or fistulae may require surgical intervention.

COMPLICATIONS AND SEQUELAE

Dissemination may occur with nephropathy, hepatomegaly, or phlebitis.

Large polypoid swellings of the vulva, anal margin, or rectal mucosa may occur.

The most common, severe morbidity results from rectal involvement; perianal abscess and rectovaginal or other fistulae are early consequences, and rectal stricture may develop 1–10 years after infection.

OTHER CONSIDERATIONS

Pregnant Women: Pregnant patients should be treated with the erythromycin regimen.

Follow-Up: Patients should be followed clinically until signs and symptoms have resolved.

Management of Sex Partners: Persons having had sexual contact with a patient who has LGV within 30 days before onset of the patient's symptoms should be examined and treated.

HIV Infection: Patients with HIV infection should be managed in the same manner as patients without HIV infection.

MOLLUSCUM CONTAGIOSUM

Etiologic Agent

Molluscum contagiosum virus
(The largest DNA virus of the poxvirus group.)

TYPICAL CLINICAL PRESENTATION

Lesions are 1–5 mm, smooth, rounded, shiny, firm, flesh-colored-to-pearly-white papules with characteristically umbilicated centers. They are most commonly seen on the trunk and anogenital region and are generally asymptomatic.

PRESUMPTIVE DIAGNOSIS

(Warrants full treatment and follow-up)

Usually diagnosed on the basis of the typical clinical presentation.

DEFINITIVE DIAGNOSIS

Microscopic examination of lesions or lesion material reveals the pathognomonic molluscum inclusion bodies.

THERAPY

Lesions may resolve spontaneously without scarring. However, they may be removed by curettage after cryoanesthesia.

Caustic chemicals (podophyllin, trichloroacetic acid, silver nitrate) and cryotherapy (liquid nitrogen) have been used successfully. If every lesion is not extirpated, the condition may recur.

COMPLICATIONS AND SEQUELAE

Secondary infection, usually with *Staphylococcus,* occurs.

Lesions rarely attain a size greater than 10 mm in diameter.

OTHER CONSIDERATIONS

Pregnant Women: Podophyllin should be avoided during pregnancy.

Follow-Up: Patients should return for re-evaluation 1 month after treatment so that any new lesions can be removed.

Management of Sex Partners: Sexual partners should be examined.

HIV Infection: Patients with HIV infection should be managed in the same manner as patients without HIV infection.

Pᴇᴅɪᴄᴜʟᴏsɪs Pᴜʙɪs

Etiologic Agent

Pthirus pubis (pubic or crab louse)

(A grayish ectoparasite that is 1–4 mm long with segmented tarsi and claws for clinging to hairs.)

TYPICAL CLINICAL PRESENTATION

Symptoms range from slight discomfort to intolerable itching. Erythematous papules, nits, or adult lice clinging to pubic, perineal, or perianal hairs are present and often noticed by patients.

PRESUMPTIVE DIAGNOSIS

(Warrants full treatment and follow-up)

A presumptive diagnosis is made when a patient with a history of recent exposure to pubic lice has pruritic, erythematous macules, papules, or secondary excoriations in the genital area.

DEFINITIVE DIAGNOSIS

A definitive diagnosis is made by finding lice or nits attached to genital hairs.

THERAPY

Lindane 1% shampoo applied for 4 minutes and then thoroughly washed off (not recommended for pregnant or lactating women or for children <2 years of age); OR

Permethrin 1% creme rinse applied to affected areas and washed off after 10 minutes; OR

Pyrethrins with piperonyl butoxide applied to the infested area and washed off after 10 minutes.

The recommended regimens should not be applied to the eyes. Involvement of the eyelashes should be treated by applying occlusive ophthalmic ointment to the eyelid margins 2 times a day for 10 days.

Clothing and linen should be disinfected by washing them in hot water, by dry cleaning them, or by removing them from human exposure for at least 72 hours.

COMPLICATIONS AND SEQUELAE

Secondary excoriations

Lymphadenitis

Pyoderma

OTHER CONSIDERATIONS

Pregnant Women: Avoid lindane in pregnant or lactating women.

Follow-Up: Patients should be evaluated after 1 week if symptoms persist. If lice are found or if eggs are observed at the hair-skin junction, retreatment may be necessary.

Management of Sex Partners: Sexual partners within the last month should be treated.

HIV Infection: Patients with HIV infection should be managed in the same manner as patients without HIV infection.

SCABIES

Etiologic Agent

Sarcoptes scabiei

(The female is 0.3–0.4 mm; the male is somewhat smaller. The female burrows under the skin to deposit eggs.)

TYPICAL CLINICAL PRESENTATION

Symptoms include itching, often worse at night, and the presence of erythematous, papular eruptions. Excoriations and secondary infections are common. Reddish-brown nodules are caused by hypersensitivity and develop 1 or more months after infection has occurred. The primary lesion is the burrow. When not obliterated by excoriations, it is most often seen on the fingers, penis, and wrists.

PRESUMPTIVE DIAGNOSIS

(Warrants full treatment and follow-up)

The diagnosis is often made on clinical grounds alone. A history of exposure to a patient with scabies within the previous 2 months supports the diagnosis.

DEFINITIVE DIAGNOSIS

Definitive diagnosis is made by microscopic identification of the mite or its eggs, larvae, or feces in scrapings from an elevated papule or burrow.

THERAPY

Recommended Regimen

Permethrin cream 5% applied to all areas of the body from the neck down and washed off after 8–14 hours; OR

Lindane (1%) 1 ounce of lotion or 30 g of cream applied thinly to all areas of the body from the neck down and washed off thoroughly after 8 hours.

Lindane should not be used following a bath, and should not be used by persons with extensive dermatitis, pregnant or lactating women, and children <2 years of age. Not recommended for pregnant or lactating women, or infants and young children.

Alternative Regimen

Crotamiton 10%, applied to the entire body nightly for 2 nights and washed off thoroughly 24 hours after the second application.

COMPLICATIONS AND SEQUELAE

Secondary bacterial infection occurs, particularly with nephritogenic strains of streptococci. Norwegian or crusted scabies (with up to 2 million adult mites in the crusts) is a risk for patients with neurologic defects and the immunologically incompetent.

OTHER CONSIDERATIONS

Pregnant Women: Avoid lindane in pregnant or lactating women.

Follow-Up: Pruritus may persist for several weeks. Retreatment should be considered in patients who are symptomatic after 1 week, especially if live mites are observed.

Management of Sex Partners: Sexual partners and close personal or household contacts within the last month should be examined and treated.

HIV Infection: Patients with HIV infection should be managed in the same manner as patients without HIV infection.

Hepatitis B

Etiologic Agent

Hepatitis B virus (HBV)
(A DNA virus with multiple antigenic components.)

Sexual transmission accounts for an estimated one-third to two-thirds of the estimated 200,000–300,000 new HBV infections that occur annually in the United States.

TYPICAL CLINICAL PRESENTATION

Hepatitis B is clinically indistinguishable from other forms of hepatitis. Most infections are clinically inapparent. Clinical symptoms and signs include various combinations of anorexia, malaise, nausea, vomiting, abdominal pain, and jaundice. Skin rashes, arthralgias, and arthritis can also occur.

PRESUMPTIVE DIAGNOSIS

(Warrants full treatment and follow-up)

HBV infection is clinically indistinguishable from other forms of viral hepatitis and many times from hepatitis caused by toxins or drugs. The diagnosis should be considered in a symptomatic patient with symptoms suggestive of an acute viral illness and with an occupational exposure or sexual history that places the patient in a high-risk group.

Groups at high risk of acquiring infection include immigrants or refugees from areas of high HBV endemicity, patients in institutions for the mentally retarded, persons with multiple sex partners, users of illicit parenteral drugs, homosexually active men, household contacts of HBV carriers, and patients of hemodialysis units.

DEFINITIVE DIAGNOSIS

Serodiagnosis of HBV infection is the only method for clinicians to reach a definitive diagnosis. A positive result for hepatitis B surface antigen (HBsAg) indicates active infection with HBV, either acute hepatitis B or the chronic carrier state. Hepatitis B e antigen (HBeAg) correlates with infectivity. Anti-HBs usually indicates past infection with present immunity.

THERAPY

No specific therapy is available for the various types of acute hepatitis, whether sexually transmitted or not. Vaccination is recommended for all persons with multiple sexual partners within the past 6 months, IV drug users, men and women diagnosed as having recently acquired another STD, and residents of correctional or long-term care facilities.

For immunization recommendations refer to Chapter 30.

COMPLICATIONS AND SEQUELAE

Long-term sequelae include chronic persistent and chronic active hepatitis, cirrhosis, hepatocellular carcinoma, hepatic failure, and death. Rarely, the course may be fulminant with hepatic failure, resulting in early death. Infectious chronic carriers may be completely asymptomatic.

OTHER CONSIDERATIONS

Pregnant Women: Pregnancy is not a contraindication to HBV or hepatitis B immune globulin (HBIG) vaccine administration.

Management of Sex Partners: Susceptible persons who have been exposed to HBV through sexual contact with a person who has acute or chronic HBV infection should receive postexposure prophylaxis. This should include 0.06 mL/kg of HBIG in a single IM dose within 14 days of their last exposure. This should be followed with the standard three-dose immunization series with HBV vaccine.

HIV Infection: Patients with HIV infection who have HBV are more likely to develop a chronic HBV state. HIV infection may also impair the response to HBV vaccine. HIV-infected persons should be tested for anti-HBs 1–2 months after the third vaccine and revaccinated with one or more doses in those who have not responded.

ENTERIC INFECTIONS

Etiologic Agents

Proctitis: *N. gonorrhoeae, C. trachomatis, T. pallidum,* and herpes simplex virus (HSV).

Proctocolities: *Campylobacter* sp., *Shigella* sp., *Entamoeba histolytica,* and rarely *C. trachomatis.*

Enteritis: *Giardia lamblia.* Among HIV-infected patients others include cytomegalovirus (CMV), *Mycobacterium avium-intracellulare, Salmonella* sp., *Cryptosporidium, Microsporidium,* and *Isospora.*

These are particularly common among persons who participate in anal intercourse (proctitis) or whose sexual practices include oral-fecal contact (enteritis).

TYPICAL CLINICAL PRESENTATION

Infections are frequently asymptomatic or minimally symptomatic. Symptoms include:

Proctitis: Anorectal pain, tenesmus, and rectal discharge.

Proctocolitis: Symptoms of proctitis plus diarrhea or abdominal cramps.

Enteritis: Diarrhea and abdominal cramping.

PRESUMPTIVE DIAGNOSIS

(Warrants full treatment and follow-up)

The typical clinical findings suggest enteric infection. Examination of a fresh stool specimen can be helpful. The finding of white cells on direct microscopy of a suspension of fresh stool or the finding of guaiac-positive or grossly bloody stools supports the diagnosis.

DEFINITIVE DIAGNOSIS

Definitive diagnostic tests vary according to the agent and site of infection involved.

THERAPY

Treatment of proctitis and enteritis should be based on etiologic diagnosis. Some asymptomatic, infected individuals for whom anal-oral contact is a sexual practice should be treated in accordance with recommendations for symptomatic individuals, as should persons whose work or social situation is associated with a likelihood of transmission (e.g., food handlers, hospital workers, day-care center employees). Until laboratory tests are available, persons with acute proctitis who have recently practiced receptive anal intercourse and have either anorectal pus on examination or PMN leukocytes on a Gram-stained smear should receive treatment for anal-genital gonorrhea and doxycycline 100 mg orally 2 times a day for 7 days.

COMPLICATIONS AND SEQUELAE

Complications and sequelae vary with the disease agent, health of the host, therapy, and other factors. Spontaneous cures are common. Morbidity may be severe, requiring hospitalization and IV hydration. Infections may become systemic (such as Gram-negative septicemia) or distantly localized (amebic hepatic cyst). Some infections may rarely be fatal (hepatitis A, disseminated bacterial disease).

OTHER CONSIDERATIONS

Follow-Up: Follow-up should be based on severity of clinical symptoms and specific etiologic agent involved.

Management of Sex Partners: Sexual partners should be evaluated for any diseases diagnosed in the index patient.

HIV Infection: Patients with HIV infection should be managed in the same manner as patients without HIV infection. HIV-infected patients are at risk for infections not commonly found in non-HIV-infected patients.

AIDS AND HIV INFECTIONS (ACQUIRED IMMUNODEFICIENCY SYNDROME)

Etiologic Agent

HIV-1 or HIV-2
(A retrovirus)

TYPICAL CLINICAL PRESENTATION

The range of symptoms associated with HIV may extend from minimal to the full clinical syndrome of AIDS. Patients with the clinical syndrome of AIDS often give a history of nonspecific symptoms for months prior to diagnosis. These symptoms may include easy fatigue, poor appetite, weight loss, lymphadenopathy, diarrhea, fever, and night sweats. Other symptoms specific to opportunistic diseases occur in patients with AIDS, such as purple to bluish skin lesions associated with Kaposi's sarcoma (KS), shortness of breath, and nonproductive cough resulting from *Pneumocystis carinii* pneumonia (PCP).

The time between infection with HIV and development of AIDS is extremely variable, ranging from a few months to 10 or more years. Once an individual is infected, current research suggests that the individual remains infected indefinitely and may transmit the infection to others. As yet unidentified factors may influence which infected individuals develop AIDS and which particular opportunistic illness may occur.

PRESUMPTIVE DIAGNOSIS

Presumptive diagnosis of HIV infection is made usually by clinical evidence, supported by serologic tests for antibodies to HIV infection.

DEFINITIVE DIAGNOSIS

Currently, isolation of the virus from body fluids is the most highly specific means to make a definitive diagnosis of HIV infection. Only a very few research laboratories have the technology to perform viral isolation. Viral antigen detection techniques are not generally available. Results from repeatably reactive enzyme-linked immunosorbent assay (ELISA) tests, Western blots, and other confirmatory tests, and a second serology, that is, examination, when combined with a careful history and physical examination, can usually resolve questionable cases.

THERAPY

To date, no treatment has been identified to eradicate the virus.

Standard therapy consists of treating opportunistic diseases aggressively as they occur. Antiretroviral therapy may play a role in treatment. However, the optimal time for initiating antiretroviral therapy has not yet been established. PCP prophylaxis should be instituted for adolescents and adults with <200 CD4+ T cells/μL. Prophylaxis should be continued for the lifetime of the patient.

COMPLICATIONS AND SEQUELAE

The outcome in patients with HIV infection is not completely understood. Most people with HIV will eventually have symptoms related to the infection. In cohort studies 70–85% of infected adults developed symptoms, and AIDS developed in 55–62% within 12 years of infection. Additional AIDS cases are expected among those who have remained AIDS-free for >12 years.

OTHER CONSIDERATIONS

Management of Sex Partners: Sexual partners should be notified by either their partners or through a referral to health department partner notification programs. Partners should receive counseling and testing.

CHAPTER 61

Gonorrhea

Gonorrhea is one of the most important sexually transmitted diseases in adolescents because of its high incidence and serious complications.

ETIOLOGY

Gonorrhea is a sexually transmitted disease caused by *Neisseria gonorrhoeae*, which has the following characteristics:

1. The organisms are spherical or oval cocci, occurring in pairs, with abutting flattened sides.
2. The organisms are Gram-negative and are usually located within polymorphonuclear leukocytes.
3. The organisms grow optimally at 35–37°C, with an ambient carbon dioxide concentration of 3–5%.
4. The organisms produce cytochrome oxidase, which is helpful in identification. *N. gonorrhoeae* can be differentiated from other *Neisseria* species, in that it ferments glucose but not maltose, sucrose, or lactose.
5. Types of organisms: *N. gonorrhoeae* species have been differentiated by several characteristics:
   a. Presence or absence of pili: The presence of pili is associated with small colonies and increased virulence in males.
   b. Opaque or transparent: Opaque growing colonies have an outer membrane protein termed protein II.
   c. Auxotyping: This is determined by the nutritional requirements of the organism.
   d. Serotyping

EPIDEMIOLOGY

Incidence

1. While gonorrhea remains one of the most common reportable diseases in the United States, the total number of cases have declined markedly over the past 15 years. This decline is disproportionately represented by the nonadolescent population. About 350,000 cases are currently reported per year in the United States. However, reported cases may only represent 50% or less of all cases.
2. Adolescents aged 15–19 account for about 30% of cases and adolescent females aged 15–19 for almost 35% of reported cases in women. Sixty percent of cases occur between the ages of 15 and 24.
3. The 20- to 24-year-old age group has the highest number of cases, and the 15- to 19-year-old age group is second. However, almost twice as many individuals are sexually active

in the 20- to 24-year-old age group as in the 15- to 19-year-old age group. When the incidence rate is corrected for this bias, the incidence in sexually active 15- to 19-year-olds is twice that of the 20- to 24-year-old age group.

4. The reasons for the high incidence in adolescents include:
   a. The increased sexuality rates that have occurred in this age group
   b. The low consistent use of condoms and foam in adolescents, which can partially protect against a sexually transmitted disease
   c. The larger degree of cervical ectopy in adolescents: *N. gonorrhoeae* preferentially infects columnar epithelial cells. Adolescents have more of this tissue exposed on the ectocervix.
   d. Lack of clinical services in settings convenient to adolescents
   e. The high incidence of asymptomatic carriers and the low use by adolescents of preventive medical care to detect these carriers

5. Seasonal variation: Higher incidence rates occur in late summer.

6. Prevalence: The prevalence rates vary on routine screening for gonorrhea, depending on the reporting facility:
   a. Sexually transmitted disease clinics: Fifteen percent or greater are positive for gonorrhea.
   b. Health departments: About 3% are positive for gonorrhea.
   c. Student health centers: Less than 1–2% are positive for gonorrhea.
   d. Adolescent clinics: Approximately 3–6% are positive for gonorrhea.

7. Correlation with drug use: Schwarcz et al. (1992) found that 32% of female adolescents with gonorrhea in San Francisco had received money or drugs in exchange for sex compared to no cases of gonorrhea in a control group of female adolescents who had not reported exchanging sex for drugs or money. In addition, 89% of these teens who had received money or drugs in exchange for sex reported using crack cocaine.

8. Trends: The number of cases and incidence have fallen in the past 10 years to less than half the cases in 1978, as shown in Table 61.1. However, a disproportionate contributor of this change has been in the nonadolescent population.

9. Race: About 61% of the reported cases occurred in the African-American population. Incidence rates in the African-American population have fallen since the late 1970s and early 1980s from over 2000 cases per 100,000 to about 1200 per 100,000, still about six times the overall national rate. The incidence in Hispanic, white, and other populations are each under 200 per 100,000.

10. Geography: The incidence rates of gonorrhea vary widely by state from rates of 300–400 per 100,000 in each of the southeastern states except Florida to 274 in Maryland, 171 in Texas, 166 in New York, and 97 in California. States with rates of 10 per 100,000 or less include Montana, Maine, Vermont, and New Hampshire. Examples of rates per 100,000 from other states include:

Florida, 175.8	Ohio, 203
Illinois, 244.5	Pennsylvania, 151
Massachusetts, 51.8	Rhode Island, 229.6
Michigan, 191	Virginia, 188
Missouri, 253	Washington, 73.1
Nevada, 139.7	

TABLE 61.1.   Cases and Incidence of Gonorrhea in United States, 1978–1995

	1978	1985	1988	1990	1992	1994	1995
Cases	1,013,436	911,419	688,087	609,169	501,409	413,647	348,137
Incidence (per 100,000)	468.3	384.5	298.7	276.6	201.6	168.4	NA[a]

[a]NA, not available.

Host

Humans are the only natural host for N. *gonorrhoeae*.

Transmission

Transmission is virtually exclusively through oral, vaginal, or anal sexual contact. The exception is gonococcal ophthalmia, which usually occurs in newborns but has been reported in physicians or laboratory technicians when direct contact of the organisms with the eye through hand transmission has occurred.

PATHOPHYSIOLOGY

N. *gonorrhoeae* causes disease by direct invasion and spread on mucosal and glandular structures lined by columnar epithelium. Adherence of the organism to the mucosa, mediated by pili and surface proteins, is followed by mucosal invasion within 24–48 hours. This results in an inflammatory response characterized by localized capillary dilation, edema, and polymorphonuclear leukocytes. Transmission to the upper genital tract may occur via adherence to sperm or with refluxed blood during menses. The loss of the endometrium and cervical mucous plug during menses may also contribute to the spread into the upper genital tract.

Virulence

The virulence of the infection may be related to certain characteristics of the organism:

1. Pili: Gonococcal pili are the main mediators of adherence of the organism to epithelial cells. Organisms with pili attach more successfully than nonpiliated forms to vaginal epithelial cells, neutrophils, and sperm.
2. Colony morphology: Cells with protein II have an "opaque" colony morphology, whereas strains without protein II are "transparent." Opaque colonies are more often found in specimens from men with gonococcal urethritis and in cervical isolates obtained from women at about midcycle. Transparent colonies are usually found in cervical cultures from women at other times than midcycle and in isolates from blood, synovial fluid, and fallopian tubes. Transparent colonies appear to be the invasive form. Colonies can shift phenotypes from opaque to transparent in vivo.
3. Auxotype: Growth requirements of N. *gonorrhoeae* organisms may relate to pathogenicity. Strains requiring arginine, hypoxanthine, and uracil are associated with asymptomatic urethral infection in males, disseminated gonococcal infection, and increased susceptibility to penicillin.

Table 61.2 outlines characteristics related to pathogenicity.

TABLE 61.2.   *Neisseria gonorrhoeae:* Characteristics Related to Pathogenicity

Characteristic	PID Associated	Urethral Associated	Disseminated Disease
Auxotype	Prototrophs	Varied	Arginine⁻, hypoxanthine⁻, uracil⁻, or proline⁻
Penicillin susceptibility	Relatively resistant	Varied	Very susceptible
Colony characteristics	Transparent	Opaque	Transparent
Stereotypes	1, 2	Varied	1

Adapted from McGee ZA. Gonococcal pelvic inflammatory disease. In: Holmes KK, Mardh PA, Sparling PF, Wiesner PJ, eds. Sexually transmitted diseases. New York: McGraw-Hill, 1986.

Clinical Manifestations

Clinical manifestations are similar to those caused by *Chlamydia trachomatis,* and both *C. trachomatis* and *N. gonorrhoeae* occur frequently together in the same individual. Susceptible sites are usually mucosal columnar epithelial areas. Both organisms produce a urethritis in males and a dysuria-pyuria syndrome and cervicitis in females. In both sexes a proctitis and conjunctivitis can occur. Both *N. gonorrhoeae* and *C. trachomatis* cause bartholinitis, endometritis, salpingitis, and perihepatitis. In prepubertal females both organisms can infect vaginal epithelium, causing a vaginitis. In addition, both organisms can cause a systemic arthritis-dermatitis syndrome and a neonatal conjunctivitis. The spectrum of gonorrhoeae infections includes:

1. Asymptomatic infections: Asymptomatic urethral and cervical infections may persist for months if untreated. Since symptomatic individuals seek treatment and most asymptomatic individuals do not, asymptomatic individuals accumulate in the population and probably account for at least 50% of infections. In the military 68% of males have been reported to be asymptomatic. In homosexual males up to 78% of pharyngeal infections and 18–23% of rectal infections are asymptomatic. Asymptomatic infections include infections of the:
   a. Urethra
   b. Endocervix
   c. Rectum
   d. Pharynx
2. Symptomatic uncomplicated infections include:
   a. Urethritis
   b. Cervicitis
   c. Proctitis
   d. Pharyngitis
   e. Bartholinitis
   f. Conjunctivitis
3. Local complications include:
   a. Salpingitis
   b. Epididymitis
   c. Bartholin's gland abscess
   d. Lymphangitis
   e. Penile edema
   f. Periurethral abscess
   g. Prostatitis
4. Disseminated gonorrhea

Genitourinary Infections   The most common clinical manifestation of gonorrhea is a genitourinary infection.

Males

1. Urethritis
   a. Follows a 2- to 6-day incubation period
   b. Dysuria
   c. Purulent urethral discharge, most marked in the morning
2. Infection can spread and cause prostatitis, epididymitis, seminal vesiculitis, and periurethral abscess or fistula.

    a. Epididymitis: Ten percent to 30% of untreated men develop this complication. Epididymitis is manifested by:
- Scrotal pain and tenderness
- Scrotal swelling
- Pain in the inguinal area and lower abdomen
- Pain, tenderness, or swelling of the lower pole of the epididymis
- Chills, fever, and malaise

    b. Prostatitis: Prostatitis is a rare complication of gonorrhea. Signs and symptoms include:
- May be asymptomatic
- Chills and fever
- Rectal pain and discomfort
- Lower back pain
- Pain on defecation
- Dysuria, urinary frequency, and, occasionally, acute urinary retention

3. Risk of infection: Risk of infection is 20–35% for a male after a single exposure with an infected female.

Females   Signs and symptoms are less specific in females than in males. Often the teen may complain of vaginal discharge, dysuria, or frequency. Common local problems include:

1. Endocervicitis
    a. Increased vaginal discharge, often purulent
    b. Dyspareunia
    c. Erythema and friability of cervix
    d. Risk of infection: Sixty percent to 90% for a female after a single exposure to an infected male
2. Urethritis
    a. Dysuria
    b. Urinary frequency
    c. Exudate from urethra or Bartholin's gland
3. Labial swelling and tenderness
4. Bartholin's gland infection: The most common complication in females apart from pelvic inflammatory disease (PID) is abscess of the Bartholin's gland.
5. Spread of infection can extend into:
    a. Uterus: Endometritis
    b. Fallopian tubes: Salpingitis (see Chapter 63). Salpingitis occurs in as many as 15–30% of women with urogenital gonorrhea. Strains causing PID vary; some are more likely to have auxotypes different from cervical or disseminated infections, some are more likely to be resistant to penicillin than disseminated strains, and others almost always grow in transparent colonies.
    c. Upper abdomen: Perihepatitis (Fitz-Hugh and Curtis syndrome)

Extragenital Sites

1. Pharyngitis
    a. Pharyngeal involvement is usually asymptomatic in over 90% of infected individuals.
    b. Pharyngitis may be manifested by a sore throat 3–7 days after exposure.
    c. Positive pharyngeal cultures are found in 3–7% of heterosexual males, 10–20% of heterosexual females, and 10–25% percent of homosexual males with genital gonorrhea, but the pharynx is the sole site of infection in less than 5% of individuals, re-

gardless of gender or sexual orientation. The infection is transmitted to the pharynx by orogenital sexual contact. Such transmission to sex partners is infrequent, with fellatio being a more effective mode of transmission than cunnilingus. In a study of pharyngeal gonorrhea in female adolescents, Brown et al. (1989) found positive pharyngeal cultures in none of 240 adolescents from a hospital adolescent clinic and 3.4% in a group of adolescents from a sexually transmitted disease public health clinic. In only 2 of 20 adolescents with pharyngeal gonococcal infection was the pharynx the only infected site. There was a significant relationship between concurrent pharyngeal and genital gonorrhea.

   d. Spontaneous elimination of the organism usually occurs in 10–12 weeks.

   e. Significance of infection: The clinical significance is controversial. However, infected individuals may be at risk for dissemination of gonorrhea.

2. Rectal gonorrhea

   a. Prevalence rates

     — Rectal cultures are positive in 35–50% of females and homosexual males with gonorrhea. The rectum is the only infected site in about 5% of females and 40% of homosexual males. Rectal infections are uncommon in heterosexual males. Most anorectal infections in females occur without a history of anogenital sexual contact and are thought to be related to infected perineal secretions.

   b. Rectal gonorrhea can produce:

     — Proctitis with anal discharge

     — Rectal bleeding

     — Anorectal pain

     — Tenesmus

     — Constipation

   c. Most anorectal infections in females are asymptomatic.

     The examination may show a purulent exudate, erythema, edema, and friability or other inflammatory changes of the rectal mucosa. The differential diagnosis for infections involving the first 5–10 cm of the rectum is *Chlamydia,* herpes, and syphilis. Inflammation extending more than 15 cm is usually caused by either *Shigella, Campylobacter, Entamoeba histolytica,* or lymphogranuloma venereum.

3. Conjunctivitis

4. Otitis externa (Pareek, 1979)

Disseminated Disease   About 0.5–1.0% of individuals with gonorrhea develop disseminated disease, with infections three times more prevalent in females and with pregnant females being at the highest risk. Other risk factors for dissemination include pharyngeal gonorrhea, complement deficiency disease, and other immune-altering disease states such as lupus erythematosus. Commonly, disseminated disease develops in individuals with asymptomatic pharyngeal or anogenital infections.

Arthritis Syndrome

1. Arthritis syndrome is the most common systemic complication of *N. gonorrhoeae,* occurring in 1–3% of infected individuals and usually within 1 month of exposure. Dissemination may arise from male or female genitourinary tract infections or infections of the rectum or pharynx. Factors involved in dissemination of gonorrhea include abnormalities in one of the complement components and hormonal influences during the menstrual cycle and pregnancy.

2. Arthritis syndrome has a higher incidence in females than males.

3. Sixteen percent of the arthritis-dermatitis infections occur in the 10- to 19-year-old age group.
4. Two patterns exist: Arthritis-dermatitis syndrome and a septic joint.
5. Arthritis-dermatitis syndrome
   a. Fever (57%)
   b. Chills (23%)
   c. Arthritis or tenosynovitis (100%): Most commonly involves the wrists, dorsum of the hands, knees, or ankles
   d. Skin lesions (55%)
      — Start as pinpoint macules that turn into pustules on broad erythematous bases and necrotic centers
      — Often tender
      — Usually less than 20 lesions on the body
      — Frequently occur on trunk and upper extremities
      — Gram stain results and culture are usually negative, but direct immunofluorescent stains in research studies on biopsy specimens of skin identify gonorrhea in more than half the specimens.
   e. Positive cultures from blood in 20–50% of patients: With tenosynovitis and dermatitis there is greater likelihood of positive blood cultures and a negative joint culture.
6. Monoarticular septic arthritis
   a. Monoarticular septic arthritis may present as an arthritis-dermatitis syndrome and then localize in one joint.
   b. Monoarticular septic arthritis may present as an isolated septic arthritis.
   c. Knees are the most frequently involved joints, followed by the elbows, ankles, wrists, and small joints of the hands and feet.
   d. Synovial fluid cultures are positive in about 30–50% of patients. Blood cultures are rarely positive by the time the infection is in a joint.
   e. Monoarticular septic arthritis is more likely than tenosynovitis to have a negative blood culture and a positive joint culture. Cultures are usually negative from synovial fluid containing less than 20,000 leukocytes/mm^3 and are more often positive if over 80,000 leukocytes/mm^3.
7. Differential diagnosis of gonococcal arthritis includes:
   a. Infections: Meningococcemia, bacteremias, endocarditis, infectious arthritis, and infectious tenosynovitis
   b. Seronegative arthritides: Reiter's syndrome, ankylosing spondylitis, psoriatic arthritis
   c. Lupus erythematosus

Differentiating features of acute gonococcal arthritis and acute Reiter's syndrome are included in Table 61.3.

Other sites of dissemination include:

1. Perihepatitis: May be a complication of salpingitis, but occasionally may be caused by hematogenous dissemination of the disease
2. Gonococcal meningitis (Sayeed et al., 1972): Rare complication that can be indistinguishable clinically from meningococcal infection
3. Gonococcal osteomyelitis (Gantz et al., 1976)
4. Complete heart block (Gann et al., 1977)
5. Gonococcal endocarditis (Cooke et al., 1979)
6. Pericarditis
7. Pneumonia
8. Adult respiratory distress syndrome (Belding and Carbone, 1991)

TABLE 61.3. Comparison of Acute Gonococcal Arthritis and Acute Reiter's Syndrome

Characteristic	Acute Gonococcal Arthritis (%)	Acute Reiter's Syndrome (%)
Back pain	0	20
Urethritis	28	76
Migratory arthralgias	83	10
Chills	33	0
Temperature greater than 39.4°C	27	39
Skin lesions	Isolated papules and pustules on extremities and trunk	Balanitis; keratoderma blennorrhagica; buccal mucosal lesions
Sacroiliac involvement	3	30
Wrist involvement	67	30
Heel involvement	7	67
Antigen HLA-B27	Usually negative	>90+

TABLE 61.4. Sensitivity and Specificity of Gram-Stained Smears

Site	Sensitivity (%)	Specificity (%)
Men with symptomatic urethritis	90–95	95–100
Men with asymptomatic urethral infection	50–70	95–100
Endocervix		
Uncomplicated gonorrhea	50–70	95–100
Pelvic inflammatory disease	60–70	95–100
Anorectum		
Blind swabs	40–60	95–100
Anoscopically obtained specimens	70–80	95–100

Adapted from Handsfield HH. Gonorrhea and uncomplicated gonococcal infection. In: Holmes KK, Mardh PA, Sparling PF, Wiesner PJ, eds. Sexually transmitted diseases. New York: McGraw-Hill, 1986.

DIAGNOSIS

Gonococcal Urethritis

1. Microscopic demonstration of typical Gram-negative intracellular diplococci on smear of urethral exudate constitutes sufficient basis for diagnosis of gonorrhea. Sensitivity of a Gram-stained specimen approaches 100% in symptomatic men, but is 60% or less for asymptomatic infections. Specificity is greater than 95%. Sensitivity and specificity of Gram-stained smears are reviewed in Table 61.4.
2. If the Gram stain result is negative or if urethral exudate is absent, a culture of a specimen taken from the anterior urethra should be done. One should use a sterile calcium alginate urethral swab inoculating a modified Thayer-Martin (MTM) medium culture plate. Sites that are normally colonized by other organisms (i.e., rectum, pharynx, or endocervix) should be cultured on selective medium (Thayer-Martin), while cultures obtained from sterile areas (i.e., blood, spinal fluid, or synovial fluid) can be plated onto nonselective, chocolate agar. Growth of oxidase-positive, Gram-negative diplococci is sufficient evidence for a diagnosis. DNA probe techniques are also be used to diagnose urethral infections.
3. An additional method of diagnosis is to culture the first 10–20 mL of uncentrifuged first-voided urine on MTM medium. This has been reported by Feng et al. (1977) as having a 94% sensitivity.
4. The homosexual male adolescent should also have cultures obtained from the rectum and pharynx.

5. In asymptomatic males the urinary leukocyte esterase dipstick on a first-catch urine can be a valuable screening technique. The sensitivity of this test for detecting individuals with a positive culture for *N. gonorrhoeae* or *C. trachomatis* varies from 72% (Shafer et al., 1989) to 83% (Sadof et al., 1987) with a specificity of 93–100%.

Gonococcal Endocervicitis

1. Cultures should be obtained from the endocervical and anal canals and inoculated separately on MTM medium to diagnose gonorrhea. Do not use a lubricant during the pelvic examination, as this may be toxic to organisms. Place a swab in the cervical os for 20–30 seconds and rotate. For screening purposes, only endocervical cultures are recommended. A single culture is 80–95% sensitive in detecting gonorrhea. If gonorrhea is suspected, a separate swab should be used in the anal canal. About 5–10% of females have positive culture from this site only. The swab should be inserted about 2 cm, avoiding fecal mass, and moved side to side for 20–30 seconds.
2. Gram-stained smears from the endocervix are not recommended except as an adjunct to culture or in symptomatic females. Such smears are only 55–65% sensitive in asymptomatic females.
3. Newer diagnostic methods include detection of gonococcal enzymes and DNA probe assays in clinical specimens. The DNA probe assay is proving to be a sensitive and specific alternative test to the culture for infections of the endocervix, urethra, pharynx, and rectum. Sensitivities as compared to cultures are in the 85% to 95% range, and specificities are in the 95% to 100% range. In one study comparing DNA probe and culture from genital infections in males and females, the overall concordance was 98.4% (Stary et al., 1993). All positive culture specimens were found to be positive by the DNA probe. Eight (14.3%) of the positive specimens by DNA probe were found to be negative by culture. Of these, three were determined to be false positive, and five were true positives.

Anorectal Gonorrhea

Positive cultures from the rectum are required for diagnosis of anorectal gonorrhea. The DNA probe may be used as an alternative test.

Gonococcal Pharyngitis

1. Diagnosis requires a positive culture from the pharynx. Alternatively, DNA probe tests have a high sensitivity and specificity for diagnosis in the pharynx.
2. Sugar fermentation should be used to confirm the diagnosis of gonorrhea when oxidase-positive, Gram-negative diplococci are cultured from sources other than the rectum or genitals.
3. Several studies have indicated that routine pharyngeal screening in adolescents is not cost effective (Brown et al., 1989; Roochvarg et al., 1991). It is probably more cost effective to treat adolescents with genital infections with medications that treat both genital and pharyngeal gonorrhea.

Systemic Infection

1. Typical signs such as tenosynovitis and classic skin lesions
2. Positive cultures or DNA tests from the urethra, endocervix, pharynx, rectum, skin lesions, synovial fluid, or blood

THERAPY

Treatment of gonorrhea should take into account that strains of *N. gonorrhoeae* resistant to traditional treatment are rising, that chlamydial infections often coexist with gonorrhea, and that serious complications can arise from both gonococcal and chlamydial infections.

Resistance

The incidence of isolates of *N. gonorrhoeae* resistant to antibiotics has increased dramatically since the early 1980s. The forms of antibiotic resistance include:

1. Plasmid mediated
   a. Penicillin: Penicillinase-producing *N. gonorrhoeae* (PPNG)
   b. Tetracycline: Tetracycline-resistant *N. gonorrhoeae* (TRNG)
2. Chromosomally mediated resistant *N. gonorrhoeae* (CMRNG)
   a. Penicillin
   b. Tetracycline
   c. Cefoxitin
   d. Spectinomycin

In 1976 PPNG was first recognized in the United States. The mechanism of acquisition was a new plasmid that carried genes for producing a β-lactamase capable of breaking the essential penicillin β-lactam ring. This problem rose slowly until 1980, at which time cases increased dramatically. PPNG became endemic in many parts of the United States, especially in New York, California, and Florida, but other areas were affected as well. Over 20% of gonococcal isolates taken from individuals who live in major urban areas are now PPNG. Another form of plasmid-mediated resistance, first isolated in 1985, is to tetracycline (TRNG).

CMRNG was the reason for the rising doses of penicillin required between 1950 and the 1970s. However, in 1983 a higher level of this resistance was described to penicillin and tetracycline. The mechanism of resistance involves multiple chromosomal mutations that cause alterations in the cell membrane to antibiotics and changes in penicillin-binding proteins. CMRNG also involves some second-generation cephalosporins and spectinomycin (rare in the United States). *N. gonorrhoeae* isolates, which require 1 μg/mL or more of penicillin for inhibition and which do not produce β-lactamase, have been designated as CMRNG.

In 1988 the Gonococcal Isolate Surveillance Project found that 21% of isolates collected from patients at 21 clinic sites were resistant to penicillin, tetracycline, cefoxitin, or spectinomycin (Schwarcz et al., 1990). They also noted that the percent of PPNG, TRNG, and CMRNG, although widespread, varied widely from city to city. PPNG was noted to be highest in coastal areas, with the highest reports coming from West Palm Beach, Florida; Long Beach, California; Honolulu, Hawaii; and Fort Brag, North Carolina. Isolates of TRNG were more prevalent in cities east of the Mississippi River, with the highest prevalences found in Baltimore, Maryland (21.1%); Philadelphia, Pennsylvania (13.1%); New Orleans, Louisiana (9.0%); Birmingham, Alabama (6.5%); and Fort Bragg, North Carolina (5.4%). CMRNG was most common in Baltimore Maryland; Denver, Colorado; Fort Bragg, North Carolina; Long Beach, California; and West Palm Beach, Florida.

Treatment Recommendations

Recommendations from the 1993 Centers for Disease Control (CDC) sexually transmitted disease guidelines include:

1. Uncomplicated urethral, endocervical, or rectal infections in adolescents and adults:
   a. Recommended regimen
       Ceftriaxone 125 mg intramuscularly (IM) at one time; OR
       Cefixime 400 mg orally in a single dose; OR
       Ciprofloxacin 500 mg orally in a single dose; OR
       Ofloxacin 400 mg orally in a single dose; PLUS
       A regimen effective against possible coinfection with *C. trachomatis* such as doxycycline 100 mg orally two times a day for 7 days or azithromycin 1 g.

       Each of the above regimens appear to cure more than 95% of anal and genital infections.

       Cefixime has the advantage of a one-time oral dose. The serum levels are not as high as with ceftriaxone nor as sustained. Its effectiveness against incubating syphilis is not known.

       Ciprofloxacin has been used at both 250- and 500-mg doses, but the 500-mg dose is recommended due to problems with decreasing susceptibility to some quinolones.

       Quinolones are contraindicated for pregnant or nursing females and for persons under 18 years of age.

       125 mg of ceftriaxone appears to be as effective as 250 mg, and no ceftriaxone-resistant strains of *N. gonorrhoeae* have been reported.
   b. Alternative regimens
       — Spectinomycin 2 g IM in a single dose: Disadvantages include the expense, injectable use only, and inactivity against syphilis.
       — Injectable cephalosporins such as ceftizoxime 500 mg IM in a single dose; cefotaxime 500 mg IM in a single dose; cefotetan 1 g IM in a single dose; and cefoxitin 2 g IM in a single dose: None offer any significant advantage compared with ceftriaxone.
       — Oral cephalosporins other than cefixime 400 mg: This includes cefuroxime axetil 1 g orally in a single dose and cefpodoxime proxetil 200 mg orally in a single dose. These appear to have less antigonococcal activity than cefixime 400 mg.
       — Quinolones other than ciprofloxacin 500 mg and ofloxacin 400 mg: These include enoxacin 400 mg orally in a single dose; lomefloxacin 400 mg orally in a single dose; and norfloxacin 800 mg orally in a single dose. None appear to offer any advantage over ciprofloxacin 500 mg or ofloxacin 400 mg.

       The above regimens should be followed with a therapy that treats *Chlamydia*. Azithromycin 1 g as a single dose is being investigated as a single drug to treat both uncomplicated gonococcal and nongonococcal infections (Odugbemi et al., 1993).
2. Special considerations
   a. Individuals with gonorrhea should have a serologic test for syphilis. In addition, the practitioner should consider offering testing for human immunodeficiency virus (HIV) infection.
   b. Incubating syphilis may be cured with regimens that include ceftriaxone or a 7-day course of either doxycycline or erythromycin. Adolescents who have documented syphilis coexistent with gonorrhea should have the syphilis treated with a regimen outlined in Chapter 64. Spectinomycin and the quinolines (ciprofloxacin, norfloxacin) have no activity against incubating syphilis. If these drugs are used, the teen should have a second serologic test for syphilis in 1 month.
   c. Some practitioners mix 1% lidocaine with ceftriaxone to reduce the discomfort associated with the injection.
3. Treatment of sexual partners: All adolescents exposed to gonorrhea should be examined, cultured, and treated presumptively. The sex partner(s) of symptomatic patients should

be evaluated and treated if their last sexual contact with the patient was within 30 days of onset of the patient's symptoms. This period should be extended to 60 days if the index patient is asymptomatic. Teens should be told to refer sex partners for evaluation and treatment. Teens should avoid sexual intercourse until patient and partner(s) are cured.

4. Follow-up: Because of the efficacy of recommended regimens, routine follow-up cultures are not needed for persons treated for uncomplicated gonorrhea. Adolescents should be told to return for an examination if symptoms or signs persist after therapy. These individuals should be evaluated by culture for *N. gonorrhoeae* including testing for antimicrobial susceptibility. Most treatment failures are due to reinfection.

5. Pharyngeal gonococcal infection: Use either ceftriaxone 125 mg IM once or ciprofloxacin 500 mg orally in a single dose.

6. Treatment in pregnant adolescents: Pregnant adolescents should be screened for gonorrhea, *Chlamydia,* and syphilis at the first prenatal care visit, with tests repeated in the third trimester. Quinolones and tetracyclines should be avoided during pregnancy. *N. gonorrhoeae* should be treated with one of the recommended cephalosporin regimens. Spectinomycin 2 g IM can be used alternatively. Erythromycin is recommended to treat *C. trachomatis* during pregnancy.

7. HIV infection: Teens infected with HIV and *N. gonorrhoeae* should receive the same treatment as those not infected with HIV.

8. Acute salpingitis: See Chapter 63.

9. Acute epididymitis: In sexually active adolescents, epididymitis is most likely caused by *N. gonorrhoeae* or *C. trachomatis.* Recommended therapy after appropriate cultures for gonorrhea and *Chlamydia* includes:
    a. Ceftriaxone 250 mg IM once; PLUS
    b. Doxycycline 100 mg two times a day for 10 days.
    Alternatively, ofloxacin 300 mg orally two times a day for 10 days can be used in individuals who are 18 years or older.

10. Disseminated gonococcal infection (DGI): Hospitalization for intravenous treatment (IV) is recommended for initial therapy. This is particularly important in individuals who have an uncertain diagnosis, in adolescents where there is uncertain compliance with therapy, and in teens with purulent synovial effusions or other serious complications.
    a. Recommended initial regimen
       — Ceftriaxone 1 g IM or IV every 24 hours
    b. Alternative initial regimens
       — Ceftizoxime 1 g IV every 8 hours; OR
       — Cefotaxime 1 g IV every 8 hours.
       — Spectinomycin 2 g IM every 12 hours should be used in those adolescents allergic to β-lactam drugs.
    c. Duration of therapy: Adolescents may be discharged 24–48 hours after resolution of symptoms to finish a week total of antibiotic therapy with an oral regimen of either:
       — Cefixime 400 mg orally two times a day; OR
       — Ciprofloxacin 500 mg orally two times a day (not to be used in pregnant and lactating women and those under 18 years of age).

11. Meningitis and endocarditis: These serious complications require high-dose IV therapy with an antibiotic effective against the causative strain. The recommended initial regimen is 1–2 g of ceftriaxone IV every 12 hours. Although optimal duration is not known, most authorities treat gonococcal meningitis for 10–14 days and endocarditis for at least 4 weeks.

12. Adult gonococcal ophthalmia: For adolescents and children weighing more than 20 kg, the treatment includes ceftriaxone 1 g IM once, and eye irrigation once with buffered ophthalmic solution should be performed to help clear the discharge. All these indi-

viduals should be followed by careful ophthalmologic examination, including slit-lamp examination. Simultaneous infection with *C. trachomatis* should be considered if the individual does not respond to antibiotics.

13. Doses in adolescents: Adolescents weighing more than 45 kg should be treated with the adult doses, as already outlined above. Adolescents who weigh less than 45 kg should be treated as follows:

   a. For uncomplicated vulvovaginitis, cervicitis, urethritis, pharyngitis, and proctitis:
   — Ceftriaxone 125 mg IM once; OR, if not tolerated,
   — Spectinomycin 40 mg/kg IM (maximum 2 g) once.
   — Adolescents and children over 8 years of age should be given doxycycline 100 mg two times a day for 7 days in addition to the above regimen.
   b. For bacteremia or arthritis:
   — Ceftriaxone 50 mg/kg as a single dose (maximum 1 g) IV for 7 days
   c. For meningitis:
   — Ceftriaxone 50 mg/kg as a single daily dose (maximum 2 g) IV for 10–14 days

Adolescents with documented gonorrhea but no history of sexual activity should be carefully evaluated for sexual abuse.

Public Health Issues

1. Relative high prevalence in adolescents as compared to other age groups
2. High prevalence in certain groups including inner-city populations, adolescent females, men in their early twenties, prostitutes, and substance-abusing individuals
3. High coinfection rates with other sexually transmitted diseases, especially *C. trachomatis*
4. Rapid emergence of multiple types of antibiotic resistance to gonorrhea
5. Large number of asymptomatic gonococcal infections, with a growing number in males

BIBLIOGRAPHY

Addison LA, Koneman EW, Yungbluth MM. Improving your lab workup for gonorrhea. Patient Care 1985; 19:85.

Belding ME, Carbone J. Gonococcemia associated with adult respiratory distress syndrome. Rev Infect Dis 1991;13:1105.

Boslego JW, Tramont EC, Takafuji ET, et al. Effect of spectinomycin use on the prevalence of spectinomycin-resistant and of penicillinase-producing *Neisseria gonorrhoeae*. N Engl J Med 1987;317:272.

Brandt KD, Cathcart ES, Cohen AS. Gonococcal arthritis: clinical features correlated with blood, synovial fluid, and genitourinary cultures. Arthritis Rheum 1974;17:503.

Braverman PK, Strasburger VC. Sexually transmitted diseases. Clin Pediatr (Phila) 1994;33:26.

Britigan BE, Cohen MS, Sparling PF. Gonococcal infection: a model of molecular pathogenesis. N Engl J Med 1985;312:1683.

Brogadir SP, Schimmer BM, Myers AR. Spectrum of the gonococcal arthritis-dermatitis syndrome. Semin Arthritis Rheum 1979;8:177.

Brown RT, Lossick JG, Mosure DJ, et al. Pharyngeal gonorrhea screening in adolescents: is it necessary? Pediatrics 1989;84:623.

Bruins SC, Tight RR. Laboratory-acquired gonococcal conjunctivitis. JAMA 1979;241:274.

Bryant DK, Fox AS, Spigland I, et al. Comparison of rapid diagnostic methodologies for *Chlamydia* and gonorrhea in an urban adolescent population: a pilot study. J Adolesc Health 1995;16:324.

Centers for Disease Control. Chromosomally mediated resistant *Neisseria gonorrhoeae* United States. MMWR 1984;33:408.

Centers for Disease Control. Penicillinase-producing *Neisseria gonorrhoeae* United States, Florida. MMWR 1986;35:12.

Centers for Disease Control. Antibiotic-resistant strains of *Neisseria gonorrhoeae*: policy guidelines for detection, management, and control. MMWR 1987;36 (5s, suppl):1S–18S.

Centers for Disease Control. 1993 Sexually transmitted diseases treatment guidelines. MMWR 1993;42 (RR–14).

Centers for Disease Control. Selected notifiable diseases, 1995. MMWR 1996;45:23.

Cooke DB, Arensberg D, Felner JM, et al. Gonococcal endocarditis in the antibiotic era. Arch Intern Med 1979;139:1247.

Duvauchelle DA, Pien FD. Gonococcal osteomyelitis:

report of a penicillin-resistant strain. Orthopedics 1994;17:719.

Feng WC, Medeiros AA, Murray ES. Diagnosis of gonorrhea in male patients by culture of uncentrifuged first-voided urine. JAMA 1977;237:896.

Fiumara NJ. Gonorrhea, part II: complications of gonorrhea. Medical Aspects of Human Sexuality 1987;(February):79.

Frewen TC, Bannatyne RM. Gonococcal vulvovaginitis in prepubertal girls. Clin Pediatr (Phila) 1979;18:491.

Gann D, Narula OS, Kaplan S, et al. Complete heart block with gonococcal septicemia. Ann Intern Med 1977;86:749.

Gantz NM, McCormack WM, Laughlin LW, et al. Gonococcal osteomyelitis: an unusual complication of gonococcal arthritis. JAMA 1976;236:2431.

Gilbaugh JH, Fuchs PC. The gonococcus and the toilet seat. N Engl J Med 1979;301:9193.

Handsfield HH. Gonorrhea and uncomplicated gonococcal infection. In: Holmes KK, Mardh PA, Sparling PF, Wiesner PJ, eds. Sexually transmitted diseases. New York: McGraw-Hill, 1986.

Handsfield HH, McCormack WM, Hook EW III, et al. A comparison of single-dose cefixime with ceftriaxone as treatment for uncomplicated gonorrhea. N Engl J Med 1991;325:1337.

Hanks JW, Scott CT, Butler CE, et al. Evaluation of a DNA probe assay (Gen-Probe PACE 2) as the test of cure for *Neisseria gonorrhoeae* genital infections. J Pediatr 1994;125:161.

Hawley HB. Gonorrhea: finding and treating a moving target. Postgrad Med 1993;94:105.

Hook EW III, Handsfield HH. Gonococcal infections in the adult. In: Holmes KK, Mardh PA, Sparling PF, Wiesner PJ, eds. Sexually transmitted diseases. 2nd ed. New York: McGraw-Hill Information Services, 1990.

Hook EW III, Holmes KK. Gonococcal infections. Ann Intern Med 1985;102:229.

Hook EW III, Jones RB, Martin DH, et al. Comparison of ciprofloxacin and ceftriaxone as single-dose therapy for uncomplicated gonorrhea in women. Antimicrob Agents Chemother 1993;37;1670–1673.

Hutt DM, Judson FN. Epidemiology and treatment of oropharyngeal gonorrhea. Ann Intern Med 1986;104:655.

Johnson J, Neas B, Parker DE, et al. Screening for urethral infection in adolescent and young adult males. J Adolesc Health Care 1993;14:356.

Lewis JS, Fakile O, Foss E, et al. Direct DNA probe assay for *Neisseria gonorrhoeae* in pharyngeal and rectal specimens. J Clin Microbiol 1993;31:2783.

Odugbemi T, Oyewole F, Isichei CS, et al. Single oral dose of azithromycin for therapy of susceptible sexually transmitted diseases: a multicenter open evaluation. West Afr J Med 1993;136.

Panke ES, Yang LI, Leist PA. Comparison of Gen-Probe DNA probe test and culture for the detection of *Neisseria gonorrhoeae* in endocervical specimens. J Clin Microbiol 1991;29:883.

Pareek SS. Gonococcal otitis externa. N Engl J Med 1979;300:1490.

Pellerano RA, Bishop V, Silber TJ. Gonococcal conjunctivitis in adolescents. Recognition and management. Clin Pediatr (Phila) 1994;33:114.

Quinn TC, Stamm WE, Goodell SE, et al. The polymicrobial origin of intestinal infections in homosexual men. N Engl J Med 1983;309:576.

Roochvarg LB, Lovchik JC. Screening for pharyngeal gonorrhea in adolescents. A reexamination. J Adolesc Health 1991;12:269.

Sadof MD, Woods ER, Emans SJ. Dipstick leukocyte esterase activity in first-catch urine specimens: a useful screening testing for detecting sexually transmitted diseases in the adolescent male. JAMA 1987;258:1932.

Sayeed ZA, Bhaduri U, Howell E, et al. Gonococcal meningitis. JAMA 1972;219:1730.

Schwarcz SK, Bolan GA, Fullilove M, et al. Crack cocaine and the exchange of sex for money or drugs. Risk factors for gonorrhea among black adolescents in San Francisco. Sex Transm Dis 1992;19:7.

Schwarcz SK, Zenilman JM, Schnell D, et al. National surveillance of antimicrobial resistance in *Neisseria gonorrhoeae*: the Gonococcal Isolate Surveillance Project. JAMA 1990;264:1413.

Schaefer RA, Enzenauer RJ, Pruitt A. Acute gonococcal flexor tenosynovitis in an adolescent male with pharyngitis. A case report and literature review. Clin Orthop 1992;281:212.

Shafer MA, Schachter J, Moscicki AB. Urinary leukocyte esterase screening test for asymptomatic chlamydial and gonococcal infections in males. JAMA 1989;262:2562.

Smith JA, Linder CW, Jay S, et al. Isolation of *Neisseria gonorrhoeae* from the urethra of asymptomatic adolescent males. Clin Pediatr (Phila) 1986;25:566.

Smith MS. Left upper quadrant presentation of Fitz-Hugh–Curtis syndrome in an adolescent. West J Med 1979;130:70.

Sparling PF. Biology of *Neisseria gonorrhoeae*. In: Holmes KK, Mardh PA, Sparling PF, Wiesner PJ, eds. Sexually transmitted diseases. 2nd ed. New York: McGraw-Hill Information Services, 1990.

Stary A, Kopp W, Zahel B. Comparison of DNA-probe test and culture for the detection of Neisseria gonorrhoeae in genital samples. Sex Transm Dis 1993;20:243.

Verdon MS, Doublas JM Jr, Wiggins SD, et al. Treatment of uncomplicated gonorrhea with single doses of 200 mg cefixime. Sex Transm Dis 1993;20:290.

Zenilman JM. Gonococcal infections in adolescents. Adolesc Med: State Art Rev 1990;1:497.

CHAPTER 62
Chlamydia trachomatis Infections

Chlamydia trachomatis has been recognized as one of the most common sexually transmitted pathogens among adolescents and young adults. Because of its potentially damaging sequelae, particularly in females and newborns, and the fact that routine screening tests are not always available, the organism is of significant concern. Until recent years, inexpensive, rapid tests were not available for screening and diagnosis. The estimated costs of health care related to chlamydial infections and complications are over $2 billion per year. This chapter's discussion focuses on non–lymphogranuloma venereum (LGV), nontrachoma-causing serotypes of *Chlamydia*.

ETIOLOGY

C. trachomatis has been classified as a nonmotile, Gram-negative, obligate intracellular bacteria, but it shares properties with viruses and bacteria. Virtually all *C. trachomatis* infections are sexually transmitted.

1. The organisms are similar to bacteria in that they contain both DNA and RNA, divide by binary fission, and have cell walls similar to Gram-negative bacteria.
2. The organisms are similar to viruses in that they are obligate intracellular organisms relying on the host cell to produce amino acids and high-energy phosphate. The organism thus can only be grown in cultured cells and not on artificial media.
3. *Chlamydia* is divided into two species: *C. trachomatis* and *C. psittaci*. *C. trachomatis* has inclusions that accumulate glycogen and thus stain with iodine; *C. psittaci* has no such inclusions. *C. trachomatis* is sensitive to sulfonamides; *C. psittaci* is not. Lastly, *C. trachomatis* is primarily a human pathogen, whereas *C. psittaci* affects humans only through animals.

Table 62.1 outlines the serotypes of *Chlamydia*.

PATHOGENESIS

The major mode of transmission of *C. trachomatis* is sexual contact. The life cycle lasts between 48 and 72 hours and is characterized by transformation between the extracellular, elementary bodies and the intracellular, initial or reticulate bodies. The infecting particle is the elementary body (300–400 nm in size), which is resistant to extracellular environment but is metabolically inactive. The elementary bodies induce active phagocytosis in the host's cell and reorganize into initial bodies. The initial bodies divert the cell's functions to the needs of the *Chlamydia* organism. By 24 hours the initial bodies divide and reorganize into many elementary bodies, which lyse the cell, causing cell death and the release of new infectious elementary bodies (Fig. 62.1). *C. trachomatis* has a predilection for columnar epithelium. The signs and symptoms associated with infection are mainly secondary to tissue necrosis and the inflammatory response.

TABLE 62.1.   Serotypes of *Chlamydia*

Species	Serotype	Disease
C. psittaci	(Many unidentified serotypes)	Psittacosis
C. trachomatis	L1, L2, L3	Lymphogranuloma venereum
C. trachomatis	A, B, Ba, C	Hyperendemic blinding trachoma
C. trachomatis	D, E, F, G, H, I, J, K	Inclusion conjunctivitis, nonngonococcal urethritis, cervicitis, proctitis, salpingitis, epididymitis, pneumonia of newborns

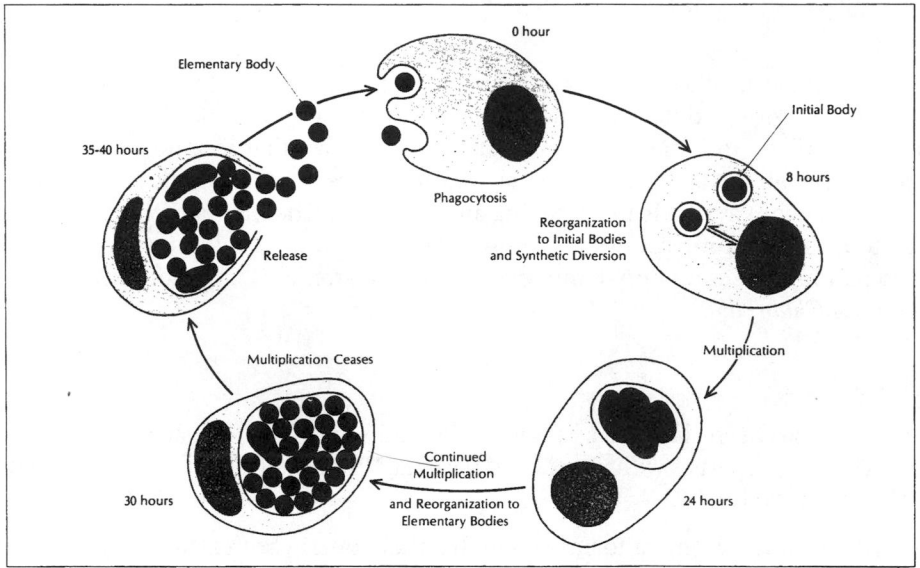

FIGURE 62.1.   Life cycle of *C. trachomatis.* (Reproduced with permission. From Alexander ER. *Chlamydia:* the organism and neonatal infection. Hosp Pract 1979;14(7):64. © 1979, The McGraw-Hill Companies. Illustration by Nancy Lou Makris.)

EPIDEMIOLOGY

Incidence

1. About 3–5 million symptomatic new cases of *C. trachomatis* infection probably occur each year in the United States. This includes an estimated 2.6 million symptomatic infections in females, 1.8 million in males, and 0.25 million in infants. These estimates do not include the large number of people with asymptomatic infection. Since it is a nonreportable disease in some states and only recently reportable in others, incidence rates and trends are only estimates. Adolescents and young adults are at substantial risk for contracting chlamydial infections and are the highest risk group of being infected.

2. Females: *C. trachomatis* is most prevalent in sexually active females between the ages of 12 and 19, with prevalence rates usually more than 10% (5% to more than 30%). The highest detection rates are in juvenile detention centers and in urban, lower socioeconomic minority, and pregnant adolescents. The predilection for younger females may be a result of increased cervical ectopy, allowing more exposure of columnar epithelium to the organism. Prevalence rates of *C. trachomatis* and of *Neisseria gonorrhoeae* among female adolescents in teenage clinics in North America include:

Study	Number of Positive Cases per Total Number in Study (%)
Anglin et al. (1981)	17/75 (22.6)
Saltz et al. (1983)	22/100 (22)
Fraser et al. (1983)	10/125 (8)
Golden et al. (1984)	19/186 (10.2)
Shafer et al. (1984)	56/366 (15.3)
Chacko and Lovchik (1984)	66/260 (25.4)
Eagar et al. (1985)	85/396 (21.5)
Neinstein and Inderlied (1986)	37/184 (20.1)
Fortenberry and Evans (1989)	563/7879 (7.1)
Hughes et al. (1989) (Canada)	66/446 (14.7)
Biro et al. (1994)	77/479 (16.0)
Symptomatic teens	52/251 (20.7)
Asymptomatic teens	25/228 (11.0)

The prevalence of *C. trachomatis* is dependent on the clinic type or site as shown by the following prevalence rates:

Sexually transmitted disease (STD) clinics	20–30%
Adolescent clinics	8–26%
Family planning clinics	6–23%
Teen pregnancy clinics	2–37%
Urban pregnant females	12% (Ferris and Litaker, 1993)
Rural pregnant females	21%
College health center	6% (Keim et al., 1992)
Enlisted U.S. Army females	8.2%

3. Males: While fewer screening studies are available for men, prevalence rates of urethral *C. trachomatis* vary from less than 5% to more than 35%. The lowest rates are in asymptomatic suburban youth, with the highest rates in symptomatic, urban, lower socioeconomic youth. The rates of *C. trachomatis* urethritis in homosexual men have been reported to be about one-third the rates in heterosexual men.

Risk Factors

Several risk factors have been associated with *C. trachomatis* infections including:

1. Age: Younger age, especially younger than 20, is the most significant risk factor for contracting chlamydial infections.
2. Prior history of STDs
3. Multiple sexual partners
4. New partner within past 2 months
5. Use of oral contraceptives: However, the use of oral contraceptives may also lower the risk of symptomatic chlamydial pelvic inflammatory disease (PID) (Wolner-Hanssen et al., 1990).
6. Use of nonbarrier contraceptives
7. Presence of exocervicitis
8. Race: There is a higher prevalence among urban, nonwhite youth and southwestern American Indians of low socioeconomic status.
9. Pregnancy

Transmission

C. trachomatis is a highly transmissible disease, with virtually all cases being sexually transmitted. In females the cervix is the usual initial site of infection; the urethra and rectum may also be infected. In males the urethra is the usual initial site of infection.

1. Seventy percent of female sex partners of males with chlamydial urethritis have positive cultures.
2. Twenty-five percent to 50% of male sex partners of females with a mucopurulent cervicitis or PID have cultures positive for *Chlamydia*.
3. Fifteen percent to 30% of males with urethritis have simultaneous gonorrhea and *Chlamydia*.

CLINICAL MANIFESTATIONS

The clinical manifestations of *C. trachomatis* are similar to those of *N. gonorrhoeae* (Table 62.2). Both tend to infect columnar or transitional epithelium to produce superficial mucosal infections. Both can invade deeper tissue, causing epididymitis or PID. PID is responsible for most of the serious acute illness and economic cost related to chlamydial infections.

Male Infections

Complications other than urethritis, epididymitis, proctitis, and Reiter's syndrome are unusual in males.

Urethritis

1. Urethritis is the most common problem associated with *C. trachomatis* in males.
2. *C. trachomatis* causes about 35–50% of urethritis cases in males.
3. Incubation period is about 7–21 days.
4. Usually dysuria and mild-to-moderate whitish or clear discharge is present.
5. Course may be asymptomatic. In one study of infected males, 25% were asymptomatic, with 33% having four or less polymorphonuclear neutrophil leukocytes (PMNs) on

TABLE 62.2. Comparison of Clinical Manifestations of *Chlamydia trachomatis* and *Neisseria gonorrhoeae*

Site of Infection	Resulting Clinical Syndrome	
	Neisseria gonorrhoeae	*Chlamydia trachomatis*
Males		
Urethra	Urethritis	Nongonococcal urethritis
Epididymis	Epididymitis	Epididymitis
Rectum	Proctitis	Proctitis
Conjunctiva	Conjunctivitis	Conjunctivitis
Systemic	Disseminated gonococcal infection	Reiter's syndrome
Females		
Urethra	Acute urethral syndrome	Acute urethral syndrome
Bartholin's gland	Bartholinitis	Bartholinitis
Cervix	Cervicitis	Cervicitis
Fallopian tube	Salpingitis	Salpingitis
Conjunctiva	Conjunctivitis	Conjunctivitis
Liver capsule	Perihepatitis	Perihepatitis
Systemic	Disseminated gonococcal infection	Arthritis-dermatitis

Gram-stained smears (Stamm, Koutsky, et al., 1984). More males with chlamydial ure-thritis have mild or absent symptoms as compared to males with gonococcal urethritis.

Epididymitis

1. *C. trachomatis* is the most frequent cause of epididymitis in sexually active males less than 35 years of age and accounts for 50% or more of the cases of epididymitis among ado-lescents and young adults.
2. Symptoms and signs include unilateral scrotal pain, swelling, tenderness, and fever.
3. Epididymitis may have an associated chlamydial urethritis.

Proctitis

1. Proctitis usually occurs in either heterosexual females or homosexual males.
2. *C. trachomatis* is responsible for up to 15% of proctitis in homosexual males.
3. LGV strains (see Chapter 68) can produce ulcerative proctitis.
4. Non-LGV strains produce milder infections ranging from asymptomatic states to symp-toms of rectal pain, bleeding, mucous discharge, and diarrhea.

Prostatitis   *Chlamydia* is a possible cause of prostatitis. While definitive studies are lack-ing, *C. trachomatis* has been isolated from some patients with prostatitis.

Reiter's Syndrome   Reiter's syndrome (conjunctivitis, dermatitis, urethritis, and arthritis [see Chapter 37]) has been associated with genital infections with *C. trachomatis*. Most indi-viduals who develop this syndrome are HLA-B27 positive.

Female Infections

Cervicitis

1. As many as 70% of adolescent females with *C. trachomatis* infections are asymptomatic, even with physical signs of a mucopurulent cervicitis. The organism may remain in the cervix as long as 15 months without symptoms.
2. Up to 50% of females with positive *C. trachomatis* cultures have signs or symptoms of a cervicitis including:
   a. Mucopurulent discharge
   b. Edematous, friable cervix
3. Cervical ectopy appears to be a risk factor for infection. Ectopy by itself is a normal find-ing in the adolescent female cervix and should not be mistaken as a cervicitis.

Urethritis

1. *C. trachomatis* can be identified from both cervix and urethra or either alone.
2. Chlamydial infection is a frequent cause of acute dysuria-pyuria syndrome (dysuria, pyuria, and <105 colonies of conventional uropathogens).

Bartholinitis   *Chlamydia, N. gonorrhoeae,* and enteric organisms can all cause bartholinitis.

Pelvic Inflammatory Disease

1. *C. trachomatis* is one of the most frequent causes of PID (see Chapter 63) in adolescent females. It is uncertain how many females with uncomplicated chlamydial infections de-

velop infections of the upper genital tract. An estimated 8% of females with *Chlamydia* have overt salpingitis. Stamm, Guinan, et al. (1984) reported that in females with both gonococcal and chlamydial infections, but who were treated only for gonorrhea, 30% developed salpingitis during follow-up. PID is the major cause of morbidity from chlamydial infections. Treatment does not always prevent sequelae such as infertility or ectopic pregnancies.

2. *C. trachomatis* has been isolated from 5% to 50% of women being evaluated for PID.
3. Symptoms and signs include lower abdominal pain, vaginal discharge, cervical motion tenderness, and uterine and adnexal tenderness.
4. Chlamydial PID may be associated with right upper quadrant pain and tenderness (perihepatitis).
5. *C. trachomatis* can produce upper genital tract infection in the endometrium of asymptomatic females. Jones et al. (1986) isolated *C. trachomatis* from the lower genitourinary tract in 43% of asymptomatic females at risk for chlamydial infections; and in 41% of those with lower genitourinary infection, *C. trachomatis* was isolated from the endometrium.
6. Postpartum and postabortion PID are potential problems in pregnant females with chlamydial infections, occurring in 19–34% of infected pregnant females who deliver vaginally. PID has also been reported in 10–28% of pregnant females with untreated *C. trachomatis* infections who had recently undergone an induced abortion (Centers for Disease Control and [CDC], 1993a & 1993b).

Perihepatitis (Fitz-Hugh and Curtis syndrome)

1. Syndrome may be associated with chlamydial and gonococcal salpingitis.
2. Signs and symptoms include right upper quadrant pain and tenderness, fever, nausea, and vomiting. Signs and symptoms of salpingitis are usually present.

Maternal Chlamydial Infections   Problems include:

1. Two-thirds of infants exposed acquire an infection (Schachter, Grossman, et al., 1986).
2. Stillbirths and neonatal death occur in up to 33% of cases.
3. One of three exposed infants have conjunctivitis. Maternal chlamydial infection is the most common cause of neonatal conjunctivitis.
4. One of six exposed infants have pneumonia. Maternal chlamydial infection is one of the most common causes of pneumonia in the first few months of an infant's life.

Reactive Arthritis   Reactive arthritis usually occurs in males but has been reported in females.

Other Infections and Complications, Male and Female

1. *C. trachomatis* is probably of no pathogenicity in the pharynx. It is present in 3.7% of males and 3.2% of females at risk, but is unassociated with signs or symptoms. In a study by Neinstein and Inderlied (1986) the organism was only isolated in 1/100 adolescents examined.
2. Rare cardiac complications include endocarditis (Dimmitt et al., 1985; Jones, Priest, et al., 1982) and myocarditis.
3. Chlamydial infections cause obstructive infertility and ectopic pregnancy in females. Undetected, untreated fallopian tube infections can be an important cause of infertility and ectopic pregnancy. Two studies of *Chlamydia* and PID in infertile females demonstrated

PID as the cause of the infertility in half the females and found that anti-chlamydial antibody was strongly associated with a tubal problem associated with infertility (Jones et al., 1982; Kelver et al., 1989). Many of these females denied a past history of salpingitis. Undetected cases of salpingitis may also be a contributor to ectopic pregnancies.

DIFFERENTIAL DIAGNOSIS

The differential diagnosis is dependent on the symptom complex of the patient (i.e., urethritis, cervicitis, epididymitis, or abdominal pain). The reader is best directed to the chapters in this book dealing with these individual problems.

The most common problem in females is a mucopurulent cervicitis, which can be caused by:

1. Infections: *N. gonorrhoeae*, *Trichomonas vaginalis*, herpes simplex, and other organisms such as *Escherichia coli*
2. Intrauterine device
3. Allergic reaction to foam or sponge
4. Idiopathic disease

The most common problem in males is a urethritis, which can also be caused by:

1. Infections: *N. gonorrhoeae*, *Ureaplasma urealyticum*, *T. vaginalis*, and herpes simplex
2. Allergic reaction to foam or sponge
3. Idiopathic disease

DIAGNOSIS

The diagnosis of *C. trachomatis* has been complicated in the past by the lack of readily available, highly sensitive, inexpensive screening tests. Today, many rapid nonculture tests have become available to fill this role. More definitive diagnostic tests include culture, fluorescent monoclonal antibody stain (DFA), enzyme immunoassay (EIA), and molecular DNA probes including nucleic hybridization tests (Gen-Probe). In addition, newer sensitive DNA techniques are becoming available such as the polymerase chain reaction (PCR) and ligase chain reaction (LCR).

C. trachomatis infections should be suspected in all sexually active adolescents, particularly those with multiple partners or signs and symptoms of urethritis, cervicitis, epididymitis, or pelvic pain. This includes females with an edematous friable cervix, mucopurulent discharge, and white blood cells on the wet mount or patients with a urethritis with Gram-negative stains or cultures for gonorrhea. In asymptomatic males the urinary leukocyte esterase dipstick on a first-catch urine sample is a good screening test for further evaluation for *C. trachomatis* or *N. gonorrhoeae.*

It must be emphasized that almost 50% or more females and 25% or more males with *Chlamydia* may be asymptomatic. By treating only presumptive cases, at least one-third of infected teenagers will be missed.

1. Considerations in collection of specimens: The accuracy of testing for *Chlamydia* is very dependent on numerous factors including the quality of the specimen collection, the transportation condition, the storage, the experience of the laboratory, and the test used.
   a. As *Chlamydia* is an obligate intracellular organism infecting columnar epithelium, the practitioner must obtain columnar epithelial cells from the endocervix or the urethra. Without appropriate collection, many specimens are likely to be unsatisfactory because they lack urethral or endocervical columnar cells.

    b. Collection site
- Females: The endocervix is the preferred site for screening specimens. When cultures are used, a specimen from the urethra increases sensitivity by as much as 23%. This has not been as well documented for nonculture techniques.
- Males: The urethra is the preferred site for screening specimens.

    c. Technique
- Females
  - (1) Obtain specimens for *Chlamydia* tests after Pap smear and *N. gonorrhoeae* culture.
  - (2) It is important to clean the cervix first to collect cell scrapings and not the discharge, as *Chlamydia* is an obligate intracellular organism.
  - (3) The appropriate swab should be inserted 1–2 cm into the endocervical canal (i.e., past the squamocolumnar junction) and rotated on the wall of the endocervical canal several times for 10–30 seconds. The swab should then be withdrawn without touching the vaginal surface.
  - (4) If a culture is performed, immediately place the swab in transport media and transport in ice.
- Urethral specimens
  - (1) If possible, avoid obtaining urethral specimens until 2 hours after voiding.
  - (2) The *Chlamydia* test should be obtained after specimens for Gram stain smear or *N. gonorrhoeae* culture.
  - (3) The urogenital swab should be gently inserted into the urethra (females: 1–2 cm; males: 2–4 cm) and rotated in one direction for at least one revolution for 5 seconds. The swab should then be placed into the appropriate transport medium (culture, EIA, or DNA probe testing) or use the swab to prepare a slide for DFA testing.
- Type of swab
  - (1) Swabs with wooden shafts should not be used because the wood may contain substances that are toxic to *Chlamydia*.
  - (2) A cytobrush may be better than Dacron swabs to collect specimens in nonpregnant women. Herold et al. (1993) found a twofold prevalence rate using the cytobrush instead of a Dacron swab in detecting *C. trachomatis* from the endocervix of a student health population. This has not been confirmed in all studies (Kellogg et al., 1992).

Further specifics of culture technique can be found in the CDC Report on chlamydial infection (CDC, 1993a).

2. Types of chlamydial tests
    a. Cytology: Cytologic tests are of little practical value because of their low sensitivity (about 40%).
    b. Serology: Serologic tests have little clinical role because of the long time interval required for results and the difficulty in differentiating between acute versus past infections. Serologic examination is useful in the diagnosis of chlamydial pneumonia in infants and for the diagnosis of LGV.
    c. Culture: The culture probably still remains the gold standard to detect *Chlamydia* and is associated with a very high specificity. The sensitivity of the culture technique has been estimated to be 70–90%. Immunoassays and DNA probe techniques, because they can detect dead organisms, may be even more sensitive in some situations. However, some of these other techniques may also be associated with false positives.
- Cultures are recommended in particular for the following specimens:
  - (1) Urethral specimens (women and asymptomatic men)

  (2) Nasopharyngeal specimens (infants)

  (3) Rectal specimens (all patients, regardless of age)

  (4) Vaginal specimens (prepubertal girls)

 — Advantages to culture include:

  (1) High sensitivity

  (2) High specificity

  (3) Preservation of organism to determine immunotype and antimicrobial susceptibility

 — Disadvantages to culture include:

  (1) Expense

  (2) Technically difficult

  (3) Strict transportation and storage requirements

  (4) At least a 48-hour incubation time required

d. Nonculture tests: Several tests are either available or in development.

 — DFA tests: These tests detect the presence of either major outer membrane protein (MOMP) or lipopolysaccharide (LPS), depending on the test used. In this test the material obtained from a swab or endocervical brush is rolled on a slide. The slide is dried and fixed and then stained by the laboratory. The stain binds to chlamydial elementary bodies, which are identified by fluorescence microscopy. The total processing time is 30–40 minutes. The anti-MOMP is specific for *C. trachomatis*, while the anti-LPS can cross-react with other chlamydial and bacterial species.

  (1) DFA advantages

   (a) Easy transport system

   (b) Rapid processing

   (c) High specificity

   (d) Low cost

  (2) DFA disadvantages

   (a) Requires high-quality equipment

   (b) Requires good laboratory technician

   (c) Variable sensitivity in different groups

 — EIA tests: These tests detect chlamydial LPS with a monoclonal or polyclonal antibody tagged with an enzyme. This enzyme leads to the conversion of a colorless material into a colored product with the intensity of the color measured quantitatively by a spectrophotometer. Specimens are collected with swabs and transported in tubes. Laboratory processing time is 3–4 hours. The use of LPS leads to cross-reaction with other organisms and other chlamydial species. The use of blocking assays to confirm initially positive tests has helped the specificity of these tests. The blocking assay uses antibodies specific for chlamydial LPS.

  (1) EIA advantages

   (a) Easy transport system

   (b) Rapid processing

   (c) Low cost

   (d) No need for specialized laboratory technicians

  (2) EIA disadvantages

   (a) Sensitivity questionable

   (b) Cannot check adequacy of the specimen

 — Nucleic acid hybridization tests (DNA probe, e.g., Gen-Probe): These tests are a recent addition for the diagnosis of chlamydial infections. In this test a chemiluminescent DNA probe complementary to a specific sequence of *C. trachomatis* ribosomal RNA (rRNA) is added to the specimen so that the probe can hybridize to any chlamydial rRNA present. The DNA:rRNA hybrids are adsorbed with magnetic particles, which can be detected using a luminometer. Many laboratories are now testing for both gonorrhea and *Chlamydia* using a single endocervical swab. Specimens should be processed within 7 days of collection. The total processing time is 2–3 hours. The assay is specific for *C. trachomatis* and does not appear to cross-react with other organisms including other chlamydial types. Newer, even more sensitive and specific, tests include the PCR and the LCR techniques. These tests use amplification techniques that can enhance sensitivity.

— Rapid *Chlamydia* tests: These tests can be completed within 30 minutes in a clinic situation without expensive equipment. They offer the advantage of giving immediate results to base clinical decisions on. However, the tests use antibodies against LPS and so a false-positive result can occur. The tests have not been evaluated extensively in clinical situations.

— Leukocyte esterase test (LET): A urine dipstick is used to screen for the presence of PMNs in the urine. The test detects enzymes produced by these cells, causing a color change on the dipstick strip. The test is only meant to be used as a screening test for urinary tract infections or a urethritis.

e. Accuracy and use of nonculture tests: Most of the published results on test accuracy have used the MicroTrak DFA (Syva), the Chlamydiazyme EIA (Abbott), and the Gen-Probe test. Other tests have been approved by the Food and Drug Administration (FDA) but have not been as extensively used in clinical studies. Because of differing techniques and sample populations, the accuracy values of different tests have varied widely from study to study.

Overall, the sensitivities of available diagnostic assays for *Chlamydia* include:

Culture	"gold standard" (about 70–90% sensitive)
DFA	60–90%
EIA	70–90%
Nucleic acid hybridization	68–96%
PCR	90–97%
LCR	93–97%
LET	40–100%
In urine:	
EIA	75–90%
PCR or LCR	93–97%

The sensitivity and specificity of the nonculture techniques seem highest in groups of adolescents with the highest risk (prevalence >10%) and lowest in groups with a low prevalence rate. The addition of blocking agents to immunoassay tests in recent years to lessen the risk of cross-reactivity with nonchlamydial flora has helped the accuracy of the immunoassay test in low-prevalence populations.

With some nonculture tests, false-positive results can be a problem, particularly in low-prevalence populations. With low-prevalence populations, as many as 50% or more of the positive results could be false positives. Nonculture positive results should be confirmed using another supplemental test, particularly if a false-positive result would lead to adverse consequences medically or socially. Confirmatory methods include culture, a different nonculture technique, or the use of an EIA-blocking antibody test.

Biro et al. (1994) compared two enzyme immunoassays and a DNA probe technique with culture for the diagnosis of endocervical *C. trachomatis* in 479 adolescent females. The following values were found:

Diagnostic Technique	Sensitivity	Specificity	Positive Predictive Value	Negative Predictive Value
Cell culture				
Asymptomatic	0.80	1.0	1.0	0.98
Symptomatic	0.75	1.0	1.0	0.94
Overall	0.77	1.0	1.0	0.96
Chlamydiazyme EIA				
Asymptomatic	0.52	1.0	1.0	0.94
Symptomatic	0.71	1.0	1.0	0.93
Overall	0.65	1.0	1.0	0.94
Microtrak EIA				
Asymptomatic	0.80	0.99	0.91	0.98
Symptomatic	0.81	0.97	0.89	0.95
Overall	0.81	0.98	0.90	0.96
PACE 2 (DNA probe)				
Asymptomatic	0.72	0.96	0.67	0.96
Symptomatic	0.65	0.96	0.81	0.91
Overall	0.68	0.96	0.75	0.94

Schubiner et al. (1990) compared the culture, DFA, EIA, and DNA probe in 200 adolescent and young adult females. The relative sensitivities, specificities, and predictive values were:

	DFA (%)	DNA Probe (%)	EIA (%)
Sensitivity	68	80	88
Specificity	98	100	99.4
Positive predictive value	85	100	95.6
Negative predictive value	95.5	97.2	98.3

Loeffelholz et al. (1992) compared a rapid PCR technique with both culture and EIA. The PCR had a sensitivity of 97% and specificity of 99.7%, while the culture had a sensitivity of 85.7% and specificity of 100%. The EIA had a sensitivity of 58.8% and specificity of 100%.

3. Accuracy in various collection sites

    a. Cervical specimen in females: The DFA and EIA have a reported sensitivity of greater than 70% in high-prevalence (>5%) populations. None of the nonculture tests have been adequately evaluated in low-prevalence populations. The specificity of nonculture tests for cervical specimens has been high (97–99%).

    b. Urethral specimens (males): The EIA and DFA tests in males with symptomatic urethritis has generally exceeded 70%. The specificities in these men have generally been high (97–99%). Nonculture techniques are not generally recommended for asymptomatic urethral infections in males, as these tests many not be sensitive enough.

    c. Urine: The LET has been used to screen sexually active adolescent males for urethritis. Positive test results require confirmation with a more specific test for *C. trachomatis* and *N. gonorrhoeae*. The LET has sensitivities of between 40% and 100% and specificities between 83% and 100%. Nonculture testing of urine sediment is being more thoroughly investigated to avoid the need for an intraurethral specimen. The EIA method on first-voided urine has a sensitivity ranging from 30% in asymptomatic males to 88% in symptomatic males with a specificity of about 97%. PCR and LCR techniques with specificities equal to culture and sensitivities higher than culture may play an expanded role in testing urine for *Chlamydia*.

   d. Rectum: The preferred method for rectal specimens is the culture. Some DFA tests have been approved for use in the rectum, but the specificity may be less than that of specimens from the cervix or urethra.

   e. Conjunctiva: Nonculture tests probably have accuracy similar to genital specimens.

   f. Sexual abuse victims: Only culture techniques should be used, as nonculture tests are not sensitive or specific enough. A second test should be done 2 weeks after the initial assault.

     Most of the nonculture tests have approval only for genital specimens in postpubertal males and females. A couple of EIA and DFA tests have approval for conjunctivitis in infants. None of the tests have approval for genital or rectal specimens from children and other victims of sexual assault. The culture technique is the most appropriate in children and abuse cases. The PCR test based on DNA amplification technology has the potential to be more sensitive than culture methods and 100% specific. The PCR test has been demonstrated to be more sensitive than culture in at least one study in women with PID (Witkin et al., 1993).

4. Screening for chlamydial infections

   a. If feasible, all sexually active teenagers should be screened for *Chlamydia*, as well as for gonorrhea. If all teenagers cannot be screened, then the following groups should have the highest priority:
     — Teens with symptoms compatible with *Chlamydia*
     — Teens attending an STD clinic who are not being treated with an anti-*Chlamydia* agent
     — All pregnant adolescents or teens attending an abortion facility
     — Teens with inconsistent use of condoms or more than one partner in the past 3 months
     Sellors et al. (1992) found that several factors were associated with a positive culture in asymptomatic females. These include cervical friability, suspicious discharge, urinary frequency, intermenstrual bleeding, and a new sex partner in the past year.

   b. Females can be screened with nonculture tests of the cervix. Positive results should be confirmed in low-risk and low-prevalence populations.

   c. Males: Because urethral specimens require an invasive examination, there has been increasing interest in using noninvasive tests. Most of the focus has been on using urine specimens. In asymptomatic males the LET test has been used (Sellors et al., 1993). Positive LET test results should be confirmed with a smear or intraurethral culture. Shafer et al. (1989) found the following values of the urinary LET among 948 asymptomatic adolescent males:
     — Sensitivity, 72%
     — Specificity, 93%
     — Positive predictive value, 58%
     — Negative predictive value, 96%
     Randolph and Washington (1990) compared the cost and benefits of screening tests for *C. trachomatis* in adolescent males. The LET urine dipstick test was the most cost effective, followed by the DFA and then the culture. For those males with a positive LET test or even for symptomatic males, EIA and DNA probe techniques applied to urine sediment are noninvasive and seem to show promising results. Hay et al. (1993) found a 90% sensitivity of the EIA test on first-catch urine sediment compared to 83% using the DFA on a urethral smear. Sanders et al. (1994) found a 85% sensitivity and 99.3% specificity using the EIA test on urine sediment in asymptomatic and symptomatic males. PCR techniques may prove to be even better.

TREATMENT

Treatment should not be dependent entirely on finding a positive chlamydial test result. Testing is not available in all sites. In is thus advised to treat all adolescents with:

1. A *Chlamydia*-associated syndrome such as mucopurulent endocervicitis, PID, gonorrhea, nongonococcal urethritis, and epididymitis
2. A positive result from *Chlamydia* culture or other chlamydial test
3. Exposure to a patient with positive culture or *Chlamydia* syndrome
4. A gonococcal infection

Regimens

Recommended Regimens   Uncomplicated urethral, endocervical, or rectal infection in adults and adolescents should be treated as follows:

1. Doxycycline 100 mg orally two times a day for 7 days; OR
2. Azithromycin 1 g orally in a single dose.

Alternative Regimens   If tetracyclines are contraindicated or not tolerated, use the following:

1. Ofloxacin 300 mg orally two times a day for 7 days; OR
2. Erythromycin base 500 mg by mouth four times a day for 7 days; OR
3. Erythromycin ethylsuccinate 800 mg by mouth four times a day for 7 days; OR
4. Sulfisoxazole 500 mg orally four times a day for 10 days (not as effective as other regimens).

Azithromycin has the advantage of single-dose administration. However, it is much more expensive than doxycycline and is not approved yet for adolescents younger than 16. Both drugs appear similar in efficacy and toxicity, but neither is approved for use during pregnancy. Ofloxacin is also very effective but is also expensive and not approved for use during pregnancy or for adolescents younger than 18. Erythromycin has more gastrointestinal toxicity but is inexpensive and can be used during pregnancy. Sulfisoxazole has the least efficacy of the regimens.

Follow-up

When taken as directed, doxycycline, azithromycin, and ofloxacin are highly effective (>95%). If one of these regimens is used, posttreatment cultures are not required unless symptoms persist or reinfection is suspected. Posttreatment cultures 3 weeks after completion of treatment should be considered if erythromycin or sulfisoxazole is used. Reculturing before 3 weeks after completion of therapy can lead to false-negative results. False-positive results from the continued presence of dead organisms may also occur if nonculture tests are done less than 3 weeks after therapy is completed. Patients with positive posttreatment cultures should be retreated with one of the preceding regimens, as resistant *Chlamydia* has not been described. Partners should also be retreated.

Adolescents with chlamydial infections are at increased risk for chlamydial infections later on. In one study of adolescents with chlamydial infections followed for up to 24 months after treatment, follow-up rates of infection were 39% (Jones, 1990).

Sex Partners

All sex partners should be referred for evaluation and treatment. The exact time intervals for exposure have not been well evaluated. The CDC recommend referring sexual partners of symptomatic patients who have had exposure within 30 days. This should be extended to 60 days if the patient is asymptomatic. The last sex partner should be treated even if the time interval is greater than 60 days. Sex partners of mothers with infected newborns should also be evaluated and treated.

Patients should avoid sexual contact until they and their partners are cured. In lieu of test-of-cure this would mean completion of therapy and lack of symptoms.

Pregnant Patients

Recommended Regimen during Pregnancy   Erythromycin base 500 mg by mouth four times a day for 7 days.

Alternative Regimens

1. Erythromycin base 250 mg by mouth four times a day for 14 days; OR
2. Erythromycin ethysuccinate 800 mg four times a day for 7 days; OR
3. Erythromycin ethylsuccinate 400 mg four times a day for 14 days.

Although not recommended by the CDC, McNeely et al. (1989) have found that 1 g/day orally of erythromycin for 7 days has a similar cure rate in pregnant women with endocervical infection as 2 g/day and is associated with fewer gastrointestinal side effects. In pregnant women who cannot tolerate erythromycin, amoxicillin 500 mg orally three times a day for 7–10 days should be used.

Doxycycline, ofloxacin, and erythromycin estolate are contraindicated during pregnancy. Sulfisoxazole is contraindicated during pregnancy near-term and for breast-feeding women. The safety of azithromycin during pregnancy and breast-feeding has not been established. However, Bush and Rosa (1994) found that azithromycin cured 100% of pregnant women in their small study and was associated with no gastrointestinal side effects. They concluded that azithromycin is a valid treatment option in pregnant patients who cannot tolerate erythromycin. Although not recommended by the CDC, clindamycin 450 mg orally four times a day for 7 days has also been found to be as effective as erythromycin in infected pregnant women (Lovchik and Alger, 1990).

HIV Infection

Adolescents with human immunodeficiency virus (HIV) infection and chlamydial infections should receive the same treatments as listed above for those without HIV infections.

PREVENTION

1. Goal
   a. To prevent overt and silent chlamydial salpingitis and its sequelae
   b. To prevent perinatal and postpartum infections
   c. To prevent adverse consequences of other chlamydial infections
2. Prevention strategies
   a. Primary prevention
      — Behavioral changes include reduction of the number of sex partners, delaying age of first intercourse, and the use of condoms. *Chlamydia* is often neglected in dis-

cussions of HIV risk and sexual behaviors. Information about *Chlamydia* should be incorporated into educational materials and discussions regarding risk behaviors. Specific areas to cover include:

(1) Rates of chlamydial infection among adolescents

(2) Adverse consequences of *Chlamydia* (e.g., PID and infertility)

(3) Clinical manifestation of chlamydial infections (and other STDs)

(4) Asymptomatic infection

(5) Treatment for sex partners

(6) Referrals on locations and telephone numbers of health-care delivery sites

— Identify and treat infected patients and their partners and also identify infected pregnant females.

b. Secondary prevention

— Screen females to identify and treat asymptomatic chlamydial infections.

— Treat partners of infected patients.

— Recognize *Chlamydia*-associated syndromes such as mucopurulent cervicitis and treat as appropriate.

3. Target populations

a. Sexually active adolescents and young adults

— Females: Females should be screened at least annually or whenever they present for a pelvic examination. In young females between 20 and 24 in lower prevalence areas, screening is advisable for those with either inconsistent use of a condom or who have a new or more than one sexual partner during the past 3 months.

— Males: The LET urine test probably can be used to screen sexually active males to identify those requiring further testing. The frequency of such testing has never been evaluated, but adolescent males infrequently seek routine health care. Thus, when sexually active males seek health care, the LET is probably a reasonable screening test.

b. Pregnant females and females undergoing an induced abortion

c. Youth, particularly females, in detention facilities or attending an STD clinic

CHLAMYDIA-ASSOCIATED SYNDROMES

Nongonococcal Urethritis

Criteria for nongonococcal urethritis (NGU) include objective evidence of urethritis in a patient with negative test results for *N. gonorrhoeae*. Stripping the urethra in suspected males by exerting pressure on the penis with the forefinger and thumb and moving from the base to the meatus three times will help demonstrate a discharge. Objective evidence of an NGU includes:

1. An abnormal discharge

2. Equal to or greater than 4 PMNs per oil immersion field in a smear from a Gram-stained intraurethral swab specimen without intracellular Gram-negative diplococci.

The LET is frequently used to screen urine from asymptomatic males for evidence of urethritis. For those adolescents with a positive LET, the diagnosis should be confirmed with a Gram-stained smear from the urethra.

As many as 50% of cases of NGU are related to *C. trachomatis*. The incubation period may vary from days to weeks. Other organisms involved include *U. urealyticum* in 20–40% of cases, *T. vaginalis* in 2–5%, and herpes simplex virus in some cases.

Treatment of Choice   Doxycycline 100 mg should be given orally twice a day for 7 days. Alternatively, erythromycin base 500 mg orally four times a day for 7 days or erythromycin ethylsuccinate 800 mg orally four times a day for 7 days could be used. If these dosages of erythromycin cannot be tolerated, the dose can be cut in half and the length extended to 14 days. The recommendations for treatment of sex partners and treatment in HIV-infected adolescents are the same as listed for chlamydial infections.

Patients should be re-evaluated if symptoms persist or recur after therapy is completed. Recurrent NGU is usually due to lack of compliance with antibiotics or to reinfection. These individuals should initially be retreated with their initial regimen. If the teen finished the initial therapy and was not re-exposed, the teen should be evaluated by an intraurethral swab for *T. vaginalis* and treated with an alternative regimen such as erythromycin base for 14 days if *T. vaginalis* is not present.

Mucopurulent Cervicitis

Mucopurulent cervicitis in many cases is caused by *C. trachomatis*. Other organisms isolated include *N. gonorrhoeae* and herpes simplex virus. However, in many other cases none of these organisms can be isolated.

Criteria for presumptive diagnosis of mucopurulent cervicitis include:

1. Mucopurulent secretion from the endocervix. Secretion is usually yellow or green, especially when viewed on a white cotton-tipped swab (positive swab test).
2. More than 10 PMNs per oil immersion field in a Gram-stained smear of endocervical secretions
3. Cervical friability (bleeding when the first swab culture is taken)
4. Erythema or edema within a zone of cervical ectopy

Mucopurulent cervicitis has been associated with adverse pregnancy outcome. Nugent and Hillier (1992) found that women with greater than or equal to 30 PMNs per high-powered oil immersion field were twice as likely to deliver a low–birth weight infant.

If *N. gonorrhoeae* is found on Gram stain or culture, a treatment regimen effective against both gonococcal and chlamydial infection should be used. When only a chlamydial infection is proven or suspected, therapy should consist of one of the regimens for chlamydial infections as outlined previously. In adolescent populations where one or both of these organisms has a high prevalence, the teen should be treated presumptively for the organism(s) that has a high prevalence rate.

Treatment of Sex Partners   Males exposed to females with mucopurulent discharge should be evaluated for an STD and treated with the same regimen as their sex partners.

Pelvic Inflammatory Disease

Since many cases of PID are caused by more than one organism, treatment regimens must include broad coverage. Evaluation and treatment of PID are discussed in detail in Chapter 63.

Acute Epididymo-Orchitis

Most epididymo-orchitis infections that affect sexually active adolescents and young adults are related to either *C. trachomatis* or to *N. gonorrhoeae* and are often associated with a urethritis. In homosexual males epididymitis may also be caused by sexually transmitted *E. coli* among the insertive partners involved in anal intercourse.

Males with epididymitis usually complain of unilateral testicular pain and tenderness, and swelling of the epididymis is usually present. The diagnosis is based on evaluating:

1. A Gram-stained intraurethral swab evaluating for Gram-negative intracellular diplococci and for more than 4 PMNs per oil immersion field
2. Culture of the urethral exudate or an intraurethral swab specimen for *N. gonorrhoeae* or *C. trachomatis.*
3. Culture and Gram-stained smear of uncentrifuged urine: Testicular torsion should be considered in the differential diagnosis of all adolescents with sudden onset of unilateral testicular pain, tenderness, and swelling. A Doppler and radionuclide scan may be required to differentiate torsion from acute epididymitis.

Treatment   Treatment should be initiated before culture results are known.

Regimen of Choice

1. Ceftriaxone 250 mg IM once; AND
2. Doxycycline 100 mg orally two times a day for 10 days.

Bed rest and elevation of the scrotum are also recommended.

Alternative Regimen   Ofloxacin 300 mg orally two times a day for 10 days is not approved for use in individuals younger than 18.

These regimens are similar in HIV-infected teens. However, in immunocompromised adolescents fungal and mycobacterial causes are more common.

Those teens who fail to respond within 3 days require close re-evaluation of the diagnosis and therapy.

Sex Partners   Sex partners should be examined for an STD and treated with a regimen effective against uncomplicated gonococcal and chlamydial infections. Both partners should avoid sexual contact until therapy is completed and both individuals are asymptomatic.

BIBLIOGRAPHY

Adger H, Sweet RL, Shafer MA, et al. Screening for *C. trachomatis* and *Neisseria gonorrhoeae* in adolescent females: value of first catch urine examination. Lancet 1984;2:944.

Alexander ER. Chlamydia: the organism and neonatal infection. Hosp Pract 1979;14:63.

Anglin TM, Brown RF, Kumar ML. *Chlamydia trachomatis* in adolescent females [Abstract]. Pediatr Res 1981; 15:440.

Barnhart KT, Sondheimer SJ. Contraception choice and sexually transmitted disease. Curr Opin Obstet Gynecol 1993;5:823.

Bevan CD, Johal BJ, Mumtaz G, et al. Clinical, laparoscopic and microbiological findings in acute salpingitis: report on a United Kingdom cohort. Br J Obstet Gynaecol 1995;102:407.

Biro FM, Reising SF, Doughman JA, et al. A comparison of diagnostic methods in adolescent girls with and without symptoms of *Chlamydia* urogenital infection. Pediatrics 1994;93:476.

Blythe MJ, Katz BP, Orr DP, et al. Historical and clinical factors associated with *Chlamydia trachomatis* genitourinary infection in female adolescents. J Pediatr 1988;112:1000.

Brunham RC, Paavonen J, Stevens CE, et al. Mucopurulent cervicitis: the ignored counterpart in women of urethritis in men. N Engl J Med 1984;311:1.

Bryant DK, Fox AS, Spigland I, et al. Comparison of rapid diagnostic methodologies for *Chlamydia* and gonorrhea in an urban adolescent population: a pilot study. J Adolesc Health 1995;16:324.

Bush MR, Rosa C. Azithromycin and erythromycin in the treatment of cervical chlamydial infection during pregnancy. Obstet Gynecol 1994;84:81.

Cates W. The epidemiology and control of sexually transmitted diseases in adolescents. Adolesc Med: State Art Rev 1990;1:409.

Catterson ML, Zaddo V. Prevalence of asymptomatic chlamydial cervical infection in active duty Army females. Milit Med 1993;158:618.

Centers for Disease Control and Prevention. Recommendations for the prevention and management of *Chlamydia trachomatis* infections, 1993. MMWR 1993a;42 (RR–12):1.

Centers for Disease Control and Prevention. 1993 Sexually transmitted diseases treatment guidelines. MMWR 1993b;42(RR–14):1.

Chacko MR, Lovchik JC. *Chlamydia trachomatis* infection in sexually active adolescents: prevalence and risk factors. Pediatrics 1984;73:836.

Chernesky MA, Mahoney JB, Mores M, et al. Detection of *Chlamydia trachomatis* antigens by enzyme immunoassay and immunofluorescein in genital specimens from symptomatic and asymptomatic men and women. J Infect Dis 1986;154:141.

Chow JM, Yonekura L, Richwald GA, et al. The association between *Chlamydia trachomatis* and ectopic pregnancy. JAMA 1990;263:3164.

Dalaker K, Gjnnaess H, Kuile G, et al. *Chlamydia trachomatis* as a cause of perihepatitis associated with pelvic inflammatory disease. Br J Vener Dis 1981;57:41.

DePunzio C, Neri E, Metelli P, et al. Epidemiology and therapy of *Chlamydia trachomatis* genital infection in women. J Chemother 1992;4:163.

Dimmitt SR, Pearman JW, Woolard KV. Chlamydial endocarditis. Aust N Z J Med 1985;15:340.

Eagar RM, Beach RK, Davidson AJ, et al. Epidemiologic and clinical factors of *Chlamydia trachomatis* in black, hispanic, and white female adolescents. West J Med 1985;143:37.

Edet EE. The prevalence of *Chlamydia trachomatis* infection among gynaecological patients. Br J Clin Pract 1993;47:21.

Falk ES, Vandbakk O. Declining trends in some sexually transmitted diseases in Norway between 1975 and 1991 with special reference to a Lapp population. Acta Derm Venereol Suppl 1993;182:15.

Ferris DG, Litaker M. Chlamydial cervical infections in rural and urban pregnant women. South Med J 1993;86:611.

Fisher MA. *Chlamydia trachomatis* genital infections. W Va Med J 1993;89:331.

Fortenberry JD, Evans DL. Routine screening for genital *Chlamydia trachomatis* in adolescent females. Sex Transm Dis 1989;16:168.

Fraser JJ, Rettig PJ, Kaplan DW. Prevalence of cervical *Chlamydia trachomatis* and *Neisseria gonorrhoeae* in female adolescents. Pediatrics 1983;71:222.

Freund KM. Chlamydial disease in women. Hosp Pract 1992;(February 15):175.

Genc M, Ruusuvaara L, Mardh PA. An economic evaluation of screening for *Chlamydia trachomatis* in adolescent males. JAMA 1993;270:2057.

Getts AG. Diagnosing *Chlamydia trachomatis* urethritis by first-catch urine enzyme immunoassay in adolescent males. J Adolesc Health Care 1989;10:209.

Golden N, Hammerschlag M, Neuhoff S, et al. Prevalence of *Chlamydia trachomatis* cervical infection in female adolescents. Am J Dis Child 1984;138:562.

Grayston JT, Mordhorst CH, Wang SP. Childhood myocarditis associated with *Chlamydia trachomatis* infection. JAMA 1981;246:2823.

Gump DW, Dickstein S, Gibson M. Endometritis related to *Chlamydia trachomatis* infection. Ann Intern Med 1981;95:61.

Hammerschlag MR. New recommendations for *Chlamydia trachomatis* infections. Infect Med 1994;11:199.

Handsfield HH, Jasman LL, Roberts PL, et al. Criteria for selective screening for *Chlamydia trachomatis* infection in women attending family planning clinics. JAMA 1986;255:1750.

Hay PE, Thomas BJ, McKenzie P, et al. Detection of *Chlamydia trachomatis* in men. Sensitive tests for sensitive urethras. Sex Transm Dis 1993;20:1.

Herold AH, Young DL, Wightman JK, et al. Comparison of the cytology brush with the Dacron swab for detecting *Chlamydia trachomatis* by enzyme immunoassay in female university students. J Am Coll Health 1993;41:213.

Horner PJ, May PE, Thomas BJ, et al. The role of *Chlamydia trachomatis* in urethritis and urethral symptoms in women. Int J STD AIDS 1995;6:31.

Hughes EG, Mowatt J, Spence JE. Endocervical *Chlamydia trachomatis* infection in Canadian adolescents. Can Med Assoc J 1989;140:297.

Jones RB. Treatment of *Chlamydia trachomatis* infections of the urogenital tract. In: Bowie WR, Caldwell HD, Jones RP, et al., eds. Chlamydial infections: proceedings of the seventh international symposium on human chlamydial infections. Cambridge: Cambridge University Press, 1990:509–518.

Jones RB, Ardery BR, Hui SL, et al. Correlation between serum antichlamydial antibodies and tubal factor as a cause of infertility. Fertil Steril 1982;38:553.

Jones RB, Mammel JB, Shepard MK, et al. Recovery of *Chlamydia trachomatis* from the endometrium of women at risk for chlamydial infection. Am J Obstet Gynecol 1986;155:35.

Jones RB, Priest JB, Kuo CC. Subacute chlamydial endocarditis. JAMA 1982;247:655.

Jones RB, Rabinovitch RA, Katz BP, et al. *Chlamydia trachomatis* in the pharynx and rectum of heterosexual patients at risk for genital infection. Ann Intern Med 1985;102:757.

Kaplan JE, Meyer M, Navin J. *Chlamydia trachomatis* infection in a male college student population. J Am Coll Health 1989;37:159.

Keim J, Woodard MP, Anderson MK. Screening for *Chlamydia trachomatis* in college women on routine gynecological exams. J Am Coll Health 1992;41:17.

Kellogg JA, Seiple JW, Klinedinst JL, et al. Comparison of cytobrushes with swabs for recovery of endocervical cells and for Chlamydiazyme detection of *Chlamydia trachomatis*. J Clin Microbiol 1992;30:2988.

Kellogg JA, Seiple JW, Murray CL, et al. Effect of endocervical specimen quality on detection of *Chlamydia trachomatis* and on the incidence of false-positive results with the Chlamydiazyme method. J Clin Microbiol 1990;28:1108.

Kelver ME, Nagamani M. Chlamydial serology in women with tubal infertility. Int J Fertil 1989;34:42.

Komaroff AL, Aronson MD, Pass TM, et al. *Chlamydia trachomatis* infection in adults with community-acquired pneumonia. JAMA 1981;245:1319.

Lee HH, Chernesky MA, Schachter J, et al. Diagnosis of *Chlamydia trachomatis* genitourinary infection in women by ligase chain reaction assay of urine. Lancet 1995;345:213.

Loeffelholz MJ, Lewinski CA, Silver SR. Detection of *Chlamydia trachomatis* in endocervical specimens by polymerase chain reaction. J Clin Microbiol 1992; 30:2847.

Lovchik JC, Alger L. Clindamycin and erythromycin compared for treatment of *Chlamydia trachomatis* infection. 29th Annual Interscience Conference on Antimicrobial Agents and Chemotherapy, Houston, 1990.

Majeroni BA. Chlamydial cervicitis: complications and new treatment options. Am Fam Physician 1994;49: 1825.

Mardh PA, Holmes KK, Oriel JD, et al. Chlamydial infections. Amsterdam: Elsevier Biomedical Press, 1982.

Mardh PA, Miller BR, Ingerselv HJ, et al. Endometritis caused by *Chlamydia trachomatis*. Br J Vener Dis 1981; 57:191.

Martin DH. Chlamydial infections. Med Clin North Am 1990;74:1367.

Martin D, Koutsky L, Eschenbach DA, et al. Prematurity and perinatal mortality in pregnancies complicated by maternal *Chlamydia trachomatis* infections. JAMA 1982;247:1585.

Martin DH, Mroczkowski TF, Dalu AZ, et al. A controlled trial of a single dose of azithromycin for the treatment of chlamydial urethritis and cervicitis. N Engl J Med 1992;327:921.

McCormack WM, Mardh PA. Fifth International Symposium on Human Chlamydial Infection. Sex Transm Dis 1982;9:216.

McCormack WM, Rosner B, McComb DE, et al. Infection with *Chlamydia trachomatis* in female college students. Am J Epidemiol 1985;121:107.

McNagny SE, Parker RM, Zenilman JM, Lewis JS. Urinary leukocyte esterase test: a screening method for the detection of asymptomatic chlamydial and gonococcal infections in men. J Infect Dis 1992;165:573.

McNeeley SG, Ryan GM, Baselski V. Treatment of chlamydial infections of the cervix during pregnancy. Sex Transm Dis 1989;16:60.

Mills RD, Young A, Cain K, et al. Chlamydiazyme plus blocking assay to detect *Chlamydia trachomatis* in endocervical specimens. Am J Clin Pathol 1992;97:209.

Moncada J, Schachter J, Bolan G, et al. Confirmatory assay increases specificity of the Chlamydiazyme test for *Chlamydia trachomatis* infection of the cervix. J Clin Microbiol 1990;28:1770.

Myhre EB, Mardh PA. *Chlamydia trachomatis* infections in a patient with meningoencephalitis. N Engl J Med 1981;304:910.

Neinstein LS, Inderlied C. Low prevalence of *Chlamydia trachomatis* in the oropharynx of adolescents. Pediatr Infect Dis J 1986;5:660.

Neinstein LS, Rabinovitz S. Detection of *Chlamydia trachomatis:* a study of the direct immunofluorescence technique and a review of diagnostic limitations. J Adolesc Health Care 1988;10:10.

Nettleman MD, Jones RB, Roberts SD, et al. Cost effectiveness of cultures for *Chlamydia trachomatis*. Ann Intern Med 1986;105:189.

Nugent RP, Hillier SL. Mucopurulent cervicitis as a predictor of chlamydial infection and adverse pregnancy outcome. The Investigators of the Johns Hopkins Study of Cervicitis and Adverse Pregnancy Outcome. Sex Transm Dis 1992;19:198.

Nuovo J, Melnikow J, Paliescheskey M, et al. Cost-effectiveness analysis of five different antibiotic regimens for the treatment of uncomplicated *Chlamydia trachomatis* cervicitis. J Am Board Fam Pract 1995;8:7.

O'Brien SF, Bell TA, Farrow JA. Use of a leukocyte esterase dipstick to detect *Chlamydia trachomatis* and *Neisseria gonorrhoeae* urethritis in asymptomatic adolescent male detainees. Am J Public Health 1988;78:1583.

Oh MK, Cloud GA, Baker SL, et al. Chlamydial infection and sexual behavior in young pregnant teenagers. Sex Transm Dis 1993;20:45.

Oh MK, Feinstein RA, Soileau EJ, et al. *Chlamydia trachomatis* cervical infection and oral contraceptive use among adolescent girls. J Adolesc Health Care 1989; 10:376.

Preece PM, Anderson JM, Thompson RG. *Chlamydia trachomatis* infection in infants: a prospective study. Arch Dis Child 1989;64:525.

Quinn TC. Update on *Chlamydia trachomatis* infections. Infect Med 1994;11:201.

Quinn TC, Goodell SE, Mkrtichian E, et al. *Chlamydia trachomatis* proctitis. N Engl J Med 1981;305:195.

Quinn TC, Warfield P, Kappus E, et al. Screening for *Chlamydia trachomatis* infection in an inner city population: a comparison of diagnostic methods. J Infect Dis 1985;152:419.

Randolph AG, Washington AE. Screening for *Chlamydia trachomatis* in adolescent males: a cost-based decision analysis. Am J Public Health 1990;80:545.

Reed BD, Huck W. Differences in the prevalence of *Chlamydia trachomatis* reported by two laboratories using direct immunofluorescence test. JAMA 1987; 257:2593.

Remafedi G, Abdalian SE. Clinical predictors of *Chlamydia trachomatis* endocervicitis in adolescent women. Looking for the right combination. Am J Dis Child 1989;143:1437.

Saltz GR, Linnemann CC Jr, Brookman RR, et al. *Chlamydia trachomatis* cervical infections in female adolescents. J Pediatr 1983;98:981.

Sanders JW, Hook EW III, Welsh LE, et al. Evaluation of an enzyme immunoassay for detection of *Chlamydia trachomatis* in urine of asymptomatic men. J Clin Microbiol 1994;32:24.

Sanders LL, Harrison HR, Washington AE. Treatment of sexually transmitted chlamydial infections. JAMA 1986;255:1750.

Schachter J. Biology of *Chlamydia trachomatis*. In: Holmes KK, Mardh PA, Sparling PF, Wiesner PJ, eds. Sexually transmitted diseases. 2nd ed. New York: McGraw-Hill Information Services, 1990.

Schachter J, Grossman M, Sweet RL, et al. Prospective study of perinatal transmission of *Chlamydia trachomatis*. JAMA 1986;255:3374.

Schachter J, Stoner E, Moncada J. Screening for chlamydia infections in women attending family planning clinics. Evaluation of presumptive indicators for therapy. West J Med 1983;138:375.

Schachter J, Sweet RL, Grossman M, et al. Experience with the routine use of erythromycin for chlamydial infection in pregnancy. N Engl J Med 1986;314:276.

Schubiner HH, Lebar W, Jemal C, et al. Comparison of three new nonculture tests in the diagnosis of *Chlamydia* genital infections. J Adolesc Health Care 1990; 11:505.

Schydlower M, Shafer MA. *Chlamydia trachomatis* infections in adolescents. Adolesc Med: State Art Rev 1990;1:615.

Scott G. Non-invasive tests for *Chlamydia trachomatis*. Lancet 1995;345:207.

Sellors JW, Mahony JB, Pickard L, et al. Screening urine with a leukocyte esterase strip and subsequent chlamydial testing of asymptomatic men attending primary care practitioners. Sex Transm Dis 1993;20:152.

Sellors JW, Pickard L, Gafni A. Effectiveness and efficiency of selective vs universal screening for chlamydial infection in sexually active young women. Arch Intern Med. 1992;152:1837.

Shafer MA, Beck A, Blain B, et al. *Chlamydia trachomatis:* important relationships to race, contraception, lower genital tract infection, and Papanicolaou smear. J Pediatr 1984;104:141.

Shafer MA, Prager V, Shalwitz J, et al. Prevalence of urethral *Chlamydia trachomatis* and *Neisseria gonorrhoeae* among asymptomatic, sexually active adolescent boys. J Infect Dis 1987;156:223.

Shafer MA, Schachter J, Moscicki AB, et al. Urinary leukocyte esterase screening test for asymptomatic chlamydial and gonococcal infections in males. JAMA 1989;262:2562.

Shafer MA, Vaughan E, Lipkin ES, et al. Evaluation of fluorescein-conjugated monoclonal antibody test to detect Chlamydia trachomatis endocervical infections in adolescent girls. J Pediatr 1986;108:779.

Shepard MK, Jones RB. Recovery of *Chlamydia trachomatis* from endometrial and fallopian tube biopsies in women with infertility of tubal origin. Fertil Steril 1989;52:232.

Skolnik NS. Screening for *Chlamydia trachomatis* infection. Am Fam Physician 1995;51:821.

Skulnick M, Small GW, Simor AE, et al. Comparison of the Clearview Chlamydia test, Chlamydiazyme, and cell culture for detection of *Chlamydia trachomatis* in women with a low prevalence of infection. J Clin Microbiol 1991;29:2086.

Stamm WE, Guinan ME, Johnson C. Effect of treatment regimens for *Neisseria gonorrhoeae* on simultaneous infection with *Chlamydia trachomatis*. N Engl J Med 1984;310:545.

Stamm WE, Harrison R, Alexander ER, et al. Diagnosis of *Chlamydia trachomatis* infections by direct immunofluorescent staining of genital secretions. A multicenter trial. Ann Intern Med 1984;101:638.

Stamm WE, Hicks CB, Martin DH, et al. Azithromycin for empirical treatment of the nongonococcal urethritis syndrome in men. A randomized double-blind study. JAMA 1995;274:545.

Stamm WE, Holmes KK. *Chlamydia trachomatis* infections of the adult. In: Holmes KK, Mardh PA, Sparling PF, Wiesner PJ, eds. Sexually transmitted diseases, 2nd ed. New York: McGraw-Hill Information Services, 1990.

Stamm WE, Koutsky LA, Benedetti JK, et al. *Chlamydia trachomatis* urethral infections in men. Prevalence, risk factors, and clinical manifestations. Ann Intern Med 1984;100:47.

Stamm WE, Running K, McKevitt M, et al. Treatment of the acute urethral syndrome. N Engl J Med 1981; 304:956.

Stamm WE, Wagner KF, Amsel R, et al. Causes of the acute urethral syndrome in women. N Engl J Med 1980;303:409.

Sweet RL, Landers DV, Walker C, et al. *Chlamydia trachomatis* infection and pregnancy outcome. Am J Obstet Gynecol 1987;156:824.

Thejls H, Rahm VA, Rosen G. Correlation between chlamydia infection and clinical evaluation, vaginal wet smear, and cervical swab test in female adolescents. Am J Obstet Gynecol 1987;157:974.

Thompson SE, Washington AE. Epidemiology of sexually transmitted *Chlamydia trachomatis* infections. Epidemiol Rev 1983;5:96.

Washington AE, Gove S, Schachter J, et al. Oral contraceptives, *Chlamydia trachomatis* infection, and pelvic inflammatory disease. A word of caution about protection. JAMA 1985;253:2246.

Washington AE, Johnson RE, Sanders LL Jr. *Chlamydia trachomatis* infections in the United States. What are they costing us? JAMA 1987;257:2070.

Webster LA, Greenspan JR, Nakashima AK, et al. An evaluation of surveillance for *Chlamydia trachomatis* infections in the United States, 1987–1991. MMWR 1993;42:21.

Werner MJ, Biro FM. Urinary leukocyte esterase screening for asymptomatic sexually transmitted disease in adolescent males. J Adolesc Health 1991;12:326.

Witkin SS, Jeremias J, Toth M, et al. Detection of *Chlamydia trachomatis* by the polymerase chain reaction in the cervices of women with acute salpingitis. Am J Obstet Gynecol 1993;168:1438.

Wolner-Hanssen P, Eschenbach DA, Paavonen J, et al. Decreased risk of symptomatic chlamydial pelvic inflammatory disease associated with oral contraceptive use. JAMA 1990;263:54.

Wolner-Hanssen P, Westrom L, Mardh PA. Perihepatitis in chlamydial salpingitis. Lancet 1980;1:901.

Wood VD, Shoroye A. Sexually transmitted disease among adolescents in the juvenile justice system of the District of Columbia. J Natl Med Assoc 1993; 85:435.

CHAPTER 63

Pelvic Inflammatory Disease

Lawrence S. Neinstein and Karen S. Himebaugh

Pelvic inflammatory disease (PID) is defined as an acute infection caused by the ascending spread of microorganisms from the lower genital tract (vagina and endocervix) to the upper genital tract (endometrium, fallopian tubes, or contiguous structures). PID has been overshadowed by the acquired immunodeficiency syndrome (AIDS) epidemic but remains one of the most serious consequences of sexual activity among adolescents. Over one-half of the adolescents in the United States are sexually active, and the rates of sexual activity have increased among younger adolescent age groups. Over 1 million women have PID each year in the United States at an estimated annual cost of over $4.2 billion. The highest prevalence of PID is in the adolescent and young adult age group. Physicians dealing with teenagers should be familiar with the disease, its presentation, and current treatment choices. Earlier diagnosis and treatment of PID may reduce the morbidity that can result from delayed or missed diagnosis. Teens with PID are at increased risk for chronic pelvic pain, ectopic pregnancy, and tubal infertility.

ETIOLOGY

Predisposing Factors

1. Number of sexual partners: The risk of PID in females with multiple partners is 4.6 times higher than for females with one partner.
2. Age at first intercourse: Earlier age is associated with increased risk.
3. Previous PID or history of prior sexually transmitted disease (STD)
   a. Females with PID are 2.3 times more likely than females without PID to have a history of previous PID.
   b. About 23% of patients with PID develop a subsequent episode.
4. Age: The highest PID rates are among females aged 15–25. Seventy percent of cases occur in females younger than 25 years old and 33% in females younger than 19 years old. In fact, gonococcal and chlamydial PID are most prevalent in sexually active females aged 16–20. Sexually active adolescents are three times more likely to have PID than women aged 25–29. Although all the reasons for the increased risk among adolescents are not known, suspected reasons include:
   a. Cervical ectopy: Adolescents have more cervical ectropion than older women. *Neisseria gonorrhoeae* and *Chlamydia trachomatis* prefer columnar epithelium. Thus, adolescents who are exposed to these organisms may be at greater risk of contracting an infection.
   b. Lack of local immunity
   c. Less use of barrier methods
   d. More risky sexual behaviors

5. Ethnicity: Nonwhite young females are at increased risk for PID compared to white young females by a factor of about 2.5:1.
6. Type of contraception
   a. Barrier methods: Condoms when used consistently and correctly throughout sexual activity are highly effective in reducing the risk of acquisition and transmission of STDs that cause PID. Condom use has increased among adolescents, but less than 50% of adolescents report consistent use in most surveys. The use of spermicides containing nonoxynol 9 can also reduce a female's risk of acquiring a bacterial STD by causing cell wall destruction of STD pathogens including *N. gonorrhoeae* and *C. trachomatis.* However, spermicide use in teens is erratic and inconsistent.
   b. Oral contraceptives: Overall, users of oral contraceptives have fewer endocervical gonococcal infections and more chlamydial endocervical infections. Oral contraceptive use seems to decrease the rates by almost 50% of both gonococcal and nongonococcal PID. This is probably related to the hormonal effects causing a decrease in menstrual blood flow and a thickened cervical mucus. In addition, the severity of the PID infection seems to be decreased in the adolescent who develops PID while using oral contraceptives. It has not been shown that oral contraceptives protect against the infertility that may be caused by subclinical infections with these organisms.
   c. Intrauterine device: A female who uses an intrauterine device (IUD) for contraception has a two to four times greater risk of developing PID. The risk factor is higher (seven to nine times increased risk) in nulliparous females. The risk of PID with IUD use is increased for both the copper-releasing IUD and the progesterone IUD system. The increased risk is mainly in the first months after insertion of an IUD, and the risks appear lower in current IUDs than in earlier types. A levonorgestrel-releasing IUD system has been studied in Europe with encouraging preliminary results showing a protective effect against PID.
7. Vaginal douching: Females who douched during the previous 3 months have a 2.1 times elevated risk of PID after controlling for other measured risk factors (Scholes et al., 1993).
8. Substance abuse: A recent survey reports that 33% of adolescents report drinking at least five drinks in one sitting within the past 2 months. Sexual disinhibition related to alcohol use or nonintravenous drug use is associated with multiple partners and failure to use condoms.
9. Bacterial vaginosis: There is an elevated risk for PID if bacterial vaginosis is present before first trimester therapeutic abortion (Larsson et al., 1992).
10. Menses: PID related to *N. gonorrhoeae* and *C. trachomatis* usually occurs within the first week after the onset of menstruation. This may relate to the loss of the protective endocervical mucous plug and the presence of menstrual blood.

Of particular concern is that many adolescent patients have several of these risk factors present.

Microbiology

1. General comments
   a. Overall, PID is polymicrobial in nature, with most cases of PID associated with more than one organism. Studies in the United States show that over 50% of females with acute PID have *N. gonorrheae* or *C. trachomatis* (or both) recoverable by culture from the endocervix. In the United States women with PID have the following organisms isolated from the upper genital tract:

N. gonorrhoeae	25–50%
C. trachomatis	10–43%
Nongonococcal, nonchlamydial	
anaerobes and aerobes	25–84%

   b. Aside from *N. gonorrhoeae* and *C. trachomatis,* the organisms isolated in the upper genital tract in females with PID include mixed anaerobic organisms (*Bacteroides* and *Peptostreptococcus* species), facultative bacteria (*Gardnerella vaginalis, Streptococcus* species, *Escherichia coli,* and *Haemophilus influenzae*), and genital tract mycoplasmas (*Mycoplasma hominis* and *Ureaplasma urealyticum*). Many individuals have both *N. gonorrhoeae* and *C. trachomatis* plus either anaerobes and aerobes. There may be a poor correlation between cervical and intra-abdominal cultures.

2. Gonococcal PID
   a. Approximately 33–50% of PID patients have gonococcal PID.
   b. About 15% of females with endocervical gonorrhea have involvement of the upper genital tract.
   c. *N. gonorrhoeae* and *C. trachomatis* occur simultaneously in about 40%.
   d. Gonococcal PID tends to produce symptoms within the *first week* of the menstrual cycle.
   e. The longer the duration of symptoms, the less chance of recovering gonorrhea. Within 24 hours of symptoms, gonorrhea is recovered in 70% of females, while after 48 hours the recovery rate drops to 19%.

3. *C. trachomatis* PID
   a. *C. trachomatis* PID is the most common bacterial STD in adolescent males and females in the United States.
   b. Thirty percent to 60% of infections may be asymptomatic.
   c. In patients with PID the onset of pain is usually the week after menses.
   d. Estimates of prevalence rates range from 8% to 39%.
   e. A threefold to sixfold increased risk for human immunodeficiency virus (HIV) seroconversion exists for women infected with *Chlamydia* as compared to those not infected.

4. Nongonococcal aerobic and anaerobic bacteria
   a. Over two-thirds of females with PID have aerobic and anaerobic bacteria on culture from culdocentesis or laparotomy specimens.
   b. Nongonococcal PID may occur following a primary gonococcal or chlamydial infection, IUD use, or a vaginal or cervical infection. The prevalence rate increases as the time from onset of symptoms to culture increases.
   c. Nongonococcal or nonchlamydial PID, with the exception of tuberculosis and mumps, seems confined to sexually active females.
   d. Severe PID associated with an abscess is invariably a polymicrobial infection with anaerobic bacteria involved (Heinonen and Miettinen, 1994).

5. *Mycoplasma hominis:* The role of the mycoplasmas in PID is still not resolved. The organism is more likely to be isolated from the cervix of females with PID than the endometrium or fallopian tubes. However, the organism has been isolated from the fallopian tubes in individuals with salpingitis and does not seem to be present in the tubes of individuals with no history of PID.

6. Other organisms: Rare causes include *Actinomyces* (mainly associated with IUD infections), *Campylobacter,* pinworms, and tuberculosis.

Pathogenesis

1. General comments: The lower genital tract (the vagina and cervix) is colonized by normal flora that include aerobic and anaerobic streptococci, coli forms, *Bacteroides* species,

lactobacilli, and genital mycoplasmas. In contrast, the upper genital tract (the uterus and fallopian tubes) is sterile. The host defenses that normally protect the spread of bacteria to the upper genital tract include an acidic vaginal pH, a thick layer of vaginal epithelial cells, and the cervical mucous plug. Also the uterotubal junction and the ampulloisthmic junction may serve as anatomic sphincterlike barriers.

2. Menstruation has been identified as a risk factor for the development of PID.
    a. Menstrual blood may serve as a carrier, as it is refluxed into the tubes.
    b. During menstruation the endocervical mucous plug is lost, allowing bacteria to enter the uterus.
    c. Menstrual blood can act as an excellent culture medium for the gonorrhea and bacteria, but this is probably not important for *Chlamydia*.
    d. Menstruation causes a loss of the endometrium, which serves as a protective barrier from infection.
3. Progression of the infection from the uterus through the fallopian tube may be facilitated by the normal ciliary activity inside the tubes. The ensuing inflammatory reaction leads to damage of the endothelial tissue, with resultant scarring and on occasion occlusion of the tubes. Previous episodes of PID may result in scarring of tubal structures, thus impairing protective mechanisms.
4. Mechanical factors such as an IUD and douching may facilitate invasion of the upper genital tract. Transport of organisms may also occur through sperm, white blood cells, or some STDs such as *Trichomonas vaginalis*. Gynecology surgery or instrumentation may also precipitate PID.

Clinical Manifestations

Symptoms

1. Abdominal pain: The pain is usually continuous, bilateral, and most severe in the lower quadrants. The pain usually increases with movement and sexual intercourse. It is usually present for less than 3 weeks.
2. Abnormal vaginal bleeding: This is present in about 35% of patients with PID. However, it may also be present in adolescents with an ectopic pregnancy or an ovarian cyst.
3. Relation of pain to menses: Gonococcal PID usually starts within 1 week of menses. Sweet et al. (1986) studied the relationship between organisms causing PID and menses. Eighty-one percent of cases of acute salpingitis that started within 7 days of menses were caused by either chlamydial or gonococcal infections, whereas 66% of cases that started after 14 days of a menstrual cycle involved only nongonococcal, nonchlamydial organisms.
4. Vaginal discharge: About 50%
5. Fever and chills: A fever over 38°C is present in about 40% of women with laparoscopically verified PID.
6. Gastrointestinal symptoms: Anorexia, nausea, vomiting; infrequent complaints
7. Right upper quadrant pain (perihepatitis): About 5–15%
8. *Chlamydia*-associated PID tends to be more subacute and smoldering than gonococcal PID.

Signs   Generally, adolescents with PID have lower abdominal pain and tenderness, cervical motion tenderness, and adnexal tenderness. A unilateral process should make the practitioner more suspicious about the diagnosis being PID.

About one-third of laparoscopically verified cases of salpingitis are associated with rectal temperatures greater than 38°C. Although 50% of individuals with PID have palpable adnexal swelling, experienced physicians have also reported adnexal swelling in 24% of individuals who have normal tubes on laparoscopy. Essentially all cases of PID should be associated with evidence of a lower genital tract infection. Almost no individuals with PID have been found to have normal smears (few or no leukocytes, dominance of Gram-positive rods, and vaginal epithelial cells). This is very helpful in excluding salpingitis.

Golden et al. (1989) compared adolescents with gonococcus-associated PID with those with *Chlamydia*-associated PID. Those with gonococcus-associated PID had a shorter duration of pain before admission, a higher mean maximum temperature, and higher leukocyte counts. Spence et al. (1990) compared 106 young adults with 65 adolescents with PID. The most significant differences were that the adolescents sought health care later in the course of the illness (7.8 days versus 5.6) and were more commonly infected with gonococcus (42% versus 28%).

DIFFERENTIAL DIAGNOSIS

There is a large differential diagnosis for PID or acute lower abdominal pain in the adolescent female. These include:

Gastrointestinal Tract

1. Acute appendicitis: One of the more difficult to distinguish from PID (Table 63.1)
2. Acute cholecystitis
3. Inflammatory bowel disease
4. Irritable bowel disease
5. Constipation
6. Gastroenteritis
7. Mesenteric lymphadenitis

Genital Tract

1. Ectopic pregnancy
2. Ovarian cyst with or without torsion

TABLE 63.1.   PID versus Acute Appendicitis

	PID	Acute Appendicitis
Age	Any after puberty	Any
Onset of symptoms	50–75% within 7 days of menses	Anytime in cycle
Pain	Dull, crampy localized to lower abdomen ± rebound	Poorly localized, periumbilical with shift to right lower quadrant, increasing severity
Vaginal discharge	55–90% present	Not associated
Menstrual pattern	Metrorrhagia	No change in usual pattern
Fever	>38°C in up to 35%	Usually <38°C; >38°C if perforation has occurred
Nausea and vomiting	<30% patients	>50%
Cervical motion tenderness	>80%	Usually none, may be present with perforation
Bowel sounds	Normal or decreased	Decreased or absent
Adnexal mass	5–60%	Not associated unless periappendiceal abscess present
Anemia	Not associated	Not associated
White blood cell count	Normal or mild elevation	Mildly elevated
Pelvic ultrasound	Common findings: cul-de-sac fluid, adnexal enlargement, complex adnexal mass	Not associated abnormalities in some cases or thickened appendiceal wall and internal debris

3. Endometriosis
4. Septic or threatened abortion
5. Pelvic thrombophlebitis
6. Dysmenorrhea
7. Mittelschmerz
8. Severe vaginal herpes simplex infection

Urinary

1. Acute pyelonephritis
2. Cystitis
3. Renal stone
4. Urethritis

Other

1. Functional pain

Diagnosis

The accurate diagnosis of PID is essential in preventing long-term sequelae. However, the diagnosis is based largely on history and physical examination, and this assessment can be difficult, especially in nonovert cases. The difficulties are demonstrated in a classic study conducted in Sweden by Jacobson and Westrom (1969) (Fig. 63.1). They performed laparoscopy on 814 consecutive patients with the clinical diagnosis of PID. Of these patients, 532 (65%) had confirmed salpingitis, 98 (12%) had another diagnosis, and 184 (23%) had a normal examination. An additional 91 patients with other clinical diagnoses were found to have salpingitis on laparoscopy. Thus, the clinical evaluation had a sensitivity of 84% and a predictive value of only 65% (532/814). The most common alternative diagnoses were ovarian cysts, ectopic pregnancy, appendicitis, and endometriosis.

No one symptom or sign is specific or pathognomonic for PID. Finding evidence of a lower genital tract infection is crucial in the diagnosis, since this is generally a prerequisite for a sexually related salpingitis. Lower abdominal tenderness, adnexal tenderness, and cervical motion tenderness are present in over 90% of women with laparoscopically documented

Acute salpingitis		532
Normal		184
Other disorders		98
Acute appendicitis	24	
Pelvic endometriosis	16	
Corpus luteum hematoma	12	
Ectopic pregnancy	11	
Ovarian tumor	7	
Chronic salpingitis	6	
Mesenteric lymphadenitis	6	
Miscellaneous	16	

Figure 63.1.   Laparosopic diagnoses in 814 women with clinically diagnosed salpingitis. (Adapted from Jacobson L, Westrom L. Objectified diagnosis of acute pelvic inflammatory disease: diagnostic and prognostic value of routine laparoscopy. Am J Obstet Gynecol 1969;105:1088–1098.)

salpingitis. However, if one were to perform laparoscopy on all women with these clinical symptoms, only about 60% will have documented salpingitis.

History

History should include:

1. Age of the adolescent
2. Sexual history including number of sexual partners, number of new partners in past 30–60 days, and symptoms in partners
3. Menstrual history including date of last menstrual period, patterns of recent menses, onset of pain in relation to menses, increased blood flow, and dysmenorrhea
4. Contraception history including use of barrier methods, IUD, or oral contraceptives
5. Drug history particularly use of illicit drugs (especially crack cocaine)
6. Vaginal douching
7. Previous STDs or PID
8. Type of pain including onset, duration, quality, and location. History of right upper quadrant pain in addition to pelvic pain suggesting perihepatitis (Fitz-Hugh and Curtis syndrome)
9. Fever or chills
10. Nausea, vomiting, or diarrhea
11. Vaginal discharge
12. Urinary symptoms (suggestive of a urethritis)
13. Dyspareunia

Abnormal uterine bleeding and dysmenorrhea can occur with salpingitis.

Physical Examination

The physical examination is critical in the diagnosis of PID. This would include careful examination of:

1. Abdomen: Look for evidence of peritoneal signs and careful palpation of the abdomen and pelvic area to help locate the source and severity of the problem. Liver tenderness in someone with presumed PID suggests Fitz-Hugh and Curtis syndrome.
2. Pelvic examination
   a. External genitalia: Look for evidence of herpes that might explain some of the pain or serve as a marker for other STDs.
   b. Vagina: Look for evidence of vaginitis.
   c. Presence of cervical motion tenderness
   d. Cervix: Mucopurulent discharge suggests cervicitis and can be marker of PID. Look for friability of cervix.
   e. Uterus: Look for presence of tenderness.
   f. Adnexa: Look for presence of tenderness or masses.
3. Gait: Many individuals with PID walk with a "PID shuffle." This is the individual who walks slightly bent over, holding the lower abdomen and shuffling the feet, while trying to move the leg and pelvis forward together with each step to minimize movement of the pelvic region.

Diagnostic Criteria

Due to the wide range of signs and symptoms of PID, diagnosis is difficult and is usually made clinically. It is better to overtreat and overdiagnose than to permit mild or atypical cases to go

Table 63.2. Diagnostic Criteria

Minimum Criteria
   Lower abdominal tenderness
   Adnexal tenderness (bilateral or unilateral)
   Cervical motion tenderness
Routine Criteria
   Oral temperature >38.3°C (100.9°F)
   Abnormal cervical or vaginal discharge
   Elevated rate of erythrocyte sedimentation or C-reactive protein
   Laboratory documentation of cervical infection with *Neisseria gonorrhoea* or *Chlamydia trachomatis*
Elaborate Criteria
   Histopathologic evidence of endometritis on endometrial biopsy
   Tubo-ovarian abscess on sonography
   Laparoscopic abnormalities consistent with PID

Adapted from Centers for Disease Control. Sexually transmitted diseases treatment guidelines, 1993. MMWR 1993;42:1.

untreated. The Centers for Disease Control (CDC) developed clinical criteria for the diagnosis (Table 63.2). The minimum criteria are intended for use in females without signs of competing diagnoses such as positive pregnancy test or evidence of appendicitis. The routine or additional criteria increase the specificity and are useful when teens present with more severe clinical signs and incorrect diagnosis and treatment could lead to unnecessary morbidity. The elaborate criteria firmly establish the diagnosis but are more expensive and often invasive. The use of any criteria serves only as a guide, since the diagnosis can be difficult to make. There are no criteria that approach anywhere near both 100% sensitivity and 100% specificity.

Laboratory Findings

Most routine laboratory findings are not of great assistance in establishing the diagnosis of PID.

1. Hematocrit: The hematocrit may be normal or low. A level below 30% suggests an ectopic pregnancy.
2. White blood cell count: This is elevated in about 56% of gonococcal PID patients and 35% of nongonococcal PID patients.
3. Sedimentation rate: A sedimentation rate greater than 15 mm/hr is found in 75% of PID patients. However, other conditions such as ectopic pregnancy and appendicitis may elevate the white blood cell count and sedimentation rate.
4. Wet mount: Wet mount is extremely useful. PID is almost always associated with evidence of a lower genital tract infection, as demonstrated by increased numbers of polymorphonuclear neutrophil leukocytes (PMNs) on a wet mount.
5. Cervical Gram stain: This may be extremely useful. A cervical Gram stain with three or more PMNs with intracellular Gram-negative diplococci is highly suggestive of gonorrhea. This test detects about two-thirds of patients with gonorrhea and is 98% specific in symptomatic females. The test is not useful in screening asymptomatic females but is helpful in the high-risk symptomatic adolescent.
6. Cervical gonorrhea and *Chlamydia* cultures: These should be routine in all sexually active adolescents at the time of the pelvic examination. However, since the results take several days, they can only be helpful in confirming a diagnosis. Treatment will usually be started before the results are known. Indirect rapid *Chlamydia* tests can be substituted for a culture in high-risk adolescents, especially if cost is a factor. The practitioner should remember that females with *Chlamydia* or gonococcal-negative endocervical cultures may have positive tubal or uterine cultures for these organisms.

7. Pregnancy test: A pregnancy test is essential to eliminate the possibility of a complication of pregnancy. It is particularly critical if a mass, unilateral pain, or a late menstrual period is present on evaluation.

8. Examination of the male partner: This can be extremely helpful if the male is found to have a discharge compatible with gonorrhea. Kamwendo et al. (1993) examined male partners of adolescent and young adult females with acute PID to determine the presence of *N. gonorrhoeae* or *C. trachomatis* infection or nonspecific urethritis (NSU) in regular sexual male partners. *N. gonorrhoeae*, *C. trachomatis*, or NSU were demonstrated in 117 (59.7%) of the 196 male partners, but only 32% of the males with *N. gonorrhoeae* or *C. trachomatis*, and 8.5% of those with NSU presented subjective symptoms of urethritis.

9. Syphilis serology: Serologic examination is recommended in individuals with PID to rule out the possibility of concomitant syphilis.

10. Culdocentesis: Culdocentesis was a common test in years past to aid in the diagnosis and as a source for cultures. The presence of fluid containing white blood cells is suggestive of PID or another source of peritonitis. If nonclotting blood is found, the culdocentesis is suggestive of ectopic pregnancy or another source of intra-abdominal bleeding. Because of vaginal contamination, the organisms grown by culdocentesis do not correlate with culture data obtained from tubal aspirates. Because of the invasiveness and unpleasantness of this test, it has fallen in use.

11. Ultrasound: Ultrasound is of diagnostic value if the pelvic examination is difficult, if there is a question of an ectopic pregnancy, or if a pelvic mass or abscess is suspected. In addition, ultrasound may detect tubo-ovarian abscesses (TOAs) in adolescents before they are clinically apparent. Golden et al. (1989) found that 19.3% of their adolescents with PID had TOAs and that in the majority of these teens the abscesses were not suspected clinically.

12. Laparoscopy: The indications for laparoscopy are controversial at present. Because of the severe prognosis of PID and the difficulty of accurately diagnosing it, some authorities advocate the liberal use of laparoscopy. However, laparoscopy is expensive, involves hospitalization, and thus is not practical on a routine basis. A more realistic approach would be to treat adolescents for a presumptive PID, especially if overt disease, a positive Gram stain, a male partner with a urethral discharge, or known STD is present. If the diagnosis is unclear or if there is treatment failure, laparoscopy should be considered.

THERAPY

As the diagnosis of PID and accurate bacteriologic diagnosis can only be made by laparoscopy, treatment must be empiric and broad-spectrum. Antibiotics should cover *N. gonorrhoeae*, *C. trachomatis*, Gram-negative organisms, anaerobes, and group B streptococci. Unfortunately, there are limited data comparing various antibiotic regimens in reducing the incidence of long-term complications such as infertility and ectopic pregnancy.

1. Indications for hospitalization: The first decision after making a tentative diagnosis of PID is whether to hospitalize the adolescent. Ideally, hospitalization is indicated whenever possible. If not possible, then indications for hospitalization include:
   a. Uncertain diagnosis when surgical emergencies such as appendicitis or ectopic pregnancy must be excluded
   b. Adnexal mass
   c. Severely ill patient or evidence of peritonitis
   d. Pregnancy
   e. Suspicion of inability of the adolescent to follow outpatient therapy

   f. Failure to respond to outpatient therapy
   g. Vomiting or intolerance of oral antibiotics
   h. Clinical follow-up within 72 hours of starting antibiotics cannot be arranged
   i. Women known to be infected with HIV
   j. Many authorities recommend that all adolescents or young women of reproductive age be hospitalized because of poor compliance with therapy and the potential for significant long-term sequelae.

2. General principles in treating acute PID
   a. Overdiagnose adolescents with PID to prevent complications and sequelae.
   b. Rule out the possibility of pregnancy.
   c. Treatment should begin early in the course and with recommended broad-spectrum regimens of antibiotics.
   d. An IUD if present should be removed once antibiotics are started.
   e. Reevaluate the adolescent in 48–72 hours after beginning treatment.
   f. Partners should be evaluated or referred and treated.
   g. Educate the adolescent regarding the use of condoms and spermicides in reducing the risk of reoccurrence of STDs and PID.

3. Inpatient therapy: Suggested regimens by the CDC include:
   a. Cefoxitin 2 g IV every 6 hours; OR cefotetan IV 2 g every 12 hours; PLUS doxycycline 100 mg every 12 hours orally or IV.

      If normal gastrointestinal function is present, doxycycline has similar bioavailability given orally as given intravenously. Other cephalosporins such as ceftizoxime, cefotaxime, and ceftriaxone with gonococcal, Gram-negative aerobic and anaerobic coverage may also be used instead of cefoxitin or cefotetan. Cefotetan has similar properties to cefoxitin but requires less frequent dosing. Less clinical data are available on the third-generation cephalosporins.

      These drugs should be given for at least 48 hours after the patient clinically improves. After discharge, continue doxycycline orally 100 mg two times a day for 10–14 days total. The teen should be re-evaluated 72 hours after discharge from the hospital.
   b. Clindamycin IV 900 mg every 8 hours; PLUS gentamicin loading dose of 2 mg/kg IV or IM and maintenance 1.5 mg/kg IV or IM every 8 hours.

      These drugs should be given for at least 48 hours after the patient clinically improves. After discharge continue either:

Doxycycline orally 100 mg two times a day until day 14 of treatment; OR clindamycin 450 mg orally four times a day until day 14 of treatment.

No data are available on the efficacy of doxycycline in treating anaerobic or Gram-negative infections when used alone after discharge from the hospital. Adding clindamycin 450 mg orally four times a day as an outpatient may be considered in some cases.

Doxycycline may prove to be unnecessary when clindamycin is used, as clindamycin appears to be an effective agent against *C. trachomatis.* In fact, Soper and Despres (1988) compared the use of cefoxitin and doxycycline versus the combination of clindamycin and amikacin. No differences were detected in the success rates. Hemsell et al. (1994) compared the response to inpatient therapy with three CDC-recommended regimens including cefoxitin plus doxycycline, clindamycin plus gentamicin, or cefotetan plus doxycycline. The three regimens produced almost identical cure rates. No serious adverse clinical or laboratory events were observed.

4. Outpatient therapy
   a. Cefoxitin 2 g IM in a single dose plus probenecid 1 g orally concurrently; OR ceftriaxone 250 mg IM; OR another third-generation cephalosporin; PLUS doxycycline 100 mg orally two times a day for 14 days.

An alternative regimen for individuals who are not able to tolerate doxycycline is erythromycin 500 mg orally four times a day for 14 days.

  b. Ofloxacin 400 mg orally two times a day for 14 days; PLUS either clindamycin 450 mg orally four times a day; OR metronidazole 500 mg orally two times a day for 14 days.

Adolescents treated as outpatients require close observation and follow-up, with hospitalization indicated if they are found unresponsive to oral therapy.

Martens et al. (1993) assessed the safety and efficacy of oral ofloxacin (400 mg twice daily for 10 days) versus cefoxitin (2 g intramuscularly) followed by doxycycline (100 mg twice daily orally for 10 days) for the outpatient treatment of uncomplicated PID. Both regimens had similar clinical effectiveness for the outpatient treatment of uncomplicated PID.

5. Follow-up
  a. Adequate treatment of adolescents with PID includes examination and appropriate treatment of their partners.
  b. In an adolescent with acute salpingitis it is advisable to remove an IUD after antibiotics are started.
  c. Follow-up examination of adolescents with acute salpingitis is essential. Patients should be reassessed approximately 48 hours after treatment is started. This should include a bimanual examination.
  d. Failure to respond to antibiotic therapy does not necessarily suggest the need to switch to another antibiotic. It is, rather, a strong indication of the need to search for an alternative diagnosis.

6. Surgery: Surgical exploration or laparoscopy is indicated for diagnosis and exclusion of surgical emergencies or for evaluation of treatment failures. In the case of an inflammatory adnexal mass, medical therapy should be tried; in 70% of cases, resolution results. However, if medical therapy fails, surgical exploration and drainage are indicated.

COMPLICATIONS AND SEQUELAE

At least one-quarter of women with acute PID experience one or more short-term or long-term sequelae. Risk factors for sequelae include the number of episodes of PID, the severity of infection as measured by the inflammatory reaction, the etiology of PID, the contraceptive method used, and the duration of the interval between the diagnosis and treatment.

Short-Term Sequelae

1. Recurrence: The recurrence rate of salpingitis has been reported to be between 12% and 33%. The prevalence is markedly higher if male partners are not examined and treated.
2. TOA: May occur in as many as a third of individuals hospitalized with salpingitis. Golden et al. (1989) found a TOA in 19.3% of their group of hospitalized adolescents. Presenting clinical findings are similar to uncomplicated salpingitis. Physical examination alone may not detect the mass because of the severe pain and tenderness obscuring a mass. Ultrasound of the pelvis is a useful test to confirm a diagnosis of a TOA when it is suspected and in following the response to therapy.

Organisms involved usually consist of a mixed flora of aerobic and anaerobic organisms. Anaerobic organisms, including *Bacteroides fragilis* and other *Bacteroides* species, are particularly prevalent. Initially during PID the purulent exudate spills into the peritoneum. With time an inflammatory mass develops in the tube, which may involve other pelvic structures such as bowel and bladder. Rupture can occur as part of this process.

Medical treatment is effective in 42–92% of cases. Regimens that include clindamycin have greater success rates, perhaps due to their superior activity against *B. fragilis*. However, cefoxitin, third-generation cephalosporins, and metronidazole may compare favorably with clindamycin. Surgical therapy is indicated for rupture or in adolescents failing to respond, as indicated by persistent fever and increasing size of the abscess. Pregnancy rates in individuals successfully treated with antibiotics for a TOA range from 9% to 50%.

3. Fitz-Hugh and Curtis syndrome: This syndrome, occurring in about 5–20% of women with acute salpingitis, consists of an acute inflammation of the hepatic capsule and peritoneum in contact with it by the organisms causing the salpingitis. The mode of spread has been proposed as either direct intraperitoneal, hematogenous, or lymphatic spread. The associated organisms are usually *N. gonorrhoeae* and *C. trachomatis*. The condition can cause acute or chronic right upper quadrant abdominal pain and can lead to chronic adhesions between the hepatic capsule and the peritoneum. The pain and tenderness may be more significant in some individuals than the pelvic signs and symptoms.

Long-Term Sequelae

1. Infertility: The infertility rate increases from approximately 13–21% with one episode of acute salpingitis, to 35% with two episodes, to about 55–75% with three or more episodes. The rate of infertility also seems to be related to the length of time between onset of symptoms and treatment. Infertility may also result from a silent infection. Up to 70% of women who are infertile because of obstructed fallopian tubes have serum antibodies to *C. trachomatis*. Many of these women have no history of clinical PID.
2. Ectopic pregnancy: There is a six to ten times greater risk than normal after one episode of PID. PID is the most common factor predisposing young women to ectopic pregnancy.
3. Chronic abdominal pain, exacerbated dysmenorrhea, and dyspareunia: This may occur in 18% of women with acute salpingitis. The symptoms may be related to adhesions surrounding the ovaries.

Buchan et al. (1993) examined the long-term morbidity in women who had previous PID diagnosis. In comparison with the controls, women with a diagnosis of PID were ten times more likely to be admitted for abdominal pain, four times more likely to be admitted for gynecological pain, six times more likely to be admitted for endometriosis, eight times more likely to be admitted for hysterectomy, and ten times more likely to be admitted for ectopic pregnancy.

Pʀᴇᴠᴇɴᴛɪᴏɴ

As clinicians caring for adolescents the goals of treatment of PID are to preserve fertility and prevent ectopic pregnancies and long-term complications. Early recognition and appropriate broad-spectrum antibiotic therapy play an important role in these goals. Another important element is evaluation and treatment as indicated of the sexual partner(s). However, another major goal should be the prevention of PID by education, screening, and treatment of STDs before an ascending infection can lead to PID. The CDC has published some guidelines for preventing STD and PID (Fig. 63.2).

Recommendations for Individuals to Prevent STD and PID

Maintain healthy sexual behavior.
- Postpone initiation of sexual intercourse until at least 2–3 years following menarche.
- Limit number of sex partners.
- Avoid "casual" sex and sex with high-risk partners.
- Question potential sex partners about STD and inspect their genitals for lesions or discharge.
- Avoid sex with infected persons.
- Abstain from sex if STD symptoms appear.

Use barrier methods.
- Use condoms, diaphragms, or vaginal spermicides for protection against STD, even if contraception is not needed.
- Use condoms consistently and correctly throughout sex.

Adopt healthy medical-care–seeking behavior.
- Seek medical evaluation promptly after having unprotected sex (intercourse without a condom) with someone who is suspected of having an STD.
- Seek medical care immediately when genital lesions or discharge appear.
- Seek routine check-ups for STD if in nonmutually monogamous relationship(s), even if symptoms are not present.

Comply with management instructions.
- Take all medications as directed, regardless of symptoms.
- Return for follow-up evaluation as instructed.
- Abstain from sex until symptoms disappear and appropriate treatment is completed.

Ensure examination of sex partners.
- When diagnosed as having an STD, notify all sex partners in need of medical assessment.
- If preferred, assist health providers in identifying sex partners.

Recommendations for Health Providers to Prevent STD and PID

Maintain up-to-date knowledge about the prevention and management of STD and PID.
- Develop an accurate base of information on the diagnosis, treatment, and prevention of STD and PID.
- Complete continuing education courses periodically to update knowledge on STD and PID prevention and management.

Provide effective patient education and counseling.
- Educate patients about STD and PID and thier potential complications.
- Encourage individuals to maintain healthy sexual behavior, use barrier methods, and adopt healthy medical-care–seeking behavior.

Provide appropriate preventive medical services.
- Screen patients for chlamydial and gonococcal infection routinely when indicated.
- Provide epidemiological treatment for STD and PID when appropriate.

Provide appropriate medical management for illness.
- Diagnose STD and PID promptly.
- Treat STD and PID promptly and with effective antibiotics.
- Encourage patients to comply with management instructions.

Ensure examination of sex partners.
- Encourage infected patients to refer all sex partners in need of medical assessment.
- Evaluate and treat sex partners appropriately.

Report all cases of STD to appropriate health authorities.

FIGURE 63.2.   CDC recommendations for preventing STD and PID. (From Centers for Disease Control. Pelvic inflammatory disease: guidelines for prevention and management. MMWR 1991;40:1.)

BIBLIOGRAPHY

Ault KA, Faro S. Pelvic inflammatory disease. Current diagnostic criteria and treatment guidelines. Postgrad Med 1993;93:85.

Bell TA. *Chlamydia trachomatis* infections in adolescents. Med Clin North Am 1990;74:1225.

Bernstine R, Stone CW, Waldron J. Post-PID sequelae and pain: assessment, management, and new findings. Medical Aspects of Human Sexuality 1987;(November):46.

Bevan CD, Johal BJ, Mumtaz G, et al. Clinical, laparoscopic and microbiological findings in acute salpingitis: report of a United Kingdom cohort. Br J Obstet Gynaecol 1995;102:407.

Bongard F, Landers DV, Lewis F. Differential diagnosis of appendicitis and pelvic inflammatory disease: a prospective analysis. Am J Surg 1985;150:90.

Bowie WR. Antibiotics and sexually transmitted diseases. Infect Dis Clin North Am 1994;8:841.

Bradley B, Hager JWD. Pelvic inflammatory disease. Hosp Med 1987;23:104.

Brauerman PK, Strasburger VC. Sexually transmitted diseases. Clin Pediatr 1994;1:26–35.

Buchan H, Vessey M, Goldacre M, et al. Morbidity following pelvic inflammatory disease. Br J Obstet Gynaecol 1993;100:558.

Bulas DI, et al. Pelvic inflammatory disease in the adolescent: comparison of transabdominal and transvaginal sonographic evaluation. Radiology 1992;183:435.

Cates W, Rolfs RT, Aral SO. Sexually transmitted disease, pelvic inflammatory disease and infertility: an epidemiologic update. Epidemiol Rev 1990;12:199.

Centers for Disease Control. Pelvic inflammatory disease: guidelines for prevention and management. MMWR 1991;40:1.

Centers for Disease Control. Premarital sexual experience among adolescent women—United States, 1970–1988. MMWR 1991;34:929.

Centers for Disease Control. Sexual behavior among high school students. United States, 1990. MMWR 1992;40:886.

Centers for Disease Control. Sexually transmitted diseases treatment guidelines, 1993. MMWR 1993;42:1.

Eschenbach DA. Epidemiology and diagnosis of acute pelvic inflammatory disease. Obstet Gynecol 1980;55(suppl):1425.

Eschenbach D, Wolner-Hanssen P. Fitz-Hugh–Curtis syndrome. In: Holmes KK, Mardh PA, Sparling PF, Wiesner PJ, eds. Sexually transmitted diseases. 2nd ed. New York: McGraw-Hill Information Services, 1990.

European Study Group: Comparative evaluation of clindamycin/gentamicin and cefoxitin/doxycycline for treatment of pelvic inflammatory disease: a multicenter trial. Acta Obstet Gynecol Scand 1992;71:129.

Forrest KA, Washington AE, Daling JR, et al. Vaginal douching as a possible risk factor for pelvic inflammatory disease. J Natl Med Assoc 1989;81:159.

Golden N, Cohen H, Gennari G, et al. The use of pelvic ultrasonography in the evaluation of adolescents with pelvic inflammatory disease. Am J Dis Child 1987;141:1235.

Golden N, Neuhoff S, Cohen H. Pelvic inflammatory disease in adolescents. J Pediatr 1989;114:138.

Grodstein F, Rothman KJ. Epidemiology of pelvic inflammatory disease. Epidemiology 1994;5:234.

Hadgu A, Westrom L, Brooks CA, et al. Predicting acute pelvic inflammatory disease: a multivariate analysis. Am J Obstet Gynecol 1986;155:954.

Heinonen PK, Miettinen A. Laparoscopic study on the microbiology and severity of acute pelvic inflammatory disease. Eur J Obstet Gynecol Reprod Biol 1994;57:85.

Hemsell DL, Little BB, Faro S, et al. Comparison of three regimens recommended by the Centers for Disease Control and Prevention for the treatment of women hospitalized with acute pelvic inflammatory disease. Clin Infect Dis 1994;19:720.

Hillis SD, Nakashima A, Marchbanks P, et al. Risk factors for recurrent *Chlamydia trachomatis* infections in women. Am J Obstet Gynecol 1994;170:801.

Howes DS, Marrazzo JM, Scott C. Recognizing pelvic inflammatory disease. Patient Care 1993;(June 15):186.

Jacobson L, Westrom L. Objectified diagnosis of acute pelvic inflammatory disease: diagnostic and prognostic value of routine laparoscopy. Am J Obstet Gynecol 1969;105:1088.

Johnson LD, Bachman JG, O'Malley PM. The 16th national survey of American high school seniors. University of Michigan Institute for Social Research press release. January 24, 1991.

Jossens MO, Sweet RL. Pelvic inflammatory disease: risk factors and microbial etiologies. J Obstet Gynecol Neonatal Nurs 1993;22:169.

Kahn JG, Walker CK, Washington AE, et al. Diagnosing pelvic inflammatory disease: a comprehensive analysis and considerations for developing a new model. JAMA 1991;226:2594.

Kamwendo F, Johansson F, Moi H, et al. Gonorrhea, genital chlamydial infection, and nonspecific urethritis in male partners of women hospitalized and treated for acute pelvic inflammatory disease. Sex Transm Dis 1993;20:143.

Katzman DK, Friedman IM, McDonald CA, et al. *Chlamydia trachomatis* Fitz-Hugh–Curtis syndrome without salpingitis in female adolescents. Am J Dis Child 1988;142:996.

Kaufman DW, Shapiro S, Rosenberg L, et al. Intra-uterine contraceptive device use and pelvic inflammatory disease. Am J Obstet Gynecol 1980;136:159.

Landers DV, Sweet RL. Current trends in the diagnosis and treatment of tubo-ovarian abscess. Am J Obstet Gynecol 1985;151:1098.

Landers DV, Wolner-Hanssen P, Paavonen J, et al. Combination antimicrobial therapy in the treatment of acute pelvic inflammatory disease. Am J Obstet Gynecol 1991;164:849.

Larsson PG, Platz-Christensen J, Thejls H, et al. Incidence of pelvic inflammatory disease after first-trimester legal abortion in women with bacterial vaginosis after treatment with metronidazole: a double-blind, randomized study. Am J Obstet Gynecol 1992;166:100.

McCormack WM. Pelvic inflammatory disease. N Engl J Med 1994;330:115.

Magnusson SS, Oskarsson T, Geirsson RT, et al. Lower genital tract infection with *Chlamydia trachomatis* and *Neisseria gonorrhoeae* in Icelandic women with salpingitis. Am J Obstet Gynecol 1986;155:602.

Martens MG, Gordon S, Yarborough DR, et al. Multicenter randomized trial of ofloxacin versus cefoxitin and doxycycline in outpatient treatment of pelvic inflammatory disease. Ambulatory PID Research Group. South Med J 1993;86:604.

Monif GRG. Significance of polymicrobial bacterial superinfection in the therapy of gonococcal endometritis-salpingitis-peritonitis. Obstet Gynecol 1980; 55(suppl):1545.

Monif GRG. Choice of antibiotics and length of therapy in the treatment of acute salpingitis. Am J Med 1985;78:188.

Paradise JE, Grant L. Pelvic inflammatory disease in adolescents. Pediatr Rev 1992;13:216.

Quan M. Pelvic inflammatory disease: diagnosis and management. J Am Board Fam Pract 1994;7:110.

Rice P, Schachter J. Pathogenesis of pelvic inflammatory disease: what are the questions? JAMA 1991;266: 2587.

Rice RJ, Coston WA, Bhoomkar A, et al. Pelvic inflammatory disease among patients in a public health practice: profile and outcomes [Letter]. Am J Public Health 1995;85:874.

Risser WL, Pokorny SF, Maklad NF. Ultrasound examination of adolescent females with lower abdominal pain. J Adolesc Health Care 1988;9:407.

Rolfs RT, Galaid EI, Zaidi AA. Pelvic inflammatory disease: trends in hospitalizations and office visits, 1979 through 1988. Am J Obstet Gynecol 1992;166: 983.

Romanowski B. Pelvic inflammatory disease. Current approaches. Can Fam Physician 1993;39:346.

Rosenfield WD. Sexually transmitted disease in adolescents: update, 1991. Pediatr Ann 1991;20:303.

Schmidt E, Nehra P. Tubo-ovarian abscess: a study of 17 patients. Am Fam Physician 1988;37:181.

Scholes D, Daling JR, Stergachis A, et al. Vaginal douching as a risk factor for acute pelvic inflammatory disease. Obstet Gynecol 1993;81:601.

Sellors J, Mahony J, Goldsmith C. The accuracy of clinical findings and laparoscopy in pelvic inflammatory disease. Am J Obstet Gynecol 1991;164:113.

Shafer MA, Irwin CE, Sweet RL. Medical progress: acute salpingitis in the adolescent female. J Pediatr 1982; 100:339.

Shafer M, Sweet RL. Pelvic inflammatory disease in adolescent females. Adolesc Med: State Art Rev 1990; 1:545.

Shafer M, Sweet RL. Pelvic inflammatory disease in adolescent females—epidemiology, pathogenesis,

diagnosis, treatment and sequelae.' Pediatr Clin North Am 1989;36:516.

Soper DE, Despres B. A comparison of two antibiotic regimens for treatment of pelvic inflammatory disease. Obstet Gynecol 1988;72:7.

Spence MR, Adler J, McLellan R. Pelvic inflammatory disease in the adolescent. J Adolesc Health Care 1990;11:304.

Strickland DM, Hauth JC, Strickland KM. Laparoscopy for chronic pelvic pain in adolescent women. Adolesc Pediatr Gynecol 1988;1:31.

Sweet RL. Pelvic inflammatory disease and infertility in women. Infect Dis Clin North Am 1987;1:199.

Sweet RL. Pelvic inflammatory disease. Hosp Pract (Off Ed) 1993;28:25.

Sweet RL, Blankfort-Doyle M, Robbie MO, et al. The occurrence of chlamydial and gonococcal salpingitis during the menstrual cycle. JAMA 1986;255: 2062.

Sweet RL, Draper DL, Hadley WK. Etiology of acute salpingitis influence of episode number and duration of symptoms. Obstet Gynecol 1981;58:62.

Sweet RL, Draper DL, Schacter J, et al. Microbiology and pathogenesis of acute salpingitis as determined by laparoscopy: what is the appropriate site to sample? Am J Obstet Gynecol 1980;138:985.

Swinker ML. Salpingitis and pelvic inflammatory disease. Am Fam Physician 1985;31:143.

Taylor-Robinson D, Thomas BJ. Laboratory techniques for the diagnosis of chlamydial infection. Genitourin Med 1991;67:256.

Thompson SE, Hager WD, Wong K, et al. The microbiology and therapy of acute pelvic inflammatory disease in hospitalized patients. Am J Obstet Gynecol 1980;136:179.

Toivonen J, Luukkainen T, Allonen H. Protective effect of intrauterine release of levonorgestrel on pelvic infection: three years' comparative experience of levonorgestrel and copper-releasing intrauterine devices. Obstet Gynecol 1991;77(2):261.

Walker CK, Kahn JG, Washington AE, et al. Pelvic inflammatory disease: metaanalysis of antimicrobial regimen efficacy. J Infect Dis 1993;168:969.

Washington AE, Sweet RL, Shafer MAB. Pelvic inflammatory disease and its sequelae in adolescents. J Adolesc Health Care 1985;6:298.

Wendel GD Jr, Cox SM, Bawdon RE, et al. A randomized trial of ofloxacin versus cefoxitin and doxycycline in the outpatient treatment of acute salpingitis. Am J Obstet Gynecol 1991;164:1390.

Westrom L. Effect of acute pelvic inflammatory disease on fertility. Am J Obstet Gynecol 1975;121:707.

Westrom L, Mardh PA. Acute pelvic inflammatory disease. In: Holmes KK, Mardh PA, Sparling PF, Wiesner PJ, eds. Sexually transmitted diseases. 2nd ed. New York: McGraw-Hill Information Services, 1990.

Wolner-Hansen P, Swensson L, Mardh PA. Laparoscopic findings and contraceptive use in women with signs and symptoms suggestive of acute salpingitis. Obstet Gynecol 1985;66:233.

CHAPTER 64

Syphilis

Syphilis is a chronic systemic infection transmitted by sexual contact.

ETIOLOGY

The agent causing syphilis is *Treponema pallidum*, a slender, spiral microorganism 5–20 mm in length. The organisms do not stain well and are best visualized by dark-field microscopy. *T. pallidum* does not grow in artificial media.

EPIDEMIOLOGY

Hosts

Human beings are the only known natural host. Experimental infections can be produced in rabbits, monkeys, and chimpanzees.

Transmission

Almost all cases are contracted during sexual contact including kissing and sexual intercourse. Rare cases occur from direct contact with infectious cutaneous or mucous membrane lesions. Rashes are not infectious if the skin is intact. Other modes of transmission include congenital and transfusion-related transmission. The estimated rate of transmission after exposure during intercourse with a person with a chancre is 30%. The risk of transmission persists during the first 4 years of untreated syphilis.

Incidence

The incidence of syphilis in the United States declined rapidly after World War II, from a peak of about 70,000 reported cases in 1948 to less than 10,000 reported cases in 1956. After 1958 the number of cases of primary and secondary syphilis increased to about 25,000 cases in the mid-1960s and again in the late 1980s to 44,600 cases in 1989. Since then the cases have fallen again to 26,498 cases of primary and secondary syphilis in 1993, 20,785 in 1994, and 15,027 in 1995.

Sample rates of primary and secondary syphilis in the United States include:

Year	Cases of Primary and Secondary Syphilis
1954	7,147
1960	16,145
1965	23,338
1970	21,982
1975	25,561

Year	Cases of Primary and Secondary Syphilis
1980	27,204
1985	27,131
1990	50,223
1992	33,973
1993	26,498
1994	20,785
1995	15,027

The largest increases in prevalence have been in California, Florida, and New York City. In selected areas of the United States the rates have approached those of the prepenicillin rates before 1943. The total cases reported in the United States in 1994 of all stages of syphilis were 81,696. The reasons for the increase in syphilis cases in the late 1980s include decreased routine screening, inadequate reporting, institution of fees in sexually transmitted disease (STD) clinics, increase in "sex for drugs," and decreased funds for contact investigation, health education staff, and materials. The actual occurrence rate is much higher, since only 12–19% of syphilis cases are reported by private physicians. After years of declining rates, congenital syphilis cases have risen since 1978 with a peak in 1991. Over 50% of the cases of congenital syphilis have been reported from Texas, Florida, California, and New York City.

Adolescents   Between 1981 and 1991, 10–12% of reported cases from primary and secondary syphilis in the United States were in the adolescent age groups. Thirty percent of primary and secondary syphilis occur in the 15- to 24-year-old age group. In the heterosexual adolescent, syphilis accounts for only about 0.5% of all STDs. The peak incidence of syphilis occurs in young adults 20–24 years old, followed by adults 25–29 years old, and then teenagers 15–19 years old. Rates in adolescents for primary and secondary syphilis rose dramatically between 1985 and 1989 but have come down somewhat since then. In adolescents the number of reported cases of primary and secondary syphilis is highest in minorities, particularly African-Americans, and is higher in females than in males.

PATHOGENESIS

T. pallidum enters the body via minute abrasions in the skin and exposure to sera of moist, mucocutaneous lesions. The infection is spread via lymphatics and blood vessels. The spirochetes cause cellular infiltrates, granuloma formation, and an obliterative endarteritis. This can lead to necrosis, with resultant ulcerations and erosions. In later stages tissue hypersensitivity becomes prominent and can lead to gummas. Syphilitic lesions heal by scar formation so that in tertiary lesions scarring is considerable.

CLINICAL MANIFESTATIONS

Syphilis in adolescents is most commonly diagnosed in asymptomatic individuals by positive serologic tests. Primary syphilitic ulcers may not be detected by the adolescent, and secondary manifestations may be mild.

Primary Syphilis

After an incubation period of 9–90 days with an average of 21 days, the primary lesions appear. Syphilis is characterized by a chancre at the point of inoculation. Characteristics of the syphilitic chancre are as follows:

1. Location
   a.   Ninety-five percent are on the external genitalia.
   b.   Usually there is a single lesion, but lesions can occasionally be multiple.
   c.   Lesions may also appear as kissing lesions, chancres that touch each other across a fold of skin.
   d.   Other primary sites include the cervix, mouth, anus, lips, face, breast, and fingers.
2. Size: Several millimeters to 1 cm
3. Typical chancre: Starts as painless papule eroding to an indurated, painless ulcer. The ulcer typically has a punched out, clean appearance, with slightly elevated edges and with a scanty yellow serous discharge.
4. Regional lymphadenopathy accompanies the lesion. The nodes are firm, nonsuppurative, bilateral, and usually painless.
5. Healing: The chancre heals in 4–6 weeks.

The primary infection may present with an inconspicuous lesion, particularly in females, and may occur with no papule or ulcer at all, particularly in previously infected patients.

Secondary Syphilis

Approximately 6–8 weeks (maximum is 6 months) after exposure or an average of 3 weeks after the onset of the chancre, the manifestations of secondary syphilis appear. During this stage *T. pallidum* can be isolated from lesions and body fluids. The signs and symptoms of secondary syphilis usually disappear after weeks or months. Most individuals remain asymptomatic after these symptoms disappear, but 25% may develop symptomatic relapses of secondary disease, with about one-fourth of these having multiple relapses. Secondary syphilis lesions are infectious if the lesions are open such as on mucous membranes or in intertriginous areas. Signs and symptoms of secondary syphilis include:

1. General skin eruption (most common manifestation affecting 90% of individuals with secondary syphilis)
   a.   Eruption involves the trunk and extremities with a predilection for palms and soles. The lesions on the palms and soles may be scaly, and hyperkeratotic and may be the last to clear.
   b.   Eruption involves skin as well as mucous membranes.
   c.   Eruption tends to follow the lines of cleavage.
   d.   Eruption is bilateral and symmetrical.
   e.   Individual lesions are sharply demarcated, 0.5–2.0 cm in diameter with a coppery hue.
   f.   Eruption is most commonly macular, papular, or papulosquamous. Less common are follicular rashes, with pustular rashes being rare.
   g.   Lesions are usually nonpruritic, but pruritus may be more common than once thought.
   h.   Eruption may last a few weeks to 12 months.
   i.   Variety: Almost any type of rash can occur with syphilis including acneform lesions, herpetiform lesions, and lesions similar to psoriasis. Lesions in intertriginous areas may erode and fissure, especially in the nasolabial folds and near the corners of the mouth. In warm, moist areas, hypertrophic granulomatous lesions (condylomata lata) may occur. These lesions usually occur near the area of the original chancre and have a broad, flat appearance.
2. General or regional lymphadenopathy (about 70%)
   a.   Nonpainful nodes

     b. Rubbery, hard feeling, discrete, with no suppuration
     c. Occasional hepatosplenomegaly
3. Flulike syndrome (about 50%)
     a. Sore throat and malaise most common
     b. Headaches
     c. Lacrimation
     d. Nasal discharge
     e. Arthralgias and myalgias
     f. Weight loss
     g. Fever
4. Syphilis alopecia (uncommon): Moth-eaten-appearing alopecia of the scalp and eyebrows
5. Other rare manifestations
     a. Arthritis or bursitis
     b. Hepatitis
     c. Iritis and anterior uveitis
     d. Glomerulonephritis

Latent Syphilis

The early latent period is defined as the first year of infection. Early syphilis includes primary, secondary, and early latent syphilis. The late latent stage refers to the period after this first year unless late (tertiary) syphilis occurs.

    Latent syphilis is characterized by:

1. Absence of clinical signs and symptoms of syphilis
2. Repeated positive serologic tests (VDRL and FTA-ABS) for syphilis
3. Negative results from serologic tests of the spinal fluid

Neurosyphilis

Neurosyphilis may develop at any time in the course of syphilis. Neurosyphilis develops in about 10–20% of patients with untreated syphilis after 2 years. Neurologic involvement although uncommon in adolescents, if occurring, is most likely to include asymptomatic neurosyphilis or acute syphilitic meningitis. Meningovascular syphilis would be much less common.

1. Asymptomatic neurosyphilis: Characterized by abnormal cerebrospinal fluid (CSF), including pleocytosis, elevated protein, and positive CSF-VDRL
2. Acute syphilis meningitis
     a. Usually occurs during secondary syphilis or the early latent period
     b. Common symptoms: Fever, headache, photophobia, and meningism
     c. Cranial nerve palsies (40%)
     d. Less frequent symptoms: Confusion, delirium, and seizures
     e. CSF: Increased protein, lymphocytic pleocytosis, and occasional lowered glucose
3. Meningovascular syphilis
     a. Infrequent in adolescents, as it occurs 5–12 years after initial infection
     b. Symptoms and signs from a syphilitic endarteritis producing local areas of infarction
     c. Symptoms: Headache, dizziness, mood changes, and memory loss
     d. Signs: Hemiparesis, hemiplegia, aphasia
     e. Other signs of parenchymal damage: Argyll Robertson pupils (accommodation, but no response to light) and injury to the posterior column of the spinal cord, causing tabes dorsalis

Late Syphilis

Signs and symptoms of late syphilis may occur 2–10 years after initial exposure in untreated or inadequately treated patients. This includes individuals with gummas and cardiovascular syphilis but not neurosyphilis. Late syphilis has not been reported in adolescents.

Cardiovascular Syphilis   Usually occurs 10–30 years after exposure. The basic lesion is aortitis, which can lead to:

1. Saccular aneurysms of ascending aorta
2. Aortic valve incompetence and regurgitation

Gummas   Gummas are granulomatous lesions of late syphilis, involving skin, soft tissue, viscera, or bones. They are usually few in number, asymmetrical, indolent, and not contagious.

Congenital Syphilis

Since adolescent pregnancy is common, it is important to be aware of the possible transmission of syphilis from an infected pregnant teenager to her developing fetus. The fetus becomes susceptible to infection after the fourth month of gestation. Thus, adequate treatment of the mother before the 16th week of gestation prevents infection of the fetus. The risk of infection of the fetus during untreated early maternal syphilis is about 80–95%. Approximately 25% of infants infected in utero die before birth, and 25% die shortly after birth, if untreated. The rest develop either early or late lesions.

1. Early congenital syphilis lesions (lesions occurring during the first 2 years of life and usually by 3 months of age)
   a. Vesicular and vesiculobullous eruptions
   b. Superficial desquamation
   c. Rhinitis
   d. Hepatosplenomegaly
   e. Hemolytic anemia, thrombocytopenia
   f. Skeletal involvement: Osteochondritis with periarticular swelling
   g. Neurosyphilis
   h. Ocular: Glaucoma, uveitis, and chorioretinitis
   i. Nephropathy: Uncommon
2. Late congenital syphilis: This type of syphilis corresponds to tertiary syphilis in adults. In 60% of cases the infection remains latent, and in the rest the lesions can be divided into:
   a. Inflammatory or hypersensitivity lesions
   b. Gummas
   c. Neurosyphilis
   d. Interstitial keratitis
   e. Clutton's joints: Symmetrical painless swelling of knees
   f. Palatal deformations
   g. Paroxysmal cold hemoglobinuria
3. Unique stigmata
   a. Hutchinson's incisors: Centrally notched screwdriver-shaped upper incisors
   b. Abnormal facies: Saddlenose, frontal bossing
   c. Eighth nerve deafness
   d. Scaphoid scapulas
   e. Hutchinson's triad: Malformed incisors, eighth nerve deafness, and interstitial keratitis

DIFFERENTIAL DIAGNOSIS

Primary Syphilis

Sexually Transmitted Causes of Genital Ulcers   The most common sexually transmitted genital ulcers in the United States are herpes, syphilis, and chancroid, in that order.

1. Herpes simplex: Usually painful, multiple lesions beginning as vesicles on an erythematous base. Primary lesions are usually bilateral, extensive, and associated with tender adenopathy, and recurrent lesions are usually unilateral without significant adenopathy. The vesicles break down into ulcers with nonindurated borders.
2. Chancroid: Usually painful lesions with a deep purulent base and often erythematous borders. Local lymph nodes are often fluctuant and tender.
3. Lymphogranuloma venereum: These lesions are rare in the United States. The primary lesion is often missed, and commonly patients present with fever and massive adenopathy (bubo).
4. Granuloma inguinale: These lesions are rare except if teen has lived or traveled to particular tropical countries such as New Guinea.

Nonsexually Transmitted Causes of Genital Ulcers   The most common nonsexually transmitted cause is trauma.

1. Traumatic lesions: There should be a history of the lesion appearing at the time of the trauma.
2. Fixed drug reaction: There may be history of similar lesion after prior drug exposure. Lesions may start as reddish plaque and become hyperpigmented, edematous, or eroded.
3. Candida balanitis
4. Behcet's syndrome: Not limited to genital area
5. Psoriasis, if excoriated
6. Lichen planus, if excoriated
7. Erythema multiforme, if excoriated
8. Cancer: Extremely rare in adolescents

Secondary Syphilis

1. Psoriasis
2. Pityriasis rosea
3. Drug eruptions
4. Tinea versicolor
5. Alopecia areata
6. Lichen planus
7. Viremia
8. Lupus erythematosus
9. Scabies
10. Pediculosis
11. Rosacea
12. Infectious mononucleosis
13. Keratoderma blennorrhagica
14. Condyloma acuminatum

Although the clinical history and appearance of these conditions can often separate them from secondary syphilis, a VDRL or RPR should be performed whenever doubt exists.

Diagnosis

Since adolescents often present with asymptomatic disease, it is essential to screen sexually active or sexually abused teens for syphilis with appropriate serologic tests. Adolescents should also be retested if they become pregnant or if they are infected with another STD.

Laboratory Findings

1. Dark-field examination: This is essential in evaluating moist ulcers and lesions such as a chancre or condyloma latum. Technique is as follows:
   a. Clean lesion with saline and gauze.
   b. Abrade with dry gauze.
   c. Squeeze lesion (with gloves) to express serous transudate. Try to avoid bleeding, which makes dark-field examination more difficult.
   d. Place a drop of transudate on a slide.
   e. Place a drop of saline on transudate and cover with a cover slip.
   f. Examine under dark-field microscope.
   g. Procedure must be repeated on 3 successive days before considered negative.
   h. For internal lesions a bacteriological loop can be used to transfer the fluid to a slide.
   i. For lymph node aspirations: Clean skin, inject 0.2 mL or less of sterile saline and aspirate the node. Place fluid on a slide.
2. Direct fluorescent antibody (DFA): Specimens from primary lesions can also be sent to reference laboratories or some state health departments for DFA staining. These specimens can be collected as above; however, saline should not be added to the slides, and they should be allowed to air-dry.

   Both dark-field microscopy and DFA staining are very specific except from oral specimens, but sensitivity is dependent on many factors including collection technique, age of lesions, and experience of laboratory personnel.
3. Serologic tests
   a. Nontreponemal antibody tests: Tests for a nonspecific antilipoidal antibody that forms in response to surface lipids on the treponeme
      — Types
         (1) Agglutination: Rapid plasma reagin (RPR, qualitative test)
         (2) Flocculation: VDRL (quantitative test) used for screening or to follow therapy
      — Use: Nontreponemal tests should be used for screening and to follow treatment success. Nontreponemal test titers correlate with disease activity and fall after treatment. If a positive qualitative test is confirmed by a treponemal test, a quantitative VDRL should be obtained, titered out to the highest point, and followed over time. A fourfold change in titer, equivalent to a change of two dilutions (e.g., from 1:8 to 1:32 or 1:16 to 1:4) demonstrates a substantial change if the same serologic test is used.
   b. Specific treponemal antibody tests
      — Types
         (1) Immunofluorescence: Fluorescent treponemal antibody absorption (FTA-ABS) is used to confirm a positive result from RPR or VDRL.
         (2) Microhemagglutination: *T. pallidum* tests (MHA-TP) have replaced the FTA-ABS test in many laboratories as the specific treponemal test to confirm a positive result from VDRL.
         (3) Immobilization: *T. pallidum* immobilization (TPI)
      — Use: Treponemal tests are specific and sensitive, but because of their expense and more difficult technical requirement are used to confirm positive results from a

TABLE 64.1.   Frequency of Positive Test Results in Untreated Syphilis

	Test			
	VDRL (%)	FTA-ABS (%)	TPI (%)	MHA-TP (%)
Primary syphilis	72	91	46	69
Secondary syphilis	100	100	98	100
Latent syphilis	73	97	95	98
Late syphilis	77	100	95	100

Adapted from Holmes KK. In: Isselbacher KJ, Adams RD, Braunwald E, et al., eds. Harrison's principles of internal medicine. New York: McGraw-Hill, 1980.

screening test. Once an individual tests positive on treponemal tests, the individual usually remains positive for life, with titers being unrelated to disease activity or treatment. Treponemal antibody titers thus should not be quantitated but recorded as reactive, nonreactive, or minimally reactive. Minimally reactive test results may represent a false positive, and the tests should be repeated.

c. Tests in development: These include treponeme-specific immunoglobulin M (IgM) antibody tests and polymerase chain reaction (PCR) tests.

d. Frequency of positive test results in untreated syphilis is indicated in Table 64.1. VDRL results are positive in about 25% of cases at onset of primary chancre. Two weeks after chancre appearance, 50% of individuals are positive; 3 weeks after chancre appearance, 75% are positive; and 4 weeks after chancre appearance, 100% are positive.

e. False-positive serology test results: About 20–40% of all positive nontreponemal test results are false positives with a nonreactive treponemal test. Most false-positive nontreponemal tests results show a low titer (dilution < 1:8). The causes of false-positive test results include:

— Acute infections: Viral infections, chlamydial infections, Lyme disease, *Mycoplasma* infections, nonsyphilitic spirochetal infections, and various bacterial, fungal, and protozoal infections
— Connective tissue diseases
— Narcotic addiction
— Aging
— Hashimoto's thyroiditis
— Sarcoidosis
— Lymphoma
— Leprosy
— Cirrhosis of the liver
— Human immunodeficiency virus (HIV) infection: Can lead to unusually high, unusually low, or fluctuating titers

False positives can occasionally arise in treponemal tests. However, most of these are reported as borderline and not positive. Only a positive TPI provides conclusive proof of past or present infection. The TPI, however, is reserved for research purposes and difficult diagnostic cases.

The tests most commonly used are:

1. RPR (screening purposes)
2. VDRL (quantitative measurement to assess clinical activity and response to therapy or qualitative test for screening)
3. MHA-TP or FTA-ABS (to confirm diagnosis in a patient with a positive result from VDRL or RPR)

Diagnosis by Stage

Primary Syphilis

1. Definitive diagnosis of early syphilis requires positive dark-field examination or DFA test of lesion exudate or tissue.
2. Presumptive diagnosis relies on positive nontreponemal test (VDRL or RPR) and positive treponemal test (e.g., FTA-ABS or MHA-TP) results.

Adolescents with positive dark-field examination results, a history of exposure, or a typical lesion plus a positive serologic test result should be treated. If the initial serologic test result is negative, it should be repeated 1 week, 1 month, and 3 months later in suspected cases. An FTA-ABS or MHA-TP should be used to confirm a positive VDRL result.

Controversy exists regarding the role for the CSF examination in early syphilis. This is based on the possibility of asymptomatic syphilis being missed and inadequately treated. At present, lumbar puncture is not recommended for routine evaluation of early syphilis, unless clinical signs and symptoms of neurological involvement are present. This is even more controversial when dealing with individuals with early syphilis who also are infected with HIV, as more aggressive therapy may be needed.

Secondary Syphilis

1. Dark-field examination of material from lesions or lymph nodes
2. VDRL or RPR

An adolescent should be treated if:

1. Dark-field examination result is positive.
2. Patient has typical findings of secondary syphilis and a positive result from VDRL or RPR. Adolescents with atypical findings or a VDRL titer less than 1:16 should have a second VDRL and an FTA-ABS or MHA-TP. Positive VDRL tests should be confirmed with an FTA-ABS test or MHA-TP.

Neurosyphilis

1. The standard test for CSF is the VDRL. It is a specific but not a sensitive test for active neurosyphilis. On the other hand the FTA-ABS is sensitive but not specific for neurosyphilis. Serum antibody may diffuse into the CSF and may not be reflective of active central nervous system (CNS) disease. However, a nonreactive FTA-ABS probably indicates the absence of active neurosyphilis. Pleocytosis in the CSF is another good indicator of active disease.
   a. The Centers for Disease Control (CDC), in their 1993 STD recommendations, list the following indications for CSF examination:
      — Neurological signs or symptoms
      — Treatment failure
      — Serum reagin titer greater than or equal to 1:32 unless duration of infection is known to be less than 1 year
      — Other evidence of active syphilis (aortitis, gumma, iritis)
      — Nonpenicillin therapy planned unless duration of infection is known to be less than 1 year
      — HIV infection
2. Spinal fluid tests should include cell count, protein, and VDRL. There are no perfect tests for evaluating neurosyphilis. The cell count is usually elevated in the presence of neu-

rosyphilis and is an excellent marker in assessing treatment. The VDRL is the standard and most specific test on spinal fluid, but it only has a 60–70% sensitivity. Although the FTA-ABS is highly sensitive, it may have 6% or more false positives, owing to transfer of antibodies across the blood-brain barrier. Some experts order both tests. If the FTA-ABS result is negative, the likelihood of neurosyphilis is very small.

Latent and Late Syphilis

1. A VDRL and FTA-ABS: The FTA-ABS is essential in latent and late syphilis because the VDRL has only a 70% sensitivity in these states. The adolescent should be treated if the FTA-ABS result is positive.
2. Examining spinal fluid in individuals with late latent syphilis and a negative neurologic examination is controversial. If a spinal tap is not performed, the concern is whether the standard 3-week treatment for latent syphilis is adequate in the treatment of asymptomatic neurosyphilis.

Syphilis in Pregnancy   All pregnant adolescents should be screened early in pregnancy. Seropositive females should be considered infected unless a prior history documents recent treatment and serologic titers have appropriately declined. Screening should be repeated in the third trimester and again at delivery in areas or populations with a high prevalence of syphilis. A female delivering a stillborn infant after 20 weeks' gestation should also be tested for syphilis.

Congenital Syphilis

1. Evaluation recommendations: Who? The CDC recommends evaluating infants born to seropositive mothers who either:
   a. Have untreated syphilis
   b. Had treated syphilis in pregnancy but the treatment was less than 1 month before delivery, involved a nonpenicillin regimen, or was accompanied by a lack of appropriate decrease in serologic titers.
   c. Do not have a well-documented history of syphilis treatment
   d. Have a documented treatment regimen but undocumented serologic follow-up after therapy
2. Evaluation recommendations: How? The CDC recommends the following evaluation of infants born to women in the preceding situations:
   a. Thorough physical examination, looking for evidence of congenital syphilis
   b. Quantitative nontreponemal serologic test for syphilis performed on the infant's sera (not cord blood)
   c. CSF analysis for cells, protein, and VDRL
   d. Long bone x-ray examination
   e. Other tests if clinically indicated (e.g., chest x-ray examination, complete blood count (CBC), liver function tests)
   f. For infants who have no evidence of congenital syphilis by this evaluation, determination of the presence of specific antitreponemal IgM antibody by a CDC-recognized method
   g. Pathological examination of the placenta or amniotic cord using specific fluorescent antitreponemal antibody staining.
3. Treatment recommendations: Who? The CDC recommends treating infants if they have any of the following:
   a. Clinical evidence of active disease

   b. X-ray evidence of active disease
   c. Reactive CSF-VDRL
   d. Abnormal CSF findings such as elevated cell count or protein even in the presence of
       nonreactive CSF-VDRL for infants born to seroreactive mothers
   e. Quantitative nontreponemal serologic titers fourfold higher than their mother
   f. Specific antitreponemal IgM antibody detected by a testing method given provisional
       or standard status by CDC
   g. Mother with untreated early syphilis or who had evidence of relapse or reinfection af-
       ter treatment

Syphilis and HIV   Many researchers believe that ulcerative lesions such as syphilitic
chancres increase the risk of transmission of HIV. McCabe et al. (1993) examined the prevalence of HIV positivity in a group of adolescents with syphilis. Of 59 adolescents with
syphilis, 15.3% were HIV positive. There is also evidence that infection with HIV may alter
the serologic response to syphilis. There have been reports of patients with coinfections with
HIV and syphilis who have unusual serologic responses. Many of these reports involve higher
than expected serologic titers, but false-negative serologic test results have also been reported.
Most treponemal and nontreponemal serologic tests for syphilis are accurate for the majority of individuals with both syphilis and HIV infections. If serologic tests are not consistent
with clinical findings, alternative tests such as biopsy and DFA staining of lesion material
should be considered. HIV-infected individuals with neurological disease should be evaluated for neurosyphilis.

Problem Sera

1. Positive VDRL and negative FTA-ABS results
    a. False-positive VDRL results
    b. Technical error leading to false-negative FTA-ABS results
2. Negative VDRL and positive FTA-ABS results
    a. Early and late syphilis: May have negative VDRL results

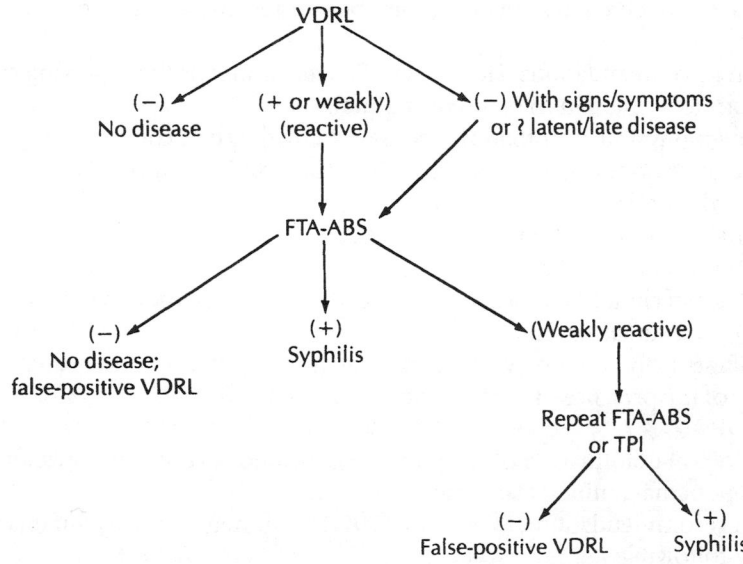

FIGURE 64.1.   Flow chart of syphilis diagnosis.

b. Adequately treated syphilis: Eighty-five percent of patients will remain FTA-ABS test positive for life after adequate treatment.
c. False-positive FTA-ABS results: Rare
3. Negative VDRL and negative FTA-ABS results
a. Absence of disease
b. Incubating or early syphilis
4. Persistently positive VDRL results
a. Untreated or inadequately treated syphilis
b. Adequately treated patients who have positive serologic test results
5. Borderline FTA-ABS results
a. May indicate syphilis or false positive.
b. Test should be repeated. If results are still borderline, TPI should be performed.

Figure 64.1 is a flow chart of syphilis diagnosis.

THERAPY

Penicillin is the optimal drug for treating syphilis. It is the only proven therapy for neurosyphilis, congenital syphilis, and syphilis during pregnancy. For individuals in these categories with a history of penicillin allergy, skin testing and desensitization, if indicated, are recommended. No adequately controlled comparative trials have been conducted to guide optimal penicillin regimens, including dose, duration, and preparation. The doses of penicillin have become controversial in certain situations, particularly in regard to CNS involvement and in individuals who are immunocompromised. The cure of syphilis is probably dependent on therapy plus an intact immune system. Less data are available on nonpenicillin regimens. Adolescents treated for gonorrhea with ceftriaxone and doxycycline are probably covered for incubating syphilis. If a different antibiotic regimen is used to treat gonorrhea, the teen should have a second serologic test for syphilis in 3 months.

Primary and Secondary Syphilis

1. Benzathine penicillin G: The total recommended dose is 2.4 million units intramuscularly (IM) at a single session.
2. Penicillin-allergic nonpregnant patients: Doxycycline 100 mg orally two times a day for 2 weeks or tetracycline 500 mg orally four times a day for 2 weeks is recommended. In penicillin-allergic nonpregnant patients who cannot tolerate tetracycline or doxycycline, three options exist:
a. Refer the patient for penicillin skin testing.
b. Prescribe erythromycin 500 mg four times a day for 2 weeks if compliance and follow-up are assured. Erythromycin is less effective than other recommended regimens.
c. Ceftriaxone 250 mg IM daily for 10 days is probably effective, but careful follow-up is mandatory. Optimal dose and duration have not been established, and experience has been limited.
3. Other considerations
a. All patients with syphilis should be tested for HIV. For high-risk patients or in high-prevalence areas, patients with primary syphilis should be retested for HIV after 3 months.
b. Those individuals with signs or symptoms that suggest neurologic disease or ophthalmic disease should be evaluated for neurosyphilis and eye disease (CSF analysis and slit-lamp examination). Routine lumbar puncture is not recommended for indi-

viduals with primary or secondary syphilis unless clinical signs and symptoms suggest neurologic involvement.

4. Follow-up: Infected individuals should be re-examined clinically and serologic test results should be rechecked at 3 and 6 months. The VDRL should be used for follow-up, as the FTA-ABS results usually remain positive throughout the individual's life. If signs or symptoms persist or nontreponemal antibody titers have not decreased fourfold by 6 months, the individual should have a CSF examination and HIV test and be retreated. Most individuals with primary syphilis are seronegative by 3-12 months, while 75–95% of individuals with secondary syphilis are seronegative by 1 year. The drops in titers for primary and secondary syphilis apply only to first episodes of primary or secondary syphilis. Those with reinfections have less predictable serologic drops.

Individuals are at risk for treatment failure if their nontreponemal titers have not declined fourfold by 3 months after treatment for primary or secondary syphilis. HIV testing should be performed at 3 months in these individuals.

Retreatment should probably include three weekly injections of benzathine penicillin G 2.4 million units IM unless neurosyphilis is present.

Latent Syphilis

Latent syphilis includes infection with *T. pallidum,* positive serology, but no other clinical evidence of disease. Early latent syphilis describe disease in individuals who have acquired the disease during the past year based on documented seroconversion, a fourfold or greater increase in titer of a nontreponemal serologic test, history of primary or secondary, syphilis symptoms, or a history of a sex partner with primary, secondary, or early latent syphilis.

These two regimens are for patients who are not allergic to penicillin and who have normal CSF examinations.

1. Early latent syphilis: Benzathine penicillin G 2.4 million units IM in a single dose.
2. Late latent syphilis or latent syphilis of unknown duration: Benzathine penicillin G 7.2 million units total administered as three doses of 2.4 million units IM each at 1-week intervals.
3. Penicillin-allergic patients: No clinical data exist that adequately document the efficacy of drugs other than penicillin for syphilis of more than 1 year's duration. CSF examinations should be performed before therapy with these regimens. Suggested regimens include:
   a. Doxycycline 100 mg orally two times a day; OR
   b. Tetracycline 500 mg orally four times a day.
   Both are given for 2 weeks for individuals with early latent syphilis and 4 weeks for other individuals. If the CSF examination shows any evidence of neurosyphilis, individuals should be treated for neurosyphilis. See page 932 for indications for CSF evaluation.
4. Other considerations
   a. All individuals with latent syphilis should be evaluated for tertiary disease including neurosyphilis, aortitis, iritis, and gummas. Indications for CSF examination are listed on page 932.
   b. All patients with syphilis should be tested for HIV.
5. Follow-up: Quantitative nontreponemal serologic titers should be done at 6 and 12 months after treatment. If titers increase fourfold or initial high titers (≥1:32) fail to decrease fourfold (two dilutions) within 12–24 months, or signs or symptoms of syphilis occur, the individual should be evaluated for neurosyphilis and retreated appropriately.

Approximately 75% of the patients with early latent disease (duration 4 years or less) become seronegative by 5 years. The remaining 25% have positive serology for life.

Late Syphilis

Late syphilis describes patients with gumma disease or cardiovascular involvement but not neurosyphilis.

1. Recommended regimen: Benzathine penicillin G 7.2 million units total should be administered as three doses of 2.4 million units IM at 1-week intervals.
2. Penicillin-allergic patients: Treat with regimens similar to those listed for late latent syphilis.
3. Other considerations
   a. Individuals with symptomatic late syphilis should have CSF examination before therapy.
   b. All patients with syphilis should have HIV testing.
   c. Approximately 25% of the patients with late disease become seronegative within 5 years, and the rest remain seropositive for life.

Neurosyphilis

Neurosyphilis can occur during any stage of syphilis. Patients with syphilitic eye involvement should be treated with regimens covering neurosyphilis. Individuals with neurologic symptoms should have a CSF examination (see guidelines on page 932).

1. Recommended regimen for neurosyphilis or syphilitic eye disease in individuals nonallergic to penicillin: Aqueous crystalline penicillin G 12–24 million units daily administered as 2–4 million units IV every 4 hours for 10–14 days.
2. Alternative regimen if compliance is a problem: Procaine penicillin G IM 2.4 million units daily, plus probenecid 500 mg orally four times a day, both for 10–14 days.
   Some experts add benzathine penicillin G 2.4 million units IM after completion of either of these two regimens.
3. Penicillin-allergic patients: Patients should be desensitized to penicillin, if necessary, and treated with penicillin. No alternatives have been adequately evaluated.
4. Follow-up: If the initial CSF examination showed an increased cell count, the examination should be repeated every 6 months until the cell count is normal. If the count has not decreased at 6 months or is not normal by 2 years, retreatment should be strongly considered.

Syphilis in Pregnancy

All pregnant women should receive penicillin doses appropriate for their stage of syphilis. While penicillin is effective in preventing transmission to the fetus and in treating infections in the fetus, the exact optimal penicillin regimens have not been adequately studied. Some experts recommend additional therapy such as a second dose of benzathine penicillin G 2.4 million units IM 1 week after the first dose, particularly in women in their third trimester with secondary syphilis. Tetracycline should not be used, as it is contraindicated in pregnancy. Erythromycin has a high risk of failure to cure the fetus. Thus, pregnant women with a history of an allergy to penicillin should be skin tested and either treated or desensitized. A Jarisch-Herxheimer reaction during the second half of pregnancy can induce premature labor or fetal distress.

Congenital Syphilis

Treatment should consist of:

1. Aqueous crystalline penicillin G 100,000–150,000 units/kg/day (50,000 units/kg IV every 12 hours during the first 7 days of life and every 8 hours thereafter) for 10–14 days; OR
2. Procaine penicillin G 50,000 units/kg/day (IM once a day) for 10–14 days (14 days if neurosyphilis is present).
   a. If more than 1 day of therapy is missed, the course should be restarted.
   b. If findings from the infant's evaluation are normal but the mother was either (*a*) treated for syphilis during pregnancy with erythromycin, (*b*) treated for syphilis less than 1 month before delivery, or (*c*) treated with penicillin appropriately but did not have an adequate serologic response, the infant should be treated with 50,000 units/kg of benzathine penicillin G IM in a single dose.
3. Penicillin-allergic children: These individuals should be treated with penicillin after desensitization, if necessary.
4. Follow-up
   a. Seropositive infants untreated during the perinatal period: These infants must be followed closely 1, 2, 3, 6, and 12 months after therapy. Nontreponemal titers should decline by 3 months of age and be absent by 6 months. If antibody titers do not follow this pattern, the child should be re-evaluated, including CSF examination, and treated.
   b. Treated infants: These infants also must be followed closely every 2–3 months. The titers should become nonreactive by 6 months of age but may fall more slowly in infants treated after the neonatal period. Infants with cells in the CSF on initial examination should have a second CSF examination at 6 months or until the cell count is normal. The infant should be retreated if the cell count does not show a downward trend or is not normal by 2 years. The CSF-VDRL should also be checked at 6 months and the infant retreated if the test is still reactive.

Management of Sex Partners

1. Persons exposed to an individual with primary, secondary, or latent (duration <1 year) syphilis within the preceding 90 days should be treated presumptively. These individuals might be infected even if seronegative. If exposed over 90 days before examination, the persons should be treated presumptively if serologic tests results are not immediately available and follow-up is uncertain.
2. Partners should be notified and treated, if affected patients have syphilis of unknown duration and high nontreponemal serologic test titers (≥1:32).
3. Sex partners of patients with late syphilis should be evaluated both clinically and serologically for syphilis.
4. Identification of at-risk sex partners: Time periods used to determine partners at risk include:
   a. Three months plus duration of symptoms for primary syphilis
   b. Six months plus duration of symptoms for secondary syphilis
   c. One year plus duration of symptoms for early latent syphilis

HIV-Infected Individuals

There have been reports among HIV-positive individuals of higher rates of neurological complications and treatment failures with traditional regimens for syphilis. There have also been cases in HIV-positive patients of rapid progress of syphilis into secondary and tertiary stages. However, no treatment regimens have, as yet, been demonstrated to be more effective in treating HIV-infected individuals than those used in patients without HIV infection. HIV-positive patients with syphilis require careful evaluation for late and unusual manifestations of syphilis, including CSF evaluation. These individuals require careful follow-up after therapy.

1. Penicillin regimens should be used whenever possible. Skin testing and desensitization can be used as appropriate.
2. Primary and secondary syphilis in HIV-infected patients: The CDC recommend no change in therapy for early syphilis for HIV-coinfected patients. Some experts recommend adding multiple doses of benzathine penicillin G similar to the dosages used to treat late syphilis or adding other antibiotics.
   a. Because of the confusing CSF findings and difficulty in definitively diagnosing neurosyphilis, some authorities recommend CSF examination in all individuals who are HIV infected and altering treatment accordingly.
   b. Follow-up: HIV-infected adolescents should have follow-up serologic testing at 1, 2, 3, 6, 9, and 12 months. Those individuals with treatment failure should have a CSF examination and be retreated similarly to those who are not HIV infected. If the CSF is normal most experts would retreat with benzathine penicillin G 7.2 million units as three weekly doses of 2.4 million units each.
3. Latent syphilis
   a. Patients with HIV and latent syphilis should have a CSF examination before treatment.
   b. Treatment in those individuals with abnormal CSF should include benzathine penicillin G 7.2 million units (as three weekly doses of 2.4 million units each).

Jarisch-Herxheimer Reaction A dramatic reaction occurs within 2 hours after treatment in 50% of patients with primary syphilis, 90% with secondary syphilis, and 25% with early latent syphilis. The reaction consists of:

1. Fever and chills
2. Myalgias
3. Headache
4. Elevated neutrophil count
5. Tachycardia

The duration of symptoms is 12–24 hours, and treatment is reassurance, bed rest, and aspirin. The reaction can induce transient uterine contractions in pregnant women.

PREVENTION

To prevent the rising spread of syphilis, recommendations include screening in the following high-risk groups:

1. All women of childbearing age: In high-risk areas pregnant women should be screened several times: at first visit, third trimester, and at time of delivery. A cord blood sample should also be drawn and held pending maternal results.
2. All sexually active teens: Especially at risk are those with multiple partners, those with a substance abuse history, and those with another STD.
3. All men and women with two or more sex partners in 6 months
4. All persons who use illicit drugs
5. All persons who have had sexual contact with prostitutes

6. All patients with other STDs or who are HIV positive: Positive cases should be reported to the local health department.

To prevent congenital syphilis, recommendations include:

1. All pregnant women, especially those with no history of prenatal care and women using illicit drugs, should be tested. High-risk mothers should be screened as already outlined here.
2. A postpartum mother should not be released from the hospital until the serological results have been reviewed.
3. The diagnosis of syphilis should be considered in any stillbirth or miscarriage and in any infant with symptoms, including snuffles, steochondritis or periostitis, hepatosplenomegaly, rash, pneumonia, failure to thrive, jaundice, lymphadenopathy, neurologic signs, fissures of the lips or other cutaneous lesions, or rhinitis.
4. All infants of women diagnosed with syphilis within 1 year of delivery should be evaluated for congenital syphilis. Conversely, mothers of infants diagnosed with congenital syphilis should be evaluated and treated for syphilis.
5. All pregnant women with positive results from serologic examination and confirmed cases of congenital syphilis should be reported to the local health department.
6. HIV testing should be considered for all women and children diagnosed with syphilis. This is because more aggressive treatment may be required in patients who are immunocompromised.

BIBLIOGRAPHY

Brown ST, Zeidi A, Larsen SA, et al. Serological response to syphilis treatment: a new analysis of old data. JAMA 1985;253:1296.

Campisi D, Whitcomb C. Liver disease in early syphilis. Arch Intern Med 1979;139:365.

Centers for Disease Control. Congenital syphilis United States, 1983–1985. MMWR 1986;35:625.

Centers for Disease Control. Increases in primary and secondary syphilis United States. MMWR 1987;36:393.

Centers for Disease Control. 1993 sexually transmitted diseases treatment guidelines. MMWR 1993;42 (RR–14):1.

Centers for Disease Control. Surveillance for gonorrhea and primary and secondary syphilis among adolescents, United States—1981–1991. MMWR 1993;42:1.

Centers for Disease Control. Selected notifiable diseases, 1995. MMWR 1996;45:23.

Cox JM, d'Angelo LJ, Silber TJ. Substance abuse and syphilis in urban adolescents: a new risk factor for an old disease. J Adolesc Health 1992;13:483.

Emmons WW III, Church LW. Syphilitic uveitis. West J Med 1994;161:168.

Felman YM. Lumbar puncture in asymptomatic neurosyphilis. Arch Intern Med 1985;145:422.

Goens JL, Janniger CK, De-Wolf K. Dermatologic and systemic manifestations of syphilis. Am Fam Physician 1994;50:1013.

Gordon SM, Eaton ME, George R, et al. The response of symptomatic neurosyphilis to high-dose intravenous penicillin G in patients with human immuno-deficiency virus infection [see comments]. N Engl J Med 1994;331:1516.

Guinan ME. Treatment of primary and secondary syphilis: defining failure at three and six month follow-up. JAMA 1987;257:359.

Holmes KK, Lukehart SA. Syphilis. In: Braunwald E, Isselbachen KJ, Petersdorf RG, et al., eds. Harrison's principles of internal medicine. 11th ed. New York: McGraw-Hill, 1987.

Hook EW III, Marra CM. Acquired syphilis in adults. N Engl J Med 1992;326:1060.

Hutchinson CM, Hook EW III, Shepherd M, et al. Altered clinical presentation of early syphilis in patients with human immunodeficiency virus infection. Ann Intern Med 1994;121:94.

Jaffe HW. Management of the reactive serology. In: Holmes KK, Mardh PA, Sparling PF, eds. Sexually transmitted diseases. New York: McGraw-Hill, 1986.

Jones BV, Lichtenstein JE. Gastric syphilis: radiologic findings. AJR 1993;160:59.

LaGuardia KD, White MH, Saigo PE, et al. Genital ulcer disease in women infected with human immunodeficiency virus. Am J Obstet Gynecol 1995;172:553.

Larsen SA, Steiner BM, Rudolph AH. Laboratory diagnosis and interpretation of tests for syphilis. Clin Microbiol Rev 1995;8:1.

Lukehart SA. Syphilis. Curr Opin Infect Dis 1990;3:3.

Lukehart SA, Hook EW III, Baker-Zander SA, et al. Invasion of the central nervous system by *Treponema pallidum:* implications for diagnosis and treatment. Ann Intern Med 1988;109:855.

McCabe E, Jaffe LR, Diaz A. Human immunodeficiency virus seropositivity in adolescents with syphilis. Pediatrics 1993;92:695.

McKown RR, Kapernick PS. Syphilis in pregnancy. South Med J 1988;81:447.

Malone JL, Wallace MR, Hendrick BB, et al. Syphilis and neurosyphilis in a human immunodeficiency virus type-1 seropositive population: evidence for frequent serologic relapse after therapy. Am J Med 1995;99:55.

Markovitz DM, Beutner KR, Maggio RP, et al. Failure of recommended treatment for secondary syphilis. JAMA 1986;255:1767.

Mindel A, Tovey SJ, Timmins DJ, et al. Primary and secondary syphilis, 20 years' experience. II. Clinical features. Genitourin Med 1989;65:1.

Musher DM. Biology of *Treponema pallidum.* In: Holmes KK, Mardh PA, Sparling PF, Wiesner PJ, eds. Sexually transmitted diseases. 2nd ed. New York: McGraw-Hill Information Services, 1990.

Pandhi RK, Singh N, Ramam M. Secondary syphilis: a clinicopathologic study. Int J Dermatol 1995;34:240.

Peterman TA, Zaidi AA, Lieb S, et al. Incubating syphilis in patients treated for gonorrhea: a comparison of treatment regimens. J Infect Dis 1994;170:689.

Rolfs RT, Goldberg M, Charrar RG. Risk factors for syphilis. Cocaine use and prostitution. Am J Public Health 1990;80:853.

Romanowski B, Sutherland R, Fick GH, et al. Serologic response to treatment of infectious syphilis. Ann Intern Med 1991;114:1005.

Schulz KF, Murphy FK, Patamasucon P, Meheus AZ. Congenital syphilis. In: Holmes KK, Mardh PA, Sparling PF, Wiesner PJ, eds. Sexually transmitted diseases. 2nd ed. New York: McGraw-Hill Information Services, 1990.

Shafer MA, Hilton JF, Ekstrand M, et al. Relationship between drug use and sexual behaviors and the occurrence of sexually transmitted diseases among high-risk male youth. Sex Transm Dis 1993;20:307.

Shew ML, Fortenberry JD. Syphilis screening in adolescent. J Adolesc Health 1992;13:303.

Sparling PF. Natural history of syphilis. In: Holmes KK, Mardh PA, Sparling PF, Wiesner PJ, eds. Sexually transmitted diseases. 2nd ed. New York: McGraw-Hill Information Services, 1990.

Swartz MN. Neurosyphilis. In: Holmes KK, Mardh PA, Sparling PF, Wiesner PJ, eds. Sexually transmitted diseases. 2nd ed. New York: McGraw-Hill Information Services, 1990.

Syphilis: The great imitator: Medical Staff Conference. West J Med 1981;134:424.

Thin RN. Early syphilis in the adult. In: Holmes KK, Mardh PA, Sparling PF, Wiesner PJ, eds. Sexually transmitted diseases. 2nd ed. New York: McGraw-Hill Information Services, 1990.

Tramont EC. Syphilis in the AIDS era. N Engl J Med 1987;316:1600.

Webster LA, Berman SM, Greenspan JR. Surveillance for gonorrhea and primary and secondary syphilis among adolescents, United States 1981–1991. MMWR 1993;42:1.

Wiesel J, Rose DN, Silver AL, et al. Lumbar puncture in asymptomatic late syphilis: an analysis of the benefits and risks. Arch Intern Med 1985;145:465.

Winters HA, Notar-Francesco V, Bromberg K, et al. Gastric syphilis: five recent cases and a review of the literature. Ann Intern Med 1992;116:314.

Wood VD, Nichols AP. Characteristics of high-risk adolescent outpatients with treponemal antibody. J Natl Med Assoc 1992;84:793.

Zenker PN. Syphilis. Adolesc Med: State Art Rev 1990; 1:511.

CHAPTER 65

Herpes Genitalis

Linda E. Schack and Lawrence S. Neinstein

Herpes genitalis lesions are caused by a large DNA virus, herpes simplex. Approximately 85–90% of genital infections are caused by herpes simplex type 2 virus (HSV-2) and the rest by herpes simplex type 1 (HSV-1). These viruses have the ability to become latent and then recur. The prevalence of herpes genitalis has increased dramatically in the past 30 years.

EPIDEMIOLOGY

Incidence and Prevalence

1. Herpes simplex virus is the cause of 90% of all vesiculoulcerative lesions of the genitalia. After human papilloma virus, it is the second most prevalent sexually transmitted disease (STD).
2. In the United States there are over 30 million people infected with genital herpes, and 500,000 more acquire the infection every year. Most of these infections are asymptomatic.
3. There has been a marked increase in the incidence of clinical herpes. In 1966 there were fewer than 18,000 visits to physicians for first episodes of herpes infections; in 1988 there were more than 160,000. The annual incidence of clinically apparent infections is 50 per 100,000 adults.
4. Adolescents may account for 25–50% of all patients with genital herpetic infection (Oill and Mishell, 1980). A study in Minnesota demonstrated that patients 15–24 years of age accounted for 47% of genital herpes infections in Rochester, Minnesota (Chuang et al., 1983). The incidence of infection increases rapidly after puberty, reaching a peak in the third decade of life.
5. Herpes labialis: Sixteen percent to 45% of all adults report at least one episode during their lifetime, with 28% having recurrences at least twice a year. Infection is most prevalent in the 2- to 4-year-old age group.
6. Herpes genitalis: At least 20% of the U.S. population have antibodies to HSV-2. Antibodies are present in 20% of sexually experienced female college students, 50% of female STD clinic patients, 80% of homosexual male STD clinic patients, and 80% of female prostitutes. More nonwhites are infected than whites (30–60% versus 20–40%). The prevalence in females is 5–10% higher than in males.

Transmission

Transmission is through sexual contact, either genital-genital or oral-genital, and by mucosal contact with infected secretions. Humans are the sole known reservoir of infection. Viral shedding is highest while genital lesions are present. Asymptomatic salivary excretion of HSV-1 occurs in about 2–9% of adults and 5–8% of children.

Brock et al. (1990) examined the frequency of asymptomatic shedding of HSV in women with genital herpes. Cultures were obtained on a daily basis from 27 women with recurrent genital herpes. Asymptomatic HSV shedding was documented on 1% of the days on which cultures were taken. However, the rate is much higher after initial episodes of herpes. A study by Koelle et al. (1992) detected viral shedding in 11.9% of women with primary HSV-1, 18.3% of women with primary HSV-2, and 22.9% of women with nonprimary first episode HSV-2 after their symptoms had resolved. The shedding was three times more frequent during the first 3 months after resolution of symptoms. A 1992 study of 144 heterosexual couples by Mertz et al. looked at transmission from source partners with recurrent genital HSV to susceptible partners. Transmission occurred in 14 (9.7%) couples after one year, and was higher with the male as the source partner (16.9% versus 3.8%).

Court cases in eight states have established that physicians have an obligation to inform their patients about the risk of transmitting HSV during asymptomatic periods. Patients also have a legal duty to disclose a history of herpes infection to prospective sexual partners.

SEROLOGIC TYPES

1. HSV-1: Primary infections with HSV-1 usually cause herpetic gingivostomatitis.
2. HSV-2: This type most commonly causes genital herpes. Antibodies are not routinely detected until puberty, at which time antibody levels correlate with past sexual activity.
3. Primary genital infections: Two-thirds of primary infections are caused by HSV-2, and one-third are caused by HSV-1.
4. Recurrent infections: Seventy percent to 90% of patients infected with HSV-2 will have a recurrence versus 50% of those infected with HSV-1. Recurrences vary by site and viral type. About 97% of recurrent genital infections are caused by HSV-2 and 3% by HSV-1.

Benedetti et al. (1994) examined recurrence rates of genital herpes after symptomatic first-episode infection. In this study of 457 patients with HSV-2, 89% had at least one recurrence during follow-up with a median monthly recurrence rate of 0.34. Thirty-eight percent had at least 6 recurrences during the first year, and 20% had more than 10 recurrences. Twenty-six percent of women and 8% of men had no or 1 recurrence in year 1 of follow-up. Patients who had severe primary HSV-2 infection (duration, ≥35 days) had recurrences nearly twice as often. Men with genital HSV-2 infection have about 20% more recurrences than do women.

PATHOGENESIS

Virus particles can be shed in salivary, cervical, and seminal secretions of infected individuals. The virus gains entry to the body via mucosal surfaces or abraded skin and replicates in the epidermal and dermal cells of a susceptible host. After replication, the virus spreads via contiguous cells to mucocutaneous projections of sensory nerves.

In oral herpes the virus lodges in the trigeminal ganglion; in genital herpes the sacral dorsal root (S2 to S4) ganglion is the target site. Centrifugal spread can then occur through peripheral sensory nerves back to the skin surface; thus, large areas may be involved.

After resolution of the primary disease the virus becomes latent. Latency appears to be lifelong but is interrupted by periods of viral reactivation, leading to silent viral shedding or clinically apparent recurrence. Reactivation of latent virus leads to transport of viral genomes to the skin surface, where replication occurs in the dermis and epidermis. Factors involved in activating latent virus may include fever, local trauma, exposure to sunlight, and stress.

Clinical Manifestations

Definition of Terms

1. Primary infection: Genital herpes in a patient seronegative for antibody to HSV-1 or HSV-2
2. Nonprimary first episode: First clinically noted infection in an individual seropositive for HSV-1 or HSV-2
3. First clinical episode: Both primary infections and nonprimary first episodes; this term should be used when the practitioner cannot clinically classify the patient's infection as a primary infection or a nonprimary first episode.
4. Recurrence: Return of genital HSV lesions in a patient with a previously documented episode of symptomatic genital herpes

Primary Infection

1. Incubation period: 1–45 days, average 6–8 days
2. Duration
   a. Time from onset of lesions to complete healing is approximately 3 weeks.
   b. Viral shedding: 11 days (median), can be much longer.
3. Symptoms start with paresthesias or burning sensations in the genital area, followed by the appearance of 1–2 mm vesicles on erythematous bases.
4. Herpetic lesions can be extensive and involve the vulva, perineum, vagina, cervix, or in males, large areas of the penis. Early lesions are vesicular and then erode to become shallow ulcers. The lesions may coalesce, producing large ulcerated areas with surrounding edema, erythema, and secondary infection. Painful lesions are present in 95% of men and 99% of women with primary HSV infection.
5. Healing follows crusting of unbroken lesions and re-epithelialization of ulcers.
6. Primary infections are usually more severe. They are characterized by significant local symptoms, multiple lesions (generally six or more), and enlarged tender regional nodes. Lesions in primary infections will be bilateral, while those appearing in recurrences tend to be unilateral.
7. Constitutional symptoms occur in over half of patients with primary infection. Systemic complaints including fever, malaise, and myalgias are reported in nearly 40% of men and 70% of women with primary HSV-2 disease. Neurological signs and symptoms (headaches, stiff neck, photophobia) are also common.
8. Dysuria, urinary retention, and dyspareunia may occur. Dysuria appears in 83% of women and 44% of men. Urethral discharge and dysuria are noted in about one-third of men with primary HSV-2 infection. Herpes can be misdiagnosed as urinary tract infection (UTI). Therefore, inquire about genital sores and pain in a teen presenting with UTI symptoms.
9. Cervical involvement occurs in 90% of primary infections and 12–20% of recurrences. Rarely, a primary infection is manifested by necrotizing cervicitis.
10. Course: Systemic symptoms appear early, peak within the first 3–4 days, and recede over the next several days. The clinical symptoms of pain and irritation increase over the first 6–7 days, are maximal between days 7–11, and recede over the second week. Lesions persist 4–15 days, ending with crusting and re-epithelialization. Scarring is uncommon. Tender inguinal adenopathy usually appears during the second and third week and is often the last symptom to resolve. Total duration is about 21 days, with a gradual worsening over the first 10 days and a 12-day healing period. Primary episodes of type 1 genital infection are similar in duration and character to those of type 2 genital infection.

Recurrent Episodes

1. The herpes virus lies dormant in the sensory neurons of the involved area until reactivation. This can occur frequently, infrequently, or never. The primary infection is the most severe, but recurrences are more likely to cause chronic anxiety and sexual dysfunction.
2. Duration
   a. Average time from onset of symptoms to complete resolution is one week.
   b. Viral shedding lasts 2–7 days.
3. Symptoms: About 50% of infected individuals have prodromal symptoms, ranging from mild tingling sensations to shooting pains in the buttocks, legs, or hips, hours to days prior to eruption. Lesions are similar to those seen in primary infection but are smaller in size and number. They tend to occur unilaterally, with the involved area being smaller, about one-tenth the area of the primary infection. Systemic signs are minimal. Pain, lesion size, and virus shedding peak within 2 days of onset.
4. The typical course is 2–4 days of worsening symptoms, followed by 4–5 days of healing.
5. Recurrent herpes, as with primary herpes, tends to be more severe in females.
6. Characteristics of recurrent episodes include predominantly nonmucosal skin involvement, small numbers of lesions (less than three), clustering of lesions, and resolution in 5–10 days.
7. Median number of recurrences of genital herpes during the first year is about four for HSV-2 and less than one for HSV-1. After the first year, recurrences tend to decrease in frequency.

Table 65.1 shows a comparison of initial infections and reactivation, and Table 65.2 shows a comparison of serologic types.

TABLE 65.1. Comparison of Initial Infections and Reactivation of Herpes Genitalis

	Initial	Reactivation
Frequency in practice	−	+
Historical data		
Previous history	−	+
Recent exposure	+	−
Precipitating factors (stress, premenstrual syndrome)	−	+
Prodromal symptoms	+	+
Severe pain	+	+/−
Systemic	+	−
Physical findings		
Mucosal	+	−
Skin sites (i.e., labia, perianal, buttocks, penile shaft, scrotum)	−	+
Widespread lesions	+	−
Local involvement	−	+
Asymptomatic	−	+
Evolution of lesions	+	+
Grouping of lesions	+/−	+
Edema	+	+/−
Tenderness of lesions	+	+
Localized lymphadenopathy	+	+/−
Fever	+	−
Unilateral	−	+
Bilateral	+	−
Prolonged course	+	−
Accelerated course	−	+
Complications	+	−

TABLE 65.2.   Comparison of Primary HSV-1, Primary HSV-2, and Nonprimary HSV-2 Infections

	Primary HSV-1 N = 20	Primary HSV-2 N = 189	Nonprimary HSV-2 N = 76
Percentage with systemic symptoms	58.0	62.0	16.0
Mean duration local pain (days)	12.5	11.8	8.7
Mean number of lesions	24.3	15.5	9.5
Percentage with bilateral lesions	100.0	82.0	55.0
Percentage forming new lesions during course of disease	68.0	75.0	45.0
Mean duration viral shedding from genital lesions (days)	11.1	11.4	6.8
Mean duration lesions (days)	22.7	18.6	15.5

Adapted from Corey L. Genital herpes. In: Holmes KK, Mardh PA, Sparling PF, Wiesner PJ, eds. Sexually transmitted diseases. 2nd ed. New York: McGraw-Hill Information Services, 1990.

DIFFERENTIAL DIAGNOSIS

Herpes genitalis lesions must be differentiated from early syphilis, chancroid, lymphogranuloma venereum, granuloma inguinale, excoriations, allergic and irritant contact dermatitis, molluscum contagiosum, warts, scabies, pediculosis, and genital lesions of Behcet's syndrome.

DIAGNOSIS

1. Clinical history and examination: Presence of symptoms and typical lesions. A history of prior episodes or recent contact with an infected partner is helpful but not necessary to establish the diagnosis.
2. Dark-field examination and syphilis serology should be obtained if ulcers have an atypical appearance.
3. Laboratory diagnosis
    a. Tzanck smear showing multinucleated giant cells is inexpensive and rapid, but sensitivity ranges from 30–80%, depending on the type of lesion and experience of the observer. Technique is reviewed in detail by Cohen (1994).
    b. Pap smear is also rapid and inexpensive but only 40% sensitive.
    c. Viral culture is the gold standard of diagnosis at present, and differentiates between HSV-1 and HSV-2. As the lesions progress through pustule, ulcer, and crusting, the sensitivity falls. Sensitivities in various stages are maculopapular, 25%; vesicular, 94%; pustular, 87%; ulcer, 70%; crusting, 27%. In clinically obvious cases of herpes, a viral culture is not absolutely necessary. However, knowledge of infection type (HSV-1 versus HSV-2) is helpful in predicting recurrences. In addition, most patients appreciate having a confirmed laboratory diagnosis, so cultures should be obtained when feasible.

        Method of obtaining HSV cultures:
        — *If intact vesicles are present:* Aspirate vesicle fluid using a fine-gauge needle (best yield) or if vesicles are too small to aspirate, gently unroof the vesicle and swab fluid and debris. Use cotton or Dacron swabs rather than calcium alginate, which inactivates the virus. Immediately place in transport medium.
        — *Pustules:* Unroof pustule and wash away purulent material with sterile saline, then swab base of lesion.
        — *To culture a ruptured vesicle or ulcers:* Swab base of lesion.
        — *If lesion is crusted:* Wash away necrotic debris with sterile saline, then swab lesion base.

- When swabbing the base of a lesion, remember that friction must be used to obtain cells. Avoid contaminating the specimen with alcohol, soap, blood, or stool. If transport medium is not available, substitute sterile distilled water (minimally decreased yield). Leave the swab in the transport medium if transport time is under 8 hours. If transport time is longer, swirl the swab vigorously in the medium and remove. If a laboratory courier is used, refrigerate the specimen prior to pickup.
- With high-titer virus specimen cultures, results may be positive in 24–48 hours, but with lower titers the culture may require up to 7 days. Since cultures can be negative in the presence of herpes, use caution in reporting negative results to patients.

d. An enzyme-linked immunosorbent assay (ELISA) is available, with a sensitivity of 70–90% compared with viral isolation. ELISA does not reliably differentiate between virus types.

e. Immunofluorescence techniques can differentiate between HSV-1 and HSV-2, have excellent sensitivity and specificity, and are rapid, but they require an experienced technician. These techniques are most often used when immediate diagnosis is needed.

f. DNA probes and polymerase chain reaction (PCR) techniques are also being developed that promise to be highly sensitive and specific.

g. Serology titers are available but are mainly used for epidemiological studies. Serology can be used to diagnose primary infection; but since acute and convalescent specimens are required, this method is not helpful in managing an acute episode.

In most cases practitioners should use viral culture when lesions are present and a diagnostic test is desired. If financial resources are limited, Tzanck smears can be used.

THERAPY

Acyclovir (Zovirax)

1. Indications: Oral acyclovir is indicated for the treatment of initial episodes and the management of recurrences in certain individuals. Patients with primary episodes are more likely to benefit if the treatment is started promptly and if the episode is severe. Treatment is also suggested for patients with six or more recurrences per year. Topical acyclovir ointment is substantially less effective than oral administration.

2. Drug action: Acyclovir is a guanosine analog that inhibits viral replication of HSV-1 and HSV-2 by interfering with viral DNA polymerase. There is little or no effect on human DNA.

3. Efficacy
   a. First clinical episodes: Acyclovir decreases:
      - Duration of viral shedding: Shortened by about 10 days
      - New lesion formation: Forty-four percent of those taking a placebo develop new lesions versus 4% of those taking acyclovir.
      - Period and severity of pain: Duration of pain is decreased by about 2 days.
      - Time to healing (crusting) is reduced by 4–9 days.
      - Proctitis symptoms: Rompalo et al. (1988) examined the effect of acyclovir in the first episode of HSV proctitis and found the median duration of rectal lesions and viral excretion to be significantly shorter in treated patients. Duration of local signs and symptoms of proctitis was also shorter.
      - There is no effect on the subsequent rate of recurrences of herpes infections treated with acyclovir.

  b. Recurrent episodes
    — Viral shedding: Reduced by approximately 1 day with acyclovir
    — Healing time: Reduced by an average of 1 day. A more pronounced effect is noted when therapy is self-initiated early in the course of a recurrent episode.
    — Duration of symptoms: Slightly shortened, but this effect is not statistically significant.
    — Recurrent episodes are not prevented if acyclovir is used only on a periodic basis.
    — Suppressive therapy: There is a significant reduction in frequency and duration of recurrent episodes when used in a prophylactic fashion. With daily use, recurrent infections are prevented in 60–90% of patients. Using suppressive therapy in individuals with six or more episodes of genital herpes, the mean number of recurrences per year was 1.8 compared with 11.4 using episodic therapy.

4. Dose
  a. Initial episodes
    — Genital herpes: Acyclovir 400 mg three times a day orally for 7–10 days or until clinical resolution occurs
    — Herpes labialis (oral herpes): Acyclovir 400 mg three times a day orally for 7–10 days.
    — Immunocompromised patient: Acyclovir 400 mg five times a day orally for 7–14 days or 5 mg/kg intravenously (IV) every 8 hours
    — Proctitis: Acyclovir 400 mg five times a day orally for 10 days or until clinical resolution occurs
    — For severe disease or complications requiring hospitalization (e.g., pneumonitis, hepatitis): Acyclovir 5–10 mg/kg IV every 8 hours for 5–7 days or until clinical resolution occurs
    — Encephalitis: Acyclovir 10 mg/kg IV every 8 hours for 14–21 days
    — Acyclovir-resistant: Foscarnet (Foscavir) 40 mg/kg IV every 8 hours
  b. Recurrent episodes: Acyclovir 400 mg three times a day orally for 5 days. For herpes labialis (oral herpes), 3 or 4 days of treatment is usually adequate.
  c. Suppressive therapy (consider suppressive therapy if the patient is having six or more recurrences per year): Acyclovir 400 mg twice daily is usually adequate. A small number of patients require higher dosing. Since recurrences tend to decrease over time, try discontinuing the medication annually and observe.

5. Toxicity: Excellent safety profile and remarkably well tolerated. Acyclovir-resistant strains are not commonly recovered from immunocompetent patients during acyclovir therapy, nor does there seem to be a high frequency of resistance after 4 months of suppressive therapy. Safety and efficacy have been demonstrated in individuals receiving suppressive therapy for up to 5 years. Other treatment considerations:
  a. Keep lesions clean and dry.
  b. Tap water compresses or sitz baths are soothing in the vesicular and pustular stages. A light application of petroleum jelly may relieve the discomfort of crusting and fissuring.
  c. Use acyclovir early in primary infections.
  d. Avoid lesion contact with fingers or eyes.
  e. Avoid sexual activity for at least 10 days after lesions heal and preferably until lesions have completely re-epithelialized (about 16–20 days).

Valacyclovir (Valtrex)

Valacyclovir is the most recent herpes antiviral agent to receive approval from the Food and Drug Administration. It has current approval for episodic treatment of *recurrent* genital herpes simplex in otherwise healthy adults. In clinical trials, valacyclovir shortened the healing time of genital herpes sores by 33% (4 days versus 6 days) on average compared to a placebo. In addition, the duration of pain associated with genital herpes was reduced by 25% (3 days versus 4 days) in patients who received valacyclovir as opposed to a placebo. Valacyclovir also stopped viral shedding 50% (2 days versus 4 days) faster on average than a placebo.

Dose: 500 mg twice a day orally for 5 days.

Valacyclovir has a more convenient administration schedule than acyclovir. Valacyclovir HCl is the hydrochloride salt of the L-valyl ester of acyclovir. This formulation was designed to improve on the relatively low bioavailability of acyclovir after oral administration. Valacyclovir is administered orally, rapidly absorbed from the gastrointestinal tract, and rapidly and almost totally converted to acyclovir and L-valine by first-pass metabolism in the intestines or liver, or both. The enhanced pharmacokinetics of valacyclovir suggest the potential for superior clinical efficacy over oral acyclovir.

Other Antiviral Agents

Famciclovir, penciclovir, and other investigational drugs have superior bioavailability to acyclovir and may be approved for treatment of herpes in the future.

PREVENTION

Patients with active lesions during a first or recurrent episode should abstain from intercourse until the lesions are clearly healed. Since viral shedding can occur in the absence of lesions, recommend regular use of condoms to any patient who has had an episode of genital herpes. Vaccines for genital herpes appear promising and are currently in phase 3 clinical trials.

COMPLICATIONS

1. Significant psychological distress: Initially, denial, shock, fear, guilt, feelings of social isolation, and anger at the partner are common. Anxiety and depression also occur and may persist in some patients, especially with recurrences.
2. Local complications: These include secondary bacterial infection of lesions, phimosis (males) or labial adhesions (females), urinary retention, constipation, and impotence. Sacral radiculopathy can also occur, causing paresthesias in the lower extremities.
3. Proctitis: Common in homosexual men. Presenting complaints may include rectal bleeding, mucoid discharge, constipation, myalgias, fever, and occasionally impotence.
4. Herpes keratitis: Predominantly associated with HSV-1 infection
5. Encephalitis and meningitis: Encephalitis is primarily caused by HSV-1 infection, with about 250–500 cases per year in the United States. The case fatality rate exceeds 70% if untreated. Aseptic meningitis and transverse myelitis occurs in as many as 36% of women and 13% of men with primary genital HSV-2 infections. However, hospitalization is required for clinically overt aseptic meningitis in a minority of these cases.
6. Neonatal herpes virus infection
   a. Neonatal infection is most commonly caused by HSV-2, with a case fatality rate of about 50%. There are an estimated 1000 cases per year in the United States. The mechanisms of infection include spread from the lower to upper genital tract, delivery through an infected birth canal, and transmission from nursery personnel with recurrent labial disease. Most babies born vaginally to mothers with primary genital herpes acquire disseminated infection.

b. Infants of pregnant women with primary herpes infections are at much greater risk than those born to mothers who have recurrences.
   — Initial infections: Brown et al. (1987) examined the effects on infants of initial episodes of genital herpes infections during pregnancy. In mothers with a primary first episode of genital HSV-2, six out of 15 infants had serious perinatal morbidity, while zero out of 14 infants with mothers who had nonprimary first episodes were affected. Asymptomatic cervical shedding of HSV-2 was detected in 10.6% of weekly visits made after a primary first episode but in only 0.5% of visits after a nonprimary first episode.
   — Recurrent infections: Prober et al. (1987) studied infants born to mothers with recurrent genital HSV infections and exposed to virus at delivery: Zero out of 34 such infants acquired an HSV infection, and 33 out of 33 possessed neutralizing antibody to HSV-2. Practitioners should reassure pregnant patients with recurrent infections that the risk of neonatal herpes is very small and that most infants can be safely delivered vaginally.
   Of those infants with neonatal herpes, 35% have no history of an infection in their mother or father; and in 90% of such infants there are no signs or symptoms in their mother at delivery.
   Although preliminary data appear favorable, acyclovir has not been conclusively shown to be safe during pregnancy. It should therefore be reserved for disseminated maternal herpes simplex infections. Use of acyclovir to treat recurrent genital herpes episodes or as suppressive therapy is not recommended during pregnancy.
c. Congenital HSV results from intrauterine infection. The syndrome is well described but rare and includes skin lesions and scars, chorioretinitis, and central nervous system involvement (microcephaly or hydranencephaly).

OBSTETRIC MANAGEMENT

Viral cultures during pregnancy do not predict viral shedding at delivery and are not routinely indicated. Women without signs and symptoms of herpes at the time of delivery may deliver the infant vaginally. Cultures of the birth canal at delivery may be useful in managing the infant. If the cultures are positive, the pediatrician should be informed and the parents or caregivers educated to observe the infant for lethargy, poor feeding, fever, or lesions. Roberts et al. (1995) found that adoption of the 1988 American College of Obstetricians and Gynecologists (ACOG) herpes guidelines resulted in a 37% decrease in the use of cesarean delivery for women with genital herpes infections at their hospital. Most of this decrease was because the new guidelines eliminated the need for a confirmatory negative herpes culture before permitting vaginal delivery. No neonatal herpes infections occurred as a result of implementing the ACOG recommendations.

PATIENT RESOURCES

1. Wellcome DIALOG, Burroughs Wellcome: A patient information booklet, including opportunity to receive periodic mailings regarding support groups, health tips, and advances in herpes research. For copies, call: 1-800-843-8889.
2. The Herpes Resource Center: A program of the American Social Health Association (ASHA). Information for physicians and patients. Telephone: 919-361-8485. To order pamphlets: 919-361-8400.
3. National Herpes Hotline: A service of ASHA. For patients with questions about any aspect of herpes. Telephone: 919-361-8488.

4. STD Hotline: Nationwide support group referrals. Telephone: 800-227-8922.
5. *Managing Herpes: How to Live and Love with a Chronic STD* (224 pages). Available through ASHA. Telephone: 800-230-6039.

SUGGESTIONS FOR MANAGING A FIRST EPISODE OF GENITAL HERPES

1. Obtain a culture if possible.
2. Screen for other STDs. Cervical sampling in female patients may need to be deferred to a subsequent visit due to pain. Human immunodeficiency virus (HIV) testing should be suggested, but it may be desirable to discuss this at the follow-up visit.
3. Briefly explain how the virus is transmitted, the possibility of recurrences, and treatment. Anticipate that the patient will be upset by the diagnosis; take time to comfort him or her and answer questions.
4. Prescribe analgesics, tap water compresses or sitz baths, and topical petrolatum if fissures or crusting are bothersome. Advise keeping lesions clean and dry.
5. If within 6 days of onset, prescribe acyclovir, 400 mg orally t.i.d. for 7–10 days.
6. Advise abstaining from sex while lesions are present.
7. Give the patient written information to take home.
8. Recommend a follow-up visit in 1 week. Suggest that the patient bring a list of questions and that the partner attend the visit if possible.

At the follow-up visit:

1. Confirm the diagnosis.
2. Assess the need to continue antiviral medication.
3. Ask about the patient's emotional state.
4. Answer questions and review information about transmission and recurrence.
5. Discuss the need for safer sex to prevent acquiring other STDs as well as transmission of herpes.
6. Suggest that the partner have an examination.

BIBLIOGRAPHY

Abramowicz M, ed. Drugs for non-HIV viral infections. Medical Lett Drug Ther 1994;36:27.

Adimora AA, Hamilton H, Holmes KK, et al. Genital herpes. In: Sexually transmitted diseases [Companion handbook]. 2nd ed. New York: McGraw-Hill, 1994.

American Academy of Pediatrics. Herpes simplex. In: Peter G, ed. 1994 red book: report of the committee on infectious diseases. 23rd ed. Elk Grove Village, Illinois: American Academy of Pediatrics, 1994:242.

Andrews EB, Tilson HH, Hurn BAL, et al. Acyclovir in Pregnancy Advisory Committee, Acyclovir in pregnancy registry: an observational epidemiologic approach. Am J Med 1988;85(suppl 2A):123.

Benedetti J, Corey L, Ashley R. Recurrence rates in genital herpes after symptomatic first-episode infection. Ann Intern Med 1994;121:847.

Benedetti JK, Zeh J, Selke S, et al. Frequency and reactivation of nongenital lesions among patients with genital herpes simplex virus. Am J Med 1995;98:237.

Bergfled WF, Munnings F. How to manage herpes in active patients. Phys Sportsmed 1994;22:71.

Bierman SM. Genital herpes: a pervasive psychological disorder. Arch Dermatol 1985;121:513.

Boehm FH, Estes W, Wright PF, et al. Management of genital herpes simplex virus infections occurring during pregnancy. Am J Obstet Gynecol 1981;141:735.

Brock BV, Selke S, Benedetti J, et al. Frequency of asymptomatic shedding of herpes simplex virus in women with genital herpes. JAMA 1990;263:418.

Brown ZA, Vontver LA, Benedetti J, et al. Effects on infants of a first episode of genital herpes during pregnancy. N Engl J Med 1987;317:1246.

Bryson YJ. Genital herpes in adolescents and young adults. In AIDS and other sexually transmitted diseases. Adolesc Med: State Art Rev 1990;1:471.

Bryson Y, Dillon M, Lovett M, et al. Treatment of first episodes of genital herpes simplex virus infection with oral acyclovir: a randomized double-blind controlled trial in normal subjects. N Engl J Med 1983;308:916.

Centers for Disease Control. Genital herpes infection United States, 1966–1979. MMWR 1982;31:137.

Centers for Disease Control. 1991 division of STD/HIV prevention annual report. Atlanta, Georgia: Center for Prevention Services, Centers for Disease Control, US Department of Health and Human Services, 1992:167.

Centers for Disease Control. 1993 sexually transmitted diseases treatment guidelines. MMWR 1993;42 (RR–14).

Chuang TY, Daniel WP Jr, Perry MO, et al. Incidence and trend of herpes progenitalis: a 15-year population study. Mayo Clin Proc 1983;58:436.

Clark JL, Tatum NO, Noble SL. Management of genital herpes. Am Fam Physician 1995;51:175.

Cohen PR. Tests for detecting herpes simplex virus and varicella-zoster virus infections. Dermatol Clin 1994;12:51.

Cohen PR, Young AW Jr. Herpes simplex: Update on diagnosis and management of genital herpes infection. Medical Aspects of Human Sexuality 1988; 22:93.

Committee on Fetus and Newborn, Committee on Infectious Disease. Perinatal herpes simplex virus infections. Pediatrics 1980;66:147.

Cone RW, Hobson AC, Brown Z, et al. Frequent detection of genital herpes simplex virus DNA by polymerase chain reaction among pregnant women. JAMA 1994;272:792.

Corey L. Genital herpes. In: Holmes KK, Mardh PA, Sparling PF, Wiesner PJ, eds. Sexually transmitted diseases. 2nd ed. New York: McGraw-Hill Information Services, 1990.

Corey L, Adams MG, Brown ZA, et al. Genital herpes simplex virus infections: clinical manifestations, course, and complications. Ann Intern Med 1983; 98:958.

Corey L, Holmes KK. Genital herpes simplex virus infections: current diagnosis, therapy, and prevention. Ann Intern Med 1983;98:973.

Corey L, Nahmias AJ, Guinan ME, et al. A trial of acyclovir in genital herpes simplex virus infections. N Engl J Med 1982;306:1313.

Corey L, Spear PG. Infections with herpes simplex viruses. N Engl J Med 1986;314:686 & 749.

Dorsky DI, Crumpacker CS. Drugs five years later: acyclovir. Ann Intern Med 1987;107:859.

Douglas JM, Critchlow C, Benedetti J, et al. A double-blind study of oral acyclovir for suppression of recurrences of genital herpes simplex virus infection. N Engl J Med 1984;310:1551.

Epstein E. Herpes simplex. In: Common skin disorders. 4th ed. Philadelphia: WB Saunders, 1994.

Gany FM, Retano MV, Morley AP. Managing genital herpes: a case resource guide. Professional Postgraduate Services, 1993.

Gibson JJ, Hornung CA, Alexander GR, et al. A cross-sectional study of herpex simplex virus types 1 and 2 in college students: occurrence and determinants of infection. J Infect Dis 1990;162:306.

Goldberg LH, Kaufman R, Kurtz TO, et al. Acyclovir Study Group. Long-term suppression of recurrent genital herpes with acyclovir: a 5-year benchmark. Arch Dermatol 1993;129:582.

Grossman JH, Wallen WC, Sever JL. Management of genital herpes simplex virus infection during pregnancy. Obstet Gynecol 1981;58:1041.

Guinan ME, MacCalman J, Kern ER, et al. The course of untreated recurrent genital herpes simplex in 27 women. N Engl J Med 1981;304:759.

Hirsch MS, Schooley RT. Treatment of herpesvirus infections, part I and part II. N Engl J Med 1983; 309:963 & 1986;309:1034.

Kinghorn GR. Genital herpes: natural history and treatment of acute episodes. J Med Virol 1993;(suppl 1):33.

Koelle DM, Benedetti J, Langenberg A, et al. Asymptomatic reactivation of herpes simplex virus in women after the first episode of genital herpes. Ann Intern Med 1992;116:433.

Kulhanjian JA, Soroush V, Au DS, et al. Identification of women at unsuspected risk of primary infection with herpes simplex virus type 2 during pregnancy. N Engl J Med 1992;326:916.

Lafferty WE, Coombs RW, Benedetti J, et al. Recurrences after oral and genital herpes simplex virus infection: influence of site of infection and viral type. N Engl J Med 1987;316:1444.

LaGuardia KD, White MH, Saigo PE, et al. Genital ulcer disease in women infected with human immunodeficiency virus. Am J Obstet Gynecol 1995;172:553.

Laskin OL. Acyclovir: pharmacology and clinical experience. Arch Intern Med 1984;144:1241.

Leads from the MMWR: genital herpes United States, 1966–1984. JAMA 1986;256:575.

Lehrman SN, Doublas JM, Corey L, et al. Recurrent genital herpes and suppressive oral acyclovir therapy: relation between clinical outcome and in vitro drug sensitivity. Ann Intern Med 1986;104:786.

McKendrick MW, McGill JI, White JE, et al. Oral acyclovir in acute herpes zoster. Br Med J 1986;293: 1529.

Mertz GJ, Benedetti J, Ashley R, et al. Risk factors for the sexual transmission of genital herpes. Ann Intern Med 1992;116:197.

Mertz GJ, Critchlow CW, Benedetti J, et al. Double-blind placebo-controlled trial of oral acyclovir in first-episode genital herpes simplex virus infection. JAMA 1984;252:1147.

Mertz GJ, Jones CC, Mills J, et al. Long-term acyclovir suppression of frequently recurring genital herpes simplex virus infection. JAMA 1988;260:201.

Mindel A. Long-term clinical and psychological management of genital herpes. J Med Virol 1993;(suppl 1):39.

Nahass GT, Goldstein JBA, Zhu WY, et al. Comparison of Tzanck smear, viral culture and DNA diagnostic methods in detection of herpes simplex and varicella-zoster infection. JAMA 1992;268:2541.

Nahmais AJ, Dowdle WR, Schinazi RF, eds. The human herpes virus: an interdisciplinary perspective. New York: Elsevier Press, 1981.

Oill PA, Mishell DR Jr. Venereal diseases in adolescents and contraception in teenagers. West J Med 1980; 132:39.

Prober CG. Herpetic vaginitis in 1993. Clin Obstet Gynecol 1993;36:177.

Prober CG, Corey L, Brown ZA, et al. The management of pregnancies complicated by genital infections with herpes simplex virus. Clin Infect Dis 1992;15: 1031.

Prober CG, Sullender WM, Yasukawa LL, et al. Low risk of herpes simplex virus infections in neonates exposed to the virus at the time of vaginal delivery to mothers with recurrent genital herpes simplex virus infections. N Engl J Med 1987;316:240.

Reeves WC, Corey L, Adams HG, et al. Risk of recurrence after first episodes of genital herpes—relation to HSV type and antibody response. N Engl J Med 1981;305:315.

Reichman RC, Badger GJ, Mertz GJ, et al. Treatment of recurrent genital herpes simplex infections with oral acyclovir: a controlled trial. JAMA 1984;251:2103.

Roberts JSW, Cox SM, Dax J, et al. Genital herpes during pregnancy: no lesions, no cesarean. Obstet Gynecol 1995;85:261.

Rompalo AM, Mertz GJ, Davis G, et al. Oral acyclovir for treatment of first-episode herpes simplex virus proctitis. JAMA 1988;259:2879.

Rooney JF, Felser JM, Ostrove JM, et al. Acquisition of genital herpes from an asymptomatic sexual partner. N Engl J Med 1986;24:1561.

Rubsamen DS, ed. Civil liability and the symptom-free herpes carrier. Professional Liability Newsletter 1990;20:11.

Spear PG. Biology of the herpesviruses. In: Holmes KK, Mardh PA, Sparling PF, Wiesner PJ, eds. Sexually transmitted diseases. 2nd ed. New York: McGraw-Hill Information Services, 1990.

Straus SE, Rooney JF, Sever JL, et al. Herpes simplex virus infection: biology, treatment, and prevention. Ann Intern Med 1985;103:404.

VanderPlate C, Aral SO. Psychosocial aspects of genital herpes virus infection. Health Psychol 1987;6:57.

Whitley RJ, Gnann JW. Acyclovir: a decade later. N Engl J Med 1992;327:782.

CHAPTER 66

Human Papilloma Virus and Molluscum Contagiosum

Anita Nelson and Lawrence S. Neinstein

HUMAN PAPILLOMA VIRUS

Human papilloma virus (HPV) is the most prevalent viral sexually transmitted disease. HPV has been identified as a necessary precondition for a wide range of epithelial disruptions varying from condyloma acuminata of the vulva, vagina, cervix, anus, buccal mucosa, and larynx to cervical dysplasia and cervical cancer. The association between HPV and cervical dysplasia is strong enough to assign causality due to the strength and consistency of the association, the time association, and the consistency with known biological facts. Southern blot techniques have enabled researchers to identify HPV DNA strands integrated into the genome of the host in virtually every primary squamous cell carcinoma of the cervix. Similar evidence has been found in metastatic lesions of cervical cancer.

HPV infection and its sequelae are critical health issues for adolescents because adolescent women are physiologically more vulnerable to acquire cervical HPV infection if exposed to the virus. Furthermore, with the more virulent subtypes of HPV, cervical cancer deaths now occur in 20- and 30-year-old women. This makes it imperative that early precursor lesions, such as cervical dysplasia, be identified and treated during the adolescent years.

Description

HPV is a small nonenveloped double-stranded DNA virus of the PAPOVA group. The viruses are tropic for epithelium, infecting surface epithelia and mucous membranes, and often producing warts or epithelial proliferations at the site of infection.

Currently, about 70 different genotypes of HPV have been identified. The genotype number (not serotype because the classification is based on DNA composition not antigenicity) is designated according to the order of discovery. Different genotypes must share less than 50% homology of the 7800–7900 base sequence. The various genotypes have considerable specificity for the epithelium they infect and the morphology of lesions that they produce. Approximately 22 types affect the genital tract including types of 6, 11, 16, 18, 31, 33, 35, 39, 41–45, 51, 52, 56, 63, 66, and 68.

The clinical significance of each of the viral types differs (Table 66.1). In general, the viral types with low oncogenic potential remain in episomal form independent of the host DNA. They are more likely to result in condyloma or koilocytosis. The oncogenic subtypes 16 and 18 integrate into the chromosomes of the infected cell near key sites such as the epidermal growth factor gene, producing immortal cell lines. Type 16 in particular has been noted to have rapid progression to advanced disease. In one study, 26% of patients with cervical intraepi-

TABLE 66.1.   Clinical Presentation of Human Papilloma Virus Infection by Type

Type	Clinical Presentation	Pap Smear Finding	Cervical Cancer Potential
6 or 11, 42–44	Condylomata acuminata or subclinical lesion	Koilocytosis or low-grade SIL[a]	Low
31, 33, 35, 39, 51–53, 55, 58, 59, 63, 66, 68	Subclinical or condyloma-tous lesions	Usually low-grade SIL, occasionally high-grade SIL	Intermediate
16 or 18, 45, 46	Papular or subclinical lesion cervix	Low- to high-grade SIL, invasive carcinoma	High

[a]SIL, squamous intraepithelial lesion.

thelial neoplasia grade 1 (CIN 1) lesions and HPV 16 infection progressed to CIN 3 within 18 months. Relative risks for CIN 3 lesions with HPV 16 range from 170 to 1200.

Epidemiology

1. Prevalence: HPV is epidemic. Exact incidence and prevalence data are not well quantified because the infection is not well documented and is not reportable. However, many surveys indicate the magnitude of the problem. Between the years 1966 and 1982 there was a 12-fold increase in office visits for HPV-related infections. In 1987 HPV infections or genital warts were visualized in 2% of the sexually active population; Pap smears detected an additional 4% of women with HPV infection, and up to 10% of sexually active men and women carried HPV DNA detected by polymerase chain reaction (PCR) technology. Each percentage point represents 1 million people.

   Studies indicate that 15–20% of adolescents and young adults seeking routine gynecologic care have HPV infections of the cervix. Using Southern blot technique, HPV DNA has been detected in 13% of female teens. Rosenfeld et al. (1987) found a prevalence of HPV of 31% in 51 teens receiving a Pap smear for routine care. DNA amplification techniques such as PCR have demonstrated HPV in 46% in one study population of college students.

2. Transmission: Transmission of the HPV types that cause genital infection is primarily through sexual contact. Infectivity rate of contacts is high. In a prospective study after the Korean war of presumably HPV-uninfected women, 85% developed genital warts within 8 months after sexual contact with returning infected soldiers. High-power magnification examination of male partners of HPV-infected women will reveal HPV infections of the penis or anus in 50–80% of cases. External genital condylomata may be contracted by autoinoculation or inoculation with HPV DNA from skin warts and from viral exposure during delivery. The virus is recoverable from fomites such as tanning couches, underwear, examination gloves, biopsy forceps, and smoke plumes; transmission has now been demonstrated from sauna benches. Condylomata acuminata have been reported in premenarcheal children and nonsexually active adolescents. However, the evidence for nonsexual transmission of condylomata acuminata in most cases is questionable. Young people with infections should be questioned and examined for evidence of sexual abuse.

3. Incubation period: Incubation period is 3 weeks to 8 months or longer, with an average of 2–3 months. Clinical expression of subclinical infections can be delayed for unpredictable periods of time.

4. Predisposing factors

   a. Multiple sexual partners: The risk of genital HPV infections increases with the number of sexual partners. There is a 5.4 times greater relative risk in individuals with three to five partners as compared to individuals with one. There should be almost no risk in nonsexually active individuals or in strictly monogamous couples. Similar patterns are seen for cervical dysplasia, that is, the risk of cervical dysplasia increases with increasing numbers of sexual partners.

b. Immunocompromise: Immunocompromise from diabetes mellitus, pregnancy, HIV infection, steroid use, or immunosuppressive drug therapy can be a factor.

c. Early age at first coitus: This is a marker for multiple sexual partners and also reflects the young woman's vulnerability to cervical infection with HPV. Shew et al. (1994) examined the relationship of HPV infection and the interval between menarche and first intercourse. The prevalence of HPV infection was 19.2% in the 108 adolescents. First sexual intercourse within 18 months of menarche was associated with a significant elevation of risk of HPV infection, in comparison with that in adolescents who postpone first intercourse for 3–4 years after menarche.

d. Smoking: Women who smoke develop cervical dysplasias at twice the rate of nonsmokers.

Pathophysiology

HPV infects the basal layer of epithelial cells. The virus seems to require access to actively dividing epithelial basal cells. Areas where such activity predominates include the transformation zone of the cervix and genital areas susceptible to microtrauma during sexual activity (Table 66.2). The infection produces characteristic morphological changes including koilocytosis (vacuolated cells), nuclear atypia, perinuclear halos, nuclear wrinkling, and hyperchromasia. There is continuum between these changes and progressive degrees of cytonuclear atypia in the basal cells and bizarre morphological changes in the surface koilocytes. These changes most likely progress to undifferentiated cells, consistent with severe dysplasia and carcinoma in situ (CIS).

Clinical Manifestations

External Genitalia

Genital Warts

1. Four major types of venereal warts occur:
   a. *Classic soft sessile or pedunculated growths:* These are usually 2–3 mm in diameter and 10–15 mm in height, with multiple fingerlike projections, and occur most frequently in moist areas such as the vaginal introitus and vagina.
   b. *Small flat-topped warts:* These are usually 1- to 4-mm papules, often located at the transformation zone of the cervix. These may be all but invisible without a colposcope or acetic acid staining, which causes them to have a blanched white appearance.

TABLE 66.2.   Distribution of Genital Human Papilloma Virus Infection in Infected Individuals by Gender

Women		Men	
Site	(%)	Site	(%)
Cervix	70	Inner surface of prepuce	70
Vulva	25	Frenulum, corona	10
Anus	20	Penile shaft, glans, and scrotum	10
Vagina	10	Anus	10
Urethra	5		

   c. *Squared-off keratotic papules:* These papules are usually 4–10 mm in diameter and typically occur in nonmucosal dry skin areas.

   d. *Giant condylomata acuminata:* These are larger, rounded soft papules and nodules with a pebbly, strawberry-like surface.

2. Location: Usually multifocal (Table 66.2)
3. Color: Pinkish, red, gray, or white
4. Symptoms: Usually asymptomatic but may cause pruritus or burning or become painful if superinfected
5. Aggravating factors: Pregnancy, skin moisture, and a vaginal or anal discharge
6. Bleeding: Anal warts may bleed during bowel movements or anal coitus; cervical or vulvar lesions may bleed in pregnancy or with coitus. Advanced cases may bleed with wiping.
7. Differential diagnosis
   a. Micropapillomatosis labialis of labia minora: Lesions with separate bases that do not converge as do the papillae of condylomata acuminata
   b. Condylomata lata: Secondary syphilis with positive dark-field examination and serology
   c. Molluscum contagiosum: Dome-shaped globular lesion with central umbilication that contains expressible cheesy material
   d. Granuloma inguinale: Rare disease; Donovan bodies found in crushed tissue smears
   e. Seborrheic keratosis
   f. Intraepithelial and invasive neoplasia
   g. Benign neoplasias: Including fibromas, lipomas, hidradenomas, and adenomas
   h. Pink pearly papules (in males): Parallel rows of lesions at the corona of the penis that demonstrate hypertrophic papillae histologically; normally present in approximately 15% of the male population

Subclinical Infections

1. Epidemiology: Sixty percent of external HPV infections
2. Presentation: Slightly elevated, well-demarcated acetowhite lesions with no distinctive surface contours
3. Color: May blend with secondary tissue but will turn white when soaked for 5 minutes with 5% acetic acid
4. Symptoms: Usually asymptomatic
5. Differential diagnosis (based on acetowhite changes): Candidiasis, folliculitis, contact dermatitis, psoriasis, and intraepithelial and invasive neoplasia
6. Diagnosis: Made by ruling out other infections' causes and confirmed by microscopy and obtaining punch biopsy

Long-term Sequelae of Superficial Infections   A strong association exists between HPV infections and malignant changes of the cervix, vulva, and penis. Over 98% of individuals with malignant and premalignant changes of the cervix have HPV DNA or antigens demonstrated in the neoplastic tissue. Although HPV is the probable carcinogen, other cofactors such as smoking or HIV are required for malignant transformation to occur.

   Approximately 30% of vulvar carcinomas are associated with current or past condylomata. Not only are these infections multifocal, they are also multicentric, so that a woman with vulvar condylomata has a 30% chance of having cervical dysplasia. Male homosexuals with a history of anal condylomata have a 50-fold increased risk of developing anal carcinoma.

   There seems to be a strong relationship between the HPV genotype and its location and association with malignant changes. Of genital malignancies, 60% are related to HPV 16;

15% are related to HPV 18; 20% are related to other genotypes in the 30s, 40s, and 50s; and less than 5% have not been typeable. HPV types 16, 18, 31, and 35 often cause unifocal lesions on the cervix, and are the types that are usually associated with CIN or penile dysplastic lesions. Types 16 and 18 are found in 65% of CIN 2 and 3. Type 18 seems especially virulent, whereas type 16 seems to be more prevalent. Conversely, HPV types 6 and 11 are usually associated with condylomata acuminata, particularly of the external genitalia, and are not usually found in lesions with grades higher than CIN 1. It is likely that CIN 1 associated with type 6 or 11 will not progress. However, this has not yet been proved in a large study population.

Therapy for Lesions of External Genitalia

1. Eliminate predisposing factors.
   a. Treat vaginitis and cervicitis.
   b. Decrease tissue trauma at coitus.
   c. Keep genital area dry.
   d. Keep diabetes mellitus under tight control.
2. Treatment of the vulvar lesions should be guided by the number, size, and keratinization of the lesion(s) and by patient preference. Effectiveness for various therapies is outlined in Table 66.3. The advantages and disadvantages of the various treatment regimens are presented on Table 66.4. The choices include:
   a. Liquid nitrogen or cryotherapy: It is often the preferred method for penile lesions and resistant vulvar lesions. It can be used during pregnancy. Its use on vaginal warts should be restrained by an appreciation of the thinness of the epithelium.
   b. Topical chemotherapies: These are most effective for the sessile lesions. Older, more keratinized lesions are more refractory to topical agents.
      — Bichloroacetic acid (BCA) or trichloroacetic acid (TCA) can be used on vulvar and vaginal surfaces and during pregnancy.
         (1) Technique: Apply occlusive anesthetic ointment to the healthy tissue surrounding the lesion. Touch lesion with 50–90% acid solution to cause blanching. Dry lesion rapidly to minimize pain (blower drier helpful). Powder with baking soda to remove unreacted acid, if possible. Careful application is advised since treatment will also desiccate normal tissue on contact.
         (2) There is no need to wash off solution after treatment.
         (3) Repeat process weekly until lesion has resolved. If warts persist after several applications, other therapies should be considered.
      — Podophyllin: Podophyllin is a popular chemical agent used to treat anogenital warts. Use weekly treatments with 20–25% podophyllin in tincture of benzoin. Do not apply to mucosal surfaces.

Table 66.3. Response and Recurrence Rates for Various Treatment Modalities of Genital Warts

Agent	Response to Therapy (%)	Recurrence Rate (%)
Liquid nitrogen	73	20
Cryotherapy	70	30
Trichloroacetic acid or bichloroacetic acid	70	38
Laser vaporization, LEEP[a]	76	25
Excisional biopsy	70	30
Interferon	65–80	25

Adapted from Ferenczy A. Epidemiology and clinical pathophysiology of condylomata acuminata. Am J Obstet Gynecol 1995;172(4):1337.
[a]LEEP, loop electrocautery excision procedure.

TABLE 66.4.   Advantages and Disadvantages of Treatment Regimens for Genital Warts

Regimen	Advantages	Disadvantages
Cryotherapy or liquid nitrogen	Office treatment Well-tolerated Useful for mucosal lesions Useful for extensive disease Safe in pregnancy No anesthesia needed Minimal risk of scarring	Extended healing period with discharge
Trichloroacetic acid or bichloroacetic acid	Widely available Office treatment Easy to apply Safe in pregnancy	Pain on application Destroys normal tissue
Podophyllin or podofilox	Widely available Easy to apply Office treatment or home treatment	Pain after application Possible toxic systemic absorption Not useful for cervical or mucosal lesions or extensive disease Contraindicated in pregnancy
Carbon dioxide laser or LEEP[a]	Useful for extensive lesions Safe in pregnancy Good cosmetic results	Requires specialized training Expensive Not readily available May require general anesthesia for extensive disease Intact DNA may be liberated into air with laser vapor
Surgical removal	Useful for extensive disease Safe in pregnancy	Requires hospital setting Expensive Scarring possible Risk of bleeding

Adapted from Erlich KS, Normoyle JL. Condylomata acuminata: waging a successful fight against anogenital warts. Female Patient 1987;12:51.
[a]LEEP, loop electrocautery excision procedure.

    (1) Place occlusive ointment on the areas surrounding the lesions to protect normal skin.
    (2) Paint the lesions with podophyllin (using the back end of a cotton swab allows for precise application).
    (3) Instruct patient to wash off the podophyllin in 1–4 hours.
    (4) If lesions are resistant, one can either leave the podophyllin on longer, use a 50% podophyllin solution, or use another modality.
    (5) Podophyllin is contraindicated during pregnancy. Most experts limit its use to vulvar or penile warts.
    — Podofilox 0.5% solution for self-treatment: Patients may apply podofilox with a cotton swab to genital warts twice daily for 3 days, followed by 4 days of no therapy. This cycle may be repeated as necessary for a total of four cycles. Total wart area treated should not exceed 10 cm², and total volume of podofilox should not exceed 0.5 mL/day. Careful, concrete instruction and demonstration of how to treat and which lesions to treat is required for successful implementation. The use of podofilox is contraindicated during pregnancy.
  c. Surgical therapies include loop electrocautery excision procedure (LEEP) excision, laser ablation, and cold knife excision (rarely performed today) and are usually reserved for large or resistant lesions.
  d. Immunotherapy with intralesional injections of interferon is very expensive and perhaps best reserved for recurrent lesions or those resistant to other therapies.
 3. Vaginal, urethral and perianal warts may be treated with various topical and surgical modalities.

a. Topical agents
— 5-Fluorouracil 5% may be applied to the vagina once a week for 12 weeks. Similar application to the meatus is accepted.
— Isolated lesions near the introitus and anus may respond to TCA.
b. Cryotherapy must be used with caution, respecting the thinness of the epithelium and avoiding scarring and constriction of the meatus.
c. LEEP excision may be feasible for pedunculated lesions. Laser therapy to the vagina is challenging but, in skilled hands, may be helpful.

4. Patients must be advised that partners do require evaluation for visible lesions, but treatment of the partner does not affect the patient's response or recurrence rates.
5. Patients should be reminded that infections are forever: recurrence is possible and involvement of nonvulvar areas possible. Frequent (at least annual) Pap smears are recommended. Safer sex practices should be emphasized.

Cervical Human Papilloma Virus

Prevalence   Dysplastic changes of the cervix should not be thought of as a problem for the adult population only. Russo and Jones (1984) evaluated 1207 sexually active adolescents in a family planning clinic. One hundred and thirty-two (11%) had abnormal findings. Of the 69 that were followed, 50 (72%) had CIN. Of these, 22 had CIN 1 (mild dysplasia), 22 had CIN 2 (moderate dysplasia), and 6 had CIN 3 (severe dysplasia or carcinoma in situ). In reviewing 19 studies of abnormal Pap smears in adolescents, Hillard (1994) found abnormally high rates ranging from 0.33 per 1000 to 85 per 1000. Her study suggested even a higher rate of 157 per 1000. It is essential that adolescents with significantly abnormal Pap smears be followed with colposcopic examination and directed biopsies.

Physiology of Cervix   The dysplastic and anaplastic changes of the cervix related to HPV infections generally occur in the transformation zone. This area of the cervix first appears during adolescence. It is useful to review the formation of this zone in understanding abnormal cervical changes.

The müllerian ducts originally form the tubes, uterus, and vagina. These structures in the fetus are lined by immature cuboidal epithelium (which becomes columnar epithelium) from the uterus to the hymenal ring. At 6–16 weeks of embryonic life the urogenital sinus epithelium grows up the vaginal vault and replaces the native epithelium up to the ectocervix with squamous epithelium. Columnar epithelium remains internally up to the ectocervix. Replacement of columnar epithelium by squamous epithelium is most rapid laterally, less rapid posteriorly, and least rapid anteriorly. Thus, most of the remaining columnar epithelium is anteriorly placed on the ectocervix, forming the ectropion, which is prominent in adolescent women.

The *original squamocolumnar junction (SCJ)* is the location on the cervix of the junction of the squamous and columnar epithelium before puberty. Before puberty the vagina is alkaline, encouraging the growth of columnar epithelia, so no metaplasia (transformation to squamous epithelium) takes place. With puberty, menarche, and rising estrogen level, several events occur:

1. Connective tissue and elastic fibers of the cervix are rearranged so that the lips of the cervix evert and bring more columnar epithelium into the vagina.
2. The pH of the vagina drops. This is a result of glycogen production by squamous cells. The glycogen provides a source of carbohydrate for the vaginal flora. Vaginal bacteria proliferate, and the lactobacilli convert glycogen to lactic acids, resulting in a lowered pH.

Acid is injurious to columnar epithelium, allowing metaplasia to occur. Metaplasia may occur from either immature undifferentiated cells in the columnar epithelium differentiating into squamous epithelium or by the ingrowth of squamous epithelium at the SCJ.

Native squamous epithelium appears as smooth, pink, and featureless epithelium. It covers the vagina and most of the cervix. *Native columnar epithelium* is a single layer, mucus-producing, tall epithelium extending between the endometrium and the SCJ. This area has an irregular surface with long papillae and deep clefts. It has a grapelike appearance after acetic acid is applied. With conversion of the columnar epithelium to squamous epithelium, a *transformation zone* is created. The transformation zone, or "T-zone," is the area between the original SCJ and the current SCJ. A physiological T-zone is normal and has some filmy whitening. This is normal metaplasia. Because the conversion of columnar epithelium to squamous epithelium is not 100% efficient, the examiner can often see small glands in these areas. When these gland openings become completely closed by squamous epithelium, the mucus-secreting epithelium may continue to produce mucus. If that mucus becomes inspissated, the gland dilates and a Nabothian cyst results. Nabothian cysts eventually self-destruct from the pressure of the inspissated mucus. In adolescents, it is uncommon for the metaplastic process or T-zone to extend into the endocervical canal because that tissue is protected by the alkaline endocervical mucus.

The T-zone is the area of the cervix most prone to dysplastic changes. Young metaplastic cells in the T-zone have phagocytic properties and can ingest potential mutagens in the vagina. Without mutagenic agents, a well-differentiated mature squamous epithelium develops. This area is then no longer at risk for dysplastic changes. If a mutagen, such as HPV DNA, is present during metaplasia, neoplasia can occur. Usually an area of dysplasia is located within the T-zone, with one border on the SCJ.

Cervical Dysplasia

Impact of Cofactors   HPV infection, as described, is clearly a causative factor for cervical dysplasia. However, the presence of HPV is not sufficient. Other cofactors are needed to cause dysplastic transformation. One such cofactor is tobacco smoking. Even when adjusted for numbers of sexual partners, women who smoke have at least twice the risk of developing cervical dysplasia than nonsmokers. There is a close relationship between smoking and cervical dysplasia. Heavier smokers tend to develop more severe dysplasia. The impact of smoking extends to cervical cancer; smokers have 10–15% higher complication rates than nonsmokers. Another cofactor is human immunodeficiency virus (HIV) infection. Patients with HIV typically have more advanced disease and even after initially successful treatment experience a 100% recurrence at 2 years.

Cervical Screening Tests   Current recommendations for Pap smear testing are that a female start having Pap smears when she first becomes sexually active or at age 18 whichever occurs first. After a female has had three consecutive annual tests that are read as normal, she may be screened less frequently if she continues to be at low risk for sexually transmitted diseases. Estimates are that less than 15% of sexually active teens are receiving Pap smears in accordance with practice guidelines.

Most cytologists have adopted the Bethesda reporting system and now will provide more descriptive reports of their findings after screening of the specimen for adequacy and correct preparation. If either of the latter is found to be wanting, the cytologist now will not provide an evaluation. A summary of the Bethesda system findings is found on Figure 66.1. The follow-up evaluation required for abnormal Pap smear findings not associated with neoplastic

STATEMENT ON SPECIMEN ADEQUACY
- Satisfactory for interpretation
- Less than optimal
- Unsatisfactory

EXPLANATION FOR LESS THAN OPTIMAL OR UNSATISFACTORY SPECIMEN
- Scant cellularity
- Porr fixation or preservation
- Presence of foreign material (e.g., lubricant)
- Partially or completely obscuring inflammation
- Partially or completely obscuring blood
- No endocervical component in a premenopausal woman who has a cervix
- Not representative of the anatomic site
- Other

GENERAL CATEGORIZATION
- Within normal limits
- Other
  - See "Descriptive Diagnoses"
  - Further action recommended

DESCRIPTIVE DIAGNOSES
Infection
- **Fungal**
  - Fungal organisms morphologically consistent with *Candida* species
  - Other
- **Bacterial**
  - Microorganisms morphologically consistent with *Gardnerella* species
  - Microorganisms morphologically consistent with *Actinomyces* species
  - Cellular changes suggestive of *Chlamydia* species infection, subject to confirmatory studies
  - Other
- **Protozoan**
  - *Trichomonas vaginalis*
  - Other
- **Viral**
  - Cellular changes associated with cytomegalovirus
  - Cellular changes associated with herpes virus simplex
  - Other

(Note: For human papilloma virus [HPV], refer to "Epithelial Cell Abnormalities, Squamous Cell.")

Reactive and Reparative Changes
- **Inflammation**
  - Associated cellular changes
  - Follicular cervicitis
- **Miscellaneous (as related to patient history)**
  - Effects of therapy
  - Ionizing radiation
  - Chemotherapy
  - Effects of mechanical devices (e.g., intrauterine contraceptive device)
  - Effects of nonsteroidal estrogen exposure (e.g., diethylstilbestrol)
  - Other

Fɪɢᴜʀᴇ 66.1.   The Bethesda System for reporting cervical or vaginal cytological diagnoses.

Epithelial Cell Abnormalities
- **Squamous cell**
  - Atypical squamous cell of undetermined significance
    - Consistent with reactive reparative changes
    - Consistent with dysplastic changes
  - Squamous intraepithelial lesion (comment on presence of cellular changes associated with HPV, if applicable)
    - Low-grade squamous intraepithelial lesion, encompassing:
      - Cellular changes associated with HPV
      - Mild (slight) dysplasia or cervical intraepithelial neoplasia grade 1 (CIN 1)
    - High-grade squamous intraepithelial lesion, encompassing:
      - Moderate dysplasia (CIN 2)
      - Severe dysplasia (CIN 3)
      - Carcinoma in situ (CIN 3)
- **Glandular cell**
  - Presence of endometrial cells in one of the following circumstances:
    - Out of phase in a menstruating woman
    - In a postmenopausal woman
    - No menstrual history available
  - Atypical glandular cells of undetermined significance (recommended follow-up or type of further investigation: Specify):
    - Endometrial
    - Endocervical
    - Not otherwise specified
  - Adenocarcinoma
    - Specify probable site of origin: Endocervical, endometrial, extrauterine
    - Not otherwise specified
  - Other epithelial malignant neoplasm: Specify

Nonepithelial Malignant Neoplasm: Specify Hormonal Evaluation (Applies to Vaginal Smears Only)
- Hormonal pattern compatible with age and history
- Hormonal pattern compatible with age and history: Specify
- Hormonal evaluation not possible
  - Cervical specimen
  - Inflammation
  - Insufficient patient history

Other

FIGURE 66.1. *continued*

changes is shown in Table 66.5. The follow-up necessary to evaluate dysplastic or predysplastic Pap smear findings is more controversial. There are three categories:

1. Atypical squamous cells of undetermined significance (ASCUS)
   a. Nearly one-fourth of patients with ASCUS have dysplasia, but it is usually mild. Patients followed for 8 months with colposcopically verified ASCUS have no progression, and many regress to normal. A wide range of follow-up strategies is possible:
      — Repeat Pap smear at 1 year. Refer only if squamous intraepithelial lesion (SIL) develops.
      — Repeat Pap smear in 4–6 months and refer for colposcopy only if abnormality such as ASCUS persists.

TABLE 66.5.   Follow-up Evaluation Recommendations for Abnormal Pap Smear Findings

Pap Smear Finding	Recommendation
Insufficient quantity	Repeat Pap smears in 2–3 months.
Poor specimen	Repeat Pap smears in 2–3 months.
Air drying artifact	Repeat Pap smears in 2–3 months.
No endocervical cells	No need to repeat Pap smear if patient has previously normal test results and is compliant with therapy. If not, repeat in 2–3 months.
Endometrial cells	Normal if near menses or while using oral contraceptives or intrauterine devices. Otherwise, recall and evaluate endometritis.
Trichomoniasis	Recall patient, perform sexually transmitted disease evaluation, treat patient and partner.
Yeast or *Gardnerella*	Review chart. If no symptoms, no need to follow up (not equivalent to bacterial vaginosis).
Inflammation	Consider recent coitus, infection.
Reactive, reparative changes	Identify irritant, if possible. Essentially normal.

— Evaluate with other tools, such as speculoscopy, to determine triage and follow-up schedule. Speculoscopy is a system with a 6X magnifying lens and a chemoluminescent light source (Speculite). The light is absorbed by healthy tissue and reflected by unhealthy tissue in the cervix. The system provides immediate visual indication of any affected areas, but does not grade the severity of the problem. Patients identified as having problems after speculoscopy may be triaged to colposcopy; those not so identified may be followed with Pap smears every 4–6 months until there is some worsening of the findings. Speculoscopy has been advocated as an adjunct to be performed at the time of the initial Pap smear to help improve the sensitivity of that screening test. High-risk adolescents may well benefit from dual screening.

2. Low-grade SIL: This category includes evidence of early HPV infection (koilocytosis) and CIN 1 lesions merged together to reflect the technical difficulties in artificially distinguishing between them and to reflect the fact that very few of these lesions have any oncogenic potential.

   The original intent of the developers of the Bethesda system was to permit more conservative management of patients with low-grade lesions. However, many practitioners are concerned that as many as 25–30% of patients with low-grade SIL on Pap smears actually harbor more advanced disease, usually high-grade SIL. For that reason, many recommend colposcopic evaluation and directed biopsy(ies) to fully evaluate the woman's cervix. With compliant patients, others use protocols that follow such patients with Pap smears until they develop high-grade SIL. Lonky et al. (1995) evaluated 1454 women with abnormal cytologic screening results: 782 with ASCUS (atypia), 355 with low-grade SIL determined by the presence of HPV alone, and 317 with low-grade SIL determined by the presence of cytologic evidence of mild dysplasia CIN 1 devoid of HPV cytopathologic features. Women from the low-grade SIL CIN 1 group were significantly more likely to harbor biopsy-proven dysplasia than were those from the ASCUS and low-grade SIL HPV groups. Adjunctive evaluation tools, such as speculoscopy, might be helpful in triaging these patients, especially those with reported isolated HPV changes. In the future DNA typing might make a significant contribution also.

3. High-grade SIL. This category includes moderate and severe dysplasia and carcinoma in situ. High-grade SIL unequivocally requires colposcopic evaluation with directed biopsies and endocervical evaluation. Patients with these findings should also be offered HIV testing.

Therapy for Cervical Dysplasia   The colposcopically directed biopsy and the endocervical test results determine the extent of the lesion and direct therapy. The principle in developing a treatment plan is that cervical dysplasia is treated to prevent progression to cancer. No therapy can eliminate the viral infection. One practice to be avoided, especially in adolescents, is to combine the diagnostic and treatment steps by performing colposcopic examination to rule out invasion and excising the T-zone by LEEP without biopsy confirmation. This practice has proven extraordinarily expensive because nearly 40% of such referred patients have no dysplasia found on LEEP specimen. It is also excessively destructive to the patient's cervix, when dysplasia is not confirmed. Preservation of cervical integrity is important to maintain future fertility. As can be seen in Table 66.6, each of the major treatment modalities has minimal adverse impacts when used once. However, since recurrent lesions may develop and require further treatment, the cumulative effects of multiple treatments (especially of LEEP) must be considered. Hillard et al. (1991) reported on another complication of treatment of cervical dysplasia related to cryotherapy in a group of 67 adolescents. Nine percent developed pelvic inflammatory disease (PID) within 1 month of treatment, and two teens developed cervical stenosis and hematometra. In general, the following is recommended:

1. If the endocervical canal is involved with the dysplastic changes or if there is a significant discrepancy between the histological and cytological results, a diagnostic cone biopsy is necessary to rule out carcinoma and will, hopefully, extirpate the dysplasia cells. A cone biopsy can be done while the patient receives anesthesia in the operating room as a traditional surgical cold knife procedure, or it can be an office-based laser or LEEP procedure.
2. If the lesions are confined to the ectocervix, a wide range of treatment options is available (Table 66.6).
3. All women with dysplasia who smoke should be encouraged to stop smoking. Advise them that continued tobacco use increases recurrences and susceptibility to cancer.
4. Some experts recommend folic acid supplements to prevent recurrences. This may be prudent in teens who have few sources of folic acid in their diets.

After successful treatment, patients require frequent Pap smears, advice about safer sex practices, and counseling to help them see HPV changes as a chronic sexually transmitted disease from which they need to protect their future partners.

TABLE 66.6.   Cervical Dysplasia Treatment Regimen Response Rates (%)[a]

	Cryotherapy	Carbon Dioxide Laser	LEEP
Response rate (%)			
Single	80	90	95
Repeated	95	95	95
Advantages	Simple office based procedure	Rapid recovery	Rapid recovery
	Inexpensive	SCJ on ectocervix	SCJ on ectocervix
	Only mildly painful	Can tailor to lesion	Can tailor to lesion
			Provides specimen for pathology
Disadvantages	Watery vaginal discharge for 4–6 weeks	Expensive	Moderately expensive
	May not be as effective for large lesions or those at 3 and 9 o'clock	More painful	More painful
	New SCJ in endocervix	Contaminated plume	Bleeding complications
	No specimen for pathology	No specimen for pathology	

[a]LEEP, loop electrocautery excision procedure; SCJ, squamocolumnar junction.

Molluscum Contagiosum

Etiology

Molluscum contagiosum is a skin disease caused by a member of the poxvirus group.

Epidemiology

1. Transmission: Transmission is by direct person-to-person contact, with a 30-day to several month incubation period. The disease is also spread by autoinoculation.
2. Incidence: Prevalence is increasing in sexually active adolescents.

Clinical Manifestations

1. Location: The lesions commonly occur on face, arms, legs, and chest. In sexually active adolescents, the lesions are commonly seen on the genital and pubic areas.
2. Appearance
   a. Lesions are flesh-colored, raised, waxy, dome-shaped, globular nodules with central umbilication.
   b. There are usually 1–20 lesions, each 3–7 mm in diameter, that often occur in clusters.
3. Symptoms: The lesions are usually asymptomatic, but inflammatory changes can occur.

Diagnosis

1. Clinical appearance is usually diagnostic.
2. If the lesions are sprayed with ethyl chloride, a distinct central area of darkness appears that is not found in warts.
3. Expressible cheesy material on potassium hydroxide preparation or with methylene blue shows intracytoplasmic inclusions (molluscum bodies).
4. Biopsy is rarely necessary.

Therapy

1. Unroofing of lesion and expression of cheesy material or application of TCA or podophyllin to base will help.
2. Liquid nitrogen applied to lesions is an alternative.
3. Light electrodesiccation may be used.
4. Patient should be observed again in 30 days to check for incubating lesions that may develop after initial treatment.

Bibliography

Adimora AA, Quinlivan EG. Papillomavirus infection. Recent findings on progression to cervical cancer. Postgrad Med 1995;98:109.

Appleby J. Management of the abnormal Papanicolaou smear. Med Clin North Am 1995;79:345.

Barrasso R, De Brux J, Croissant O, et al. High prevalence of papillomavirus-associated penile intraepithelial neoplasia in sexual partners of women with cervical intraepithelial neoplasia. N Engl J Med 1987;317:916.

Becker TM. Genital warts—a sexually transmitted dis-

ease (STD) epidemic? Colposc Gynecol Laser Surg 1984;1:193.

Beckmann A, Daling JR, Sherman KJ, et al. Human papillomavirus infection and anal cancer. Int J Cancer 1989;43:1042.

Bistoletti P, Lidbrink P. Sexually transmitted diseases including genital papillomavirus infection in male sexual partners of women treated for cervical intraepithelial neoplasia III by conization. Br J Obstet Gynaecol 1988;95:611.

Bornstein J, Rahat MA, Abramovici H. Etiology of cervical cancer: current concepts. Obstet Gynecol Surv 1995;50:146.

Campion MJ. Clinical manifestations and natural history of genital human papillomavirus infection. Obstet Gynecol Clin North Am 1987;14:363.

Campion MJ, McCance DJ, Cuzick J, et al. Progressive potential of mild cervical atypia: prospective cytological, colposcopic, and virological study. Lancet 1986;2:237.

Campion MJ, Singer A, McCance DJ, et al. Subclinical penile human papillomavirus infection in consorts of women with cervical neoplasia: a clue to the high-risk male. Colposc Gynecol Laser Surg 1987;3:11.

Chuang T, Perry HO, Kurland LT, et al. Condylomata acuminatum in Rochester, Minn., 1950–1979. Arch Dermatol 1984;120:476.

Corey L. Warts and molluscum contagiosum. In: Isselbachker KJ, Adarms RD, Braunwald E, et al., eds. Harrison's Principles of internal medicine. 9th ed. New York: McGraw-Hill, 1980.

Davis AJ, Emans SJ. Human papillomavirus infection in the pediatric and adolescent patient. J Pediatr 1989;115:1.

Erlich KS, Normoyle JL. Condylomata acuminata: waging a successful fight against anogenital warts. Female Patient 1987;12:51.

Eron LJ, Judson F, Tucker S, et al. Interferon therapy for condylomata acuminata. N Engl J Med 1986;315:1059.

Evander M, Edlund K, Gustafsson A, et al. Human papillomavirus infection is transient in young women: a population-based cohort study. J Infect Dis 1995;171:1026.

Ferenczy A. Epidemiology and clinical pathophysiology of condylomata acuminata. Am J Obstet Gynecol 1995;172:1331.

Ferenczy A, Bergeron C, Richart RM. Human papillomavirus DNA in fomites on objects used for the management of patients with genital human papillomavirus infections. Obstet Gynecol 1989;74:950.

Ferenczy A, Choukroun D, Falcone T, et al. The effect of cervical loop electrosurgical excision on subsequent pregnancy outcome: North American experience. Am J Obstet Gynecol 1995;172(4):1246.

Ferenczy A, Mitae M, Nagai N, et al. Latent papillomavirus and recurring genital warts. N Engl J Med 1986;313:1059.

Gottlieb SL, Myskowski PL. Molluscum contagiosum. Int J Dermatol 1994;33:453.

Hillard PA. Human papillomavirus and the abnormal Papanicolaou smear in adolescents. Female Patient 1994;19:48.

Hillard PA, Biro FM, Wildey L. Complications of cervical cryotherapy in adolescents. J Reprod Med 1991;36:711.

Johnson K. Periodic health examination, 1995 update: 1. Screening for human papillomavirus infection in asymptomatic women. Canadian Task Force on the Periodic Health Examination. Can Med Assoc J 1995;152:483.

Johnstone JD, McGoogan E, Smart GE, et al. A popula-tion-based, controlled study of the relation between HIV infection and cervical neoplasia. Br J Obstet Gynaecol 1994;101:986.

Jones EED, Russo JF, Combroski RA, et al. Cervical intraepithelial neoplasia in adolescents. J Adolesc Health Care 1984;5:243.

Kiviat NB, Koutsky LA, Critchlow CW, et al. Prevalence and cytologic manifestations of human papilloma virus HPV types 6, 11, 16, 18, 31, 33, 35, 42, 44, 45, 51, 52 and 56 among 500 consecutive women. Int J Gynecol Pathol 1992;11:197.

Korkolopoulou P, Kolokythas C, Kittas C, et al. Correlation of colposcopy and histology in cervical biopsies positive for CIN and/or HPV infection. Eur J Gynaecol Oncol 1992;13:502.

Lonky NM, Navarre GL, Saunders S, et al. Low-grade Papanicolaou smears and the Bethesda system: a prospective cytohistopathologic analysis. Obstet Gynecol 1995;85:716.

Lynch PD. Condylomata acuminata. Clin Obstet Gynecol 1985;28:142.

McLachlin CM. Pathology of human papillomavirus in the female genital tract. Curr Opin Obstet Gynecol 1995;7:24.

Maymon R, Bekerman A, Werchow M, et al. Clinical and subclinical condyloma. Rates among male sexual partners of women with genital human papillomavirus infection. J Reprod Med 1995;40:31.

Moscicki AB. Genital human papillomavirus infections. Adolesc Med: State Art Rev 1990;1:451.

Moscicki AB, Palefsky JM, Gonzales J, et al. The association between human papillomavirus deoxyribonucleic acid status and the results of cytologic rescreening tests in young, sexually active women. Am J Obstet Gynecol 1991;165:67.

Rando RF, Groff DE, Chirikjian JG, et al. Isolation and characterization of the novel human papillomavirus type 6 DNA from an invasive vulvar carcinoma. J Virol 1986;57:353.

Reid R, Greenberg M, Jenson AB, et al. Sexually transmitted papillomaviral infections. I. The anatomic distribution and pathologic grade of neoplastic lesions associated with different viral types. Am J Obstet Gynecol 1987;156:212.

Reid R, Herschman BR, Crum CP, et al. Genital warts and cervical cancer: V. The tissue basis of colposcopic change. Am J Obstet Gynecol 1984;149:293.

Rosenfeld W, Burk R, Coupey S. Prevalence of human papilloma virus in sexually active adolescent females [Abstract]. J Adolesc Health Care 1987;8:301.

Russo JF, Jones DED. Abnormal cervical cytology in sexually active adolescents. J Adolesc Health Care 1984;5:269.

Shew ML, Fortenberry JD, Miles P. Interval between menarche and first sexual intercourse, related to risk of human papillomavirus infection. J Pediatr 1994;125:661.

Sidawy MK, Tabbara SO. Reactive change and atypical squamous cells of undetermined significance in Papanicolaou smears: a cytohistologic correlation. Diagn Cytopathol 1993;9:423.

Smith EM, Johnson SR, Cripe T, et al. Perinatal transmission and maternal risks of human papillomavirus infection. Cancer Detect Prev 1995;19:196.

Vermund SH, Kelley KF, Klein RS, et al. High risk of human papillomavirus infection and cervical squamous intraepithelial lesions among women with symptomatic human immunodeficiency virus infection. Am J Obstet Gynecol 1991;165:392.

Widra EA, Dookhan D, Jordan A, et al. Evaluation of the atypical cytologic smear: validity of the 1991 Bethesda system. J Reprod Med 1994;39:9 & 682.

Wright TC Jr, Gagnon S, Richart RM, et al. Treatment of cervical intraepithelial neoplasia using the loop electrosurgical excision procedure. Obstet Gynecol 1992;79:173.

CHAPTER 67

Pediculosis Pubis and Scabies

PEDICULOSIS PUBIS

Etiology

Pediculosis pubis is caused by the pubic crab louse, *Pthirus pubis*, a wingless, oval, yellow-gray insect 1–4 mm in length.

Epidemiology

1. Transmission: The parasites are transmitted by close bodily contact, chiefly by sexual contact, but can also be transmitted by clothing and bedding.
2. Life cycle: The parasite spends its life on skin and feeds on blood. It dies in about 24 hours without animal contact. The female pubic louse lays about three eggs per day, which are attached to hair shafts as nits. The nits hatch in 8–10 days. Adult life expectancy is about 1 month.

Clinical Manifestations

1. Asymptomatic: Lice are found by patient, friend, or contact.
2. Symptoms occur 1–2 weeks after contact and more rapidly if patient had prior infestation. Symptoms include:
   a. Pruritus related to a bite as a probable hypersensitivity reaction
   b. Secondary infections from scratching
3. Areas occurring: Pubic hair, hairs of abdomen, thighs, axilla, and perianal area are often affected; occasionally eyebrows and lashes are affected. Nits may appear on terminal hair on trunk, thighs, axillary region, bearded area, and eyelashes.
4. After prolonged infestation, small blue maculae may appear on thighs and abdomen. These are uncommon but specific for pubic lice. They may represent altered blood pigments or excretion from salivary gland of the louse.
5. Thirty-seven percent of cases of pediculosis pubis had coexisting sexually transmitted disease (Opaneye et al., 1993).

Diagnosis

1. Clinical history
2. Finding nits (eggs) or lice: Nits are small, yellowish-white, glistening, oval kernels attached to hair shafts. (Lice were described under "Etiology.")

Therapy

1. Recommended regimens include:
   a. Lindane 1% shampoo applied for 4 minutes and then thoroughly washed off. Not recommended for pregnant or lactating women; OR
   b. Permethrin 1% creme rinse (Nix) applied to affected area and washed off after 10 minutes; OR
   c. Pyrethrins and piperonyl butoxide (nonprescription Rid, R +C, A-200 pyrinate) applied to the affected area and washed off after 10 minutes.

   Lindane cream and lotion are no longer recommended for the treatment of pubic lice. Lindane shampoo is the least expensive treatment. The side effects of seizures and aplastic anemia have not been reported when treatment is limited to the recommended 4 minute period.
2. Retreatment is indicated after 7 days if lice are found or eggs are observed at the hair-skin junction.
3. Clothing or bed linen coming in contact with the patient within the past 2 days should be washed or dried by machine (hot cycle) or dry cleaned. Fumigation is not necessary.
4. Residual nits should be removed with a fine comb. For nits that are difficult to remove, use a solution of vinegar and water to loosen them.
5. Sexual contacts within the last month should be treated as above.
6. Pregnancy: Use permethrin or pyrethrins with piperonyl butoxide.
7. Human immunodeficiency virus (HIV) infection: Can use same therapy as in noninfected adolescents.
8. Pediculosis of eyelashes: Treat with application of occlusive ophthalmic ointment to the eyelid margins two times a day for 10 days. This will smother lice and nits. Do not apply lindane or other medications to the eyes.

SCABIES

Scabies, a highly contagious ectoparasitic infection, is a common cause of pruritus and rash in adolescents. It is one of the most widespread infestations worldwide.

Etiology

Scabies is caused by a small mite, *Sarcoptes scabiei* var. *hominis*. The adult mite has a rounded body, four pairs of legs, and measures 400 μm in length. This parasite is host-specific for humans.

Epidemiology

1. Transmission: The mite is transmitted to the host after close personal contact. Nonsexual transmission is common.
2. Life cycle: The male impregnates the female on the skin surface or in a superficial burrow. The male dies in 2–3 days. The female mite (about 0.4 mm in length) then wanders for a short distance and burrows into the skin, traveling at $^1/_2$–5 mm/day while laying two to three eggs per day. Egg laying is completed in 4–5 weeks and the adult female dies within the burrow. After 3–5 days the eggs hatch, and the larvae return to the skin surface to mature in 8–17 days. Fortunately, only 10% of eggs become adults. The average infected host has 3–50 adult female mites.
3. Age: In underdeveloped countries, scabies has the highest prevalence in preschool children and adolescents. In developed nations the prevalence is similar in all ages.

Clinical Manifestations

1. Incubation: Symptoms occur 1–2 months after first exposure and 1–2 days after re-exposure.
2. Lesions: Scabies is an intensely pruritic papular eruption. The host may present with only pruritus, which is often worse at night. The rash is usually a symmetrical polymorphous eruption, including red papules with or without excoriations, vesicles, pustules, or crusted lesions. The burrows, if seen, appear as short wavy lines a few millimeters to 1 cm in length.
3. Areas occurring: Scabies involves finger webs, flexor surfaces of wrists, axillary folds, nipples, umbilicus, belt-line area, buttocks, thighs, knees, and ankles. In the male the penis and scrotum are common areas of involvement. Scabies usually spares the face, neck, and scalp except in children.
4. Differential diagnosis: The lesions can become secondarily infected and eczematized and thus confused with eczema, atopic or contact dermatitis, and impetigo. Papulovesicular lesions may be confused with papular urticaria, chickenpox, drug eruptions, folliculitis, and dermatitis herpetiformis.

Diagnosis

1. Clinical picture of pruritus with lesions in distribution as outlined earlier: Diagnosis is often made on distribution of lesions alone. A similar clinical history in family members or close contacts is helpful. Burrows are virtually pathognomonic for human scabies.
2. Isolation of mite: Scrape lesion or burrow with a #15 blade and mineral oil. Look for ova, feces, or organism. Do not use potassium hydroxide, as it dissolves the mite's body and feces. An alternative method is a shave biopsy of the superficial layer of skin. The specimen is examined with immersion oil on low power. The shave biopsy specimen has a higher sensitivity than the skin scraping specimen.

Therapy

1. Recommended regimen
   a. Topical 5% permethrin cream (Elimite) applied to all areas of the body from the neck down and washed off by bath or shower after 8–14 hours: The teen should be careful to apply underneath fingernails and skin folds. The cream can be applied at bedtime and removed the next morning; OR
   b. Lindane (1%) 1 ounce of lotion or 30 g of cream applied thinly to all areas of the body from the neck down and washed off thoroughly after 8 hours: Include web spaces of digits and under fingernails. No preapplication shower is necessary; in fact, a shower may increase unnecessary systemic absorption. Prescribe only the required amount, which is usually 1 ounce per treatment. Do not prescribe refills.
   Lindane should not be used following a bath and not with extensive dermatitis. Pregnant or lactating women and children younger than 2 years of age should not use lindane. If the patient has a bad infestation, a second treatment is recommended 1 week later. Permethrin is highly effective and safer than lindane (Kwell) but costs more. Lindane resistance has been reported in some areas of the United States.
2. Alternative regimen: Crotamiton (10%) (Eurax) applied to the entire body from the neck down, nightly for two consecutive nights, and washed off 24 hours after the second application.

3. Bedding and clothing should be machine washed, machine dried using hot cycle, dry cleaned, or removed from body contact, set aside in sealed plastic bag for at least 72 hours. Fumigation of living areas is not necessary.

4. Follow-up: Pruritus may persist for several weeks. The practitioner may either retreat those who are symptomatic or retreat only if live mites are observed.

5. Sex partners: Sex partners, as well as close personal or household contacts within the last month, should be treated.

6. Pregnant women: Pregnant or lactating women should not use lindane but should use permethrin or crotamiton regimens.

7. Use oral steroids for severe systemic or local reactions.

8. Antipruritics (e.g., hydroxyzine [Atarax], trimeprazine tartrate [Temaril], promethazine [Phenergan]) may be used for pruritus. Crotamiton (Eurax) is also antipruritic.

9. HIV Infection: HIV-infected individuals should use the same treatment. HIV-infected individuals are at increased risk for Norwegian scabies, a disseminated infection.

   Norwegian scabies is more difficult to treat and may require, particularly in those who are immunosuppressed, several treatments with scabicides and sometimes sequential use of several agents.

Therapy Problems   Treatment problems are usually manifested by continued pruritus.

1. Examination reveals continued infestation, which could be the result of:
   a. Inadequate therapy: All skin below neck areas may not have been treated.
   b. Reinfection
   c. Resistance to therapy
   Continued infestation requires retreatment, using the same or another agent.
2. Examination suggests no scabies but dry or irritated skin, which could be the result of:
   a. Irritation or sensitization from therapy
   b. Residual sensitization from the mite or its products
   Use topical steroids or antipruritic drugs.

BIBLIOGRAPHY

Billstein SA. Human lice. In: Holmes KK, Mardh PA, Sparling PF, Wiesner PJ, eds. Sexually transmitted diseases. 2nd ed. New York: McGraw-Hill Information Services, 1990.

Brodell RT, Helms SE. Office dermatologic testing: the scabies preparation. Am Fam Physician 1991;44:505.

Buntin DM, Roser T, Lesher JT Jr, et al. J Am Acad Dermatol 1991;25:527–534.

Burkhart CG. Scabies: an epidemiologic reassessment. Ann Intern Med 1983;98:498.

Burns DA. The treatment of human ectoparasitic infection. Br J Dermatol 1991;125:89.

Centers for Disease Control. 1993 sexually transmitted diseases treatment guidelines. MMWR 1993;42 (RR–14):1.

Felman Y, Nikitas J. Scabies. Cutis 1984;33:266.

Gurevitch AW. Scabies and lice. Pediatr Clin North Am 1985;32:987.

Hogan DJ, Schachner L, Tanglertsampan C. Diagnosis and treatment of childhood scabies and pediculosis. Pediatr Clin North Am. 1991;38:941.

Lane AT. Scabies and head lice. Pediatr Ann 1987;16:51.

Levin S, Pottage JC Jr, Kessler HA, et al. The office appointment to the sexually transmitted disease: part I. Disease-A-Month 1987a;33:133.

Levin S, Pottage JC Jr, Kessler HA, et al. The office appointment to the sexually transmitted disease: part II. Disease-A-Month 1987b;33:185.

Levine GI. Sexually transmitted parasitic diseases. Prim Care 1991;18:101.

Levisohn DR. Treatment of scabies and similar infestations. West J Med 1992;156:193.

Martin DH, Mroczkowski TF. Dermatologic manifestations of sexually transmitted diseases other than HIV. Infect Dis Clin North Am 1994;8:533.

Molianari F. Update on the treatment of pediculosis and scabies. Pediatr Nurs 1992;18:600.

Moore P. Diagnosing and treating scabies. Practitioner 1994;238:632.

Opaneye AA, Jayaweera DT, Walzman M, et al. Pediculosis pubis: a surrogate marker for sexually transmitted diseases. J R Soc Health 1993;113:6.

Orkin M, Maibach HI. Scabies. In: Holmes KK, Mardh PA, Sparling PF, Wiesner PJ, eds. Sexually transmitted diseases. 2nd ed. New York: McGraw-Hill Information Services, 1990.

Orkin M, Maibach HI. Scabies therapy—1993. Semin Dermatol 1993;12:22.

Permethrin for head lice. Med Lett Drugs Ther 1986; 28:87.

Pien FD, Grekin JL. Common ectoparasites. West J Med 1983;139:382.

Rabinowitz L, Esterly N. Dermatology. In: Avery ME, First LR, eds. Pediatric medicine. Baltimore: Williams & Wilkins, 1994.

Rasmussen JE. Scabies. Pediatr Rev 1994;15:110.

Rosenfeld WD. Sexually transmitted diseases in adolescents: update 1991. Pediatr Ann 1991;20:303.

Routh HB, Mirensky YM, Parish LC, et al. Ectoparasites as sexually transmitted diseases. Semin Dermatol 1994;46:1237.

Sokoloff F. Identification and management of pediculosis. Nurse Pract 1994;19:62.

Sterling GB, Janniger CK, Kihiczak G, et al. Scabies. Am Fam Physician 1992;46:1237.

CHAPTER 68

Minor Venereal Diseases
Chancroid, Lymphogranuloma Venereum, and Granuloma Inguinale

Chancroid, lymphogranuloma venereum (LGV), and granuloma inguinale constitute the classic minor venereal diseases. In the United States most patients with genital ulcers have genital herpes, syphilis, or chancroid. Herpes is most common. About 3–10% of patients with genital ulcers have more than one of these present. Chancroid has increased in prevalence since 1985 and has become a significant sexually transmitted disease (STD) in the United States. LGV and granuloma inguinale are both uncommon in the United States but should be considered in the differential diagnosis of genital ulcers. Genital ulcerative infections are associated with increased risk for human immunodeficiency virus (HIV) infection.

CHANCROID

Chancroid is characterized by multiple genital ulcerations. The disease has become of recent concern because of its rising prevalence and local outbreaks. Another concern is that chancroid genital lesions are a well established cofactor for HIV transmission. In addition, as many as 10% of patients with chancroid may be coinfected with *Treponema pallidum* or herpes simplex virus (HSV). Chancroid must be considered in the differential diagnosis of any adolescent with a painful genital ulcer, especially if associated with enlarged, tender inguinal adenopathy.

Etiology

Chancroid is caused by *Haemophilus ducreyi*, a nonmotile, nonacid-fast, Gram-negative *Streptobacillus* with rounded ends.

Epidemiology

1. Incidence: The global incidence of chancroid exceeds that of syphilis, with the major areas of high incidence being Southeast Asia, Africa, and South America. Chancroid has been considered a disappearing disease in developing countries. However, chancroid has re-emerged in the United States during the last decade. From 1950 to 1980, cases were infrequently reported. After an epidemic in California in 1981, numbers increased, peaking in 1987 at 5035 cases. There has been a sharp decline thereafter from 4212 cases in 1990 to 773 in 1994. However, new areas continue to report outbreaks. Almost 95% of cases are reported by five states: New York, California, Florida, Georgia, and Texas.

2. Race: Increased in African-American and Hispanic patients
3. Male-to-female ratio: Ranges from 3:1 to 25:1
4. Transmission: Transmission is through sexual contact. Most of the cases have been contracted through heterosexual contact and many through prostitutes.
5. Relation to crack cocaine: A number of studies have established a link between syphilis incidence rates and cocaine use, specifically crack cocaine. A similar link appears to be present for chancroid.

Clinical Manifestations

1. Incubation period: One to 14 days, with an average of 3–5 days
2. Primary lesion: A small inflammatory papule becomes pustular and then ulcerative, with a nonindurated border, usually within about 24–48 hours. The lesions do not have a vesicular appearance. The lesions classically have scalloped edges surrounded by a red halo. The lesions bleed easily and are very painful. Multiple ulcers may occur, may become necrotic or erosive, and may merge to form giant ulcers. The base of the ulcers may be covered with a gray or yellow necrotic purulent exudate.
3. Location
   a. In male: Prepuce, coronal sulcus, and frenulum
   b. In female: Labia, clitoris, and perianal region
   c. Extragenital sites: Lip, tongue, and finger
4. Lymphadenopathy: Fifty percent of patients develop painful, tender, inguinal lymphadenopathy within 7–10 days of the primary lesion. Suppuration and spontaneous rupture may occur. The chancroidal bubo (fluctuant lymph node) is usually unilateral, painful, and unilocular, with marked redness of the overlying skin.
5. Although fever and malaise may occur, spread to distant sites is very unusual.
6. Females: Many females are carriers without disease or have asymptomatic lesions of the vagina or cervix.

Differential Diagnosis

Chancroid may be confused with or coexist with herpes genitalis, primary syphilis, LGV, traumatic lesions, Behcet's syndrome, or fixed drug eruptions. The prevalence of genital ulcers in adolescents would be in the following order: herpes, nonspecific trauma, syphilis, and then chancroid.

1. In syphilitic chancres the ulcers are nonpainful, with indurated borders. A dark-field examination and serological examination are needed for confirmation.
2. In LGV the lesions are nonpainful. The adenopathy develops after the lesions have healed.
3. In herpes, the lesions start as vesicles, are usually painful, more superficial, more numerous, and surrounded by a narrower zone of erythema. Adenopathy is usually bilateral. Smears and cultures can be used for confirmation.

Diagnosis

The diagnosis may be difficult because it is often made only on clinical grounds. All individuals with genital ulcers should receive a serologic test for syphilis and possibly other tests including a dark-field examination or direct immunofluorescence test for *T. pallidum*, a culture or antigen test for HSV, and a culture for *H. ducreyi*.

Diagnosis involves:

1. Clinical appearance
2. Smears: Direct smear from an ulcer or aspiration material from an infected lymph node (bubo) is required for diagnosis. The lesion should be cleaned thoroughly and serous exudate collected on a cotton-tipped applicator from the undermined border of an ulcer. This is carefully rolled (one direction onto a glass slide) and Gram stained. The bacteria arrange themselves in parallel short chains described as schools of fish. A promising test in the future is the immunofluorescent test of the ulcer material.
3. Culture: A culture may be attempted from lesions, buboes, or blood, but the organism is difficult to grow in vitro.
4. Immunodiagnostic, DNA probe, and polymerase chain reaction (PCR) tests are being investigated but are not routinely available.
5. Centers for Disease Control (CDC) case definition criteria for chancroid include:
   a. Definite: The recovery of *H. ducreyi* from an individual, regardless of site of recovery or symptoms.
   b. Probable: One or more painful ulcers; AND
      — No evidence of *T. pallidum* on dark-field examination or by a serologic test for syphilis performed at least 7 days after onset of ulcers; AND
      — Either the clinical presentation of the ulcer(s) is not typical of disease caused by HSV or the HSV test results are negative.
      The combination of a painful ulcer with tender inguinal adenopathy is suggestive of chancroid, and when accompanied by suppurative inguinal adenopathy is almost pathognomonic.
6. HIV testing should be considered in the management of patients with genital ulcers, especially those with syphilis or chancroid.

Therapy

1. Recommended regimens include:
   a. Azithromycin 1 g orally in a single dose; OR
   b. Ceftriaxone 250 mg intramuscularly (IM) in a single dose; OR
   c. Erythromycin base 500 mg orally four times a day for 7 days.
   Azithromycin and ceftriaxone have the advantage of single-dose therapy. Azithromycin has not been approved for adolescents younger than 16 years of age.
2. Alternative regimens
   a. Amoxicillin 500 mg plus clavulanic acid 125 mg orally three times a day for 7 days; OR
   b. Ciprofloxacin 500 mg orally two times a day for 3 days.
   These alternative regimens have not been studied as extensively as the recommended regimens. Ciprofloxacin is contraindicated for pregnant and lactating women, children, and adolescents younger than 18 years of age.
3. Aspirate fluctuant gland masses from a site of normal skin tissue. Traditionally, this technique has been advised to decrease the risk of developing chronic draining sinuses.
4. Follow-up: Follow-up with infected individuals should occur within 3–7 days after initiation of therapy and should continue weekly until resolution of signs and symptoms. There should be subjective improvement within 3 days and objective improvement within 7 days. If there is no improvement, the practitioner must consider whether the diagnosis is correct, there is a coinfection with another STD, the individual is infected with HIV, or treatment compliance is poor. Large ulcers may require more than 2 weeks to re-

solve, and fluctuant lymphadenopathy heals even more slowly than ulcers. Adenopathy may progress to fluctuation despite successful therapy and does not represent treatment failure.

5. No sexual activity while clinical disease is present
6. Sexual partners: Treat recent sexual partners. Since the incubation period is usually not longer than 10 days, treating partners within that time period is usually sufficient.
7. Pregnancy: The safety of azithromycin for pregnant and lactating women has not been established. Ciprofloxacin is contraindicated during pregnancy.
8. HIV-infected patients: These individuals may require longer courses of therapy, and healing may be slower. Treatment failures do occur. The 7-day erythromycin regimen may be better unless very close follow-up is possible.

Lymphogranuloma Venereum

LGV is a systemic infectious disease that is usually sexually transmitted. It is characterized by a primary genital or anal lesion, followed by suppuration of regional lymph nodes and constitutional signs and symptoms. The disease is of interest in the adolescent, in that it is a rare cause of genital ulcerative lesions and lymphadenopathy.

Etiology

The causative agent of LGV is an obligate intracellular organism of the genus *Chlamydia*. LGV is caused by L_1, L_2, and L_3 strains of *Chlamydia trachomatis*. Strains A–C cause trachoma and D–K cause genital infections and inclusion conjunctivitis. Strains causing LGV are more invasive in the host and thus cause systemic disease, rather than being restricted to mucous membrane surfaces.

Epidemiology

1. Frequency: About 400 reported cases in the United States each year
2. Age: Peak incidence in the third decade
3. Male-to-female ratio: 3.4:1
4. Transmission: Usually sexually transmitted but can occasionally be contracted from fomites

Clinical Manifestations

1. Incubation period: Three days to 30 days; usually 7–12 days
2. Primary lesion
   a. Usually takes one of four forms: Papule; small, painless, nonindurated ulcer on the penis, labia, vagina, or anus; herpetiform lesion; or urethritis or cervicitis. The most common of the four is a herpetiform ulcer at the site of infection.
   b. Rectal intercourse can lead to a primary rectal infection with consequent diarrhea, rectal discharge, and tenesmus.
3. Secondary manifestations
   a. Inguinal syndrome: Painful regional adenopathy is the most common manifestation of secondary disease and the most common lesion in heterosexual individuals. The syndrome usually occurs 1–6 weeks after the primary lesion. The node enlargement begins as discrete adenopathy and then the nodes can become matted and fluctuant. This produces the characteristic bubo. The skin overlying the bubo often becomes at-

tached to the underlying lymph nodes and takes on a characteristic deep reddish blue color. Inguinal adenopathy is unilateral in 70% of cases. The organism may spread and cause the following:
— Constitutional symptoms including headache, fever, chills, and myalgias: LGV can present as a fever of unknown origin.
— Systemic complications, including arthritis, meningitis, encephalitis, conjunctivitis, hepatitis, pneumonitis, erythema nodosum, and erythema multiforme

4. Late manifestations (uncommon)
   a. Proctocolitis and hyperplasia of intestinal and perirectal lymphatic tissue (lymphorrhoids): The majority of anorectal disease is in females and homosexual males.
   b. Perirectal abscesses
   c. Rectovaginal and anorectal fistulas
   d. Rectal strictures often manifested by constipation, ileus, weight loss, and abdominal distention
   e. Elephantiasis of genitals 1–20 years after onset (rare)
   f. Scarring of pelvis and resultant infertility

Differential Diagnosis

1. Genital-inguinal lesion
   a. Syphilis
   b. Herpes simplex
   c. Chancroid
   d. Granuloma inguinale
   e. Pyogenic infections
   f. Cat-scratch fever
2. Rectal fistulas
   a. Inflammatory bowel disease
   b. Chronic rectal infections: Gonorrhea, amebiasis, tuberculosis
   c. Granuloma inguinale

Diagnosis

1. Clinical manifestations
2. Culture: Culture for *Chlamydia* can be obtained from a node aspirate.
3. Complement fixation: Titers higher than 1:16 and particularly higher than 1:64 indicate active or recent infection. Acute and convalescent titers are required for complete interpretation. Titers are also positive after *Chlamydia* urethritis, psittacosis, or trachoma. The microimmunofluorescent test is more sensitive than complement fixation but is not routinely available.
4. Cytology: Direct immunofluorescent techniques are available to identify *Chlamydia*, although these are not specific for LGV strains.
5. Biopsy of node: A biopsy is useful if needed to rule out lymphoma.

Therapy

1. Recommended regimen: Doxycycline 100 mg two times a day for 21 days
2. Alternative regimens
   a. Erythromycin 500 mg orally four times a day for 21 days
   b. Sulfamethoxazole 500 mg orally four times a day for 21 days

3. Surgery: Occasionally, aspiration of a fluctuant node or incision and drainage of an abscess is required.
4. Follow-up: Patients should be followed clinically until signs and symptoms have resolved.
5. Sex partners: Sexual contacts within 30 days before onset of symptoms should be examined, tested for urethral or cervical chlamydial infection, and treated.
6. Pregnancy and lactation: Pregnant and lactating women should be treated with the erythromycin regimen.
7. HIV infection: HIV-infected adolescents should be treated with same regimens as noninfected adolescents.

GRANULOMA INGUINALE

Granuloma inguinale is extremely uncommon in the United States but is in the differential diagnosis of STDs that cause chronic progressive ulcerative disease of the genital and anal areas.

Etiology

Granuloma inguinale is caused by *Calymmatobacterium granulomatis,* a nonmotile Gram-negative coccobacillus.

Epidemiology

1. Frequency: Less than 100 cases per year in the United States
2. Sex: Male prevalence greater than female
3. Geographic prevalence: In this country, more common in the southern United States; highest prevalence in underdeveloped countries
4. Transmission: Primarily through sexual contact; only mildly contagious, requiring several exposures for clinical disease; autoinoculation also leads to spread.

Clinical Manifestations

1. Primary lesion: Indurated nodule(s) appears after an 8- to 80-day incubation period.
2. Granulomatous phase: The nodules erode to form clean granulomatous, beefy red, sharply defined lesions that are usually painless.
   a. Lesions bleed readily on contact.
   b. Lesions slowly enlarge and may spread to continuous areas.
   c. Pseudobuboes result from the granulomatous inflammation.
3. Other presentations
   a. Lymphatic obstruction with lymphedema
   b. Hematogenous spread to spine
4. Sites involved
   a. Genitalia: Ninety percent of cases
   b. Inguinal region: Ten percent of cases
   c. Anal region: Five percent to 10% of cases
   d. Distant sites: One percent to 5% of cases

Differential Diagnosis

The diagnosis may be confused in the disease's early stages with syphilis, herpes simplex, chancroid, and pyogenic infections.

Diagnosis

1. Clinical appearance is highly suggestive.
2. Giemsa or Wright's stain: A piece of clean granulation tissue is spread against a slide and strained with Giemsa or Wright's stain. Intracytoplasmic rods (Donovan bodies) in large mononuclear cells are indicative of granuloma inguinale.
3. Currently under development is a serologic test that uses an indirect immunofluorescence technique applied to paraffin-embedded tissue sections of lesions containing Donovan bodies. The test has a sensitivity of 100% and a specificity of 98%. This test may prove valuable, as there is no culture method for *C. granulomatis*.

Therapy

1. Tetracycline 500 mg orally four times a day for 2–3 weeks
2. Gentamicin 40 mg IM twice a day for 2 weeks

BIBLIOGRAPHY

Bassa AG, Hoosen AA, Moodley J, et al. Granuloma inguinale (donovanosis) in women. An analysis of 61 cases from Durban, South Africa. Sex Transm Dis 1993;20:164.

Becker LE. Lymphogranuloma venereum. Int J Dermatol 1976;15:26.

Burgoyne RA. Lymphogranuloma venereum. Prim Care 1990;17:153.

Centers for Disease Control. Chancroid, California. MMWR 1982;31:173.

Centers for Disease Control. Chancroid, Massachusetts. JAMA 1986;255:1673.

Centers for Disease Control. 1989 sexually transmitted diseases treatment guidelines. MMWR 1989;(S–8).

Centers for Disease Control. 1993 sexually transmitted diseases treatment guidelines. MMWR 1993;42 (RR–14):1.

Chancroid in Los Angeles County. Public Health Letter (Los Angeles County, Department of Health Services) 1987;9:21–22.

Chui L, Albritton W, Paster B, et al. Development of the polymerase chain reaction for diagnosis of chancroid. J Clin Microbiol 1993;31:659.

Dangor Y, Ballard RC, da L Exposto F, et al. Accuracy of clinical diagnosis of genital ulcer disease. Sex Transm Dis 1990;17:184.

Elgart ML. Sexually transmitted diseases of the vulva. Dermatol Clin 1992;10:387.

Engelkens HJ, vander Meijden WI, Stolz E. Donovanosis still exists. Int J Dermatol 1992;31:244.

Fiumara NJ. Chancroid. Medical Aspects of Human Sexuality 1986;20:75.

Freinkel AL, Dangor Y, Koornhof HJ, et al. A serological test for granuloma inguinale. Genitourin Med 1992; 68:269.

Goens JL, Schwartz RA, DeWolf K. Mucocutaneous manifestations of chancroid, lymphogranuloma venereum and granuloma inguinale. Am Fam Physician 1994;49:415.

Handsfield HH, Totten PA, Fennel CL, et al. Molecular epidemiology of *Haemophilus ducreyi* infections. Ann Intern Med 1981;95:315.

Hart G. Chancroid, granuloma inguinale, lymphogranuloma venereum [HEW Publication N7.9–8302]. Washington DC: US Department of Health, Education & Welfare, 1979.

Hart G. Donovanosis. In: Holmes KK, Mardh PA, Sparling PF, Wiesner PJ, eds. Sexually transmitted diseases. 2nd ed. New York: McGraw-Hill Information Services, 1990.

Heaton ND, Yates-Bell A. Thirty year follow-up of lymphogranuloma venereum. Br J Urol 1992;70:693.

Jones CC, Rosen T. Culture diagnosis of chancroid. Arch Dermatol 1991;127:1823.

Jordan WC. Chancroid: a review for the family practitioner. J Natl Med Assoc 1991;83:724.

Joseph AK, Rosen T. Laboratory techniques used in the diagnosis of chancroid, granuloma inguinale, and lymphogranuloma venereum. Dermatol Clin 1994; 12:1.

Kraus SJ. Diagnosis and management of acute genital ulcers in sexually active patients. Semin Dermatol 1990;9:160.

Klotz SA, Drutz DJ, Tam MR, et al. Hemorrhagic proctitis due to lymphogranuloma venereum serogroup L2. N Engl J Med 1983;308:1563.

Martin DH, CiCarlo RP. Recent changes in the epidemiology of genital ulcer disease in the United States. The crack cocaine connection. Sex Transm Dis 1994;21:S76.

Marx R, Aral SO, Rolfs RT, et al. Crack, sex and STD. Sex Transm Dis 1992;18:92.

Mroczkowski TF, Martin DH. Genital ulcer disease. Dermatol Clin 1994;12:753.

Perine PL, Osoba AO. Lymphogranuloma venereum. In: Holmes KK, Mardh PA, Sparling PF, Wiesner PJ, eds. Sexually transmitted diseases. 2nd ed. New York: McGraw-Hill Information Services, 1990.

Richens J. The diagnosis and treatment of donovanosis. Genitourin Med 1991;67:441.

Ridgway GL. Quinolones in sexually transmitted diseases. Drugs 1993;45(suppl 3):134.

Ronald AR, Albritton W. Chancroid and *Haemophilus ducreyi*. In: Holmes KK, Mardh PA, Sparling PF, Wiesner PJ, eds. Sexually transmitted diseases. 2nd ed. New York: McGraw-Hill Information Services, 1990.

Ronald AR, Plummer FA. Chancroid and *Haemophilus ducreyi*. Ann Intern Med 1985;102:705.

Rosenfeld WD. Sexually transmitted diseases in adolescents: update 1991. Pediatr Ann 1991;20:303.

Schmid GP. The treatment of chancroid. JAMA 1986; 255:1757.

Schmid GP, Sanders LL Jr, Blount JH, et al. Chancroid in the United States: reestablishment of an old disease. JAMA 1987;258:3265.

Sehgal VN, Sharma HK. Donovanosis. J Dermatol 1992;19:932.

Tal S, Nichola C. Epidemiological and clinical features in 165 cases of granuloma inguinale. Br J Vener Dis 1970;46:461.

Tyndall MW, Agoiki E, Plummer FA, et al. Single dose azithromycin for the treatment of chancroid: a randomized comparison with erythromycin. Sex Transm Dis 1994;21:231.

Drug Use and Abuse

CHAPTER 69

Overview of Drug Use and Abuse

Lawrence S. Neinstein, Drew Pinsky, and Bruce S. Heischober

Drug use among adolescents increased explosively in the 1960s and 1970s. Although drug use by teenagers declined until 1991, the use of drugs among American secondary school students has been rising since 1991 among 8th grade students and since 1992 among 10th and 12th graders. More specifically (Johnston et al., 1995a):

1. In 1995 it was estimated that more than 48% of American youth try an illicit drug before they finish high school.
2. By 12th grade nearly one-third of adolescents have illicitly used drugs other than marijuana.
3. About 4.6% of high school seniors actively smoke marijuana on a daily basis.
4. Rise in drug use: The prevalence of 8th graders taking any illicit drug in the prior 12 months has almost doubled since 1991 (from 11% to 21%). Since 1992 the prevalence for use of any illicit drugs in the prior 12 months has increased by nearly two-thirds among 10th graders (from 20% to 33%) and by nearly half among 12th graders (from 27% to 39%). The use of other drugs, including LSD, other hallucinogens, inhalants, stimulants, barbiturates, and cocaine and crack, has also begun rising gradually among students.
5. About 3.5% of high school seniors drink alcohol daily, and when surveyed, 29.8% had had five or more drinks in a row at least once in the previous 2 weeks.
6. In 1995 marijuana use, in particular, continued the strong resurgence that began in the early 1990s.

Health-care providers should be aware of drug effects, the health consequences of drugs, and the management of drug abuse. If the practitioner is uncomfortable with management, he or she should be prepared to refer the teenager to appropriate local resources.

DEFINITIONS

Some definitions of terms are useful to keep in mind when one is dealing with the issue of drugs. A task force of the Panels on Alcoholism and Drug Abuse of the American Medical Association's Council on Scientific Affairs conducted a survey of substance abuse experts to help develop standard definitions (Rinaldi et al., 1988).

1. *Drug abuse:* Any use of drugs that causes physical, psychological, economic, legal, or social harm to the individual user or to others affected by the drug user's behavior.
2. *Drug intoxication:* Changes in physiological functioning, psychological functioning, mood states, cognitive processes, or all of these, as a consequence of excessive consumption of a drug; usually disruptive.

3. *Drug addiction:* Chronic disorder characterized by the compulsive use of a substance resulting in progressive physical, psychological, or social harm to the user and by continued use despite that harm.

4. *Psychological dependence:* The emotional state of craving a drug either for its positive effect or to avoid negative effects associated with its absence.

5. *Physical dependence:* A physiological state of adaptation to a drug, usually characterized by the development of tolerance to drug effects and the emergence of a withdrawal syndrome during prolonged abstinence.

6. *Depressants:* Depressants include sedatives and minor and major tranquilizers.
   a. *Sedatives:* Drugs that reduce anxiety and induce sleep. Sedatives can lead to physical and psychological dependence.
      — Alcohol
      — Barbiturates
      — Methaqualone (Quaalude, no longer legally available)
      — Glutethimide (Doriden)
   b. *Minor tranquilizers:* Drugs that reduce anxiety. Included in this group are diazepam (Valium), alprazolam (Xanax), and chlordiazepoxide (Librium). Physical and psychological dependence commonly occurs with these drugs.
   c. *Major tranquilizers:* This group includes the phenothiazines, such as thioridazine (Mellaril), trifluoperazine (Stelazine), and chlorpromazine (Thorazine).

7. *Stimulants:* Stimulants produce tolerance and strong psychological dependence. Physical dependence was previously thought to occur only to a mild degree or not at all. It is now well established that a physical withdrawal syndrome indicating physical dependence occurs in this class of drugs. In addition, this class of drugs is clearly able to affect the mesolimbic reward systems of the central nervous system in such a way as to induce intense cravings and profoundly influence preconscious drives to use. The central-nervous-system stimulants, which cause increased alertness and activity, include:
   a. Amphetamines (methamphetamine)
   b. Nicotine
   c. Caffeine
   d. Cocaine

8. *Hallucinogens:* These drugs affect sensations, emotions, and awareness, causing distortion of perceived reality. They can produce tolerance and psychological dependence but no physical dependence.
   a. LSD (D-lysergic acid diethylamide)
   b. Mescaline
   c. DMT (dimethyltryptamine)
   d. DOM (2.5-dimethoxy-4-methylamphetamine)
   e. PCP (phencyclidine hydrochloride)
   f. Psilocybin/psilocin
   g. MDA (methylene dioxyamphetamine)
   h. MDMA (methylene dioxymethamphetamine)

9. *Opiates:* Opiates are used to relieve pain. They produce tolerance and strong physical and psychological dependence. Included in this class of drugs are:
   a. Morphine
   b. Heroin
   c. Codeine
   d. Meperidine (Demerol)
   e. Methadone

10. *Volatile solvents:* These drugs have a general depressant effect on the central nervous system and may create hallucinogenic experiences. They include glue, cement, deodorant

spray, gasoline, and cleaning solution. They can produce tolerance and psychological dependence but no true physical dependence.

11. *Anabolic-androgenic steroids:* These drugs are synthetic derivatives of testosterone, engineered by chemists to have a longer half-life (testosterone activity is measured in minutes) and less androgenic activity. Most in use today are orally active alkylated testosterone analogs or injectable testosterone esters. They are used in cycles of 6–12 weeks, with combining of oral and injectable agents—called "stacking."

PREVALENCE OF DRUG USE

Most of the prevalence data on drug use during adolescence and young adulthood come from the National Institute on Drug Abuse, which has published an annual survey of high school seniors since 1975, the Monitoring the Future Study. This survey (Johnston et al., 1995a) includes approximately 50,000 students from 400 public and private high schools. In addition, since 1977, a total of 1200 college students and 11,000 young adult post–high school graduates have been followed up. In 1995 (Johnston et al., 1995a), 48.4% of teenagers had tried some illegal drug by their senior year, and about 28.1% of teenagers had tried some illicit drug other than marijuana. The incidence of drug use is the highest among 18- to 25-year-old young adults. In 1994, 45.5% of college students and almost 60% of young adults 19–28 years of age had tried some illicit drug. The onset of use is most common between the ages of 13 and 15 years. Although use of drugs such as heroin, PCP, LSD, and marijuana is highly publicized, the two most commonly used drugs and the two that have the most potential for killing and disabling youth are nicotine and alcohol.

- Table 69.1 shows the prevalence of drug use among 8th, 10th, and 12th graders in 1995.
- Figure 69.1 illustrates the lifetime prevalence and recency of use of 12 types of drugs for high school seniors in the class of 1995.
- Tables 69.2 through 69.5 illustrate the trends in the lifetime prevalence, annual prevalence, 30-day prevalence, and 30-day daily prevalence, respectively, of drug use among high school seniors.
- Table 69.6 shows trends in lifetime prevalence of various types of drugs among college students 1–4 years beyond high school.
- Figure 69.2 shows trends in lifetime prevalence of marijuana use and of any illicit drug among high school seniors.
- Figure 69.3 displays trends in the annual prevalence of illicit drug use in comparison with illicit drugs other than marijuana for the class of 1995.
- Figure 69.4 suggests some disturbing trends in the annual use of marijuana, LSD and other psychedelics, inhalants, and amphetamines.
- Figure 69.5 illustrates, for the same cohort, the trends in perceived availability, perceived risk of regular use, and prevalence of use of marijuana in 12th graders during the preceding 30 days.
- Figure 69.6 illustrates trends in perceived availability, perceived risk of trying, and prevalence of use of cocaine in 12th graders during the past year.
- Figure 69.7 compares lifetime use of selected drugs by grade in school of users, in 1995.
- Figure 69.8 shows trends in annual prevalence of use of alcohol, marijuana, and cocaine by college students.

Data are also available from the National School-Based Youth Risk Behavior Survey. Table 69.7 shows the drug use among youth aged 12–21 years in 1991.

Text continued on page 997.

TABLE 69.1.   Prevalence of Various Drug Use for 8th, 10th, and 12th Graders, 1995 (Percent)

	Ever Used	Used in Past Year	Used in Past Month	Uses Daily
Any illicit drug[a]				
8th Grade	28.5	21.4	12.4	—
10th Grade	40.9	33.3	20.2	—
12th Grade	48.4	39.0	23.8	—
Any illicit drug[a]				
Other than marijuana				
8th Grade	18.8	12.6	6.5	—
10th Grade	24.3	17.5	8.9	—
12th Grade	28.1	19.4	10.0	—
Marijuana/hashish				
8th Grade	19.9	15.8	9.1	0.8
10th Grade	34.1	28.7	17.2	2.8
12th Grade	41.7	34.7	21.2	4.6
Inhalants[b,c]				
8th Grade	21.6	12.8	6.1	0.2
10th Grade	19.0	9.6	3.5	0.1
12th Grade	17.4	8.0	3.2	0.1
Nitrites[d]				
8th Grade	—	—	—	—
10th Grade	—	—	—	—
12th Grade	1.5	1.1	0.4	0.2
Hallucinogens[c]				
8th Grade	5.2	3.6	1.7	0.1
10th Grade	9.3	7.2	3.3	*
12th Grade	12.7	9.3	4.4	0.1
LSD				
8th Grade	4.4	3.2	1.4	*
10th Grade	8.4	6.5	3.0	*
12th Grade	11.7	8.4	4.0	0.1
PCP[d]				
8th Grade	—	—	—	—
10th Grade	—	—	—	—
12th Grade	2.7	1.8	0.6	0.3

Adapted from Johnston LD, O'Malley PM, Bachman JG. Monitoring the Future Study. Ann Arbor: News and Information Services of the University of Michigan, December 1995.

Level of significance of difference between the 2 years: $s = 0.05$, $ss = 0.01$, $sss = 0.001$. *Em dash* indicates data not available. *Asterisk* indicates less than 0.05%. Any apparent inconsistency between the change estimate and the prevalence estimates for the 2 years is due to rounding error.

Approximate N: 8th Grade = 17,500 in 1995
                 10th Grade = 17,000 in 1995
                 12th Grade = 15,400 in 1995

[a]For 12th graders: Use of "any illicit drugs" includes any use of marijuana, LSD, other hallucinogens, crack, other cocaine, or heroin, *or* any use of other opiates, stimulants, barbiturates, or tranquilizers not under physician's orders. For 8th and 10th graders: The use of other opiates and barbiturates has been excluded because these younger respondents appear to overreport use (perhaps because they include the use of nonprescription drugs in their answers).

[b]For 12th graders only: Data based on five of six forms; N is five-sixths of N indicated.

[c]Inhalants are unadjusted for underreporting of amyl and butyl nitrites; hallucinogens are unadjusted for underreporting of PCP.

[d]For 8th, 10th, and 12th graders: Data based on one form; N for 12th graders is one-sixth of N indicated and N for 8th and 10th graders is one-half of N indicated.

[e]For 12th graders only: Data based on four of five forms; N is four-sixths of N indicated.

[f]In 1995 the heroin question was changed in half of the questionnaire forms. Separate questions were asked for use with injection and without injection. Data presented here represents the combined data from all forms.

[g]Only drug use which was not under a doctor's orders is included here.

[h]For 12th graders: Data based on two of six forms; N is two-sixths of N indicated.

[i]For all grades: In 1993 the question text was changed slightly in half of the forms to indicate that a "drink" meant "more than a few sips." The data in the upper line for alcohol came from forms using the original wording, while the data in the lower line came from forms using the revised wording. In 1993, each line of data was based on one of two forms for the 8th and 10th graders and on three of six forms for 12th graders. N is half of N indicated for all groups. Data for 1994–1995 were based on all forms for all grades.

TABLE 69.1.   *continued*

	Ever Used	Used in Past Year	Used in Past Month	Uses Daily
Cocaine				
8th Grade	4.2	2.6	1.2	0.1
10th Grade	5.0	3.5	1.7	0.1
12th Grade	6.0	4.0	1.8	0.2
Crack[e]				
8th Grade	2.7	1.6	0.7	*
10th Grade	2.8	1.8	0.9	*
12th Grade	3.0	2.1	1.0	0.1
Heroin[f]				
8th Grade	2.3	1.4	0.6	*
10th Grade	1.7	1.1	0.6	*
12th Grade	1.6	1.1	0.6	0.1
Other opiates[g]				
8th Grade	—	—	—	—
10th Grade	—	—	—	—
12th Grade	7.2	4.7	1.8	0.1
Stimulants[g]				
8th Grade	13.1	8.7	4.2	0.2
10th Grade	17.4	11.9	5.3	0.2
12th Grade	15.3	9.3	4.0	0.3
Ice[h]				
8th Grade	—	—	—	—
10th Grade	—	—	—	—
12th Grade	3.9	2.4	1.1	0.1
Barbiturates[g]				
8th Grade	—	—	—	—
10th Grade	—	—	—	—
12th Grade	7.4	4.7	2.2	0.1
Tranquilizers[g]				
8th Grade	4.5	2.7	1.2	0.1
10th Grade	6.0	4.0	1.7	*
12th Grade	7.1	4.4	1.8	0.1
Alcohol[i]				
Any use				
8th Grade	54.5	45.3	24.6	0.7
10th Grade	70.5	63.5	38.8	1.7
12th Grade	80.7	73.7	51.3	3.5
5+ Drinks in last 2 weeks				
8th Grade	—	—	—	14.5
10th Grade	—	—	—	24.0
12th Grade	—	—	—	29.8
Been drunk[h]				
8th Grade	25.3	18.4	8.3	0.2
10th Grade	46.9	38.5	20.8	0.6
12th Grade	63.2	52.5	33.2	1.3
Cigarettes				
Any use				
8th Grade	46.4	—	19.1	9.3
10th Grade	57.6	—	27.9	16.3
12th Grade	64.2	—	33.5	21.6
1/2 pack+/day				
8th Grade	—	—	—	3.4
10th Grade	—	—	—	8.3
12th Grade	—	—	—	12.4
Smokeless tobacco[d]				
8th Grade	20.0	—	7.1	1.2
10th Grade	27.6	—	9.7	2.7
12th Grade	30.9	—	12.2	3.6
Steroids[h]				
8th Grade	2.0	1.0	0.6	*
10th Grade	2.0	1.2	0.6	0.1
12th Grade	2.3	1.5	0.7	0.2

TABLE 69.2. Long-Term Trends in *Lifetime* Prevalence of Various Types of Drugs for 12th Graders

Percent Ever Used

	Class of 1975	Class of 1976	Class of 1977	Class of 1978	Class of 1979	Class of 1980	Class of 1981	Class of 1982	Class of 1983	Class of 1984	Class of 1985	Class of 1986	Class of 1987	Class of 1988	Class of 1989	Class of 1990	Class of 1991	Class of 1992	Class of 1993	Class of 1994	Class of 1995	1994–1995 Change
Approximate N =	9,400	15,400	17,100	17,800	15,500	15,900	17,500	17,700	16,300	15,900	16,000	15,200	16,300	16,300	16,700	15,200	15,000	15,800	16,300	15,400	15,400	
Any illicit drug[a,b]	55.2	58.3	61.6	64.1	65.1	65.4	65.6	64.4	62.9	61.6	60.6	57.6	56.6	53.9	50.9	47.9	44.1	40.7	42.9	45.6	48.4	+2.8
Any illicit drug other than marijuana[a,b]	36.2	35.4	35.8	36.5	37.4	38.7	42.8	41.1	40.4	40.3	39.7	37.7	35.8	32.5	31.4	29.4	26.9	25.1	26.7	27.6	28.1	+0.5
Marijuana/hashish	47.3	52.8	56.4	59.2	60.4	60.3	59.5	58.7	57.0	54.9	54.2	50.9	50.2	47.2	43.7	40.7	36.7	32.6	35.3	38.2	41.7	+3.5s
Inhalants[c]	—	10.3	11.1	12.0	12.7	11.9	12.3	12.8	13.6	14.4	15.4	15.9	17.0	16.7	17.6	18.0	17.6	16.6	17.4	17.7	17.4	−0.3
Inhalants, adjusted[a,c,d]	—	—	—	—	18.2	17.3	17.2	17.7	18.2	18.0	18.1	20.1	18.6	17.5	18.6	18.5	18.0	17.0	17.7	18.3	17.8	−0.5
Amyl and butyl nitrites[e,f]	—	—	—	—	11.1	11.1	10.1	9.8	8.4	8.1	7.9	8.6	4.7	3.2	3.3	2.1	1.6	1.5	1.4	1.7	1.5	−0.2
Hallucinogens	16.3	15.1	13.9	14.3	14.1	13.3	13.3	12.5	11.9	10.7	10.3	9.7	10.3	8.9	9.4	9.4	9.6	9.2	10.9	11.4	12.7	+1.3
Hallucinogens, adjusted[g]	—	—	—	—	17.7	15.6	15.3	14.3	13.6	12.3	12.1	11.9	10.6	9.2	9.9	9.7	10.0	9.4	11.3	11.7	13.1	+1.4
LSD	11.3	11.0	9.8	9.7	9.5	9.3	9.8	9.6	8.9	8.0	7.5	7.2	8.4	7.7	8.3	8.7	8.8	8.6	10.3	10.5	11.7	+1.2
PCP[e,f]	—	—	—	—	12.8	9.6	7.8	6.0	5.6	5.0	4.9	4.8	3.0	2.9	3.9	2.8	2.9	2.4	2.9	2.8	2.7	−0.1
Cocaine	9.0	9.7	10.8	12.9	15.4	15.7	16.5	16.0	16.2	16.1	17.3	16.9	15.2	12.1	10.3	9.4	7.8	6.1	6.1	5.9	6.0	+0.1
Crack[h]	—	—	—	—	—	—	—	—	—	—	—	—	5.4	4.8	4.7	3.5	3.1	2.6	2.6	3.0	3.0	0.0
Other cocaine[i]	—	—	—	—	—	—	—	—	—	—	—	—	14.0	12.1	8.5	8.6	7.0	5.3	5.4	5.2	5.1	−0.1
Heroin	2.2	1.8	1.8	1.6	1.1	1.1	1.1	1.2	1.2	1.3	1.2	1.1	1.2	1.1	1.3	1.3	0.9	1.2	1.1	1.2	1.6	+0.4s
Other opiates[k]	9.0	9.6	10.3	9.9	10.1	9.8	10.1	9.6	9.4	9.7	10.2	9.0	9.2	8.6	8.3	8.3	6.6	6.1	6.4	6.6	7.2	+0.6
Stimulants[b,k]	22.3	22.6	23.0	22.9	24.2	26.4	32.2	27.9	26.9	27.9	26.2	23.4	21.6	19.8	19.1	17.5	15.4	13.9	15.1	15.7	15.3	−0.4
Crystal meth. (ice)[j]	—	—	—	—	—	—	—	—	—	—	—	—	—	—	—	2.7	3.3	2.9	3.1	3.4	3.9	+0.5
Sedatives[k,m]	18.2	17.7	17.4	16.0	14.6	14.9	16.0	15.2	14.4	13.3	11.8	10.4	8.7	7.8	7.4	7.5	6.7	6.1	6.4	7.3	7.6	+0.3
Barbiturates[k]	16.9	16.2	15.6	13.7	11.8	11.0	11.3	10.3	9.9	9.9	9.2	8.4	7.4	6.7	6.5	6.8	6.2	5.5	6.3	7.0	7.4	+0.4
Methaqualone[b,m]	8.1	7.8	8.5	7.9	8.3	9.5	10.6	10.7	10.1	8.3	6.7	5.2	4.0	3.3	2.7	2.3	1.3	1.6	0.8	1.4	1.2	−0.2
Tranquilizers[k]	17.0	16.8	18.0	17.0	16.3	15.2	14.7	14.0	13.3	12.4	11.9	10.9	10.9	9.4	7.6	7.2	7.2	6.0	6.4	6.6	7.1	+0.5
Alcohol[n]	90.4	91.9	92.5	93.1	93.0	93.2	92.6	92.8	92.6	92.6	92.2	91.3	92.2	92.0	90.7	89.5	88.0	87.5	87.0	80.4	80.7	+0.3
Been drunk[l]	—	—	—	—	—	—	—	—	—	—	—	—	—	—	—	—	—	—	80.0	—	—	+0.3
Cigarettes[l]	73.6	75.4	75.7	75.3	74.0	71.0	71.0	70.1	70.6	69.7	68.8	67.6	67.2	66.4	65.7	64.4	63.1	61.8	61.9	62.0	64.2	+2.2s
Smokeless tobacco[e]	—	—	—	—	—	—	—	—	—	—	—	31.4	32.2	30.4	29.2	—	—	32.4	31.0	30.7	30.9	+0.2
Steroids[l]	—	—	—	—	—	—	—	—	—	—	—	—	—	—	3.0	2.9	2.1	2.1	2.0	2.4	2.3	−0.1

From Johnston LD, O'Malley PM, Bachman JG. Monitoring the Future Study. Ann Arbor: News and Information Services of the University of Michigan, December 1995.

Level of significance of difference between the two most recent classes: $s = 0.05$, $ss = 0.01$, $sss = 0.001$. *Em dash* indicates data not available.

[a]Use of "any illicit drugs" includes any use of marijuana, hallucinogens, cocaine, or heroin, or any use of other opiates, stimulants, barbiturates, methaqualone (excluded since 1990), or tranquilizers not under a physician's orders.

[b]Beginning in 1982 the question about stimulant use (i.e., amphetamines) was revised to get respondents to exclude the inappropriate reporting of nonprescription stimulants. The prevalence rate dropped slightly as a result of this methodological change.

[c]Data based on four of five forms in 1976–1988; N is four-fifths of N indicated. Data based on five of six forms in 1989–1995; N is five-sixths of N indicated.

[d]Adjusted for underreporting of amyl and butyl nitrites. See text for details.

[e]Data based on a single questionnaire form; N is one-fifth of N indicated in 1979–1988 and one-sixth of N indicated in 1989–1995.

[f]Question text changed slightly in 1987.

[g]Adjusted for underreporting of PCP. See text for details.

[h]Data based on one of five forms in 1986; N is one-fifth of N indicated. Data based on two questionnaire forms in 1987–1989; N is two-fifths of N indicated in 1987–1988 and two-sixths of N indicated in 1989. Data based on six questionnaire forms in 1990–1995.

[i]Data based on a single questionnaire form in 1987–1989; N is one-fifth of N indicated in 1987–1988 and one-sixth of N indicated in 1989. Data based on four of six forms in 1990–1995; N is four-sixths of N indicated.

[j]In 1995 the heroin question was changed in half of the questionnaire forms. Separate questions were asked for use with injection and without injection. Data presented here represents the combined data from all forms.

[k]Only drug use that was not under a physician's orders is included here.

[l]Data based on two of six forms; N is two-sixths of N indicated. Steroid data based on one of six forms in 1989–1990; N is one-sixth of N indicated in 1989–1990. Steroid data based on two of six forms since 1991; N is two-sixths of N indicated since 1991.

[m]Sedatives: Data based on five questionnaire forms in 1975–1988, six questionnaire forms in 1989, one questionnaire form in 1990 (N is one-sixth of N indicated in 1990), and six questionnaire forms beginning in 1991. Methaqualone: Data based on five forms in 1975–1988, six forms in 1989, and one of six forms beginning in 1990 (N is one-sixth of N indicated beginning in 1990).

[n]Data based on five questionnaire forms in 1975–1988 and on six questionnaire forms in 1989–1992. In 1993 the question text was changed slightly in three forms to indicate that a "drink" meant "more than a few sips." The data in the upper line for alcohol came from the three forms using the original wording; the data in the lower line came from the three forms using the revised wording (N is three-sixths of N indicated). Data for 1994–1995 were based on all six forms.

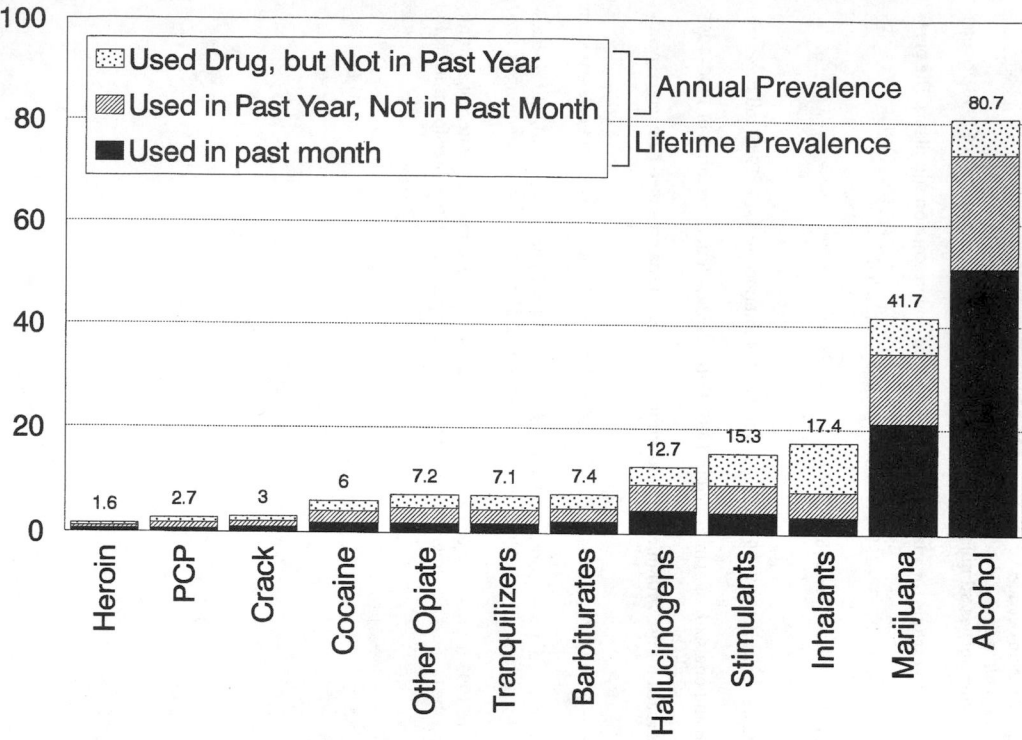

Figure 69.1.   Prevalence and recency of use of 12 types of drugs, class of 1995. (Adapted from Johnston LD, O'Malley PM, Bachman JG. Monitoring the Future Study. Ann Arbor: News and Information Services of the University of Michigan, December 1995).

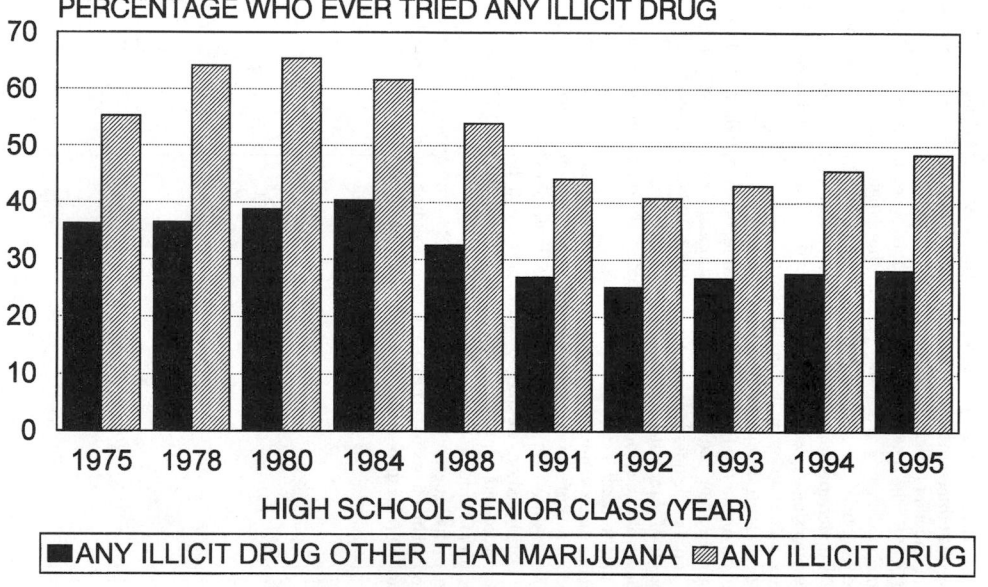

Figure 69.2.   Trends in lifetime prevalence of marijuana use and of any illicit drug among high school seniors (Adapted from Johnston LD, O'Malley PM, Bachman JG. Monitoring the Future Study. Ann Arbor: News and Information Services of the University of Michigan, December 1995).

TABLE 69.3. Long-Term Trends in *Annual* Prevalence of Various Types of Drugs for 12th Graders

Percent Who Used in Past 12 Months

	Class of 1975	Class of 1976	Class of 1977	Class of 1978	Class of 1979	Class of 1980	Class of 1981	Class of 1982	Class of 1983	Class of 1984	Class of 1985	Class of 1986	Class of 1987	Class of 1988	Class of 1989	Class of 1990	Class of 1991	Class of 1992	Class of 1993	Class of 1994	Class of 1995	1994–1995 Change
Approximate N =	9400	15,400	17,100	17,800	15,500	15,900	17,500	17,700	16,300	15,900	16,000	15,200	16,300	16,300	16,700	15,200	15,000	15,800	16,300	15,400	15,400	
Any illicit drug[a,b]	45.0	48.1	51.1	53.8	54.2	53.1	52.1	49.4	47.4	45.8	46.3	44.3	41.7	38.5	35.4	32.5	29.4	27.1	31.0	35.8	39.0	+3.2s
Any illicit drug other than marijuana[a,b]	26.2	25.4	26.0	27.1	28.2	30.4	34.0	30.1	28.4	28.0	27.4	25.9	24.1	21.1	20.0	17.9	16.2	14.9	17.1	18.0	19.4	+1.4
Marijuana/hashish	40.0	44.5	47.6	50.2	50.8	48.8	46.1	44.3	42.3	40.0	40.6	38.8	36.3	33.1	29.6	27.0	23.9	21.9	26.0	30.7	34.7	+4.0ss
Inhalants[c]	—	3.0	3.7	4.1	5.4	4.6	4.1	4.5	4.3	5.1	5.7	6.1	6.9	6.5	5.9	6.9	6.6	6.2	7.0	7.7	8.0	+0.3
Inhalants, adjusted[c,d]	—	—	—	—	8.9	7.9	6.1	6.6	6.2	7.2	7.5	8.9	8.1	7.1	6.9	7.5	6.9	6.4	7.4	8.2	8.4	+0.2
Amyl/butyl nitrites[e,f]	—	—	—	—	6.5	5.7	3.7	3.6	3.6	4.0	4.0	4.7	2.6	1.7	1.7	1.4	0.9	0.5	0.9	1.1	1.1	0.0
Hallucinogens	11.2	9.4	8.8	9.6	9.9	9.3	9.0	8.1	7.3	6.5	6.3	6.0	6.4	5.5	5.6	5.5	5.8	5.9	7.4	7.6	9.3	+1.7ss
Hallucinogens, adjusted[g]	—	—	—	—	11.8	10.4	10.1	9.0	8.3	7.3	7.6	7.6	6.7	5.8	6.2	6.0	6.1	6.2	7.8	7.8	9.7	+1.9ss
LSD	7.2	6.4	5.5	6.3	6.6	6.5	6.5	6.1	5.4	4.7	4.4	4.5	5.2	4.8	4.9	5.4	5.2	5.6	6.8	6.9	8.4	+1.5ss
PCP[e,f]	—	—	—	—	7.0	4.4	3.2	2.2	2.6	2.3	2.9	2.4	1.3	1.2	2.4	1.2	1.4	1.4	1.4	1.6	1.8	+0.2
Cocaine	5.6	6.0	7.2	9.0	12.0	12.3	12.4	11.5	11.4	11.6	13.1	12.7	10.3	7.9	6.5	5.3	3.5	3.1	3.3	3.6	4.0	+0.4
Crack[h]	—	—	—	—	—	—	—	—	—	—	—	4.1	3.9	3.1	3.1	1.9	1.5	1.5	1.5	1.9	2.1	+0.2
Other cocaine[i]	—	—	—	—	—	—	—	—	—	—	—	4.1	9.8	7.4	5.2	4.6	3.2	2.6	2.9	3.0	3.4	+0.4
Heroin[j]	1.0	0.8	0.8	0.8	0.5	0.5	0.5	0.6	0.6	0.5	0.6	0.5	0.5	0.5	0.6	0.5	0.4	0.6	0.5	0.6	1.1	+0.5sss
Other opiates[k]	5.7	5.7	6.4	6.0	6.2	6.3	5.9	5.3	5.1	5.2	5.9	5.2	5.3	4.6	4.4	4.5	3.5	3.3	3.6	3.8	4.7	+0.9ss
Stimulants[h,k]	16.2	15.8	16.3	17.1	18.3	20.8	26.0	20.3	17.9	17.7	15.8	13.4	12.2	10.9	10.8	9.1	8.2	7.1	8.4	9.4	9.3	−0.1
Crystal meth. (ice)	—	—	—	—	—	—	—	—	—	—	—	—	—	—	—	1.3	1.4	1.3	1.7	1.8	2.4	+0.6
Sedatives[k,m]	11.7	10.7	10.8	9.9	9.9	10.3	10.5	9.1	7.9	6.6	5.8	5.2	4.1	3.7	3.7	3.5	3.6	2.9	3.4	4.2	4.9	+0.7s
Barbiturates[k]	10.7	9.6	9.3	8.1	7.5	6.8	6.6	5.5	5.2	4.9	4.6	4.2	3.6	3.2	3.3	3.4	3.4	2.8	3.4	4.1	4.7	+0.6
Methaqualone[k,m]	5.1	4.7	5.2	4.9	5.9	7.2	7.6	6.8	5.4	3.8	2.8	2.1	1.5	1.3	1.3	0.7	0.5	0.6	0.2	0.8	0.7	−0.1
Tranquilizers[k]	10.6	10.3	10.8	9.9	9.6	8.7	8.0	7.0	6.9	6.1	6.1	5.8	5.5	4.8	3.8	3.5	3.6	2.8	3.5	3.7	4.4	+0.7s
Alcohol[n]	84.8	85.7	87.0	87.7	88.1	87.9	87.0	86.8	87.3	86.0	85.6	84.5	85.7	85.3	82.7	80.6	77.7	76.8	76.0	73.0	73.7	+0.7
Been drunk[l]	—	—	—	—	—	—	—	—	—	—	—	—	—	—	—	—	52.7	50.3	49.6	51.7	52.5	+0.8
Steroids[l]	—	—	—	—	—	—	—	—	—	—	—	—	—	—	1.9	1.7	1.4	1.1	1.2	1.3	1.5	+0.2

From Johnston LD, O'Malley PM, Bachman JG. Monitoring the Future Study. Ann Arbor: News and Information Services of the University of Michigan, December 1995.
Level of significance of difference between the two most recent classes: s = 0.05, ss = 0.01, sss = 0.001. *Em dash* indicates data not available. See Table 69.2 for relevant footnotes.

TABLE 69.4. Long-Term Trends in *30-Day* Prevalence of Various Types of Drugs for 12th Graders

Percent Who Used in Last 30 Days

	Class of 1975	Class of 1976	Class of 1977	Class of 1978	Class of 1979	Class of 1980	Class of 1981	Class of 1982	Class of 1983	Class of 1984	Class of 1985	Class of 1986	Class of 1987	Class of 1988	Class of 1989	Class of 1990	Class of 1991	Class of 1992	Class of 1993	Class of 1994	Class of 1995	1994–1995 Change
Approximate N =	9400	15,400	17,100	17,800	15,500	15,900	17,500	17,700	16,300	15,900	16,000	15,200	16,300	16,300	16,700	15,200	15,000	15,800	16,300	15,400	15,400	
Any illicit drug[a,b]	30.7	34.2	37.6	38.9	38.9	37.2	36.9	32.5	30.5	29.2	29.7	27.1	24.7	21.3	19.7	17.2	16.4	14.4	18.3	21.9	23.8	+1.9
Any illicit drug other than marijuana[a,b]	15.4	13.9	15.2	15.1	16.8	18.4	21.7	17.0	15.4	15.1	14.9	13.2	11.6	10.0	9.1	8.0	7.1	6.3	7.9	8.8	10.0	+1.2s
Marijuana/hashish	27.1	32.2	35.4	37.1	36.5	33.7	31.6	28.5	27.0	25.2	25.7	23.4	21.0	18.0	16.7	14.0	13.8	11.9	15.5	19.0	21.2	+2.2s
Inhalants[c]	—	0.9	1.3	1.5	1.7	1.4	1.5	1.5	1.7	1.9	2.2	2.5	2.8	2.6	2.3	2.7	2.4	2.3	2.5	2.7	3.2	+0.5
Inhalants, adjusted[c,d]	—	—	—	—	3.2	2.7	2.5	2.5	2.5	2.6	3.0	3.2	3.5	3.0	2.7	2.9	2.6	2.5	2.8	2.9	3.5	+0.6
Amyl/butyl nitrites[e,f]	—	—	—	—	2.4	1.8	1.4	1.1	1.4	1.4	1.6	1.3	1.3	0.6	0.6	0.6	0.4	0.3	0.6	0.4	0.4	0.0
Hallucinogens	4.7	3.4	4.1	3.9	4.0	3.7	3.7	3.4	2.8	2.6	2.5	2.5	2.5	2.2	2.2	2.2	2.2	2.1	2.7	3.1	4.4	+1.3sss
Hallucinogens, adjusted[g]	—	—	—	—	5.3	4.4	4.5	4.1	3.5	3.2	3.8	3.5	2.8	2.3	2.9	2.3	2.4	2.3	3.3	3.2	4.6	+1.4sss
LSD	2.3	1.9	2.1	2.1	2.4	2.3	2.5	2.4	1.9	1.5	1.6	1.7	1.8	1.8	1.8	1.9	1.9	2.0	2.4	2.6	4.0	+1.4sss
PCP[f]	—	—	—	—	2.4	1.4	1.4	1.0	1.3	1.0	1.6	1.3	0.6	0.3	1.4	0.4	0.5	0.6	1.0	0.7	0.6	-0.1
Cocaine	1.9	2.0	2.9	3.9	5.7	5.2	5.8	5.0	4.9	5.8	6.7	6.2	4.3	3.4	2.8	1.9	1.4	1.3	1.3	1.5	1.8	+0.3
Crack[h]	—	—	—	—	—	—	—	—	—	—	—	—	1.3	1.6	1.4	0.7	0.7	0.6	0.7	0.8	1.0	+0.2
Other cocaine[i]	—	—	—	—	—	—	—	—	—	—	—	—	4.1	3.2	1.9	1.7	1.2	1.0	1.2	1.3	1.3	0.0
Heroin[j]	0.4	0.2	0.3	0.3	0.2	0.2	0.2	0.2	0.2	0.3	0.3	0.2	0.2	0.2	0.3	0.2	0.2	0.3	0.2	0.3	0.6	+0.3sss
Other opiates[k,m]	2.1	2.0	2.8	2.1	2.4	2.4	2.1	1.8	1.8	1.8	2.3	2.0	1.8	1.6	1.6	1.5	1.1	1.2	1.3	1.5	1.8	+0.3
Stimulants[j,k]	8.5	7.7	8.8	8.7	9.9	12.1	15.8	10.7	8.9	8.3	6.8	5.5	5.2	4.6	4.2	3.7	3.2	2.8	3.7	4.0	4.0	0.0
Crystal meth. (ice)[l]	—	—	—	—	—	—	—	—	—	—	—	—	—	—	—	0.6	0.6	0.5	0.6	0.7	1.1	+0.4
Sedatives[k,m]	5.4	4.5	5.1	4.2	4.4	4.8	4.6	3.4	3.0	2.3	2.4	2.2	1.7	1.4	1.6	1.4	1.5	1.2	1.3	1.8	2.3	+0.5s
Barbiturates[k]	4.7	3.9	4.3	3.2	3.2	2.9	2.6	2.0	2.1	1.7	2.0	1.8	1.4	1.2	1.4	1.3	1.4	1.1	1.3	1.7	2.2	+0.5ss
Methaqualone[k,m]	2.1	1.6	2.3	1.9	2.3	3.3	3.1	2.4	1.8	1.1	1.0	0.8	0.6	0.5	0.6	0.2	0.2	0.4	0.1	0.4	0.4	0.0
Tranquilizers[k]	4.1	4.0	4.6	3.4	3.7	3.1	2.7	2.4	2.5	2.1	2.1	2.1	2.0	1.5	1.3	1.2	1.4	1.0	1.2	1.4	1.8	+0.4s
Alcohol[n]	68.2	68.3	71.2	72.1	71.8	72.0	70.7	69.7	69.4	67.2	65.9	65.3	66.4	63.9	60.0	57.1	54.0	51.3	51.0	50.1	51.3	—
Been drunk[l]	—	—	—	—	—	—	—	—	—	—	—	—	—	—	—	—	—	—	48.6	50.1	51.3	+1.2
Cigarettes	36.7	38.8	38.4	36.7	34.4	30.5	29.4	30.0	30.3	29.3	30.1	29.6	29.4	28.7	28.6	29.4	28.3	27.8	28.9	30.8	33.2	+2.4
Smokeless tobacco[e]	—	—	—	—	—	—	—	—	—	—	—	11.5	11.3	10.3	8.4	—	—	11.4	10.7	31.2	33.5	+2.3s
Steroids[l]	—	—	—	—	—	—	—	—	—	—	—	—	—	—	0.8	1.0	0.8	0.6	0.7	0.9	0.7	-0.2

From Johnston LD, O'Malley PM, Bachman JG. Monitoring the Future Study. Ann Arbor: News and Information Services of the University of Michigan, December 1995.
Level of significance of difference between the two most recent classes: $s = 0.05$, $ss = 0.01$, $sss = 0.001$. Em dash indicates data not available. See Table 69.2 for relevant footnotes.

TABLE 69.5. Long-Term Trends in 30-Day Prevalence of *Daily* Use of Various Types of Drugs for 12th Graders

Percent Who Used Daily in Last 30 Days

	Class of 1975	Class of 1976	Class of 1977	Class of 1978	Class of 1979	Class of 1980	Class of 1981	Class of 1982	Class of 1983	Class of 1984	Class of 1985	Class of 1986	Class of 1987	Class of 1988	Class of 1989	Class of 1990	Class of 1991	Class of 1992	Class of 1993	Class of 1994	Class of 1995	1994–1995 Change
Approximate N =	9400	15,400	17,100	17,800	15,500	15,900	17,500	17,700	16,300	15,900	16,000	15,200	16,300	16,300	16,700	15,200	15,000	15,800	16,300	15,400	15,400	
Marijuana/hashish	6.0	8.2	9.1	10.7	10.3	9.1	7.0	6.3	5.5	5.0	4.9	4.0	3.3	2.7	2.9	2.2	2.0	1.9	2.4	3.6	4.6	+1.0ss
Inhalants[c]	—	*	*	0.1	*	0.1	0.2	0.1	0.1	0.1	0.2	0.2	0.1	0.2	0.2	0.3	0.2	0.1	0.1	0.1	0.1	+0.1
Inhalants, adjusted[c,d]	—	—	—	—	0.1	0.2	0.2	0.2	0.2	0.2	0.4	0.4	0.4	0.3	0.3	0.3	0.5	0.2	0.2	0.2	0.2	—
Amyl/butyl nitrites[e,f]	—	—	—	—	*	0.1	0.1	0.0	0.2	0.1	0.3	0.5	0.3	0.3	0.3	0.1	0.5	0.2	0.2	0.2	0.2	-0.1
Hallucinogens	0.1	0.1	0.1	0.1	*	0.1	0.1	0.1	0.1	0.1	0.1	0.1	0.1	*	0.1	0.1	0.1	0.1	0.1	0.1	0.1	0.0
Hallucinogens, adjusted[g]	—	—	—	*	0.2	0.2	0.1	0.2	0.2	0.2	0.3	0.3	0.2	*	*	0.1	0.1	0.1	0.1	0.1	0.1	0.0
LSD	*	*	*	*	*	*	0.1	*	0.1	0.1	0.1	*	0.1	0.1	*	0.1	0.1	0.1	0.1	0.3	0.3	0.0
PCP[e,f]	—	—	—	—	0.2	0.2	0.3	0.2	0.1	0.1	0.4	0.3	0.3	0.3	0.2	0.1	0.1	0.1	0.1	0.2	0.2	0.0
Cocaine	0.1	0.1	0.1	0.1	0.2	0.2	0.3	0.2	0.2	0.2	0.4	0.4	0.3	0.2	0.3	0.1	0.1	0.1	0.1	0.1	0.2	+0.1
Crack[h]	—	—	—	—	—	—	—	—	—	—	—	—	0.1	0.1	0.1	0.1	0.1	0.1	0.1	0.1	0.1	0.0
Other cocaine[i]	—	—	—	—	—	—	—	—	—	—	—	—	0.2	0.2	0.1	0.1	0.1	*	0.1	0.1	0.1	+0.1
Heroin[j]	0.1	*	*	*	*	*	*	*	0.1	*	*	*	*	0.1	0.1	*	0.1	*	*	*	0.1	0.0
Other opiates[k]	0.1	0.1	0.2	0.1	0.1	0.1	0.1	0.1	0.1	0.1	0.1	0.1	0.1	0.1	0.2	0.2	0.1	0.2	0.2	0.1	0.3	+0.1
Stimulants[k]	0.5	0.4	0.5	0.5	0.6	0.7	1.2	0.7	0.8	0.6	0.4	0.3	0.3	0.3	0.3	0.2	0.2	0.2	0.2	0.2	0.3	0.0
Crystal meth. (ice)[l]	—	—	—	—	—	—	—	—	—	—	—	—	—	—	—	0.1	0.1	0.1	0.1	*	0.1	+0.1
Sedatives[k,m]	0.3	0.2	0.2	0.2	0.1	0.2	0.2	0.2	0.2	0.1	0.1	0.1	0.1	0.1	0.1	0.1	0.1	0.1	0.1	*	0.1	+0.1
Barbiturates[k]	0.1	0.1	0.2	0.1	*	0.1	0.1	0.1	0.1	*	0.1	0.1	0.1	*	0.1	0.1	0.1	0.1	0.1	*	0.1	+0.1
Methaqualone[b,m]	*	*	*	*	0.1	0.1	0.1	0.1	*	*	*	*	*	0.1	*	*	*	0.1	0.0	0.1	0.1	0.0
Tranquilizers[k]	0.1	0.2	0.3	0.1	0.1	0.1	0.1	0.1	0.1	0.1	*	*	0.1	*	0.1	0.1	0.1	*	*	0.1	0.1	0.0
Alcohol																						
Daily[n]	5.7	5.6	6.1	5.7	6.9	6.0	6.0	5.7	5.5	4.8	5.0	4.8	4.8	4.2	4.2	3.7	3.6	3.4	2.5	2.9	3.5	+0.6ss
Been drunk daily[l]	—	—	—	—	—	—	—	—	—	—	—	—	—	—	—	—	0.9	0.8	0.9	1.2	1.3	+0.1
5+ drinks in a row in last 2 wk	36.8	37.1	39.4	40.3	41.2	41.2	41.4	40.5	40.8	38.7	36.7	36.8	37.5	34.7	33.0	32.2	29.8	27.9	27.5	28.2	29.8	+1.6
Cigarettes																						
Daily	26.9	28.8	28.8	27.5	25.4	21.3	20.3	21.1	21.2	18.7	19.5	18.7	18.7	18.1	18.9	19.1	18.5	17.2	19.0	19.4	21.6	+2.2s
Half-pack or more per day	17.9	19.2	19.4	18.8	16.5	14.3	13.5	14.2	13.8	12.3	12.5	11.4	11.4	10.6	11.2	11.3	10.7	10.0	10.9	11.2	12.4	+1.2
Smokeless tobacco[e]	—	—	—	—	—	—	—	—	—	—	—	4.7	5.1	4.3	3.3	—	—	4.3	3.3	3.9	3.6	-0.4
Steroids[l]	—	—	—	—	—	—	—	—	—	—	—	—	—	—	0.1	0.2	0.1	0.1	0.1	0.4	0.2	-0.2

From Johnston LD, O'Malley PM, Bachman JG. Monitoring the Future Study. Ann Arbor: News and Information Services of the University of Michigan, December 1995.
Level of significance of difference between the two most recent classes: s = 0.05, ss = 0.01, sss = 0.001. *Em dash* indicates data not available. *Asterisk* indicates less than 0.05%. Any apparent inconsistency between the change estimate and the prevalence estimates for the two most recent classes is due to rounding error. See Table 69.2 for relevant footnotes.

TABLE 69.6. Trends in Lifetime[e] Prevalence of Various Types of Drugs among College Students 1–4 Years beyond High School

Percent Who Used in Lifetime

	1980	1981	1982	1983	1984	1985	1986	1987	1988	1989	1990	1991	1992	1993	1994	1993–1994 Change
Approx. Wtd. N =	(1040)	(1130)	(1150)	(1170)	(1110)	(1080)	(1190)	(1220)	(1310)	(1300)	(1400)	(1410)	(1490)	(1490)	(1410)	
Any illicit drug[f]	69.4	66.8	64.6	66.9	62.7	65.2	61.8	60.0	58.4	55.6	54.0	50.4	48.8	45.9	45.5	-0.4
Any illicit drug[f] other than marijuana	42.2	41.3	39.6	41.7	38.6	40.0	37.5	35.7	33.4	30.5	28.4	25.8	26.1	24.3	22.0	-2.4
Marijuana	65.0	63.3	60.5	63.1	59.0	60.6	57.9	55.8	54.3	51.3	49.1	46.3	44.1	42.0	42.2	+0.2
Inhalants[b]	10.2	8.8	10.6	11.0	10.4	10.6	11.0	13.2	12.6	15.0	13.9	14.4	14.2	14.8	12.0	-2.8s
Hallucinogens	15.0	12.0	15.0	12.2	12.9	11.4	11.2	10.9	10.2	10.7	11.2	11.3	12.0	11.8	10.0	-1.8
LSD	10.3	8.5	11.5	8.8	9.4	7.4	7.7	8.0	7.5	7.8	9.1	9.6	10.6	10.6	9.2	-1.4
Cocaine	22.0	21.5	22.4	23.1	21.7	22.9	23.3	20.6	15.8	14.6	11.4	9.4	7.9	6.3	5.0	-1.4
Crack[c]	NA	NA	NA	NA	NA	NA	NA	3.3	3.4	2.4	1.4	1.5	1.7	1.3	2.1	-0.4
MDMA ("ecstasy")[g]	NA	NA	NA	NA	NA	NA	NA	NA	NA	3.8	3.9	2.0	2.9	2.3	2.1	-0.2
Heroin	0.9	0.6	0.5	0.3	0.5	0.4	0.4	0.6	0.3	0.7	0.3	0.5	0.5	0.6	0.1	-0.5s
Other opiates[a]	8.9	8.3	8.1	8.4	8.9	6.3	8.8	7.6	6.3	7.6	6.8	7.3	7.3	6.2	5.1	-1.1
Stimulants[a]	29.5	29.4	30.1	27.8	27.8	25.4	22.3	19.8	17.7	14.6	13.2	13.0	10.5	10.1	9.2	-0.9
Stimulants, adjusted[a,d]	NA	NA	NA	NA	NA	NA	NA	NA	NA	NA	NA	NA	NA	NA	NA	NA
Crystal meth. (ice)[h]	NA	NA	NA	NA	NA	NA	NA	NA	NA	NA	1.0	1.3	0.6	1.6	1.3	-0.4
Sedatives[a]	13.7	14.2	14.1	12.2	10.8	9.3	8.0	6.1	4.7	4.1	NA	NA	NA	NA	NA	NA
Barbiturates[a]	8.1	7.8	8.2	6.6	6.4	4.9	5.4	3.5	3.6	3.2	3.8	3.5	3.8	3.5	3.2	-0.3
Methaqualone[a]	10.3	10.4	11.1	9.2	9.0	7.2	5.8	4.1	2.2	2.4	NA	NA	NA	NA	NA	NA
Tranquilizers[a]	15.2	11.4	11.7	10.8	10.8	9.8	10.7	8.7	8.0	8.0	7.1	6.8	6.9	6.3	4.4	-1.9s
Alcohol[i]	94.3	95.2	95.2	95.0	94.2	95.3	94.9	94.1	94.9	93.7	93.1	93.6	91.8	91.2	—	—
More than a few sips	NA	NA	NA	NA	NA	NA	NA	NA	NA	NA	NA	NA	NA	87.1	88.1	+1.0
Cigarettes	NA	NA	NA	NA	NA	NA	NA	NA	NA	NA	NA	NA	NA	NA	NA	NA

From Johnston LD, O'Malley PM, Bachman JG. The Monitoring the Future Study. Vol. II: college students and young adults. Ann Arbor: News and Information Services of the University of Michigan, 1994.

Level of significance of difference between the two most recent years: $s = 0.05$, $ss = 0.01$, $sss = 0.001$. Any apparent inconsistency between the change estimate and the prevalence estimates for the two most recent years is due to rounding. An *asterisk* indicates a percentage of less than 0.05%. NA indicates data not available.

[a]Only drug use which was not under a physician's orders is included here.

[b]This drug was asked about in four of the five questionnaire forms in 1980–1989, and in five of the six questionnaire forms in 1990–1994. Total N in 1994 (for college students) is 1175.

[c]This drug was asked about in two of the five questionnaire forms in 1987–1989, and in all six questionnaire forms in 1990–1994.

[d]Based on the data from the revised question, which attempts to exclude the inappropriate reporting of nonprescription stimulants.

[e]Data are uncorrected for cross-time inconsistencies in the answers.

[f]Use of "any illicit drug" includes any use of marijuana, hallucinogens, cocaine, and heroin, or any use of other opiates, stimulants, barbiturates, methaqualone (until 1990), or tranquilizers not under a physician's orders.

[g]This drug was asked about in two of the five questionnaire forms in 1989, and in two of the six questionnaire forms in 1990–1994. Total N in 1994 (for college students) is 470.

[h]This drug was asked about in two of the six questionnaire forms. Total N in 1994 (for college students) is 470.

[i]In 1993, the question text was changed slightly in three of the questionnaire forms to indicate that a "drink" meant "more than a few sips." The data in the upper line came from forms using the original wording (N was approximately 750 in 1993), while the data in the lower line came from forms using the revised wording. Data is based on all six forms again in 1994, using the revised question wording.

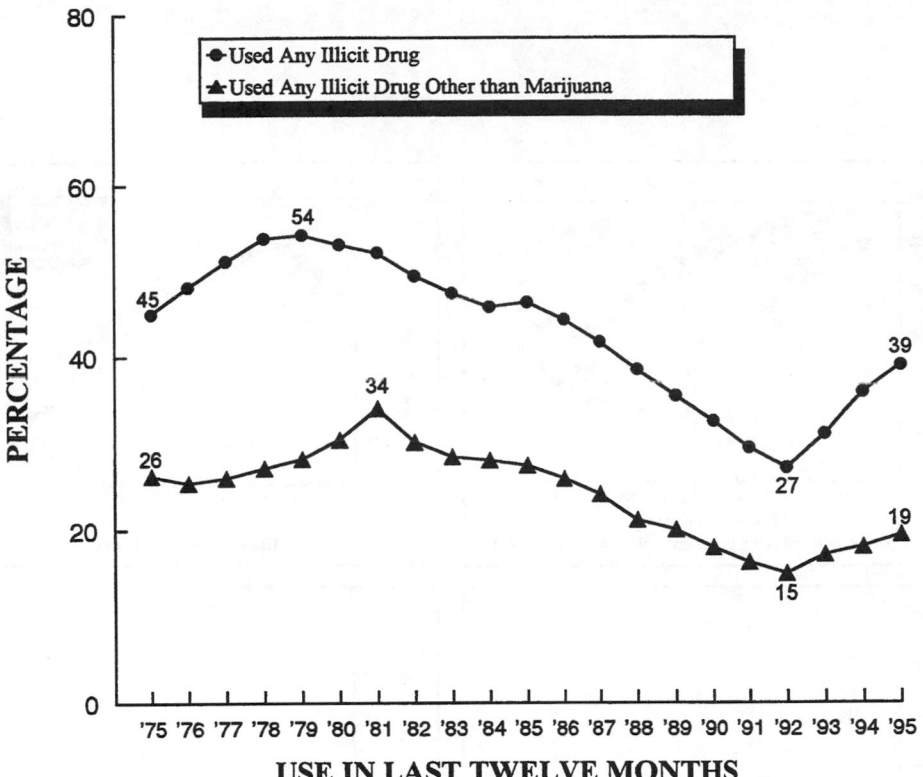

FIGURE 69.3.   Trends in annual prevalence of an illicit drug use index for 12th graders. Notes: Use of "any illicit drugs" includes any use of marijuana, hallucinogens, cocaine, and heroin, or any use not under a physician's orders of other opiates, stimulants, barbiturates, methaqualone (excluded since 1990), or tranquilizers. Beginning in 1982 the question about stimulant use (i.e., amphetamines) was revised to get respondents to exclude the inappropriate reporting on nonprescription stimulants. The prevalence rate dropped slightly as a result of this methodological change. (From Johnston LD, O'Malley PM, Bachman JG. Monitoring the Future Study. Ann Arbor: News and Information Services of the University of Michigan, December 1995.)

Cigarette Use

Cigarette use among teenagers was fairly steady for a decade but has been increasing for several years (21.6% daily use in 1995). Thirty percent of high school seniors currently smoke, a figure that has not fallen since 1979. There are currently about an equal number of adolescent female and adolescent male smokers. The rate of daily smoking rose significantly in all three grade levels in 1992 through 1995. In the past 3 years, personal disapproval of smoking has fallen in all grades. Because much of adolescent behavior is influenced by peer norms, this portends a continued rise in smoking (Johnston et al., 1995b).

Alcohol Use

Alcohol use underwent little change from 1991. Even though rates are lower than at their peak in the late 1970s, current statistics reveal that alcohol use is still common at all three grade levels. More than 14% of 8th graders, 24% of 10th graders, and 29.8% of high school seniors in 1995 had had five or more drinks in a row at least once in the previous 2 weeks.

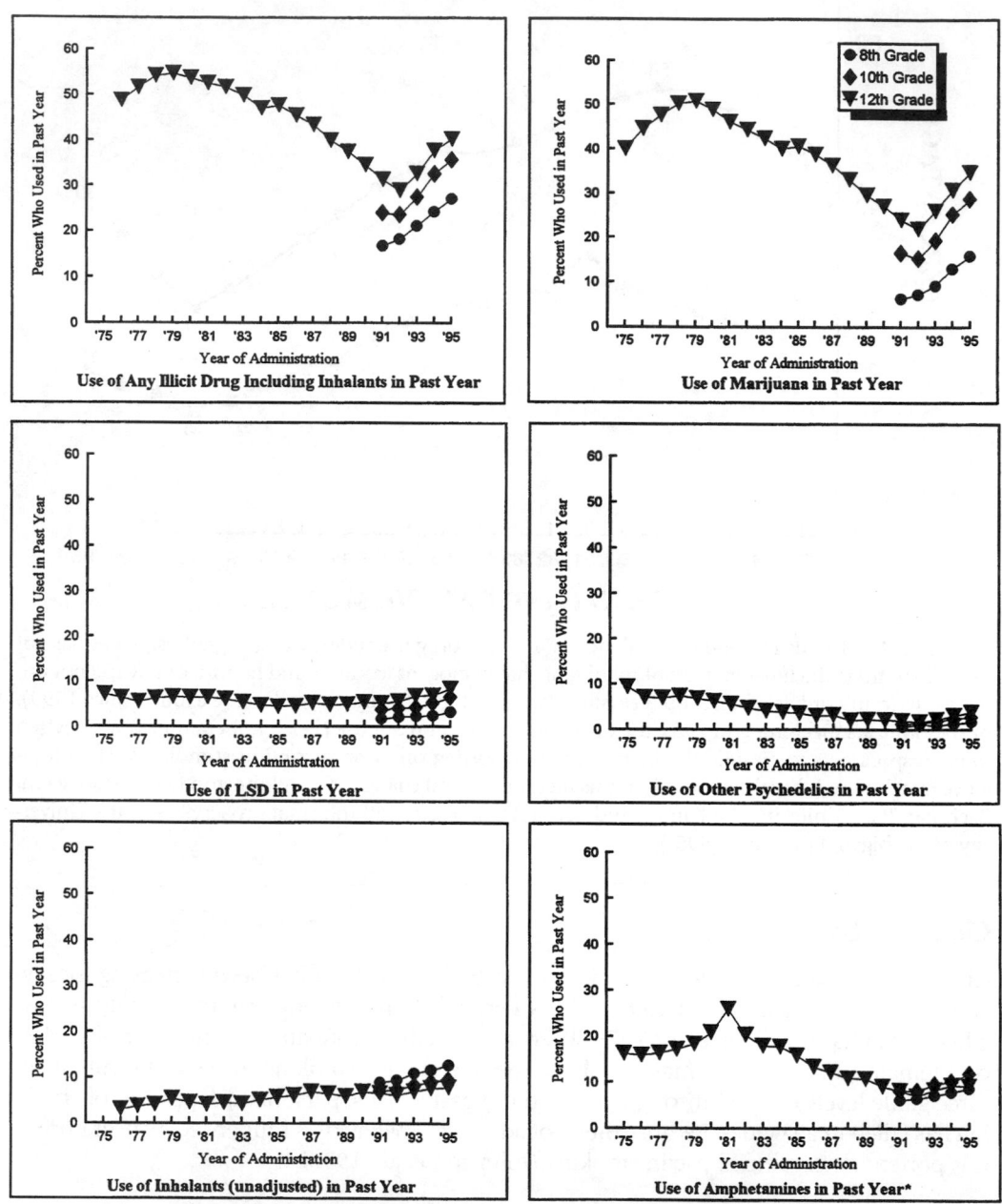

FIGURE 69.4.   Trends in annual use of selected drugs by grade, 1975–1995. *Beginning in 1982, the question about stimulant use (i.e., amphetamines) was revised to get respondents to exclude the inappropriate reporting of nonprescription stimulants. The prevalence dropped slightly as a result of this methodological change. (From Johnston LD, O'Malley PM, Bachman JG. Monitoring the Future Study. Ann Arbor: News and Information Services of the University of Michigan, December 1995.)

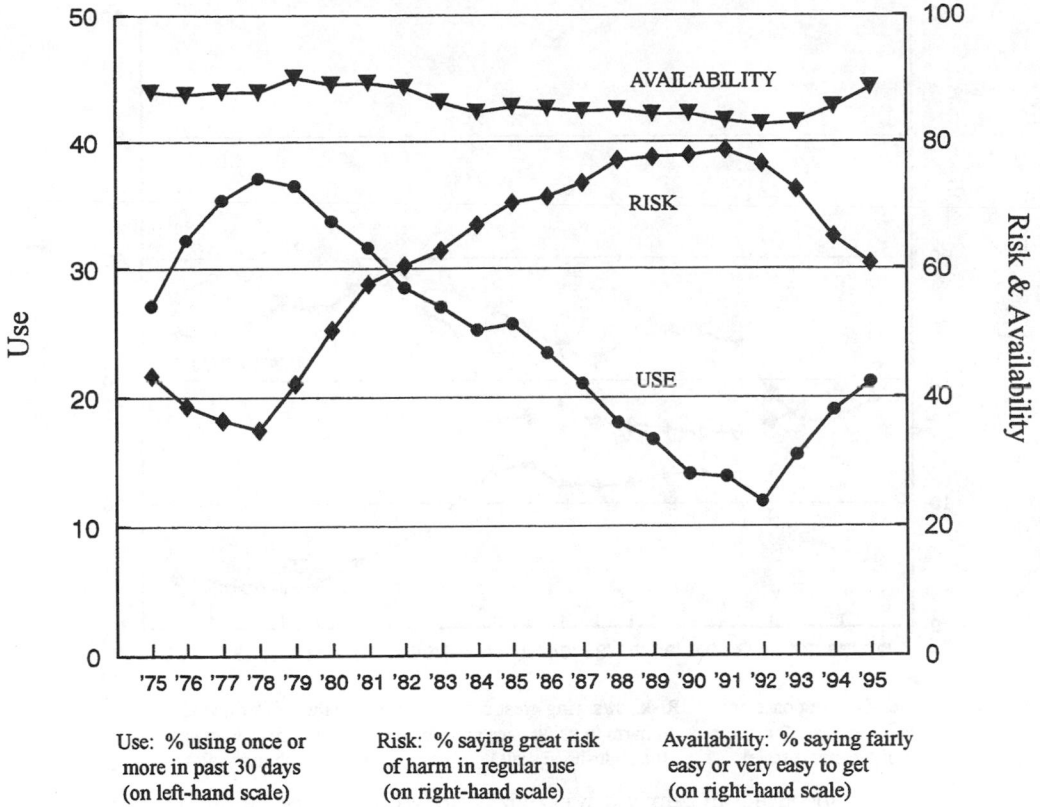

FIGURE 69.5.   Marijuana: trends in perceived availability, perceived risk of regular use, and prevalence of use in past 30 days for 12th graders. (From Johnston LD, O'Malley PM, Bachman JG. Monitoring the Future Study. Ann Arbor: News and Information Services of the University of Michigan, December 1995.)

The 1994 survey revealed that more than 40% of college students had had five or more drinks in a row in the previous 2 weeks (Johnston et al., 1994). These statistics reveal that episodes of heavy drinking are still common. More than 80% of the senior class of 1995 had used alcohol at least once in their lifetime (Johnston et al., 1995).

Marijuana Use

Marijuana use rose sharply until about 1979, at which point the use seemed to peak. The trend toward declining use persisted until 1992, when a sharp reversal developed. This reversal appears to be a current trend. In 1995, 41.7% of high school seniors reported past or current use of marijuana—a distinct increase from 35%, reported just 2 years earlier. The proportion of seniors who reported marijuana use in the past 12 months declined from 50.8% in the class of 1979, to 22% in the class of 1992, only to increase to 26% in 1993 and 34.7% in 1995. In 1995, the proportion of students reporting any use of marijuana in the past 12 months was 15.8% for 8th graders, 28.7% for 10th graders, and 34.7% for 12th graders. Reviewing data on 8th and 10th graders for the past 3 years also reveals disturbing trends. During the past 3 years, annual use of marijuana doubled in 8th and 10th graders and grew by over 50% among 12th graders.

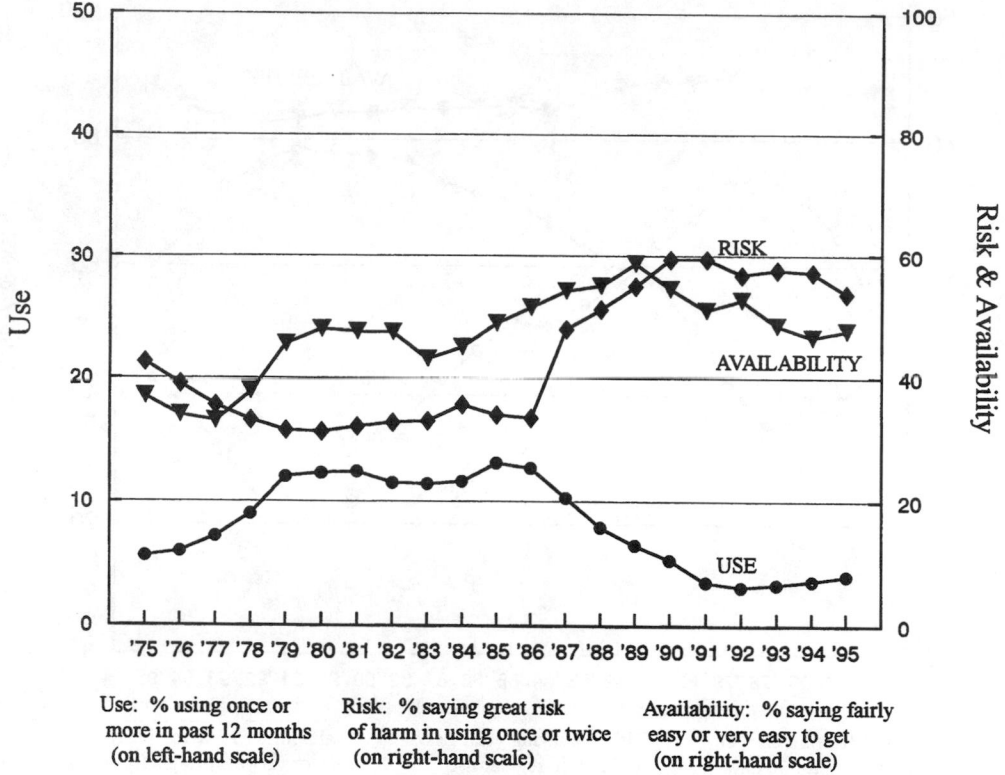

FIGURE 69.6.   Cocaine: trends in perceived availability, perceived risk of regular use, and prevalence of use in past 30 days for 12th graders. (From Johnston LD, O'Malley PM, Bachman JG. Monitoring the Future Study. Ann Arbor: News and Information Services of the University of Michigan, December 1995.)

Other Drugs

Nearly 28% of 1995 high school seniors had used some illicit drug other than marijuana. The overall prevalence rate for use of any drug had declined, from a peak level of 65.6% in 1981 to a nadir of 40.7% in 1992. This trend has reversed in the past several years, with the prevalence increasing in the class of 1995 to 48.4%. Other than marijuana, the most prevalent illicit drugs used by adolescents include stimulants, inhalants, cocaine, hallucinogens, tranquilizers, and sedatives. The prevalence of cocaine use among high school seniors has fallen off steadily since 1986. In 1994 the prevalence of cocaine use reached a low of 5.9%, which remained almost unchanged in the 1995 study group (6.0%). Current use (within the past 30 days) dropped from a peak level of 6.7% in 1985 to 1.3% in 1993 but rose to 1.8% in 1995. The proportion of seniors who had used cocaine at least once in the previous year declined from 13.1% in 1985 to just more than 3% in 1991 but has since risen to 4.0% in 1995. Data collected for the first time in 1986 on the lifetime prevalence of crack cocaine use showed an increase among seniors from 4% in 1986 to 5.6% in 1987, with a decrease to 2.6% in 1993 and a slight increase to 3.0% in 1995. The more recent downward trend in the use of stimulants, which began in 1982, continued to a low in 1992, subsequent to which a sudden reversal developed. Sedative use had declined steadily from 1975 to 1992, at which point lifetime prevalence for 12th graders was found to be 6.1%. In 1995 the prevalence rose to 7.6%. Methaqualone use, which had risen sharply from 1976 until 1981, has continued to decline since 1982 (1.2% in 1995). Hallucinogen use declined from

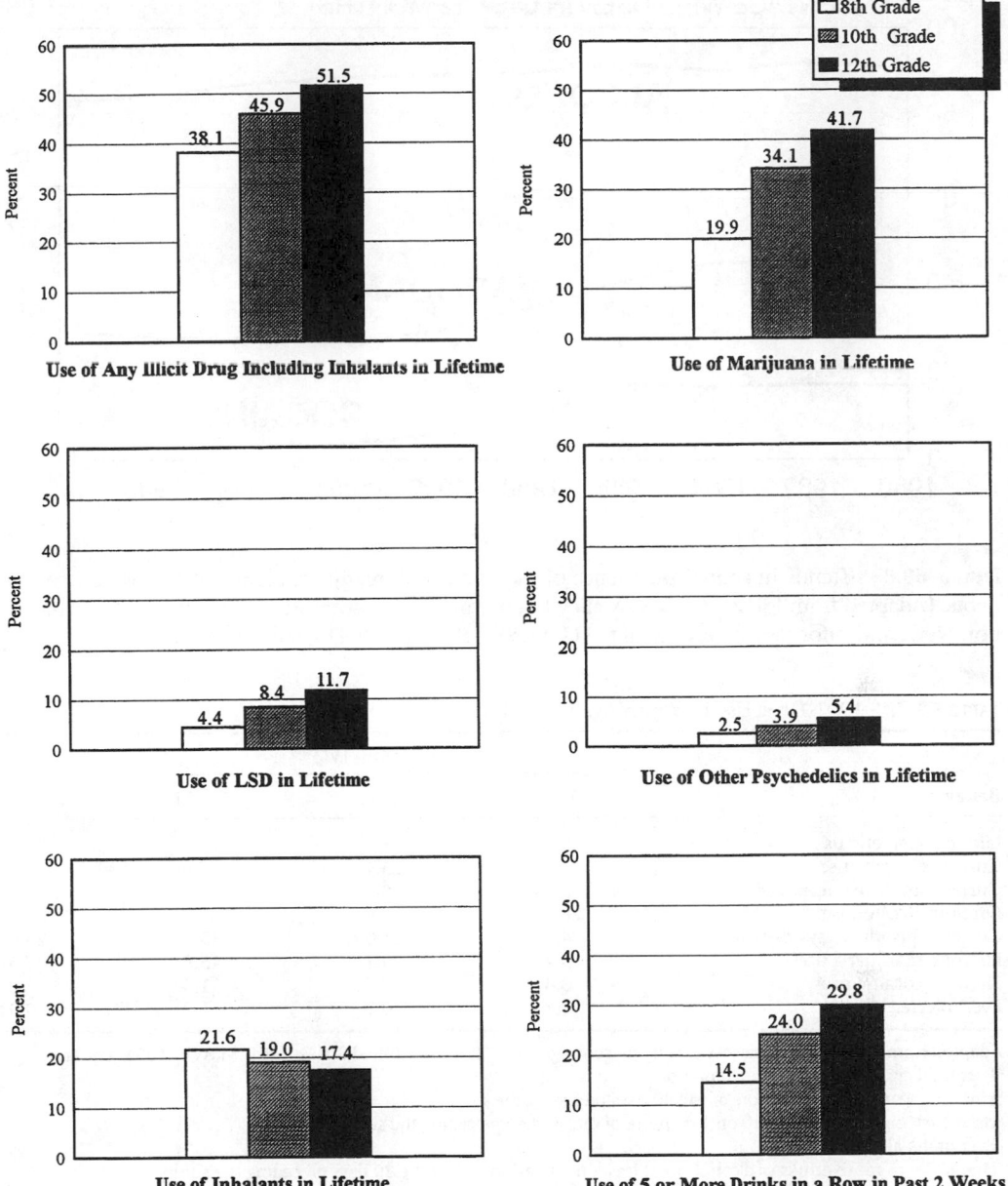

FIGURE 69.7. Lifetime use of selected drugs by grade in 1995 (From Johnston, LD, O'Malley PM, Bachman JG. Monitoring the Future Study. Ann Arbor: News and Information Services of the University of Michigan, December 1995.)

1975 to 1988; however, in 1989 there was a slight increase in use, and 1995 data reveal the highest levels seen in over a decade. The use of LSD continued to rise in all 8th, 10th, and 12th graders in 1995.

Clearly a new trend is evolving; it reverses the past decade's decline in the use of illicit substances. This trend appears to be largely the result of increased use of hallucinogens (primarily LSD), marijuana, inhalants, and stimulants other than cocaine.

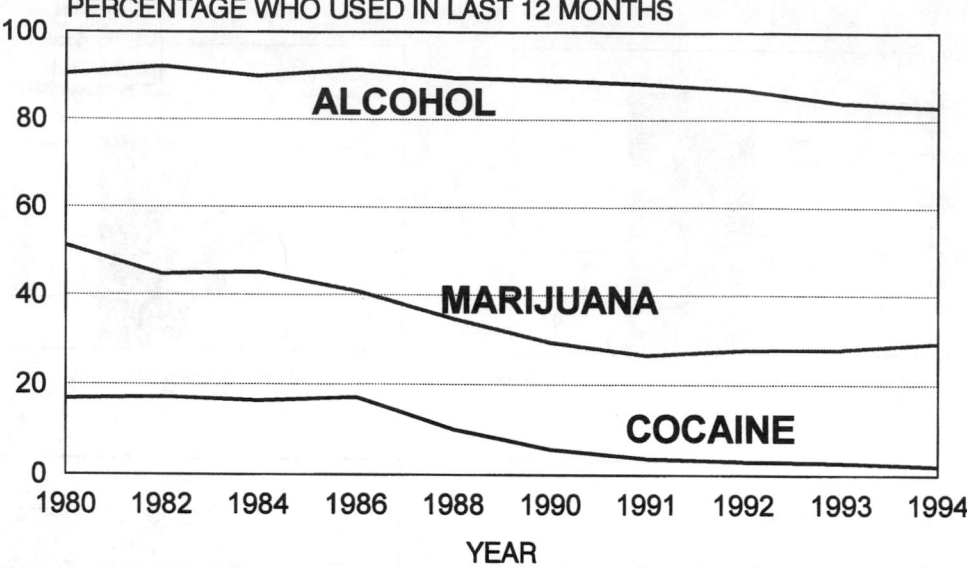

Figure 69.8.   Trends in annual prevalence of use of alcohol, marijuana, and cocaine by college students. (Adapted from Johnston LD, O'Malley PM, Bachman JG. Monitoring the Future Study. Ann Arbor: News and Information Services of the University of Michigan, December 1995).

Table 69.7.   1991 Drug Use in Youth Aged 12–21 Years

Behavior	Age Group (yr)			
	12–13	14–17	18–21	Total
Lifetime cigarette use[a]	29.9	58.0	76.9	60.4
Current cigarette use[b]	7.7	25.4	37.6	27.0
Current smokeless tobacco[c]	2.7	8.8	8.5	7.5
Lifetime alcohol use[d]	28.0	65.6	86.7	67.3
Current episodic heavy drinking[e]	4.3	21.0	39.7	25.6
Lifetime marijuana use[f]	3.4	20.4	45.8	27.5
Lifetime cocaine use[g]	0.4	2.5	11.4	5.8
Ever injected drugs	0.1	0.9	1.2	0.9

Adapted from Health risk behaviors among persons aged 12–21 years—United States, 1991. MMWR 1994;43:231.
[a]Ever tried cigarette smoking, even one or two puffs.
[b]Smoked cigarettes on 1 or more of the 30 days preceding the survey.
[c]Used chewing tobacco or snuff on 1 or more of the 30 days preceding the survey.
[d]Ever drank alcohol.
[e]Drank five or more drinks of alcohol on at least one occasion during the 30 days preceding the survey.
[f]Ever used marijuana.
[g]Ever used cocaine.

Daily Use

The 30-day prevalence of daily use of drugs among high school seniors in 1995 includes the following percentages:

Cigarettes	21.6%
Alcohol	3.5%
Marijuana	4.6%
Inhalants	0.1%

Cocaine	0.2%
Stimulants	0.3%
Hallucinogens	0.1%
Sedatives	0.1%
Tranquilizers	<0.05%
Heroin	0.1%

Age and Drug Use

Table 69.1 and Figure 69.7 illustrate the relationship between grade in school and drug use. According to the table, the majority of experimentation with illicit drugs occurs during high school. However, for marijuana, alcohol, and cigarettes, many of the initial experiences take place before high school. Inhalant users, in particular, often have their first experience before the 10th grade. Initial experience with cocaine is more common in the 10th grade and beyond.

DRUG BELIEFS AMONG ADOLESCENTS

Harmfulness of Drugs

The majority of high school seniors perceive *regular* use of illicit drugs as entailing a great risk to the user. The percentages of seniors responding in such a manner were (Johnston et al., 1995):

Heroin	87.2%
LSD	78.1%
Cocaine	87.9%
Barbiturates	61.6%
Amphetamines	65.9%

Regular use of cigarettes was judged to be a great risk to the user by 65.6% of the respondents, and 60.8% believed regular use of marijuana to be a great risk. Only 24.8% considered one or two daily alcoholic drinks to carry great risk, and only 45% considered five or more drinks once or twice a weekend to carry great risk.

Attitudes about the potential risks to users have shown a tendency toward decreasing perceived risk (Fig. 69.5). This is particularly evident with marijuana, methamphetamine, LSD, and cocaine, especially when perceptions about occasional use are the focus. This shift toward attitudes and beliefs that favor drug use appear to have contributed to a recent resurgence in the use of marijuana and methamphetamine. There is growing concern that 1994 and 1995 data reflecting a decrease in the perceived risk of using cocaine may presage a trend toward increasing use of this drug.

Extent of Disapproval

The great majority of high school seniors do not approve of the regular use of any illicit drug. The percentages that disapprove of the regular use of various drugs are outlined in Table 69.8. Seventy-three percent of high school seniors disapproved of taking one or two drinks nearly every day. The overall trend in all categories is toward diminished disapproval of drug use, particularly in relation to marijuana, LSD, and stimulants (including cocaine) (Table 69.9). The environment of decreased perceived risk and less disapproval from peers correlates with increasing patterns of substance use. In terms of alcohol use, there has been a reversal of the

TABLE 69.8.   High School Seniors Disapproving of Regular Use of Illicit Drugs

Drug	Percentage Disapproving		
	Regular Use	Use	Trial Use
Marijuana	81.9		56.7
LSD	92.5		81.1
Cocaine	96.1		90.3
Heroin	96.4		92.8
Amphetamines	94.3		82.2
Barbiturates	95.2		87.3
Steroids		91.0	
Try one or two drinks of alcoholic beverage		27.3	
Take one or two drinks nearly every day		73.3	
Take four or five drinks nearly every day		88.8	
Have five or more drinks once or twice each weekend		66.7	

Adapted from Johnston LD, O'Malley PM, Bachman JG. Monitoring the Future Study. Ann Arbor: News and Information Services of the University of Michigan, December 1995.

trend toward increasing disapproval that occurred in the 1980s. This is especially evident in disapproval of taking one or two drinks nearly every day and having five or more drinks once or twice each weekend (Johnston et al., 1995a).

REASONS FOR DRUG USE

Self-report

Adolescents and researchers report a multitude of reasons for the use of drugs by teenagers. These include:

1. Use of the drugs by family and peers
2. Exploration and experimentation
3. To gain social acceptance
4. As a result of low self-esteem
5. To seek a change in consciousness or in perceptions or mood
6. To enhance the ability to act socially
7. To relieve a stressful situation
8. As a challenge to parents or authority
9. As a response to messages in the media regarding tobacco and alcohol that convey the idea that these drugs are important for one's body image and sexual identity
10. As a rite of passage
11. To enhance one's sexuality
12. As a reaction to boredom

Correlates to Drug Use

In fact, it may not be possible to pinpoint exactly why any particular teenager uses drugs; however, certain correlates have been found among drug users (Bachman et al., 1981).

1. Sex: Cigarette smoking is more prevalent among females, whereas alcohol use is more prevalent among males. Other drug use is about equal between the sexes.
2. Truancy: There is a highly positive correlation between a history of the use and abuse of drugs and truancy.

TABLE 69.9. Long-Term Trends in *Disapproval* of Drug Use by 12th Graders

| | Percent "Disapproving"[a] | | | | | | | | | | | | | | | | | | | | | |
Q. Do you disapprove of people (who are 18 or older) doing each of the following?[b]	Class of 1975	Class of 1976	Class of 1977	Class of 1978	Class of 1979	Class of 1980	Class of 1981	Class of 1982	Class of 1983	Class of 1984	Class of 1985	Class of 1986	Class of 1987	Class of 1988	Class of 1989	Class of 1990	Class of 1991	Class of 1992	Class of 1993	Class of 1994	Class of 1995	1994–1995 Change
Try marijuana once or twice	47.0	38.4	33.4	33.4	34.2	39.0	40.0	45.5	46.3	49.3	51.4	54.6	56.6	60.8	64.6	67.8	68.7	69.9	63.3	57.6	56.7	-0.9
Smoke marijuana occasionally	54.8	47.8	44.3	43.5	45.3	49.7	52.6	59.1	60.7	63.5	65.8	69.0	71.6	74.0	77.2	80.5	79.4	79.7	75.5	68.9	66.7	-2.2
Smoke marijuana regularly	71.9	69.5	65.5	67.5	69.2	74.6	77.4	80.6	82.5	84.7	85.5	86.6	89.2	89.3	89.8	91.0	89.3	90.1	87.6	82.3	81.9	-0.4
Try LSD once or twice	82.8	84.6	83.9	85.4	86.6	87.3	86.4	88.8	89.1	88.9	89.5	89.2	91.6	89.8	89.7	89.8	90.1	88.1	85.9	82.5	81.1	-1.4
Take LSD regularly	94.1	95.3	95.8	96.4	96.9	96.7	96.8	96.7	97.0	96.8	97.0	96.6	97.8	96.4	96.4	96.3	96.4	95.5	95.8	94.3	92.5	-1.8s
Try cocaine once or twice	81.3	82.4	79.1	77.0	74.7	76.3	74.6	76.6	77.0	79.7	79.3	80.2	87.3	89.1	90.5	91.5	93.6	93.0	92.7	91.6	90.3	-1.3
Take cocaine regularly	93.3	93.9	92.1	91.9	90.8	91.1	90.7	91.5	93.2	94.5	93.8	94.3	96.7	96.2	96.4	96.7	97.3	96.9	97.5	96.6	96.1	-0.5
Try crack once or twice	—	—	—	—	—	—	—	—	—	—	—	—	—	—	—	92.3	92.1	93.1	89.9	89.5	91.4	+1.9
Take crack occasionally	—	—	—	—	—	—	—	—	—	—	—	—	—	—	—	94.3	94.2	95.0	92.8	92.8	94.0	+1.2
Take crack regularly	—	—	—	—	—	—	—	—	—	—	—	—	—	—	—	94.9	95.0	95.5	93.4	93.1	94.1	+1.0
Try coke powder once or twice	—	—	—	—	—	—	—	—	—	—	—	—	—	—	—	87.9	88.0	89.4	86.6	87.1	88.3	+1.2
Take coke powder occasionally	—	—	—	—	—	—	—	—	—	—	—	—	—	—	—	92.1	93.0	93.4	91.2	91.0	92.7	+1.7
Take coke powder regularly	—	—	—	—	—	—	—	—	—	—	—	—	—	—	—	93.7	94.4	94.3	93.0	92.5	93.8	+1.3
Try heroin once or twice	91.5	92.6	92.5	92.0	93.4	93.5	93.5	94.6	94.3	94.0	94.0	93.3	96.2	95.0	95.4	95.1	96.0	94.9	94.4	93.2	93.2	-0.4
Take heroin occasionally	94.8	96.0	96.0	96.4	96.8	96.7	97.2	96.9	96.9	97.1	96.8	96.6	97.9	96.9	97.2	96.7	97.3	96.8	97.0	96.2	95.7	-0.5
Take heroin regularly	96.7	97.5	97.2	97.8	97.9	97.6	97.8	97.5	97.7	98.0	97.6	97.6	98.1	97.2	97.4	97.5	97.8	97.2	97.5	97.1	96.4	-0.7
Try amphetamines once or twice	74.8	75.1	74.2	74.8	75.1	75.4	71.1	72.6	72.3	72.8	74.9	76.5	80.7	82.5	83.3	85.3	86.5	86.9	84.2	81.3	82.2	+0.9
Take amphetamines regularly	92.1	92.8	92.5	93.5	94.4	93.0	91.7	92.0	92.6	93.6	93.3	93.5	95.4	94.2	94.2	95.5	96.0	95.6	96.0	94.1	94.3	+0.2
Try barbiturates once or twice	77.7	81.3	81.1	82.4	84.0	83.9	82.4	84.4	83.1	84.1	84.9	86.8	89.6	89.4	89.3	90.5	90.6	90.3	89.7	87.5	87.3	-0.2
Take barbiturates regularly	93.3	93.6	93.0	94.3	95.2	95.4	94.2	94.4	95.1	95.1	95.5	94.9	96.4	95.3	95.3	96.4	97.1	96.5	96.1	96.1	95.2	-0.9
Try one or two drinks of an alcoholic beverage (beer, wine, liquor)	21.6	18.2	15.6	15.6	15.8	16.0	17.2	18.2	18.4	17.4	20.3	20.9	21.4	22.6	27.3	29.4	29.8	33.0	30.1	28.4	27.3	-1.1
Take one or two drinks nearly every day	67.6	68.9	66.8	67.7	68.3	69.0	69.1	69.9	68.9	72.9	70.9	72.8	74.2	75.0	76.5	77.9	76.5	75.9	77.8	73.1	73.3	+0.2
Take four or five drinks nearly every day	88.7	90.7	88.4	90.2	91.7	90.8	91.8	90.9	90.0	91.0	92.0	91.4	92.2	92.8	91.6	91.9	90.6	90.8	90.6	89.8	88.8	-1.0
Have five or more drinks once or twice each weekend	60.3	58.6	57.4	56.2	56.7	55.6	55.5	58.8	56.6	59.6	60.4	62.4	62.0	65.3	66.5	68.9	67.4	70.7	70.1	65.1	66.7	+1.6
Smoke one or more packs of cigarettes per day	67.5	65.9	66.4	67.0	70.3	70.8	69.9	69.4	70.8	73.0	72.3	75.4	74.3	73.1	72.4	72.8	71.4	73.5	70.6	69.8	68.2	-1.6
Take steroids	—	—	—	—	—	—	—	—	—	—	—	—	—	—	—	90.8	90.5	92.1	92.1	91.9	91.0	-0.9
Approx. N =	2677	2957	3085	3686	3221	3261	3610	3651	3341	3254	3265	3113	3302	3311	2799	2566	2547	2645	2723	2588	2603	

From Johnston LD, O'Malley PM, Bachman JG. Monitoring the Future Study. Ann Arbor: News and Information Services of the University of Michigan, December 1995.
Level of significance of difference between the two most recent classes: s = 0.05, ss = 0.01, sss = 0.001. Em dash indicates data not available.
[a]Answer alternatives were: (1) Don't disapprove, (2) Disapprove, and (3) Strongly disapprove. Percentages are shown for categories (2) and (3) combined.
[b]The 1975 question asked about people who are "20 or older."

3. Work experience: There is a positive correlation between number of hours worked and drug use.
4. Lifestyle: Strong religious commitment has been found to be negatively correlated to drug use. Adolescents with more liberal or radical political views and teenagers with more social lifestyles have a higher prevalence of drug use.
5. Demographics: Urban teenagers and adolescents living in the northeastern United States have a higher prevalence of drug use, whereas teenagers in the South exhibit lower use.

Newcomb et al. (1986) found 10 risk factors to correlate with adolescent drug use, in increasing order of correlation: poor self-esteem, psychological distress, poor academic achievement, low degree of religiosity, poor relationship with parents, sensation seeking, early alcohol use, adult drug use, deviance, and peer drug use. The single most predictive variable for drug use in an adolescent is drug use in that adolescent's closest friend.

STAGES OF DRUG USE

MacDonald (1987) suggested five stages of adolescent substance abuse, as follows:

Stage 0: Showing curiosity. At this stage the teen is usually normal but may have low self-esteem and a strong desire for peer acceptance. Given the teen's natural curiosity and tendency to exhibit a sense of immortality, he or she decides to try a mood-altering chemical. Often feeling good and suffering no dire consequences, the teen enters stage 1.

Stage 1: Learning about the drug-induced mood swings. The teen learns more about use of drugs, but use is limited to group settings, usually on weekends. Peer pressure is frequently intense and is a prime reason for continuance. The teen's discomfort with family, school, or social problems is often relieved temporarily by the drug use.

Stage 2: Seeking the drug-induced mood swings. Having learned that these drugs can alleviate perceived pain and anxiety, the adolescent now seeks the highs of drug use. The teen may acquire a supply of drugs and paraphernalia. The drugs are now used more to relax than as part of the social scene. The teen becomes a regular weekend and occasional weekday user. Behavioral changes may occur during this stage, including a decrease in school performance and abandonment of extracurricular interests.

Stage 3: Being preoccupied with the drug-induced mood swings. The teen loses control of his or her life and is concerned only with getting high. The behavioral changes are more pronounced and more obvious. New behaviors may also include stealing, school truancy, and lying. Drug dealing, to obtain the money necessary for continued drug use, may start.

Stage 4: Burnout. At this point the teen is using drugs just to feel normal. Drugs may no longer produce euphoria. "Zombies" and "space cadets" are common terms used by adolescents to describe this group.

Chapters 70 through 74 of this book focus on specific drugs, concentrating on drug-use patterns and effects on health. Chapter 75, the final chapter in this section, discusses approaches to managing drug abuse.

BIBLIOGRAPHY

Abelson HJ, Fishburne PM, Cisin IH. National Survey on Drug Abuse: 1977; vol 1: Main findings. Washington, D.C.: National Institute on Drug Abuse, 1977.

Bachman JG, Johnston LD, O'Malley PM. Smoking, drinking and drug use among American high school students: correlates and trends, 1975–1979. Am J Public Health 1981;71:59.

Frances R, Miller SI. Clinical textbook of addiction disorders. New York: The Guildford Press, 1991.

Franklin JE. Addiction medicine. JAMA 1995;273:1656.

Harrison PA, Luxenberg MG. Comparisons of alcohol and other drug problems among Minnesota adolescents in 1989 and 1992. Arch Pediatr Adolesc Med 1995;149:137.

Jalali B, Jalali M, Crocetti G, et al. Adolescents and drug use: toward a more comprehensive approach. Am J Orthopsychiatry 1981;51:120.

Johnston LD, O'Malley PM, Bachman JG. National trends in drug use and related factors among American high school students and young adults, 1975–1986. (Publication No. 87–1535.) Washington, D.C.: U.S. Department of Health and Human Services, 1987a.

Johnston LD, O'Malley PM, Bachman JG. Psychotherapeutic, licit, and illicit use of drugs among adolescents: an epidemiological perspective. J Adolesc Health Care 1987b;8:36.

Johnston LD, O'Malley PM, Bachman JG. Drug use, drinking, and smoking: national survey results from high school, college and young adult populations, 1975–1988. (Publication No. [ADM] 89–1638.) Washington, D.C.: U.S. Department of Health and Human Services, 1989.

Johnston LD, O'Malley PM, Bachman JG. The Monitoring the Future Study. Vol. II: college students and young adults. Ann Arbor: News and Information Services of the University of Michigan, 1994.

Johnston LD, O'Malley PM, Bachman JG. Drug use rises again in 1995 among American teens. Ann Arbor: News and Information Services of the University of Michigan, December 11, 1995a.

Johnston LD, O'Malley PM, Bachman JG. Cigarette smoking among American teens rises again in 1995. Ann Arbor: News and Information Services of the University of Michigan, December 11, 1995b.

Konings E, DuboiArber F, Narring F, et al. Identifying adolescent drug users: results of a national survey on adolescent health in Switzerland. J Adolesc Health 1995;16:240.

Los Angeles Street Drug Identification Program: Monthly reports. Los Angeles: Department of Health Services, County of Los Angeles, 1981.

Lowinson JH, Ruiz P, Millman RB, Langroid JG, eds. Substance abuse: a comprehensive textbook. 2nd ed. Baltimore: Williams & Wilkins, 1992.

Lowry R, Holtzman D, Truman BI, et al. Substance use and HIV-related sexual behaviors among U.S. high school students: are they related? Am J Public Health 1994;84:1116.

MacDonald DI. Drugs, drinking, and adolescents. Chicago: Year Book Medical Publishers, 1984.

MacDonald DI. Patterns of alcohol and drug use among adolescents. In: Rogers PD, ed. Symposium on chemical dependency. Pediatr Clin North Am 1987;34:275.

MacDonald DI. High school cocaine use declines. JAMA 1988;259:1615.

MacKenzie RG, Jacobs EA. Recognizing the adolescent drug abuser. Primary Care 1987;4:225.

Newcomb MD, Maddahian E, Bentler PM. Risk factors for drug use among adolescents: concurrent and longitudinal analyses. Am J Public Health 1986;76:525.

O'Malley PM, Bachman JG, Johnston LD. Period, age, and cohort effects on substance use among young Americans: a decade of change, 1976–1986. Am J Public Health 1988;78:1315.

O'Malley PM, Johnston LD, Bachman JG. Adolescent substance use: epidemiology and implications for public policy. Pediatr Clin North Am 1995;42:241.

Patton LH. Adolescent substance abuse. Risk factors and protective factors. Pediatr Clin North Am 1995;42:283.

Rinaldi RC, Steindler EM, Wilford BB, Goodwin D. Clarification and standardization of substance abuse terminology. JAMA 1988;259:555.

Skinner WF. The prevalence and demographic predictors of illicit and illicit drug use among lesbians and gay men. Am J Public Health 1994;84:1307.

Warner LA, Kessler RC, Hughes M, et al. Prevalence and correlates of drug use and dependence in the United States: results from the National Comorbidity Survey. Arch Gen Psychiatry 1995;52:219.

Wright JD, Pearl L. Knowledge and experience of young people regarding drug misuse, 1969–94. Br Med J 1995;310:20.

Yesalis CE, Kennedy NJ, Kopstein AN, et al. Anabolic-androgenic steroid use in the United States. JAMA 1993;270:1217.

CHAPTER 70

Alcohol

Lawrence S. Neinstein and Drew Pinsky

Alcohol is the most widely used drug in the United States. Readily available and inexpensive, it has been used by about 80% to 90% of adolescents by age 18 years. The monthly prevalence of alcohol use among high school seniors was 51% in 1995 and over 67% for college students. More than 3% of high school seniors used alcohol daily in 1995 (Johnston et al., 1995). Almost one third of high school seniors drank over five drinks in a row in the prior 2 weeks. About 3.8% of college students drank alcohol daily in 1994. An estimated 4.6 million adolescents aged 14–17 years have alcohol problems. Motor vehicle accidents as a result of driving under the influence are the leading cause of death among the 15- to 24-year-old age group. Alcohol-related motor vehicle accidents result in 8000 adolescent deaths and 45,000 injuries each year. Alcohol use is also involved in approximately 40% of the 10,000 annual nonautomotive accidental deaths of adolescents, and in a significant number of the 5500 suicides and 5000 homicides of adolescents each year. Health-care providers should not underestimate the effects of alcohol use on adolescents or its consequences.

ALCOHOL AND ITS EFFECTS

Although alcohol is a central-nervous-system-depressant, at low doses it has behavioral stimulant properties, particularly for persons with an alcoholic diathesis. The principal ingredient of all alcoholic beverages is ethanol. Most beers and wines contain between 3% and 20% alcohol. Moderate doses of alcohol in the nontolerant individual induce sedation, euphoria, decreased inhibitions, and impaired coordination. As the dose and resulting blood alcohol level increase, ataxia, decreased mentation, poor judgment, labile mood, and slurred speech occur. Heavy use of alcohol may induce unconsciousness, anesthesia, respiratory failure, coma, and death.

Although alcohol may adversely affect multiple organ systems of the body, adolescent alcohol abusers usually are spared the complications of prolonged alcohol use such as cirrhosis, alcoholic hepatitis, or pancreatitis. Acute withdrawal symptoms such as delirium tremens (DTs) or seizures also are unusual in adolescents. Farrow et al. (1987) examined the health and nutritional status of adolescent alcohol abusers. Any significant health or nutritional disability from the abuse related primarily to poor dietary habits. These teens' hematological status, liver function, and growth parameters were normal.

FACTORS CONTRIBUTING TO TEENAGE ALCOHOL USE

Adolescent alcohol use is an individual as well as a social problem. Available literature points to several variables that appear to be associated with the use of alcohol by adolescents. Although the conclusions reached in these studies sometimes differ, the hypothesized contributing factors include:

1. Family and parental factors
   a. Genetic: Twin adoption studies support a genetic predisposition for alcoholism.
   b. Parents as role models: Parental attitudes about alcohol and parental drinking practices influence adolescent alcohol use, especially during early adolescence.
   c. Style of parenting: Extreme parenting styles (authoritarian or permissive) and inconsistent discipline seem to contribute to increased alcohol use among adolescents.
   d. Perceived family support: High levels of perceived family support are correlated with low levels of alcohol and drug use. Cohen et al. (1994) demonstrated that children who reported that parents spent more time with them and communicated with them more frequently had lower onset rates of using alcohol and tobacco in the preceding month.
2. Peer influence
   a. Peer pressure to maintain alcohol abuse: Although parental factors contribute to initiation of alcohol use, peer attitudes and behavior contribute even more significantly to the maintenance of alcohol use and abuse.
   b. Group acceptance: As adolescents separate from their family, they often associate with peers who have attitudes and beliefs similar to their own. Studies indicate that an individual's alcohol and drug use closely parallels that of his or her peer group.
   c. Group norms: There is a tendency within certain peer groups to excuse drunken behavior and to minimize the physical consequences of heavy drinking. These groups also tend to negate any fear of consequences or punishment.
3. Desire to attain adult status: The adolescent's desire to imitate adult behavior and society's identification of drinking as an adult privilege contribute to adolescent alcohol abuse. In addition, alcohol use is often seen as a rite of passage to achieve adult status.
4. Sexuality socialization: As adolescents learn to establish relationships and explore their sexuality, they simultaneously become concerned with body image, social behavior, and developing sexual arousal. Alcohol lessens inhibitions, enabling the adolescent to focus less on being socially incompetent and facing possible rejection. Alcohol use also enables the adolescent to blame any social awkwardness on his or her drinking. However, alcohol use leaves the adolescent less able to make complex decisions regarding his or her sexuality.
5. Psychological problems, including low self-esteem and personality disorders (e.g., antisocial personality)
6. Curiosity
7. Lack of church involvement
8. Timing of sexual maturation: Earlier puberty is associated with a younger age at onset of both drinking and smoking among adolescent girls (Wilson et al., 1994).

Among these factors contributing to teen alcohol use, family and parental factors, peer influences, desire to attain adult status, and sexuality socialization seem to be the major contributing factors. Societal support and tolerance of alcohol use and abuse exacerbate the problem. The easy availability of alcohol and society's perception that alcohol is not a drug also contribute to adolescent alcohol use.

REASONS FOR DRINKING

Teenagers give the following reasons for drinking (Rachal et al., 1975):

1. Curiosity
2. Peer conformity
3. Enjoyment
4. Escape
5. Parental encouragement to take first drink to celebrate a special occasion

PROBLEM DRINKING AMONG ADOLESCENTS

Problem drinking has been defined as having been drunk six or more times in the past year or acknowledging problems in three out of the following areas because of drinking:

1. Trouble with a teacher or principal
2. Difficulties with friends
3. Driving after drinking
4. Criticism by dates
5. Trouble with the police

Incidence of Adverse Consequences of Alcohol Use

Nearly half of male high school seniors can be described as problem drinkers (MacDonald, 1986). Nearly one-fourth of female seniors who have ever consumed alcohol report that they are also problem drinkers. It is estimated that nearly one-third of adolescents ages 14–17 have alcohol problems. By age 15, one-fifth of the boys and one-sixth of the girls report that they are problem drinkers. These statistics do not include school dropouts, and there is evidence that dropouts use alcohol more heavily than their counterparts who have stayed in school. Problem drinking can seriously interfere with the successful completion of the psychological developmental tasks of adolescence, resulting in a maturational arrest.

Harrison and Luxenberg (1995) reported on alcohol and drug use among Minnesota adolescents. They found a continued trend in the proportion of students who reported at least three adverse consequences of alcohol and drug use, including 1% of 6th graders, 7% of 9th graders, and 16% of 12th graders. Alcohol was the primary substance of abuse among students. The most commonly reported consequences include tolerance, blackouts, violence, and school or job absenteeism. The problem users were about two to seven times more likely than comparable students with a lesser or no drug history to report parental alcohol or other drug problems, physical abuse, and sexual abuse. They were also 2 to 15 times more likely to have low self-esteem and emotional distress, to exhibit antisocial behavior, and to have made suicide attempts.

Binge Drinking

Binge drinking is defined as five or more consecutive drinks within the prior 2 weeks. The 1995 high school senior survey data indicate that 29.8% of 12th graders are binge drinkers. Wechsler et al. (1994), in a national survey of college students, reported that 44% were binge drinkers, including almost one-fifth of the students who were frequent binge drinkers. Other studies have also demonstrated high levels of college binge drinking. In the college survey, almost half (47%) of the frequent binge drinkers had five or more different drinking-related problems, including having had injuries and having engaged in unplanned sex, since the beginning of the school year. This group of drinkers are three times as likely as nonbinge drinkers to engage in unplanned sexual activity, six times as likely to drive after consuming large amounts of alcohol, and twice as likely to ride with an intoxicated driver. Male bingers are four times as likely to be involved in arguments or fights.

DIAGNOSIS

The medical practitioner must be acutely aware of the differing patterns of use manifested in adolescence so as to be able to formulate accurate diagnostic impressions and thereby use therapeutic interventions with the greatest likelihood of improving outcome. Alcoholism and problem drinking during adolescence may have similar manifestations and consequences. Problem drinking can develop as an attempt to escape the psychic distress resulting from a distinct primary psychiatric disorder such as major depression. It may result in acting out in response to unique psychodynamic circumstances or an evolving personality disorder. In these circumstances the use will generally subside if the primary disorder is properly identified and treated. If, however, the adolescent does, in fact, have alcoholism, attempts to treat the secondary psychiatric manifestations will do little or nothing to prevent the evolution of this progressive disorder. Because the manifestations of alcoholism in adolescence may be only very subtly distinguished from problem drinking, it is exceedingly important to have a clear understanding of the defining features of the diagnosis of alcoholism.

Alcoholism is a primary, chronic disease with genetic, psychosocial, and environmental factors influencing its development and manifestations.

Characteristics of Alcoholism

1. The disease is often progressive and may be fatal.
2. The individual has impaired control over drinking, progressive preoccupation with alcohol use despite significant adverse consequences, and distortions in thinking, most notably denial.
3. Adverse consequences include impairments in work or school functioning, negative influences on interpersonal relationships, and legal or health-status ramifications.
4. A family history of alcoholism is present in the majority of cases.
5. Research suggests that genetics is a major determinant in the risk of alcoholism. Further recent information shows that the biologic features of these genetic determinants create an environment in the dopaminergic meso-limbic reward systems that may predispose a person to progressive use of alcohol and, in addition, may facilitate potent biological reinforcement by substances other than alcohol that also stimulate this region of the brain. Cocaine and amphetamines are two such compounds with a great potential for dependency. Similarly, there appear to be unique elements of the endorphin system in the alcoholic brain that may result in a predisposition to opiate dependency. Although alcoholism is not the only route to dependency on these substances, experimentation with these drugs by an adolescent with suspected alcoholism suggests a more treacherous clinical circumstance and a need for immediate intervention by the health-care provider.

The biopsychosocial consequences of drug use during adolescence are often the same, whether or not addictions are present. The natural history of the clinical situation and the effectiveness of specific treatments, however, are clearly a function of the specificity of the diagnostic circumstances.

Further confounding diagnostic accuracy is the fact that adolescents who use large amounts of alcohol generally deceive the physicians with whom they come in contact. Because of the teen's (and family's) denial, the physician often does not recognize the alcohol dependence. The serious medical illnesses and somatic complaints associated with long-term adult drug or alcohol use are generally not available as clues when one is assessing the adolescent. Thus the physician is largely dependent on the history in recognizing and diagnosing adolescent alcohol abuse.

Behavioral Changes

The following behavioral changes (Table 70.1) can arouse the suspicion of alcohol or other drug abuse (but none of them is an absolute indicator of excessive drinking):

TABLE 70.1. Developing Signs of Alcoholism in Teenagers

Social/Psychological Signs	Classroom Behavior	Physical Signs
Personality change when drinking	Attendance	A change in tolerance to
Blackouts or temporary amnesia during	Misses Monday mornings	alcohol, either an increase
and after drinking episodes	Late after lunch	or a decrease
Loss of control of drinking	Leaves school early on Fridays	Hangovers
Drinks more than peers and more often	Frequent absences	Marked weight gain or loss
Morning drinking to overcome hangover	General	Repeated minor injuries
effects	Works below expected potential	Sexual activity beyond
Drinking-related arrests	level	standard of peer group
Defensiveness about alcohol usage	Inconsistency in aggressiveness	Characteristics of final
Obsession with consumption of next drink	and passivity in classroom	phases—obvious and
Mixing of alcohol with drugs for a better	participation	tragic:
high	Drinks at school, hides alcohol	Extended binges
Need to drink before going to a party	in locker	Physical tremors
Feeling of remorse about drinking	Boasts about drinking	Hallucinations
Occurrence of fights when drinking	Alcohol on breath	Deliria
Development of elaborate system of lies,	Change in peer group affiliation	Convulsions
alibies, and excuses to cover up drinking	Sleeps during classes	
	General troubles in school	

Adapted from the National Council on Alcoholism of San Fernando Valley, California.

1. Changes in activity such as loss of interest in school, play, home, or work
2. Changes in sleeping patterns
3. Changes in eating patterns
4. Changes in personality: May be reflected in mood changes, fighting with friends and with family members, or truancy
5. Manifestations of depression, such as poor attention span, difficulties in concentrating, lack of interest, and boredom
6. Trouble with law enforcement
7. Multiple or frequent accident-related injuries
8. School failure
9. Blackouts

Screening Instruments

Determining the extent of alcohol abuse and diagnosing alcoholism in the adolescent is crucial. The HEADSS psychosocial profile, as outlined in Chapter 3, is a helpful interview technique in eliciting a history of substance abuse. Several screening devices are also available to help make this diagnosis. The Michigan Alcoholism Screening Test (MAST) (Fig. 70.1) is the most widely used screening test. A shorter instrument is the CAGE questionnaire (Fig. 70.2). Other available instruments include:

1. Adolescent Alcohol Involvement Scale (AAIS)
2. Drinking Analysis Questionnaire (DAQ)
3. Adolescent Alcohol Abuse Questionnaire
4. MacAndrew Alcoholism Scale
5. Addiction Severity Index (ASI)
6. Severity of Alcohol Dependence Questionnaire (SADQ)
7. Perceived Benefit of Drinking Scale

Many of these screening instruments are compiled in the *NIAAA Treatment Handbook, Series 2: Alcoholism Treatment Assessment Research Instruments* (Lettieri et al., 1987). A family his-

Circle "Yes" or "No," depending on whether the statement says something true or not true about you. Please answer all questions. The test can be scored to let you know where you lie on a scale from social drinker to addictive drinker. (Underlined answers count for score; in the questionnaire given to the patient, no yes or no answers are underlined.)

1.	Do you feel you are a normal drinker?	Yes	<u>No</u>	2
2.	Have you ever awakened on the morning after some drinking the night before and found you couldn't remember a part of the evening?	<u>Yes</u>	No	2
3.	Do your friends or family ever worry or complain about your drinking?	<u>Yes</u>	No	1
4.	Can you stop drinking without a struggle after one or two drinks?	Yes	<u>No</u>	2
5.	Do you ever feel bad about your drinking?	<u>Yes</u>	No	1
6.	Do friends or relatives think you are a normal drinker?	Yes	<u>No</u>	2
7.	Do you ever try to limit your drinking to certain times of the day or to certain places?	<u>Yes</u>	No	1
8.	Are you always able to stop drinking when you want to?	Yes	<u>No</u>	2
9.	Have you ever attended a meeting of Alcoholics Anonymous (AA)?	<u>Yes</u>	No	5
10.	Have you gotten into fights when drinking?	<u>Yes</u>	No	1
11.	Has your drinking ever created problems with your friends or family?	<u>Yes</u>	No	2
12.	Have your friends or any family member ever gone to anyone for help about your drinking?	<u>Yes</u>	No	2
13.	Have you ever lost friends or spouse because of your drinking?	<u>Yes</u>	No	2
14.	Have you ever gotten into trouble at work or school because of your drinking?	<u>Yes</u>	No	2
15.	Have you ever lost a job because of your drinking?	<u>Yes</u>	No	2
16.	Have you ever neglected your obligations, your family, or your school work for 2 or more days in a row because you were drinking?	<u>Yes</u>	No	2
17.	Do you ever drink before noon?	<u>Yes</u>	No	2
18.	Have you ever been told you have liver trouble?	<u>Yes</u>	No	1
19.	After heavy drinking, have you ever had delirium tremens (DTs) or severe shaking, heard voices, or seen things that were not there?	<u>Yes</u>	No	5
20.	Have you ever gone to anyone for help about your drinking?	<u>Yes</u>	No	5
21.	Have you ever been in a hospital because of your drinking?	<u>Yes</u>	No	5
22.	Have you ever been a patient in a psychiatric hospital or on a psychiatric ward of a general hospital when drinking was part of the problem?	<u>Yes</u>	No	2
23.	Have you ever been seen at a psychiatric or mental health clinic or gone to a doctor, social worker, or clergyman for help with an emotional problem in which drinking played a part?	<u>Yes</u>	No	2
24.	Have you ever been arrested, even for a few hours, because of drunk behavior?	<u>Yes</u>	No	2
25.	Have you ever been arrested for drunk driving or driving after drinking?	<u>Yes</u>	No	<u>2</u>
			TOTAL	57

Your score is _____

0–3	Probably not alcoholic
5–10	80% risk of alcoholism
10 or more	Definitely alcoholic

FIGURE 70.1. Michigan Alcoholism Screening Test (MAST) questionnaire on drinking habits. (Adapted from Selzer ML. The Michigan Alcoholism Screening Test: the quest for a new diagnostic instrument. Am J Psychol 1971;127:89.)

1. Have you ever felt you ought to Cut down on your drinking?
2. Have people Annoyed you by criticizing your drinking?
3. Have you ever felt bad or Guilty about your drinking?
4. Have you ever had a drink first thing in the morning to steady your nerves or to get rid of a hangover (Eye opener)?

Two or more affirmative answers is considered probable alcoholism on this 4-point scale.

Figure 70.2.   CAGE questionnaire for alcoholism. (From Ewing JA. Detecting alcoholism: the CAGE questionnaire. JAMA 1985;252:14.)

tory of alcoholism or addiction also places the adolescent at high risk of abusing an addictive substance and having a subsequent addiction for the reasons described above. The Children of Alcoholics Screening Test (CAST) (Dinning and Dark, 1989) may help to identify the adolescent child of an alcoholic or addict and may give reason for increased suspicion that the adolescent may have or may develop an alcohol or other drug problem.

Werner et al. (1994) examined several scales and variables in an attempt to predict problem drinking among female college freshman. The CAGE questions, the Perceived-Benefit-of-Drinking Scale, the student's tobacco use, the student's best friend's drinking pattern, and the age at which the student first started drinking showed some potential, as a group, to be a clinically useful screening measure for predicting subsequent problem drinking.

Consequences of Heavy Drinking

Physical Consequences

The following may result from the intake of large amounts of alcohol at a single setting:

1. Acute intoxication
2. Acute gastritis
3. Acute pancreatitis
4. Decrease in sexual functioning
5. Blackouts (amnesia)
6. Motor vehicle accidents: Blood alcohol concentration less than 0.05% considered "legally safe" for driving; 0.08% to 0.15% considered "legally intoxicated" in some states
7. Nonautomotive accidents and trauma
8. Coma and death

Alcohol use can also interfere with the treatment of chronic medical conditions such as diabetes mellitus and seizure disorders. Furthermore, it can interfere with medications that the adolescent may be taking.

Fetal Alcohol Syndrome

Fetal alcohol syndrome is the most common cause of teratogenic mental retardation and is also the most preventable. *There is no known safe level of alcohol use during pregnancy.* Alcohol readily crosses the placenta and can result in the fetal alcohol syndrome, which is characterized by:

1. Abnormal facies: Microcephaly; short, upturned nose; thin upper lip; short palpebral fissures; and hypoplastic maxilla

2. Cardiac abnormalities: Especially atrial and ventricular septal defects
3. Renal abnormalities: Deformed kidneys
4. Genital abnormalities: Hypospadias and labial hypoplasia
5. Skeletal abnormalities: Contractures of the extremities; pectus excavatum
6. Hirsutism
7. Central-nervous-system abnormalities: Electroencephalographic changes; mental retardation
8. Abnormal size: Small for gestational age
9. Behavior: Irritability in infancy; hyperactivity in childhood

TREATMENT

The initial stages of treatment are usually difficult. Early intervention by the provider of primary health care for problems with alcohol includes screening, assessment, referral services, and, in some instances, brief behavioral interventions. Health-care providers who care for adolescents should possess the basic skills to communicate effectively with adolescents and their parents about alcohol and other drug-use problems and concerns. The provider should also be able to provide appropriate referrals for substance abuse services in the community.

Naltrexone, an opiate antagonist, has been advocated as a useful adjunct in the treatment of alcoholism early in recovery. The alcoholic person appears to have unique genetically determined biological potential for highly reinforcing euphorigenic effects of alcohol on the endorphin axis. Naltrexone blocks these effects and seems to decrease the probability of a sustained relapse early in recovery. Use of this medication thus far has been studied in adult populations. It tends to be expensive and carries the potential for hepatotoxic effects.

Components of successful treatment of adolescent alcohol abuse and dependence include:

1. Accurate diagnosis and assessment: Treatment of any primary psychiatric disturbances should they be identified. If the patient meets criteria for a diagnosis of alcoholism or addiction, then proceed with interventions listed below. If the diagnosis is uncertain, always proceed with these suggestions. Reassessment of psychiatric symptoms should be undertaken after a minimum of 30 days. Very often, prominent psychiatric symptoms will remit spontaneously with abstinence.
2. Acknowledgment: Breaking down the denial that a problem exists is crucial in allowing the adolescent to recover.
3. Disease concept of recovery: Viewing alcoholism as a primary progressive disease implies a long-term, ongoing recovery process requiring abstinence and learning to live without alcohol and drugs. The recovery process also helps to expose and deal with accumulated feelings of guilt and shame, while rebuilding coping skills and self-esteem.
4. Positive alternatives: Treatment requires that the adolescent learn substitute activities that provide pleasure and reward to replace the "highs" of drug use. These activities should be realistic and attainable.
5. Support systems: Sober peer-support systems are essential for recovery. Alcoholics Anonymous, Cocaine Anonymous, and Narcotics Anonymous provide 12-step programs useful for recovering adolescents.
6. Family involvement: Alcoholism is a family illness. The substance abuse of one member of the family system affects the other members. Dysfunctional coping trends are established. Recovery and treatment should help establish a new, healthier equilibrium. Family members should be encouraged to attend Alanon or Alateen, which are 12-step self-help groups for family members.

BIBLIOGRAPHY

Blanken AJ. Measuring use of alcohol and other drugs among adolescents. Public Health Rep 1993;108:25.

Bowen OR, Sammons JH. The alcohol-abusing patient: a challenge to the profession. JAMA 1988;260:2267.

Brust J. Other agents: phencyclidine, marijuana, hallucinogens—neurologic complications of drugs and alcohol abuse. Neurol Clin 1993;11:555.

Centers for Disease Control and Prevention. Update: trends in fetal alcohol syndrome—United States, 1979–1993. JAMA 1995;273:1406.

Chang G, Astrachan BM. The emergency department surveillance of alcohol intoxication after motor vehicle accidents. JAMA 1988;260:2533.

Cohen DA, Richardson J, LaBree L. Parenting behaviors and the onset of smoking and alcohol use: a longitudinal study. Pediatrics 1994;94:368.

Cohen S. The bottle babies, adolescent alcoholism. Transitions 1980(December);3:7.

Council on Scientific Affairs. Alcohol and the driver. JAMA 1986;255:522.

Cyr MG, Wartman SA. The effectiveness of routine screening questions in the detection of alcoholism. JAMA 1988;259:51.

Decker MD, Graitcer PL, Schaffner W. Reduction in motor vehicle fatalities associated with an increase in the minimum drinking age. JAMA 1988;260:3604.

Dinning WD, Dark LA. The Children of Alcoholics Screening Test: relationship to sex, family environment, and social adjustments in adolescents. J Clin Psychol 1989;45:335.

Donovan JE, Jessor R. Adolescent problem drinking: psychosocial correlates in a national sample study. J Stud Alcohol 1978;39:1506.

Donovan JE, Jessor R, Jessor L. Problem drinking in adolescence and young adulthood: a follow-up study. J Stud Alcohol 1983;44:109.

Ewing JA. Detecting alcoholism; the CAGE questionnaire. JAMA 1985;252:14.

Farrow JA, Rees JM, Worthington-Roberts BS. Health, developmental, and nutritional status of adolescent alcohol and marijuana abusers. Pediatrics 1987;79:218.

Fleming JP, Kellam SG, Brown CH. Early predictors of age at first use of alcohol, marijuana, and cigarettes. Drug Alcohol Depend 1982;9:285.

Forney PD, Forney MA, Ripley WK. Alcohol and adolescents: knowledge, attitudes, and behavior. J Adolesc Health Care 1988;9:194.

Frances R, Miller SI. Clinical textbook of addiction disorders. New York: The Guildford Press, 1991.

Gitlow SE, Hennecke L. Etiology of alcoholism: a new theoretic mosaic. Semin Adolesc Med 1985;4:235.

Grube JW, Wallack L. Television beer advertising and drinking knowledge, beliefs, and intentions among schoolchildren. Am J Public Health 1994;84:254.

Hall W. The health risks of cannabis. Aust Fam Physician 1995;24:1237.

Harrison PA, Luxenberg MG. Comparisons of alcohol and other drug problems among Minnesota adolescents in 1989 and 1992. Arch Pediatr Adolesc Med 1995;149:137.

Hawkins RO Jr. Adolescent alcohol abuse: a review. J Dev Behav Pediatr 1982;2:83.

Hingson R, Merrigan D, Heeren T. Effects of Massachusetts raising its legal drinking age from 18 to 20 on deaths from teenage homicide, suicide, and nontraffic accidents. Pediatr Clin North Am 1985;32:221.

Hingson R, Heeren T, Winter M. Lower legal blood alcohol limits for young drivers. Public Health Rep 1994;109:738.

Johnston LD, O'Malley PM, Bachman JG. Drug use, drinking, and smoking: national survey results from high school, college, and young adults populations, 1975–1988. (DHHS Publication No. [ADM] 89–1638.) Washington, D.C.: U.S. Department of Health and Human Services, 1989.

Johnston LD, O'Malley PM, Bachman JG. Illicit drug use by American high school seniors in 1989. Ann Arbor: News and Information Services of the University of Michigan, February 13, 1993.

Johnston LD, O'Malley PM, Bachman JG. Monitoring the Future Study. Ann Arbor: News and Information Services of the University of Michigan, December 1995.

Jones JW. Children of Alcoholics Screening Test: test manual. Chicago: Camelot Unlimited, 1985.

Jones KL, Smith DW, Hanson JW. The fetal alcohol syndrome: clinical delineation. Ann NY Acad Sci 1976;273:130.

Kandel DB. On processes of peer influences in adolescent drug use: a developmental perspective. Advances in Alcohol Substance Abuse 1985;4:139.

Kinney J, Leaton G. Loosening the grip: a handbook of alcohol information. St. Louis: CV Mosby, 1983.

Kruse J. Alcohol use during pregnancy. Am Fam Physician 1984;29:199.

Lang RM, Borow KM, Neumann A, et al. Adverse cardiac effects of acute alcohol ingestion in young adults. Ann Intern Med 1985;102:742.

Lettieri DJ, Nelson JE, Sayers MA, eds. NIAAA treatment handbook, series 2: alcoholism treatment assessment research instruments. (DHHS Publication No. 87–1380.) Washington, D.C.: U.S. Department of Health and Human Services, 1987.

Lewis DD, Woods SE. Fetal alcohol syndrome. Am Fam Physician 1994;50:1035.

Lieber CS. Medical disorders of alcoholism. N Engl J Med 1995;333:1058.

MacDonald DI. Drugs, drinking, and adolescents. Chicago: Year Book Medical Publishers, 1984.

MacDonald DI. How you can help prevent teenage alcoholism. Contemp Pediatr 1986;November:50.

Marden PG, Kolodner K. Alcohol use and abuse among adolescents. Rockville, Maryland: National Council on Alcoholism. National Institute on Alcohol Abuse and Alcoholism, 1977.

Meeks J. Adolescents at risk for drug and alcohol abuse. Semin Adolesc Med 1985;1:231.

Meyer R, Neuropharmacology of ethanol. Boston: Birkhauser, 1991.

Midanik LT, Clark WB. The demographic distribution of U.S. drinking patterns in 1990: description and trends from 1984. Am J Public Health 1994;84:1218.

Monforte R, Estruch R, Valls-Sole J, et al. Autonomic and peripheral neuropathies in patients with chronic alcoholism: a dose-related toxic effect of alcohol. Arch Neurol 1995;52:45.

Morrison SF, Rogers PD, Thomas MH. Alcohol and adolescents. Pediatr Clin North Am 1995;42:371.

Morse RM, Flavin DK. The definition of alcoholism. JAMA 1992;268:1012.

Pandina RJ, White HR. Patterns of alcohol and drug use of adolescent students and adolescents in treatment. J Stud Alcohol 1981;42:441.

Rachal JV, Williams JR, Brehm ML, et al. A national study of adolescent drinking behavior, attitudes, and correlates [conducted by Research Triangle Institute for the National Institute on Alcohol Abuse and Alcoholism]. Washington, D.C.: U.S. Department of Health, Education, and Welfare, 1975. [Available from National Technical Information Service, Springfield, Va.]

Rogers PD, Hanio J, Jarmuskewicz J. Alcohol and adolescence. Pediatr Clin North Am 1987;34:289.

Schonberg SK. Guidelines for the treatment of alcohol- and other drug–abusing adolescents. Rockville, Maryland [Rockwall II, 5600 Fishers Lane, Rockville 20857]: U.S. Department of Health and Human Services, Public Health Service, Substance Abuse and Mental Health Services Administration, Center for Substance Abuse Treatment, 1993.

Schwartz RH, Hayden GF, Getson PR, et al. Drinking patterns and social consequences: a study of middle-class adolescents in two private pediatric practices. Pediatrics 1986;77:139.

Selzer ML. The Michigan Alcoholism Screening Test: the quest for a new diagnostic instrument. Am J Psychol 1971;127:89.

Skinner HA, Holt S, Schuller R. Identification of alcohol abuse using laboratory tests and a history of trauma. Ann Intern Med 1984;101:847.

Stephenson JN, Moberg P, Daniels BJ, et al. Treating the intoxicated adolescent: a need for comprehensive services. JAMA 1984;252:1884.

Sutocky JW, Shultz JM, Kizer KW. Alcohol-related mortality in California, 1980 to 1989. Am J Public Health 1993;83:817.

Swadi H. Alcohol abuse in adolescence: an update. Arch Dis Child 1993;68:341.

U.S. Public Health Service. Alcohol and other drug abuse in adolescents. Am Fam Physician 1994;50:1737.

Volpicelli JR. Naltrexone in alcohol dependence. Lancet 1995;346:456.

Wechsler H, Isaac N. "Binge" drinkers at Massachusetts colleges: prevalence, drinking style, time trends, and associated problems. JAMA 1992;267:2929–2931.

Wechsler H, Davenport A, Dowdall G, et al. Health and behavioral consequences of binge drinking in college: national survey of students at 140 campuses. JAMA 1994;272:1672.

Werner MJ. Principles of brief intervention for adolescent alcohol, tobacco, and other drug use. Pediatr Clin North Am 1995;42:335.

Werner MJ, Walker LS, Greene JW. Longitudinal evaluation of a screening measure for problem drinking among female college freshmen. Arch Pediatr Adolesc Med 1994;148:1331.

Williams CL, Perry CL, Wagenaar AC, et al. Where and how adolescents obtain alcoholic beverages. Public Health Rep 1993;108:459.

Wilson DM, Killen JD, Hayward C, et al. Timing and rate of sexual maturation and the onset of cigarette and alcohol use among teenage girls. Arch Pediatr Adolesc Med 1994;148:789.

CHAPTER 71

Tobacco

Lawrence S. Neinstein and Drew Pinsky

Cigarette smoking has been listed as the most important source of preventable morbidity and premature death in every report by the surgeon general of the United States since 1964. Cigarette use by the adolescent should be of major concern to the health-care practitioner, particularly because cigarette smoking is rising among young Americans. This chapter reviews tobacco use among teenagers and its health consequences.

PREVALENCE

By late adolescence a sizable proportion of young people have developed regular cigarette smoking habits, despite the demonstrated known risks. Since 1975, when the study of American high school students was started (Johnston et al., 1994), tobacco in the form of cigarettes has been the substance most frequently used on a daily basis. Although the prevalence rates for high school students smoking on a daily basis dropped during the 1977–1981 period (from 29% to 20%; peaked in 1976 and 1977), there has been little decrease since 1981 in either the prevalence of those smoking daily or those having smoked in the past 30 days. In fact, the rates for 8th and 10th graders have been increasing in recent years. Among both 8th and 10th graders, the prevalence of those smoking in the 30 days prior to the Monitoring the Future Study has increased by one-third from 1991 to 1995. About 19% of the 8th graders and 28% of the 10th graders now report this level of use. Since 1992 the smoking rate has risen by over one-fifth among high school seniors, with a rate of one in three who now have smoked in the 30 days prior to the survey (Johnston et al., 1995b). The rate of daily smoking rose in all grade levels studied between 1992 and 1995, from 7% to 9.3% among 8th graders, from 12.3% to 16.3% among 10th graders, and from 17.2% to 21.6% among 12th graders. The study also shows that teenagers greatly underestimate the dangers of smoking, with only about half of the 8th graders believing that smokers run a great risk of harming themselves by smoking a pack or more daily. The increases in smoking affect many broad groups of adolescents, including males and females, all three of the largest racial/ethnic groups, all socioeconomic levels, those planning to go to college and those not, those living in all regions of the country, and those living in cities as well as rural areas.

Before 1970, males smoked considerably more than female adolescents. Currently rates are about equal between male and female adolescents. Trends in smoking rates among teenagers are shown in Table 71.1 and Figures 71.1 and 71.2.

Other data are available from the National Household Survey on Drug Abuse. Nelson et al. (1995) reviewed the trends in persons aged 12–19 between 1974 and 1991. Overall smoking prevalence declined much more rapidly from 1974 through 1980 (1.9 percentage points annually among younger adolescents) than from 1985 through 1991 (0 to 0.5 percentage points annually among all adolescents). Since 1980, smoking has declined at a slightly faster

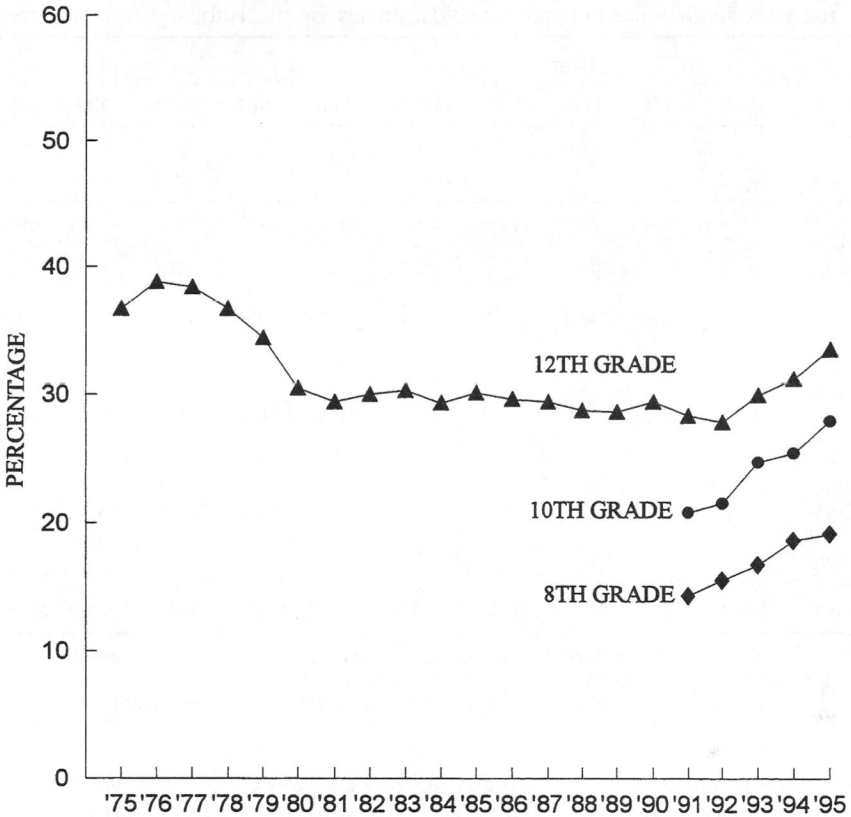

FIGURE 71.1. Thirty-day prevalence of cigarette smoking for 8th, 10th, and 12th graders. (From Johnston LD, O'Malley PM, Bachman JG. Cigarette smoking among American teens rises again in 1995. Ann Arbor: News and Information Services of the University of Michigan, December 11, 1995.)

rate among older female adolescents than among male adolescents. Though only minimal declines have occurred among white adolescents since 1985, smoking among African-American adolescents of all ages declined in nearly every survey population during each study period. For African-American adolescents, between 1974 and 1985 the range of decline was 1.0 to 2.9 percentage points and between 1985 and 1991, 0.7 to 1.5 percentage points annually.

REASONS THAT TEENAGERS SMOKE

The reasons teenagers give for smoking are similar to those they give for use of any drug: curiosity, independence, imitation, media influence, peer pressure, conformity, pleasure, rebellion, habit, and to enhance a feminine or masculine image. Among the risk determinants for teenagers who smoke are the following (National Clearinghouse for Smoking and Health, 1974):

1. Peer use: Estimated 90% chance that adolescent will smoke if his or her best friend smokes—perhaps the best predictor of smoking habits in an adolescent
2. Sibling use
3. Parental use: If one parent, doubles risk that teenager will smoke; if both parents or one parent and a sibling, increases risk three to four times
4. Amount of free money available to spend

TABLE 71.1.   Long-Term Trends in Prevalence of Cigarettes for 8th, 10th, and 12th Graders

	1975	1976	1977	1978	1979	1980	1981	1982	1983	1984	1985
Lifetime											
8th Grade											
10th Grade											
12th Grade	73.6	75.4	75.7	75.3	74.0	71.0	71.0	70.1	70.6	69.7	68.8
Thirty-Day											
8th Grade											
10th Grade											
12th Grade	36.7	38.8	38.4	36.7	34.4	30.5	29.4	30.0	30.3	29.3	30.1
Daily											
8th Grade											
10th Grade											
12th Grade	26.9	28.8	28.8	27.5	25.4	21.3	20.3	21.1	21.2	18.7	19.5
$1/2$ pack+/day											
8th Grade											
10th Grade											
12th Grade	17.9	19.2	19.4	18.8	16.5	14.3	13.5	14.2	13.8	12.3	12.5
Approximate Ns:											
8th Grade											
10th Grade											
12th Grade	*9400*	*15,400*	*17,100*	*17,800*	*15,500*	*15,900*	*17,500*	*17,700*	*16,300*	*15,900*	*16,000*

From Johnston LD, O'Malley PM, Bachman JG. Cigarette smoking among American teens rises again in 1995. Ann Arbor: News and Information Services of the University of Michigan, December 11, 1995.
[a]Level of significance of difference between the two years indicated: $s = 0.05$, $ss = 0.01$, $sss = 0.001$.

Besides the recent increase in smoking, adolescents appear to begin smoking at an earlier age. Initiation of tobacco use increases rapidly after age 11 and peaks between ages 17 and 19. There seems to be a strong cohort effect: if a group of teens has a high rate of smoking, this group will maintain a high rate in future years.

Attempts to Stop Smoking

Once started, smoking is hard to stop. It has been reported that more than 50% of teens in high school who smoke half a pack or more per day cannot stop after trying. Of those in high school who smoke on a daily basis, three-fourths are smoking on a daily basis 7–9 years later. The strength of nicotine addiction is such that as many as 85% of adolescents who smoke two or more cigarettes completely and overcome the initial discomfort will go on to become regular smokers.

Despite all the adverse publicity regarding smoking, the proportion of seniors who perceive smoking a pack a day as a great risk has fallen since 1993 (Johnston et al., 1995b) (Table 71.2 and Fig. 71.3). Even though most adolescents believe that smoking is a hazard to health, few consider it a threat to their own health. The personal disapproval of smoking fell from 1991 to 1993, suggesting that peer norms toward smoking are becoming less restrictive.

Other Correlates to Smoking in Adolescents

1. Academic performance: There is a negative relationship of tobacco use to academic performance (Tables 71.3 and 71.4).
2. Positive association with the use of other illicit drugs and alcohol: Among adolescents who smoke a pack per day, 95% have used another drug, 81% have used another drug besides marijuana, and 26% are daily users of some illicit drug.

Table 71.1. *continued*

1986	1987	1988	1989	1990	1991	1992	1993	1994	1995	1994–1995 Change[a]	1991–1995 Change[a]
					44.0	45.2	45.3	46.1	46.4	+0.3	+2.4
					55.1	53.5	56.3	56.9	57.6	+0.7	+2.5
67.6	67.2	66.4	65.7	64.4	63.1	61.8	61.9	62.0	64.2	+2.2s	+1.1
					14.3	15.5	16.7	18.6	19.1	+0.5	+4.8ss
					20.8	21.5	24.7	25.4	27.9	+2.5ss	+7.1sss
29.6	29.4	28.7	28.6	29.4	28.3	27.8	29.9	31.2	33.5	+2.3s	+5.2sss
					7.2	7.0	8.3	8.8	9.3	+0.5	+2.1ss
					12.6	12.3	14.2	14.6	16.3	+1.7s	+3.7sss
18.7	18.7	18.1	18.9	19.1	18.5	17.2	19.0	19.4	21.6	+2.2s	+3.1ss
					3.1	2.9	3.5	3.6	3.4	−0.2	+0.3
					6.5	6.0	7.0	7.6	8.3	+0.7	+1.8ss
11.4	11.4	10.6	11.2	11.3	10.7	10.0	10.9	11.2	12.4	+1.2	+1.7s
					17,500	*18,600*	*18,300*	*17,300*	*17,500*		
					14,800	*14,800*	*15,300*	*15,800*	*17,000*		
15,200	*16,300*	*16,300*	*16,700*	*15,200*	*15,000*	*15,800*	*16,300*	*15,400*	*15,400*		

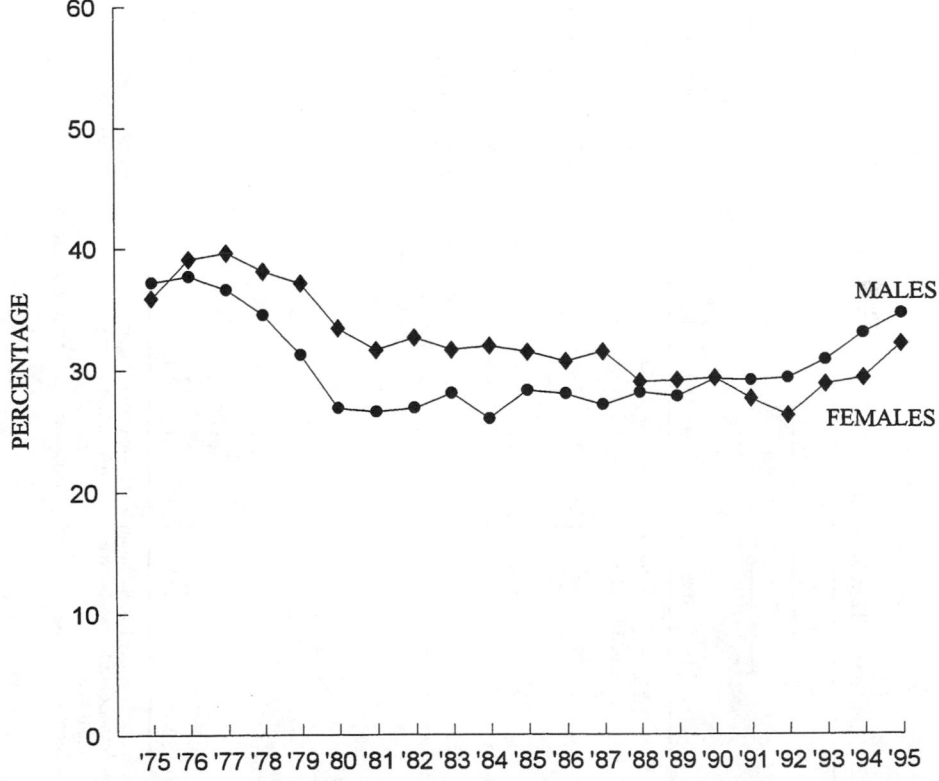

Figure 71.2. Trends in 30-day prevalence of cigarette use by gender among 12th graders. (From Johnston LD, O'Malley PM, Bachman JG. Cigarette smoking among American teens rises again in 1995. Ann Arbor: News and Information Services of the University of Michigan, December 11, 1995.)

TABLE 71.2.   Cigarettes: Trends in 30-Day Prevalence by Subgroups for 8th, 10th, and 12th Graders[a]

| | **Percent Who Smoked in Last 30 Days** | | | | | | | | | | | | | | | | | | | | |
| | **8th Grade** | | | | | | | **10th Grade** | | | | | | | **12th Grade** | | | | | | |
	1991	1992	1993	1994	1995	1994–1995 Change	1991–1995 Change	1991	1992	1993	1994	1995	1994–1995 Change	1991–1995 Change	1991	1992	1993	1994	1995	1994–1995 Change	1991–1995 Change
Approximate N =	*17,500*	*18,600*	*18,300*	*17,300*	*17,500*			*14,800*	*14,800*	*15,300*	*15,800*	*17,000*			*15,000*	*15,800*	*16,300*	*15,400*	*15,400*		
Total	14.3	15.5	16.7	18.6	19.1	+0.5	+4.8sss	20.8	21.5	24.7	25.4	27.9	+2.5ss	+7.1sss	28.3	27.8	29.9	31.2	33.5	+2.3s	+5.2sss
Sex																					
Male	15.5	14.9	17.2	19.3	18.8	-0.5	+3.3sss	20.8	20.6	24.6	26.6	27.7	+1.1	+6.9sss	29.0	29.2	30.7	32.9	34.5	+1.6	+5.5sss
Female	13.1	15.9	16.3	17.9	19.0	+1.1	+5.9sss	20.7	22.2	24.5	23.9	27.9	+4.0ss	+7.2sss	27.5	26.1	28.7	29.2	32.0	+2.8s	+4.5ss
College plans																					
None or under 4 yr	29.2	31.9	34.1	36.6	36.5	-0.1	+7.3ss	36.5	35.0	41.9	42.2	46.3	+4.1s	+9.8sss	38.1	38.6	37.3	40.9	43.5	+2.6	+5.4ss
Complete 4 yr	11.8	13.1	14.3	16.1	16.8	+0.7	+5.0sss	17.3	18.6	21.0	21.7	24.7	+3.0ss	+7.4sss	24.2	23.8	27.3	28.0	29.9	+1.9	+5.7sss
Region																					
Northeast	13.7	14.4	15.0	17.8	18.6	+0.8	+4.9s	22.4	21.9	27.1	24.5	27.8	+3.3	+5.4s	30.5	29.6	34.2	33.2	34.4	+1.2	+3.9
North Central	15.5	16.5	16.3	18.5	20.9	+2.4	+5.4ss	22.9	24.3	26.0	28.8	30.1	+1.3	+7.2ss	34.6	31.7	33.2	36.2	37.8	+1.6	+3.2
South	15.7	17.0	18.2	19.5	19.4	-0.1	+3.7s	21.2	19.8	24.0	25.7	30.8	+5.1ss	+9.6sss	25.4	26.4	29.0	30.7	33.5	+2.8	+8.1sss
West	10.0	12.2	16.4	18.0	16.5	-1.5	+6.5sss	16.7	20.2	21.2	20.1	19.6	-0.5	+2.9	23.2	22.8	22.9	24.0	26.5	+2.5	+3.3
Population density																					
Large MSA[b]	12.8	15.0	14.1	15.5	16.5	+1.0	+3.7s	19.7	21.6	22.5	22.3	23.3	+1.0	+3.6	26.2	25.6	29.5	29.0	33.9	+4.9ss	+7.7sss
Other MSA	14.9	15.3	17.8	20.7	19.4	-1.3	+4.5ss	20.3	20.3	23.8	26.3	28.9	+2.6	+8.6sss	29.3	26.9	29.8	31.1	31.7	+0.6	+2.4
Non-MSA	14.8	16.4	17.9	17.8	21.5	+3.7s	+6.7ss	22.7	23.7	28.2	26.7	31.3	+4.6s	+8.6sss	28.6	31.5	30.3	33.8	36.2	+2.4	+7.6ss
Parental education[c]																					
1.0–2.0 (Low)	26.2	24.1	23.3	26.1	25.3	-0.8	-0.9	23.5	28.4	29.5	26.4	30.9	+4.5	+7.4ss	31.3	27.1	26.5	26.2	31.2	+5.0	-0.1
2.5–3.0	16.4	16.9	19.8	20.6	22.7	+2.1	+6.3sss	24.1	23.3	28.0	29.1	33.2	+4.1ss	+9.1sss	28.7	30.3	30.4	32.8	35.0	+2.2	+6.3sss
3.5–4.0	13.9	14.9	17.4	20.1	20.8	+0.7	+6.9sss	20.4	20.6	24.8	26.0	27.8	+1.8	+7.4sss	28.4	27.8	29.9	31.4	33.2	+1.8	+4.8ss
4.5–5.0	10.1	13.3	12.5	14.9	14.9	0.0	+4.8sss	18.5	19.5	20.1	22.6	25.9	+3.3s	+7.4sss	26.9	25.8	30.1	32.0	32.6	+0.6	+5.7sss
5.5–6.0 (High)	11.3	11.5	13.3	15.1	14.5	-0.6	+3.2s	18.5	18.9	21.4	20.7	21.8	+1.1	+3.3	27.1	25.5	30.5	30.4	34.0	+3.6	+6.9ss

From Johnston LD, O'Malley PM, Bachman JG. Cigarette smoking among American teens rises again in 1995. Ann Arbor: News and Information Services of the University of Michigan, December 11, 1995.
[a]Level of significance of difference between the two indicated years: $s = 0.05$, $ss = 0.01$, $sss = 0.001$.
[b]MSA, Metropolitan statistical area.
[c]Parental education is an average score of mother's education and father's education.

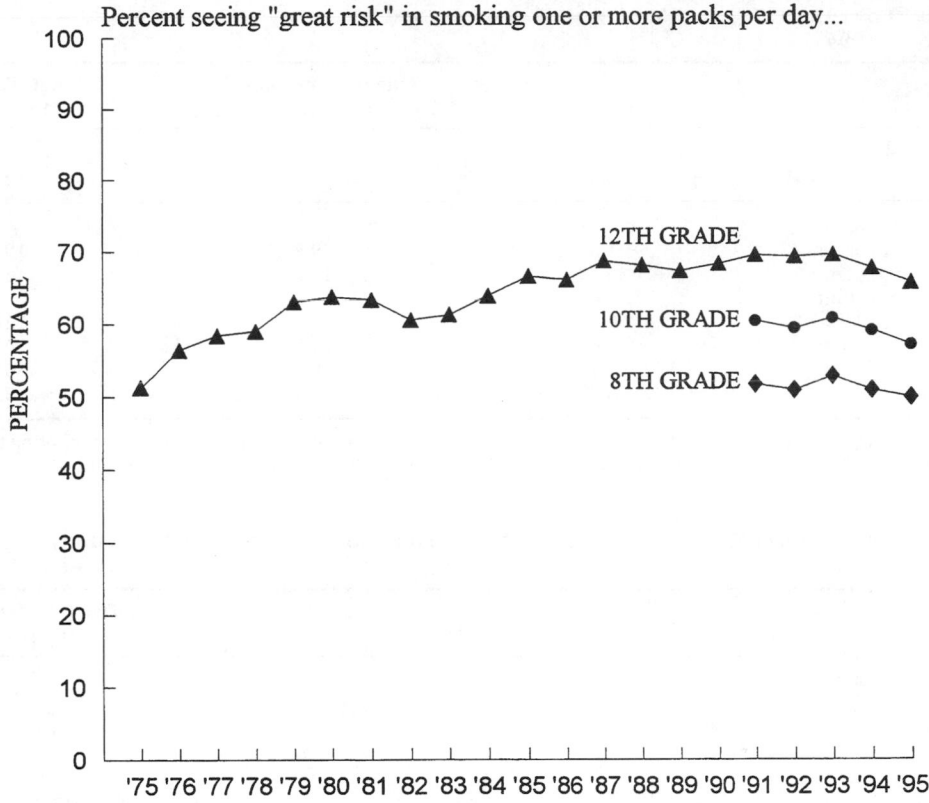

Percent seeing "great risk" in smoking one or more packs per day...

FIGURE 71.3. Trends in perceived harmfulness of smoking for 8th, 10th, and 12th graders. (From Johnston LD, O'Malley PM, Bachman JG. Cigarette smoking among American teens rises again in 1995. Ann Arbor: News and Information Services of the University of Michigan, December 11, 1995.)

3. Parental behaviors and styles: Cohen et al. (1994) found that children who reported that parents spent more time with them and communicated with them more frequently had lower onset rates of using alcohol and tobacco in the preceding month.
4. Pubertal development: Wilson et al. (1994) found that patterns of pubertal progression—early versus late puberty and fast versus slow progression—are associated with the age at which girls start to drink alcohol and smoke cigarettes. In this study of 1463 female students, 10.7–18.2 years of age, girls with earlier puberty (midpoint <12.2 years) first reported smoking cigarettes at a median age of 12.8 years, 0.6 year younger than girls with later puberty.
5. History of substance abuse: Substance-abusing teens smoke at rates far above those of the general adolescent population (Myers and Brown, 1994). These teens also appear at an increased risk of having negative health consequences regardless of posttreatment drug and alcohol use.
6. Exposure to cigarette advertising: Adolescents with high exposure to cigarette advertising are significantly more likely to be smokers than are those with low exposure to cigarette advertising (Botvin et al., 1993).

HEALTH CONSEQUENCES

Nicotine is a highly addictive compound. Its action is largely mediated through nicotinic acetylcholine receptors. These receptors, although primarily on cholinergic neurons, are lo-

Table **71.3.**   Cigarette Use Related to Sex, Education, and Region of the Country in 12th Graders, 1994

	Ever Used	One or More Daily in Past 30 Days	Half-Pack or More Daily
Sex			
Males	63.0	20.4	12.7
Females	60.6	18.1	9.5
College plans			
None or <4 yr	71.2	29.8	19.6
4-Yr program	59.1	15.7	8.2
Region of country			
Northeast	65.1	21.3	12.2
North Central	64.4	23.8	15.3
South	61.7	19.3	10.8
West	56.7	12.4	5.9

Adapted from Johnston LD, O'Malley PM, Bachman JG. National survey results on drug use from the Monitoring the Future Study, 1975–1994. (NIH publication No. 95–4026.) Washington, D.C.: National Institutes of Health, 1995.

Table **71.4.**   Smokeless Tobacco Use Related to Sex, Education, and Region of the Country, in 12th Graders, 1994

	Ever Used	30-Day Prevalence of Daily Use
Sex		
Males	47.4	7.2
Females	15.6	0.3
College plans		
None or <4 yr	38.1	6.6
4-Yr program	28.1	2.8
Region of country		
Northeast	29.2	4.5
North Central	35.6	4.7
South	29.3	3.5
West	28.3	3.2

Adapted from Johnston LD, O'Malley PM, Bachman JG. National survey results on drug use from the Monitoring the Future Study, 1975–1994. (NIH publication No. 95–4026.) Washington, D.C.: National Institutes of Health, 1995.

cated on a variety of noncholinergic presynaptic and postsynaptic sites throughout the brain. This allows nicotine to affect a variety of neuronal pathways involved in behavioral reward and arousal processes. Nicotine releases endogenous opiates and leads to an increase in the secretion of growth hormone, cortisol, and vasopressin. There is a rapid onset of action, 7.5 seconds after inhalation. Nicotine causes:

1. Increased pain threshold and tolerance
2. Decreased craving for sweets
3. Improved performance in some tasks that demand alertness

Cigarette smoking causes the largest group of preventable deaths. It is estimated that a period of $5\frac{1}{2}$ minutes is lost for each cigarette smoked, equaling a loss of 4.6 years of life during 25 years of smoking a pack per day. The estimated number of deaths from preventable causes is about 400,000, or 19% of total preventable deaths. The health risks to children and adolescents, reviewed by the American Heart Association (1994), include effects on the cardiovascular system, the respiratory system, and the fetus and neonate, as well as risk-taking behaviors of adolescents. Other potential risks may extend to other areas, including reports that cigarette smoking decreases breast-milk production in mothers, by-products of tobacco use are transmitted in breast milk, exposure to passive smoking may alter children's intelligence and behavior, and passive smoke exposure in childhood may be a risk factor for the development of lung cancer as an adult.

Cardiovascular Consequences

1. Increased risk of premature coronary artery disease and a greater mortality rate from coronary artery disease: Approximately one-fifth of deaths from cardiovascular disease are attributable to smoking. In 1990, smoking caused almost 180,000 deaths from cardiovascular disease. Passive smoking caused 53,000 deaths, of which 37,000 were related to heart disease.
2. Increased risk of cardiomyopathies
3. Increased risk of stroke
4. Negative cardiovascular effects of cigarette smoke include:
   a. Endothelial damage: Damage to the vascular endothelium caused by components of cigarette smoke; may lead to atherosclerosis
   b. Coronary vaso-occlusive factors: Platelet aggregation and vasomotor reactivity; prothombotic state
   c. Increased carbon monoxide production
   d. Increased plasma viscosity
   e. Increased plasma fibrinogen
   f. Nicotine effects: Increase in heart rate, blood pressure, cardiac output, and myocardial oxygen consumption, as well as formation of arrhythmias; possible serious consequences in anyone with underlying cardiovascular disease
   g. Increase in total cholesterol concentration; reduction in concentrations of high-density lipoproteins

Cancer

1. Lung cancer: Smoking is responsible for more than 85% of lung cancers. The risk of squamous-cell carcinoma is increased 10 times in smokers. Lung cancer among females is now increasing because of the increased prevalence of smoking among females. Approximately 80–85% of lung cancer deaths are related to smoking.
2. Other cancers
   a. Smoking has also been linked to cancer of the mouth, larynx, pharynx, esophagus, stomach, pancreas, uterine cervix, kidneys, ureters, and bladder.
   b. Approximately 30% of all cancer deaths are due to smoking.
      — An estimated 82% of laryngeal cancer deaths
      — About 93% of oral-cavity tumors in men and 61% of such cancers in women
      — About 80% of esophageal cancer deaths
      — An estimated 14% of all leukemias
   c. Overall rates of death from cancer are twice as high among smokers as among non-smokers; heavier smokers have rates that are four times greater.
   d. A synergistic interaction between tobacco and alcohol is thought to exist. Alcohol and tobacco account for 75–95% of all oral, esophageal, and laryngeal cancers.

Pulmonary Disease

Cigarette smoking is the most important factor in the development of chronic obstructive pulmonary disease. Smokers have increased mortality rates for chronic bronchitis and emphysema. Even smokers without clinical pulmonary disease have changes in small airways, as measured by pulmonary function tests. Approximately 80–90% of deaths caused by chronic obstructive lung disease are in smokers.

Gastrointestinal Disorders

The risk of having peptic ulcer disease is increased 1.5 to 2 times in smokers.

Dermatological Disorders

Investigators have recently found evidence of premature wrinkling of the skin in smokers.

Pregnancy Complications

Cigarette smoking has been linked to an increased rate of stillbirths, lower-than-average birth weight for gestational age, and an increased mortality rate in the neonatal period. Because the health risk seems to be greatest when a pregnant female smokes after the fourth month of gestation, preventive discussions during prenatal visits are especially important before the fourth month. Cornelius et al. (1995) examined the effects of tobacco on the offspring of 310 adolescents. Maternal tobacco use before delivery was associated in the infants with reduced birth weight, length, head and chest circumferences, and ponderal index, but not with younger gestational age at birth or number of morphological abnormalities. Cornelius et al. found that the effects of prenatal tobacco and marijuana use by adolescent mothers were prominent despite lower levels of prenatal exposure in their offspring than in the offspring of adult mothers who attended the same clinic. Young maternal age may increase the offspring's risk of negative effects from prenatal tobacco and marijuana exposure.

Adverse Effects of Smokeless Tobacco

Another serious health hazard to adolescents is smokeless (chewing) tobacco. These products are proven carcinogens but are perceived by many adolescents as being safe. In addition, there are few government regulations regarding sales and advertising.

There are approximately 10–12 million users of smokeless tobacco in the United States, 3 million of whom are less than 21 years of age, with an especially large group in adolescent males. Sixteen percent of adolescent males 12–17 years of age have used smokeless tobacco in the past year, and of these, one-third use it at least once a week. A recent review of the literature reveals that the groups at highest risk of regularly using smokeless tobacco are white youth and young adults aged 10–30, with the most vulnerable living in the southern United States.

Smokeless tobacco is known to increase the risk of oral cancer of the pharynx and hypopharynx and can lead to gingival recession and oral leukoplakia. In female users, it can also lead to low birth weight in their infants and to early delivery.

The American Academy of Pediatrics (Committee on Environmental Hazards, 1985) has recommended that:

1. Practicing pediatricians should take action to require placement of strong health warnings on all smokeless tobacco products and to ban all advertising and free giveaways of smokeless tobacco products.
2. The U.S. Federal Trade Commission and the U.S. Congress should take regulatory and legislative action to require placement of strong health warnings on all packages of all smokeless tobacco products and to ban all advertising of such products.

3. The Federal Trade Commission should sponsor counteradvertisements that accurately inform the public of the dangers of smokeless tobacco.
4. Congress should empower the U.S. Food and Drug Administration to set limits on nitrosamines in smokeless tobacco products.
5. Congress should reinstate the federal excise tax on smokeless tobacco and set the tax high enough to deter youngsters from purchasing smokeless tobacco products.
6. The players' associations of the major professional sports should discourage their member athletes from appearing in smokeless-tobacco advertising.

TREATMENT AND PREVENTION

Stopping cigarette smoking in adolescents who already smoke on a regular basis is difficult. Primary prevention before smoking has started is the most effective strategy to decrease the prevalence of smoking. Secondary prevention is also important, because children and adolescents whose parents smoke are exposed to health risks and are also more likely themselves to become smokers in the future. A comprehensive strategy that includes health-professional interventions, policy changes, advertising restrictions, comprehensive school-based programs, community activities, and advocacy approaches is needed. Physicians and other health professionals have major roles in each of these interventions

Bruvold (1993) conducted a meta-analysis of adolescent smoking prevention programs. Evaluations of 94 separate interventions were included. Behavioral effects were found to be greatest for interventions with a social-reinforcement orientation.

Educational Measures

1. Information approach: Although information is an important aspect of preventing and treating cigarette smoking, it is not sufficient. Adolescents usually understand the health risks of smoking but often cannot relate to distant health risks. Providing information, by itself, has usually failed.
2. Social and psychological approaches: Giving adolescents skills to cope with social pressures may bring added success to informational sessions.

Parental Involvement

The importance of parents as role models for their children cannot be overemphasized. Convincing parents to stop smoking can have a tremendous impact on the number of adolescents who smoke.

Research into Motivational Factors

Research into the motivation for smoking may provide new clues to successful treatment and prevention methods.

Early Intervention

The smoking habit is formed early, often by 10–12 years of age or less. Kelder et al. (1994) found that there is clear tracking of smoking behaviors in childhood. The early consolidation of health behaviors suggests that interventions should begin before the 6th grade in school—before the prevalence of smoking increases to 10% or more. Early intervention within a primary-health-care setting for problems with tobacco and other drugs includes screening, assessment, and referral services, and cognitive and behavioral brief interventions (Werner, 1995). Health-care providers who care for adolescents should possess basic skills in communicating with adolescents and young adults and with parents about their concerns about tobacco and other drug use. The providers should also be able to identify appropriate substance-abuse services in their communities and be able to decide the appropriate referral options for given adolescent patients. More research and options are needed to determine the most cost-effective approaches to tobacco cessation in the office practice.

Identification of High-Risk Groups

Several groups of adolescent smokers are at special risk: oral contraceptive users, pregnant adolescents, drug abusers, and hypertensive adolescents. A concerted effort should be made to encourage these adolescents, particularly, to eliminate their cigarette habit.

Antismoking Legislation

Continued state and federal legislation in the form of advertisement restrictions and increased taxes on cigarettes should be supported. A model proposed by DiFranza et al. (1987) suggests that:

1. Possession of tobacco by children should be prohibited. Many children believe that smoking cannot be that bad if cigarettes are not illegal for children.
2. Possession or use of tobacco by students should be specifically prohibited on school property.
3. The sale of all tobacco products to individuals younger than age 21 years should be prohibited.
4. Signs warning that it is illegal for minors to buy tobacco should be conspicuously visible to both employees and customers.
5. State law should require public schools to provide education about the health effects of tobacco use.
6. Cigarette vending machines should be prohibited, just as alcohol vending machines are prohibited.
7. All free distributions of tobacco should be prohibited.
8. All vendors of tobacco products should be licensed annually.
9. Penalties for the sale of tobacco to minors must be stringent enough to deter would-be offenders.

Smoking Cessation Techniques

Smoking-cessation suggestions for individual adolescents are as follows:

1. Set a date to quit.
2. Identify in a diary the situations that can trigger smoking, and plan to avoid them.
3. Get rid of tobacco products and paraphernalia.
4. Make a contract to quit and a plan for rewarding your success.
5. Suggest substitute activities such as chewing gum or munching on carrots or celery.
6. Anticipate withdrawal symptoms and discuss them with the adolescent. They include irritability, headaches, insomnia, drowsiness, constipation, diarrhea, and increased appetite. These effects usually are transient, lasting up to 4 weeks.
7. Suggest an increase in exercise, relaxation techniques, or both.
8. Spend more time with nonsmoking peers.

9. If an adolescent has a strong desire to stop smoking but is having difficulties despite repeated attempts, a nicotine-replacement system can be tried.

A nicotine gum (Nicorette) is a cation exchange resin with 2 mg of nicotine in a sugar-free, flavored gum. About 90% of the nicotine is absorbed during a 30-minute period. The teen should slowly chew one piece for 15–30 minutes whenever the urge for a cigarette occurs, using no more than 30 pieces per day. The usual requirement is about 10–15 pieces per day. The use of nicotine gum is usually associated with 50–100% higher quit rates. The gum should be avoided by pregnant teens, those with cardiovascular disease, and those with temporomandibular joint dysfunction. The gum can exacerbate existing hypertension, peptic ulcer disease, diabetes mellitus, hyperthyroidism, and esophagitis.

Transdermal nicotine has shown similar efficacy. A variety of products are available, the primary difference among them being the duration of nicotine delivery. The patches typically come in three dosage levels for titration and weaning purposes. The same relative contraindications apply as for nicotine gum. Great care should be taken to stress to the adolescent that he or she should not smoke while using the patch, because major cardiac events have been reported in that circumstance.

Smoking Cessation Resources

1. American Academy of Family Physicians (800-274-2237): AAFP Stop Smoking Kit (address: Health Education Department, Box 8723, Kansas City, MO 64114-0723); provides instructions and other materials necessary for establishing office-based smoking cessation program
2. U.S. Office of Smoking and Health: *Smoking and Health Bulletin* (address: Park Building, Suite I-58, 12429 Parklawn Dr., Rockville, MD 20857); other references and self-help materials also available
3. American Lung Association (contact local office)
    a. A Healthy Beginning Counseling Kit: Kit for health-care providers, including guidebook on counseling about passive smoking, waiting room poster, tent card, and sample parent's packet
    b. *Freedom From Smoking in 20 Days:* Available from local chapters of the American Lung Association
4. American Cancer Society (contact local office)
    a. Tobacco-Free Young America: A Kit for Busy Practitioners
    b. Fresh Start: Kit available from local chapters of the American Cancer Society; contains no-smoking prescription pads, buttons, and self-help materials
5. National Cancer Institute (800-4-CANCER)
    a. *The Smoking Digest: A Progress Report on the Nation, Kicking the Habit;* compendium on all aspects of smoking, from effects to cessation methods (address: Publications Orders, Office of Cancer Communications, National Cancer Institute, National Institutes of Health, Bldg. No. 31, Room 10A18, Bethesda, MD 20205 [Publication No. 79-1549, 1979]).
    b. Helping Smokers Quit Kit (address: Publications Orders, Office of Cancer Communications, National Cancer Institute, National Institutes of Health, Bldg. No. 31, Room 10A18, Bethesda, MD 20205)
6. National Heart, Lung, and Blood Institute (202-783-3238): *Clinical Opportunities for Smoking Intervention: A Guide for the Busy Physician* (National Institutes of Health publication No. 86-2178).
7. American Medical Association (312-464-0500): Creating a Tobacco Free Society: A Physician Leadership Kit (address: 515 North State St., Chicago, IL 60610.)

BIBLIOGRAPHY

American Heart Association. Active and passive tobacco exposure: a serious pediatric health problem. (A statement from the Committee on Atherosclerosis and Hypertension in Children, Council on Cardiovascular Disease in the Young, American Heart Association.) Circulation 1994;90:2581.

Bartechhi CE, MacKenzie TD, Schrier RW. The human costs of tobacco use [two parts]. N Engl J Med 1994; 330:907, 975.

Benowitz NL. Drug therapy: pharmacologic aspects of cigarette smoking and nicotine addiction. N Engl J Med 1988;319:1319.

Benowitz NL, Hall SM, Herning RI, et al. Smokers of low-yield cigarettes do not consume less nicotine. N Engl J Med 1983;309:139.

Benowitz NL, Jacob P III, Yu L, et al. Reduced tar, nicotine, and carbon monoxide exposure while smoking ultralow- but not low-yield cigarettes. JAMA 1986; 256:241.

Berenson JGS, Johnson CC. Attitudes of southern adolescents toward smoking South Med J 1995;88:601.

Botvin GJ, Goldberg CJ, Botvin EM, et al. Smoking behavior of adolescents exposed to cigarette advertising. Public Health Rep 1993;108:217.

Bruvold WH. A meta-analysis of adolescent smoking prevention programs. Am J Public Health 1993;83: 872.

Centers for Disease Control. Cigarette smoking in the United States, 1986. MMWR 1987;36:581.

Centers for Disease Control and Prevention. Changes in the cigarette brand preferences of adolescent smokers—United States, 1989–1993. JAMA 1994a;272:843.

Centers for Disease Control and Prevention. Minors' access to cigarette vending machines—Texas. JAMA 1994b;272:1402.

Centers for Disease Control and Prevention. Reasons for tobacco use and symptoms of nicotine withdrawal among adolescent and young adult tobacco users—United States, 1993. JAMA 1994c;272:1648.

Centers for Disease Control and Prevention. Cigarette smoking among adults—United States, 1993. JAMA 1995;273:369.

Cohen DA, Richardson J, LaBree L. Parenting behaviors and the onset of smoking and alcohol use: a longitudinal study. Pediatrics 1994;94:368.

Colditz GA, Bonita R, Stampfer MJ, et al. Cigarette smoking and risk of stroke in middle-aged women. N Engl J Med 1988;318:937.

Committee on Environmental Hazards; American Academy of Pediatrics. Smokeless tobacco: a carcinogenic hazard to children. Pediatrics 1985;76:1009.

Connolly GN, Winn DM, Hecht SS, et al. The reemergence of smokeless tobacco. N Engl J Med 1986;314: 1020.

Consensus Panel. Health applications of smokeless tobacco use. JAMA 1986;255:1045.

Cornelius MD, Taylor PM, Geva D, et al. Prenatal tobacco and marijuana use among adolescents: effects on offspring gestational age, growth, and morphology. Pediatrics 1995;95:738.

Council on Scientific Affairs. Health effects of smokeless tobacco. JAMA 1986;255:1038.

Cummings SR. Kicking the habit: benefits and methods of quitting cigarette smoking. West J Med 1982;137: 443.

DiFranza JR, Norwood BD, Garner DW, et al. Legislative efforts to protect children from tobacco. JAMA 1987;257:3387.

Epps RP, Manley MW, Glynn TJ. Tobacco use among adolescents: strategies for prevention. Pediatr Clin North Am 1995;42:389.

Escobedo LG, Anda RF, Smith PF, et al. Sociodemographic characteristics of cigarette smoking initiation in the United States. JAMA 1990;264:1550.

Evans RI. Smoking in children: developing a social psychological strategy of deterrence. Prev Med 1976;5: 122.

Fielding JE. Smoking: health effects and control [Parts 1 and 2]. N Engl J Med 1985;313:491, 555.

Fiore MC, Novotny TE, Pierce JP, et al. Methods used to quit smoking in the United States: do cessation programs help? JAMA 1990;263:2760.

Fletcher DJ. Kicking the nicotine habit. Postgrad Med 1985;77:123.

Hartz AJ, Anderson AJ, Brooks HL, et al. The association of smoking with cardiomyopathy. N Engl J Med 1984;311:1201.

Hughes JR, Miller SA. Nicotine gum to help stop smoking. JAMA 1984;252:2855.

Husten CG, Manley MW. How to help your patients stop smoking. Am Fam Physician 1990;42:1017.

Janerich DT, Thompson WD, Varela LR, et al. Lung cancer and exposure to tobacco smoke in the household. N Engl J Med 1990;323:632.

Johnston LD, O'Malley PM, Bachman JG. National trends in drug use and related factors among American high school students and young adults, 1975–1986. (DHHS publication No. 87-1535.) Washington, D.C.: U.S. Department of Health and Human Services, 1987.

Johnston LD, O'Malley PM, Bachman JG. Drug use, drinking, and smoking: national survey results from high school, college, and young adults populations, 1975–1988. (DHHS publication No. [ADM] 89-1638.) Washington, D.C.: U.S. Department of Health and Human Services, 1989.

Johnston LD, O'Malley PM, Bachman JG. Drug use rises again in 1995 among American teens. Ann Arbor: News and Information Services of the University of Michigan, December 11, 1995a.

Johnston LD, O'Malley PM, Bachman JG. Cigarette smoking among American teens rises again in 1995. Ann Arbor: News and Information Services of the University of Michigan, December 11, 1995b.

Kaufman DW, Helmrich SP, Rosenberg L, et al. Nicotine and carbon monoxide content of cigarette smoke and the risk of myocardial infarction in young men. N Engl J Med 1983;308:409.

Kelder SH, Perry CL, Klepp KI, et al. Longitudinal tracking of adolescent smoking, physical activity, and food choice behaviors. Am J Public Health 1994;84:1121.

Kessler DA. Nicotine addiction in young people. N Engl J Med 1995;333:186.

Leventhal H, Glynn K, Fleming R. Is the smoking decision an informed choice? JAMA 1987;257:3373.

MacKenzie TD, Bartecchi CE, Schrier RW. The human costs of tobacco use. N Engl J Med 1994;330:975.

Marcus SE, Giovino GA, Pierce JP, et al. Measuring tobacco use among adolescents. Public Health Rep 1993;108(suppl 1):20.

McIlvain H, Susman JL, Cavis C, et al. Physician counseling for smoking cessation: is the glass half empty? J Fam Pract 1995;40:148.

Mittelmark MB, Murray DM, Luepker RV, et al. Predicting experimentation with cigarettes: the Childhood Antecedents of Smoking Study (CASS). Am J Public Health 1987;77:206.

Myers MG, Brown SA. Smoking and health in substance-abusing adolescents: a two-year follow-up. Pediatrics 1994;93:561.

Nelson DE, Giovino GA, Shopland DR, et al. Trends in cigarette smoking among U.S. adolescents, 1974 through 1991. Am J Public Health 1995;85:34.

Ockene JK, Ockene IS. 9 Ways to help your patients stop smoking. Your Patient and Cancer 1982;(January):47.

O'Connell DL, Alexander HM, Dobson AJ, et al. Cigarette smoking and drug use in school children. II. Factors associated with smoking. Int J Epidemiol 1981;10:223.

Palmer AB. Some variables contributing to the onset of cigarette smoking among junior high school students. Soc Sci Med 1970;4:359.

Pederson LL, Baskerville JC, Lefcoe NM. Change in smoking status among school-aged youth: impact of a smoking awareness curriculum—attitudes, knowledge, and environmental factors. Am J Public Health 1981;71:1401.

Pierce JP, Lee L, Gilpin EA. Smoking initiation by adolescent girls, 1944 through 1988. JAMA 1994;271:609.

Rosencransn JA. Neurobehavioral mechanisms of nicotine action: role in the initiation and maintenance of tobacco dependence. J Subst Abuse Treat 1993;10:161.

Sherin K. Smoking cessation. Postgrad Med 1982;72:99.

Silagy C, Mant D, Fowler G, et al. Meta-analysis on efficacy of nicotine replacement therapies in smoking cessation. Lancet 1994;343:139.

Silvis GL, Perry CL. Understanding and deterring tobacco use among adolescents. Pediatr Clin North Am 1987;34:363.

Tonnesen P, Fryd V, Hansen M, et al. Effect of nicotine chewing gum in combination with group counseling on the cessation of smoking. N Engl J Med 1988;318:15.

U.S. Public Health Service. Teenage smoking: national patterns of cigarette smoking, age 12 through 18, in 1972 and 1974. (DHEW publication No. [NIH] 76-931.) Washington, D.C.: U.S. Department of Health, Education, and Welfare, 1974.

U.S. Public Health Service. Cigarette smoking among teenagers and young women. (DHEW publication No. 77-1203.) Washington, D.C.: U.S. Department of Health, Education and Welfare, 1977a.

U.S. Public Health Service. Smoking and health; vols 1, 2. Modifying the risk for the smokers: health consequences, education, cessation activities, and social action. Proceedings of the Third World Conference. (DHEW publication No. [NIH] 77-1143.) Washington, D.C.: U.S. Department of Health, Education, and Welfare, 1977b.

U.S. Public Health Service. Smokeless tobacco or health. (NIH publication No. 93-3461, September 1992.) Washington, D.C.: National Institutes of Health, 1993.

Wang MQ, Fitzhugh EC, Green L, et al. Tobacco use among American adolescents: geographic and demographic variations. South Med J 1994;87:607.

Warner KE, Goldenhar LM, McLaughlin CG. Cigarette advertising and magazine coverage of the hazards of smoking. N Engl J Med 1992;326:305.

Werner MJ. Principles of brief intervention for adolescent alcohol, tobacco, and other drug use. Pediatr Clin North Am 1995;42:335.

Wilson DM, Killen JD, Hayward C, et al. Timing and rate of sexual maturation and the onset of cigarette and alcohol use among teenage girls. Arch Pediatr Adolesc Med 1994;148:789.

CHAPTER 72

Marijuana

Lawrence S. Neinstein, Bruce S. Heischober, and Drew Pinsky

Marijuana remains the most widely abused illicit drug in the United States. A consistent decline was noted between 1979 and 1992 in marijuana use. A trend toward increasing use has now been documented in all ages studied. In 1992, 22% of high school seniors reported having used marijuana in the previous 12 months. This percentage increased to 26% in 1993, 31% in 1994, and 34.7% in 1995. The lifetime prevalence increased from 32.6% in 1992 to 41.7% in 1995. During the period between 1992 and 1995 the annual use of marijuana more than doubled among 8th graders (to 15.8%), grew by two-thirds among 10th graders (to 28.7%), and grew by over two-fifths among 12th graders (to 34.7%). Of particular concern is the rise in daily use of marijuana. Active daily use of marijuana more than doubled to 4.6% among high school seniors in 1995. About 1 in every 35 10th graders (2.8%) is a daily user.

Marijuana is no longer considered a benign drug. It has been shown to have negative effects on both physical and psychological health. The frequent use and abuse of marijuana must be taken seriously.

THE DRUG

Marijuana is derived from the flowering tops and leaves of the plant *Cannabis sativa*.

1. Preparations
   a. Joint: This form of marijuana usually consists of chopped-up leaves and stems of the plants, which are rolled into cigarettes and smoked.
   b. Cookies and brownies: Marijuana is sometimes baked into cookies or brownies and ingested orally.
   c. Pipe: Loose marijuana is often smoked in pipes or bongs, sometimes in combination with other drugs such as cocaine or phencyclidine (PCP).
   d. Hashish: This preparation is the strongest form of marijuana. It is composed of a pure resin derived from the leaves and flowers of the female plant and is usually pressed into a "brick" and smoked.
2. Slang names: *Grass, pot, weed, dope, bud, endo,* and *blunts* (hollowed-out small cigars, refilled with marijuana)
3. Active ingredient: Δ-9-Tetrahydrocannabinol (THC) is the active ingredient in all forms of marijuana.
4. Potency: In the 1960s the average potency was 0.1–0.5% THC. Recent analysis shows that today most marijuana averages 4–5% THC. Samples of sensimilla, a potent marijuana cultivated to obtain high THC levels, average 7–9% but have tested as high as 14%. Hash oil may contain 20–30% THC. This increase in potency may be a factor in the recent increase in reports of side effects.

5. Metabolism: THC is primarily metabolized in the liver. The drug is fat soluble and thus can accumulate for long periods in the body. Smoked marijuana has 5 to 10 times the bioavailability of the ingested drug.
6. Excretion: Cannabinoid metabolites are carried by the enterohepatic circulation to the intestinal lumen and excreted in the feces (65%) or are carried through the renal circulation and excreted in the urine (35%).

    Carboxy and hydroxy cannabinoids are the major metabolites detected in urine drug screens. The cannabinoid metabolites may be detected for 3–10 days in the occasional user and for 1–2 months in chronic users. Because this compound is stored in fat tissue, changes in activity or diet that mobilize fat may cause sudden increases in levels of cannabinoids detected in urine. Interpretation of the urine drug screen depends somewhat on the level detected.

    Level <20 ng/mL: Considered negative
    Level of 20–50 ng/mL: May not distinguish recent use in the occasional user from past use in long-term users
    Level >50 ng/mL: May be detected in long-term users for up to 2 weeks after last use
    Level >400 ng/mL: Indicates recent heavy use

7. Effects of intoxication
    a. Physical reactions: Increase in heart rate, a reddening of the conjunctivae, dry mouth and throat, dilated pupils, sleepiness
    b. Distortion of time sense
    c. Auditory and visual enhancement or distortions
    d. Impaired learning and cognitive functions
    e. Increase in appetite
    f. Low to moderate dose: Euphoria, time distortion, increased talking, and the reactions described above (item a)
    g. High dose: Mood fluctuations, depersonalization, and hallucinations
    h. Potential toxic reactions: Anxiety, panic, organic brain syndrome, psychoses, delusions, hallucinations, and paranoia
    i. Seizures: Marijuana may precipitate seizures in epileptic individuals.
    j. Psychosis: Marijuana may precipitate psychotic episodes in schizophrenic individuals.

ADVERSE EFFECTS

Despite the prevalence of marijuana use, it is only in recent years that the potential medical consequences have been more intensively studied. The risk of adverse effects increases with increased potency, amount used, frequency of use, and length of exposure to marijuana. Early age at onset also increases the risk of negative effects. Although some side effects are known, others are postulated but not yet conclusively documented in well-controlled studies.

Pulmonary Effects

1. Marijuana smoking results in a substantially greater respiratory burden of carbon monoxide and tar than does cigarette smoking (Wu et al., 1988).
2. Non-tobacco-smoking heavy marijuana smokers have functional impairment of airway conductance (Tashkin et al., 1980; Tashkin et al., 1993).
3. Chronic marijuana use leads to bronchoconstriction and bronchitis with cough, increased sputum production, and wheezing (Cohen, 1983).

4. Animal studies show extensive tissue damage with heavy use and cytotoxic effect on alveolar macrophages (Tashkin et al., 1976). However, Sherman et al. (1991) found that pulmonary alveolar macrophages of marijuana-only smokers do not produce increased amounts of oxidants in comparison with macrophages of nonsmoking subjects.
5. Human studies demonstrate a decrease in forced expiratory volume in 1 second (FEV_1), a decrease in maximal midexpiratory flow rate (MMFR), and an increase in airway resistance. These effects wear off after the drug is discontinued (Tashkin et al., 1976).
6. Metaplastic cellular changes have been observed in dogs and humans (Tashkin et al., 1976; Nahas and Latour, 1992).
7. A link between chronic marijuana smoke exposure and lung cancer in humans has been postulated (Ferguson et al., 1989). There has now been a series of reports suggesting a link between heavy marijuana smoking and cancers of the head and neck and the upper airways.

Cardiovascular Effects

1. Tachycardia (Tashkin et al., 1976)
2. Mild decrease in exercise capacity, which could be potentially harmful in cardiac patients (Tashkin et al., 1976)

Endocrine and Immune Function Effects

1. Antagonistic effects on insulin: These effects could potentially cause problems, including ketoacidosis, in adolescents with diabetes (Lantner et al., 1980).
2. Menstrual function: An increase in anovulatory cycles occurs in heavy users, increasing the risk of menstrual disorders and infertility (Smith et al., 1979; Mueller et al., 1990).
3. Abortions: Monkeys have an increased rate of abortions with moderate to heavy use (40% with use versus 8% without) (Sassenrath et al., 1979).
4. Male fertility: Heavy use of marijuana causes a decrease in sperm count and motility and an increase in the number of sperm with abnormal morphologic features (Hembree et al., 1979).
5. Testosterone levels: A drop in testosterone level may occur as a result of marijuana's effects on luteinizing hormone or on Leydig's cells in the testes. This has not been confirmed by all researchers (Kolodny et al., 1974; Mendelson et al., 1974).
6. Gynecomastia is a well-known complication of heavy marijuana use, particularly in the younger adolescent population.
7. Immune suppression: Concern has been reported about a suppression of immune function with heavy doses of tetrahydrocannabinol. Trisler and Specter (1994) reported a decrease in cytolytic function with marijuana.

Seizures

THC causes convulsions in dogs and can interact with anticonvulsant medications. Caution should be advised in adolescents with seizure disorders who use marijuana (Lantner et al., 1980).

Behavioral Changes

1. Intellectual changes
   a. Short-term use can lead to a decrease in reading comprehension and in problem-solving ability (Lantner et al., 1980; Miller et al., 1977).

b. Long-term use may impair memory, learning ability, and perception (Dupont, 1985; Miller et al., 1977).

2. Social changes
   a. There is a high correlation between heavy marijuana use, truancy, and poor academic achievement (Schwartz et al., 1987; Smith and Fogg, 1978).
   b. Heavy use in monkeys leads to a decrease in social interaction (Chapman et al., 1979).
   c. A study of human couples revealed that marijuana use led to a decrease in interpersonal skills between the pairs studied (Janowsky et al., 1979).
   d. A study of marijuana-dependent adolescents found increased disruptions in family harmony associated with long-term marijuana use, as evidenced by problems in getting along with parents, violent family arguments, and runaway behavior (Schwartz et al., 1987).
   e. Depression, suicidal ideation, drug-related accidents and injuries, legal problems, and unhealthy sexual behaviors were associated with marijuana dependence (Schwartz et al., 1987).

3. Amotivational syndrome: A syndrome associated with chronic heavy marijuana use and consisting of a state of passive withdrawal from usual work and recreational activities, with seven components (outlined by Schwartz [1987a])
   a. Loss of interest, general apathy, and passivity
   b. Loss of desire to work consistently and loss of productivity, accompanied by a lack of concern about the poor work performance
   c. Loss of energy and tiredness
   d. Moodiness, sullenness, and inability to handle frustration
   e. Impairment in concentration and inability to process new material
   f. Slovenly habits and appearance
   g. A lifestyle revolving around procurement and use of marijuana and other drugs

4. Cannabis psychosis: There is little evidence for the existence of a cannabis psychosis. However, the drug may precipitate several types of mental dysfunction in susceptible individuals, including a brief toxic psychosis resembling the delirium of a high fever, a short-lived acute anxiety state, and an acute depressive reaction.

Controversy exists over the presence of these behavioral changes, including the amotivational syndrome. Since heavy drug users may already have underlying behavioral problems and may already be depressed, alienated, or bored, it is difficult to distinguish whether marijuana is the cause or whether the behaviors are preexistent. In one long-term study, Shedler and Block (1990), examined this issue in 101 children who were followed and given personality tests at 7, 11, and 18 years of age. By the end of the study, three groups could be distinguished: abstainers, experimenters (tried marijuana no more than once a month), and frequent users (smoked marijuana at least once a week and had used at least one other drug). The study demonstrated marked personality differences among the three groups, with many of these changes noted long before any drug use occurred. The frequent users got along poorly with other children, lacked self-confidence, and were insecure, alienated, impulsive, and unpredictable. The abstainers were more inhibited, conventional, shy, neat, and anxious. The experimenters were more likely to be responsive, curious, active, and open.

Pope et al. (1995) reviewed the neuropsychological effects of cannabis. Their review included both "drug-administration" studies in which known amounts of cannabis were administered to volunteers and "naturalistic" studies in which heavy marijuana users were tested after some period of abstinence. This review suggested a "drug residue" effect on attention, psychomotor tasks, and short-term memory during the 12–24 hour period immediately after cannabis use. However, the evidence was not yet sufficient to support or refute either a more prolonged drug residue effect or a toxic effect on the central nervous system that persisted even after drug residues had left the body.

Motor Performance

Marijuana causes a decrease in both psychomotor functions and reaction times. This poses a dangerous problem for the adolescent who drives after getting high (*Marijuana and Health*, 1981). Specific functions related to driving skills that are impaired include:

1. Tracking: The ability to follow a moving object and to control the position of a car in relation to the highway
2. Signal detection: The ability to quickly notice and respond to lights or other unpredictable stimuli
3. Glare recovery time: The ability to see clearly after exposure to bright lights such as headlights

The impairment of these driving skills, in conjunction with marijuana-induced decreased judgment, impaired time and distance estimation, and impaired motor performance, makes driving under the influence of marijuana dangerous. There is good evidence that marijuana causes lingering effects on memory and coordination. Striking changes in the ability of pilots to operate a landing simulator persisted 24 hours after exposure to cannabis, during which time the pilots reported no awareness of marijuana aftereffects (Leirer and Yesavage, 1991).

Drug Interactions

1. Potentiates sedation when used with alcohol, diazepam, antihistamines, phenothiazines, barbiturates, and narcotics
2. Potentiates stimulation when used with cocaine and amphetamines
3. Antagonistic with the effects of phenytoin, propranolol, and insulin

TREATMENT

Treatment of marijuana use in the adolescent involves differentiation between the experimental or occasional use and the abuse of marijuana. After initially experimenting with marijuana, many adolescents do not use it again or use it very infrequently. However, physicians should not overlook the negative effects of marijuana use in adolescence. Frequent marijuana use can interfere with the cognitive, emotional, and social development of adolescence. Deterioration in school performance, family and social problems, accidents, and legal difficulties suggest the need for intervention and treatment. Chapter 75 discusses management in more detail.

BIBLIOGRAPHY

Bachman JG, Johnston LD, O'Malley PM, et al. Explaining the recent decline in marijuana use: differentiating the effects of perceived risks, disapproval, and general lifestyle factors. J Health Soc Behav 1988;29:92.

Chait LD. Subjective and behavioral effects of marijuana the morning after smoking. Psychopharmacology 1990;100:328.

Chait LD, Perry JL. Acute and residual effects of alcohol and marijuana, alone and in combination, on mood and performance. Psychopharmacology 1994;115:340.

Chapman LF, Sassenrath EN, Goo GP. Social behavior of rhesus monkeys chronically exposed to moderate amounts of delta-9-tetrahydrocannabinol. In: Nahas

GG, Paton WDM, eds. Marijuana: biological effects. Oxford, England: Pergamon Press, 1979.

Cohen MI. Marijuana: What is really known? In: Adolescent substance abuse: a report of the 14th Ross Roundtable. Columbus, Ohio: Ross Laboratories, 1983.

Dupont RL. Marijuana, alcohol, and adolescence: a malignant synergism. Semin Adoles Med 1985;1:311.

Farber SJ, Huertas VE. Intravenously injected marijuana syndrome. Arch Intern Med 1976;136:337.

Farrow JA, Rees JM, Worthington-Roberts BS. Health, developmental, and nutritional status of adolescent alcohol and marijuana abusers. Pediatrics 1987;79: 218.

Ferguson RP, Hasson J, Walker S. Metastatic lung cancer in a young marijuana smoker. JAMA 1989;261:41.

Fisher M, Glassroth J. The respiratory effects of marijuana and hashish. Intern Med 1988;9:140.

Gash A, Karliner JS, Janowsky D, et al. Effects of smoking marijuana on left ventricular performance and plasma norepinephrine. Ann Intern Med 1978;89: 448.

Gil E, Chen B, Kleerup E, et al. Acute and chronic effects of marijuana smoking on pulmonary alveolar permeability. Life Sci 1995;56:2193.

Grinspoon L, Bakalar JB. Marijuana. In: Lowinson JH, Ruiz P, Millman RB, eds. Substance abuse: a comprehensive textbook. 2nd ed. Baltimore: Williams & Wilkins, 1992.

Heath RG, Fitzjarrell AT, Garey RE. Chronic marijuana smoking: its effects on function and structure of the primate brain. In: Nahas GG, Paton WDM, eds. Marijuana: biological effects. Oxford, England: Pergamon Press, 1979.

Hembree WC, Nahas GG, Huang HFS. Changes in human spermatozoa associated with high-dose marijuana smoking. In: Nahas GG, Paton WDM, eds. Marijuana: biological effects. Oxford, England: Pergamon Press, 1979.

Hingson R, Zuckerman B, Amaro H, et al. Maternal marijuana use and neonatal outcome: uncertainty posed by self-reports. Am J Public Health 1986;76:667.

Jalali B, Jalali M, Crocetti G, et al. Adolescents and drug use: toward a more comprehensive approach. Am J Orthopsychiatry 1981;51:120.

Janowsky DS, Clopton PL, Leichner PP, et al. Interpersonal effects of marijuana, Arch Gen Psychiatry 1979;36:781.

Johnston LD, O'Malley PM, Bachman JG. Drug use, drinking, and smoking: national survey results from high school, college, and young adult populations, 1988. (DHHS publication No. [ADM] 89–1638.) Washington, D.C.: U.S. Department of Health and Human Services, 1989.

Johnston LD, O'Malley PM, Bachman JG. Drug use rises again in 1995 among American teens. Ann Arbor: News and Information Services of the University of Michigan, December 11, 1995.

Joesoef MR, Beral V, Aral SO, et al. Fertility and use of cigarettes, alcohol, marijuana, and cocaine. Ann Epidemiol 1993;3:592.

Kolodny RC, Masters WH, Kolodner RM, et al. Depression of plasma testosterone levels after chronic intensive marijuana use. N Engl J Med 1974;290:872.

Lantner IL, O'Brien JE, Voth HM. Answering questions about marijuana use. Patient Care 1980;May 30:112.

Leirer VO, Yesavage JA. Marijuana carry-over effects on aircraft pilot performance. Aviat Space Environ Med 1991;62:221.

Marijuana and health. Institute of Medicine. Washington, D.C: National Academy Press, 1981.

Mendelson JH, Kuehnle J, Ellingboe J, et al. Plasma testosterone levels before, during, and after chronic marijuana smoking. N Engl J Med 1974;291:1051.

Miller L, Cornett T, Drew W. Marijuana: dose-response effects on pulse rate, subjective estimates of potency, pleasantness, and recognition memory. Pharmacology 1977;15:268.

Mohs ME, Watson RR, Leonard-Green T. Nutritional effects of marijuana, heroin, cocaine, and nicotine. J Am Diet Assoc 1990;90:1261.

Moyer TP, Palmen MA, Johnson P, et al. Marijuana testing: how good is it? Mayo Clin Proc 1987;62:413.

Mueller BA, Daling JR, Weiss NS, et al. Recreational drug use and the risk of primary infertility. Epidemiology 1990;1:195.

Nahas GG. Current status of marijuana research. JAMA 1979;242:2775.

Nahas G, Latour C. The human toxicity of marijuana. Med J Aust 1992;156:495.

National Household Survey on Drug Abuse: main findings, 1985. (DHHS publication No. 163MP.) Washington, D.C.: National Institute on Drug Abuse, 1988.

Pope HG Jr, Gruber AJ, Yugelun-Todd D. The residual neuropsychological effects of cannabis: the current status of research. Drug Alcohol Depend 1995;38:25.

Sassenrath EN, Chapman LF, Goo GP. Reproduction in rhesus monkeys chronically exposed to delta-9-tetrahydrocannabinol. In: Nahas GG, Paton WDM, eds. Marijuana: biological effects. Oxford, England: Pergamon Press, 1979.

Schwartz RH. Frequent marijuana use in adolescence. Am Fam Physician 1985;31:210.

Schwartz RH. Marijuana: an overview. Pediatr Clin North Am 1987a;34:305.

Schwartz RH. Are you ready to deal with the pot-smoking patient? Contemporary Pediatrics 1987b;April:84.

Schwartz RH, Hoffman NG, Jones R. Behavioral, psychosocial, and academic correlates of marijuana usage in adolescence. Clin Pediatr 1987;26:264.

Shedler J, Block J. Adolescent drug use and psychological health: a longitudinal inquiry. Am Psychol 1990; 45:612.

Sherman MP, Roth MD, Gong H Jr, et al. Marijuana smoking, pulmonary function, and lung macrophage oxidant release. Pharmacol Biochem Behav 1991;40:663.

Shiono PH, Klebanoff MA, Nugent RP, et al. The impact of cocaine and marijuana use on low birth weight and preterm birth: a multicenter study. Am J Obstet Gynecol 1995;172:19.

Silber TJ, Getson P, Ridley S, et al.. Adolescent marijuana use: concordance between questionnaire and immunoassay for cannabinoid metabolites. J Pediatr 1987;2:299.

Smith CG, Smith MT, Besch NT. Effects of Δ-9-tetrahyrocannabinol (THC) on female reproduction function. In: Nahas GG, Paton WDM, eds. Marijuana: biological effects. Oxford, England: Pergamon Press, 1979.

Smith GM, Fogg CP. Psychological predictors of early use, late use, and nonuse of marijuana among teenage students. In: Kandel DB, ed. Longitudinal research on drug use: empirical findings and methodological issues. New York: Halstead Press, 1978.

Tashkin DP. Pulmonary complications of smoked substance abuse. West J Med 1990;152:525.

Tashkin DP, Calvarese BM, Simmons MS, Shapiro BJ. Respiratory status of seventy-four habitual marijuana smokers. Chest 1980;78:699.

Tashkin DP, Fligiel S, Wu JTC, et al. Effects of habitual use of marijuana and/or cocaine on the lung. NIDA Research Monograph 1990;99:63.

Tashkin DP, Shapiro BS, Lee PE, Harper CE. Subacute effects of heavy marijuana smoking on pulmonary function in healthy men. N Engl J Med 1976;294: 125.

Tashkin DP, Simmons MS, Chang P, et al. Effects of smoked substance abuse on nonspecific airway hyperresponsiveness. Am Rev Respir Dis 1993;147:97.

Tashkin DP, Soares JR, Hepler RS, Shapiro BJ, Rachelefsky GS. Cannabis, 1977. Ann Intern Med 1978;89: 539.

Trisler K, Specter S. Delta-9-tetrahydrocannabinol treatment results in a suppression of interleukin-2–induced cellular activities in human and murine lymphocytes. Int J Immunopharmacol 1994;16:593.

Wilson WH, Wllinwood EH, Mathew RJ, et al. Effects of marijuana on performance of a computerized cognitive-neuromotor test battery. Psychiatry Res 1994; 51:115.

Wu T, Tashkin DP, Djahed B, Rose JE. Pulmonary hazards of smoking marijuana as compared with tobacco. N Engl J Med 1988;318:347.

Yesavage JA, Leirer VO, Denari M, et al. Carryover effects of marijuana intoxication on aircraft pilot performance: a preliminary report. Am J Psychiatry 1985; 142:1325.

CHAPTER 73

Hallucinogens

Lawrence S. Neinstein and Bruce S. Heischober

The hallucinogen class of drugs includes LSD (D-lysergic acid diethylamide tartrate), peyote, mescaline, psilocybin, certain mushrooms, DMT (dimethyltryptamine), morning-glory seeds, MDMA (methylene dioxymethamphetamine), STP (dimethoxy-4-methylamphetamine; serenity-tranquility-peace pill), jimsonweed, and PCP (phencyclidine). The term *hallucinogen* is actually a misnomer, because these drugs produce illusions or distortions of perceived reality rather than hallucinations. True hallucinations do occur with the use of volatile solvents (e.g., gasoline). Set (user's attitudes and expectations) and setting (drug-taking environment) greatly influence the user's experience with this class of drugs. With the exception of the hallucinogenic amphetamines, physical withdrawal does not occur.

PREVALENCE

Overall, the prevalence of hallucinogen use decreased in the late 1970s and early 1980s and then began a slow but definite rise in the late 1980s that has continued into the 1990s. Approximately 12.7% of the 1995 seniors in the Monitoring the Future Study of high school seniors had used hallucinogens; 11.7% had used LSD; and 2.7% had used PCP (Johnston et al., 1995). The lifetime prevalence rates for college students in 1994 were 10% for hallucinogens and 9.2% for LSD (Johnston et al., 1994). The 1992 National Household Drug Survey showed the following hallucinogen prevalence rates for ever using and trends:

Age	1979	1985	1988	1992
12–17 yr	7.1	3.3	3.5	2.6
18–25 yr	25.1	11.3	13.8	13.4

The 1992 National Household Survey also showed the following trends for hallucinogen use comparing sex and ethnic group:

Age	Total	Male	Female	White	African-American	Hispanic
12–17 yr	2.6	2.4	2.9	3.2	0.2	2.8
18–25 yr	13.4	15.9	11.1	16.5	3.0	8.1

Two trends emerging from the "pop culture" scene are partially responsible for the resurgence of LSD and the emergence of the use of MDMA, or ecstasy, a hallucinogenic methamphetamine derivative. "Rave" or "house" parties involve alternative forms of rock music played in coordination with colorful, pulsating light effects and augmented by the use of LSD or MDMA. Frequently the drugs are supplied as part of the admission price or by the organizers of the event. The parties commonly are held in an abandoned house or industrial building, and maps are made available or sold at some time shortly before the event. These parties may last 12 hours or longer, attaining a type of trance state being desirable. Devotees of such events frequently emphasize the absence of alcohol and clearly feel that they are not abusing drugs in this context. There has also been a revival of interest in the 1960s psychedelic movement, from music to memorabilia, dress, and lifestyle.

It is important to emphasize that one should not label an adolescent because of his or her dress or music; yet, especially in early adolescence, information about the peer group can give insights into the thinking and behaviors of the identified patient. There is also the suggestion that familiarity with an adolescent's music preference can open avenues of communication, allowing more effective data collection by the clinician.

An extremely important fact should be remembered in regard to the current wave of LSD use. In the 1960s, doses of up to 500 µg were not unusual. According to Drug Enforcement Agency (DEA) and Sheriff's Crime Laboratory data, the average current dose is in the 25–50 µg range. Most users today describe a seemingly mild "trip" with colorful visual "tracers," enhancement of sound, and light sensations. Psychiatric emergency services are not seeing the same level of acuity as was seen in the 1960s. There is clearly a disregard for and underestimation of the dangers of LSD because of the lower dose. However, even at this lower dosage level, one is at risk of having chronic psychiatric problems, acute physical trauma, and other consequences of risk-taking behaviors that might occur under the influence of the drug.

LSD

Although LSD (D-lysergic acid diethylamide tartrate) peaked in popularity in the 1960s, the drug was tried by more than 11% of high school seniors in 1995. In the 1995 Monitoring the Future Study of high school seniors (Johnston et al., 1995), 8.4% of seniors had used LSD in the previous year, 4.0% had used LSD in the 30 days before the survey, and 0.1% used LSD daily. Among college students, 9.2% had used LSD at least once, 5.2% in the past year, and 1.8% in the past 30 days. LSD is making a comeback nationwide among white middle-class high school and college students. Compared to the rates between 1985 to 1990, an approximately 25% increase in lifetime-, annual-, and monthly-use rates of LSD occurred in 1995. An increase has also been noted in LSD-related arrests, as well as in seizures of larger quantities of LSD. LSD-related visits to emergency departments by adolescents has increased, and LSD-related violent behavior, including suicide, homicide, and accidental death, were higher than in the previous 5-year period. The risk attributed to occasional use of LSD by high school students has fallen.

The most common hallucinogen identified among samples submitted to the Los Angeles County Street Drug Identification Program in 1980 was LSD. From time to time the sale of LSD as decals or stickers of popular cartoon characters recurs, with unfortunate results. This colorful vehicle has the potential to appeal to younger children, who may unknowingly take the LSD.

Origin

LSD is derived from an alkaloid found in rye fungus. It is made by mixing lysergic acid with diethylamide, freezing the mixture, and then extracting the resulting LSD. The procedure is not easy; thus much of the LSD sold on the street is either adulterated or contains no LSD. In one survey of LSD submitted to the Los Angeles County Street Drug Identification Program, 11% contained no LSD.

Action

LSD is the most potent psychoactive drug. It inhibits the release of serotonin and gives rise to a nonspecific stress response and autonomic changes. The drug is rapidly absorbed from the gastrointestinal tract, with onset of action in 30–40 minutes. LSD has a half-life of 3 hours and is not detected on standard urine drug screens. Tolerance develops rapidly but is short-lived. Some daily users of LSD describe the practice of "doubling up" (doubling the previous day's dose when using on consecutive days) to counteract tolerance.

1. Physiological effects: These occur within 30 minutes to several hours after use and usually resolve within 6 hours. Included are:
   a. Conjunctival injection
   b. Ataxia
   c. Increase in blood pressure, heart rate, and temperature
   d. Mydriasis, lacrimation, and piloerection
   e. Flushing
   f. Decrease in urine output
   g. Decrease in appetite
   h. Dry mouth
2. Psychological effects: The major effects of LSD and the reason for its abuse are the psychological effects, which may last up to 14 hours or longer and may include:
   a. Depersonalization
   b. Loss of time sense and of the relationship between current impressions and past experience
   c. Loss of ego boundaries between the user and his or her surroundings
   d. Loss of muscle coordination and pain perception
   e. Decrease in judgment
   f. Visual and auditory illusions; synesthesias (a secondary sensation caused by an actual perception of a different sense; e.g., sound producing the sensation of color)
   g. Impairment of attention, motivation, and concentration
   h. Depression, paranoia, confusion, and fragmentation may occur.

A fairly typical description of the effects of LSD is given by its discoverer, Dr. Albert Hoffman, a Swiss chemist, who reported:

> I lost all control of time. Space and time became more and more disorganized, and I was overcome with fears that I was going crazy. The worst part of it was I was clearly aware of my condition, though I was not able to stop it. Often I felt that I was outside of my body. I thought I had died. My ego was suspended somewhere in space, and I thought my body was lying dead on the sofa. I observed and registered clearly that my "alter ego" was moving about the room moaning. . . . I became dizzy and delirious with fantastic visions of extraordinary vividness accompanied by a kaleidoscopic play of intense coloration.
>
> *Albert Hoffman, quoted by Jenkins and Brody, 1974*

Dr. Hoffman's description of the sense of being an observer is frequently reported by LSD users and distinguishes LSD psychosis from schizophrenia.

Dose

The usual dose of LSD is between 25 and 100 µg. Anything more than 250 µg is considered especially dangerous. The drug is commonly distributed as a soluble powder or liquid. It is usually colorless, odorless, and tasteless in its manufactured state, but is most often colored when sold. It is sold as cylindrical tablets or gelatin squares, or is applied to small pieces of paper known on the street, respectively, as microdots, windowpanes, and blotters. As mentioned earlier, it is also sold as decals or stickers.

Slang Names

Slang names for LSD include acid, beast, Big "D," black, blue barrels, blotters, blue cheer, brown dot, cubes, fry, microdots, orange sunshine, panes, sugar, sunshine, trips, white lightning, and window panes.

Effects

1. Symptoms of intoxication
   a. General: Anorexia, nausea, flushing, elevated temperature
   b. Neurological: Dizziness, paresthesia, dilated pupils, hyperactive reflexes, tremor
   c. Psychiatric: Labile affect, anxiety, body image changes, euphoria, floating feeling, illusions, restlessness, sleep disturbance, paranoia, and depersonalization
   d. Cardiovascular: Elevated blood pressure, tachycardia
2. Symptoms of overdose
   a. General: Dry mouth, perspiration, elevated temperature, flushing
   b. Neurological: Grand mal seizures, dilated pupils, hyperactive reflexes, tremor, dizziness, coma
   c. Psychiatric: Toxic psychosis, suspiciousness, anxiety, body distortions, irritability, delirium, illusions
   d. Cardiovascular: Tachycardia, hypertension, circulatory collapse
   e. Gastrointestinal: Anorexia, nausea, vomiting, abdominal cramps
   f. Hematological: Coagulopathies
3. Tolerance and psychological dependence; no physical dependence
4. Bad trips: Bad trips are negative emotional responses, often triggered by environmental factors (setting) or feelings within the user (set). These responses terrify the user and may produce a sense of panic, fragmentation, and a sense of "going crazy."
5. Flashbacks: Recurrence of LSD-induced state after effects of the drug have worn off. They may occur spontaneously for variable lengths of time after original drug ingestion. Concurrent use of selective serotonin reuptake inhibitor agents may induce or worsen the LSD flashback syndrome (Markel et al., 1994), possibly as a result of the similarity in neuroreceptor physiology for both LSD and serotonin.
6. Chronic adverse effects: May include psychosis, depression, and personality changes

Treatment of a Bad Trip and of Overdose

Treatment of a bad trip should be done by someone with experience in this area. Important components include the following:

1. Provide an appropriate setting. Often the setting, such as a room with loud music, will induce a bad trip. Changing the setting to a peaceful, calm area will often alleviate the problem.
2. Help to restore contact with reality. The person dealing with the user should try to calm the user by talking to him or her about familiar things. The user should be reassured that his or her unusual sensations will cease when the drug wears off. The helping individual should listen carefully to the user and respond sympathetically. If the user is high on PCP, then talking the user down will be counterproductive and should be avoided (see section on PCP in this chapter).
3. Avoid the use of any medications, if possible.
4. Avoid discussing reasons for use of the drug or personal problems of the user during a bad trip.
5. Support respiration and circulation as needed.

6. Treat hyperthermia.
7. Treat seizures.
8. Treat hypertension.
9. Look for other causes of symptoms—an overdose of LSD is not common.

MDMA

Methylenedioxymethamphetamine (MDMA), better known as "X" or ecstasy, has gained in popularity during the past decade. This and other related drugs (such as methylene-dioxyethamphetamine [MDEA]) have been termed "designer drugs." In the early 1980s the drug was not a controlled substance, and anecdotal reports in the psychiatric literature led some therapists to recommend/"prescribe" it, particularly in couples therapy. It was reported to increase empathy and even the feeling of physically merging with the significant other. By 1985 this drug and related chemicals were classified as Schedule I drugs by the DEA.

MDMA has physiological effects similar to those of the other amphetamines; in the overdose situation, users are treated identically. Clinically the drug has mild euphorigenic properties, similar to amphetamine and methamphetamine, mediated through the norepinephrine-dopamine neurotransmitters. The mild hallucinogenic properties are attributed to interaction with serotoninergic neurons in the central nervous system. In studies of monkeys treated with MDMA, damage was found in serotonin-mediated neurons.

PEYOTE AND MESCALINE

Peyote is a cactus (*Lophophora*) that grows in the southwestern United States and in Mexico. The tops of the cactus contain numerous alkaloids including mescaline (3,4,5-trimethoxyphenethylamine). Although many drugs are sold as mescaline, of the 459 samples submitted to the Los Angeles County Street Drug Identification Program in 1980, 96% contained no mescaline. Most mescaline capsules contain either LSD or both LSD and PCP. Peyote is sold either as buttons derived from the cactus or as capsules containing ground peyote. Street names include big chief, buttons, cactus, mesc, and mescal.

Action

Mescaline has its onset of action within 30 minutes to 2 hours after use, with effects lasting about 6–12 hours. The mescaline high differs from the LSD high in several ways:

1. LSD creates a more intense experience than mescaline does.
2. Mescaline intensifies body sense, whereas LSD tends to have a stronger effect on the mind.
3. Mescaline is less disorienting than LSD.
4. Mescaline use is frequently accompanied by unpleasant side effects such as nausea and vomiting.

Doses

The usual human dose ranges from 100 to 500 mg.

Side Effects

Tolerance and psychological dependence can occur with mescaline, but no physical addiction occurs. Bad trips are less severe and less frequent with mescaline than with LSD.

Psilocybin

Mushrooms containing psilocybin and psilocin produce effects similar to those of the other hallucinogens. The mushrooms are ingested orally, and there is a rapid onset of effects in about 15 minutes. The effects peak at 90 minutes, begin to wear off in about 2–3 hours, and disappear after about 5–6 hours. The average dose is 4–10 mg of psilocybin.

In a statewide survey of California high school students completed in 1986, Schwartz and Smith (1988) found that the use of hallucinogenic mushrooms exceeded that of LSD by 7th, 9th, and 11th graders. Street names for psilocybin mushrooms include shrooms, mushrooms, Silly Putty, magic Mexican mushrooms, and psychedelic mushrooms.

DMT

DMT (dimethyltryptamine) is a natural constituent of the seeds of several plants found in the West Indies and South America. DMT is usually prepared as an orange liquid in which either tobacco, marijuana, or parsley is soaked and then smoked; it is inactive orally. This drug has effects similar to those of other hallucinogens, except that the "trip" is short, lasting only 1–3 hours. DMT is known on the street as businessman's special or businessman's lunch.

Morning-Glory Seeds

The seeds of some members of the bindweed family, including the morning glory (*Rivea corymbosa* and *Ipomoea*), have been used for centuries for their hallucinogenic effects. Morning-glory seeds are legally available on seed racks but, to prevent spoilage, are usually coated with dangerous chemicals such as methyl mercury. The active principal ingredient in the seeds is similar to LSD but is about one-tenth as potent. The effects of morning-glory seeds are similar to those of LSD; however, there is an increase in side effects such as nausea, dizziness, and diarrhea, and an extremely bitter taste.

Nutmeg

Nutmeg is extracted from the dried seed kernels of an evergreen tree found in the South Pacific Islands. This common spice is ubiquitous in household pantries, and outbreaks of its use usually follow media reports of its hallucinogenic properties; it has long been used by prison inmates. Nutmeg contains lysergide as well as several other hallucinatory alkaloids The presence of an extremely potent emetic, geraniol, has discouraged widespread use.

STP

STP (*serenity-tranquility-peace* pill, dimethoxy-4-methylamphetamine) is related to mescaline but is about 100 times more potent. Its effects are also similar to the rest of the hallucinogenic drugs, with the exception that with STP the incidence of unpleasant sensations is increased and the effects seem to last longer, up to 72 hours.

Jimsonweed

Jimsonweed (*Datura stramonium*) has anticholinergic and hallucinogenic properties. It grows wild throughout the United States but especially in the Southwest. Adolescents make tea from the seeds. Users may have an anticholinergic syndrome at presentation for medical evaluation.

PCP

The use of phencyclidine (PCP) steadily declined in the 1980s. The 1995 Monitoring the Future Study of high school seniors (Johnston et al., 1995) found that 2.7% of the seniors had used PCP at some time, 1.8% in the past year, and that 0.6% were current users (within the previous 30 days). Daily use occurred among 0.3% of the seniors. These data have shown no statistically significant change in the 1990s. Data from the most recent Drug Abuse Warning Network (DAWN) survey, which monitors drug-related emergency department visits at representative hospitals across the United States, showed a significant increase for PCP in 1992.

PCP was introduced in the 1950s as a general anesthetic. Clinical trials revealed PCP to be an effective anesthetic, but during surgical recovery it caused excessive agitation, excitement, and disorientation. In 1965, the drug was discontinued as an investigational drug for human use. In the late 1960s, its use increased in San Francisco as an experimental psychedelic drug, called the peace pill. It was unpopular at that time, because of excessive reports of bad trips. However, during the mid and late 1970s its popularity increased tremendously, and the drug became one of the nation's major drugs of abuse. Until 1978 the drug was still legally manufactured as Sernylan for veterinary anesthesia. PCP is still an unsafe and commonly abused drug among adolescents, especially in urban areas.

Metabolism

PCP is the hydrogen chloride salt of phencyclidine. It is related to the anesthetic ketamine. The drug is rapidly inactivated by hepatic metabolism and excreted in the urine as the monopiperidine conjugate. Because PCP is fat soluble, it has the ability to remain in the body for prolonged periods. Its urinary excretion is highly dependent on urine pH, with significantly higher excretion rates at an acidic pH. The half-life of PCP is 3 days. The active ingredient is the phencyclidine itself, not the metabolites.

Action

PCP is a dissociative anesthetic with analgesic, stimulant, depressant, and hallucinogenic properties. The drug acts on the thalamus, midbrain, and sensory cortex to impair proprioception and the brain's ability to organize input. Its physiological effects are more fully discussed in the Clinical Manifestations section, below. PCP generally induces one of several clinical states:

1. Acute intoxication
2. Acute or prolonged delirium: Disorientation, clouded consciousness, and abnormal cognition
3. Schizophreniform psychosis: Hallucinations, thought disorder, and delusions
4. Mania: Hallucinations, elevated mood, and elevated self-attitude
5. Depressive reactions: May occur after long-term use of PCP

Dose

PCP may be packaged as a liquid, powder, tablet, leaf mixture, or rock crystal. It can be used intravenously, intramuscularly, or orally, or it can be snorted or smoked. Examples of methods of using the drug and associated doses are listed as follows:

	Average Dose
Smoking (joint)	3 mg
Snorting (powder)	5 mg
Swallowing (tablet)	5 mg
Injection (liquid)	10 mg
Eyedrops (liquid)	Unknown
Rectally (liquid)	Unknown
Vaginally (liquid)	Unknown

Dose ranges may vary tremendously. In Los Angeles the amount of PCP per joint ranges from 0.1 to 161 mg (Los Angeles County Street Drug Identification Program, 1980). In addition, approximately 20% of PCP sold contains no PCP. In terms of potency, less than 5 mg is considered a low dose, 5–10 mg a moderate dose, and greater than 10 mg a high dose.

Street Names

Street names for PCP include the following:

angel dust	dust	lovely	scaffle
angel mist	elephant tranquilizer	lovely dust mist	shermans
animal	embalming fluid	magic dust	sherms
animal tranquilizer	flakes	mist	snorts
aurora borealis	goon	monkey dust	soma
busy bee	goon dust	orange crystal	star dust
Cadillac	gorilla biscuits	parsley	super grass
CJ	green tea	peace	super joint
columbo	hog	peace pill	super weed
crystal	jet fuel	Peter Pan	super X
crystal joints	juice	pip	surfer
cyclones	kaps	pits	whack whack
Detroit pink	KJ crystal	polvo	worm
devil's dust	kool S	porker	zombie weed
dipper	Lemmon 714	puffy	zoom
dummy dust	live ones	rocket fuel	

Clinical Manifestations

The clinical symptoms of PCP use vary with the dose, the route of administration, and the experience of the user. Intravenous, intramuscular, and oral routes of administration are more difficult to regulate than the smoking of PCP. In addition, inexperienced users have more side effects than experienced users. Following are clinical manifestations by dosage:

Low Dose (less than 5 mg)

1. Blank stare
2. Horizontal and vertical nystagmus
3. Gait ataxia
4. Increased blood pressure
5. Increased deep-tendon reflexes
6. Decreased proprioception and sensations

7. Miosis or midposition, reactive pupils
8. Diaphoresis
9. Flushing
10. Behavioral disorders
    a. Disorganized thought processes
    b. Distortion of one's body image and of objects
    c. Amnesia
    d. Agitated or combative behavior
    e. Unresponsive behavior
    f. Disinhibition of underlying psychopathology
    g. Schizophrenic reactions
    h. Catalepsy, catatonia
    i. Illusions
    j. Anxiety, excitement

Moderate Dose (5–10 mg)

1. Hypertension
2. Vertical and horizontal nystagmus
3. Myoclonus
4. Midposition pupil size
5. Dysarthria
6. Diaphoresis
7. Fever
8. Hypersalivation
9. Mutism
10. Amnesia
11. Anxiety, excitement
12. Delusions
13. Behavior: May be stuporous or extremely agitated; violent or psychotic behavior can occur

High Dose (>10 mg)

1. Unresponsive, immobile state
2. Eyes that may remain open during coma
3. Hypertension
4. Arrhythmias
5. Increased deep-tendon reflexes
6. Muscle rigidity
7. Decerebrate posturing
8. Convulsions
9. Spontaneous nystagmus
10. Miosis
11. Decreased urine output
12. Dysarthria
13. Diaphoresis and flushing
14. Fever
15. Amnesia
16. Mutism

Massive Oral Overdose (>500 mg)

1. Prolonged coma
2. Extensor posturing
3. Seizures
4. Hypoventilation
5. Hypertension or hypotension
6. Prolonged and fluctuating confusional state after recovery from coma

Recovery

Recovery usually occurs within 24 hours but can proceed for days, depending on the dose and the acidity of the urine. With higher doses the coma can last 5–6 days, followed by a prolonged recovery marked by behavioral disorders. Cognitive, memory, and speech disorders may last up to a year after the last use of PCP. Flashbacks may occur, as with LSD.

Diagnosis

The diagnosis of PCP use should be suspected in all adolescents with a distorted thought process, especially when there is evidence of analgesia or nystagmus. Any individual with open-eye coma, horizontal and vertical nystagmus, hypertension, and rigidity should be considered to have taken PCP.

1. Common symptoms for diagnosis
   a. Nystagmus: Vertical and horizontal
   b. Ataxia
   c. Miotic but reactive pupils
   d. Disorientation with either a catatonic or an agitated state
   e. Increased blood pressure
   f. Increased deep-tendon reflexes
   g. Severe intoxication: Seizure, coma, rigidity, and decerebrate posturing
2. Identification: PCP can be found in the blood, urine, and gastrointestinal secretions. The best fluid to sample is the urine.
   a. Blood level: A level of 25–100 ng/mL may be found in an acute confusional state; a level of more than 100 ng/mL may be found in patients in a comatose state.
   b. Urinary level: Levels may vary in different clinical states. Excretion in the urine is highly pH dependent and will decrease dramatically as the pH becomes alkaline. It is important to determine the pH of urine sent for analysis.
   c. Method: PCP can be detected by gas chromatography, thin-layer chromatography, and gas chromatography—mass spectrometry. The latter method is the most accurate.
3. Differential diagnosis: Table 73.1 compares PCP overdose with that of other drugs.

Complications

1. Death can occur during PCP use. Death is usually caused by injuries sustained during periods of analgesia and of aggression directed at self or others. Death can also occur as a result of convulsions and cerebral hemorrhage.
2. Seizures: Generalized motor seizures may be early or delayed in appearance (Burns and Lerner, 1976).
3. Hypertension: Usually the hypertension is mild, but there has been a reported case of hypertensive cerebral hemorrhage in a 13-year-old adolescent (Eastman and Cohen, 1975).

TABLE 73.1.   Comparing PCP Overdose with Overdose of Major Types of Drugs

Signs and Symptoms	PCP	Stimulants	Other Hallucinogens	Sedatives	Narcotics
Aggressive and violent behavior	+[a]	+			
Ataxia	+		+	+	+
Coma	+			+	+
Confusion	+		+	+	+
Convulsions	+	+			
Drowsiness				+	+
Hallucinations	+	+	+		
Hyperreflexia	+	+	+		
Hypertension	+	+	+		
Nystagmus	+			+	
Dilated pupils		+	+		
Pinpoint pupils					+
Paranoia	+	+	+		
Psychosis	+	+	+		
Respiratory depression				+	+
Slurred speech	+			+	+

[a]+, Sign or symptom present.

4. Renal failure: This complication can occur as a result of rhabdomyolysis and myoglobinuria (Cogen et al., 1978; Patel et al., 1979).
5. Fetal effects: One case report has described an infant with abnormal behavior and abnormal facies born to a mother who used PCP (Golden et al., 1980).
6. Psychosis: This can last several weeks in patients with PCP overdose and is usually more common in adolescents who have underlying psychological problems.

Treatment

1. Use extreme caution: PCP users are unpredictable, often having little awareness of the consequences of their behavior.
2. Reduce stimulation: Reducing the level of light, sound, and other external stimulation can rapidly bring down a PCP user. In an emergency, one can cover the user with a blanket.
3. Remove all hazards; however, do not forcibly take an object from a PCP user.
4. Do not enter water to save a PCP user; use some other first-aid technique such as a life preserver.
5. Do not use mace.
6. Do not corner or touch a PCP user.
7. Restraints are not recommended; they may cause the PCP user to harm himself or herself in an attempt to escape.
8. Do not attempt to talk to a patient who has recently used PCP.
9. Try to avoid administering other medications, but if necessary, diazepam, 2.5 mg given intravenously, or ativan, 1 to 2.0 mg given intramuscularly or intravenously, can be used to treat seizures.
10. Theoretically, acidification of the urine increases elimination, but possible renal complications outweigh the small possible benefit.
11. Support respiratory and cardiovascular functions if necessary.
12. Besides basic cardiopulmonary resuscitation, it is essential to check for signs of head, neck, back, or internal injuries. Because of the behavioral effects of the drug, such injuries can occur. Unconscious victims should be placed on their side so that aspiration does not occur.

13. Treat hypertension with nitroprusside, labetalol, or phentolamine (see Chapter 74).
14. Severe agitation and psychosis can be treated with haloperidol. Avoid phenothiazine use because of the risk of excessive orthostatic hypotension and the potential for enhancing the cholinergic imbalance. As noted in the sections on cocaine and amphetamines, there are some authorities who recommend that neuroleptic agents be avoided in favor of benzodiazepines alone. If the agitation is severe, then the differential diagnosis and initial management should be the same as for the delirious patient (see cocaine treatment section in Chapter 74).
15. Treat hyperthermia as indicated.
16. Use intravenously administered diphenhydramine for dystonias.
17. Excessive salivation may need suctioning.
18. Diuresis: Although there is no evidence to support diuresis, some authors recommend use of furosemide (40–20 mg) and intravenous administration of fluids to maintain urine output at greater than 250 mL/hr.
19. During the recovery phase, an adolescent may have paranoia, regressive behavior, and a slow phase of reintegration. Adolescents may need inpatient psychiatric support through this period.
20. Referral to a drug rehabilitation program is indicated for any adolescent whose drug use causes significant life problems.

SUMMARY

It is important to remember that one cannot rely on history in managing patients who have allegedly taken an hallucinogen. Especially in this class of drugs, adulteration and misrepresentation of the substance are common. In addition, in the case of a patient with clouded sensorium and fever, even with a history of ingestion of LSD, the differential diagnosis must include central-nervous-system infection, endocrine disorder, drug or alcohol withdrawal syndrome, or ingestion of an unknown toxin.

Another dilemma occurs in the situation of the combative patient with a history of hallucinogen use. Although chemical and physical restraints are discouraged, if more passive means of calming the patient have not been effective, restraints must be used to facilitate further clinical evaluation and diagnostic testing. It is essential that every clinician become adept at using at least one sedative and one major tranquilizer. Ativan is probably the best suited of the benzodiazepines because it can be given intramuscularly, intravenously, or orally and is more effective than diazepam (Valium) as an anticonvulsant. Haloperidol (Haldol) and droperidol are superior to the phenothiazines because they have fewer cardiovascular side effects such as hypotension. Recently, droperidol has come into favor because of its more rapid onset of action and shorter half-life and because it is approved for intravenous use. It is also more sedating than haldolperidol. All major tranquilizers lower the seizure threshold.

BIBLIOGRAPHY

Abraham HD, Aldridge AM. Adverse consequences of lysergic acid diethylamide. Addiction 1993;88:1327.

Baldrige EB, Bessen HA. Phencyclidine. Emerg Med Clin North Am 1990;8:541.

Balster RL, Chait LD. The behavioral pharmacology of phencyclidine. Clin Toxicol 1976;9:513.

Beebe DK, Walley E. Substance abuse: the designer drugs. Am Fam Physician 1991;43:1689.

Bolter A, Heminger A, Martin G, et al. Outpatient clinical experience in a community drug abuse program with phencyclidine abuse. Clin Toxicol 1976;9:593.

Brown RT, Braden NJ. Hallucinogens. Pediatr Clin North Am 1987;34:341.

Brust J. Other agents: phencyclidine, marijuana, hallucinogens—neurologic complications of drugs and alcohol abuse. Neurol Clin 1993;11:555.

Burns RS, Lerner SE. Perspectives: acute phencyclidine intoxication. Clin Toxicol 1976;9:477.

Burns RS, Lerner SE, Corrado R. Phencyclidine states of acute intoxication and fatalities. West J Med 1975; 123:345.

Cogen FC, Rigg G, Simmons JL, et al. Phencyclidine-associated acute rhabdomyolysis. Ann Intern Med 1978;88:210.

Cohen S. The angel dust states: phencyclidine toxicity. Pediatr Rev 1979;1:17.

Crosley CJ, Finet EF. Cerebrovascular complications in phencyclidine intoxication. J Pediatr 1979;94:316.

Eastman JW, Cohen SN. Hypertensive crisis and death associated with phencyclidine. JAMA 1975;231: 1270.

Fauman B, Aldinger G, Fauman M, et al. Psychiatric sequelae of phencyclidine abuse. Clin Toxicol 1976;9: 529.

Giannini AJ. PCP: detecting the abuser. Medical aspects of human sexuality 1987;21:100.

Gold MS, Schuchard K, Gleaton T. LSD use among U.S. high school students. JAMA 1994;271:426.

Golden NL, Sokol RJ, Rubin L. Angel dust: possible effects on the fetus. Pediatrics 1980;65:18.

Jalali B, Jalali M, Crocetti G, et al. Adolescents and drug use: toward a more comprehensive approach. Am J Orthopsychiatry 1981;51:120.

Jenkins DP, Brody P. Facts about commonly used drugs. 3rd ed. Phoenix: Do It Now Foundation, 1974.

Johnston LD, O'Malley PM, Bachman JG. Drug use, drinking, and smoking: national survey results from high school, college, and young adults populations, 1975–1988. (DHHS publication No. [ADM] 89–1638.) Washington, D.C.: U.S. Department of Health and Human Services, 1989.

Johnston LD, O'Malley PM, Bachman JG. The Monitoring the Future Study. Vol II: college students and young adults. Ann Arbor: News and Information Services of the University of Michigan, 1994.

Johnston LD, O'Malley PM, Bachman JG. Drug use rises again in 1995 among American teens. Ann Arbor: News and Information Services of the University of Michigan, 1995.

Los Angeles County Street Drug Identification Program. Los Angeles: Department of Health Services, County of Los Angeles, 1980.

Luisada PV, Brown BI. Clinical management of phencyclidine psychosis. Clin Toxicol 1976;9:539.

Markel H, Lee A, Holmes RD, et al. LSD flashback syndrome exacerbated by selective serotonin reuptake inhibitor antidepressants in adolescents. J Pediatr 1994;125:817.

Milhorn HT Jr. Diagnosis and management of phencyclidine intoxication. Am Fam Physician 1991;43: 1293.

Patel R, Ansari A, Hughes JI. Myoglobinuric acute renal failure associated with phencyclidine abuse. West J Med 1979,131.244.

Price WA, Giannini AJ. Management of PCP intoxication. Am Fam Physician 1985;32:115.

Schuckit MA, Morrissey ER. Propoxyphene and phencyclidine use in adolescents. J Clin Psychiatry 1978; 39:7.

Schwartz RH. LSD. Its rise, fall, and renewed popularity among high school students. Pediatr Clin North Am 1995;42:403.

Schwartz RH, Hoffmann NG, Smith D, et al. Use of phencyclidine among adolescents attending a suburban drug treatment facility. J Pediatr 1987;110:322.

Schwartz RH, Smith DE. Hallucinogenic mushrooms. Clin Pediatr 1988;27:70.

Stockard JJ, Werner SS, Aalbers JA, et al. EEG findings in phencyclidine intoxication. Arch Neurol 1976;33:200.

Varipapa RJ. PCP treatment. Clin Toxicol 1977;10:353.

Werner MJ. Hallucinogens. Pediatr Rev 1993;14:466.

Wilkinson P. The young and the reckless. Rolling Stone Magazine, May 5, 1994.

Wong LK, Bieman J. Metabolites of phencyclidine. Clin Toxicol 1976;9:583.

50 Years of LSD: State of the art and perspectives of hallucinogens. Symposium of the Swiss Academy of Medical Sciences, Lugano, Switzerland, October 21–22, 1993. Jahresber Schweiz Akad Med Wiss 1993;109:23.

CHAPTER 74

Miscellaneous Drugs
Stimulants, Inhalants, Opiates, Depressants, and Anabolic Steroids

Lawrence S. Neinstein and Bruce S. Heischober

STIMULANTS

Stimulants include drugs such as nicotine (see Chapter 71), caffeine, cocaine, and amphetamines. Cocaine and amphetamines are discussed in this section.

Cocaine

Cocaine is a stimulant made from an alkaloid contained in the leaves of the coca bush, *Erythroxylon coca*. Its use goes back to the Inca Indians 3000 years ago. Crack and rock cocaine are ready-to-smoke, potent, relatively inexpensive, and highly addictive freebase forms of cocaine popular with adolescents and young adults. The use of crack by adolescents is associated with rapid addiction and with serious behavioral and medical complications.

    Prevalence   Cocaine has been tried by about 6.0% of the class of 1995 (1995 national survey results on drug use from the Monitoring the Future Study [Johnston et al., 1995]), a decrease from 17.3% in 1985 and 15.2% in 1987. However, the use in the past year and 30-day use has increased slightly in the past several years. Annual use for seniors went from 3.1% in 1992 to 4.0% in 1995. Thirty-day use changed from 1.3% in 1992 and 1993 to 1.5% in 1994 and then to 1.8% in 1995. See Figure 74.1 for trends by region of the country. Of the seniors, 1.8% had used cocaine in the 30 days before the survey, and 0.2% had used cocaine daily in the 30-day period before the survey. Crack cocaine had been used by 3.0% of this group. The 1992 National Household Survey on Drug Abuse (1992), found that 1.7% of adolescents 12–17 years old had tried cocaine (down from 6.5% in the 1982 survey and 3.4% in 1988). Current use among young people aged 18–25 years decreased from 6.8% in 1982 to 4.5% in 1988 and to 15.8% in 1992. Data from the Youth Risk Behavior Survey, conducted as part of the 1992 National Health Interview Survey revealed lifetime cocaine use at 2.5% for the 14- to 17-year-old group and 11.4% for the 18- to 21-year-old group (Centers for Disease Control, 1994).

    Action, Routes of Administration, Street Names, and Clinical Use

1. Cocaine has three major pharmacological actions
   a. Potent stimulant of the central and peripheral nervous systems

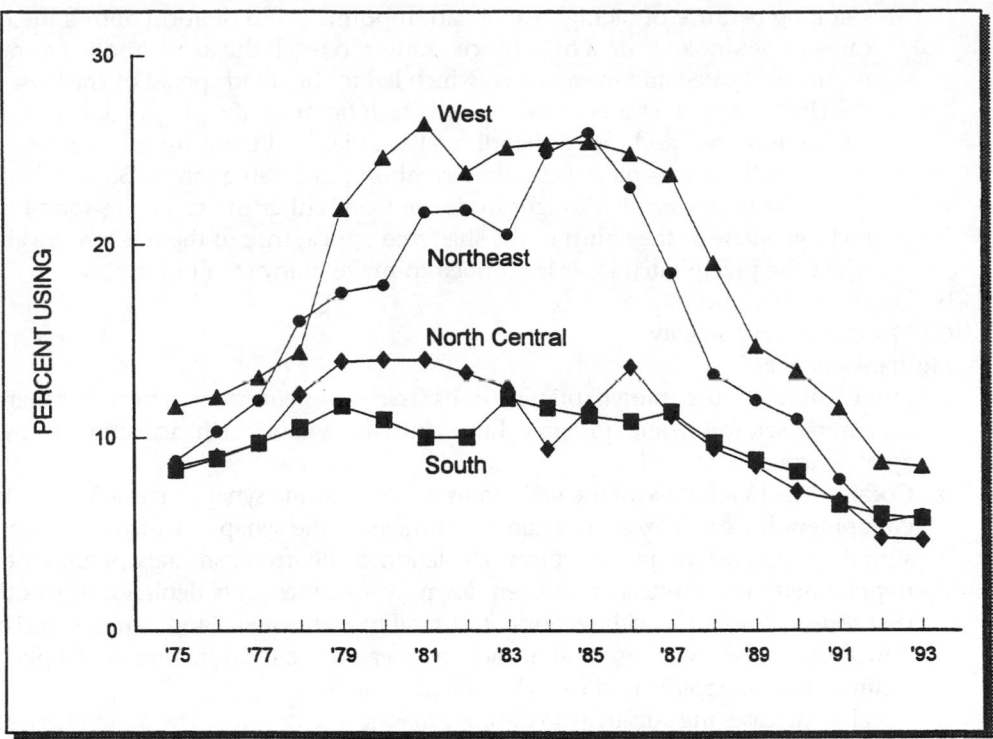

FIGURE 74.1.   Trends in seniors' lifetime prevalence of cocaine use by region of the country. (From Johnston LD, O'Malley PM, Bachman JG. National survey results on drug use from the Monitoring the Future Study, 1975–1993; vol 1: Secondary school students. [NIH publication No. 94-3809.] Washington, D.C.: U.S. Department of Health and Human Services, 1994.)

— This profound stimulation has greatly contributed to cocaine's abuse potential.

— Cocaine is cut into grams or spoons (half grams) and is usually adulterated with mannitol, lactose, or sucrose. Caffeine, amphetamines, phenylpropanolamine, procaine, and lidocaine have all been substituted for cocaine.

— Cocaine hydrochloride powder is usually chopped with a razor blade into "lines" on a piece of glass; a line is then snorted, often through a rolled piece of paper or dollar bill.

— A large shift has occurred in the distribution of cocaine, from selling cocaine hydrochloride powder to selling freebase cocaine in small chunks, or rocks (crack). Freebase cocaine is a more purified form of cocaine. The older method of making freebase involved mixing cocaine with an alkaline solution and adding a solvent such as ether. The solution would separate into two layers, with the top layer containing freebase cocaine dissolved in the solvent. The solvent would then be evaporated, leaving relatively pure cocaine crystals. These crystals can be smoked in a cigarette or water pipe. Crack is another form of cocaine that involves converting cocaine hydrochloride to a freebase state. Crack is extracted from cocaine powder by using baking soda, heat, and water. This method is safe and simple compared with making freebase cocaine with ether. With cocaine hydrochloride powder, the drug's effects would be lost during

smoking because of its high vaporization point. The base form allows the cocaine to be smoked and a high concentration to reach the user. Producing crack is uncomplicated and inexpensive, which led to the rapid spread of crack use in the United States. Dealers prefer to sell crack because of its high addiction potential, low cost, and ease of handling. Each vial sold typically contains one or more small, cream-colored chunks resembling rock salt at about $5 to $10 per rock. The term *crack* is thought to derive from either the crackling sound the rocks generate as they burn or the shattered appearance of the freebase cocaine when the precipitated layer is dropped to make many small pieces.
- b. Local anesthetic activity
- c. Vasoconstrictive activity
2. Mechanisms of action
- a. Stimulation of the presynaptic neurons releases neurotransmitters (primarily dopamine, serotonin, and norepinephrine) into the synaptic cleft, activating postsynaptic neurons.
- b. Cocaine blocks reuptake of the neurotransmitters, causing synaptic entrapment. This entrapment leaves an excess of neurotransmitters in the synapse, which continue to stimulate the postsynaptic receptors. Depletion of neurotransmitters occurs as entrapped neurotransmitters are broken down by enzymes. This depletion leaves the user feeling dysphoric, with feelings of irritability, restlessness, and depression. This downside can be so intense that it leads to repeated use to overcome the dysphoric feeling. This can rapidly lead to cycles of highs and lows.
- c. Cocaine increases the sensitivity of the postsynaptic receptor sites. The central-nervous-system stimulation leaves the user alert, full of self-confidence, and feeling immune to outside influences.
3. Routes of administration (Table 74.1)
4. Street names: Coke, Bernice, blow, Charlie, flake, nose candy, rock, toot, base, snow, crack, and gold dust
5. Combinations
- a. Speedball: Heroin and cocaine, taken intravenously
- b. Primo: Cocaine and marijuana, smoked
- c. Space base: Cocaine and phencyclidine (PCP), smoked
- d. Caviar or champagne: Rock or crack cocaine and marijuana, smoked
- e. Jim Jones: Marijuana cigarette laced with cocaine dipped in PCP
- f. Snowcap: Cocaine sprinkled on a bowl of marijuana

TABLE 74.1.   Cocaine: Routes of Administration

Method	Peak High	Duration of Effects	Amount Entering Bloodstream (%)	Side Effects
Freebase smoking	Seconds to 1 min	4–15 min	80	Burns, explosions, pulmonary edema, direct lung toxin, decreased air exchange
Intravenous	30 sec–2 min	12–30 min	100	Embolism, thrombosis, infection, anaphylactic reactions leading to shock and death
Snorting	2–30 min	30 min–1 hr	65	Nasal septum perforation, nosebleeds

Other routes of administration include eye drops and enemas.

g. Space basing: Rock or crack cocaine with PCP and tobacco
h. Speedball: Heroin and cocaine, injected
i. Whacking: Rock or crack cocaine with PCP and tobacco, smoked
6. Clinical use: Cocaine is primarily used by otolaryngologists, plastic surgeons, and emergency medicine physicians to provide local anesthesia and vasoconstriction of mucous membranes.

Effects

1. Symptoms of intoxication
    a. General: Hyperalert state, increased talking, restlessness, elevated temperature, anorexia, nausea, dry mouth, dilated pupils, sweating
    b. Neurological: Seizures, dizziness, paresthesias, hyperactive reflexes, tremor
    c. Psychiatric: Labile affect, insomnia, delirium, aggression, elation, euphoria, hallucinations, agitation, irritability, anxiety, skin picking (the act of picking at imagined bugs under the skin, formication), suspicious feelings
    d. Cardiac: Arrhythmias, hypertension, tachycardia
2. Symptoms of overdose
    a. General: Dry mouth, nausea, vomiting, anorexia, dilated pupils, excessive sweating, increased talking, flushing, increased temperature, respiratory failure
    b. Neurological: Seizures, paresthesias, hyperactive reflexes, tremor, pinprick analgesia, facial grimaces, headache, coma
    c. Psychiatric: Toxic psychosis, skin picking, paranoid behavior, anxiety, delirium, body image change, hallucinations, irritability
    d. Cardiac: Tachycardia, angina, arrhythmias, chest pain, hypertension, cardiovascular collapse
3. Complications: Until recent years, cocaine overdose was thought to be rare. However, particularly with the advent of crack use, many deaths caused by cardiovascular or respiratory collapse have been reported. The pathogenesis of these cardiovascular complications has not been fully elucidated but may be related to a combination of the sympathomimetic and membrane anesthetic effects of cocaine. Complications include:
    a. Cardiovascular: Chest pain, arrhythmias, hypertension, myocardial infarction, cardiomyopathy, myocarditis, stroke
    b. Psychiatric: Depression, schizophreniform psychosis, toxic delirium, anxiety, paranoia, suicide
    c. Neurological: Seizures, headaches, cerebral hemorrhage, cerebral infarctions, cerebral vasculitis
    d. Malnutrition
    e. Hyperpyrexia
    f. Obstetric: Placental abruption, lower infant weight, prematurity, microcephaly
    g. Pulmonary: Pneumothorax, pneumomediastinum, pneumopericardium, pulmonary edema, pulmonary hemorrhage
    h. Skin: Burns and skin infarction
    i. Head and neck: Erosion of dental enamel, gingival ulceration, keratitis, chronic rhinitis, perforated nasal septum, midline granuloma, altered olfaction, optic neuropathy, osteolytic sinusitis
    j. Sexual dysfunction
    k. Renal: Rhabdomyolysis
    l. Endocrine: Hyperprolactinemia

m. Gastrointestinal
— Acute ischemic syndromes are the most prominent gastrointestinal complication of cocaine use. Severe ischemia can result from intense activation of α-adrenergic receptors in the mesentery. This can lead to gastropyloric ulcerations, gangrene and perforation of both small and large intestines, and colitis.
— Massive overdose has occurred as a result of the rupture of small bags of cocaine swallowed by the individual in an attempt to transport the cocaine. Overdose caused by the rupture of these bags has been called "body packer syndrome."
— Several cases of acute hepatotoxic effects and hepatocellular necrosis from cocaine use have also been reported (Gourgoutis, 1994).

4. Symptoms of post-cocaine-use dysphoria: Depression, sadness, crying spells, suicidal ideation, melancholia, apathy, inability to concentrate, delusions, anorexia, insomnia, paranoia (especially regarding police)

5. Symptoms of cocaine abstinence or withdrawal
a. These symptoms include depression, anhedonia, irritability, aches and pains, restless but protracted sleep, tremors, nausea, weakness, intense cravings for more cocaine, slow comprehension, suicidal ideation, lethargy, and hunger.
b. Cocaine causes strong dependence, as evidenced by the resulting cravings to alleviate depression and irritability when the drug's effects wear off.

6. Tolerance
a. Because of cocaine's powerful euphoriant effects and its short half-life, repeated use leads to rapid development of tolerance. Addicts can progress from small doses to large daily quantities in short periods.
b. No tolerance develops to the cardiovascular side effects.

Treatment of Cocaine Toxicity

1. Support respiratory and cardiovascular functions. Individuals should have frequent monitoring of vital signs, and a cardiac monitor should be used.
2. Treat arrhythmias. Controversial treatment includes sedation (benzodiazepines) and the use of labetalol. Ventricular arrhythmias in the setting of chest pain with suspected ischemia should be treated with lidocaine (follow advanced cardiac life support protocols).
3. Treat severe hypertension that does not respond to initial benzodiazepine therapy with nitroprusside, labetalol, or phentolamine.*
4. Treat chest pain with nitrates (calcium-channel blockers—conflicting data on animal models*).
5. Treat agitation and psychosis with haloperidol or droperidol. (Avoid chlorpromazine [Thorazine] because of the possibility of a severe drop in blood pressure or anticholinergic crisis.) However, when the agitation is severe enough to warrant use of a major tranquilizer, initial management protocols for acute delirium should be considered: immediate measurement of blood sugar and arterial blood gases, or pulse oximetry, followed by thiamine, high-flow O_2, ampule of D50, lumbar puncture, computed tomography scan, and so on. Some authorities oppose the use of neuroleptic agents and recommend benzodiazepines (Ativan or Valium) only.
6. Treat seizures with diazepam or lorazepam (Ativan) (which can be given intramuscularly).
7. Treat hyperthermia with cooling blanket.
8. Treat hypoglycemia.
9. Maintain calm, supportive environment.
10. Monitor suicide potential after toxic reaction.

*Pure β-blockers are no longer recommended because of the unopposed α-stimulation that may result; labetalol is a combination α- and β-blocker, though β-blockade predominates. In animal models, calcium-channel blockers have been shown to protect against cocaine-induced arrhythmias, and another study showed an increased incidence of seizures in animals receiving them. Benzodiazepines are useful in decreasing the central sympathetic overactivity responsible for many of the cardiovascular side effects of cocaine. In addition, when there is evidence of ischemia, aspirin and heparin therapy should be initiated to oppose cocaine's direct effect on platelet aggregation.

COCAETHYLENE

When individuals combine alcohol and cocaine, a third substance, cocaethylene is formed in the body (Rose, 1994). This substance has been associated with the higher incidence of cardiovascular side effects when these substances are used together. The half-life is 2 hours—versus 38 minutes for cocaine.

AMPHETAMINE/METHAMPHETAMINE AND "LOOK-ALIKES"

Amphetamines are central-nervous-system stimulants and work as a sympathomimetic drug. Amphetamines act on the central nervous system to cause the release of neurotransmitters from presynaptic neurons, and directly stimulate postsynaptic catecholamine receptors. They also prevent reuptake of neurotransmitters and act as a mild monoamine oxidase inhibitor. Routes of administration include oral, snorting, and intravenous. The characteristics of amphetamines are similar to those of cocaine.

By the late 1970s it was thought that the vast majority of street methamphetamine was actually "look-alike" methamphetamine comprising caffeine, ephedrine, and phenylpropanolamine. "Biker speed," or "crank," was produced and distributed on the West Coast in limited quantities. During the early 1980s a process using ephedrine to synthesize methamphetamine became popular. This relatively simple process results in a high yield of D-methamphetamine. The D-isomer is cortically more active than the L-isomer (the active ingredient in Vicks Inhaler). Methamphetamine HCl is much more versatile than the hydrochloride salt of cocaine. It has high bioavailability in the salt form by any route of administration, such as snorting, smoking, ingesting by mouth, or passing across other mucous membranes such as the vaginal mucosa. "Ice" actually consists of pure crystals of D-methamphetamine; there is no difference between smoking street speed or ice. Today there are many areas in the western and southwestern United States, where methamphetamine is the predominant stimulant of abuse. There is concern that because of its ease of production, longer half-life than cocaine, and favorable physical properties, use will spread to other areas of the United States. Look-alikes containing combinations of caffeine, ephedrine, and phenylpropanolamine are particularly dangerous. A much larger dose is necessary to achieve the same level of cortical stimulation as with an amphetamine. This combination has greater cardiovascular stimulation to begin with, so abuse of look-alikes puts the individual at great risk of stroke, myocardial infarction, or hypertensive crisis.

Dose, Medical Use, and Street Names

1. Dosage forms: The most common types of amphetamines include:
    a. Dextroamphetamine sulfate (Dexedrine): Orange, heart-shaped tablets, often referred to as hearts, oranges, or "dexies"
    b. Methamphetamine (Desoxyn): Often referred to as speed, crystal, or "meth"
    c. Amphetamine sulfate (Benzedrine sulfate): Rose-colored, heart-shaped tablets, often called hearts or peaches; also come as oval tablets called footballs

  d. Benzphetamine (Didrex): Yellow (25 mg) or pink (50 mg) tablets
  e. Most "cross-tops": Now actually ephedrine
  f. Smoking form
     — Smoking methamphetamine is becoming very common. On the streets, this form is sometimes referred to as ice, or as croak when it is mixed with crack cocaine. Smoking crystal methamphetamine ("ice") may be more addictive and more potent than snorting or ingesting it; it produces higher concentrations of drug in the brain for a shorter period.
  2. Medical use: Forms of amphetamines have been used for weight loss, behavioral disorders of children, and narcolepsy. Their efficacy for weight loss is highly questionable, and they are overused in the treatment of behavioral disorders.
  3. Street names: Street names include A's, meth, speed, crystal, cartwheel, copilots, footballs, magnums, powder, twenty-twenty, whites, white crosses, crank, ice, ups, dexies, bombido, bennies, black beauties, splash, crosses, and crossroads.

Prevalence

The 1995 Monitoring the Future Study (Johnston et al., 1995) found that 15.3% of high school seniors had tried stimulants. The prevalence in the past year was 9.3%; 4.0% had used a stimulant in the past month, and 0.3% of seniors had used stimulants daily in the 30 days before the survey. The 1992 National Household survey showed the following trends in stimulant use:

Age (yr)	1979	1985	1988	1992
12–17	3.4	5.6	4.2	2.1
18–25	17.0	18.2	17.1	6.8

Effects

  1. Symptoms of intoxication, overdose, and abstinence are similar to those of cocaine.
  2. Tolerance and dependence can occur.
  3. Stimulant psychosis remits with abstinence. The psychosis is indistinguishable from schizophrenia, mania, and delusional disorders. Psychosis recurs at lower doses for a shorter period.
  4. As with cocaine, postuse dysphoria occurs because of depletion of neurotransmitters.
  5. Complications of amphetamine overdose resemble those of cocaine. They include coma, circulatory collapse, arrhythmias, cerebral hemorrhage, hypertension, seizures, and hyperthermia. Note, however, that cocaine and the amphetamines are structurally dissimilar. Cocaine is an ester of benzoic acid and, as a local anesthetic, has pronounced effects on nerve membrane and therefore conduction. Amphetamines are phenylisopropylamines with no direct cell membrane effects. Arrhythmias, seizures, and other medical complications are not as common with amphetamines, though addiction potential is no less.

Treatment of Amphetamine Toxicity

  1. Support respiratory and circulatory function.
  2. When clinical presentation suggests significant ingestion or possible coingestion, aggressive use of a large-bore (40 French) orogastric tube and of multiple-dose activated charcoal (1 g/kg body weight) is mandatory.
  3. Treat hypertension and arrhythmias. Arrhythmias are not as common or severe as cocaine-related disorders. Generally the hypertension and arrhythmias respond to sedation (e.g., Ativan or Valium).
  4. Treat hyperthermia with a cooling blanket.

5. Treat agitation and paranoid delusions with haloperidol or droperidol. Avoid Thorazine because of the possibility of a severe drop in blood pressure, anticholinergic crisis, or seizure activity (also see cocaine toxicity treatment section, above). Beyond 5–10 mg of haloperidol or droperidol, the sedating benefit is minimal and benzodiazepines should be added.
6. Treat seizures with diazepam or Ativan (which can be used intramuscularly).
7. Maintain a calm, supportive environment with avoidance of external stimulation.
8. Monitor suicide potential after toxic condition has lessened.
9. Avoid acidification of the urine; the drug may cause precipitation of myoglobin in renal tubules in the presence of rhabdomyolysis
10. Methylenedioxymethamphetamine (MDMA): See Chapter 73. Overdoses of 3,4-methylenedioxyamphetamine (MDA) (MDMA, and N-methyldiethanolamine (MDEA) are treated identically to other amphetamine overdoses.

KHAT (METHCATHINONE, CATHINONE, EPHEDRINE)

When ephedrine is reduced, the hydroxy group is lost and methamphetamine results. When this group is oxidized, methcathinone is produced. This is the active ingredient in khat leaves (*Catha edulis*), used as a tea or chewed for its euphoriant and stimulant effects in Africa and the Middle East. In Russia, methcathinone is third, after alcohol and tobacco, as a drug of abuse. Clandestine laboratories producing this substance have appeared in the midwestern United States recently, and this drug is now gaining in popularity because of the same effects produced by methamphetamine.

INHALANTS

Inhalants can be classified as volatiles, aerosols/propellants, and anesthetics. Included are spray paints, plastic cement (model-airplane glue), rubber cement, typewriter-correction fluid, gasoline, nitrites, and nitrous oxide, to name a few. Fluorinated propellants are no longer used in hair sprays and deodorants, though other propellants have been abused (e.g., isobutane). They are often the first mood-altering substance used by children. Use of inhalants decreases with increasing age, but studies show that inhalant abusers are at increased risk of abusing alcohol and illicit drugs.

Prevalence

The 1995 national survey on drug use from the Monitoring the Future Study (Johnston et al., 1995) found that 17.4% of the 12th graders had tried using inhalants, with 8.0% having used them in the past year and 3.2% in the month before the survey. Daily use in the 30 days before the survey was 0.1%. The annual use was highest in the 8th graders—12.8%, which was a marked increase in the past year for these younger individuals (9.0% in 1991; 9.5% in 1992; 11.0% in 1993; and 11.7% in 1994). The use of inhalants from the National Household Survey showed that 5.7% of 12- to 17-year-old adolescents had ever used and 12.5% of 18- to 25-year-old young people had ever used. "Fad" use also occurs sporadically and may follow news reports of a certain trend or a media portrayal of inhalant use.

Pathophysiology

Inhalants are attractive to adolescents because of their rapid onset of action, low cost, and easy availability. They are typically used by inhaling from a plastic bag containing the substance ("bagging") or by inhaling a cloth saturated with the substance ("huffing"). The initial effect is stimulation and excitation, which then progresses to a depressant effect on the central nervous system.

Of the myriad products and substances abused, toluene is the most common volatile component. It is present in spray paint, airplane glues and rubber cement, cleaning fluids, inks (magic markers), and lacquer thinner.

Symptoms of Intoxication

1. General: Lacrimation, rhinorrhea, salivation, irritation of the mucous membranes, anorexia, vomiting, sleepiness
2. Neurological: Dizziness, headaches, slurred speech, ataxia, diplopia
3. Psychiatric: Euphoria, decreased inhibition, decreased judgment

Symptoms Caused by Specific Inhalant Groups

1. Solvents: Bronchitis, liver damage, renal damage, central nervous system damage, coma, cardiac arrhythmias
2. Amyl and butyl nitrites: Methemoglobinemia
3. Gasoline: Lead poisoning
4. Aerosol sprays: Giddiness and hallucinations lasting 5–10 minutes

Trauma and Accidental Injury   Trauma and accidental injury may also occur during inhalant abuse.

Symptoms of Overdose

1. Slow and shallow respirations
2. Delirium
3. Arrhythmias
4. Stupor
5. Seizures
6. Loss of consciousness
7. Cardiopulmonary arrest and death
8. Sudden sniffing-death syndrome
   a. Not associated with toluene.
   b. Has occurred after inhalation of fluorocarbons or halogenated hydrocarbons.
   c. Postulated mechanism involves sensitization of the myocardium by the solvent to the arrhythmogenic effects of epinephrine and increased sympathetic outflow, which occurs during the initial brief excitatory phase of intoxication.

Treatment

Treatment is aimed at control of arrhythmias and respiratory and circulatory support. Although tolerance to inhalants may develop, withdrawal symptoms do not usually occur.

NITROUS OXIDE

Also known as laughing gas, nitrous oxide has long been abused by health-care personnel. More recently it has seen a resurgence of interest in the adolescent population. It is most commonly sold in small balloons or inhaled from whipped-cream cans, in which it is used as a propellant. Occasionally, individuals will gain access to a tank of nitrous oxide. Deaths have occurred after prolonged inhalation of 100% N$_2$O in a closed space.

NITRITES

Amyl, butyl, and isobutyl nitrite are examples of nitrites. They are volatile liquids abused for their vasodilatory action and subjective feeling of light-headedness (known as the "rush"). Amyl nitrite requires a prescription and is currently indicated in cyanide poisoning to produce methemoglobin. Butyl and isobutyl nitrite are available over the counter (commonly available in "head shops") as room deodorizer, cologne, or liquid incense.

Individuals abusing nitrites rarely seek medical attention for complications of abuse. The most common side effects are severe headache, dizziness, orthostatic hypotension, and occasionally syncope. These effects are a result of smooth-muscle relaxation. Clinically significant methemoglobinemia is extremely rare as a complication of nitrite abuse. Definitive evidence linking nitrites, immunosuppression, Kaposi's sarcoma, and infection with human immunodeficiency virus are lacking.

OPIOIDS

Opium has been known and used for centuries. The term *opioid* refers to all drugs, natural and synthetic, with morphinelike activity, and antagonists that bind to opioid receptors. All the opiates are derived from the opium poppy, *Papaver somniferum*. The plant is primarily grown in the Middle East and the Far East. Crude opium is obtained from the seed pods of the poppy. From this crude opium, morphine, codeine, and heroin are manufactured. The cost of heroin addiction in the United States is greater than $3 billion per year. In general, the drug is unpopular among adolescents; however, the recent trend of smoking heroin provides a route of administration that is familiar to many, and heroin usage appears to be on the increase. Heroin dependence, regardless of the chosen route of administration, creates intense addictive disease and carries at best a guarded prognosis.

HEROIN

Action, Dose, and Street Names

1. Action: Heroin is morphine treated with acetic acid. It has a stronger and faster onset of action than morphine and acts on both the central nervous system and the peripheral nervous system to:
   a. Induce analgesia
   b. Cause sedation, narcosis, or stupor
   c. Act as a respiratory depressant
   d. Block the cough reflex
   e. Cause vasodilation, with a resultant fall in blood pressure
   f. Increase nonpropulsive contractions of the intestines
   g. Induce constriction of the pupils
2. Dose: Heroin in the United States is generally only about 5% pure. It is commonly mixed with sugar, talcum powder, Epsom salt, or quinine. This mixture is usually heated into a solution and injected intravenously. Besides leg and arm veins, the veins between the toes, the veins under the tongue, and the dorsal vein of the penis are often used for injection. Heroin is sometimes injected under the skin (skin popping) or is snorted in the same manner as cocaine; the effect is less intense with any of these methods than with

intravenous use. The duration of the effects of intravenously injected heroin is 3 to 6 hours.

3. Street names: Heroin is also called smack, scat, junk, horse, H. Jones, shit, hard stuff, brown, chiva, do-jee, estuffa, hombre, mud, polvo, and stofa.

Prevalence

Although actual numbers are small, there has been a trend toward increased use of snorting and smoking opiate derivatives among adolescents. Casual users of opiates outnumber addict users 10 to 1. In the 1995 Monitoring the Future Study (Johnston et al., 1995), 1.6% of high school seniors had previously tried heroin, 1.1% had used heroin in the past year; and 0.6% had used it in the past month. These rates are almost double those of 1994.

Effects

1. Symptoms of intoxication include: Anxiety, slow comprehension, euphoria, floating feeling, flushing, hypotonia, pinpoint pupils, skin picking, sleepiness, and constipation.
2. Newer synthetic narcotics are 80 times more potent than morphine (fentanyl) and pose an increased danger of death by overdose. Symptoms of narcotic overdose include:
   a. General: Pinpoint pupils, slow and shallow respirations, decreased temperature, pulmonary edema, constipation, cyanosis
   b. Neurological: Pinprick analgesia, ataxia, stupor, slow comprehension, hypotonia, diminished reflexes, coma
   c. Psychiatric: Delirium
   d. Cardiac: Circulatory collapse and hypotension
3. Symptoms of withdrawal include:
   a. General: Muscle aches, chills, coryza, flulike symptoms, lacrimation, muscle spasms, nausea, vomiting, piloerection, sweating, increased respiratory rate and temperature, yawning, hot and cold flashes
   b. Neurological: Paresthesia, tremors, ejaculation/orgasm, mydriasis
   c. Psychiatric: Anxiety, sleep disturbances, supplicating behavior, irritability, restlessness
   d. Cardiac: Hypertension, tachycardia
   e. Gastrointestinal: Abdominal cramps, diarrhea
4. Protracted abstinence syndrome includes miosis, hyposensitive respiratory center, decreased pulse, decreased blood pressure, decreased temperature, poor stress tolerance, decreased self-image, weakness, depression, fatigue, and hyposensitivity to carbon dioxide.

Complications

1. Pronounced tolerance: Physical and psychological dependence
2. Cutaneous: Abscesses, cellulitis, lymphadenitis, phlebitis, and tongue and penile lesions from injections
3. Pulmonary: Foreign fibers (talc, cotton), arteritis and thrombosis of the pulmonary vessels, septic emboli, lung abscesses, pulmonary fibrosis, pulmonary hypertension, pneumonia, and respiratory depression
4. Cardiac: Pulmonary edema, arrhythmias caused by quinine, and bacterial endocarditis
5. Infections: Hepatitis, endocarditis, septic arthritis, osteomyelitis, tetanus, tuberculosis, and acquired immunodeficiency syndrome (AIDS)
6. Myositis ossificans: Extraosseous metaplasia of muscle caused by needle manipulation

7. Neurological: Coma, seizures, transverse myelitis, polyneuropathy, cerebrovascular accidents, deafness, and infections (abscesses, meningitis, mycotic aneurysm)
8. Crush injuries caused by immobility
9. Renal lesions: Nephrotic syndrome caused by hepatitis or foreign injected matter and focal glomerulosclerosis
10. Endocrine: Increased incidence of amenorrhea and infertility
11. Immunological: Hypergammaglobulinemia, false-positive VDRL test result in 23% of addicts, false-positive latex fixation result in 21% of addicts, and a defect in cellular immunity characterized by a decrease in lymphocyte responsiveness
12. Chronic constipation
13. Fetal effects
    a. Opiate withdrawal during pregnancy threatens viability of fetus.
    b. Methadone maintenance is recommended.
14. Neonatal effects
    a. Withdrawal in 70% of neonates, manifested by tremors, jitters, seizures, and tachypnea
    b. Forty percent prevalence of low birth weight in neonates
    c. Respiratory compromise at birth

Treatment

1. Treatment of heroin overdose
    a. Support respiratory and circulatory function.
    b. Treat hypoxia.
    c. Treat pulmonary edema with positive pressure.
    d. Treat hypotension with volume expanders and pressors.
    e. Treat arrhythmias.
    f. Give naloxone (Narcan), 0.4 mg intravenously; dose may be repeated every 3 to 10 minutes if no reaction occurs, up to 10 mg for 30 minutes. Repeated doses may be needed in 2–3 hours as the naloxone wears off. Naloxone does not reverse hypotension that is caused by opiate-induced histamine release. Always observe the patient for at least 6 hours after the initial response to naloxone, because opiates, especially propoxyphene and methadone, have a longer half-life. The patient should be admitted to the hospital for observation. Longer-acting opiate antagonists will be available soon.
    g. Look for evidence of other drug involvement.
    h. Treat hypoglycemia, if present, with 50 mL of 50% glucose solution given intravenously.
    i. Look for and treat any infectious complications.
2. Treatment of withdrawal
    a. General support and reassurance
    b. Several detoxification protocols
       — Methadone substitution with gradual detoxification
       — Clonidine detoxification; after 10 days, follow with naltrexone
       — Clonidine detoxification without naltrexone
    c. Symptomatic treatment of abdominal cramping (with dicyclomine [Bentyl]), bone pain, and insomnia
    d. Supportive treatment of chemical dependency with 12-step meetings, group therapy (see Chapter 75)

3. Methadone
   a. The use of methadone is strictly regulated by the federal government. The U.S. Food and Drug Administration requires that detoxification, rather than methadone maintenance, be used for patients who have been dependent on opiates for less than 1 year. Patients who have been dependent on heroin for more than 1 year are eligible for methadone maintenance. Methadone should, however, be reserved for the most recalcitrant cases. The methadone withdrawal syndrome is protracted and extremely unpleasant. Perhaps not unjustifiably, methadone-dependent patients have a pathological fear of withdrawal. It is difficult to treat the methadone-dependent patient. Many patients will also continue to use heroin, further confounding the potential for successful treatment. With the advent of AIDS, there has been a renewed public-health interest in methadone programs. In some cities, clean needles, bleach, and condoms have been distributed in an attempt to curb the spread of AIDS among abusers of intravenous narcotics.
   b. Goals of methadone maintenance include:
      — Suppression of abstinence syndrome
      — Avoidance of euphoria and sedation
      — Inclusion of the individual in the treatment effort
      — Removal of the individual from criminal activity
      — Improvement of health status
      — Reduction of the risk of infection (AIDS, hepatitis)
   c. Methadone maintenance is the treatment of choice for the person with intractable addiction.
   d. Methadone is the safest opiate during pregnancy.

DEPRESSANTS

The central-nervous-system depressants include the barbiturates; the nonbarbiturate hypnotic drugs such as glutethimide (Doriden) and methaqualone (Quaalude); the major tranquilizers (phenothiazines) and minor tranquilizers (benzodiazepines), and the carbamates such as meprobamate (Equanil and Miltown).

Barbiturates

Barbiturates are hypnotic and sedative drugs derived from barbituric acid. More than 50 types of pills containing barbiturates are available in the United States. The most frequently abused barbiturates are secobarbital and pentobarbital.

Action, Dose, Type, and Street Names

1. Action: Barbiturates are central-nervous-system depressants. Low doses result in mild sedation, higher doses result in hypnosis, and still higher doses result in anesthesia and possible death. Long-acting barbiturates have a strong anticonvulsant action and are thus a popular antiseizure medication (phenobarbital).
2. Dose: Barbiturates are generally taken orally, although some users inject them intravenously. Many of the pills are made in Mexico and contain varying amounts of secobarbital.
3. Type: Barbiturates are divided into ultrashort-acting, short-acting, intermediate-acting, and long-acting types.

   a. Ultrashort acting: Thiopental (Pentothal) and methohexital (Brevital), usually used for anesthesia

   b. Short acting: Secobarbital (Seconal) and pentobarbital (Nembutal), usually used as sleeping pills

   c. Intermediate acting: Amobarbital (Amytal) and butabarbital (Butisol)

   d. Long acting: Phenobarbital (Luminal)

4. Street names: Street names include reds, red devils, yellow jackets, rainbows, tooies, blue heavens, purple hearts, Mexican reds, nebbies, nimbies, bluebirds, blue devils, blues, yellows, Christmas trees, trees, barbs, beans, goofballs, and stumblers.

Prevalence   The 1995 Monitoring the Future Study (Johnston et al., 1995) found that 7.4% of the seniors had used barbiturates at some time in their life. Of reporting seniors, 4.7% had used barbiturates during the previous 12 months; 2.2% had used them in the previous 30 days; and 0.1% had used them daily during the previous 30 days. The 1992 National Household Survey showed the following sedative use among adolescents and young adults:

Age (yr)	Total	Male	Female	White	African-American	Hispanic
12–17	1.5	0.9	2.1	1.5	1.1	1.5
18–25	3.2	4.4	2.1	3.8	0.6	2.7

Side Effects

1. Symptoms of intoxication include:
   a. General: Muscle aches, anorexia, fatigue, floating feeling, sleepiness, yawning
   b. Neurological: Ataxia, slow comprehension, diplopia, dizziness, dysmetria, hypotonia, poor memory, lateral nystagmus, slurred speech
   c. Psychiatric: Anxiety, delirium, depressed mood, euphoria, irritability, "toxic" psychosis, violent behavior
   d. Cardiac: Orthostatic hypotension

2. Symptoms of overdose include pinprick analgesia, ataxia, slow comprehension, delirium, orthostatic hypotension, hypotonia, irritability, lateral nystagmus, slow and shallow respirations, and bradycardia. Coma, shock, and death are possible.

3. Physical dependence occurs with a severe withdrawal syndrome after the drug is stopped. The withdrawal syndrome can be fatal. The severity of the withdrawal syndrome parallels the strength of the drug, the dose used, and the duration of prior abuse. Withdrawal symptoms include:
   a. General: Abdominal cramps, flushing, nausea, sweating, increased temperature, weakness
   b. Neurological: Convulsions, headaches, grand mal seizures, hyperactive reflexes, tremor
   c. Psychiatric: Anxiety, delirium, hallucinations, irritability, "toxic" psychosis, sleep disturbance
   d. Cardiac: Tachycardia, orthostatic hypotension, circulatory collapse

4. Tolerance to barbiturates occurs through increased metabolism of the drug and by adaptation of the central nervous system to the drug's effects. However, the lethal dose does not increase. Cross-tolerance to other depressant drugs can also be seen.

5. Synergism: When barbiturates are used in combination with other depressants such as alcohol, the effect of both is potentiated and lethal overdoses may occur more easily.

6. Allergic reactions: Asthma, urticaria, dermatitis, fever, and angioneurotic edema can be caused by barbiturates.

7. Dermatological reactions: Cutaneous lesions and bullae are possible side effects.

Treatment of Overdose

1. Maintain adequate airway, respirations, and circulation. Use mechanical ventilation and treat shock as necessary. Supportive care is outlined in the Management of Drug Overdose section in Chapter 75.
2. Remove unabsorbed toxins by gastric lavage if ingestion is recent; then use activated charcoal.
3. Remove absorbed toxins by alkaline diuresis or dialysis.
4. Consider using naloxone (Narcan) to treat any possible coexisting narcotic overdose.
5. Avoid central-nervous-system stimulants.
6. Lethal dose
   a. Short-acting barbiturates: Ingestion of more than 3 g, or blood level greater than 2 mg/dL.
   b. Long-acting barbiturates: Ingestion of more than 6 to 9 g, or blood level greater than 11–12 mg/dL.

Treatment of Withdrawal

1. Give supportive care as needed.
2. The goal of treatment is to relieve symptoms of withdrawal and prevent progression of the withdrawal. Wesson and Smith (1977) recommended the following protocol:
   a. Give a 200 mg oral pentobarbital challenge dose and assess neurological changes in 60 minutes.
   b. The daily (24-hour) pentobarbital requirement is calculated on the basis of the neurological examination:

Neurological Examination after 60 Minutes	*24-Hour Pentobarbital Requirement*
Asleep but arousable	None
Drowsy; slurred speech; coarse nystagmus; ataxia; marked intoxication	400–600 mg
Comfortable; fine lateral nystagmus as the only sign of intoxication	800 mg
No signs of drug effects; no intoxication	1000–1200 mg or more

   c. Convert the 24-hour pentobarbital requirement to phenobarbital, substituting 30 mg of phenobarbital for every 100 mg of pentobarbital. This is given in four divided doses.
   d. After the 24-hour phenobarbital requirement is determined (not more than 600 mg/day), the patient's condition is stabilized for 24 to 48 hours at the initial dose.
   e. After stabilization, detoxification begins by tapering of the phenobarbital dose by 10–20% per day (approximately 30 mg/day).
3. Other detoxification protocols are also available.

Nonbarbiturate Hypnotic Drugs

This group includes drugs such as glutethimide (Doriden) and methaqualone (Quaalude) that are similar in effect to short-acting barbiturates. These drugs have high abuse potential and are not good therapeutic agents. Tolerance and psychological and physical dependence can all occur. The effects of the drugs include a sense of euphoria, a loss of concern for self, and withdrawal from reality. Heavy use leads to intoxication, with unsteadiness, tremors, loss of memory, irritability, and delirium and may result in coma and cardiovascular and respiratory failure. Withdrawal from these drugs is dangerous and can result in seizures, coma, and death. Treatment is similar to that of barbiturate abuse.

Tranquilizers

Tranquilizers include the major tranquilizers, such as the phenothiazines, and the minor tranquilizers, such as diazepam (Valium) and alprazolam (Xanax). The major tranquilizers are not frequent drugs of abuse among adolescents. The minor tranquilizers have the potential for psychological and physical dependence. However, abuse of these drugs is more common in adults than in adolescents. The minor tranquilizers are fairly safe with regard to overdose, with minimal serious side effects after ingestions of 50–100 times the daily dosage. However, these drugs have serious lethal potential when combined with alcohol, barbiturates, or other drugs with depressant effects.

Detoxification   Detoxification from benzodiazepine dependence can be accomplished in several ways:

1. Slow, gradual outpatient detoxification lasting 2 to 3 months; decreasing the dose by one-sixth every 10 days
2. Rapid inpatient detoxification using the phenobarbital substitution method for 10–14 days
3. Rapid inpatient detoxification using long-acting benzodiazepines such as chlordiazepoxide for 10 to 14 days

Benzodiazepine Receptor Antagonist   Flumazenil is the first specific benzodiazepine receptor antagonist to become available. It is an imidazobenzodiazepine available for intravenous injection only. Indications include benzodiazepine overdose. It is given in incremental doses of 0.2 mg/min. If a clinical effect is not seen after 5 mg is given, it is unlikely that higher doses will be helpful. In patients who have been long-term users and those who have taken an overdose of an agent with a long half-life, redosing may be necessary. Deaths have occurred in overdose patients when antidote half-life was not compared with the effective half-life of drug "on board."

In mixed overdoses involving tricyclic antidepressants, flumazenil is contraindicated. In this setting it can cause seizure activity. It is also contraindicated in individuals who are physically dependent on benzodiazepines. This dependence can occur rapidly. In one study of healthy adults treated for 2 weeks with therapeutic doses of lorazepam, use of flumazenil precipitated a full-blown benzodiazepine-withdrawal state (agitation, tremor, flushing).

An antidote is at best an adjunct in the management of the overdose patient. A secure airway, intravenous access, cardiac monitoring, and pulse oximetry are never to be overlooked.

ANABOLIC STEROIDS

Anabolic steroids are synthetic derivatives of testosterone. Though a steroid-dependence syndrome is not listed in the *Diagnostic and Statistical Manual of Mental Disorders*, 4th edition (DSM-IV), abusers of this class of drug exhibit tolerance, withdrawal, and psychological dependence. Treatment may require detoxification and a rehabilitation phase comparable to traditional drug treatment.

The numerous agents fit into two basic categories: the oral agents are 17α methyl derivatives of testosterone, and the injectable agents are esters of testosterone and 19-nortestosterone. The ideal anabolic steroid would have minimal androgenic activity and a longer half-life than the parent compound, testosterone. The 17α alkylated steroids have a half-life of approximately 8–10 hours, whereas the injectable forms have half-lives in the range of 21 days. Though these agents have less androgenic activity in lower dosage ranges, this activity is lost at higher doses. Many abusers use 10 times the usual therapeutic dose and use combinations of oral and injectable agents concurrently in 6- to 12-week cycles (called "stacking").

Prevalence

The Monitoring the Future Study for 1995 found a lifetime prevalence in seniors of 2.3%; however, other studies have reported lifetime prevalence rates in male high school seniors as high as 11%.

Side Effects

1. Cardiovascular
   a. Decreased high-density lipoprotein and increased low-density lipoprotein cholesterol
   b. Increased systolic blood pressure
2. Endocrine
   a. Premature epiphyseal closure
   b. Female virilization
   c. Hypogonadism
3. Hepatic: Hepatocellular carcinoma
4. Psychiatric
   a. Psychosis
   b. Mania
   c. Mood swings
   d. Violence syndrome (hyperaggressiveness)
   e. Depression during withdrawal
5. Addictive: Dependence syndrome, including:
   a. Tolerance
   b. Withdrawal symptoms
   c. Inability to cut down or control use
   d. Continued use despite adverse consequences

Treatment of Withdrawal or Dependence

Patients exhibiting psychotic behavior or severe depression will require inpatient care. Appropriate pharmacological intervention with antipsychotic, antidepressant, and anxiolytic agents may be indicated, usually for a short period.

For the patient meeting DSM-IV criteria (3 of 12 listed) for substance dependence, a traditional drug treatment approach is indicated. Attendance at 12-step meetings attendance and "working a program" are ideal in providing the adolescent with a conceptual framework to work through this problem.

Designer Drugs

"Designer drug" is an imprecise term originating with a fentanyl analog that was synthesized in a clandestine laboratory and sold on the street as heroin. The intent of the "chemists" was to synthesize a substance closely related to the controlled substance and yet technically legal.

Legislation has closed this loophole, but the term "designer drug" persists. Common designer drugs include:

Drug	Method of Use	Effects
Dextromethamphetamine	Smoked	Impulsiveness, fearlessness, paranoia
MDA ("love drug")	Oral	Feelings of euphoria and empathy without hallucinations
MDMA ("ecstasy" or "Adam") and MDEA ("Eve")	Oral	Feelings of euphoria and empathy, mild visual hallucinations, increased self-esteem, anorexia, bruxism, hypertension, tachycardia, diaphoresis, ataxia
α-Methylfentanyl ("synthetic heroin," "china white")	Injected	Analgesia, miosis, central nervous depression, respiratory depression

A survey in a large private Southern university of illicit drug use by undergraduate students found a significant drop in amphetamine use, but a large increase in mescaline and MDMA use from 16% in 1986 to 24% in 1990 (Cuomo, 1994).

BIBLIOGRAPHY

Arruda JA, Kurtzman NA, Pillay KG. Prevalence of renal disease in asymptomatic heroin addicts. Arch Intern Med 1975;135:535.

Cantwell JD. Cocaine and cardiovascular events. Physician Sportsmed 1986;14:77.

Centers for Disease Control. Health risk behaviors among persons age 12–21 years—United States, 1992. MMWR 1994;43:231.

Chakko S, Myerburg RJ. Cardiac complications of cocaine abuse. Clin Cardiol 1995;18:67.

Chambers HF, Morris L, Tauber MG, et al. Cocaine use and the risk for endocarditis in intravenous drug users. Ann Intern Med 1987;106:833.

Cicero TJ, Bell RD, Wiest WG, et al. Function of the male sex organs in heroin and methadone users. N Engl J Med 1975;292:882.

Cone EJ, Holicky BA, Grant TM, et al. Pharmacokinetics and pharmacodynamics of intranasal "snorted" heroin. J Anal Toxicol 1993;17:327.

Council on Scientific Affairs. Clinical aspects of amphetamine abuse. JAMA 1978;240:2317.

Crack. Medical Lett Drugs Ther 1986;28:69.

Cuomo MJ, Dyment PG, Gammino VM. Increasing use of "ecstasy" (MDMA) and other hallucinogens on a college campus. J Am Coll Health 1994;42:271.

Das G. Cocaine abuse and reproduction. Int J Clin Pharmacol Ther 1994;32:7.

Diagnostic and statistical manual of mental disorders. 4th ed. Washington, DC: American Psychiatric Association, 1994.

Dinwiddie SH. Abuse of inhalants: a review. Addiction 1994;89:925.

Dole VP. Implications of methadone maintenance for theories of narcotic addiction. JAMA 1988;260:3025.

DuRant RH, Escobedo LG, Heath GW. Anabolic-steroid use, strength training, and multiple drug use among adolescents in the United States. Pediatrics 1995; 96:23.

DuRant RH, Rickert VI, Ashworth CS, et al. Use of multiple drugs among adolescents who use anabolic steroids. N Engl J Med 1993;328:922.

Evanko D. Designer drugs. Postgrad Med 1991;89:67.

Fox CH. Cocaine use in pregnancy. J Am Board Fam Pract 1994;7:225.

Garber MW, Flaherty D. Cocaine and sudden death. Am Fam Physician 1987;36:227.

Gawin FH, Ellinwood EH Jr. Cocaine and other stimulants: Actions, abuse, and treatment. N Engl J Med 1988;318:1173.

Gold MS. Crack abuse: its implications and outcomes. Medical Times 1987;April:27.

Gold MS, Semlitz L, Dackis CA, et al. The adolescent cocaine epidemic. Semin Adolesc Med 1985;1:303.

Goldstein FJ. Cocaine: clinical pharmacology and toxicology. Medical Times 1988;March:123.

Gottlieb LS, Boylen TC. Pulmonary complications of drug abuse. West J Med 1974;120:8.

Gourgoutis G, Das G. Gastrointestinal manifestations of cocaine addiction. Int J Clin Pharmacol Ther 1994;32:136.

Gray JD. Medical consequences of cocaine. Can Fam Physician Med Fam Can 1993;39:1975.

Grinspoon L. Cocaine: a drug and its social evolution. New York: Basic Books, 1985.

Haddad LM. Cocaine abuse: background, clinical presentation, and emergency treatment. Internal Medicine for the Specialist 1986;7:67.

Haim DY, Lippmann ML, Goldberg SK, et al. The pulmonary complications of crack cocaine: a comprehensive review. Chest 1995;107:233.

Hall J. Rophies: foreign sedative abused by local groups. Dade County Information for Action Drug Surveillance News 1994;1(3).

Heilpern KL, Karras DJ. Cocaine-induced cardiopulmonary disease. Emergency Medicine Reports 1994; 15(2).

Heischober B, Miller MA. Methamphetamine abuse in California. NIDA Res Monogr 1991;115:72–83.

Henry JA, Jeffreys KJ, Dawling S. Toxicity and deaths from 3,4-methylenedioxymethamphetamine ("ecstasy"). Lancet 1992;340:384.

Hollander JE, Burstein JL, Hoffman RS, et al. Cocaine-associated myocardial infarction. Clinical safety of thrombolytic therapy. Cocaine Associated Myocardial Infarction (CAMI) Study Group. Chest 1995; 107:1237.

Holzman C, Paneth N. Maternal cocaine use during pregnancy and perinatal outcomes. Epidemiol Rev 1994;16:315.

Isner JM, Estes M III, Thompson PD, et al. Acute cardiac events temporally related to cocaine abuse. N Engl J Med 1986;315:1438.

Jalali B, Jalali M, Crocetti G, et al. Adolescents and drug use: toward a more comprehensive approach. Am J Orthopsychiatry 1981;51:120.

Jatlow P. Cocaethylene: pharmacologic activity and clinical significance. Ther Drug Monit 1993;15: 533.

Johnson S, Michals TJ, Turnball JM, et al. Detecting cocaine abuse in a patient. Medical Aspects of Human Sexuality 1986;20:66.

Johnston LD, O'Malley PM, Bachman JG. Drug use, drinking, and smoking: national survey results from high school, college, and young adults populations, 1975–1988. (DHHS publication No. [ADM] 89-1638.) Washington, DC: U.S. Department of Health and Human Services, 1989.

Johnston LD, O'Malley PM, Bachman JG. National survey results on drug use from the Monitoring the Future Study, 1975–1993; vol 1: Secondary school students. (NIH publication No. 94–3809.) Washington, D.C.: U.S. Department of Health and Human Services, 1994.

Johnston LD, O'Malley PM, Bachman JG. Drug use rises again in 1995 among American teens. Ann Arbor: News and Information Services of the University of Michigan, 1995.

Kalix P. Khat, an amphetamine-like stimulant. J Psychoactive Drugs 1994;26:69.

Khantzian EJ, McKenna GJ. Acute toxic and withdrawal reactions associated with drug use and abuse. Ann Intern Med 1979;90:361.

King GS, Smialek JE, Troutman WG. Sudden death in adolescents resulting from the inhalation of typewriter correction fluid. JAMA 1985;253:1604.

King P, Coleman JH. Stimulants and narcotic drugs. Pediatr Clin North Am 1987;34:349.

Kirn TF. Methadone maintenance treatment remains controversial even after 23 years of experience. JAMA 1988;260:2970.

Lange WR, White N, Robinson N. Medical complications of substance abuse. Postgrad Med 1992;92: 205.

Lowinson JH, Ruiz P, Millman RB, Langroid JG, eds. Substance abuse: a comprehensive textbook. Baltimore: Williams & Wilkins, 1992.

Manschreck TC. Cocaine abuse: Medical and psychopathologic effects. Drug Ther 1988;18(Aug):26.

Mathias DW. Cocaine-associated myocardial ischemia: review of clinical and angiographic findings. Am J Med 1986;81:675.

McCarron MM, Wood D. The cocaine body packer syndrome. JAMA 1983;250:1417.

McCune J, Golbus J. Rheumatic manifestations of intravenous drug abuse. Internal Medicine for the Specialist 1987;8:72.

McHugh MJ. The abuse of volatile substances. Pediatr Clin North Am 1987;34:333.

Mofensen HC. Cocaine and crack: the latest menace. Contemp Pediatr 1986;44(Oct).

Mouhaffel AH, Madu EC, Satmary WA, et al. Cardiovascular complications of cocaine. Chest 1995;107: 1426.

National Institute on Drug Abuse. National Household Survey on Drug Abuse: main findings, 1985. (DHHS publication No. 163MP.) Washington, D.C.: U.S. Department of Health and Human Services, 1988.

National Survey on Drug Abuse: main findings. Rockville, Maryland: National Institute on Drug Abuse, 1989.

Neuspiel DR. Behavior in cocaine-exposed infants and children: association versus causality. Drug Alcohol Depend 1994;36:101.

O'Connor B. Hazards associated with the recreational drug "ecstasy." Br J Hosp Med 1994;52:507.

O'Donnell AE, Selig J, Aravamuthan M, et al. Pulmonary complications associated with illicit drug use. An update. Chest 1995;108:460.

Pope HG Jr, Katz DL. Psychiatric and medical effects of anabolic-androgenic steroid use. Arch Gen Psychiatry 1994;51(5):375–382.

Randall T. Cocaine, alcohol mix in body to form even longer lasting, more lethal drug. JAMA 1992;257: 1043.

Rollingher IM, Belzber AS, Macdonald IL. Cocaine-induced myocardial infarction. Can Med Assoc J 1986;135:45.

Rose JS. Cocaethylene: a current understanding of the active metabolite of cocaine and ethanol. Am J Emerg Med 1994;12:489.

Roth D, Alarcon FJ, Fernandez JA, et al. Acute rhabdomyolysis associated with cocaine intoxication. N Engl J Med 1988;319:673.

Rowbotham MC. Neurologic aspects of cocaine abuse. West J Med 1988;149:442.

Savoy-Moore RT, Church MW, Dombrowski MP, et al. Cocaine use and reproductive function. The Female Patient 1992;17:109.

Schnoll SH, Daghestani AN, Hansen TR. Cocaine dependence. Resident and Staff Physician 1984;30:24.

Schulz JE. Illicit drugs of abuse. Primary Care 1993;20: 221.

Schwartz RH, Luxenberg MG, Hoffmann NG. Crack use by American middle-class adolescent polydrug abusers. J Pediatr 1991;118:150.

Shiono PH, Klebanoff MA, Nugent RP, et al. The impact of cocaine and marijuana use on low birth weight and preterm birth: a multicenter study. Am J Obstet Gynecol 1995;172:19.

Siegel R. Cocaine smoking disorders: diagnosis and treatment. Psychiatr Ann 1984;14:728.

Smith DE. Diagnostic, treatment, and aftercare approaches to cocaine abuse. J Subst Abuse Treat 1984; 1:5.

Smith HWB III, Liberman HA, Brody SL, et al. Acute myocardial infarction temporally related to cocaine use: clinical, angiographic, and pathophysiologic observations. Ann Intern Med 1987;107:13.

Tanner SM, Miller DW, Alongi C. Anabolic steroid use by adolescents: prevalence, motives, and knowledge of risks. Clin J Sports Med 1995;5:108.

Tarr JE, Marklin M. Cocaine. Pediatr Clin North Am 1987;34:319.

U.S. Department of Commerce. Statistical Abstract of the United States, 1994. 114th ed. Washington, D.C.: the Department, 1994.

Van Dyke C, Byck R. Cocaine. Sci Am 1982;246:128.

Warner EA. Cocaine abuse. Ann Intern Med 1993;119: 226.

Warner EA. Is your patient using cocaine? Clinical signs that should raise suspicion. Postgrad Med 1995;98: 173.

Washton AM, Gold MS, Pottash AC. Crack: early report on a new drug epidemic. Postgrad Med 1986;80:52.

Washton AM, Stone-Washton N. Outpatient treatment of cocaine and crack addiction: a clinical perspective. NIDA Res Monogr 1993;135:15.

Webb D, Thadepalli H. Skin and soft tissue polymicrobial infections from intravenous abuse of drugs. West J Med 1979;130:200.

Willens HJ, Chakko SC, Kessler KM. Cardiovascular manifestations of cocaine abuse: a case of recurrent dilated cardiomyopathy. Chest 1994;106:594.

Woods JH, Katz JL, Winger G. Use and abuse of benzodiazepines: issues relevant to prescribing. JAMA 1988;260:3476.

Yesalis CE, Kennedy NJ, Kopstein AN, et al. Anabolic-androgenic steroid use in the United States. JAMA 1993;270:1217.

Zamora-Quezada JC, Dinerman H, Stadecker MJ, et al. Muscle and skin infarction after free-basing cocaine (crack). Ann Intern Med 1988;108:564.

CHAPTER 75

Approaches to the Management of Drug Abuse

Lawrence S. Neinstein, Drew Pinsky, and Bruce S. Heischober

The management of drug abuse in adolescents is complex and always requires the cooperation of a multidisciplinary team or a residential treatment center. In an assessment of an adolescent for drug abuse, it is essential to evaluate certain areas during the history taking and physical examination.

PHYSICIAN'S RESPONSIBILITIES

The physician's responsibilities in dealing with drug-abusing adolescents are:

1. To be well informed regarding current drugs of abuse and their pharmacology
2. To understand one's own limitations and use community resources as needed
3. To be aware of available community resources for emergency medical services, crisis intervention, residential treatment programs, counseling services, legal services, vocational counseling, and housing and recreational facilities
4. To develop relationships with emergency departments at local hospitals, working with them on identification and referral of adolescents at high risk of substance abuse or identified as abusing substances
5. To become familiar with laws related to drug abuse
6. To be able to manage acute drug ingestion
7. To provide drug education to schools, youth organizations, adolescents, and parents
8. To provide supportive counseling to the adolescent
9. To be aware of the unique problems of chemically dependent adolescents who are in recovery
10. To recognize the child or adolescent at high risk of chemical dependency and to intervene appropriately

HISTORY TAKING

In taking the adolescent's history, the health-care provider should keep the following points in mind:

1. Be supportive, nonthreatening, open, and honest.
2. The history is best taken in a quiet area, especially if the adolescent is in the emergency department.
3. If an adolescent is under the influence of mood-altering chemicals, do not attempt or expect to get an accurate history.

4. Assess:
   a. Level of chemical use (i.e., experimental use, regular use, daily preoccupation, or dependence)
   b. What drugs are being used, their frequency, and route of administration
   c. Age at onset of drug use and current emotional and physical development of the adolescent
   d. Whether drug use has caused significant life problems in any area of the adolescent's life (i.e., family, school, legal, health, social, or financial)
   e. Whether there is evidence of chemical dependency (i.e., cravings, blackouts, loss of control, continued use despite significant life problems, unsuccessful attempts to quit using)
   f. Stress factors in the family, peers, or school
   g. Family history of chemical dependency
   h. Peer group level of substance use
   i. Whether the individual is in a category of persons at high risk for chemical dependency. Adolescents at risk include:
      — Child of alcoholics or addicts
      — Physically disabled
      — Gay
      — Engaged in other high-risk behavior (gang, crime, prostitution)
      — A history of depression; a learning disability; hyperactivity; peers or siblings who use drugs; low self-esteem; physical or sexual abuse; runaway behavior; participation in an antisocial peer group; a significant loss, such as a divorce or death in the family or a move to a new community; a psychiatric disorder
5. Use questionnaires. A few standard questionnaires to measure drug and alcohol dependency, such as the Michigan Alcoholism Screening Test (MAST) (Selzer, 1971), have been developed. The MAST has been tested in older adolescents, but many other questionnaires have not been tested in adolescents. Leccese and Waldron (1994) reviewed measurement instruments used in assessing substance abuse in adolescents.
6. Other questionnaires include the Adolescent Assessment/Referral System (AARS) and the Problem-Oriented Screening Instrument for Teenagers (POSIT) (Rahdert, 1991).
7. Assess for evidence of associated medical problems.

PHYSICAL EXAMINATION

1. General appearance: Look for evidence of malnutrition and infection.
2. Vital signs: Check the following:
   a. Blood pressure: Increased with amphetamines, phencyclidine (PCP), D-lysergic acid diethylamide (LSD), and drug withdrawals; decreased with narcotic use.
   b. Pulse: Increased with hallucinogens, stimulants, and drug withdrawal.
   c. Respiration: Depressed with barbiturates, opiates, and tranquilizers.
   d. Temperature: Increased with PCP and amphetamines; decreased with morphine or barbiturates.
3. Skin: Assess for evidence of needle tracks in the antecubital fossa, inguinal and jugular areas, and dorsal vein of the penis. Assess for nodules, abscesses, and cigarette stains and burns. Pustular acne may occur with the use of barbiturates, LSD, and amphetamines, cyanosis with opiates and sedatives, and flushed skin with PCP and LSD. Burns on lips may occur as a result of smoking marijuana or cocaine. Because of formication, methamphetamine abusers have multiple small ulcerations in various stages of healing.

4. Lymphatic vessels: Explore for lymphadenopathy caused by the injection of foreign material. Look for evidence of lymphangitis caused by injected substances.

5. Eyes: Tennant (1988) described a rapid eye test to detect current drug intoxication:

   a. General observation: Look for redness of sclera, ptosis, retracted upper lid (white sclera is visible above the iris, causing the appearance of a blank stare), glazing, excessive tearing of eyes, and swelling of eyelids.

   b. Pupil size: Look for dilation (>6.5 mm) or constriction (<3.0 mm).

   c. Pupil reaction to light: Look for slow, sluggish, or absent response.

   d. Nystagmus: Hold examining finger in a vertical position and then have teen follow the finger as it is moved to the side, in a circle, and up and down. Positive test result is failure to hold gaze or jerkiness of eye movements.

   e. Convergence: The teen is unable to track or hold the cross-eyed position after an examining finger is moved from 1 foot away from teen's nose to 1 inch and held there for 5 seconds.

   f. Corneal reflex: Decreased rate of blinking occurs after the cornea is touched with a strand of cotton or thread.

   g. Rapid eye test: Results are considered suggestive of drug influence only if two or more of the five primary eye signs (ptosis, abnormal pupil size, nonreactive pupil, nystagmus, and nonconvergence) are present. The following list of common eye signs to determine the use of various drugs is adapted from Tennant (1988):

   — *Marijuana*
     (1) Normal-sized pupil
     (2) Slow or no reaction of pupil to light
     (3) Nonconvergence
     (4) Redness of sclera
     (5) Glazing of cornea
     (6) Horizontal nystagmus
     (7) Swollen eyelids
     (8) Watering

   — *Heroin*
     (1) Constricted pupil
     (2) Nonreactive pupil
     (3) Ptosis
     (4) Glazing of cornea
     (5) Decreased corneal reflex
     (6) Swollen eyelids

   — *Alcohol/benzodiazepines*
     (1) Normal-sized pupil
     (2) Slow or no reaction of pupil to light
     (3) Nystagmus
     (4) Redness of sclera
     (5) Glazing of cornea
     (6) Nonconvergence

   — *Cocaine/amphetamine*
     (1) Dilated pupil
     (2) Slow or no reaction of pupil to light
     (3) Decreased corneal reflex

   — *Phencyclidine (PCP)*
     (1) Normal-sized pupil
     (2) Slow or no reaction of pupil to light

(3) Vertical and horizontal nystagmus
(4) Retracted upper eyelid
(5) Decreased corneal reflex
(6) Swollen eyelids
— *Amphetamines*
(1) Dilated pupils
(2) Nonreactive pupil
— *Barbiturates*
(1) Lateral nystagmus

6. Nasopharynx: Check for nasal mucosal injury and perforation caused by nasal insufflation of drugs: methamphetamine, heroin, cocaine. Also check for bruxism (amphetamines).
7. Cardiorespiratory system: Explore for evidence of pneumonitis caused by aspiration or infection, pulmonary hypertension, arrhythmias, or signs of endocarditis.
8. Gastrointestinal system: Check for the following:
   a. Weight loss: Amphetamines and cocaine
   b. Vomiting: Opiates and peyote
   c. Constipation: Opiates
   d. Diarrhea: Marijuana or opiate withdrawal
   e. Abdominal pain: Hallucinogens or amphetamines; opiate withdrawal
9. Musculoskeletal system: Check for the following:
   a. Tremors: Hallucinogens or stimulants; long-term use of alcohol, sedatives, or opiates
   b. Rigidity: PCP
10. Central nervous system: Check for the following:
   a. Seizures: Can occur during withdrawal from barbiturates, glutethimide, or tranquilizers, or as a result of intoxication with amphetamines
   b. Slurred speech: Caused by barbiturates, opiates, and solvents
   c. Hyperreflexia: Caused by hallucinogens and stimulants
   d. Hyporeflexia: Caused by sedatives and narcotics
   e. Truncal ataxia: Caused by PCP
   f. Mental status: Overt psychoses with hallucinogens and amphetamines; depression resulting from barbiturates and withdrawal from stimulants; hallucinations from LSD, PCP, barbiturates, and stimulants; panic states caused by marijuana, stimulants, and hallucinogens

DIAGNOSTIC CLUES BY DRUG CLASS (TOXIDROMES, OR POISONING SYNDROMES)

1. Sympathomimetics: Delusions, paranoia, restlessness, agitation, tachycardia, hypertension, hyperpyrexia, diaphoresis, mydriasis and hyperreflexia, dry mouth, diarrhea, sweating
2. Sedative-hypnotics: Respiratory depression, miosis and lateral nystagmus, drowsiness, lethargy, coma, hypotension, and fluctuating levels of consciousness with glutethimide; mydriasis with barbiturates
4. Hallucinogens: Bizarre behavior, psychosis, hallucinations
5. Opiates: Coma, hypotension, bradycardia, hypothermia, hyporeflexia, miotic pupils, depressed respiration, coma, needle marks
6. Phenothiazines: Miosis, hypotension, tremors, extrapyramidal movements, cardiac arrhythmias
7. Anticholinergics (e.g., tricyclics, antidepressants, jimsonweed): Delirium with mumbling speech, tachycardia, dry flushed skin, dilated pupils, myoclonus, decreased bowel sounds,

hypotension, arrhythmias, increased QRS-complex duration, choreoathetoid movements, urinary retention ("mad as a hatter, blind as a bat, red as a beet, hot as a hare, and dry as a bone")

8. Cholinergics (e.g., *Amanita muscaria* mushrooms): SLUDGE = *s*alivation, *l*acrimation, *u*rination, *d*efecation, *g*astrointestinal upset, and *e*mesis; also miosis, confusion, seizures, or coma

DRUG SCREENING

The technology for drug screening and identification has greatly expanded in recent years. Inexpensive, reliable, and rapid tests are currently available. Drug testing can provide reliable and useful information in the diagnosis and management of substance abuse in adolescents. However, the practitioner should keep in mind that false-positive and false-negative results do occur and that positive results on screening tests should be confirmed with more specific tests. The practitioner faces many dilemmas with drug testing. Questions such as the circumstances in which it is ethical to order such tests, the confidentiality of the results, and the action plan for handling positive test results are often more difficult than the actual technical aspects of the tests. Occupational, school, and sports-participation drug screening tests are becoming more common.

Resources

Practitioners involved in drug screening may wish to consult the following resources:

1. For urine collection: *Drug Testing Procedures Handbook* (U.S. Department of Transportation publication No. S/N 050-000-00538-1). Available from the Superintendent of Documents, U.S. Government Printing Office, P.O. Box 371954, Pittsburgh, PA 15250.
2. Medical review officer activities: *Medical Review Officer Manual* (U.S. Department of Health and Human Services, National Institute on Drug Abuse). Available free from the Division of Workplace Programs, Room 9A-54, 5600 Fishers Lane, Rockville, MD 20857.
3. Seminars for prospective medical review officers. Contact the American Society of Addiction Medicine, 5225 Wisconsin Ave., N.W., Suite 409, Washington, DC 20015.

Indications for Testing

1. Psychiatric symptoms
2. Significant changes in performance or behavior in daily activities or school
3. Sudden changes in behavior
4. Recurrent unexplained accidents
5. Recurrent unexplained respiratory ailments
6. Monitoring of compliance during recovery program
7. Emergency department evaluations of trauma victims, automobile accidents, or unexplained illness in an adolescent with risk factors

Testing should always be undertaken with a clear plan of action in mind, including appropriate referrals. A single positive test result cannot be ignored but does not determine the frequency and extent of drug use.

There is no universal agreement about screening suspected adolescent substance abusers without their knowledge. The American Academy of Pediatrics (1989) issued a statement that involuntary drug tests should not be ordered for competent older adolescents unless they have been informed of the procedure. The American Academy of Child and Adolescent Psychiatry (1991) issued the following statement: "Confidentiality is not unconditional when the child's mental status is severely impaired or when the adolescent is judged to be in a life-threatening situation."

Techniques

The best time to collect urine specimens is early morning. Monday morning is a good time, although Sunday collections might be even more revealing. Suspected teens may need to be observed during the collection to prevent substitution or addition of liquids.

1. Types of tests
   a. Color spot: Rapid but not highly sensitive or specific
   b. Immunoassay screening tests such as: Enzyme-multiplied immunoassay technique (EMIT), radioimmunoassay (RIA), fluorescent polarization immunoassay (FIPA), and latex agglutination test. The EMIT is the most widely used immunoassay method and is a good screening test, but positive results should be confirmed by a more specific technique. There are also a variety of new specific assays such Ontrak, a second-generation latex agglutination immunoassay that is simple to perform and does not require expensive instrumentation.
   c. Thin-layer chromatography (TLC): Widely used technique for drug screening. Problems can occur with the sensitivity and specificity.
   d. Gas-liquid chromatography (GLC): Used primarily for identification of volatile compounds.
   e. High-performance liquid chromatography (HPLC): Mainly used for determination of serum levels of therapeutic agents, but increasingly used for identification of illicit drugs.
   f. Gas chromatography–mass spectrometry (GC-MS): Used for confirmation of positive screening results; highly sensitive and specific.
2. Duration of detectability of drugs in the urine

Drug or Drug Class	Duration (hr)
Alcohol	12
Amphetamine and methamphetamine	48
Barbiturates	
Pentobarbital	24
Secobarbital	24
Phenobarbital	900
Benzodiazepines	
Oxazepam	72
Cocaine	
As benzoylecgonine	96–144
Codeine	48
Heroin	24
Propoxyphene	48
Marijuana	
Single dose	120
Daily use	240
Long-term daily use	336–720
Methaqualone	112–570
Phencyclidine	200

Management

1. In the treatment of drug abuse, it is important to remember:
   a. Chemical dependency is a disease, not a moral weakness.
   b. Chemical dependency is treatable but not curable. Recovery is ongoing.
   c. Adolescents may use drugs for self-medication to deal with negative feelings or to treat underlying psychiatric conditions. In this setting, treating the primary condition is essential. Substance use may subside if the appropriate primary condition is properly treated.
   d. It is difficult to get an adolescent to stop abusing drugs unless his or her denial is broken and alternative solutions are offered.
   e. Well-meaning family members may unknowingly enable an adolescent to continue abusing drugs by rescuing him or her from the consequences of drug use.
2. Involvement with an outpatient drug clinic or residential treatment program is often required for the drug-abusing adolescent. Residential treatment programs are indicated when:
   a. An adolescent is unable to stop using drugs in an outpatient setting
   b. An adolescent's behavior is out of control
   c. An adolescent has significant life problems warranting intervention
   d. Legal involvement dictates residential treatment as a condition of probation
   e. An adolescent's home environment is not supportive of stopping drug use

Selection of Drug Treatment Program

The American Academy of Pediatrics Committee on Substance Abuse (1985) listed suggestions for selection of a drug treatment program:

1. A program's staff should view drug and alcohol use as the primary disease and not as a symptom of some other emotional problem. Direct attention should be given to the child's drug use.
2. The program should maintain an abstinence contract. Any use is abuse.
3. A drug-free environment is essential.
4. Support groups such as Alcoholics Anonymous (AA), Narcotics Anonymous (NA), Cocaine Anonymous (CA), ALANON, and ALATEEN should be incorporated into the treatment program before the youngster leaves treatment.
5. Drug or alcohol addiction is a family disease, so the program must include involvement and treatment of the whole family if at all possible.
6. The Alcoholics Anonymous 12-step program is a fundamental part of the program because it provides the teen with good tools for change during and after treatment.
7. A locally based program should be chosen if a good one exists.
8. Intimate teen-counselor interaction should be considered; a ratio of no larger than 1:6 should be maintained.
9. Cost of the program should be considered.
10. Inquiry should be made into the type of therapy used.
11. An aftercare program should be an integral part of the program.
12. The program should assist adolescents in progressively reconstructing each area of life, including family, school, friendships, and leisure-time activities.
13. Separate units for adolescents and adults are desirable.
14. A school program should be an integral part of the program.

Components of Drug Treatment Program

Treatment of chemical dependency involves abstinence, rehabilitation, the use of tools for recovery, and extended care. Necessary components include:

1. Abstinence from all mood-altering substances is essential because of cross-addiction and cross-tolerance.
2. The teen should become actively involved in a 12-step program such as AA, NA, or CA. These programs offer a sponsor who acts as a guide to recovery and a source of support and encouragement for the adolescent. If the patient has bona fide addiction, involvement in such a program is essential to avoid the progressive natural history of addiction.
3. Positive alternative activities to drug use that are attainable and agreeable to the adolescent, such as sports, dancing, camping, skating, and relaxation or meditation, should be offered.
4. Vocational and educational assistance is needed because drug use can interfere with achievement.
5. Contact between the adolescent and non-drug-using peers should be encouraged. Outpatient treatment programs, 12-step programs, and activities such as "sober" dances are sources of new friends for the recovering adolescent.
6. Family therapy is needed because chemical dependency in one family member has an impact on other family members. Family members should also be required to go to a 12-step program such as ALANON or ALATEEN.
7. The parents and the adolescent should have a contract specifying expected behavior on the part of the teen, with appropriate privileges and consequences.
8. Individual therapy should be given to the teen for work on self-esteem, assertiveness skills, and expression of feelings.
9. The severity of illness should determine the type and intensity of treatment rendered. Assessment of illness severity based on a biopsychosocial view of addiction includes evaluation for:
   a. Acute intoxication and or withdrawal
   b. Biomedical conditions and complications
   c. Emotional and behavioral conditions or complications
   d. Treatment resistance versus acceptance
   e. Relapse potential
   f. Recovery environment to which the adolescent is returning

Third-party payers use these assessment dimensions to determine "medical necessity" for specified levels of intensity of treatment. Addiction treatment today involves placing patients on a continuum of care from comprehensive inpatient to outpatient modalities. A quality program should assist in determining the appropriate level of care and moving the patient as seamlessly as possible through levels of care, always matching the intensity of service to the particular patient's needs.

Practitioners should remember that treatment for adolescent substance abuse does work. Studies have demonstrated clear improvements in substance-use frequency and in the number of substances used 1 year after treatment and also have shown sharp reductions in school and legal problems (Bergmann et al., 1995). However, substance-abuse treatment must entail more than the formal treatment episode, such as continuing attendance at support groups, family support, and help with reentry at school. Identification of adolescent substance abuse and referral are key roles for primary care providers.

EARLY INTERVENTION

Early intervention is another area of substance-abuse intervention that is being implemented and evaluated. Unlike prevention, which is directed at the general population, early intervention targets individuals who are just beginning to have problems relating to their substance abuse or a family member's abuse. Unlike treatment, early intervention provides low-intensity service to individuals who are experimenting with substances and who have substance-related problems that are not yet severe. Early intervention programs and strategies are being implemented across the United States, but evaluation has not been extensive. Effectiveness of the programs has not been well demonstrated, and the potential for labeling some adolescents inappropriately as substance abusers is a consideration.

STREET NAMES FOR DRUGS

In treating adolescents for drug use, it is important for the practitioner to be familiar with drug slang. Drug slang constantly changes, and no listing is ever up-to-date. In addition, communities often have their own terms for drugs, and the translation may vary from one locality to another. Following is a listing of slang words that seem to be used widely and frequently.

Slang	*Translation*
A's	amphetamine
Acapulco gold	high-grade marijuana
acid	LSD, D-lysergic acid diethylamide tartrate
adam	methylenedioxymethamphetamine (MDMA) (psychedelic)
angel dust	dimethyltryptamine (DMT) or PCP sprinkled over parsley or tobacco
babo	Nalorphine
bag	packet of drugs
bagging	sniffing glue in a bag
bams	meprobamate
barbs	barbiturates
base	cocaine
Beast (The)	LSD
bennies	Benzedrine (brand of amphetamine sulfate)
Bernice	cocaine
bhang	marijuana
big chief	mescaline
Big "D"	LSD
black	LSD
black beauty	methamphetamine
blow	cocaine
blue angels	
bluebirds	
blue devils	amobarbital sodium
blue heaven	
blues	
Blue Cheer	type of LSD
blue racers	barbiturates
blues-and-reds	(*see* rainbows)
blue velvet	paregoric in combination with amphetamine or antihistamine such as Pyribenzamine (brand of tripelennamine)
bombers	large marijuana cigarettes
bombido	injectable amphetamine
boo	marijuana
booze	alcohol
brown	heroin

Slang	*Translation*
brown dot	LSD
BT-72s	phenylpropanolamine
buds	marijuana
bullets	Seconal (brand of secobarbital sodium)
buscuso	coca paste
bush	marijuana
businessman's trip	DMT
buttons	dried tops of the *Lophophora* cactus (peyote)
cactus	mescaline
candy	barbiturates
cap	capsule
cartwheel	white, round, double-scored amphetamine tablet
caviar	rock or crack cocaine with marijuana, smoked
chalk	methamphetamine hydrochloride, powder form
champagne	rock or crack cocaine with marijuana, smoked
Charlie	cocaine
Chicano green	type of dark green marijuana
china white	heroin, fentanyl
chipping	periodic use of intravenously used drugs
Christmas tree	Tuinal (brand of amobarbital sodium and secobarbital sodium)
coke	cocaine (extract of dried leaves of *Erythroxylon coca*)
cokie	cocaine addict
Coolie	PCP
copilots	amphetamines
crank	methamphetamine hydrochloride
crap	heroin
Cristina	methamphetamine hydrochloride
crosses	amphetamines
crystal	methamphetamine hydrochloride, powdered or crystalline form
cubes	LSD
DET	diethyltryptamine
dexies	Dexedrine (brand of dextroamphetamine sulfate)
DMT	dimethyltryptamine
dollies	Dolophine (brand of methadone hydrochloride) tablets
DOM	dimethoxymethylamphetamine (*see also* STP)
doobie	marijuana cigarette
downers	nonnarcotic central-nervous-system depressants
dust	cocaine, PCP
dynamite	high-grade heroin
ecstasy	dimethoxymethamphetamine
Eve	freebase cocaine
flake	cocaine
footballs	amphetamine tablets (oval shaped)
gage	marijuana (term seldom used)
ganja	hashish
gee-head	paregoric user
geeze	inject heroin
gold dust	cocaine

Slang	*Translation*
goofballs	barbiturates
grass	marijuana (dried leaves, seeds, and stems of *Cannabis sativa*)
greenies	ethchlorvynol
H	heroin (diacetyl morphine)
Harry	heroin (diacetyl morphine)
Harvey Wallbanger	STP-LSD (*see* STP)
hash	hashish (resin from *Cannabis*)
hay	marijuana
hearts	Dexedrine (brand of dextroamphetamine sulfate)
hog	PCP
honk	spray-paint inhalation
horse	heroin (diacetyl morphine)
hyke	Hycodan (brand of hydrocodone)
ice	methamphetamine (crystal)
J	marijuana cigarette
Jim Jones	marijuana cigarette laced with cocaine dipped in PCP
joint	marijuana cigarette
jug	ampule of injectable drugs
juice	PCP
junk	heroin (diacetyl morphine)
junkie	heroin user
key	kilogram of marijuana
KJ	marijuana and PCP
lemons	methaqualone
lid	one ounce of marijuana (approximately)
Llesea	Mexican term for marijuana
locoweed	jimsonweed (*Datura stramonium*)
ludes	Quaalude methaqualone
M	morphine sulfate
mad dog	cheap wine
magic mushroom	mushroom (*Psilocybe mexicana*) containing psilocybin
magnums	amphetamines
mesc	mescaline
mese	mescaline (resin from *Lophophora* cactus—peyote)
meth	methamphetamine
Mexican brown	brown marijuana from Mexico
Mickey, or Mickey Finn	combination of alcohol and chloral hydrate
Miss Emma	morphine sulfate
MJ	marijuana
mota	Mexican term for good marijuana
mushroom	psilocybin (psychedelic)
nembies	pentobarbital sodium
number	marijuana cigarette
orange	STP-LSD (*see also* STP)
orange sunshine	form of LSD
Panama red	potent grade of marijuana from Panama
pasta	coca paste

Slang	*Translation*
peace pill	Sernylan (brand of phencyclidine [PCP]), an anesthetic originally for dogs
peanuts	barbiturates
PG	paregoric
piece of stuff	one ounce of heroin
pinks	secobarbital sodium
pitillo	coca paste
popper	amyl nitrate in ampule form (generally sniffed)
pot	marijuana
powder	amphetamine sulfate in powder form
primo	marijuana cigarette laced with cocaine
purple	STP-LSD (*see also* STP)
purple hearts	Dexamyl (brand of dextroamphetamine sulfate and amobarbital sodium)
pussy juice	alcohol and metronidazole
rainbows	Tuinal (brand of amobarbital sodium and secobarbital sodium; red-and-blue capsules)
red devils	secobarbital
reds	secobarbital
reds and blues	(*see* rainbows)
roach	butt of marijuana cigarette
roaches	Librium
rock	cocaine
rope	hashish
rosie	alcohol
scag	heroin (diacetyl morphine)
scat	heroin (diacetyl morphine)
schoolboy	codeine
seven fourteens	methaqualone
sherms	PCP
shit	heroin or marijuana
shrooms	hallucinogenic mushrooms
Simple Simon	psilocybin from the Mexican mushroom (*Psilocybe mexicana*)
six pack	fentanyl
skag	heroin
smack	heroin (diacetyl morphine)
snow	cocaine
snowcap	cocaine sprinkled on a bowl of marijuana
spacebasing	rock or crack cocaine with PCP and tobacco
speed	methamphetamine
speedball	heroin and cocaine injected
splash	methamphetamine
STP	dimethoxymethylamphetamine (*see also* DOM) (serenity-tranquility-peace)
stuff	heroin (diacetyl morphine)
sugar	LSD
sunshine	LSD
surfer	phencyclidine (PCP)

Slang	Translation
tea	marijuana
toot	cocaine
trips	LSD
T's	Talwin (brand of pentazocine)
T's and blues	pentazocine and tripelennamine
T's and B's	pentazocine and tripelennamine
twenty-twenty	amphetamine
uppers	CNS stimulants
Water	PCP
weed	marijuana
whacking	rock or crack cocaine with PCP and tobacco, smoked
Whites	amphetamines
white crosses	amphetamines
white lemons	methaqualone
white lightening	alcohol
white mole	amphetamine
window panes	LSD in gelatin sheets
yellow jackets	pentobarbital sodium
yellows	pentobarbital sodium
zonkers	barbiturates

MANAGEMENT OF DRUG OVERDOSE

Support of Vital Functions

1. Establish and maintain a clear airway.
2. Provide ventilatory support if necessary.
3. Assess and support cardiovascular status.
   a. Hypotension should be treated with volume expansion as necessary or with drugs, if refractory to volume.
   b. Determination of cardiac rate and rhythm is essential.
4. Monitor urinary output through a urinary catheter in comatose patients.
5. Monitor vital signs frequently, including temperature and respiratory rate.
6. Monitor O_2 tension with pulse oximetry.
7. Unconscious patients and those having seizures should receive dextrose, naloxone, and oxygen. The initial dose of naloxone to an unconscious adolescent or adult is 2 mg. If the individual is a known narcotics addict, the dose can be lowered to 0.2–0.4 mg.

Prevention of Further Absorption

Though debate continues as to the use of gastric lavage and whether it is of benefit in overdose situations, the following reasoning is prudent. Unless one is absolutely sure as to the agent(s) ingested, entertaining the possibility of an unknown ingestion should dictate the use of gastric lavage and evacuation with a large-bore (40 French) orogastric tube and repeated doses of activated charcoal (1 g/kg body weight). Moreover, aggressive airway management is critical; therefore, if the level of consciousness is thought to be decreasing, it may be wise to intubate prior to instituting gastric emptying and lavage and administering charcoal, even if a gag reflex is still present.

Removal of Toxins Already Absorbed

1. Forced diuresis: This measure is helpful mainly for drugs that are excreted unchanged in the urine, especially for aspirin and barbiturate overdoses. It is essential to follow volume status, electrolyte values, and urine output closely when one is proceeding with this treatment.
2. Alkalinization of the urine: This measure is beneficial in the treatment of aspirin and phenobarbital overdoses.
3. Hemodialysis: This is used to treat patients with severe intoxication, clinical instability, or coexistent hepatic or renal failure, or when the patient has ingested a potentially lethal dose and the drug is diffusible across dialysis membranes. Dialysis may help in the treatment of severe overdoses of lithium, amphetamines, aspirin, long-acting barbiturates, and alcohol.

Specific Measures

1. Acetaminophen (Tylenol): *N*-Acetylcysteine (Mucomyst) has been shown to be effective when given within 24 hours of ingestion.
2. Amphetamines: Lorazepam (Ativan) or haloperidol (Haldol) is useful for agitation. Severe hypertension can be treated with nitroprusside; avoid β-blockers. (Hemodialysis has been used in severe overdose.)
3. Barbiturates: Consider whether barbiturate is long or short acting.
   a. Long acting: Use forced diuresis, alkalinization of the urine, charcoal hemoperfusion, or hemodialysis.
   b. Short acting: Use charcoal hemoperfusion for severe overdoses.
4. Ethchlorvynol (Placidyl): Lethal levels require hemodialysis or charcoal perfusion.
5. Glutethimide (Doriden): Alkaline lavage of the stomach and charcoal can be used to impede absorption of the drug. Dialysis and hemoperfusion, when indicated, can improve clearance.
6. Methaqualone (Quaalude): Treatment is mainly supportive. When indicated, charcoal hemoperfusion can be used.
7. Narcotics: Naloxone can reverse the respiratory and CNS depressive action of the opiates. Be prepared to give additional doses as necessary. The starting dose is 2 mg. More may be needed for an overdose, and less may be necessary to avoid precipitating withdrawal symptoms in a known addict.
8. Phenothiazines: For dystonic reactions, diphenhydramine (Benadryl), 25–50 mg given intravenously, will reverse reactions. Treatment of overdoses should include lavage and forced diuresis.
9. Tricyclic antidepressants, including Amitriptyline (Elavil, Triavil), imipramine (Tofranil), and doxepin (Sinequan): Gastric emptying is clearly of benefit within the first 1–2 hours, and probably later because of delayed gastric emptying caused by anticholinergic effects. This should be followed by the use of activated charcoal. The mainstay of treatment is alkalinization of the blood with $NaHCO_3^-$. A dose of 1–2 mmol/kg given intravenously for significant cardiac conduction delay or ventricular dysrhythmias. Physostigmine should be avoided. In significant ingestions, early agitation may proceed rapidly to coma; elective early intubation is prudent.
10. Lithium: Treatment includes gastric lavage, sodium as intravenously administered normal saline solution, urine alkalinization, and, in severe cases, hemodialysis.
11. Benzodiazepines: Give flumazenil, 0.2 mg over 30 seconds. Another 0.3 mg can be given over 30 seconds if there is no response after the first 30 seconds. If there is no response after another 30 seconds, give 0.5 for 30 seconds at 1-minute intervals, up to a total dose of 3 mg.

BIBLIOGRAPHY

American Academy of Child and Adolescent Psychiatry. Position statement: drug and alcohol screening. AACAP Newsletter. 1991;Summer:31.

American Academy of Pediatrics. A guide to acute medical management of intoxication in adolescents. Adolescent Health Update 1994;6:1.

American Academy of Pediatrics Committee on Adolescence, Committee on Bioethics and Provisional Committee on Substance Abuse. Screening for drugs of abuse in children and adolescents. Pediatrics 1989;84:396.

American Academy of Pediatrics Committee on Substance Abuse, California Chapter 2. Recommended criteria for selection of drug treatment program. Los Angeles Pediatric Society Newsletter 1985;January:11.

Anglin TM. Interviewing guidelines for the clinical evaluation of adolescent substance abuse. In: Rogers PD, ed. Symposium on Chemical Dependency. Pediatr Clin North Am 1987;34:381.

Belfer ML. Substance abuse with psychiatric illness in children and adolescents: definitions and terminology. Am J Orthopsychiatry 1993;63:70.

Bergmann PE, Smith MB, Hoffmann NG. Adolescent treatment: implications for assessment, practice guidelines, and outcome management. Pediatr Clin North Am 1995;42:453.

Blum RW. Adolescent substance abuse: diagnostic and treatment issues. In: Rogers PD, ed. Symposium on Chemical Dependency. Pediatr Clin North Am 1987;34:523.

Canay EC, Decker CE, Schnoll SH. Emergency treatment of the drug-abusing patient for treatment staff physicians. (Medical monograph series V. 1, NO4.) Rockville, Maryland: U.S. Department of Health and Human Services, Public Health Service, Alcohol, Drug Abuse and Mental Health Administration, 1980.

Cherubin CE, Sapira JD. The medical complications of drug addiction and the medical assessment of the intravenous drug user: 25 years later. Ann Intern Med 1993;119:1017.

Cohen S. Alternatives to adolescent drug abuse. JAMA 1977;238:1561.

Farrow JA, Deisher RA. Practical guide to the office assessment of adolescent substance abuse. Pediatr Ann 1986;15:675.

Felter R, Izsak E, Lawrence SH. Emergency department management of the intoxicated adolescent. In: Rogers PD, ed. Symposium on Chemical Dependency. Pediatr Clin North Am 1987;34:399.

Floren AE. Urine drug screening and the family physician. Am Fam Physician 1994;49:1441.

Frances R, Miller SI. Clinical textbook of addiction disorders. New York: The Guildford Press, 1991.

Franklin JE. Addiction medicine. JAMA 1995;273:1656.

Fretthold DW. Drug-testing methods and reliability. J Psychoactive Drugs 1990;22:419.

Fuller PG JR, Cavanaugh RM Jr. Basic assessment and screening for substance abuse in the pediatrician's office. Pediatr Clin North Am 1995;42:295.

Godley SH, Godley MD, Pratt A, et al. Case management services for adolescent substance abusers: a program description. J Subst Abuse Treat 1994;11:309.

Hoffmann NG, Mee-Lee D, Arrowood AA. Treatment issues in adolescent substance use and addictions. Adolesc Med State Arts Rev 1993;4:371.

Huberty DJ, Huberty CE, Flanagan-Hobday K, et al. Family issues in working with chemically dependent adolescents. In: Rogers PD, ed. Symposium on Chemical Dependency. Pediatr Clin North Am 1987;34:507.

Jalali B, Jalali M, Crocette G, et al. Adolescents and drug use: toward a more comprehensive approach. Am J Orthopsychiatry 1981;51:120.

Johnson RL. Drug abuse. Pediatr Rev 1995;16:197.

Kaminer Y, Adolescent substance abuse: a comprehensive guide to theory and practice. New York: Plenum Medical, 1994.

Kandel DB, Davies M, Karus D, et al. The consequences in young adulthood of adolescent drug involvement: an overview. Arch Gen Psychiatry 1986;43:746.

Klitzner M, Fisher D, Stewart K, et al. Substance abuse: early intervention for adolescents. Princeton, New Jersey: Pacific Institute for Research and Evaluation, Robert Wood Johnson Foundation, 1993.

Kulberg A. Substance abuse: clinical identification and management. Pediatr Clin North Am 1986;33:325.

Kulig K. Initial management of ingestions of toxic substances. N Engl J Med 1992;326:1677.

Lange WR, White N, Robinson N. Medical complications of substance abuse. Postgrad Med 1992;92:205.

Leccese M, Waldron HB. Assessing adolescent substance use: a critique of current measurement instruments. J Subst Abuse Treat 1994;11:553.

Long WA Jr, Brown RC, Jenkins RR, et al. The role of the pediatrician in substance abuse counseling. Pediatrics 1983;72:251.

Lowinson JH, Ruiz P, Millman RB, Langroid JG, eds. Substance abuse: a comprehensive textbook. Baltimore: Williams & Wilkins, 1992.

MacKenzie R, Cheng M, Haftel A. The clinical utility and evaluation of drug screening techniques. Pediatr Clin North Am 1987;34:423.

MacKenzie RG, Jacobs R. Recognizing the adolescent drug abuse. Primary Care 1987;14:225.

McLellan AT, Arndt IO, Metzger DS. The effects of psychosocial services in substance abuse treatment. JAMA 1993;269:1953.

Morrison MA. Addiction in adolescents. West J Med: Addiction Medicine (Special Issue) 1990;152:543.

Muramoto ML, Leshan L. Adolescent substance abuse: recognition and early intervention. Primary Care 1993;20:141.

Newcomb M.D, Bentler PM. Frequency and sequence of drug use: a longitudinal study from early adolescence to young adulthood. J Drug Educ 1986;16:101.

Nowinski J. Substance abuse in adolescents and young adults: a guide to treatment. New York: Norton, 1990.

Petraitis J, Flay BR, Miller TQ. Reviewing theories of adolescent substance use: organizing pieces in the puzzle. Psychol Bull 1995;117:67.

Rahdert ER, ed. The Problem-Oriented Screening Instrument for Teenagers. (Publication No. ADM 91-1735.) Washington, D.C.: Alcohol, Drug Abuse, and Mental Health Administration, U.S. Department of Health and Human Services, 1991.

Reuter P, Caulkins JP. Redefining the goals of national drug policy: recommendations from a working group. Am J Public Health 1995;85:1059.

Riggin OZ. Adolescent substance abuse: prevalence, assessment, prevention, and treatment. Nurse Pract Forum 1993;4:207.

Rogers PD, Speraw SR, Ozbek I. Assessment of the identified substance-abusing adolescent. Pediatr Clin North Am 1995;42:351.

Sanders JM Jr. Adolescents and substance abuse. Pediatrics 1985;76:630.

Sanders JM Jr. Identifying substance abuse in adolescents. Postgrad Med 1988;84:123.

Saxon AJ, Calsyn DA, Hauer VM, et al. Clinical evaluation and use of urine screening for drug abuse. West J Med 1988;149:296.

Schwartz JG, Zollars PR, Okorodudu AO, et al. Accuracy of common drug screen tests. Am J Emerg Med 1991;9:166.

Schwartz RH. Why drug screening belongs in your practice. Patient Care 1994;April 30:46.

Selzer M. The Michigan Alcoholism Screening Test: the quest for a new diagnostic instrument. Am J Psychiatry 1971;127:1653.

Tennant F. Is your patient abusing drugs? Postgrad Med 1988;84:107.

Valentine JL, Komoroski EM. Use of a visual panel detection method for drugs of abuse: clinical and laboratory experience with children and adolescents. J Pediatr 1995;126:135.

Werner MJ. Principles of brief intervention for adolescent alcohol, tobacco, and other drug use. Pediatr Clin North Am 1995;42:335.

Westreich LM, Rosenthal RN. Physical examination of substance abusers. Postgrad Med 1995;97:111.

Wheeler K, Malmquist J. Treatment approaches in adolescent chemical dependency. In: Rogers PD, ed. Symposium on Chemical Dependency. Pediatr Clin North Am 1987;34:437.

Woolf AD, Shannon MW. Clinical toxicology for the pediatrician. Pediatr Clin North Am 1995;42:317.

Zaret D, Hawkins DJ, Rogers PD. Risk factors for adolescent substance abuse: implications for pediatric practice. In: Rogers PD, ed. Symposium on Chemical Dependency. Pediatr Clin North Am 1987;34:481.

Psychosocial Problems and Concerns

CHAPTER 76

Common Concerns of Adolescents and Their Parents

Lawrence S. Neinstein, Maria A. Juliani, and Joan Shapiro

During the adolescent years, teenagers and their families face a myriad of issues and concerns. As stated earlier in this book, what seems important to the adolescent may not seem important to his or her parents, and vice versa. Often, the issues that concern adolescents are resolved by the teens themselves or with the help of friends or family and are never brought to the physician's attention. In cases where the physician is involved, he or she may be asked to answer questions such as, Am I normal? Is my teen normal? or, What can I do about this problem? Occasionally, the issue becomes severe enough to create family disruption. And in the extreme, issues or problems may lead to truancy, juvenile delinquency, substance abuse, or suicide.

Just what is normal adolescent behavior? Chapter 2 dealt with many aspects of normal psychosocial development in the adolescent. This chapter emphasizes common psychosocial concerns to which parents and physicians should be especially sensitive. Unfortunately, there are no clear-cut answers to what is normal. It is important for physicians to remember their own adolescence but not necessary to rely purely on their own experiences to determine what is expected adolescent behavior. In assessing issues that trouble adolescents or their families the health-care provider must consider:

1. The severity of the problem: Is this behavior usual for the adolescent or is there a marked change?
2. The chronicity of the problem: Has the problem been present for days or for months or years?
3. The adolescent's development in regard to independence, body image, peers, school, and identity: Is the behavior consistent with the developmental stage of the adolescent?
4. Daily functioning: Are the problems severe enough to interfere with the daily functioning of the adolescent in areas such as school and social activities?

Any concern of an adolescent or parent deserves assessment. While some topics such as daydreaming or pubertal gynecomastia can be handled by discussion and reassurance, other issues such as family conflicts, psychosomatic illnesses, or depression may require several or more sessions with the adolescent and family. When the problem involves severe or chronic disorders or violent behavior, referral is usually indicated. Indications in considering a referral include:

1. Suicidal behavior
2. Substance abuse
3. Psychotic or other severe psychiatric symptoms
4. Developmental delay or learning disabilities
5. Behavioral problems that have been present since childhood

TABLE 76.1. Common Adolescent Behavior, Trouble Sign, or Problem Behavior

Not a Significant Concern	Trouble Sign	Problem Behavior
One or two minor nonviolent violations of the law or school regulations	Repeated violation of the law or school regulations	Any violent act or crime
Sexual activity in the context of a loving relationship	Sexual provocativeness	Sexual promiscuity
Leaving home for a day and in particular running away to a familiar home once	Running away more than once in 3 months	Running away to the streets
Skipping school or missing a class once	Skipping school more than once in 3 months	Chronic absenteeism from school
Occasional experimentation with alcohol or drugs	Regular use of drugs and alcohol	Addiction to drugs or drug dealing
Occasional arguing with parents and other adults	Aggressive outbursts	Oppositionalism leading to violence at home or suspension from school

Adapted from Steinberg L, Levine A. You and your adolescent: a parent's guide for ages 10–20. New York: Harper & Row, 1990.

6. Problems that have persisted despite extensive interventions by the primary caregiver
7. Problems felt to be beyond the skills of the practitioner
8. Adolescents with a problem but practitioner is unsure what it is (i.e., the adolescent with no friends who is socially withdrawn)
9. Severe stress in the family such as death, divorce, or suicide of parent or sibling
10. School behavior and performance that has changed dramatically
11. Runaway behavior
12. Frequent fights

Types of behaviors that may indicate common adolescent behavior, a trouble sign, or a problem behavior are shown in Table 76.1.

REFERRALS

When the practitioner decides that a referral is necessary, several considerations are important:

1. Motivation: Are the teen and parent(s) motivated to attend counseling sessions? Without such motivation, compliance is extremely poor.
2. Do the teen and family understand the reason for the referral?
3. Is the referral appropriate for the problem? Many options exist for referrals for psychosocial problems, including psychologists, psychiatrists, vocational counselors, youth programs (Big Brothers/Big Sisters, YMCA), and residential or vocational programs such as the Job Corps.

Several interventions may help in making the referral:

1. The practitioner should reassure the adolescent that the primary health-care practitioner will continue to follow the adolescent and will be very much involved in his or her care.
2. The practitioner should explain that as part of the total evaluation and treatment of the adolescent's problem, a psychological or psychiatric evaluation is important. If, despite a negative medical evaluation, the teen or family feels strongly that the problem is organic, the practitioner can still explain that the psychological evaluation is important in the diagnostic workup. The teen and family should also be advised that even if the problem turns out to be organic, the counseling could still help the teen cope better with the symptoms.
3. The practitioner should explain his or her concerns to the adolescent and family. As part of this explanation, the health-care practitioner could ask the teen whether he or she thinks that things could be going better. If the teen answers yes, the practitioner can state that counseling is one way to help make things go better.

4. The practitioner should reassure the adolescent that the counseling will usually be arranged for a limited time and that if counseling does not work out the teen or family can stop.
5. The adolescent should be aware that seeing a psychologist or psychiatrist does not mean that the teen is crazy. Counseling should be explained as an opportunity to make the adolescent feel better and to enhance family or interpersonal relations.
6. It is necessary for the physician and the parents to distinguish the adolescent from his or her behavior. While we may find the adolescent's behavior negative or unhealthy, we must convey acceptance of the adolescent himself or herself.

CONCERNS OF TEENAGERS

Common concerns of teenagers include:

1. Parental conflicts: Rules (curfew, driving), privacy, expectations, and peer relationships
2. Sibling conflicts
3. School: Popularity, academic pressures, teachers, and adjustment to a new school
4. Peers: Dating concerns regarding relationships and sexuality
5. Identity: Who am I? Concerns surrounding body image, loneliness, and shyness
6. Medical concerns: Menstrual disorders, short stature, acne, weight disorders, and pubertal gynecomastia
7. Psychosomatic problems: Headaches, stomach pains, and insomnia
8. Situational anxiety
9. Mild depression
10. Safety concerns: Violence in the environment, community, home, school
11. Prospects for the future: Economic realities, pregnancy, and particularly human immunodeficiency virus (HIV).

CONCERNS OF PARENTS

Common concerns of parents with regard to their teenage son or daughter include:

1. Adolescent rebellion: Mild rebellion is common in early and middle adolescence. Marked rebellion, however, may be an indication of family dysfunction.
2. Wasting time by the adolescent, especially daydreaming: Parents should be reassured that this is usually a normal part of adolescent development.
3. Risk-taking behavior: Risk taking is a common part of the early and middle adolescent process. Life-threatening, risk-taking behavior requires family sessions for the purposes of educating and limit setting and evaluation of any associated unmet needs of the adolescent.
4. Mood swings: Assessment of the severity, including detailed description of the moods and changes, is required.
5. Drug experimentation: Evaluation of the type and degree of drug use is required.
6. School problems: Evaluation of the type and severity of the problem is required.
7. Psychosomatic problems: Medical evaluation that explores the source of any stress is required.
8. Sexual activity: Definition of the parents' concern is required. The need for confidentiality between teen and practitioner should be explained to the parents, but discussion between teen and parent should be encouraged.
9. Eating disorders
10. Safety issues, violence in the environment, driving safety (e.g., teen or other motorists driving under the influence)

CHAPTER 77

High-Risk and Out-of-Control Behavior

Lawrence S. Neinstein and Richard MacKenzie

Changes in society over the past 25–30 years have significantly influenced the adolescent years. The educational experience has been prolonged and the job market reduced. Adaptation to intrinsic psychological developmental triggers must be made in an environment of increasing drug use, sexual activity, media stimulation, and weakened family structure. Attempts by adolescents to cope with these pressures often result in social behaviors that are associated with inherent but inconstant degrees of risk to health. The consequences of this health risk may be immediate or long-range. Consider the following. In the United States it is estimated that:

- Every 31 seconds a teenager becomes pregnant.
- Every 1–2 minutes a teen gives birth.
- Every 78 seconds a teen attempts suicide.
- Every 20 minutes a teen is killed in a car accident.
- Every 90 minutes a teen is murdered and another commits suicide.

The major causes of death and disability among the approximately 40 million American youth have essentially social and behavioral issues at their root. This chapter focuses on risk-taking behavior among adolescents in general, as well as on specific out-of-control, high-risk activities.

EPIDEMIOLOGY OF RISK-TAKING BEHAVIOR

Mortality

Motor vehicle accidents, suicide, and homicide comprise the three chief causes of death among adolescents (see Chapter 5). Many of these events are drug or alcohol related. Not included in mortality figures is the subsequent disability associated with these leading causes of mortality.

Morbidity

It is estimated that 20% of U.S. teenagers have great difficulty making the transition from childhood to adulthood and that this difficulty is often reflected in their risk behaviors. The frequency of these morbidities correlates with the teen's biobehavioral risk profile. The latter is directly dependent on the frequency and number of risky behaviors that the teenager uses to resolve psychological and social developmental needs. Frequent subsequent problems include:

1. Pregnancy: In the United States more than 1 million teens become pregnant each year (Hayes, 1987), with approximately 450,000 giving birth. Teenage pregnancies, often due to the lack of regular prenatal care, are associated with a high rate of complications. Factors increasing pregnancy and parenting risks include poverty, poor intellect, low motivation and expectations, lower status employment and wages, reliance on public assistance, inadequate literacy and work skills, substance or emotional or sexual abuse, difficulty obtaining child care, and increased number of children. Fifty-one percent of adolescents use no contraception during first intercourse, and 20% of adolescent pregnancies occur within 1 month of first intercourse.

2. Sexual activity: About 43% of adolescents between 14 and 17 have been sexually active and about 82% of 18- to 21-year-old adolescents and young adults surveyed in the 1992 Youth Risk Survey (CDC, 1994) have had sexual intercourse. Sexually transmitted diseases (STDs) are epidemic in this age group, with adolescents having the highest prevalence of any age group nationally, if prevalence is expressed only for those who are sexually active.

3. Substance abuse: Estimates for problem alcohol use in senior high school students run as high as 30%. About 1 in 30 high school seniors drinks alcohol daily, and when surveyed, 29.8% had five or more drinks in a row at least once in the previous 2 weeks. In 1994 it was estimated that more than 48% of American youth tried an illicit drug before they finished high school. Nearly one-third of adolescents by 12th grade have illicitly used drugs other than marijuana. A rise in illicit drug use, particularly marijuana, occurred starting in about 1992 in eighth-graders and 1993 in older students.

4. Runaway behavior: Over 1 million teens run away each year (Deisher and Farrow, 1986), with an estimated 10–25% of these becoming long-term street youth. These youth usually survive through criminal activity such as prostitution, burglary, or drug dealing.

5. Suicide: Since 1950 suicide rates have increased four to five times for male adolescents and doubled for female adolescents. Between 1980 and 1992 the rate of suicides declined among persons under age 25 years from 5.7 per 100,000 persons to 5.4. For persons aged 20–24 the suicide rate declined 7.2% (16.1 to 14.9). However, the rate increased among persons aged 15–19 years by 28.3% (8.5 to 10.9) and among persons aged 10–14 years by 120% (0.8 to 1.7). For African-American males ages 15–19 the rate increased by 165.3%.

   Twenty-five percent of males and 42% of females report that they have seriously considered committing suicide at some time in their life (Centers for Disease Control, 1989). Lifetime prevalence of suicide attempts in older adolescents is approximately 7%. Rates are significantly higher for females (10%) versus males (3.8%).

6. School dropout: The dropout rate for high school students is approximately 25%, with rates as high as 50–80% in some inner cities (Scales, 1988).

7. Crime: In the 1992 Health Risk Behaviors Survey among persons aged 12–21 years (Centers for Disease Control, 1994), the following was found:

Behavior	*12–13 yr*	*14–17 yr*	*18–21 yr*	*Total*
Participated in a physical fight	49.0	43.8	29.4	38.8
Carried a weapon	12.6	17.1	13.6	14.8

In the National Adolescent Student Health Survey (NASHS) study (Centers for Disease Control, 1989), 49% of boys and 28% of girls reported having been in at least one physical fight in the past year; 34% reported being threatened, and 14% robbed. Age-specific arrest rates for burglary, robbery, and aggravated assault peak between 17 and 21 years of age.

Factors Involved in Risk-Taking Behavior

Childhood and adolescence are continuous events in the life cycle. The manner in which the developmental challenges of adolescence are expressed is dependent on, if not largely determined by, personality traits and other characteristics established in childhood. The physical, psychological, and social maturational forces of development combine to determine behavior at any moment. During adolescence these behaviors may be perceived by those close to the teenagers as a problem, since they may constitute a health risk. Viewed developmentally, however, these behaviors serve a purpose (i.e., that of a developmental task accomplishment). Often the adolescent does not perceive risk-taking behavior as a problem but, rather, as a solution. This paradox helps explain the behavior and also the difficulty of managing youth who engage in high-risk behaviors.

General characteristics about risk-taking behaviors in adolescents include:

1. Many behaviors that affect health, both positively and negatively, throughout an individual's life, are first tried out during the teenage years (e.g., cigarette smoking, sexual activity, exercise and physical conditioning, dietary changes, and study habits).
2. The risk that any behavior has to health may be immediate (e.g., drinking and driving), delayed (e.g., pregnancy and education), or remote (e.g., smoking and lung cancer). The more immediate the consequence of behavior to health, the greater the likelihood of effecting change through intervention.
3. Consequences of risk behaviors may be universal and invariant (risk from crack), related to specific factors (environment, gender, and situations), or related to intensity of involvement (dieting and anorexia nervosa).
4. Factors that influence health-related behaviors are usually acquired or consolidated during adolescence (e.g., values, beliefs, attitudes, motivations, self-concept, and general lifestyle).
5. Problem behaviors that contribute to risk tend to occur in combinations or clusters (e.g., smoking, drinking, interpersonal violence, suicidal ideation, school dropout, family discord, and drug use).
6. Risk at any developmental period reflects the number of risk factors present during that period and the cumulative effects of risk factors occurring early in life. The effect may not only be cumulative but may be compounded and lead to other risk behaviors (e.g., the effect of long-term alcohol or drug use on driving or suicidal ideation). High-risk adolescents usually have multiple social and psychological handicaps, which amplifies the severity of reaction and limits the options for problem solving and task accomplishment.

Biopsychosocial Factors

Many factors have been suggested as contributing to the problem behaviors among youth in the United States. Although biological maturational forces have remained relatively constant, pubertal timing and social environment have changed. This has put increased pressure on the individual for adaptation. These factors include:

1. *Menarche occurs earlier, marriage has been delayed, and values have changed regarding premarital sexual intercourse.* Incongruence between biological development and psychoemotional preparedness enhances the potential for high-risk behaviors or personal stressful responses.
2. The U.S. population has become more *urbanized*, with lack of purposeful work for youth.
3. The American family has *increased mobility*, with a subsequent need for teens to re-establish social relations at a time when social skills are often poorly developed.

4. *Breakdown of the family* includes a proliferation of single parents and working parents, lack of an extended family, and the interposition of the media as an arbiter of family values.

5. The foundation of the adolescent experience, *the educational process, has become more prolonged* to prepare the individual for a high-tech society. This has resulted in an increased risk for mainstream adolescents to drop out.

6. A shift has occurred in *how society views its young,* from being an economic asset to being an economic liability.

7. Western cultures tend to expose rather than protect adolescents from *environmental influences* (e.g., drugs and alcohol; automobiles; violent behaviors).

8. *Change occurs rapidly* during adolescence, and pressures for adaptation are great.

Certain youth are predisposed to having difficulty with the transition from childhood to adulthood. This group includes:

1. Youth reared in a context of poverty
2. Youth with a chronic illness
3. Youth who have been physically, sexually, or emotionally abused as children
4. Youth living with extreme family pathology, parental mental illness, or substance abuse
5. Youth with educational handicaps
6. Youth with a gay or lesbian sexual orientation

In summary, high-risk and out-of-control behaviors require prompt evaluation and attention. They encompass a wide spectrum of behaviors, including runaway behavior, truancy, theft, vandalism, substance abuse, sexual promiscuity, and suicide. Loss of parental control must be assessed along with what has been tried to regain control. The practitioner must evaluate what are the greatest influences on the teen's present behavior and how those influences are related to developmental needs. Underlying issues often involve autonomy, low self-esteem, frustration, or depression.

ADOLESCENT DEPRESSION

An often unrecognized common characteristic of the acting-out or out-of-control adolescent is underlying depression. In the NASHS (Centers for Disease Control, 1989), many of the 8th and 10th grade students reported depression and coping difficulties. In fact, 61% reported feeling sad and hopeless, 36% reported having nothing to look forward to, 45% expressed difficulty coping with home and work, and 34% expressed serious thoughts of attempting suicide. The depression may vary from common adolescent mood swings or short-lived situational episodes to chronic recurring feelings of worthlessness, helplessness, and hopelessness.

1. Factors associated with adolescent depression
   a. Decreased self-esteem: The adolescent's perceived sense of self falls short of expectation.
   b. Significant loss
      — Death of or rejection by a loved relative or boyfriend or girlfriend
      — Separation or divorce of parents
      — Loss of boundaries and guidelines within the family
      — Perception of not being normal (e.g., physical illness)
   c. Inability to cope with adolescent developmental tasks
   d. Parental depression or substance abuse
   e. Family conflicts or poor communication
   f. Learning disability
   g. Unrealistic parental expectations
   h. Problems in peer relationships

2. Clinical manifestations: Adolescent depression is characterized by a range of psychological, behavioral, and physiological changes or problems.
   a. Psychological
      — Lowered self-esteem and self-concept
      — Hopelessness, with negative views of the future
      — Helplessness, with negative views of the world and of the adolescent's relationship to it: The slightest challenge may be overwhelming for the depressed adolescent.
      — Dysphoria: A state of general dissatisfaction or unhappiness
      — Feelings of inappropriate guilt or worthlessness
      — Pessimism
      — Excessive self-criticism
   b. Behavioral
      — Changes in academic performance
      — Acting-out behavior, including truancy, runaway behavior, sexual promiscuity, and theft
      — Substance abuse
      — Social isolation
      — Decreased motivation
      — Loss of interest in usual activities
      — Taking unnecessary risks
      — Suicidal gestures
   c. Physiological
      — Fatigue and poor energy
      — Insomnia, especially sleep induction problems
      — Changes in eating patterns, especially anorexia
      — Weight loss or weight gain
      — Menstrual irregularities
      — Headaches and abdominal pain
3. Types of depression: Depression can occur as a primary disorder, as part of an organic disease, or in response to an adverse situation. Major types of depression during adolescence as defined in *Diagnostic and Statistical Manual of Mental Disorders* (DSM-IV; American Psychiatric Association, 1994) include:
   a. Major depressive episode
      — At least five of the following symptoms are present for a 2-week period and represent a change from previous functioning. At least one of the symptoms is either depressed mood or loss of interest or of pleasure.
        (1) Depressed or irritable mood most of the day, nearly every day
        (2) Markedly diminished interest or pleasure in all or most activities of the day nearly every day
        (3) Significant weight loss or weight gain when not dieting or decrease or increase in appetite
        (4) Insomnia or hypersomnia nearly every day
        (5) Psychomotor agitation or retardation nearly every day
        (6) Fatigue or loss of energy nearly every day
        (7) Feelings of worthlessness or excessive or inappropriate guilt nearly every day
        (8) Diminished ability to think or concentrate nearly every day
        (9) Recurrent thoughts of death, suicidal ideation, or suicide attempt
      — The depression is not related to an organic factor, nor is it a normal reaction to a death.

— There is no evidence of delusions or hallucinations, schizophrenia, schizophreniform disorder, psychotic disorder, or delusional disorder.

— No history of a manic episode exists.

b. Bipolar disorder, depressed: The individual is having a major depressive episode as just defined, with the exception that the adolescent has previously had one or more manic episodes.

c. Dysthymic disorder: This is mainly a chronic disturbance of mood, involving primarily a depressed or irritable mood for most days for at least 1 year (in adolescents). Dysthymia differs from major depression in that the former is usually associated with milder symptoms for a longer period of time. A major depression is usually associated with discrete episodes of more severe depression that can be distinguished from the person's usual functioning. Criteria of dysthymia in adolescents include:

— Depressed or irritable mood for most of the day, for most days, for at least 1 year

— Presence, while depressed, of at least two of the following symptoms:

(1) Poor appetite or overeating

(2) Insomnia or hypersomnia

(3) Fatigue

(4) Low self-esteem

(5) Poor concentration

(6) Feelings of helplessness

— Never without a depressed or irritable mood for more than 2 months in a 1-year period

— No evidence of a major depressive episode during the 1 year

— Never has had a manic episode

— No evidence of a chronic psychotic disorder

— No evidence of an organic factor involved

d. Adjustment disorder with depressed mood

— A depressive reaction to an identifiable psychosocial stressor(s) occurs within 3 months of onset of the stressor(s).

— Reaction includes either:

(1) Impairment in occupational or school functioning or in usual social activities; OR

(2) Symptoms are in excess of normal and expectable reaction to the stressor(s).

— The reaction has lasted over 6 months.

— The reaction is not just one instance of a pattern of overreaction to stress.

— The reaction does not meet the criteria for any specific mental disorder, including uncomplicated bereavement.

e. Organic affective syndrome, depressed

— Prominent and persistent depressed mood

— Evidence from history, physical examination, or laboratory tests of a specific etiologic factor, including endocrine disorders such as hyperthyroidism and hypothyroidism; pheochromocytoma and hypercortisolism; hallucinogens; brain tumors; and collagen vascular diseases

f. Uncomplicated bereavement: Depression is secondary to stressful loss. Although poor appetite, weight loss, and insomnia are common, feelings of worthlessness, low self-esteem, and marked psychomotor retardation are uncommon. The reaction usually starts within the first 2 or 3 months of the death and may last as long as a year.

4. Comparison of adult and adolescent depression

a. Similarities in the depression of adults and adolescents include similar mood changes and feelings of hopelessness and worthlessness.

b. Differences include:
   — Depressed adolescents often look less depressed and appear more angry or rebellious.
   — Acting-out behaviors, including suicide attempts, are more common among adolescents.
   — Adult depression often meets with sympathy from friends and relatives, while depressed adolescents who act out are greeted by anger.

INCARCERATED YOUTH OR JUVENILE DELINQUENCY

Definition

A juvenile delinquent is a person less than 17 years old who commits any criminal offense as defined by state or local laws. These individuals are subject to the regulations of the juvenile or family court, with a goal of rehabilitation and not punishment. Many states have excluded offenses such as murder and assault with a deadly weapon. These fall under the jurisdiction of the adult criminal court. A "status offender" is a juvenile younger than 17 who is regularly disobedient to his or her parents or guardians and is beyond their disciplinary control or has run away from home or is unlawfully absent from school. The offense that was committed is not illegal if carried out by an adult. Examples include truancy, runaway behavior, and curfew violation. These adolescents are often referred to as *persons, children, juveniles,* or *minors in need of supervision* (PINS, CHINS, JINS, or MINS, respectively). In some states, juvenile delinquents and status offenders are still grouped together. Increasingly, states and local agencies are separating these two groups; however, an effective system to deal with status offenders is lacking in most areas. Many of these young people are referred to mental health or social service agencies by the court. A "youthful offender" is an individual 17–21 years of age who commits an illegal act. These individuals are tried in the criminal court system but are usually separated from adults while serving their sentence.

Youth may become incarcerated for numerous reasons including illegal activity, status offenses, or the need for protection and guardianship. The placement of many of these youth, particularly in adult facilities, places them at risk of abuse and the risk of coming in contact with other criminals.

Epidemiology

1. Prevalence: Each year, more than 590,000 children are incarcerated in public and private juvenile facilities including jails, detention centers, camps, and ranches. Another 90,000 are placed in adult jails each year. According to the U.S. Department of Justice, about one-third of all reported arrests for major crimes are youth under the age of 18, with about 58% being under the age of 21. Almost 13% of arrests for major crimes are of individuals under the age of 15. The most frequent crimes include theft, motor vehicle theft, burglaries, robberies, and aggravated assaults. Over the past 25 years the number of arrests for juvenile crime has increased approximately sixfold, with a marked increase in violent crime. However, in the 1980s, there was a decrease in juvenile arrest rates.
2. Characteristics
   a. Sex: Males account for 78% of juvenile arrests and 92% of juvenile arrests for violent crimes. Females are more likely to be arrested for prostitution or running away. During the 1950s most of the attention on juvenile delinquency concen-

trated on males. Recently, however, the incidence of female delinquency has escalated. Over the past 10 years the rate of arrest of females has increased six times more than that of males. While female delinquency in the 1950s and 1960s centered mainly on sexual misconduct, today, more females are involved in armed robbery, gang activity, drug trafficking, burglary, weapons possession, aggravated assault, and prostitution.

b. Race: Minorities account for 31% of juvenile arrests. Minorities, especially African-Americans, are disproportionately both the victims and perpetrators of crime in the United States. The arrest rate leading to incarceration is increasing rapidly among Hispanic youth. Minorities account for 58% of juvenile arrests for violent crimes.

c. Age: Peak age for juvenile arrests is 15–16 years of age, while 18 years is the peak age for violent crimes (homicide, rape, and assault).

d. Medical precursors
— XYY syndrome
— Klinefelter's syndrome
— Frontal or temporal lobe epilepsy
— Learning disability or attention deficit disorder

e. Social and environmental determinants
— Low socioeconomic status
— Lack of employment
— Sense of failure and low self-esteem
— Family conflicts
— School difficulties
— Peer-group involvement with delinquent adolescents
— Disorganization within the environment
— Lack of sense of belonging
— Lack of appropriate role models
— Family history of alcoholism, criminal behavior, or psychiatric conditions
— History of physical or sexual abuse

f. Seriously delinquent adolescents: Those youth with a higher prevalence of more violent or sexually assaultive behavior have a higher prevalence of violent behavior in childhood, a history of perinatal trauma, and more frequent head and facial trauma. Psychopathology, mostly characterized as conduct disorder, is common.

g. Incarcerated delinquents: Such individuals are reported to have had a higher prevalence of perinatal difficulties, child abuse, and history of severe head or face injury. Major depression and suicide attempts are common in this group.

h. Recurrence: A subgroup of adolescents accounts for the majority of juvenile crime. In one study, 54% of juvenile delinquents were repeaters and accounted for 85% of crimes committed, while a subgroup of 6.3% committed 52% of the crimes (Wolfgang et al., 1972).

Legal Rights

1. Judicial rights: Adolescents are generally processed through a civil proceeding, without a jury trial. However, they have the right to legal counsel, the right to notice of charges, the right to remain silent, the right to confrontation with the accuser, and the right to proof of guilt beyond a reasonable doubt.

2. Treatment rights: Many laws have been enacted in the past 15 years regarding areas of care for juvenile delinquents. These laws have covered specific issues such as staffing requirements and guidelines for the use of psychiatric medication.

Health Problems

A comprehensive review of health and medical issues of institutional youth is beyond the scope of this book. However, the health-care provider should keep in mind that approximately 1 million adolescents live away from home and that about one-half of these are in institutions for juvenile offenders. Forty percent to 80% of these adolescents have medical problems that include:

1. Problems inherent to adolescents living in poverty
   a. Unmet nutritional needs
   b. Problems common to adolescents in general, including acne, scoliosis, weight control problems, minor trauma, short stature, and gynecological problems
   c. Pre-existing conditions that have been undetected due to poor access to medical care: Hernias, undescended testes, and congenital heart disease
2. Problems related to delinquent behaviors and lifestyle
   a. Injuries: Four to eight times more common
   b. Substance abuse
   c. STDs and pregnancy
3. Health problems associated with delinquency (e.g., learning disabilities and attention deficit disorders): Some researchers postulate a subpopulation of adolescents in whom learning disabilities precede the onset of delinquency and who undergo a downward spiral of school failure, frustration, anger, and more failure, leading to lowered self-esteem, truancy, and social isolation.
4. Health problems attributable to the social and physical environment
   a. Suicide
   b. Institutional violence
   c. Depression

Morris et al. (1995) reviewed the health risk behaviors of youth in juvenile correctional facilities. They found that risky behavior began early with initiation plateauing at age 15 or 16. Male and female youth reported comparable rates of drinking, binge drinking, and illicit drug use. North American Natives began drinking at earlier ages, had more binge drinking, more illegal drug use, and the most fight-related behavior. By age 12, 62% reported a history of sexual intercourse, and by age 14 89% were sexually active. The onset of sexual intercourse was at an average age of 12. Fighting was common, with 25% reporting fight-related injuries in the past year. Almost one-half of the group were in a gang. Suicide had been contemplated by 22%. STDs were common, and less than half of the group used a condom at last intercourse.

Incarcerated youth should have a health screening as part of the intake procedures. In addition, short-term care facilities should be available.

RUNAWAY BEHAVIOR

Definition

Runaway behavior is defined as an unauthorized absence from home.

Epidemiology

1. Incidence: Approximately 500,000 to 1 million adolescents run away each year (Carper, 1979).
2. Age: Mean age is 15 years, with almost all runaways between the ages of 14 years old and 17 years old (Carper, 1979).

3. Race: A majority of runaways are white suburban adolescents (Carper, 1979).
4. Length of time away from home
   a. Less than 3 days: 72%
   b. Four to 14 days: 15%
   c. More than 14 days: 13%
5. Return behavior
   a. Return home on their own: 50%
   b. Return home through parental or peer involvement: 30%
   c. Return home through police intervention: 14%
   d. Never return home: 6%

Types of Runaways

1. Abortive: No actual runaway behavior; just a fantasy
2. Crisis: A short stay away from home secondary to an acute problem
3. Casual: The streetwise adolescent with frequent runaway episodes

Reasons for Running Away

Many reasons exist for runaway behavior, including lack of communication between parents and the adolescent, school failure, overly strict or overly permissive parents, experimentation, escape from a hopeless situation, being thrown out of the house, and the simultaneous crises of adolescence, parental middle-age crisis, and elderly grandparents. Other reasons include depression, revenge, and imitation of peers. Not infrequently, incestuous family incidents and other episodes of physical or sexual abuse are the precipitants for running away.

For those adolescents who become homeless, the situation is aggravated by decreased access to food, shelter, medical services, social supports, and so forth. A common characteristic of homeless youth is a lack of a mainstream social network. They often therefore create their own social network within their environment.

Runaway or homeless youth are at increased risk for many health problems including STDs, suicidal ideation, substance abuse, and human immunodeficiency virus (HIV) infection. Allen et al. (1994) reported HIV prevalence rates among homeless youth of 0–7.3% (median, 2.3%). Rotheram-Borus (1993) reported a rate of suicide attempts in runaway youth of 37%, with 44% of the attempters having made an attempt within the previous month. Females were significantly more likely than males to have attempted suicide and to be depressed. Runaways with histories of attempting suicide were significantly more likely to be currently suicidal and depressed.

SUICIDE

(See Chapter 79.)

SUBSTANCE ABUSE

(See Chapters 69–75.)

INTERVENTIONS

For the primary care physician, the contact point with youth engaging in high-risk behavior is often the presentation of a medical problem. However, rather than merely treating the medical problem, the physician who desires to intervene effectively with youth with high-risk behaviors must explore further. A brief psychosocial or lifestyle interview must be conducted prior to or during the medical examination. One such method is the HEADSS Adolescent Risk Profile (home, education, activities, drugs, sex [activity, orientation, and sexual abuse], and Suicide) discussed in Chapter 3. The HEADSS evaluation not only assesses risk but also provides an opportunity to educate the adolescent with regard to health-compromising behaviors or practices. The assessment should include:

1. Medical evaluation
2. Psychosocial evaluation (HEADSS)
3. Family assessment
4. Vocational assessment
5. School assessment

Important considerations include:

1. High-risk youth with multiple problems are best dealt with by a multidisciplinary team, functioning in an interdisciplinary manner. Without allied health professionals the physician must have a comprehensive listing of local resources. Effective referral, particularly with high-risk youth, is best accomplished through a telephone call to a specific contact person, who should be identified while the adolescent is still in the office.
2. Basic needs such as food, shelter, and safety must be addressed before considering major psychotherapeutic interventions.
3. Every effort should be made to draw on the adolescent's own resources or options for change (i.e., to find alternate solutions). Interventions must be both feasible and practical (i.e., within the realm of possibility for that particular teen and capable of serving the appropriate developmental function).
4. Family involvement, when indicated, may optimize the intervention strategy, but if such intervention is not done skillfully, the adolescent's problems may simply be compounded. The ability to educate a family for change is inversely proportional to the degree of dysfunction.
5. Risk profiles may be modified by direct or indirect interventions. An example of a direct intervention would be a stop-smoking education program, while an indirect method would be increasing a health-enhancing behavior, such as jogging or running to discourage smoking.
6. Characteristics of health professionals that enhance their ability as vehicles for change include:
   a. Ability to develop trust through establishment of a confidential relationship
   b. Willingness to see the youth's viewpoints as real
   c. Ability to listen
   d. Unconditional positive regard for the adolescent in his or her struggle
   e. Knowledge of self
7. The opportunity to change a system (individual or family) is greatest when the system is unbalanced or in transition. Staff availability during a crisis may be more effective than traditionally scheduled counseling or psychotherapy.

BIBLIOGRAPHY

Adams GR, Gullotta T, Clancy MA. Homeless adolescents: a descriptive study of similarities and differences between runaways and throwaways. Adolescence 1985;21:715.

Adams PF, Schoenborn CA, Moss AJ, et al. Health-risk behaviors among our nation's youth: United States, 1992. Vital Health Stat 10 1995;192:1.

Allen DM, Lehman JS, Green TA, et al. HIV infection among homeless adults and runaway youth, United States, 1989–1992. Field Services Branch. AIDS 1994; 8:1593.

Andrews JA, Lewinsohn PM. Suicidal attempts among older adolescents: prevalence and co-occurrence with psychiatric disorders. J Am Acad Child Adolesc Psychiatry 1992;31:655-662.

American Psychiatric Association. Diagnostic and statistical manual of mental disorders, 4th revised ed. Washington DC: American Psychiatric Association, 1994.

Angold A. Childhood and adolescent depression. I. Epidemiological and etiological aspects. Br J Psychiatry 1988;152:601.

Barnum R. Clinical evaluation of juvenile delinquents facing transfer to adult court. J Am Acad Child Adolesc Psychiatry 1987;26:922.

Beeferman D, Orvaschel H. Group psychotherapy for depressed adolescents: a critical review. Int J Group Psychother 1994;44:463.

Bewley B. The epidemiology of adolescent behavior problems. Br Med Bull 1986;42:200.

Brage DG. Adolescent depression: a review of the literature. Arch Psychiatr Nurs 1995;9:45.

Brent DA, Kolko DJ, Wartells ME, et al. Adolescent psychiatric inpatients' risk of suicide attempts at 6 month follow-up. J Am Acad Child Adolesc Psychiatry 1993;32:95–105.

Brickman AS, McManus M, Grapentine WL. Neuropsychological assessment of seriously delinquent adolescents. J Am Acad Child Adolesc Psychiatry 1984; 23:453.

Calhoun G, Jurgens J, Chen F. The neophyte female delinquent: a review of the literature. Adolescence 1993;28:461.

Cappelli M, Clulow MK, Goodman JT, et al. Identifying depressed and suicidal adolescents in a teen health clinic. J Adolesc Health 1995;16:64.

Carlson GA, Cantwell DP. Unmasking masked depression in children and adolescence. Am J Psychiatry 1980;137:445.

Carper JM. Emergencies in adolescents: runaways and father-daughter incest. Pediatr Clin North Am 1979; 26:883.

Caton CL. The homeless experience in adolescent years. New Dir Ment Health Serv 1986;30:63.

Centers for Disease Control. National Adolescent Student Health Survey (NASHS), 1987. MMWR 1989; 38:147.

Centers for Disease Control. Health risk behaviors among persons age 12–21 years—United States, 1992. MMWR 1994;43:231.

Compas BE, Ey S, Grant KE. Taxonomy, assessment, and diagnosis of depression during adolescence. Psychol Bull 1993;114:323.

Deisher RW, Farrow JA. Recognizing and dealing with alienated youth in clinical practice. Pediatr Ann 1986;15:759.

Donovan JE, Jessor R. Structure of problem behavior in adolescence and young adulthood. J Consult Clin Psychol 1985;53:890.

Englander SW. Some self-reported correlates of runaway behavior in adolescent females. J Consult Clin Psychol 1984;52:484.

Farrow J, ed. Health and health needs of homeless and runaway youth—position paper of the Society for Adolescent Medicine. J Adolesc Health Care 1993; 13:717.

Flowers, Ronald B. The adolescent criminal: an examination of today's juvenile offender. Jefferson, North Carolina: McFarland, 1990.

Friedman SB, Sarles RM. Out of control behavior in adolescents. Pediatr Clin North Am 1980;27:97.

Garland EJ. Adolescent depression. Part 1. Diagnosis. Can Fam Physician 1994a;40:1583.

Garland EJ. Adolescent depression. Part 2. Treatment. Can Fam Physician 1994b;40:1591.

Hamer DL. Adolescents in the juvenile justice system. In: Shearin RB, Wientzen RL, eds. Clinical adolescent medicine. Boston: GK Hall Medical Publishers, 1983.

Hayes CD, ed. Risking the future: adolescent sexuality, pregnancy and child bearing, vol 1. Washington DC: National Academy Press, 1987.

Hofmann AD, Greydanus DE. Adolescent medicine. 2nd ed. Norwalk, Connecticut: Appleton & Lange, 1989.

Hollander HE, Turner FD. Characteristics of incarcerated delinquents: relationship between development disorders, environmental and family factors, and patterns of offense and recidivism. J Am Acad Child Adolesc Psychiatry 1985;24:221.

Hsu LKG, Wisner K, Richey ET. Is juvenile delinquency related to an abnormal EEG? J Am Acad Child Adolesc Psychiatry 1985;24:310.

Irwin CE Jr, Millstein SG. Biopsychosocial correlates of risk-taking behaviors in adolescence: can the physician intervene? J Adolesc Health Care 1986;7(suppl): 82S.

Jessor R. Adolescent development and behavioral health. In: Matarazzo JD, Weiss SM, Herd JA, Miller NE, eds. Behavioral health: a handbook of health enhancement and disease prevention. New York: Wiley, 1984.

Kipke MD, O'Connor S, Palmer RF, MacKenzie RG. Street youth in Los Angeles: profile of a group at high risk for HIV. Arch Pediatr Adolesc Med 1995;149: 513.

Levine MD, Karniski WM, Palfrey JS. A study of risk factor complexes in early adolescent delinquency. Am J Dis Child 1985;139:50.

Lewis DO, Feldman M, Barrengos A. Race, health, and delinquency. J Am Acad Child Psychiatry 1985;24: 161.

Lewis DO, Pincus JH, Lovely R. Biopsychosocial characteristics of matched samples of delinquents and nondelinquents. J Am Acad Child Adolesc Psychiatry 1987;26:744.

Litt IF, Cohen MI. Prisons, adolescents, and the right to quality care: the time is now. Am J Public Health 1974;64:894.

Luger M, Goddard MS. Juvenile delinquency and juvenile justice. In Shen JTY, ed. The clinical practice of adolescent medicine. New York: Appleton-Century-Crofts, 1980.

MacDonald NE, Fisher WA, Wells GA, et al. Canadian street youth: correlates of sexual risk-taking activity. Pediatr Infect Dis J 1994;13:690.

MacKenzie RG. At-risk youth. In: McAnarney ER, Kreipe RE, Orr DP, Comerci GD, eds. Textbook of adolescent medicine. Philadelphia: WB Saunders, 1992.

MacKenzie RG. Considerations in developing a system of health care for adolescents. In: Tonkin RS, ed. Clinical pediatrics—international practice and research. Current issues in the adolescent patient. London: Bailliere Tindall, 1994.

McConville BJ, Bruce RT. Depressive illnesses in children and adolescents: a review of current concepts. Can J Psychiatry 1985;30:119.

McManus M, Alessi NE, Grapentine WL. Psychiatric disturbance in serious delinquents. J Am Acad Child Adolesc Psychiatry 1984;23:602.

McManus M, Brickman A, Alessi NE. Neurological dysfunction in serious delinquents. J Am Acad Child Adolesc Psychiatry 1985;24:481.

Middleman AB, Faulkner AH, Woods ER, et al. High-risk behaviors among high school students in Massachusetts who use anabolic steroids. Pediatrics 1995;96:268.

Moretti MM, Fine S, Haley G. Childhood and adolescent depression: child-report versus parent-report information. J Am Acad Child Adolesc Psychiatry 1985; 24:298.

Morgan IS. Recognizing depression in the adolescent. MCN Am J Matern Child Nurs 1994;19:148.

Morris RE, Harrison EA, Knox GW. Health risk behaviorial survey from 39 juvenile correctional facilities in the United States. J Adolesc Health 1995; 17:334.

Myers K, Troutman B. Developmental aspects of child and adolescent depression. Curr Opin Pediatr 1993; 5:419.

National Research Council. Losing generations: adolescents in high risk settings. Washington DC: National Academy Press, 1993.

Perry CL, Jessor R. The concept of health promotion and the prevention of adolescent drug abuse. Health Educ Q 1985;12:169.

Petersen AC, Compas BE, Brooks-Gunn J, et al. Depression in adolescence. Am Psychol 1993;48:155.

Pfeffer CR. Attempted suicide in children and adolescents: causes and management. In: Lewis M, ed. Child and adolescent psychiatry: a comprehensive textbook. Baltimore: Williams & Wilkins, 1991.

Pratt W, Mosher W, Hoon M. Understand U.S. fertility: findings from the National Survey of Family Growth, Cycle III. Popul Bull 1984;39:1.

Rivara FP, Farrington DP. Prevention of violence. Arch Pediatr Adolesc Med 1995;149:421.

Robbins DM, Beck JC, Pries R. Learning disability and neuropsychological impairment in adjudicated, unincarcerated male delinquents. J Am Acad Child Adolesc Psychiatry 1983;22:40.

Rotheram-Borus MJ. Suicidal behavior and risk factors among runaway youths. Am J Psychiatry 1993;150:103.

Scales P. Helping adolescents create their futures. FL Educator 1988;(Fall):4.

Schoenbach VJ, Garrison GZ, Kaplan BH. Epidemiology of adolescent depression. Public Health Rev 1984;12:159.

Shamsie SJ. Violence and youth. Can J Psychiatry 1985; 30:498.

Shanok SS, Lewis DO. Medical histories of female delinquents. Arch Gen Psychiatry 1973;29:56.

Shanok SS, Malani SC, Ninan OP. A comparison of delinquent and nondelinquent adolescent psychiatric inpatients. Am J Psychiatry 1983;140:582.

Steinberg L. Familial factor in delinquency. J Adolesc Res 1987;2:255.

Stierlin H. A family perspective on adolescent runaways. Arch Gen Psychiatry 1973;29:56.

Stumphauzer JS. Behavioral approaches to juvenile delinquency: future perspectives. In: Michaelson L, Herson M, Turner SM, eds. Future perspectives in behavior therapy. New York: Plenum Press, 1981.

Tolan PH, Cromwell RE, Brasswell M. Family therapy with delinquents: a critical review of the literature. Fam Process 1986;25:619.

Warren JK, Gary F, Moorhead J. Self-reported experiences of physical and sexual abuse among runaway youths. Perspect Psychiatr Care 1994;30:23.

Wittchen HU, Knauper B, Kessler RC. Lifetime risk of depression. Br J Psychiatry Suppl 1994;26:16.

Wolfgang ME, Figlio RM, Sellin T. Delinquency in a birth cohort. Chicago: University of Chicago Press, 1972.

Woolf AD. Delinquency and the pediatrician. Pediatr Rev 1988;9:249.

Woolf A, Funk SG. Epidemiology of trauma in a population of incarcerated youth. Pediatrics 1985;75:463.

Yancy WS. Juvenile delinquency: considerations for pediatricians. Pediatr Rev 1995;16:12.

Yates GL, MacKenzie RG, Pennbridge J, et al. A risk profile comparison of runaway and nonrunaway youth. Am J Public Health 1988;78:820.

Young RL, Godfrey W, Mathews B. Runaways: a review of negative consequences. Fam Relations 1983;32:275.

CHAPTER 78
Youth Violence

Curren Warf

Violence is a pervasive problem in American society. It is of particular significance for the adolescent, who more than anyone else, is likely to be the victim. Violence takes many forms: homicide and assault, sexual assault, battering in intimate relationships, child abuse, and hate crime violence. Suicide as well may be considered a violent act turned toward oneself. Violent behavior is a complex phenomenon that is stimulated by multiple factors including poverty, racism, alcohol and drug use, and early childhood exposure to violence, including media violence. The consequences of violent behavior are made vastly more lethal with the presence of a firearm, especially a handgun. Violence results in death, disability, emotional traumatization, and tremendous financial cost for our society. Its presence affects all of us both as citizens and health-care providers, and confronts health-care providers with particular challenges. Young perpetrators of violence may have their lives destroyed and wasted in the criminal justice system. Public attitudes about violence have recently shifted from considering it entirely a criminal justice matter to appreciating the important public health aspects. This chapter outlines the epidemiology, etiology, risk factors, and potential prevention strategies.

Several characteristics of adolescents make them vulnerable to involvement in violence. Adolescence is characterized by increasingly close identification with peers, a sense of invincibility, and risk taking and impetuosity. Adolescent thinking tends to be concrete, especially in the younger teen, with an inability to appreciate long-term consequences; the young teen may also be susceptible to the dichotomous, simplistic moral code often found in gangs emphasizing loyalty to one's group and rejection of one's "enemies" or rivals.

EPIDEMIOLOGY

1. Homicide rates: Reasonably good statistics are available for homicide victimization throughout the United States. However, much less is known about the epidemiology of other categories of violent behavior: assaults, sexual assault, intimate battering, and hate crime violence.
   a. U.S. homicide rates: The United States has the highest homicide rate in the world among industrialized countries (Fig. 78.1). The United States is the only industrialized country to have a homicide rate among young men (16–24) over 5 per 100,000; many countries have a rate under 1 per 100,000. The U.S. rate among adolescent males in 1992 was 37.3 per 100,000. In fact, over 90% of all homicides in the industrialized world take place in the United States. The homicide rates among American youth are not evenly distributed, with significantly higher rates among inner-city, African-American youth (see ethnicity below).
   b. Trends: From 1979 to 1989 homicide rates for persons 15–19 years old increased 61% from 6.9 to 11.1 per 100,000, the largest increase for any age group. It is inter-

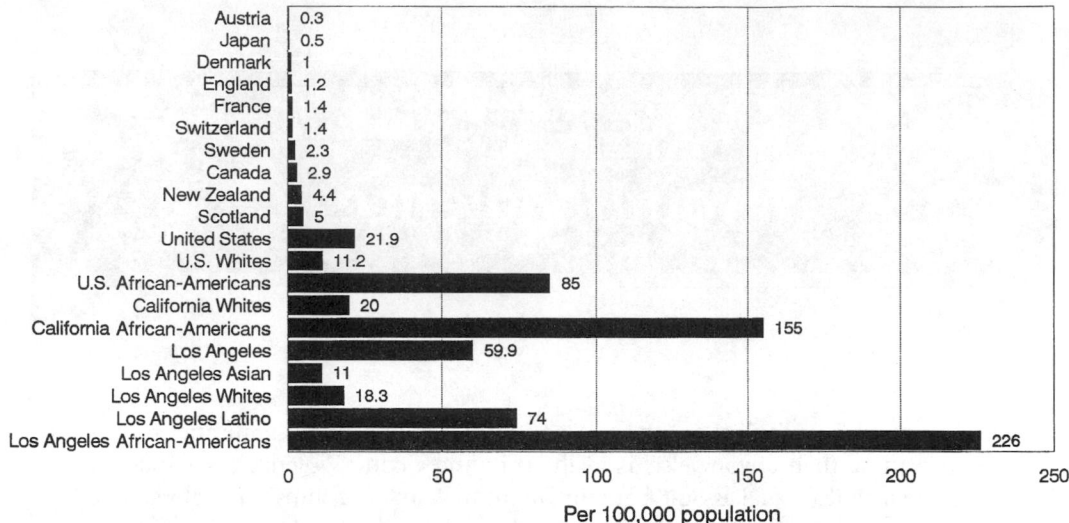

Figure 78.1.   Homicide victimization per 100,000 males 15–24 years old in selected nations, California, and Los Angeles County, 1986–1989. (Compiled from L.A. County Department of Health Services; Fingerhut L, Kleinman J. International and interstate comparisons of homicide among young males. JAMA 1990;263:3292; and Fingerhut LA, Ingram DD, Feldman JJ. Firearm homicide among black teenage males in metropolitan counties. Comparison of death rates in two periods, 1983 through 1985 and 1987 through 1989. JAMA 1992;267:3054.)

esting that during this same period the nonfirearm rate decreased 29%, indicating that the *increase in homicide rate resulted entirely from firearm use.* Homicide victimization rates affecting young urban African-American males have increased rapidly during the decade of the 1980s, doubling or tripling in many cities (Fig. 78.2).

   c. Firearm deaths: There has been a steadily increasing proportion of total mortality attributable to firearms. As of 1991, firearm-related deaths equaled or excelled automobile accident deaths in seven states (California, Louisiana, Maryland, Nevada, New York, Texas, and Virginia) and the District of Colombia. It is projected that by the year 2003 firearm deaths may become the leading cause of injury-related death in the country. In every urban center and for every ethnic group, firearm homicides exceed nonfirearm homicides. In these areas firearm homicide victimization rates are highest for African-American males and lowest for white females. In addition to the mortality problem, for every young person killed with a firearm there is an additional individual who is maimed and left permanently disabled, mainly from neurological injuries. There are also thousands of victims who survive firearm injuries but suffer lesser injuries.

2. Violent crime rate trends: There has been a growing escalation of youth involvement in violent crime over the last decade or more, and in 1990 the United States experienced its highest juvenile (aged 10–17) violent crime (murder, forcible rape, robbery, and aggravated assault) arrest rate in history, 430 per 100,000, 27% higher than the 1980 rate. The arrest rate for white youth was almost 300 per 100,000, for African-American youth over 1400 per 100,000. It should be remembered that youth frequently are in groups when crimes are committed and that multiple individuals may be arrested for single events. Arrest rate, then, may give an inflated impression of the incidence of assaultive events.

    Most disturbing, during the 1980s the country experienced a 145% increase in the homicide arrest rate for African-American youth, whereas the rate for white youth rose

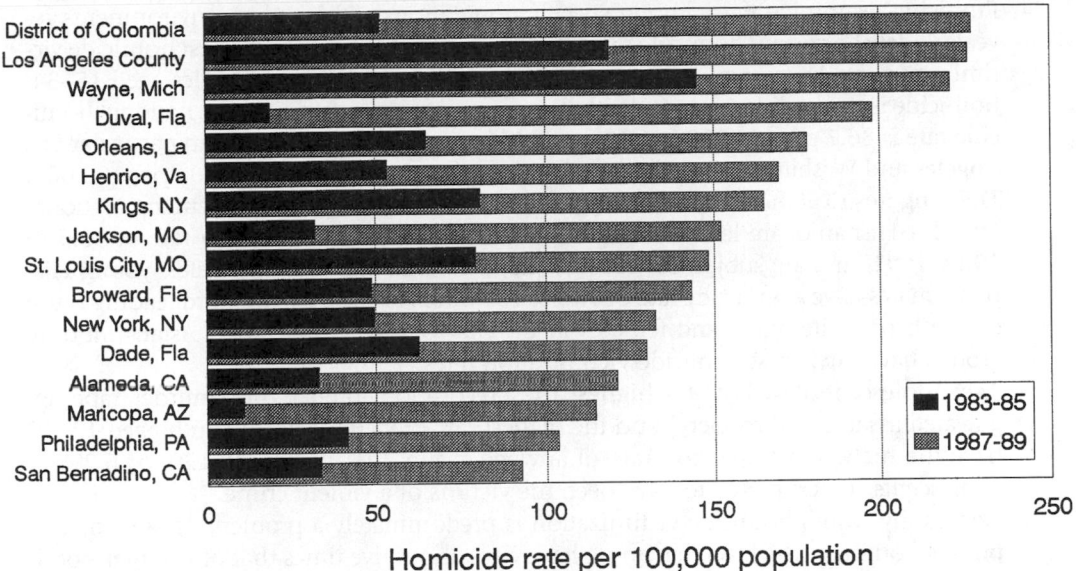

FIGURE 78.2.   Comparison of firearm homicide rates for adolescent African-American males, aged 15–19 years, 1983–1985 and 1987–1989. (Adapted from Fingerhut LA, Ingram DD, Feldman JJ. Firearm homicide among black teenage males in metropolitan counties. Comparison of death rates in two periods, 1983 through 1985 and 1987 through 1989. JAMA 1992;267:3054.)

48% and for other races declined 45%. During the last decade the proportion of juveniles who commit murder with guns has increased 79% so that now three out of four juvenile homicides are committed with firearms. Historically, from 1960 to 1990 the juvenile murder arrest rate increased 332%.

There have been remarkable increases in arrest rates for all other violent crimes as well. The rate for forcible rape more than doubled from 10.9 per 100,000 in 1965 to 21.9 per 100,000 in 1990; robbery arrest rates achieved an all-time high of 156.2 per 100,000 in 1990; aggravated assault, with the highest rate for any violent crime of almost 250 per 100,000, showed increases among white youth of 59% and among African-American youth of 89% for the decade 1980 to 1990. Weapon law violations (151 per 100,000) reached the highest level in history, representing a 58% increase for whites and a 103% increase for African-Americans.

3. Gender
   a. Homicide victims: Teenage males outnumber females as victims of homicide by a factor of over 6:1. Young males are more likely to be victims of violent crimes of all categories, except sexual assault.
   b. Adolescent homicide offenders: Ninety-four percent of those under 18 years old who are convicted of murder are male.
   c. Sexual assault: Female adolescents have the highest risk of any age group for being subjected to sexual assault. Because of the difficulty in obtaining reliable data, the incidence of adolescent sexual assault is not known. Though less common, male adolescents may also be subjected to sexual assault.

The reasons for male preponderance both as victims and perpetrators of homicides are controversial. Probable factors include cultural values that reward aggressive behavior of children, the absence of nurturance and nonviolent male role models for many youth, and the physiological effects of male sex hormone.

4. Ethnicity: Examining rates among specific populations within urban environments reveals widely discrepant homicide rates. African-Americans have the highest homicide victimization rate by far, and for young African-American males and females aged 15–34, homicide is the leading cause of death. For young African-Americans, the national homicide rate is 86.7 per 100,000 (154.4 for males); in many urban centers, in particular Los Angeles and Washington DC, the homicide rate for males is well over 200 per 100,000. These figures rival mortality rates experienced by combat soldiers in Vietnam. National rates for Hispanics are less well known but appear to be lower, with a rate of 30.5 in 1989–1991, and are subject to wide geographic variation. In Los Angeles, young Hispanic males have a homicide rate of 74 per 100,000. Homicide is the third leading cause of death of white males and females in the 15- to 24-year age range. Asian minority groups have the lowest homicide victimization rates.

5. Age: Adolescents have both the highest arrest record for violent crime (murder, rape, aggravated assault, and robbery) and the highest rate of victimization. Youth aged 12–19 have the highest victimization rate of any age group. In 1987, 1,728,120, or 6.2% of adolescents, are estimated to have been the victims of a violent crime.

6. Geography: Youth homicide victimization is predominately a problem of large metropolitan counties, which on the whole have rates about five times that of nonmetropolitan counties. Five states (California, Michigan, Missouri, Florida, and New York) and Washington DC account for the majority of homicides of African-American youth. However, violence is not only an inner-city problem of African-Americans and Latino males. Poverty and residence in a low-income neighborhood are stronger predictors of violence in adolescents than race or ethnicity. In addition, suburban schools have also reported significant increases in violence in recent years.

7. Relationship of offender to victim: The most common misconception is that intentional violence is a premeditated event that is randomly directed toward innocent bystanders. The opposite is true, with the vast majority of violent encounters occurring between friends and acquaintances and within families. Among males of all ethnic groups the most common relationship between offender and victim is that of a friend or acquaintance. In about 25% of youth homicides the victim is the initiator of violence. For adolescent female victims the most common perpetrator is a boyfriend, mirroring the situation for adult females, for whom the most common perpetrator is a family member or intimate partner. Ninety percent of females are murdered by males. Youth homicide overwhelmingly takes place between members of the same ethnic groups. In cases where the perpetrator is known, about 93% of homicides of young African-American males are committed by other young African-American males. Among whites, about 85% of murders are committed by other white youth. In large urban centers there has been an increase in drive-by shooting. These events are largely gang related and appear to be motivated by a desire for retribution for a perceived wrong. However, victims are frequently unrelated to the perceived problems. The presumption encountered that young victims of violence are themselves perpetrators is usually unjustified.

8. Method of homicide: The large majority (over 80%) of successful adolescent homicides involve the use of a handgun. Among 15- to 19-year-olds firearm homicide is the most rapidly increasing cause of death. There are estimated to be about 200 million firearms in civilian hands in the United States. About 60 million of these are handguns. About 43% of homes have one or more handguns; at least 30% of gun owners with children keep one or more loaded guns in the home. Consequently, about 9 million adolescents have access to handguns in their own homes. When a teenager fires a gun at home, the most common victim is himself, the second most common victim is a friend. When

there is a handgun in a home, a household member is roughly 43 times more likely to be the victim of the firearm than an intruder.

Among high school–aged students, carrying a gun and hanging out with friends who carry guns stand out as the two most important modifiable risk factors for being murdered or otherwise victimized by gun violence. Despite the fact that most teens who carry guns do so for a sense of security, the reality is that this act puts them at greatly increased risk. The principal effect of having a gun is to worsen the outcomes of violent encounters: fistfights or assaults become murders, attempted rapes and robberies are completed, suicidal gestures are completed. The single most important factor in all sorts of firearm injuries is the accessibility of firearms themselves.

9. Precipitating events: Precipitating events leading to assault include a desire for retaliation or revenge for previous perceived verbal or physical insult, escalation of showing-off contests, and jealousy. Homicides by adolescents are usually impetuous acts that are instantly regretted. The large majority of youth homicides take place between friends and acquaintances and are not gang related. In fact, adolescent homicide can almost be defined as "a fistfight with a gun in the fist." Nationally, about 4% of youth homicides are gang related. However, in inner-city environments, in regions where gangs are prevalent, gang violence may account for as much as 30–40% or more of young homicide victims.

10. Other risk factors for violence
    a. Alcohol and drug use: Half or more of violent encounters among adolescents involve drug or alcohol use. This may be directly through disinhibition by the intoxicants or indirectly through involvement in the drug trade.
    b. Media violence: Over 1200 studies now confirm the association between higher levels of viewing violence and increased acceptance of aggressive attitudes and increased aggressive behavior. The most significant impact on later behavior appears to be exposure to violence as a young child. Decreasing early childhood exposure to violent television and film is an integral component of effective violence prevention.
    c. Child abuse: Experiencing child abuse is a well-documented risk factor for later participation in violent behavior. An interesting longitudinal study designed to examine long-term effects of abuse and neglect found that both physical abuse and neglect (but not sexual abuse) increased the likelihood of arrest as a juvenile by over 50%, arrest as an adult by 38%, and arrest for a violent crime by 38%, as compared with a matched comparison group (Widom, 1992).
    d. Environment: Witnessing violence in the family environment as a young child, in particular spousal battery, has in a number of studies been found to correlate with later violent behavior both in intimate relationships and in society at large.
    e. Social factors include:
       — Poverty, unemployment, sense of hopelessness about the future
       — Racism, a sense of being excluded from the justice system
       — Poor schools and recreational opportunities

ASSESSMENT OF RISK

To implement interventions to decrease the risk of violence, it is recommended that healthcare providers assess the risk of the youth's involvement with violence, including taking a thorough history of the teens involvement with violence as an aggressor, a victim, a witness to violence in the community, a nonviolent problem solver, and a participant in gender role–related violence. In assessing risk, as with other situations, it is important to be cognizant of the developmental stage of the youth. Open-ended, nonthreatening, nonjudgmental questions should be used such as:

"Many young people I talk to have been affected by community violence, how have you
  been affected?"
"Do you feel safe in the community where you live and go to school?"
"Have you ever been in a serious fight?"
"Do you know anyone who has been seriously injured or killed by violence? How many?
  Were any of them close friends? Did you witness any of these events?"
"Have you ever been threatened with a weapon? Shot at?"
"Do you have friends that carry guns?"

PREVENTION AND INTERVENTION

Recently there has been a proliferation of violence prevention programs; however, evaluations of efficacy are exceedingly difficult. Promising approaches begin as early in life as
possible and enhance nurturant and nonviolent parenting methods.

Primary prevention strategies are approaches directed at either the entire population or
focused on selected populations at greatest risk. Any serious strategy of violence prevention
must include efforts directed at young children, when basic values and approaches to frustration and conflict are learned. Particular issues to be addressed include familial violence,
corporal punishment, and child abuse, which are known to correlate with later violent behavior of children. Apparently effective strategies include:

1. Identification of young, stressed, and most especially, socially isolated parents, and providing them with home visitation and early intervention parenting training programs
2. Increasing financial stability of impoverished families at risk, in particular families
   headed by single parents
3. Identification and referral of pregnant and parenting teenagers and their partners to teen
   parenting and support groups
4. Preschool programs that address intellectual, emotional, and social needs of young children and encourage the development of nonviolent conflict resolution skills
5. Reduction of early childhood exposure to media violence, including cartoon violence
6. Engaging teens, especially young teens, in supervised recreational activities
7. Improving the quality of the school environment
8. Prevention of school truancy and dropout
9. Employment programs, particularly for young people who are out of school

In addition, curricula for conflict resolution have been developed for use in secondary
schools. Specific curricula approaches that appear to be effective are:

1. Alternative solution generation
2. Self-esteem enhancement
3. Peer negotiation skills
4. Problem-solving skills training
5. Anger management

Effective primary prevention programs must be developmentally appropriate and comprehensive in approach (especially those involving teenagers) and must include multiple components, reinforcing nonviolent behaviors in a variety of contexts such as the family, school,
peer groups, and the media. These approaches attempt to provide access to ongoing relationships with nonviolent, caring adult mentors, particularly for those teens from stressed, or
single-parent families. Through reducing risk factors, children and youth are empowered to
resist effects of detrimental life circumstances.

Firearms

Removal of firearms from the environment of youth through legislation, strict enforcement of existing laws, and removal of firearms from the home environment is of essential importance in prevention of the grave consequences of violent behavior. Recommendations include:

1. Parents of adolescents and children should be encouraged to remove firearms from their homes. This is consistent with the recommendations of the American Academy of Pediatrics (1994). Attempts at interventions less than removal have not been shown to reduce mortality. Parents who keep loaded firearms at home should be informed that this is extremely dangerous for their children, and they may be held legally culpable for any adverse consequences. Parents must be made aware that, if they keep a gun at home, the most likely victim is their teenage son and that firearms at home are far more likely to be used to shoot a friend or a family member than an intruder. Additionally, parents may inquire about the presence of loaded firearms in the homes of their children's friends and require that they be eliminated before children can play in the area.
2. Locked containers: If parents are unwilling to remove firearms from the home, they should be advised to separate ammunition from the weapons and keep both in separate securely locked containers. Trigger locks should be placed on all firearms. It must be emphasized, however, that teenagers have manual dexterity equal to that of adults and these measures may have little impact on the youth's ability to obtain and use a firearm if he desires to do so.
3. Safety classes: Since accidental discharges make up a minority of firearm injuries, safety classes in use of firearms have never been shown to reduce the risk associated with firearm ownership.
4. Strict laws: Most states have laws making it an offense for a minor to be in possession of a firearm under most circumstances. These laws must be enforced.
5. Handgun bans: The American Academy of Pediatrics (1994) and many other medical and health organizations recommend that handguns be banned. Bans on handguns and restrictions on handgun manufacturers may, over time, reduce the number of handguns in circulation.

Secondary Interventions

Secondary interventions may be directed at youth who have been identified after risk behaviors have become apparent. These may include:

1. Intensive individual or family psychotherapy
2. Enhancement of the school environment with smaller class size and supervised after-school activities
3. Providing caring, nonviolent adult mentors
4. Integrating youth into activities with nondisturbed peers

Health practitioners who are affiliated with inner-city hospitals may be in a pivotal position to identify youth who have survived gunshot wounds or other assaults and initiate secondary intervention programs. The "patch them up and get them out" approach essentially sends identified very high-risk youth back into the same dangerous environment to either be further victimized or to seek retribution and perpetuate a cycle of violence.

It must be remembered that youth (aged 11–24) are the most likely age group to be victims of violent crime, which can initiate a vicious cycle of crime-retaliation-crime. It is important then to educate youth in how to avoid becoming victims, including the victims of other adolescents. This may be through avoiding particularly unsafe environments, developing after-school activities, and avoiding hanging out with youth with guns.

Although the causes of juvenile violence are not completely understood and programs designed to prevent delinquency have not been thoroughly evaluated, successful approaches to intervention appear to have the following characteristics:

1. They are appropriately supportive of children and adolescents and their families.
2. They are intensive (i.e., they involve the commitment of considerable time, personnel, and effort).
3. They are broad based (i.e., they intervene in a number of the systems [including family, school, and peer] in which the child or adolescent is involved and use multiple services [e.g., educational, health, and social] as appropriate for the individual child or adolescent).

Tertiary Intervention

Tertiary intervention takes place after a youth has become embroiled in violent activities and may occur largely through the juvenile justice system. Goals of the juvenile justice system include rehabilitation, punishment, deterrence, and public safety. The effectiveness of punishment on antisocial behavior is of significant debate, and there is no clear evidence that punishment leads to improvement. Almost nothing is known about the effectiveness of the juvenile justice system in reducing subsequent delinquency among teenagers. Parenthetically, health care for teens in juvenile confinement is a serious concern in that incarcerated youth have a greater than average number of health problems that may worsen during confinement, and only 1% of eligible juvenile justice facilities have been accredited as meeting existing voluntary standards for providing health care.

BIBLIOGRAPHY

American Academy of Pediatrics, Center to Prevent Handgun Violence. Steps to prevent firearm injury. Elk Grove, Illinois: The Academy, 1994.

American Academy of Pediatrics, Committee on Communications. Media violence. Pediatrics 1995;95:949.

American Medical Association. Adolescents as victims of family violence. JAMA 1993;270:1850.

American Psychological Association. Violence and youth: psychology's response. Washington, DC: American Psychological Association, 1993.

Bureau of Justice Statistics. Violent crime in the United States, 1990. Washington, DC: US Department of Justice, 1991.

Centers for Disease Control. Weapon carrying among high school students—United States, 1990. MMWR 1991;40:681.

Centers for Disease Control and Prevention. Violence-related attitudes and behaviors of high school students—New York City, 1992. JAMA 1993;270:2032.

Centerwall BS. Race, socioeconomic status, and domestic homicide, Atlanta, 1971–72. Am J Public Health 1984;74:813.

Centerwall BS. Homicide and the prevalence of handguns: Canada and the United States, 1976 to 1980. Am J Epidemiol 1991;134:1245.

Centerwall BS. Television and violence. The scale of the problem and where to go from here. JAMA 1992; 267:3059.

Clancy TV, Misick LN, Covington D, et al. The financial impact of intentional violence on community hospitals. J Trauma 1994;37:1.

Coben JH, Weiss HB, Dearwater SR. A primer on school violence prevention. J Sch Health 1994;64:309.

Cotten NU, Resnick J, Browne DC, et al. Aggression and fighting behavior among African-American adolescents: individual and family factors. Am J Public Health 1994;84:618.

Dolins JC, Christoffel KK. Reducing violent injuries: priorities for pediatrician advocacy. Pediatrics 1994; 94:638.

DuRant RH, Cadenhead C, Pendergrast RA, et al. Factors associated with the use of violence among urban black adolescents. Am J Public Health 1994;84:612.

Eron LD. Media violence. Pediatr Ann 1995;24:84.

Fingerhut LA, Ingram DD, Feldman JJ. Firearm homicide among black teenage males in metropolitan counties. Comparison of death rates in two periods, 1983 through 1985 and 1987 through 1989. 1992; 267:3054.

Fingerhut L, Kleinman J. International and interstate comparisons of homicide among young males. JAMA 1990;263:3292.

Garbarino J, Dubrow N, Kostelny K, et al. Children in danger: coping with the consequences of community violence. San Francisco: Jossey Bass Publishers, 1992.

Garrett D. Violent behaviors among African-American adolescents. Adolescence 1995;30:209.

Golding AM. Leading article—understanding and preventing violence: a review. Public Health 1995; 109:91.

Goodwillie S. Voices from the future, our children tell us about violence in America. Children's express. New York: Crown Publishers, 1993.

Groves BM, Zuckerman B, Marans S. Silent victims. Children who witness violence. JAMA 1993;269:262.

Hammond WR, Yung B. Psychology's role in the public health response to assaultive violence among young African-American men. 1993;48:142.

Hausman AJ, Spivak H, Prothrow-Stith D. Adolescents' knowledge and attitudes about and experience with violence. J Adolesc Health 1994;15:400.

Issacs M. The impact of community violence on African American children and families, collaborative approaches to prevention and intervention. National Center for Education in Maternal and Child Health, 1992.

Jaffe PG. Children of battered women. Newbury Park: Sage Publications, 1990.

Johnson EM, Belfer ML. Substance abuse and violence: cause and consequence. J Health Care Poor Underserved 1995;6:113.

Kellerman AL, Reay DT. Protection or peril? An analysis of firearms-related deaths in the home. N Engl J Med 1986;314:1557.

Kellerman AL, Rivarra FP, Somes G, et al. Suicide in the home in relation to gun ownership. N Engl J Med 1992;327:467.

Mondragon D. Clinical assessment of gang violence risk through history and physical exam. J Health Care Poor Underserved 1995;6:209.

National Research Council, Commission on Behavioral and Social Sciences and Education. Losing generations, adolescent in high-risk settings. Washington, DC: National Academy Press, 1993.

O'Donnell L, Cohen S, Hausman A. Forum on youth violence in minority communities. Evaluation of community-based violence prevention programs. Public Health Rep 1991;106:276.

Prothrow-Stith DB. The epidemic of youth violence in America: using public health prevention strategies to prevent violence. J Health Care Poor Underserved 1995;6:95.

Prothrow-Stith D. Deadly consequences. New York: Harper Collins Publishers, 1991.

Prothrow-Stith D. Violence prevention, curriculum for adolescents. Teenage health teaching modules. Newton, Massachusetts: Education Development Center.

Rachuba L, Stanton B, Howard D. Violent crime in the United States. An epidemiologic profile. Arch Pediatr Adolesc Med 1995;149:953.

Rivara FP, Farrington DP. Prevention of violence. Role of the pediatrician. Arch Pediatr Adolesc Med 1995; 149:421.

Rodriguez MA, Brindis CD. Violence and Latino youth: prevention and methodological issues. Public Health Rep 1995;110:260.

Ropp L, Visintainer P, Uman J, et al. Death in the city. An American childhood tragedy. JAMA 1992;267:2905.

Rosenberg ML. Academic medical centers have a major role in preventing violence. Acad Med 1993;68:268.

Seltzer F. Trend in mortality from violent deaths: unintentional injuries, United States, 1960–1991. Stat Bull Metrop Insur Co 1995;76:19.

Sheley JF, McGee ZT, Wright JD. Gun-related violence in and around inner-city schools. Am J Dis Child 1992; 146:677.

Singer MI, Anglin TM, Song LY, et al. Adolescents' exposure to violence and associated symptoms of psychological trauma. JAMA 1995;273:477.

Slaby RG, Stringham P. Prevention of peer and community violence: the pediatrician's role. Pediatrics 1994;94:608.

Sloan JH, Kellermann AL, Reay DT, et al. Handgun regulations, crime, assaults, and homicide. A tale of two cities. N Engl J Med 1988;319:1256.

Tomes H. Research and policy directions in violence: a developmental perspective. J Health Care Poor Underserved 1995;6:146.

US Department of Justice. Crime in the United States, uniform crime reports. Washington, DC: Federal Bureau of Investigation, August 30, 1992.

Waller JA, Skelly JM, Davis JH. Characteristics, costs, and effects of violence in Vermont. J Trauma 1994; 37:921.

Webster DW, Wilson ME. Gun violence among youth and the pediatrician's role in primary prevention. Pediatrics 1994;94:617.

Weil DS, Hemenway D. Loaded guns in the home: analysis of a national random sample of gun owners. JAMA 1992;267:3033.

White MP. A comprehensive approach to violence prevention. J Health Care Poor Underserved 1995;6: 254.

Widom C. The cycle of violence. National Institute of Justice, Research in Brief, US Department of Justice, October, 1992.

Wilson-Brewer R, Spivak H. Violence prevention in schools and other community settings: the pediatrician as initiator, educator, collaborator, and advocate. Pediatrics 1994;94:623.

CHAPTER 79

Suicide

Lawrence S. Neinstein, Maria A. Juliani, and Joan Shapiro

Although adolescence is a relatively healthy age, the 15- to 24-year-old age group is the only age group where the mortality rate has not decreased significantly since 1960. This is secondary to the continued significant death rates from violent causes: accidents, homicides, and suicides. Suicides are the third leading cause of death among the male population in the 15- to 24-year-old age group and the fourth highest cause of death in this age group among the female population. For the adolescent, a suicide attempt may represent either a help-seeking gesture or the ultimate symbol of depression and resignation. For the family, suicide imposes grief at the loss, rage at the act of suicide, and guilt for having failed. And for the health-care professional, a suicide attempt presents a crisis that he or she may feel totally inadequate to handle based on prior training. This chapter discusses the dynamics of adolescent suicide and suicide attempts—epidemiology, risk profile, etiology, warning symptoms, evaluation, and treatment.

EPIDEMIOLOGY

1. Suicide rates: Efforts to estimate attempted and successful suicides are confounded by the fact that many suicide attempts are recorded as accidental overdoses by family physicians and, in addition, because many accidents are actually suicides. Approximately 2000 adolescents under the age of 19 commit suicide each year.
   a. Male suicide rates in the United States are indicated in Table 79.1.
   b. Female suicide rates in the United States are indicated in Table 79.2.
   c. Recent changes in suicide rates among youth between 1980 and 1992 are indicated in Table 79.3.
   d. Table 79.4 reviews the results of the Youth Risk Behavior Survey in regard to suicide risk.
      Since 1950, suicide rates have increased four to five times for male adolescents and doubled for female adolescents. Between 1980 and 1992, the number and rate of suicides declined among persons under age 25 years from 5381 (5.7 per 100,000 persons) to 5007 (5.4). For persons aged 20–24, the suicide rate declined 7.2% (16.1 to 14.9). However, the rate increased among persons aged 15–19 years by 28.3% (8.5 to 10.9) and among persons aged 10–14 years by 120% (0.8 to 1.7). For African-American males aged 15–19 the rate increased by 165.3%.
      Estimates of the ratio of suicide attempts to completions in adolescents range from 50:1 to 200:1. Based on the above figure of 2000 suicides, estimates of attempts are 100,000–400,000 per year. Rates of second attempts vary from 6% to 16% within 1 year.
2. Sex: Males outnumber females in completed suicides by 3:1, while females outnumber males in attempts by the same margin of 3:1.

TABLE 79.1. Male Suicide Rates in the United States (per 100,000)

Year and Race	Age Group (yr)		
	10–14	15–19	20–24
1950	0.5	3.5	9.3
1960	0.9	5.6	11.5
1970	0.9	8.8	19.3
1975	1.2	12.2	26.4
1986	2.3	16.4	26.6
1990	2.2	18.1	25.7
African-American	1.6	11.5	19.0
White	2.3	19.3	26.8

From US Department of Health, Education & Welfare, National Center for Health Statistics, Mortality Statistics Branch. Vital statistics of the United States, Volume 2. Mortality, Part A. Hyattsville, Maryland: National Center for Health Statistics, 1988.

TABLE 79.2. Female Suicide Rates in the United States (per 100,000)

Year and Race	Age Group (yr)		
	10–14	15–19	20–24
1950	0.1	1.8	3.3
1960	0.2	1.6	2.9
1970	0.3	2.9	5.7
1975	0.4	2.9	6.8
1986	0.7	3.8	4.9
1990	0.9	3.7	4.1
African-American	<0.1	1.9	2.6
White	0.9	4.0	4.4

From US Department of Health, Education & Welfare, National Center for Health Statistics, Mortality Statistics Branch. Vital statistics of the United States, Volume 2. Mortality, Part A. Hyattsville, Maryland: National Center for Health Statistics, 1988.

TABLE 79.3. Change in Suicide for Persons 10–24, by Age Group, from 1980 to 1992—United States

Race and Age	Male			Female		
	1980 Rate	1992 Rate	Change (%)	1980 Rate	1992 Rate	Change (%)
White						
10–14	1.4	2.6	+86	0.3	1.1	+233
15–19	15.1	18.4	+22	3.3	3.7	+12
20–24	27.7	26.6	−4	5.9	4.0	−32
African-American						
10–14	0.5	2.0	+300	0.2	0.4	+100
15–19	5.6	14.8	+164	1.6	1.9	+19
20–24	19.9	21.2	+7	3.1	2.4	−23
Other						
10–14	0.0	1.1	Undefined	0.0	0.2	Undefined
15–19	18.6	17.5	−6	3.0	5.0	+67
20–24	24.2	21.1	−13	6.3	6.2	−2
Total	14.5	15.4	6	3.1	2.8	−10

Adapted from National Center for Health Statistics. Advance report of final mortality statistics, 1992. Monthly Vital Statistics Report No. 43, 1994.

TABLE 79.4. Behavior Related to Attempted Suicide Among High School Students during 12 Months Preceding Survey, 1991 Youth Risk Behavior Survey

Category	Thought Seriously about Suicide (%)	Made Suicide Plans (%)	Attempted Suicide (%)	Suicide Attempt Required Medical Attention (%)
Sex				
Female	37.2	24.9	10.7	2.5
Male	20.8	12.5	3.9	1.0
Grade				
9	29.1	19.4	9.1	1.9
10	29.5	18.6	7.6	1.6
11	31.6	20.7	6.3	1.8
12	25.8	15.9	5.8	1.7
Race or ethnicity				
White	29.9	19.0	6.7	1.6
African-American	22.2	14.8	6.6	1.8
Hispanic	26.8	15.9	7.9	1.7
TOTAL	29.9	18.6	7.3	1.7

Adapted from Kann L, Warren W, Collins JL, et al. Results from the national school-based 1991 Youth Risk Behavior Survey and progress toward achieving related health objectives for the nation. Public Health Rep 1995;108:47.

3. Race: Suicide rates are higher in white adolescents than African-American or Hispanic (Table 79.3). White males have the highest risk. Another high-risk group are American Indians.

4. Family history: Suicidal behavior tends to "run in families." A history of suicide attempts or suicide among first- or second-degree relatives increases risk for adolescent suicide by three times.

5. Age: As outlined in Tables 79.1 and 79.2, suicide is uncommon in all adolescents less than 14 years of age, with the rates rising dramatically thereafter. The largest increase in suicide rates since 1970 has been in 15- to 19-year-old male adolescents.

6. Psychiatric comorbidity: Probable or definite personality disorders were more common in adolescent suicide victims than in controls, particularly cluster B (impulsive-dramatic) and C (avoidant-dependent disorders). Axis I psychiatric disorders have been found to be present in at least 90% of adolescent suicide victims.

7. Marital status: In the general population, suicide rates are less for married individuals, but the reverse is true in the 15- to 19-year-old population, where the rates of suicide for married individuals are increased 1.5–1.7 times over those for unmarried individuals.

8. Season: Rates are increased in the spring and fall.

9. Geographic: Rates are higher in the western United States than in other regions of the country.

10. Method used for completed suicides
    a. Firearms and explosives: In 1992, firearm-related deaths accounted for 64.9% of suicides among persons younger than 25 years. Among persons aged 15–19, firearm-related suicides accounted for 81% of the increase in the overall rate from 1980 to 1992. The use of firearms is more common in male suicides. However, firearm suicides have increased significantly in adolescent females.
    b. Poisonings: Poison is used in about 15–20% of male suicides and 25–30% of female suicides.
    c. Suffocation: Hanging, strangulation, or drowning is used in about 15–20% of male suicides and 10% of female suicides.
    d. Others: A small percentage of suicides are accomplished through piercing with a sharp instrument or jumping from a high place.

11. Suicide at college: Most studies indicate that suicide rates in college students are no higher than that in the general population for the same age group. The incidence of suicide in college students appears to be approximately 10–14 per 100,000 per year.

RISK FACTORS IN THE SUICIDAL ADOLESCENT

Although it is impossible to predict which adolescent will attempt suicide, risk factors are cited in the literature that should increase the index of suspicion for a potentially suicidal patient. These factors may also be of value in evaluating the future risk of an adolescent who has attempted suicide.

1. Abuse of alcohol or other substance: Crumley (1990) summarizes data on the relationship between adolescent suicide behavior and substance abuse. Adolescents who abuse psychoactive substances, particularly those with any type of depressive disorder, appear to be at higher risk for suicidal behavior.
2. Physical illness
3. Recent behavioral changes
4. Major psychiatric disorder
5. Feelings of hopelessness, helplessness, or low self-esteem: Swedo et al. (1991) found that adolescent suicide attempters could be differentiated from normal adolescents and at-risk adolescents without a recent suicide attempt by hopelessness and suicidal ideation.
6. Feelings of anger, rejection, social isolation, or expendability
7. Recent loss of a significant person or relationship
8. Poor school record
9. History of a broken family or family discord
10. History of prior abuse: Riggs et al. (1990) reported a five times greater risk of suicide in adolescents with a prior history of physical abuse and a threefold increase of suicide in those teens with a history of sexual abuse.
11. Alcoholic parents
12. History of suicide in the family
13. Prior attempts
14. Clear intention to repeat
15. Agent used in a past attempt: Jumping and shooting are of higher risk than ingestion or cutting.
16. Location and chance of rescue: The risk is higher with an adolescent who has attempted suicide in a remote site with no probability of discovery.
17. Presence of firearms in the house: Brent et al. (1993) found that the presence of firearms may be associated with adolescent suicide even in the absence of clear psychiatric illness.

PROCESS OF THE ADOLESCENT SUICIDE ATTEMPT

Although the history of each suicidal adolescent is different, many such adolescents exhibit a behavior pattern that can be broken down into four components:

1. Long-standing history of problems: Suicide is a deficiency disease, a deficiency of social connections. Many adolescents who attempt suicide exhibit a long history of deficiency or of problems that create an underlying vulnerability. These problems include parents or relatives who have attempted suicide; one or both natural parents absent from the home; unwanted stepparents; divorce in the family; history of family conflicts; parents with alcohol problems; history of foster placements; or marked residential mobility.

2. Escalation phase: In many adolescents who have attempted suicide, the vulnerability created during childhood increases during the adolescent period. This period of escalating problems is characterized by frequent family conflicts, as the family fails to deal adequately with the adolescent developmental process. The adolescent often begins to feel isolated from his or her family and other social structures. Significant physical or mental illness in the family may also exacerbate the adolescent's vulnerability.

3. Progressive social isolation: Failure of available adaptive techniques for coping with old and new problems often leaves the suicidal adolescent feeling progressively socially isolated. This is often associated with a significant failure of communication with parents. The adolescent seems to have lost or never developed the capability to express his or her feelings with words. Although these adolescents are often depressed, the depression may not be manifested in the typical adult behaviors of depressed affect, anorexia, weight loss, and so forth. In fact, the adolescent may appear outwardly cheerful, but the depression may manifest itself through behavior such as substance abuse, delinquency, runaway behavior, early onset of sexual activity or sexual promiscuity, or boredom.

4. Final stage: The suicide attempt is often preceded by a precipitating event that caps this long process of increasing despair. Precipitating events often include loss of a girlfriend or boyfriend, pregnancy, school problems, death of a friend or relative, or a family fight.

Prodromal Signs

Several signs in the adolescent should alert family, friends, or the health-care provider to the potential for suicide. These prodromal signs include sadness, hopelessness, emptiness, lack of energy, insomnia, eating problems, loss of interest in social life and school, boredom, loneliness, irritability, truancy, substance abuse, or a change in social behavior. Other signs include accident proneness, giving away of prized possessions, and statements such as, "My family (or the world) would be better off without me."

Assessment of the Suicidal Adolescent

1. Medical therapy: The first priority is to treat any life-threatening medical complication of the suicide attempt.

2. Physical protection: The suicidal adolescent should be provided immediate physical protection so that a reattempt does not occur.

3. Psychological intervention: As soon as the medical evaluation and therapy is completed, the adolescent requires calming down and reassurance that he or she is in a safe place. At this time an initial evaluation should be performed. This evaluation should attempt to assess:
   a. Predisposing conditions: These include:
      — Sex and age of adolescent
      — Underlying health status
      — History or evidence of prior mental disorder
      — History of family, school, or peer problems
      — History of suicide attempts or substance abuse in family members
      — History of prior suicide attempts
      — History of incest or abuse
      — History of accidents or prior self-destructive behavior
      — History of substance abuse
      — Prior use of coping strategies

— Recent experience of loss
— Presence of firearms or drugs available in the home
— Available support systems including reaction by parents and others: Do the parents take the attempt seriously, and are they supportive of seeking help? What family or peer support system will the adolescent be returning to at home?

b. State of mind: This includes evaluating the teen's:
— Level of depression
— Level of hopelessness, helplessness, and self-esteem
— Feelings of expendability (e.g., that the teen is not important to the family and that to some extent the family would be "better off" without the teen)
— Openness to further counseling
— Level of panic and disorganization
— Attitude about death

c. Suicide attempt: This includes evaluating:
— Method: Lethality and current access to method
— Timing: Sudden impulse versus well planned
— Intent: No real intention versus strong intention to die
— Desire to repeat
— Circumstances surrounding the attempt: Possibility of rescue from attempt versus an attempt carried out in isolation

Features suggesting a high risk of a second suicide attempt include lethal method, attempt carried out in isolation or precautions taken to avoid discovery, elaborate plan, history of prior attempts, high desire to repeat, marked degree of hopelessness and helplessness, sense of expendability, lack of a strong support system, and lack of desire on adolescent's part for help.

4. Disposition
Ideally all adolescents with a suicide attempt should have a mandatory short-term hospitalization to assess the adolescent and the family.

a. Indications for longer hospitalization
— Medical complications
— Psychosis
— Use of a lethal method with clear intent of suicide
— An uncommunicative adolescent or one who communicates ambivalence regarding the will to live
— Lack of family support

If the adolescent shows a high lethality index, keep the teen in a safe and secure environment under one-to-one nursing supervision. If the teen refuses voluntary admission, initiate procedures for involuntary hospitalization.

b. Conditions for sending adolescent home
— Depression is mild and fits into adolescent pattern of mood swings.
— Adolescent has a supportive family willing to help.
— No evidence of long-standing psychosis or severe depression.
— Adolescent clearly no longer feels suicidal.
— Appropriate medical and psychosocial follow-up have been arranged.
— Case has been evaluated by a psychiatrist, psychologist, or another appropriately trained health-care professional.

5. Follow-up: Every suicidal adolescent should have conscientious follow-up care by a psychiatrist, psychologist, or other mental health counselor. The continuation of collaboration of medical doctor and mental health providers is an essential component of follow-up care. Weekly or more frequent visits should be scheduled initially. During

this period the adolescent's problems can be explored in more depth, with careful attention given to the areas of school, social and family problems, and existing support mechanisms.

6. Outpatient management of at-risk adolescents: The assessment as just described should be obtained, with plans for close follow-up by the appropriate mental health counselor. A suicide prevention contract is also in order. This is a written or oral contract with the practitioner that the teen will not attempt suicide without contacting the practitioner or will contact the practitioner if the teen feels out of control. If suicidal ideation is significant or the suicide potential is judged to be high, then voluntary or involuntary hospitalization would be necessary. Parents should always be notified if a minor is considered at risk of suicide.

Suicide is a tragic but increasingly more common expression of alienation among adolescents. Every suicidal gesture and threat among adolescents must be taken seriously and evaluated in detail. Rather than a manipulative attempt to "get attention," all adolescent suicidal ideation, gestures, or attempts are cries for their problem and pain to be attended to.

PREVENTION OF ADOLESCENT SUICIDE

The Centers for Disease Control (CDC) have published suicide prevention guidelines. The suggested strategies include:

1. School gatekeeper training to help school staff identify and refer students at risk for suicide
2. Community gatekeeper training to train community members (e.g., clergy, police, recreation staff) and clinical health-care providers to identify and refer teens at risk for suicide
3. General suicide education for students to learn about suicide, its warning signs, and how to seek help for themselves or others
4. Screening programs to identify high-risk adolescents and young adults
5. Peer support programs in or outside of school to further peer relationships and competency in social skills
6. Crisis centers and hotlines
7. Restriction of access to handguns, drugs, and other common means of suicide
8. Intervention after a suicide to help prevent or contain suicide clusters and to help adolescents and young adults cope effectively with feelings of loss

BIBLIOGRAPHY

Berman AL, Jobes DA. Suicide prevention in adolescents (age 12–18). Suicide Life Threat Behav 1995; 25:143.

Bhatia SC, Khan MH, Sharma A. Suicide risk: evaluation and management. Am Fam Physician 1986;34:167.

Brent DA, Johnson B, Bartle S, et al. Personality disorder, tendency to impulsive violence, and suicidal behavior in adolesents. J Am Acad Child Adolesc Psychiatry 1993;32:69.

Brent D, Johnson B, Perper J, et al. Personality disorder, personality habits, impulsive violence and completed suicide attempts in adolescents J Am Acad Adolesc Psychiatry 1994;33:8.

Brent DA, Perper JA, Allman CJ, et al. The presence and accessibility of firearms in the homes of adolescent suicides: a case-control study. JAMA 1991;266:2989.

Brent DA, Perper JA, Moritz G. Firearms and adolescent suicide. A community case-control study. Am J Dis Child 1993;147:1066.

Cappelli M, Clulow MK, Goodman JT, et al. Identifying depressed and suicidal adolescents in a teen health clinic. J Adolesc Health 1995;16:64.

Centers for Disease Control. Suicide, United States, 1970–1980. MMWR 1985;34:353.

Centers for Disease Control. Premature mortality due to suicide and homicide, United States, 1983. MMWR 1986;35:357.

Centers for Disease Control. Youth suicide—United States, 1970–1980. MMWR 1987;36:87.

Centers for Disease Control. Programs for the prevention of suicide among adolescents and young adults. MMWR 1994;43:1.

Centers for Disease Control. Suicide among children, adolescents, and young adults—United States, 1980–1992. MMWR 1995;44:289.

Centers for Disease Control and Prevention. Fatal and nonfatal suicide attempts among adolescents—Oregon, 1988–1993. JAMA 1995;274:452.

Committee on Adolescence, American Academy of Pediatrics. Suicide and suicide attempts in adolescents and young adults. Pediatrics 1988;81:322.

Crumley FE. Adolescent suicide attempts. JAMA 1979; 241:2404.

Crumley FE. Substance abuse and adolescent suicidal behavior. JAMA 1990;263:3051.

Curran DK. Adolescent suicidal behavior. Washington DC: Hemisphere Publishing, 1987.

Deykin EY, Buka SL. Suicidal ideation and attempts among chemically dependent adolescents. Am J Public Health 1994;84:634.

Diekstra RFW, Hawton K, eds. Suicide in adolescence. Boston: Martinus Nijhoff Publishers, 1987.

Eisenberg L. Adolescent suicide: on taking arms against a sea of troubles. Pediatrics 1980;66:315.

Gispert M, Wheeler K, Marsh L, et al. Suicidal adolescents: factors in evaluation. Adolescence 1985;20: 753.

Harkavy JM, Asnis G. Suicide attempts in adolescence: prevalence and implications [Letter]. N Engl J Med 1985;313:1290.

Hergenroeder AC, Kastner L, Farrow JA, et al. The pediatrician's role in adolescent suicide. Pediatr Ann 1986;15:787.

Holinger PC, Offer D, Zola MA. A prediction model of suicide among youth. J Nerv Ment Dis 1988;176:275.

Kann L, Warren W, Collins JL, et al. Results from the national school-based 1991 Youth Risk Behavior Survey and progress toward achieving related health objectives for the nation. Public Health Rep 1995;108:47.

Kellerman AL, Rivara FP, Somes G. Suicide in the home in relation to gun ownership. N Engl J Med 1992; 327:467.

Kjelsberg E, Winther M, Dahl AA. Overdose deaths in young substance abusers: accidents or hidden suicides? Acta Psychiatr Scand 1995;91:236.

Lipschitz A. Suicide prevention in young adults (age 18–30). Suicide Life Threat Behav 1995;25:155.

Marks A. Management of the suicidal adolescent on a nonpsychiatric adolescent unit. J Pediatr 1979;95:305.

Morrissey RF, Dicker R, Abikoff H, et al. Hospitalizing the suicidal adolescent: an empirical investigation of decision-making criteria. J Am Acad Child Adolesc Psychiatry 1995;34:902.

Moscicki EK. Epidemiology of suicidal behavior. Suicide Life Threat Behav 1995;25:22.

Murphy GE, Wenzel RD. Family history of suicidal behavior among suicide attempts. J Nerv Ment Dis 1982;170:86.

National Center for Health Statistics. Advance report of final mortality statistics, 1992. Monthly Vital Statistics Report No. 43, 1994.

Neiger BL, Hopkins RW. Adolescent suicide: character traits of high-risk teenagers. Adolescence 1988;23: 469.

Pfeffer C, Normandin L, Kakuma T. Suicidal children grow up: suicidal behavior and psychiatric disorders among relatives. J Am Acad Child Adolesc Psychiatry 1994;33:8.

Phillips DP, Carstensen LL. Clustering of teenage suicides after television news stories about suicide. N Engl J Med 1986;315:685.

Phillips DP, Paight DJ. The impact of televised movies about suicide: a replicative study. N Engl J Med 1987; 317:809.

Rich CL, Young D, Fowler RC. San Diego suicide study. I. Young vs. old subjects. Arch Gen Psychiatry 1986; 43:577.

Riggs S, Alario AJ, McHomey C. Health risk behaviors and attempted suicide in adolescents who report prior maltreatment. J Pediatr 1990;116:815.

Rotheram-Borus MJ. Suicidal behavior and risk factors among runaway youths. Am J Psychiatry 1993;150: 103.

Shaffer D, Gould M, Hicks RC. Worsening suicide rate in black teenagers. Am J Psychiatry 1994;151:1810.

Smith CW Jr, Bope ET. The suicidal patient: the primary care physician's role in evaluation and treatment. Postgrad Med 1986;79:195.

Smith JA, Carter JH. Suicide and black adolescents: a medical dilemma. J Natl Med Assoc 1986;78:1061.

Sudak HS, Ford AB, Rushforth NB. Adolescent suicide: an overview. Am J Psychother 1984;38:350.

Sudak HS, Ford AB, Rushforth NB, eds. Suicide in the young. Boston: John Wright PSG. 1984b.

Swedo SE, Rettew DC, Kuppenheimer M, et al. Can adolescent suicide attemptors be distinguished from at-risk adolescents? Pediatrics 1991;88:620.

White YS. Youth suicide. Med J Aust 1995;163:146.

Woznica J, Shapiro J. An analysis of adolescent suicide attempts: the expendable child. Pediatr Psychol 1990; 15:789.

Young MA, Fogg LF, Scheftner WA, et al. Interactions of risk factors in predicting suicide. Am J Psychiatry 1994;151:434.

CHAPTER 80

School Problems

Howard Schubiner, Arthur L. Robin, and Lawrence S. Neinstein

School problems, including school phobia, truancy, dropout, academic performance problems, attention deficit hyperactivity disorders (ADHD), and learning disabilities, represent common complaints in adolescent medicine clinics. The adolescent's primary care physician can play a critical role in the evaluation and management of such problems by:

1. Evaluating the adolescent for biomedical disorders such as hearing and vision dysfunction, ADHD, subtle mental retardation, and seizure disorders
2. Screening the adolescent for emotional disorders such as depression, anxiety, family conflict, and initiating referrals as necessary
3. Assessing the impacts of chronic illness (or its treatment) on the adolescent and his or her family
4. Assessing the impact of family, school, or community factors on academic performance
5. Initiating and coordinating appropriate referrals for the psychometric testing necessary to determine the presence of learning disabilities, ADHD, and related problems
6. Demystifying learning disabilities, ADHD, and related problems, educating the adolescent and the family about such disabilities, and encouraging the adolescent to develop appropriate attitudes for coping effectively with these disabilities
7. Educating the patient and the family about the legal obligations of the public schools to meet the educational needs of youngsters with disabilities
8. Cooperating with the public schools in determining the eligibility for special education services, which requires physician certification
9. Contributing to the development and coordination of an overall school-based intervention plan and serving as an advocate for the adolescent
10. Providing short-term counseling for milder school and home-related problems and anticipatory guidance to prevent the development of additional complications (e.g., adjustment reactions, parent-teen conflict)
11. Providing medical or drug therapy for ADHD
12. Serving as a case manager with whom the adolescent can periodically "check in" to monitor the overall progress of a coordinated set of medical, school, and psychological services

SCHOOL PHOBIA

School phobia is defined as a persistent and irrational fear of going to school. The problem usually arises either because the adolescent cannot cope with the pressures and challenges at school or as a result of other stresses, typically in the family. Common stress factors include:

1. Fear of undressing in a group
2. Fear of confrontations with teachers

3. Fear of poor grades
4. Fear of being picked first or last for a team or school project
5. Fear of participation in athletics
6. Family dysfunction
7. Fear that peers will criticize (openly or otherwise) their physical appearance
8. Fear of not having enough money
9. Fear of sexual expression
10. Fear of inadequate vocational or academic preparation
11. Fear of individuating or separating from parents

The health-care provider must explore with the adolescent his or her fears and reasons for disliking school. Depending on the home situation the practitioner may recommend more parental involvement and an immediate return to school, or in overrestrictive families the physician may wish to lessen parental involvement by working out a contract regarding school attendance between the physician and the adolescent. Psychological referral may be advisable, depending on the severity and type of underlying problem (e.g., family dysfunction or clinical phobia).

SCHOOL TRUANCY AND DROPOUT

While the adolescent with school phobia has some fear of attending school, the adolescent who is truant or who drops out of school is making a conscious decision to miss school. It is now becoming accepted that school failure is one of the common precursors to truancy and school dropout. And most importantly, school dropout often precedes high-risk social behaviors such as involvement in gangs and violence, running away, sexual promiscuity, and excessive drug or alcohol use. For the clinician who sees adolescent patients, these facts are critical in reinforcing the importance of an educational history that includes academic performance and goals, as well as skipping classes or consideration of dropping out. School dropout is a major problem, particularly among lower socioeconomic classes and can reach as high as 50% in certain school districts, particularly among male students. In addition to the risk behaviors seen in dropouts, they have higher rates of unemployment and lower incomes than high school graduates.

As mentioned, one of the primary causes of truancy and dropout is poor academic performance (and all of its causes, see next section). In addition, truancy and dropout may be caused by pregnancy, marriage, or the need to work to support family members.

Primary prevention of truancy and dropout is the best way to attack this problem. For those at risk for dropping out (e.g., those with early school failure, truancy, high-risk behaviors, poor "fit" within a school system), it will be necessary to work with the adolescent and the family to identify any primary learning disabilities, ADHD, or related conditions, then establish appropriate goals for academic achievement, and define an appropriate placement. In addition, the clinician will need to assess the motivation of the adolescent and family for academic performance, their short- and long-term goals, conflicts at home or at school, relationships with peers and teachers, and medical causes of academic difficulties. This information is necessary to develop a plan to improve performance or resolve barriers to continuing involvement in school. A behavioral plan of rewards and punishments is often needed to re-establish parental control and motivate the adolescent to attend school and complete homework. The adolescent should be involved in the development of this type of plan to attempt to optimize compliance. It is critical to identify and support the academic or extracurricular strengths of an adolescent. Educational options may include work-study programs, vocational programs, independent study programs, early graduation, or adult education programs. Follow-up is essential to determine if the initial plan is working and what further steps may need to be taken.

It should be kept in mind that some of the world's most famous people had difficulties in traditional school settings, so there may be room for optimism (particularly for those who have above-average intelligence). However, the fact remains that the majority of school dropouts have a tough road ahead of them in our present economic milieu.

ACADEMIC PERFORMANCE PROBLEMS

Adolescents who are having difficulty with academic performance constitute a significant group of patients seen in the outpatient setting. During middle school and high school there is an increased need to organize materials, develop appropriate study habits, and use abstract thought processes. Therefore, it is not uncommon for academic problems to arise during these years and in fact may be the presenting issue for an office visit. In addition, there will be a number of students who have never done well in school and now that they are adolescents may have poor academic performance complicated by other health risk behaviors. An interview with a parent is crucial in uncovering academic performance problems, as the adolescent may be less concerned with a drop in grades.

Poor academic performance can be due to a wide variety of causes related to factors within the individual adolescent, the school, the family, and the community. However, it is also common to have multiple factors that coexist and make the evaluation and management more complex. The specific causes of poor academic performance are not always clear. For example, it is commonly believed that substance abuse and membership in a gang are likely causes of school failure. However, it is now believed that academic failure is more likely to precede some of these health risk behaviors, as students gravitate toward other youth who are also failing at school.

Defining and Identifying the Problem

The identification of academic performance problems is a critical step in the evaluation of every adolescent (see Chapter 4 on health screening). This is particularly important in view of the fact that school performance may be an important marker of other health risk behaviors. Therefore, the adolescent's physician should inquire about grades and absences at all routine office visits.

If a potential problem is identified, it is important to clearly define the problem.

1. Who "owns" the problem?
   a. Does the adolescent have concerns about his or her progress?
   b. Are parents concerned with "average" work that may not allow for matriculation into certain colleges?
   c. Have the teachers identified particular issues that should be resolved?
2. What is the specific problem?
   a. Has there been a drop in grades, behavior problems, inconsistent performance, emotional issues, or underachievement for the presumed level of intelligence?

It is necessary to get information from the patient, the family, and the school to understand the nature of the problem and to begin an evaluation.

Causes of Poor Academic Performance

1. Biomedical causes
   a. Hearing or vision problems: Such problems are unlikely to be the primary cause for an adolescent but may contribute to the overall picture.

    b. Mental retardation: Subtle forms of mental retardation may not have been picked up earlier. For example, patients with the fragile X syndrome (or female carriers of this syndrome), Klinefelter's syndrome, Turner's syndrome, XXX chromosome syndrome (females only), tuberous sclerosis, neurofibromatosis, or the fetal alcohol syndrome may not have been formerly diagnosed.

    c. Chronic illness: Patients with severe asthma, cystic fibrosis, diabetes mellitus, sickle cell anemia, juvenile rheumatoid arthritis, epilepsy, congenital heart diseases, or other disorders may have had sufficient absences to cause academic problems. In addition, the side effects of medications may also impair cognitive function to some degree.

    d. Neurological disorders: Certain seizure disorders such as simple generalized or partial complex seizures may be subtle enough to be missed. Borderline forms of cerebral palsy may also present difficulties in early diagnosis. Rarely, progressive neurological diseases such as Wilson's disease or subacute sclerosing panencephalitis may present as cognitive impairment.

2. ADHD: Some adolescents may not have been diagnosed as a child, while others may have been diagnosed but never treated. In particular, females with attention deficit disorder *without* hyperactivity are often not diagnosed.

3. Learning disabilities: Specific learning disabilities are common (occurring in approximately 3–5% of students) usually related to specific problems in reading, spelling, mathematics, or written expression.

4. Psychological and behavioral causes: An adolescent's school performance may be affected by depression, substance abuse, anxiety disorders, conduct disorder, or physical, sexual, or emotional abuse.

5. Family issues: A variety of family problems may affect academic performance, including parental depression, drug or alcohol abuse, and divorce; conflict within the family (parent-teen or parent-parent); or mismatches between parent-adolescent-school expectations for achievement.

6. School and peer relationships: Adolescents who have poor peer relationships or interact with a peer group that does not value academic achievement may present with academic problems. The school may not be able to meet the needs of certain students (e.g., the bright and bored, those with special needs, those who learn in different ways, or those who do not value the educational experience).

7. Cultural or environmental factors: Adolescents who have had a lack of opportunity to achieve adequately, received poor teaching, or had cultural or economic disadvantages that interfere with appropriate education may also present with academic performance problems. Children from ethnic or cultural backgrounds different than the prevailing school norm in which English is not the primary language may also experience difficulty with a standard curriculum. The practitioner should attempt to distinguish such cultural or environmental factors from all of the other previously mentioned causes of academic performance problems.

Evaluation

History   The history is the most important and often the most challenging part of the evaluation to complete. It is necessary to align with the adolescent to let him or her know that your interest is to help the adolescent achieve his or her educational goals, rather than to "take the side of the parents or the school."

1. Interview with the parents
    a. Developmental history

— Pregnancy history (use of drugs, alcohol, medications)
— Perinatal history (prematurity, birth history, sepsis, asphyxia)
— Developmental milestones (for delays in language acquisition, communications skills, other discrete areas)
— Speech, vision, or hearing problems

b. Medical history
— Chronic illnesses such as asthma, otitis media
— Neurological disorders such as head injuries, neurological symptoms
— Hospitalizations
— Family history such as neurological or psychological disorders, ADHD or learning disabilities in the family (a family history of resistance to thyroid hormone is strongly associated with ADHD)

c. Behavioral history
— Peer and family relationships
— Suspected drug or alcohol use
— Psychological symptoms
— Antisocial behaviors
— Symptoms of ADHD (inattention, impulsivity, restlessness)

d. School history (attempt to get similar information from the school)
— History of prior problems
— Behaviors reported in school
— Specific problems (i.e., which classes, which hours, which teachers, missing assignments, missing homework, poor test scores)
— Perceived motivation and goals
— Grades, attendance, suspensions
— Parents' educational level and their expectations for their adolescent
— Prior attempts to improve the situation
— Prior educational or IQ testing

2. Interview with the adolescent
a. School history
— The perspective of the adolescent on the problem or lack thereof
— Assess motivation and goals
— Likes and dislikes about school
— Specific problem areas in school (e.g., homework, tests, assignments, workload, difficulty of the work)
— Factors that prevent academic achievement
— Future plans for employment
— Specific strengths: This is a critical area to identify. If an adolescent has one strong area, you can often build self-esteem by encouraging development in that area while using it as a "hook" to keep the adolescent motivated to stay in school.

b. Medical and behavioral history
— Symptoms of acute or chronic illness
— Drug and alcohol use
— Peer support and influences
— Family conflicts or problems with parents
— Psychological symptoms

3. School records or phone interviews with teachers are helpful to obtain the perspective of the school and to identify the interventions that have been attempted.

Physical Examination

1. Height, weight, and head circumference
2. General inspection
   a. For nutritional status
   b. For minor anomalies (e.g., short palpebral fissures, epicanthal folds, thin upper lip of fetal alcohol syndrome, clinodactyly, wide set eyes, epicanthal folds of XXX syndrome)
3. Mental status for psychological problems
4. Ears, nose, and throat: For otitis, thyroid enlargement
5. Genital: For sexual maturity rating, testicular size (large testes in fragile X syndrome, small testes in Klinefelter's syndrome)
6. Neurological: Neurological examination is indicated when a neurological problem is suspected. This may include testing of cranial nerves, muscle strength and tone, gait, co-ordination, involuntary movements (particularly looking for tics), and reflexes and a sensory examination. Some recommend testing for "soft" neurological signs. These may include reflex asymmetry, strabismus, hyperkineses, co-ordination difficulties, poor fine visual-motor co-ordination, confused laterality, choreiform movements, overflow and mirror movements, and extinction to double simultaneous tactile stimulation. Five percent of normal children display one or two soft signs.

Testing

1. Audiometric testing
2. Visual acuity testing
3. Cognitive ability testing: General intellectual ability test such as the Wechsler Intelligence Scale for Children-III (WISC-III) for up to age 16 and the Wechsler Adult Intelligence Scale-Revised (WAIS-R) for over 16
4. Achievement testing: Woodcock-Johnson Psychoeducational Battery; Wechsler Individual Achievement Test; Kaufman Test of Educational Achievement
5. Learning disability analysis: Compare IQ and achievement tests, looking for significant discrepancies between average IQ and below-average achievement (usually discrepancies of at least two standard deviations). Occasionally, further educational testing of specific reading, mathematics, writing, and language skills must be done following determination that there is a significant discrepancy.
6. Neuropsychological testing: Testing is indicated if there is either an unusual pattern of functioning on IQ or achievement tests that defies a traditional learning disability explanation or if there are indications of neurological problems.
7. ADHD screening: See next section.
8. Psychopathology screening: May ask parent or youth to complete a standardized self-report measure that broadly screens for psychopathology such as the Child Behavior Checklist or the Personality Inventory for Children.
9. Family problems screening: May ask the adolescent or parent to complete a self-report screening measure of family conflict such as the Conflict Behavior Questionnaire.

ATTENTION DEFICIT HYPERACTIVITY DISORDER

ADHD is a developmental disorder affecting approximately 5% of children and adolescents, characterized by developmentally inappropriate degrees of inattention, impulsivity, and hyperactivity. It arises in early childhood, is relatively chronic and pervasive in nature, and is not accounted for on the basis of gross neurological, sensory, language, or motor impairment, mental retardation, or severe emotional disturbance. As a result of these core symptoms, ADHD adolescents have difficulty getting their schoolwork done, organizing their personal lives, resolving disputes and communicating with their parents, following rules established by adult authority figures, and maintaining good peer relationships. Eventually, such cumulative life failure thwarts them from accomplishing the developmental tasks of adolescence, including independence seeking, identity formation, mature same and opposite-sex interpersonal relationships, and vocational planning. As a result, many such adolescents develop low self-esteem and depressed affect.

Contemporary follow-up studies have suggested that ADHD is truly a life span disorder; over 80% of ADHD children continue to manifest the full clinical syndrome in adolescence, and over 50% continue to manifest the full clinical syndrome in adulthood. In adolescence, paying attention and controlling impulses remain the greatest problems, while motoric hyperactivity diminishes or transforms into mental restlessness. Those adolescents with ADHD alone are most likely to exhibit the comorbid difficulties with learning, self-esteem, depression, or other emotional problems, while those with ADHD plus oppositional defiant disorder or conduct disorder are most likely to exhibit the problems with truancy, dropout, substance abuse, and severe family conflict.

Etiology

While the exact cause of ADHD remains unknown, mounting evidence from neurochemical, neurophysiological, genetic, and family studies converges to suggest that in most cases, ADHD is an inherited condition with a biochemical basis involving deficits in the availability of neurotransmitters to the frontal-orbital circuits of the neurobehavioral regulatory systems of the brain. In short, ADHD is a biologically handicapping condition that cannot be "cured," and the goal of treatment is to maximize the quality of the adolescent's daily life and facilitate completion of the developmental tasks of adolescence through flexible combinations of medical, psychosocial, and educational interventions.

Diagnostic Criteria

The fourth edition of the *Diagnostic and Statistical Manual of Mental Disorders* (DSM-IV) includes a list of nine inattention criteria and a list of nine hyperactivity-impulsivity criteria. Subtypes of ADHD are based on various combinations of these lists (1a and 1b), together with criteria 2–5.

1. Either (a) or (b)
   a. Inattention: At least six of the following symptoms of inattention have persisted for at least 6 months to a degree that is maladaptive and inconsistent with developmental level:
      (1) Often fails to give close attention to details or makes careless mistakes in schoolwork, work, or other activities
      (2) Often has difficulty sustaining attention in tasks or play activities
      (3) Often does not seem to listen when spoken to directly
      (4) Often does not follow through on instructions and fails to finish schoolwork, chores, or duties in the workplace (not due to oppositional behavior or failure to understand instructions)
      (5) Often has difficulty organizing tasks and activities
      (6) Often avoids, dislikes, or is reluctant to engage in tasks that require sustained mental effort (such as schoolwork or homework).
      (7) Often loses things necessary for tasks or activities (e.g., toys, school assignments, pencils, book, tools)

(8) Is often easily distracted by extraneous stimuli

(9) Is often forgetful in daily activities

b. Hyperactivity-impulsivity: At least six of the following symptoms of hyperactivity-impulsivity have persisted for at least 6 months to a degree that is maladaptive and inconsistent with developmental level:

— Hyperactivity

(1) Often fidgets with hands or feet or squirms in seat

(2) Often leaves seat in classroom or in other situations in which remaining seated is expected

(3) Often runs about or climbs excessively in situations where it is inappropriate (in adolescents or adults, may be limited to subjective feelings of restlessness)

(4) Often has difficulty playing or engaging in leisure activities quietly

(5) Is often "on the go" or often acts as if "driven by a motor"

(6) Often talks excessively

— Impulsivity

(7) Often blurts out answers before questions have been completed

(8) Often has difficulty awaiting turn

(9) Often interrupts or intrudes on others (e.g., butts into conversations or games)

2. Some symptoms that caused impairment were present since age 6 or 7.

3. Some impairment from the symptoms is present in two or more settings (e.g., at school, work, and at home).

4. There must be clear evidence of clinically significant impairment in social, academic, or occupational functioning.

5. The symptoms do not occur exclusively during the course of a pervasive developmental disorder, schizophrenia, or other psychotic disorder and are not better accounted for by another mental disorder (e.g., mood disorder, anxiety disorder, dissociative disorder, or a personality disorder).

6. DSM-IV subtypes

a. 314.01. ADHD, combined type: If both criteria 1a and 1b are met for the past 6 months

b. 314.00. ADHD, predominantly inattentive type: If criterion 1a is met but criterion 1b is not met for the past 6 months

c. 314.01. ADHD, predominantly hyperactive-impulsive type: if criterion 1b is met but criterion 1a is not met for the past six months

d. 314.09. ADHD, not otherwise specified: If prominent symptoms of inattention or hyperactivity-impulsivity are present that do not meet criteria for ADHD

The DSM-IV criteria capture the core ADHD symptoms of inattention, impulsivity, and restlessness. Practitioners should keep in mind that with adolescents, attention is a broad construct including difficulties activating or getting started with tasks, sustaining concentration, sustaining effort, remaining organized, and making transitions. In addition, it is becoming increasingly evident that impulsivity and restlessness are really parts of a single, broader dimension of impaired delayed responding or behavioral disinhibition.

Associated Features or Comorbidity

1. Oppositional defiant disorder: A pattern of negativistic, hostile, and defiant behavior lasting at least 6 months, involving loss of temper, frequent arguments with adults, refusing to comply with requests, deliberately annoying others, being angry and vindictive, and blaming others for one's own mistakes (Fischer et al., 1993). Fifty-nine percent of ADHD teens have oppositional defiant disorder.

2. Conduct disorder: A repetitive pattern of antisocial behavior violating others' basic rights or societal norms, involving physical aggression, threats, use of weapons, cruelty to people or animals, destruction of property, deceitfulness and theft, repeated running away from home, frequent truancy, or sexual assault. Forty-three percent of ADHD teens have conduct disorder (Fischer et al., 1993). There is sometimes a progression from oppositional defiant disorder to conduct disorder, and from conduct disorder in adolescence to antisocial personality disorder in adulthood.
3. Learning disabilities or academic achievement problems: A significant discrepancy between average to above-average intellectual ability and below-average academic achievement in reading, math, spelling, handwriting, or language, thought to reflect a processing deficit. Between 19% and 26% of ADHD children have learning disabilities in at least one area. Even though most ADHD adolescents do not have learning disabilities, they do consistently show academic achievement problems, with scores on standardized achievement tests lower than matched controls and a greater likelihood of grade retentions, school dropout, or expulsions.
4. Emotional complications: ADHD adolescents often show more symptoms of anxiety, depression, and poor self-esteem but do not consistently show higher rates of formally diagnosed mood or anxiety disorders.
5. Substance abuse: ADHD adolescents show more cigarette and alcohol use than matched controls, with these findings accounted for primarily by the subgroup with comorbidity for conduct disorder.
6. Driving behavior: ADHD adolescents show less sound driving skills or habits than matched control groups, with greater likelihood of accidents, more bodily injuries associated with crashes, and more traffic citations, particularly for speeding. The subgroup with comorbid oppositional defiant disorder or conduct disorder are at the highest risk for such deficient driving skills or habits.
7. Family relations: ADHD adolescents and their parents display more negative, controlling interactions, fewer positive, facilitative interactions, and more conflicts than matched controls. Mothers of ADHD adolescents report more personal psychological distress than mothers of matched controls. The adolescents themselves underestimate the degree of family conflict, compared to their mothers.
8. Other health risk behaviors: Recent findings suggest that an ADHD adolescent may be more likely to have multiple sexual partners and less likely to use contraception.

Epidemiology

1. Prevalence: Five percent to 6% of children between ages 4 and 16. Using Barkley's (1990) follow-up finding that 83% met ADHD criteria in adolescence, we would estimate that 4–5% of adolescents have ADHD.
2. Sex: Male-to-female ratio is 6:1 in clinic samples and 3:1 in community samples.
3. Age: The problem typically starts in early grade school, with an increased prevalence of school and home-based problems in adolescence. Because the transitions to middle and high school entail increased organizational demands, many brighter youngsters or less hyperactive youngsters with ADHD may first become educationally impaired by attentional problems in adolescence, resulting in diagnosis and treatment. For 50–60% of ADHD adolescents, there will be residual impairments into adulthood.

Making a Diagnosis of ADHD: Clinical Guidelines

1. Inclusion criteria: Does the adolescent meet the DSM-IV inclusion criteria for ADHD? Because of performance inconsistency, information from parents, adolescents, and teachers

is required to answer this question. Interview the parents and the adolescent concerning the DSM-IV criteria, and collect rating scales from them.

2. Differential diagnosis: If the adolescent meets the DSM-IV inclusion criteria, can alternative syndromes that look like ADHD be ruled out? Refer for psychological testing to explore learning disabilities, and conduct a thorough interview to address other psychiatric syndromes. Inquire about the major life stressors in the adolescent's history, and examine the temporal covariation between the ADHD symptoms and the major life stressors (e.g., if the onset of the inattentive symptoms are in temporal proximity to a major life stressor, the stressor might explain the symptoms).

3. Rating scales: We find it useful to give the parents, adolescents, and teachers a copy of the DSM-IV criteria and ask them to rate the presence on a four-point Likert scale. In addition, there are many psychometrically sound rating scales to choose from. Use at least one parent and one teacher rating scale, and consider an adolescent self-report scale. Look to see whether the adolescent is rated in the clinical range, usually 1.5 to 2.0 standard deviations above the normative means for non-ADHD teenagers. Our recommendations for rating scales include:

   a. Child Behavior Checklist (parents) and Teacher Report Form (teachers): Comprehensive, well-validated measures assessing attention problems, as well as a broad array of other forms of psychopathology and social competence. Easily computer scored. Look for T scores above 60 on attention scales. Available from University Associates in Psychiatry, One South Prospect Street, Burlington, VT 05401.

   b. Conners' Parent Questionnaire: At present, use the 48-item version, and compute all the factor scores and the hyperactivity index. Look for T scores over 70 on the learning problems factor score as a measure of inattention; the hyperactivity index is an impure mixture of conduct, attention, and emotional problems and will usually be elevated in youngsters who also have substantial repertoires of oppositional behavior. Conners is thoroughly revising and renorming his rating scales at the present time. Available from Multi-Health Systems, Inc., 908 Niagara Falls Boulevard., North Tonawanda, NY 14120; 1-800-456-3003.

   c. Child Attention Profile (Barkley, 1991): Brief, 12-item teacher rating scale that clearly separates inattention from overactivity. Items derived from Achenbach Teacher Report Form. Works well clinically, but published norms do not currently go through high school. Published in Barkley's (1991) workbook.

   d. Brown Attention-Activation Disorder Scale (BAADS): A 40-item self-report measure assessing five components of a broad attention-activation construct:
      (1) Activating and organizing to work
      (2) Sustaining attention and concentration
      (3) Sustaining energy and effort
      (4) Managing affective interference
      (5) Utilizing working memory and accessing recall
      T scores give an indication of how much impairment an adolescent is reporting relative to a nonclinical population. Recently normed; promising measure. Available from The Psychological Corporation, 555 Academic Court, San Antonio, TX 78204-2498; 1-800-228-0752.

   e. Continuous Performance Tests (CPTs): CPTs measure attention and distractibility for research and clinical settings. Respondents are required through the use of a computer program to press a button whenever a specific letter or number appears. The tests are presented in gamelike formats and take between 10 and 30 minutes. In preliminary studies CPTs have been shown to be specific but not particularly sensitive (i.e., positives are usually correct but some false negatives occur). They can be a useful measure to obtain in office settings and can be useful in monitoring drug treatment. Two CPTs to consider are the Gordon Diagnostic System (available from Gordon Systems, P.O. Box 746, DeWitt, NY 13214; 1-315-446-4849) and the Connors' CPT (available from Multi-Health Systems, Inc., 908 Niagara Falls Boulevard, North Tonawanda, NY 14120; 1-800-456-3003).

4. Integrate information from ratings and interview. Make a differential diagnosis and clearly present it to the family and the adolescent.

LEARNING DISABILITIES

Public schools define learning disabilities in accordance with the Individuals with Disabilities Education Act, the recertified version of PL94–142. Specific learning disabilities mean a disorder in one or more of the basic psychological processes involved in understanding or in using language, spoken or written, which may manifest itself in an imperfect ability to listen, think, speak, read, write, spell, or to do mathematical calculations. The term includes such conditions as perceptual handicaps, brain injury, minimal brain dysfunction, dyslexia, and developmental aphasia. The term does not include children who have learning problems which are primarily the result of visual, hearing, or motor handicaps, of mental retardation, of emotional disturbance, or of environmental, cultural, or economic disadvantage.

A cybernetic or information processing model can help us understand how an individual adolescent's learning disability in reading, writing, mathematics, or language is a complex interplay of four stages of cognitive processing:

1. Input: Input disabilities include visual perception problems, auditory perception problems, and sensory integration problems.
2. Integration: Integrative disabilities involve understanding information, sequencing, abstracting, and organizing.
3. Memory: Memory difficulties may involve short- or long-term memory.
4. Output: Output disabilities may involve language or writing problems and motor disabilities.

Educators commonly summarize such information processing disabilities in terms of reading, mathematics, writing, and language disorders. They commonly take the presence of a significant discrepancy between actual achievement and expected achievement for a given adolescent's intellectual ability as evidence of a learning disability. Practically, a discrepancy of two standard deviations between scores on an IQ test and scores on an achievement test is often presumptive evidence of a learning disability. For example, an individual with a full-scale IQ score of 100 with a reading achievement test score of 78 would qualify (assuming these tests have a mean of 100 with a standard deviation of 10).

Reading Disorders

Reading involves (*a*) decoding (the act of transcribing a printed word back into speech) and (*b*) comprehension (the act of interpreting the message or meaning of the text). With dyslexia, the most common reading disorder, the adolescent's decoding skills are impaired, but comprehension is intact. Common clinical indicators of decoding difficulties include guessing at words, having trouble with sound-letter combinations, and making spelling errors involving mispronunciations of words. In addition, dyslexic teens may have trouble sequencing speech into words, syllables, and phonemes, and rearranging sounds into spoken words. If decoding is intact, but comprehension is impaired, this relatively rare reading disability is called hyperlexia. The hyperlexic adolescent can read any text but not understand what has been read; they often also have oral language disabilities.

Math Disorders

The terms *dyscalculia* and *acalculia* are often applied to teenagers with impairment in the ability to do arithmetic computations or develop number and spatial concepts, resulting in math achievement far below that expected for grade and intellectual level. Such youngsters have trouble learning to use number words and facts and difficulty applying math to common life problems. One subgroup of dyscalculic adolescents also have pervasive learning disorders in reading and spelling. However, Rourke (1989) has further identified a second group with low math achievement and poor spatial skills, who have average to superior reading achievement and verbal abilities. IQ testing reveals that these adolescents consistently show high verbal and low performance ability; neuropsychological testing confirms that their verbal abilities are intact, but their spatial abilities are deficient. Rourke has labeled such a pattern a "nonverbal learning disability," and extensively studied its assessment, prognosis, and treatment.

Writing Disorder

The term *writing disorder* refers to difficulty with spelling and other linguistic aspects of writing, such as composing and punctuating sentences and organizing cohesive paragraphs; it does not refer to difficulties with handwriting. Since writing disorders often coexist with reading disorders, dyslexic adolescents should also always be evaluated for a possible writing disorder. The adolescent with a writing disorder is capable of formulating complex thoughts but because of difficulties with spelling is unable to express them in writing at the level expected for his or her intellectual ability. Paragraphs will be poorly organized; sentences will be short with abrupt endings; and expository writing will read more like a list of answers to test questions than a fluent essay. Writing disorders become particularly debilitating in high school and college, when there are increased demands for written expression.

Management of Learning and Achievement Problems

1. Legal responsibilities of the public schools
   Children with disabilities are guaranteed a free and appropriate education by three federal laws:
   a. Individuals with Disabilities Education Act (IDEA): IDEA is the basic special education act that outlines that schools are obligated to conduct multidisciplinary evaluations for adolescents suspected of having a handicapping condition, and if the handicap is confirmed, provide special education interventions. These interventions are encoded in an individual education program (IEP) written at a team meeting including the parents. This law outlines specific types of disabilities such as learning disabilities, emotional impairment, mental impairment, and other health impairments. Recently, the other health impairment category has been interpreted as covering ADHD children with educational handicaps. IDEA has a funding stream associated with it at the local, state, and federal levels.
   b. Section 504 of the Rehabilitation of the Handicapped Law: Section 504 is a civil rights law that outlaws discrimination against handicapped individuals in federally funded programs in education and the workplace and requires schools to make reasonable accommodations to educate handicapped individuals. Any condition that interferes with a major life function such as learning may be considered such a handicap; ADHD has recently been interpreted as a handicap under Section 504. Children suspected of having a handicap must be evaluated, and if the handicap is confirmed,

reasonable accommodations are typically made first in regular education. Section 504 has no funding stream associated with it.

c. Americans with Disabilities Act: This law basically extends the protections of Section 504 to the private sector and therefore may apply to older adolescents who are working.

Also specific state laws and local policies within school districts elaborate on the federal laws. Most state education departments provide free manuals to professionals and parents explaining special education procedures. Primary care physicians should become familiar with these laws, inform parents about them, and encourage parents of adolescents suspected of having handicapping conditions to make verbal and written requests for school-based evaluations and interventions. Although an exhaustive account of educational interventions is not possible in this chapter, we will summarize a few of the most common accommodations helpful to adolescents with ADHD and learning disabilities.

ACCOMMODATIONS

Failure to complete or hand in assignments on time is a major deficit of ADHD and learning disabled teenagers. Accommodations for youth with ADHD include:

1. Modifying lesson presentation: This will make it easier for the inattentive youngster to remain on task and complete assignments. It often involves breaking lessons into short segments, frequently monitoring on-task behavior, redirecting the adolescent to the task if the adolescent's attention wanders, and providing frequent positive feedback for successful task completion. When a paper is assigned to be due in 1 month, for example, the teacher might construct intermediate steps to monitor the adolescent: (*a*) hand in a reference list; (*b*) hand in notes; (*c*) hand-in a first draft.
2. Adjusting testing procedures: Adjusting testing procedures by permitting extended time to complete examinations, providing a quiet environment, or administering oral tests is also commonly employed.
3. Organizational assistance: This may take the form of note-taking training, assignment sheets, a second set of textbooks at home, checks to make sure students have the materials they need to complete assignments, and monitoring of handing in assignments.
4. Computers: Students with writing disorders often benefit from an early emphasis on computers, using word processors in school to complete examinations and weekend assignments.
5. Weekly home or school progress reports: Co-ordinating weekly home or school progress reports, with home-based incentives for positive teacher ratings, motivates task completion and cements teacher-parent communication.

Special Education

A continuum of alternative placements for students certified as learning disabled or otherwise health impaired includes resource rooms, separate self-contained rooms, separate schools, residential placements, and even home-bound instruction. Placement is usually in the least restrictive environment to best prepare the disabled individual to live in a society with nondisabled individuals. Instructional procedures for reading, mathematics, and writing disabilities rely heavily on contemporary cognitive and developmental psychology and emphasize selecting alternative teaching methods that help the learner bypass his or her area of disability.

MANAGEMENT OF ATTENTION DEFICIT HYPERACTIVITY DISORDER

Management of ADHD usually requires a comprehensive plan that includes the adolescent in the decision-making process. A treatment plan that allows the adolescent to participate in setting goals and developing strategies is more likely to succeed. Many adolescents with ADHD have had major conflicts with their parents, and often the treatment plan includes negotiating around that conflict and helping the parents and adolescent work toward common goals. As described earlier in the chapter, many adolescents with ADHD have comorbid conditions, which should be considered in the treatment plan.

The principles of management of ADHD include education, medication, home interventions, counseling, school interventions (see above), and advocacy.

Education

Education about ADHD should be provided for the adolescent (as mentioned above), for the parents and family, often for the school, and even for the friends of the adolescent. A wide array of useful pamphlets, books, and videos is available from the ADD Warehouse (1-800-233-9273). However, it is critical to take some time to explain some of the basics in person to make sure the teenager has a clear understanding of the condition. This begins with the process of informing the adolescent and the parents of the diagnosis. It is common for adolescents to have some resistance to this diagnosis, as it may be regarded as a "psychological problem" that makes them feel different from their peers. It is important to explain the diagnosis fully and carefully to the adolescent and the parents. Blame for the condition can be deflected by describing the genetic origin and neurochemical nature of the disorder, which may make ADHD seem more acceptable to the family and adolescent.

Adolescents must know that there is hope for improved academic performance. This is important, as adolescents with ADHD often have low self-esteem due to their poor grades, frequently hearing "they could do better if they only tried," and seeing reports of "not living up to potential." If physicians take a small amount of time at each visit to offer some education about ADHD to the adolescent, they will find that the adolescent is more likely to accept the diagnosis and begin to understand why he or she may act in certain ways. This is the first step in the development of insight, which can play a crucial role in allowing the adolescent to consciously alter his or her behaviors. A useful analogy in explaining ADHD is that of poor eyesight. Poor eyesight is hereditary and not someone's "fault." It causes one to have difficulty "focusing" and therefore may cause problems in school and in overall functioning. Simple interventions, such as wearing glasses, can help one see clearly and improve academic and overall performance. ADHD is a "biochemical" problem that is inherited and causes difficulty in focusing and thinking clearly. Medical and behavioral interventions can help the person function better. If adolescents understand this line of reasoning, they will have an easier time in accepting the diagnosis and therapy. In addition, they may be less likely to feel some of the stigma that may be attached to the diagnosis.

Medication

Medication should not generally be the only treatment received by the adolescent, but it is frequently the cornerstone of treatment for ADHD, as when it is successful, it appears to correct the underlying disorder in the brain. Since about three-quarters of adolescents respond to medical therapy, a medication trial should be undertaken for almost all adolescents diagnosed with ADHD.

Stimulants   The stimulants are considered the first-line agents, as they appear to be the most effective and safe agents. They have been shown to be effective in aiding the core symptoms of ADHD. Recent studies have also shown that social interactions and academic productivity are also improved. Studies specifically looking at the response of adolescents to stimulants do not show as dramatic results as those in children, possibly due to some of the influences faced by adolescents.

Methylphenidate

DOSES   Methylphenidate (Ritalin) is used most frequently and should be started at low doses before building up to the optimal dose. The dosage range is usually from 5 to 30 mg per dose given at intervals of approximately 4 hours (a typical titration method is to start with 5 mg and increase by 5-mg doses at weekly intervals to 20-mg doses, checking weekly by telephone for positive effects and side effects). The onset of action is about 30 minutes. Doses are usually given in the morning and before lunch on school days; however, it should be recognized that ADHD affects the whole social fabric of an adolescent such as their sports performance, their relationship with friends and family, their risk for injury (from their potential inattentive or impulsive actions while bicycling, skateboarding, rollerblading, boating, or driving), and their decisions about lifestyle risks (e.g., impulsive use of drugs or alcohol). Therefore, as they mature, it makes sense to negotiate a treatment plan that considers coverage by medication throughout the day and on weekends. This is especially important for those adolescents who experience irritability when the dose "wears off." Tolerance rarely develops, and drug "holidays" are not usually required (with the exception of those few adolescents who begin to decrease their growth velocity).

SIDE EFFECTS   Serious side effects (and the relative contraindications to use) include:

1. Elevated blood pressure
2. Arrhythmias (particularly when used in association with alcohol, caffeine, or sympathomimetics)
3. Development of psychosis or tics

Patients who develop tics may have underlying Tourette syndrome (a comorbid feature of ADHD in 2–5%), and these patients should be managed in conjunction with a neurologist. When systematic observation for tics are undertaken, they are observed more frequently but usually resolve with a decrease in dosage or discontinuation of the medication.

Minor side effects of methylphenidate include:

1. Weight loss (usually mild)
2. Headaches
3. Abdominal pain
4. Dizziness
5. Dry eyes or mouth
6. Sweating
7. Irritability
8. Insomnia: Insomnia may occur if the medication is taken too late in the evening, although many patients seem to have an easier time in falling asleep while taking stimulants.

When a dosage trial is undertaken, persistent symptoms of nervousness or jitteriness and feeling "spaced out" or "overfocused" are indications that the dose is too high. Suppression of growth is rarely a problem in adolescents (especially those receiving lower doses) but should be monitored. It has been shown that ultimate height is not compromised. Finally, some patients develop symptoms of irritability and acting out when the dose of methylphenidate is wearing off. These patients should be given doses at 3 or $3\frac{1}{2}$ hours or be switched to a longer acting preparation.

Long-Acting Stimulant Medications   Longer acting stimulant medications include sustained release methylphenidate (Ritalin SR), dextroamphetamine (Dexedrine) spansules, pemoline (Cylert), and Adderall (a combination of amphetamine and dextroamphetamine).

Sustained-release methylphenidate can be useful, as its duration of action is about 6–8 hours and can be given once or twice daily. However, it only comes in a 20-mg preparation and is often not as effective as the short-acting tablet. It can be helpful for patients who require only small doses or those who experience too many "ups and downs" with the short-acting methylphenidate. Some clinicians have used both short-acting and sustained-release methylphenidate together as one would use regular and Lente insulin.

Dextroamphetamine (Spansules)   Dextroamphetamine is a much more effective long-acting preparation and is also tolerated quite well (often with less side effects than methylphenidate). It comes in 5-mg, 10-mg, and 15-mg spansules and is generally considered to be twice as potent as methylphenidate on a milligram per milligram basis. Therefore, few patients require more than 15–20 mg b.i.d. The side effect profile is similar to methylphenidate. Some clinicians feel that dextroamphetamine is more likely to be abused than is methylphenidate, and reports of abuse of methylphenidate are now common. Adolescents taking stimulants should be warned of the dangers of providing these agents to others. Recently, Adderall has been introduced as a long-acting stimulant. Although there is sparse evidence to date of its effectiveness, it appears to be effective and is used in a similar way to dextroamphetamine.

Pemoline   Pemoline is a long-acting stimulant with a different mechanism of action from those mentioned above. It comes in 18.75-mg, 37.5-mg, and 75-mg capsules. It is usually taken once a day, and the maximum daily dose is 2–3 mg/kg. Due to reports of liver toxicity, liver function tests must be monitored on a regular basis (every 3–6 months). It has the advantages of very low abuse potential and no cardiovascular side effects.

Tricyclic Antidepressants   Tricyclic antidepressants are generally considered to be second-line agents in the medical treatment of ADHD but have been shown to be effective in approximately three-quarters of patients in recent studies. They may be the medication of choice for patients who do not tolerate stimulants (generally each of the stimulants should be tried before making this determination), for those who have coexistent depression or enuresis or in whom a tic disorder has developed. Imipramine (Tofranil), desipramine (Norpramin), and nortriptyline (Pamelor) have been used successfully. A trial of 4–6 weeks at adequate doses should be attempted (blood levels are useful to confirm this as children often metabolize tricyclics faster than do adults), and ECG monitoring should be done initially to look for cardiac toxicity (heart rate >130 bpm, PR interval >0.20 seconds, QRS duration >0.12 seconds, QT_c >0.45 seconds). Relative contraindications include a history of cardiac arrythmias, heart disease, syncope, or family history of sudden death. Side effects include drowsiness, dry mouth, constipation, nausea, sweating, tremor, and postural hypotension. Rarely, neurological side effects such as seizures, an acute organic brain syndrome, and hypomania can occur. The daily dosage is approximately 3–5 mg/kg of imipramine and desipramine (and 1.5–2 mg/kg of nortriptyline). Toxicity is more likely to occur at the higher dosage ranges.

Clonidine   Clonidine (Catapres) is a central-acting α_2-agonist that has been shown to be effective for ADHD as well. It is particularly useful in the evening to help with insomnia and for patients with coexistent tic disorders. Some clinicians also use clonidine to treat aggressiveness. Carbamazepine (Tegretol) and molindone (Moban) have also been tried for such youth. Clonidine comes in tablets of 0.1 mg, 0.2 mg, and 0.3 mg, as well as skin patches of similar strengths. The tablets are taken two to three times a day (or at night only for insomnia) starting with 0.05 or 0.1 mg. The patch delivers the medication for 1 week (and can be divided to deliver smaller doses). A long-acting agent, guanfacine (Tenex), has also recently been shown to be effective.

Other Medications   Other medications that have been tried include antidepressants such as fluoxetine (Prozac) and other serotonin reuptake inhibitors, venlaflaxine (Effexor), bupropion (Wellbutrin), and β-adrenergic inhibitors such as nadolol (Corgard). Antidepressants and clonidine can be used in combination with the stimulants.

Behavioral or Psychological Interventions

While medical therapy may be effective in improving the ADHD symptoms, there are often a variety of other issues (such as conduct disorder, oppositional defiant disorder, poor self-esteem, family conflict, depression, anxiety disorders, and the use or abuse of alcohol and other drugs) that require attention. If the initial evaluation reveals a significant substance use disorder, the clinician should refer the adolescent for a substance abuse workup or treatment before undertaking any additional intervention. The presence of oppositional behavior, family conflict, peer relationship difficulties, depression, or anxiety is an indication to refer the family for behavioral or psychological interventions. The most common behavioral or psychological interventions include family therapy, individual therapy, and social skills training. It is often useful for families with newly diagnosed ADHD adolescents to have a burst of 10–15 sessions of behavioral or psychological intervention, followed by less frequent checkups. If new problems surface during a follow-up checkup, another burst of therapy may be scheduled. Individual therapy is usually helpful in building self-esteem and reducing anxiety but does not reliably result in behavior change in the classroom or at home.

Family therapy is the treatment of choice for the home-based problems and conflicts between ADHD teenagers and their parents. Early in treatment the therapist divides the family issues into two categories: (*a*) non-negotiable issues (basic rules for living in a family, e.g., no violence, drugs, alcohol) and (*b*) negotiable issues (all other independence-related conflicts, which may be subject to negotiation and compromise). Strategic structural intervention techniques are used to reinforce parental authority around the nonnegotiable issues (i.e., the therapist teaches the parents how to establish and consistently follow behavioral contracts for these basic rules). External authorities such as the juvenile justice system or mental health inpatient system are used to back up parents when they no longer have the ability to exert any control over the adolescents.

In the case of issues that can be negotiated between parents and adolescents, problem-solving communication training is used to teach parents and adolescents to work out mutually acceptable compromise solutions. The therapist instructs, models, and coaches the family to learn and practice the steps of problem solving: (*a*) clearly define the problem in a nonaccusatory fashion; (*b*) brainstorm a list of alternative solutions; (*c*) systematically evaluate the positive or negative impacts of each solution, culminating in a mutually acceptable compromise solution; and (*d*) plan the details for implementing the solution. The family resolves a number of significant conflicts with the therapist present as a coach and then is given successively more complex assignments to apply problem-solving skills at home in weekly family meetings.

As the family begins to practice problem-solving skills in the sessions and at home, the therapist targets negative communication patterns, again coaching families to replace accusatory, defensive language with more productive, goal-oriented language. In a recent study, Barkley and his colleagues (1993) compared the effectiveness of problem-solving communication training, parent contingency management, and structural family therapy for ameliorating conflict between ADHD adolescents and their parents. They found that all three treatments proved equally effective, but only 25–33% of the families reported clinically significant change (compared to much higher rates in children), indicating we have a long way to go in improving such treatment programs.

As part of an overall family intervention, it is also useful to teach parents the effective use of behavior modification techniques, as Barkley (1990) did in his parent contingency management condition. These techniques are crucial for parents of ADHD adolescents to help them teach their children to stay motivated to complete homework assignments and household chores. Setting up explicit rewards for appropriate activities and punishments for pro scribed activities is a cornerstone of behavioral management. Clinicians can help parents with home interventions by offering advice on how to carry out simple behavioral contracts.

SUMMARY

In summary, clinicians can best help adolescents with ADHD and learning disabilities by encouraging them, believing that they can succeed, helping them to understand their disorder and how it affects them, mediating conflict between them and their parents, finding the optimal medication regimen (if appropriate), and helping them obtain the services they require through their school system.

BIBLIOGRAPHY

Achenbach T. Manual for the child behavior checklist and revised child behavior profile. Burlington, Vermont: TM Achenbach, 1991.

Ahmann PA, Waltonen SJ, Olson KA, et al. Placebo-controlled evaluation of Ritalin side effects. Pediatrics 1993;91:6.

Ambrosini PJ, Bianchi MD, Rabinovich H, et al. Antidepressant treatments in children and adolescents. II. Anxiety, physical, and behavioral disorders. J Am Acad Child Adolesc Psychiatry 1993;32:3.

American Psychiatric Association. The diagnostic and statistical manual of mental disorders, 4th ed. Washington DC: American Psychiatric Association, 1994.

Barkley R. Attention deficit hyperactivity disorder: a handbook for diagnosis and treatment. New York: Guilford Press, 1990.

Barkley R. Attention deficit hyperactivity disorder: a clinical workbook. New York: Guilford Press, 1991.

Barkley RA, Guevremont DC, Anastopoulos AD, et al. Driving-related risks and outcomes of attention deficit hyperactivity disorder in adolescents and young adults: a 3- to 5-year follow-up survey. Pediatrics 1993;92:2.

Biederman J, Baldessarini RJ, Goldblatt A, et al. A naturalistic study of 24-hour electrocardiographic recordings and echocardiographic findings in children and adolescents treated with Desipramine. J Am Acad Child Adolesc Psychiatry 1993;32(4): 805–813.

Biederman J, Baldessarini RJ, Wright V, et al. A double-blind placebo controlled study of Desipramine in the treatment of ADD. 1. Efficacy. J Am Acad Child Adolesc Psychiatry 1989;28(5):777–784.

Carlson GA, Ranade L, Qadir A. Management of psychopharmacologic agents in children and adolescents. Psychiatr Q 1992;63:4.

Conners CK, Wells KC. ADD-H adolescent self-report scale. Psychopharmacol Bull 1985;21:921–922.

DePaul GJ, Stoner G. ADHD in the schools: assessment and intervention strategies. New York: Guilford Press, 1994.

Dodick D, Adler CH. Tourette's syndrome: current approaches to recognition and management. Postgrad Med 1992;92:5.

Dworkin PH. School failure. Pediatr Rev 1989;10:10.

Faigel HC, Sznajderman S, Tishby O, et al. Attention deficit disorder during adolescence: a review. J Adol Health 1995;16:174–184.

Fischer M, Barkley RA, Fletcher K, et al. The adolescent outcome of hyperactive children: predictors of psychiatric, academic, social, and emotional adjustment. J Am Acad Child Adolesc Psychiatry 1993; 32:2.

Gadow KD, Sverd J, Sprafkin J, et al. Efficacy of methylphenidate for attention-deficit hyperactivity disorder in children with tic disorder. Arch Gen Psychiatry 1995;52:444–455.

Goyette CH, Conners CK, Ulrich RF. Normative data on revised Conners parent and teacher rating scales. J Abnorm Child Psychol 1978;6:221–236.

Illingworth, R. Early failure of the famous. Pediatrician 1986;13:70–73.

Kalscheur JA. Benefits of the Americans With Disabilities Act of 1990 for children and adolescents with disabilities. Am J Occup Ther 1992;46:5.

Kelly DP, Aylward GP. Attention deficits in school-aged children and adolescents. Pediatr Clin North Am 1992;39:3.

Klein RG. Prognosis of attention deficit disorder and its management in adolescence. Pediatr Rev 1987;8: 216.

Klein RG. Clinical efficacy of methylphenidate in children and adolescents. L'Encephale 1993;19:89–93.

Landman GB. Preventing school failure: the physician as child advocate. Pediatr Clin North Am 1986;33:4.

Levy HB, Harper CR, Weinberg WA. A practical approach to children failing in school. Pediatr Clin North Am 1992;39:4.

Lipkin PH, Goldstein IJ, Adesman AR. Tics and dyskinesias associated with stimulant treatment in attention-deficit hyperactivity disorder. Arch Pediatr Adolesc Med 1994;August:148.

Reiff MI, Banez GA, Culbert TP. Children who have attentional disorders: diagnosis and evaluation. Pediatr Rev 1993;14:12.

Robin AL. Training families with ADHD adolescents. In: Barkley R, ed. Attention deficit hyperactivity disorder: a handbook for diagnosis and treatment. New York: Guilford Press, 1990:462–497

Robin AL. ADHD in adolescence: the next step [Educational videotape]. Worcester, Massachusetts: Practice Development Workshops, 1993.

Robin AL, Foster SL. Negotiating parent-adolescent conflict: a behavioral family systems perspective. New York: Guilford Press, 1989.

Rourke BP. Nonverbal learning disabilities. New York: Guilford Press, 1989.

Rubenstein JS, Hastings EM. School refusal in adolescence: understanding the symptom. Adolescence 1980;15:775.

Silver L (ed.) Learning disabilities. Child Adolesc Psychiatr Clin North Am 1993;April:2.

Spencer T, Biederman J, Wilens T. Tricyclic antidepressant treatment of children with ADHD and tic disorders. J Am Acad Child Adolesc Psychiatry 1994;33:8.

Steingard R, Biederman J, Spencer T, et al. Comparison of clonidine response in the treatment of attention-deficit hyperactivity disorder with and without comorbid tic disorders. J Am Acad Child Adolesc Psychiatry 1993;32(2):350–353.

Weiss G, Hechtman L. Hyperactrive children grown up, 2nd ed. New York: Guilford Press, 1993.

Wilens TE, Biederman J, Geist DE, et al. Nortriptyline in the treatment of ADHD: a chart review of 58 cases. J Am Acad Child Adolesc Psychiatry 1993;32:3.

Wilens TE, Biederman J, Spencer T. Clonidine for sleep disturbances with attention-deficit hyperactivity disorder. J Am Acad Child Adolesc Psychiatry 1994;33:3.

Wilens TE, Spencer T, Biederman J, et al. Combined pharmacotherapy: an emerging trend in pediatric psychopharmacology. J Am Acad Child Adolesc Psychiatry 1995;34:1.

Youngs BB. School phobia. Medical Aspects of Human Sexuality 1983;17:244.

CHAPTER 81
Rape and Sexual Abuse

Lawrence S. Neinstein, Maria A. Juliani, Joan Shapiro, and Curren Warf

RAPE

Rape is defined as sexual intercourse involving force or the threat of force without a person's consent; or as sexual intercourse involving a person incapable of giving consent due to mental illness, intoxication, and so forth. The act of being raped is one of the most devastating encounters a person can experience. The victim, most often a female, is the object of a hostile, dehumanizing attack that may have long-lasting effects on the victim's self-worth and identity. This is especially true for the adolescent who is still dealing with the issues of separation, independence, and the development of sexual identity. Rape, as a first or early sexual experience, may jeopardize future sexual adjustment. Attempted sexual assaults may be deeply traumatizing for young people as well.

Rape is a serious medical and psychological emergency. Any physician willing to devote the time and support needed can examine the rape victim. It bears emphasizing here that the future psychological impact of the rape will likely depend more on the care and attitudes of the treatment team, police, and family than on the physical act of rape itself.

There are three main categories of rape that vary in relationship to the perpetrator.

1. Stranger rape: Stranger rape is the most traumatizing and most likely to be associated with other injuries, use of a weapon, or threat to life. This is the least common category, but the most highly associated with grave medical and psychological consequences.
2. Acquaintance rape: Acquaintance rape may be extremely confusing to the young woman and, though less likely to be associated with serious physical injury, may be associated with a great deal of self-blame and guilt. This is the most common type of sexual assault.
3. Statutory rape: Statutory rape is a legal category that encompasses unlawful sexual activity between a minor female under the age of 18 and a male over the age of 18 that is activity that is unlawful only because of the age or status of those involved. Rape in this instance is something of a misnomer in that no assault or lack of consent is implied. In most states it is not reportable.

Legal Issues

State codes vary in requirements of physicians reporting responsibilities. In general, rape cases occurring within 72 hours in which evidence is gathered or medical treatment provided must be reported. It is important for practitioners to become familiar with local laws. Usually in cases of rape, the patient may limit his or her consent to a confidential report that includes only the victim's name, address, type of crime, and extent of injuries. The victim usually also has the option to consent to the collection of evidence, in which case a full report and specimens are released to the police.

The physician's legal responsibility is limited to examination, treatment, and reporting of the case. It is not the physician's responsibility to determine whether an assault occurred; that is a legal decision. The physician can help legal authorities most by keeping accurate and thorough medical records.

Epidemiology of Forcible Rape

1. Incidence
   a. In 1960, 9.6 rapes per 100,000 U.S. population were reported.
   b. In 1977, 29.1 rapes per 100,000 U.S. population, or 63,000 rapes, were reported. Of these, 74% were completed rapes, and 26% were attempted rapes.
   c. In 1986, 37.5 rapes per 100,000 U.S. population were reported. Rate for females is 73 per 100,000 reported rapes.
   d. In 1991, 42.3 rapes per 100,000 U.S. population were reported. Rate for females is 83 per 100,000 reported rapes.
   e. In the National Adolescent Student Health Survey (American School Health Association et al., 1989), 12% of 8th and 10th graders reported that someone raped or tried to rape them outside of a school. Eighteen percent reported that during the past year, someone tried to force them to have sex against their wishes.
   f. In a national sample of college students (DeKeseredy, 1988), 54% of women reported some form of sexual victimization.
2. Reportability: Unreported cases range from an estimated 39% to as high as 90% of all rapes in the United States. Reasons for not reporting include fear of stigmatization by family and friends, fear of being blamed, desire to protect perpetrator (if he is friend, boyfriend, or family member), and fear of retaliation by perpetrator or perpetrator's friends.
3. Arrests: Fifty percent of reported cases of rape in the United States lead to arrests.
4. Convictions: Two-thirds of those arrested and booked for rape are prosecuted, and 47% of those prosecuted are found guilty. Thus, for every 100 reported cases of rape, there are 16 convictions. In 1991, 13.3% of closed rape cases involved victims under 18 years old.
5. Demographic characteristics
   a. Age
      — Rapist: The most common age in the United States is 16–20 years of age; 40% of rapists fall into this age range. Twenty-six percent of rapists are 20–24 years of age.
      — Victim: Fifty percent of victims are less than 18 years old. Peak age for victimization is age 16–19.
   b. Sex
      — Rapist: Eighty-one percent of rapists are male, and 19% are female.
      — Victim: Ninety-six percent of victims are female, and 4% are male.
   c. Victim-offender relations: The rapist has been variously reported to be a total stranger 36–91% of the time (average is 50%). The remaining cases are between acquaintances or family members. It is important to remember that victims often underreport offenses in direct relationship to the degree of acquaintance with the rapist.
   d. Other risk factors: Irwin et al. (1995) reported that young women who had been raped in an urban community had a higher prevalence of a recent sexually transmitted disease (STD) and have other human immunodeficiency virus (HIV) risk behavior. Rape was not independently associated with HIV, syphilis, or herpes simplex virus 2 (HSV-2) infections.
6. Temporal distribution: The incidence of reported rapes is higher during the summer months, on weekends, and from the hours of 8:00 PM to 2:00 AM.

7. Resistance: Zoucha-Jansen et al. (1993) found that forceful verbal resistance, physical resistance, and fleeing were all associated with rape avoidance, whereas nonforceful verbal resistance and no resistance were associated with being raped. Injury rates were no higher in women who used forceful resistance.

Myths and Realities

Myth	*Fact*
Rape is a sexual act.	Rape is a violent assault acted out sexually. It violates a victim's sense of integrity and control.
Rape is a nonviolent crime.	Rape is a violent crime. Eighty-seven percent of rapists carry a weapon or threaten violence against the victim.
Women ask for rape.	Rapists look for available, vulnerable targets, not sexily dressed young females. No person asks to be hurt or degraded.
Rapists are easy to spot.	Most rapists appear normal. Most are young and married.
Most rapes are a "spur of the moment" act occurring in a dark alley by a stranger.	Most rapes are planned; 50% are committed by an acquaintance. Fifty-seven percent occur in the victim's or rapist's house.
Rape only happens to young women.	Rape occurs at all ages and in both sexes. The range reported is 4 months to 92 years of age.
Most rapes are interracial.	Most rapes involve persons of the same race or culture.
It is impossible to really rape a nonconsenting adult female.	It is possible to rape a nonconsenting adult female. An erect penis can penetrate any oral, genital, or anal opening.

Effects of Rape

Rape is a terrifying experience for the adolescent, with the threat of injury or death often present. The rape often disrupts the adolescent's sense of equilibrium and growing sense of identity. In the aftermath of being raped, an adolescent may act in a bizarre or inappropriate manner; for example, he or she may be aggressive or withdrawn. Several stages of emotional responses, called the *rape trauma syndrome* (Burgess and Holstrom, 1974), have been observed in rape victims:

1. Early acute stage
   a. Disorientation is characterized by shock, terror, and disruption of behavior.
   b. Victim may act hysterical or stoical.
   c. Insomnia, anorexia, and vomiting are common.
2. Second stage (lasts days to weeks)
   a. Victim seems to adjust to normal life.
   b. Denial and suppression are common.
   c. Mistrust of men (by female victims) and friends is common.
   d. Adolescents often withdraw from their peer group.
3. Third stage
   a. Mild to serious depression often occurs.
   b. Slow integration of rape experience into victim's self-image.

Common postrape feelings include:

1. Fear
   a. Fear of being alone
   b. Fear of crowds
   c. Fear of the rapist returning
   d. Global fear
   e. Fear of men (by female victims)
   f. Fear of others finding out
2. Powerlessness, helplessness, loss of control
   a. A feeling that privacy and right to choose have been taken away
   b. A feeling of inability to change the situation or to stop crying
3. Guilt
   a. Guilt for "causing" the rape
   b. Guilt for not fighting back
   c. Guilt "for being stupid and getting into that situation"
4. Shame, embarrassment
   a. Feeling dirty
   b. Feeling judged
5. Anger
   a. Anger at the rapist
   b. Anger at oneself
6. Wanting to forget
7. Disruption of normal sex life
8. Depression

Special Considerations for Adolescent Victims and Their Families   Data are scarce on particular concerns of adolescent rape victims. Table 81.1 outlines concerns of 122 sexually abused adolescents and their families, as reported in a study by Mann (1981). In this study, the impact of the rape was severe in 80% of parents and only 37% of the adolescents. Although a majority of teenagers expressed concern about bodily safety, guilt, and peer relations, parents were more often concerned with retaliation, sexual aspects, and future problems. Eighty percent of the adolescents in the study experienced problems with their parents after the rape, whereas only 20% of adolescents found their parents supportive and understanding. Twenty-five percent of adolescents felt their parents overreacted; 24% found their parents overprotective; and 24% felt rejected by their parents.

Peipert and Domalgalski (1994) compared adolescent rape victims with victims over 20 years of age. Adolescent victims were more likely to be assaulted by an acquaintance or rela-

TABLE 81.1.   Concerns of 122 Sexually Abused Adolescents and Their Families

Concern	Victims (%)	Parents (%)
Fear of safety	65	50
Self-blame, shame	59	17
Irrational bodily fears (of infertility, abnormal genital development)	45	67
Fear of pregnancy	48	79
Anger at assailant	45	67
Fear of venereal disease	34	52
Fear of future sexuality	21	66
Anger at victim	0	41

Data adapted from Mann EB. Self-reported stresses of adolescent rape victims. J Adolesc Health Care 1981;2:29.

tive (77% versus 56%) and to delay medical evaluation. Cunningham et al. (1994) found that a history of physical abuse, sexual abuse, or rape is related to engaging in a variety of HIV risk behaviors, with an increase in these behaviors between adolescence and young adulthood.

Commonly, teenage girls and their parents are concerned about what a sexual assault means regarding their state of virginity. In some cultural groups this may have tremendous significance, and the young woman may be further victimized by being viewed as "spoiled goods" and have great anxiety about her ability to marry. It is important to state that being victimized by sexual assault does not affect the state of virginity, and that rape is a violent act, not a sexual one.

Special Considerations for Mental Retardation Victims   Furey et al. (1994) examined sexual abuse in the mentally retarded population. Most of the victims were women (72%) who mostly had no problems communicating verbally and few secondary disabilities. The majority of the perpetrators were men (88%) and included other individuals with mental retardation, paid staff, family members, and others. Most sexual abuse occurred in the victim's residence, and in 92% the victim knew the abuser.

Special Considerations for Male Victims   Male adolescents who have been sexually abused are probably the least reported and least studied group of abused victims. Most studies are weighted toward younger children or females. However, as reported by Deisher and Bidwell (1987), male sexual abuse is not uncommon and is significantly underreported. Males may be embarrassed by the homosexual aspect of an assault and by disclosure of such details. In addition, practitioners may fail to recognize and pursue this possibility because of their lack of awareness of this problem.

There are no precise epidemiological data. Finkelhor (1984) estimated that there is about one abused male for every two abused females. In large studies of sexual abuse, male victims have composed 8–14% of the total abused individuals. Spencer and Dunklee (1986) evaluated males in the San Diego program and found that males composed 11% of abused children. In this study, 68% of the males had physical evidence of abuse. Fifty-three percent gave a history of anal penetration, 46% of fellatio, and 25% a history of the perpetrator ejaculating. Five percent had an STD. Another study of male victims by Anderson et al. (1981) reported the following types of abuse: 33% fondling, 42% oral-genital contact, 31% anal-penile contact, 14% forced masturbation, and 4% other.

The offenders are usually known to the male victim, and 98% of the time the perpetrators are male. In one study 21% of the perpetrators were parental figures, 31% were acquaintances, 22% were others known to the victim, and 22% were strangers (Anderson et al., 1981). Most of the abuse occurred as a result of coercion by the perpetrators through their role as authority figures. Force was used in 8% of the cases if the perpetrator was a family member and in 28% of cases if the perpetrator was a nonfamily member.

Two patterns of abuse have been noted:

1. Abuse that is continuous in nature, beginning early in childhood and persisting into adolescence or stopping before adolescence, with acting-out behavior noted during adolescence

2. Episodic abuse beginning in adolescence: This second type is less frequently seen in family settings and often begins after a youth has run away from home. Adolescents are often reluctant to report such behavior.

Male adolescents who have been abused are often recognized in one of four settings: the criminal justice system, the mental health system, emergency medical care settings, and in retrospective studies of middle-class college populations. However, abused male adolescents can also be diagnosed in the course of providing outpatient services if the practitioner is able to recognize the subgroups that are at particular risk for abuse and the signs of abuse.

Subgroups

1. Street youth: Boyer (1986) reported that 75% of adolescent female prostitutes and 63% of adolescent male prostitutes had been sexually abused.
2. Homosexual male adolescents: Many homosexual male adolescents are often forced out of their homes at an early age when their orientation becomes known or are subjected to stigma associated with homosexuality subverting their self-esteem. This may result in damaging and abusive lifestyles and relationships.
3. Youth with a parental history of physical or sexual abuse

Struckman-Johnson et al. (1994) reported on forced sexual contact since the age of 16 among a predominantly heterosexual group of college students. They found that 34% reported coercive sexual contact, 24% from women, 4% from men, and 6% from both. In 12% the sexual contact was forced through physical restraint, physical intimidation, threat of harm, or harm. In 77% of the incidents that contact was initiated by an acquaintance.

Possible signs of abuse are discussed later in this chapter.

Medical Evaluation and Treatment

1. The examination is best conducted by physician comfortable with adolescents.
2. Obtain details of the assault, other recent sexual experiences, and a history of previous STDs.
3. Perform a complete physical examination with attention to bruises, scars, and abrasions.
4. Perform a thorough examination of genitals, perineum, anus, rectum, and pharynx, explaining rationale for each step.
5. Take photographs of any area of trauma.
6. Obtain VDRL and cultures for gonorrhea and *Chlamydia* at all appropriate sites. Do not use nonculture techniques for *Chlamydia* or gonorrhea, as they have inadequate specificity for forensic use. Discuss possible testing for HIV, including appropriate pretest counseling. VDRL should be repeated after 1 month.
7. Other legally mandated tests for evidence collection may include foreign hair collection, clothing, blood from victim for typing, filter paper disk with saliva from victim, and swabs from perianal, anal verge, and rectal canal for presence of acid phosphatase. The "chain of evidence" must be maintained when collecting forensic specimens by strictly following rape kit protocols or evidence will not be of value in criminal prosecution.
8. Treat acute injuries and administer tetanus and STD prophylaxis. Evidence of trauma has been found in about 20–37% of adolescent male victims. In victims of long-term abuse the trauma may be less obvious.
9. Provide information sheet or manual. The availability of a survivor manual or booklet is helpful to victims. The Los Angeles County survivor manual has a special section for male victims (Fig. 81.1).
10. Provide counseling follow-up.

Management of Rape Victim

General Approach   The following are important considerations for the practitioner to keep in mind:

1. Need of privacy: The medical history should be taken and the examination performed in a quiet, private area of the facility.

You have survived a violent attack. Some of your feelings may be the same as those of a female sexual assault survivor.

You may feel:
- Guilt
- Powerlessness
- Concern regarding your safety

However, there are special issues that may be different for you:
- Sexuality-masculinity
- Medical procedures
- Reporting to law enforcement
- Telling others
- Finding resources and support

You need to know that strong or weak, outgoing or withdrawn, homosexual or heterosexual, old or young, attractive or unattractive, you have done nothing that justifies this violent attack. At no point and under no circumstances does anyone have the right to violate or control another's body. Sexual assault is a crime of violence and power, not of lust or passion.

The special support you may need as a man may include:
- Calling a crisis line anonymously and requesting a male counselor
- Requesting an older or male nurse
- Finding a support group of male survivors

As a man, many factors or fears may influence your decision to report or not to report to law enforcement. There are both advantages and disadvantages if you choose to report.

Advantages:
- You may apply for Victims of Violent Crimes Compensation
- Collection of medical evidence will be paid for
- Your report may help protect others

Disadvantages:
- You may be treated in an unpleasant manner
- You may not be believed
- The chances of prosecution are slim

Feeling responsible is a normal reaction to sexual assault. However, sexual assault is never the responsibility of the survivor. You did nothing to deserve this. You may want to talk to someone about your feelings. Below are resources to call.

[List of local resources]

FIGURE 81.1.   "I am a male survivor" information sheet for male victim of sexual assault. (Reproduced from Survivor, Los Angeles Commission on Assaults against Women, 543 North Fairfax Avenue, Los Angeles, CA 90036, 1985.)

2. Need of an experienced practitioner: The interview and examination should preferably be conducted by a physician experienced in caring for rape victims.
3. Presence of a companion: A sympathetic friend or family member should be allowed to stay with the victim if he or she so desires. A companion can be extremely important to help the young person negotiate through interactions with the police and judicial system. If a friend or family member is not available, many communities have support agencies that can provide a trained person.
4. Need of emotional support: Crisis intervention begins when the rape victim enters the health facility. The treating physician should:
   a. Endeavor to take into account possible pre-existing emotional problems in the victim.

     b. Allow the victim time to express his or her feelings.
     c. Urge the victim to get immediate emotional support through rape crisis centers, rape hotlines, and psychosocial follow-up. In addition, when possible, a friend or family member should accompany the victim home.
     d. Discuss with the victim the possibility of nightmares, psychosexual disturbances, or depression. The victim should understand that such problems are natural and that help is available. It is also important to eradicate myths the teenager may have about rape.
5. Reporting: After taking the history, the practitioner should inform the victim that rape is a reportable crime by law (true in most areas; the practitioner should check local laws). The victim usually has the right to consent to examination and treatment without collection of evidence. It is recommended that the victim be encouraged to allow collection of legal evidence; this is mandatory if legal charges are contemplated.
6. Police: The police should not be present in the examination room.
7. Issue of control: It is important for the physician to help the victim regain a sense of control over his or her body by encouraging the victim to make as many decisions during the examination as possible. During the examination it is crucial that the victim be told that he or she is in control of what will be done. The victim has the right to refuse examination or treatment and can stop the examination at any time.

History   The history should include:

1. Length of time between alleged assault and the examination
2. The manner of the alleged assault: Inquire whether or not the perpetrator used a condom; inquire regarding injuries sustained at the time of attack.
3. Date of last menses
4. Use of oral contraceptive or intrauterine device
5. Date and time of last voluntary coitus
6. Any significant actions after alleged assault, such as showering or douching
7. Parity

Examples of medical report forms for suspected sexual assault and suspected child sexual abuse are included as Figures 81.2 and 81.3, respectively.

Examination

1. Recommended techniques for the examining physician include:
     a. Explain in detail what you will be doing and why; obtain consent for the examination.
     b. Reassure the adolescent victim that he or she will be in control.
     c. Keep personal contact with the adolescent, both through verbal and eye contact.
     d. For the internal examination of a female, use a warmed speculum, without lubrication.
     e. Proceed slowly, allowing the victim to relax.
     f. During the examination, remark on the normal findings, so the victim can feel that he or she is still normal.
2. Physical findings
     a. General appearance, emotional state, and behavior should be recorded.
     b. Condition of patient's clothing should be observed and mentioned.
     c. All areas of body should be explored for signs of trauma. Look closely at the neck and upper arms, where bruises resulting from forced restraint are apt to appear.

Text continued on page 1162.

State of California

MEDICAL REPORT—SUSPECTED SEXUAL ASSAULT

Patients requesting examination, treatment and evidence collection: Penal Code § 13823.5 requires every physician who conducts a medical examination for evidence of a sexual assault to use this form to record findings. Complete each part of the form and if an item is inapplicable, write N/A.

Patients requesting examination and treatment only: Penal Code § 11160–11161 requires physicians and hospitals to notify a law enforcement agency by telephone and in writing if treatment is sought for injuries inflicted in violation of any state penal law. If the patient consents to treatment only, complete Part A #1 and 2, Part B #1, and Part E #1–10 to the extent it is relevant to treatment, and mail this form to the local law enforcement agency.

Minors: Civil Code § 34.9 permits minors, 12 years of age or older, to consent to medical examination, treatment, and evidence collection related to a sexual assault without parental consent. Physicians are required, however, to attempt to contact the parent or legal guardian and note in the treatment record the date and time the attempted contact was made including whether the attempt was successful or unsuccessful. This provision is not applicable if the physician reasonably believes the parent or guardian committed the sexual assault on the minor. If applicable, check here ( ) and note the date and time the attempt to contact parents was made in the treatment record.

Liability and release of information: No civil or criminal liability attaches to filling out this form. Confidentiality is not breached by releasing it to law enforcement agencies.

A. GENERAL INFORMATION   Name of Hospital:
(print or type)

1. Name of patient					Patient ID number			
2. Address			City		County	State	Phone (W) (H)	
3. Age	DOB	Sex	Race	Date/time of arrival	Date/time of exam	Date/time of discharge	Mode of transportation	

4. Phone report made to law enforcement agency:
Name of officer   Agency   ID number   Phone

5. Responding officer   Agency   ID number   Phone

B. PATIENT CONSENT

1. I understand that hospitals and physicians are required by Penal Code § 11160–11161 to report to law enforcement authorities cases in which medical care is sought when injuries have been inflicted upon any person in violation of any state penal law. The report must state the name of the injured person, current whereabouts, and the type and extent of injuries.

Patient/Parent/Guardian (circle)

2. I understand that a separate medical examination for evidence of sexual assault at public expense can, with my consent, be conducted by a physician to discover and preserve evidence of the assault. If conducted, the report of the examination and any evidence obtained will be released to law enforcement authorities. I understand that the examination may include the collection of reference specimens at the time of the examination or at a later date. Knowing this, I consent to a medical examination for evidence of sexual assault. I understand that I may withdraw consent at any time for any portion of the evidential examination.

Patient/Parent/Guardian (circle)

3. I understand that collection of evidence may include photographing injuries and that these photographs may include the genital area. Knowing this, I consent to having photographs taken.

Patient/Parent/Guardian (circle)

4. I have been informed that victims of crime are eligible to submit crime victim compensation claims to the State Board of Control for out-of-pocket medical expenses, loss of wages, and job retraining and rehabilitation. I further understand that counseling is also a reimbursable expense.

Patient/Parent/Guardian (circle)

C. AUTHORIZATION FOR EVIDENTIAL EXAM
I request a medical examination and collection of evidence for suspected sexual assault of the patient at public expense.

Law Enforcement Officer

Agency   ID Number   Date

DISTRIBUTION OF OCJP 923 FOR EVIDENTIAL EXAMS ONLY | **HOSPITAL IDENTIFICATION INFORMATION**

ORIGINAL TO LAW ENFORCEMENT;
PINK COPY TO CRIME LAB (SUBMIT WITH EVIDENCE);
YELLOW COPY TO HOSPITAL RECORDS

OCJP 923   86 96699

FIGURE 81.2.   Example of medical form for suspected sexual assault. (Reproduced from State of California, Office of Criminal Justice Planning.)   *Figure continues through page 1155.*

D. OBTAIN PATIENT HISTORY. RECORDER SHOULD ALLOW PATIENT OR OTHER PERSON PROVIDING HISTORY TO DESCRIBE INCIDENT(S) TO THE EXTENT POSSIBLE AND RECORD THE ACTS DESCRIBED BELOW. DETERMINE AND USE TERMS FAMILIAR TO THE PATIENT. FOLLOW-UP QUESTIONS MAY BE NECESSARY TO ENSURE THAT ALL ITEMS ARE COVERED.

1. Name of person providing history	Relationship to patient	Date/time of assault(s)

2. Location and physical surroundings of assault (bed, field, car, rug, floor, etc.)

3. Name(s), number and race of assailant(s)

4. Acts described by patient
(Any penetration, however slight, of the labia or rectum by the penis or any penetration of a genital or anal opening by a foreign object or body part constitutes the act. Oral copulation and masturbation only require contact.)

	Yes	No	Attempted	Unsure	If more than one assailant, identify person.
Penetration of vagina by					
Penis					
Finger					
Foreign object					
Describe the object					
Penetration of rectum by					
Penis					
Finger					
Foreign object					
Describe the object					
Oral copulation of genitals					
of victim by assailant					
of assailant by victim					
Oral copulation of anus					
of victim by assailant					
of assailant by victim					
Masturbation					
of victim by assailant					
of assailant by victim					
other					
Did ejaculation occur outside a body orifice?					
if yes, describe the location on the body.					
Foam, jelly, or condom used (circle)					
Lubricant used					
Fondling, licking or kissing (circle)					
If yes, describe the location on the body.					
Other acts					

5. Physical injuries and/or pain described by patient

	Yes	No
Lapse of consciousness:		
Vomited:		
Pre-existing physical injuries:		

If yes, describe: _____

8. Pertinent medical history

Last menstrual period: _____

Any recent (60 days) anal-genital injuries, surgeries, diagnostic procedures, or medical treatment which may affect physical findings? ( ) Yes ( ) No

If yes, record information in separate medical chart.

Consenting intercourse within past 72 hours? ( ) Yes ( ) No

Approximate date/time: _____

DO NOT RECORD ANY OTHER INFORMATION REGARDING SEXUAL HISTORY ON THIS FORM.

6. Methods employed by perpetrator

	Yes	No	Area of body
Weapon inflicted injuries			
Type of weapon(s)			
Physical blows by hands or feet (circle)			
Grabbing/grasping/holding (circle)			
Physical restraints Type(s) used			
Bites			
Choking			
Burns (including chemical/toxic)			
Threat(s) of harm			
To whom:			
Type of threat(s)			
Other method(s) used Describe:			

7. Post-assault hygiene/activity
( ) Not applicable if over 72 hours

	Yes	No
Urinated		
Defecated		
Genital wipe/wash		
Bath/shower		
Douche		
Removed/inserted tampon, sponge, diaphragm (circle)		
Brushed teeth		
Oral gargle/swish		
Changed clothing		

HOSPITAL IDENTIFICATION INFORMATION

OCJP 923

86 96699

FIGURE 81.2.   *continued*

E. CONDUCT A GENERAL PHYSICAL EXAM AND RECORD FINDINGS. COLLECT AND PRESERVE EVIDENCE FOR EVIDENTIAL EXAM.

1. Blood pressure	Pulse	Temperature	Respiration	2. Height	Weight	Eye color	Hair color

3. Note condition of clothing upon arrival (rips, tears, presence of foreign materials)

4. Collect outer and underclothing worn during or immediately after assault.

5. Collect fingernail scrapings, if indicated.

6. Record general physical appearance:

- Record injuries and findings on diagrams: erythema, abrasions, bruises (detail shape), contusions, induration, lacerations, fractures, bites, burns, and stains/foreign materials on the body.
- Record size and appearance of injuries. Note swelling and areas of tenderness.
- Collect dried and moist secretions, stains, and foreign materials from the body including the head, hair, and scalp. Identify location on diagrams.
- Scan the entire body with a Wood's Lamp. Swab each suspicious substance or fluorescent area with a separate swab. Label Wood's Lamp findings "W.L."
- Collect the following reference samples at the time of the exam if required by crime lab: saliva, head, hair, and body/facial hair from males.
- Record specimens collected on Section 11.

7. Examine the oral cavity for injury and the area around the mouth for seminal fluid. Note frenulum trauma.
- If indicated by history: Swab the area around the mouth. Collect 2 swabs from the oral cavity up to 6 hours post-assault for seminal fluid. Prepare two dry mount slides.
- If indicated by history, take a GC culture from the oropharynx and offer prophylaxis. Take other STD cultures as indicated.
- Record specimens collected on Section 11.

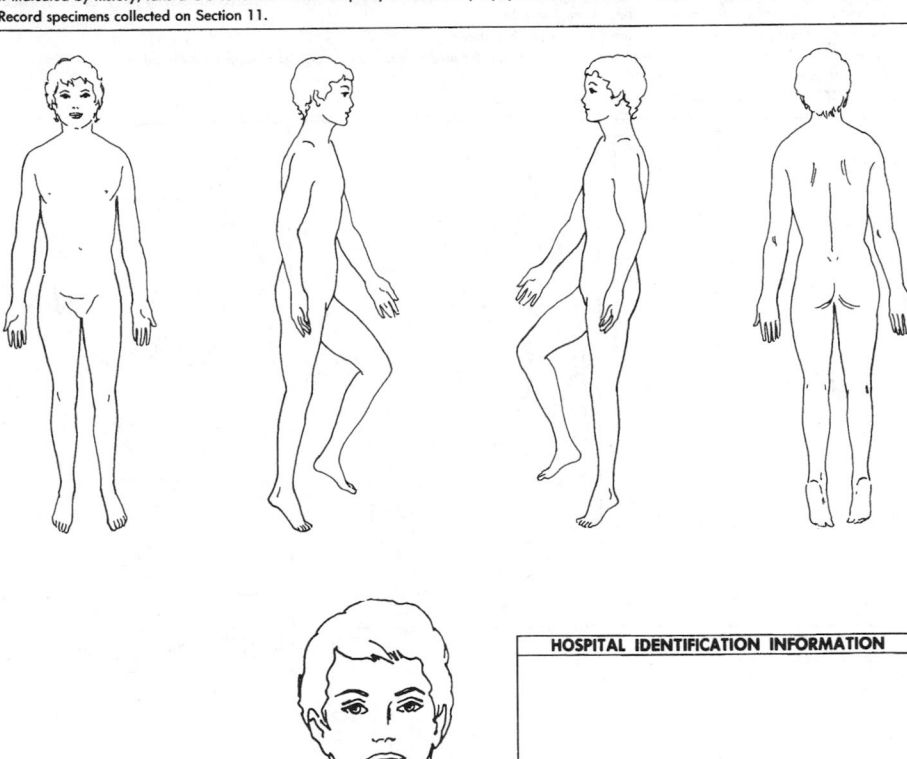

HOSPITAL IDENTIFICATION INFORMATION

OCJP 923

86 96699

8. External genitalia
- Examine the external genitalia and perianal area including the inner thighs for injury and foreign materials.
- Collect dried and moist secretions and foreign materials. Identify location on diagrams.
- Cut matted pubic hair. Comb pubic hair to collect foreign materials.
- Scan area with Wood's Lamp. Swab each suspicious substance or fluorescent area. Label Wood's Lamp findings "W.L."
- Collect pubic hair reference samples at time of exam if required by crime lab.
- For males, collect 2 penile swabs if indicated. Collect one swab from the urethral meatus and one swab from the glans and shaft. If indicated by history, take a GC culture from the urethra and offer prophylaxis. Take other STD cultures as indicated.
- Record specimens collected on Section 11.

9. Vagina and cervix
- Examine for injury and foreign materials.
- Collect 3 swabs from vaginal pool. Prepare 1 wet mount and 2 dry mount slides. Examine wet mount for sperm. Take a GC culture from the endocervix and offer prophylaxis. Take other STD cultures as indicated.
- If the assault occurred more than 24 hours prior to the exam, collection of cervical swabs may be indicated up to 2 weeks post-assault if no possibility exists of contaminating the specimen with semen from previous coitus. Label cervical swabs and slides to distinguish them from the vaginal swabs and slides.
- Aspirate/washings to detect sperm are optional.
- Record specimens collected on Section 11.
- Obtain pregnancy test (blood or urine).

10. Anus and rectum
- Examine the buttocks, perianal skin, and anal folds for injury.
- Collect dried and moist secretions and foreign materials. Foreign materials may include lubricants and fecal matter.
- If indicated by history and/or findings: Collect 2 rectal swabs and prepare 2 dry mount slides. Avoid contaminating rectal swabs by cleaning the perianal area and dilating the anus using an anal speculum.
- Conduct an anoscopic or proctoscopic exam if rectal injury is suspected.
- If indicated by history, take a GC culture from the rectum and offer prophylaxis. Take other STD cultures as indicated.
- Record specimens collected on Section 11.
- Take blood for syphilis serology. Offer prophylaxis.

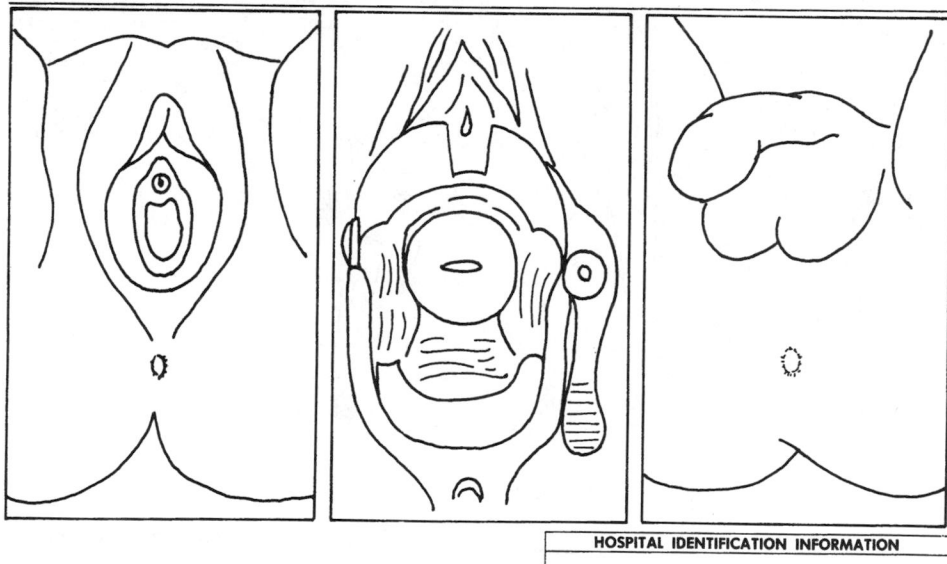

HOSPITAL IDENTIFICATION INFORMATION

OCJP 923   86 96699

FIGURE 81.2.   *continued*

11. Record evidence and specimens collected.

ALL SWABS AND SLIDES MUST BE AIR DRIED PRIOR TO PACKAGING (PENAL CODE § 13823.11). AIR DRY UNDER A STREAM OF COOL AIR FOR 60 MINUTES. Swabs and slides must be individually labeled, coded to show which slides were prepared from which swabs, and time taken. All containers (tubes, bindles, envelopes) for individual items must be labeled with the name of the patient, contents, location of the body where taken, and name of hospital. Package small containers in a large envelope and record chain of custody. See the State of California Medical Protocol for Examination of Sexual Assault and Child Sexual Abuse Victims published by the state Office of Criminal Justice Planning, 1130 K Street, Sacramento, CA 95814 (916) 324-9100 for additional information.

SPECIMENS FOR PRESENCE OF SEMEN, SPERM MOTILITY, AND TYPING TO CRIME LAB

	Swabs	Dry mount slides	Yes	No	N/A	Taken by	Time
Oral							
Vaginal							
Rectal							
Penile							
Aspirate/washings (optional)							
Vaginal wet mount slide examined for spermatozoa, dried, and submitted to crime lab							
Motile sperm observed							
Non-motile sperm observed							

OTHER EVIDENCE TO CRIME LAB

	Yes	No	N/A	Taken by
Clothing				
Fingernail Scrapings				
Foreign materials on body				
Blood				
Dried secretions				
Fiber/loose hair				
Vegetation				
Dirt/gravel/glass				
Matted pubic hair cuttings				
Pubic hair combings				
Comb				
Swabs of bite marks				
Control swabs				
Photographs				
Area of the body _____				
Type of camera _____				
Other _____				

REFERENCE SAMPLES AND TOXICOLOGY SCREENS TO CRIME LAB

Reference samples and toxicology screens can only be collected with the consent of the patient. Reference samples can be collected at the time of the exam or at a later date according to crime lab policies. Toxicology screens should be collected at the time of the exam upon the recommendation of the physical examiner or law enforcement officer.

Reference samples

	Yes	No	N/A	Taken by
Blood typing (yellow top tube)				
Saliva				
Head hair				
Pubic hair				
Facial/body hair				

Toxicology screens

Blood/alcohol toxicology (grey top tube)				
Urine toxicology				

EXAM INFORMATION (print)

Anoscopic exam				
Proctoscopic exam				
Genital exam done with:				
Direct visualization				
Colposcope				
Hand held magnifier				

PERSONNEL INVOLVED (print) | PHONE

	PHONE
History taken by:	
Physical examination performed by:	
Specimens labeled and sealed by:	
Assisting nurse:	

FINDINGS

Report of sexual assault, exam reveals:

☐ PHYSICAL FINDINGS
  ☐ Exam consistent with history
  ☐ Exam inconsistent with history

☐ NO PHYSICAL FINDINGS
  ☐ Exam consistent with history
  ☐ Exam inconsistent with history

SUMMARY OF FINDINGS

PHYSICAL EXAMINER

Print name of physical examiner

Signature of physical examiner

License number of physical examiner

LAW ENFORCEMENT OFFICER

I have received the indicated items as evidence and the original of this report.

Law enforcement officer

Law enforcement agency   ID number   Date

HOSPITAL IDENTIFICATION INFORMATION

ARRANGE FOLLOW-UP FOR STD, PREGNANCY, INJURIES, AND PROVIDE REFERRALS FOR PSYCHOLOGICAL CARE.

OCJP 923   86 96699

State of California   Office of Criminal Justice Planning (OCJP) 925

MEDICAL REPORT—SUSPECTED CHILD SEXUAL ABUSE

Record examination findings: Penal Code § 13823.5 requires every physician who conducts a medical examination for evidence of child sexual abuse to use this form to record findings. Complete each part of the form and if an item is inapplicable, write N/A.

Child abuse reporting law: Penal Code § 11166 requires all professional medical personnel to report suspected child abuse, defined by Penal Code § 11165, immediately by telephone and submit a written report (DOJ SS 8572) within 36 hours to the local law enforcement agency, county department of social services or probation department. Professional medical personnel means any physician and surgeon, psychiatrist, psychologist, dentist, resident, intern, podiatrist, chiropractor, licensed nurse, dental hygienist, or any other person who is currently licensed under Division 2 (commencing with Section 500) of the Business and Professions Code.

Minors: Civil Code § 34.9 permits minors, 12 years of age or older, to consent to medical examination, treatment, and evidence collection related to a sexual assault without parental consent. Physicians are required, however, to attempt to contact the parent or legal guardian and note in the treatment record the date and time the attempted contact was made including whether the attempt was successful or unsuccessful. This provision is not applicable if the physician reasonably believes the parent or guardian committed the sexual assault on the minor. If applicable, check here ( ) and note date and time attempt to contact parents was made in the treatment record.

Liability and release of information: No civil or criminal liability attaches to filling out this form. Confidentiality is not breached by releasing this form or other relevant information contained in the medical records to law enforcement or child protective agencies (Penal Code § 11167).

A. AUTHORIZATION FOR EXAM REQUESTED BY PATIENT/PARENT/GUARDIAN (Note: Parental consent for an evidential examination is not required in cases of known or suspected child abuse. Contact a law enforcement or child protective service agency.)

I hereby request a medical examination for evidence of sexual abuse and treatment for injuries. I understand that collection of evidence may include photographing injuries and these photographs may include the genital area. I further understand that hospitals and physicians are required to notify child protective authorities of known or suspected child abuse and if child abuse is found or suspected, this form and any evidence obtained will be released to a child protective agency.

_____
Patient/Parent/Guardian (circle)

I have been informed that victims of crime are eligible to submit crime victim compensation claims to the State Board of Control for out-of-pocket medical expenses, loss of wages, and job retraining and rehabilitation. I further understand that counseling is also a reimbursable expense.

_____
Patient/Parent/Guardian (circle)

B. AUTHORIZATION FOR EVIDENTIAL EXAM REQUESTED BY CHILD PROTECTIVE AGENCY

I request a medical examination and collection of evidence for suspected sexual abuse of the patient at public expense.

Law enforcement officer or child protective services	Agency	ID number	Date

C. GENERAL INFORMATION   Name of Hospital:
(print or type)

1. Name of patient	Patient ID number

2. Address	City	County	State	Phone

3. Age	DOB	Sex	Race	Date/time of arrival	Date/time of exam	Date/time of discharge

4. Name of: ( ) Mother ( ) Stepmother ( ) Guardian Address	City	County	State	Phone (W) (H)

5. Name of: ( ) Father ( ) Stepfather ( ) Guardian Address	City	County	State	Phone (W) (H)

6. Siblings: Name	DOB	Name	DOB	Name	DOB

7. Phone report made to: ( ) Law enforcement agency

Name	Agency	ID number	Phone

( ) Child protective services

Name	Agency	ID number	Phone

8. Responding officer	Agency	ID number	Phone

DISTRIBUTION OF OCJP 925	**HOSPITAL IDENTIFICATION INFORMATION**
ORIGINAL TO CHILD PROTECTIVE AGENCY REQUESTING EXAM; PINK COPY TO CRIME LAB (SUBMIT WITH EVIDENCE); YELLOW COPY TO HOSPITAL RECORDS	

OCJP 925   86 96698

FIGURE 81.3.   Example of medical report form for suspected child sexual abuse. (Reproduced from State of California, Office of Criminal Justice Planning.)

D. OBTAIN PATIENT HISTORY. RECORDER SHOULD ALLOW PATIENT OR OTHER PERSON PROVIDING HISTORY TO DESCRIBE INCIDENT(S) TO THE EXTENT POSSIBLE AND RECORD THE ACTS AND SYMPTOMS DESCRIBED BELOW. DETERMINE AND USE TERMS FAMILIAR TO THE PATIENT. FOLLOW-UP QUESTIONS MAY BE NECESSARY TO ENSURE THAT ALL ITEMS ARE COVERED.

1. Name of person providing history	Relationship to child	Address	City	County	State	Phone (W) (H)

2. Chief complaint(s) of person providing history

3. Chief complaint(s) in child's own words

4. ☐ Less than 72 hours since incident(s) took place Date/time/location	☐ Over 72 hours since incident(s) took place Date(s) or time frame/location

5. Identity of alleged perpetrator(s), if known	Age	Sex	Race	Relationship to child

6. Acts described by patient and/or other historian

	Described by patient			Described by historian		
	Yes	No	Unk	Yes	No	Unk
Vaginal contact						
Penis						
Finger						
Foreign object						
Describe the object						
Anal contact						
Penis						
Finger						
Foreign object						
Describe the object						
Oral copulation of genitals						
of victim by assailant						
of assailant by victim						
Oral copulation of anus						
of victim by assailant						
of assailant by victim						
Masturbation						
of victim by assailant						
of assailant by victim						
other						
Did ejaculation occur outside a body orifice?						
If yes, describe the location on the body:						
Foam, jelly, or condom used (circle)						
Lubricant used						
Fondling, licking or kissing (circle)						
If yes, describe the location on the body:						
Other acts:						

Was force used upon patient?
If yes, describe:

7. Post-assault hygiene/activity
( ) Not applicable if over 72 hours

	Described by patient			Described by historian		
	Yes	No	Unk	Yes	No	Unk
Urinated						
Defecated						
Genital wipe/wash						
Bath/shower						
Douche						
Removed/inserted tampon						
Brushed teeth						
Oral gargle/swish						
Changed clothing						

8. Symptoms described by patient and/or other historian

	Described by patient			Described by historian		
	Yes	No	Unk	Yes	No	Unk
Physical symptoms						
Abdominal/pelvic pain						
Vulvar discomfort or pain						
Dysuria						
Urinary tract infections						
Enuresis (daytime or nighttime)						
Vaginal itching						
Vaginal discharge						
Describe color, odor and amount below.						
Vaginal bleeding						
Rectal pain						
Rectal bleeding						
Rectal discharge						
Constipation						
Incontinent of stool (daytime or nighttime)						
Lapse of consciousness						
Vomiting						
Physical injuries, pain, or tenderness. Describe below.						
Behavioral/emotional symptoms						
Sleep disturbances						
Eating disorders						
School						
Sexual acting out						
Fear						
Anger						
Depression						
Other symptoms						

Additional information:

HOSPITAL IDENTIFICATION INFORMATION

OCJP 925

86 96690

FIGURE 81.3. *continued* (Figure continues through page 1161.)

E. OBTAIN PERTINENT PAST MEDICAL HISTORY

1. Menarche age ( ) N/A	Date of last menstrual period ( ) N/A	Use of tampons ( ) Yes ( ) No ( ) N/A	History of Vaginitis ( ) Yes ( ) No ( ) N/A

2. Note pre-existing physical injuries ( ) N/A

---

3. Pertinent medical history of anal-genital injuries, surgeries, diagnostic procedures, or medical treatment? ( ) Yes ( ) No   If yes, describe

---

4. Previous history of child abuse? ( ) Yes ( ) No ( ) Unknown. If known, describe

---

F. CONDUCT A GENERAL PHYSICAL EXAM AND RECORD FINDINGS. COLLECT AND PRESERVE EVIDENCE FOR EVIDENTIAL EXAM.

1. Blood pressure	Pulse	Temperature	Respiration	Include percentiles for children under six Height Weight

2. Record general physical condition noting any abnormality   ( ) Within normal limits

---

* Record injuries and findings on diagrams: erythema, abrasions, bruises (detail shape), contusions, induration, lacerations, fractures, bites, and burns.
* Record size and appearance of injuries. Note swelling and areas of tenderness.
* Examine for evidence of physical neglect.
* Take a GC culture from the oropharynx as a base line. Take other STD cultures as indicated. Provide prophylaxis.

  IF EXAMINED WITHIN 72 HOURS OF ALLEGED INCIDENT(S):
* Note condition of clothing upon arrival (rips, tears, or foreign materials) if applicable. Use space below to record observations.
* Collect outer and underclothing if worn during or immediately after the incident.
* If applicable, collect fingernail scrapings.
* Collect dried and moist secretions, stains, and foreign materials from the body including the head, hair, and scalp. Identify location on diagrams.
* Scan the entire body with a Wood's Lamp. Swab each suspicious substance or fluorescent area with a separate swab. Label Wood's Lamp findings "W.L."
* Examine the oral cavity for injury and the area around the mouth for seminal fluid. Note frenulum trauma. If indicated by history: Swab the area around the mouth. Collect 2 swabs from the oral cavity up to 6 hours post-assault for seminal fluid. Prepare two dry mount slides.
* Collect saliva and head hair reference samples at the time of the exam if required by crime lab and if there is a need to compare them to a suspect.
* Record specimens collected on Section 7.

HOSPITAL IDENTIFICATION INFORMATION

OCJP 925   86 96698

Figure 81.3. *continued*

Optional: Take photographs of genitals before and after exam.

Record injuries and findings on anal-genital diagrams: abrasions, erythema, bruises, tears/transections, scars, distortions or adhesions, etc. Use anal-genital chart on next page to record additional descriptive information.

3. External genitalia
*   Examine the external genitalia and perianal area including inner thighs for injury.
*   For boys, take a GC culture from the urethra. Take other STD cultures as indicated. Provide prophylaxis.
    IF EXAMINED WITHIN 72 HOURS OF INCIDENT:
*   Collect dried and moist secretions and foreign materials. Identify location on diagrams.
*   Pubertal children: Cut matted pubic hair. Comb pubic hair to collect foreign materials. Collect pubic hair reference samples at time of exam if required by crime lab and if there is a need to compare them to a suspect.
*   Scan area with Wood's Lamp. Swab each suspicious substance or fluorescent area. Label Wood's Lamp findings "W L."
*   For boys, collect 2 penile swabs if indicated. Collect one swab from the urethral meatus and one swab from the glans and shaft. Take a GC culture from the urethra. Take other STD cultures as indicated. Provide prophylaxis.
*   Record specimens collected on Section 7.
4. Vagina
*   Examine for injury and foreign materials.
*   Pre-pubertal girls with intact hymen/normal vaginal orifice: No speculum exam necessary.
*   Pre-pubertal girls with non-intact hymen and/or enlarged vaginal orifice: Only conduct a speculum exam if major trauma is suspected and use pediatric speculum.
*   Take a GC culture from the vaginal introitus in pre-pubertal girls with intact hymen/normal vaginal orifice; from the vagina in pre-pubertal girls with non-intact hymen and/or enlarged vaginal orifice; and, the endocervix in adolescents. Take other STD cultures as indicated. Provide prophylaxis.
*   Obtain pregnancy test (blood or urine) from pubertal girls.
    IF EXAMINED WITHIN 72 HOURS OF INCIDENT:
*   Pre-pubertal girls with intact hymen/normal vaginal orifice: Collect 2 swabs from the vulva.
*   Adolescents or pre-pubertal girls with non-intact hymen and/or enlarged vaginal orifice: Collect 3 swabs from vaginal pool. Prepare 1 wet mount and 2 dry mount slides. Examine wet mount for sperm and trichomonas.
*   Record specimens collected on Section 7.
5. Anus and rectum
*   Examine the buttocks, perianal skin, and anal folds for injury.
*   Conduct an anoscopic or proctoscopic exam if rectal injury is suspected.
*   Take a GC culture from the rectum. Take other STD cultures as indicated. Provide prophylaxis.
*   Take blood for syphilis serology. Provide prophylaxis.
    IF EXAMINED WITHIN 72 HOURS OF ALLEGED INCIDENT:
*   Collect dried and moist secretions and foreign materials. Foreign materials may include lubricants and fecal matter.
*   If indicated by history and/or findings: Collect 2 rectal swabs and prepare 2 dry mount slides. Avoid contaminating rectal swabs by cleaning the perianal area and relaxing the anus using the lateral or knee-chest position prior to insertion of swabs.
*   Record specimens collected on Section 7.

| DRAW SHAPE OF ANUS AND ANY LESIONS ON GENITALIA, PERINEUM, AND BUTTOCKS | DRAW SHAPE OF HYMEN AND ANUS AND ANY LESIONS ON GENITALIA, PERINEUM, OR BUTTOCKS |

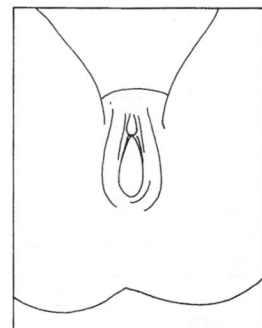

HOSPITAL IDENTIFICATION INFORMATION

OCJP 925   86 96698

FIGURE 81.3.   *continued*

6. Anal-genital chart

Female/Male General	WNL	ABN	Describe
Tanner stage			
Breast 1 2 3 4 5	☐	☐	_____
Genitals 1 2 3 4 5	☐	☐	_____
Inguinal adenopathy	☐	☐	_____
			_____
Medial aspect of thighs	☐	☐	_____
			_____
Perineum	☐	☐	_____
			_____

	Yes	No	
Vulvovaginal/urethral discharge	☐	☐	_____
			_____
Condyloma acuminata	☐	☐	_____

Female	WNL	ABN	Describe
Labia majora	☐	☐	_____
			_____
Clitoris	☐	☐	_____
			_____
Labia minora	☐	☐	_____
			_____
Periurethral tissue/ urethral meatus	☐	☐	_____
			_____
Perihymenal tissue (vestibule)	☐	☐	_____
			_____
Hymen	☐	☐	_____

Record diameter of hymen and check measurement used:

☐ Horizontal

☐ Vertical

Posteriour fourchette	☐	☐	_____
			_____
Fossa Navicularis	☐	☐	_____
			_____
Vagina	☐	☐	_____
			_____
Other			_____

Exam position used:
☐ Supine
☐ Knee chest

OCJP 925

Male	WNL	ABN	Describe
Penis	☐	☐	_____
Circumcised ☐ Yes ☐ No			_____
Urethral Meatus	☐	☐	_____
			_____
Scrotum	☐	☐	_____
			_____
Testes	☐	☐	_____
			_____

Female/Male Anus	WNL	ABN	Describe
Buttocks	☐	☐	_____
			_____
Perianal skin	☐	☐	_____
Anal verge/ folds/rugae	☐	☐	_____
			_____
Tone	☐	☐	_____

Anal spasm
☐ Yes ☐ No

Anal laxity
☐ Yes ☐ No

Note presence of stool in rectal ampulla
☐ Yes ☐ No

Method of exam for anal tone (discretion of examiner)
☐ Observation
☐ Digital exam

Exam position used:
☐ Supine
☐ Prone
☐ Lateral recumbent

Anoscopic exam
☐ Yes ☐ No ☐ N/A

Proctoscopic exam
☐ Yes ☐ No ☐ N/A

Genital exam done with:
Direct visualization   ☐
Colposcope   ☐
Hand held magnifier   ☐

86 96698

HOSPITAL IDENTIFICATION INFORMATION

FIGURE 81.3.   *continued*

7. Record evidential and specimens collected.

FOR EVIDENTIAL EXAMS CONDUCTED WITHIN 72 HOURS OF ALLEGED INCIDENT

ALL SWABS AND SLIDES MUST BE AIR DRIED PRIOR TO PACKAGING (PENAL CODE § 13823.11). AIR DRY UNDER A STREAM OF COOL AIR FOR 60 MINUTES. Swabs and slides must be individually labeled, coded to show which slides were prepared from which swabs, and time taken. All containers (tubes, bindles, envelopes) for individual items must be labeled with the name of the patient, contents, location of body where taken, and name of hospital. Package small containers in a larger envelope and record chain of custody. See the State of California Medical Protocol for Examination of Sexual Assault and Child Sexual Abuse Victims published by the state Office of Criminal Justice Planning, 1130 K Street, Sacramento, California 95814 (916) 324-9100 for additional information.

SPECIMENS FOR PRESENCE OF SEMEN, SPERM MOTILITY, AND TYPING TO CRIME LAB

	Swabs	Dry Mount Slides	Yes	No	N/A	Taken by	Time
Oral							
Vaginal							
Rectal							
Vulvar							
Penile							

Vaginal wet mount slide examined for spermatozoa and trichomonas, dried, and submitted to crime lab

Motile sperm observed

Non-motile sperm observed

OTHER EVIDENCE TO CRIME LAB

	Yes	No	N/A	Taken by
Clothing				
Fingernail scrapings				
Foreign materials on body				
Blood				
Dried secretions				
Fiber/loose hair				
Vegetation				
Dirt/gravel/glass				
Matted pubic hair cuttings				
Pubic hair combings				
Comb				
Swabs of bite marks				
Control swabs				
Photographs				
Area of body				
Type of camera				
Other				

REFERENCE SAMPLES AND TOXICOLOGY SCREENS TO CRIME LAB

Reference samples can be collected at the time of the exam or at a later date according to crime lab policies if there is a need to compare them to a suspect. Toxicology screens should be collected at the time of the exam upon the recommendation of the physical examiner, law enforcement officer, or child protective services.

Reference samples	Yes	No	N/A	Taken by
Blood typing (yellow top tube)				
Saliva				
Head hair				
Pubic hair				
Toxicology screens				
Blood/alcohol toxicology (grey top tube)				
Urine toxicology				

OCJP 925

CLINICAL EVIDENCE TO HOSPITAL LAB

	Yes	No	N/A	Taken by
Syphilis serology (red top tube)				
STD culture				
Oral				
Vaginal				
Rectal				
Penile				
Pregnancy test Blood (red top tube) or urine				

PERSONNEL INVOLVED (print)   PHONE

History taken by:

Physical examination performed by:

Specimens labeled and sealed by:

Assisting nurse:

Family assessment taken by: ( ) N/A   ( ) Report attached

Additional narrative prepared by physician: ( ) N/A   ( ) Report attached

FINDINGS AND FOLLOW-UP

Report of child sexual abuse, exam reveals:
☐ PHYSICAL FINDINGS   ☐ NO PHYSICAL FINDINGS
  ☐ Exam consistent with history   ☐ Exam consistent with history
  ☐ Exam inconsistent with history   ☐ Exam inconsistent with history

SUMMARY OF PHYSICAL FINDINGS:
☐ Oral trauma   ☐ Genital trauma
☐ Perineal trauma   ☐ Anal trauma
☐ Hymenal trauma
☐ Other findings consistent/inconsistent (circle one) with history as follows:

Follow-up arranged: ( ) Yes ( ) No
Child released to: _____

PHYSICAL EXAMINER

Print name of examiner

Signature of examiner

License number of examiner

LAW ENFORCEMENT/CHILD PROTECTIVE SERVICES

I have received the indicated items of evidence and the original of this report.

Law enforcement officer or child protective services

Agency   ID number   Date

HOSPITAL IDENTIFICATION INFORMATION

86 96698

FIGURE 81.3.   *continued*

d. Check for abdominal crepitus; this may signify vaginal or rectal laceration with intraabdominal bleeding.

e. Notice and record any areas of the body containing foreign material. Keep all such material for evidence. Do not write "no evidence of rape"; this can eliminate a case from court. Instead, if there is no evidence of trauma, write "no evidence of trauma."

3. Pelvic examination: Only after a thorough examination of the entire body is performed should the pelvic or rectal examination be performed. A primary responsibility of the physician is to avoid further trauma to the patient in performing this part of the examination. Be sure to ask the victim if he or she has ever had a pelvic or rectal examination.

a. External genitalia: Note and record signs of blood secretions and sites of hematoma, abrasions, and lacerations. Application of toluidine blue will make local injuries more apparent. In females, note the state of the hymen. In cases of prepubertal sexual trauma, a normal general and external genital examination excludes internal injuries, and a vaginal examination is not required. However, if there is pain, bleeding, a history of vaginal or rectal penetration, or sign of injury, an internal and pelvic and rectal examination must be performed. General anesthesia may be required, especially in the prepubertal female.

b. Vaginal and rectal examination: The examination should be performed with water-lubricated instruments. In females, note any injury to the vagina and cervix. In prepubertal females, digital or speculum examinations are rarely indicated unless there is active bleeding, in which case general anesthesia should be considered.

Collection of Specimens   The following list of specimens should be collected and properly labeled, including contents, site of collection, patient's name, physician's name, and the date. All specimens should be placed in separate sealed containers such as envelopes, culture tubes, or blood specimen tubes.

Other than photographs of areas of acute or chronic trauma, the following collections are for cases in which the adolescent has been sexually assaulted in the past 72 hours.

1. Clothing: The patient's clothing should be wrapped and handled as little as possible. Each article of clothing should be wrapped separately, if possible.

2. Debris: Any foreign matter, dried stains, vegetation, dirt, gravel, or loose hair should be placed in a labeled specimen container. To minimize loss, debris should be placed into a sheet of paper, which is then folded. The folded sheet is then placed in an evidence envelope.

3. Pubic combings
    a. Place clean paper under the patient's buttocks.
    b. Comb pubic hair toward paper to collect loose hairs.
    c. Fold paper and place inside a labeled envelope.

4. Dried secretions: Collect swabs of dried secretions on body.
    a. Slightly moisten a swab with distilled water.
    b. Swab each dried secretion with a separate swab (e.g., dried blood, dried semen, or bite mark).
    c. Smear the specimen onto a microscopic slide. Let it air-dry; initial and date the slide; and place slide into a slide holder.
    d. Insert swab into a tube and discard cap so as to allow the swab to air-dry. Tape the swab to the tube.
    e. Clearly label each swab and slide.

5. Collection from vagina and, if indicated, rectum and pharynx:
    a. Swab site with nylon swab.

b. Smear onto two slides: Air-dry one slide for blood typing. Examine the other slide for sperm presence and motility and then air-dry.

c. Place slides in slide holder and initial and date the slides.

d. Insert swab into a tube and discard cap to allow swab to air-dry. Tape swab to tube.

e. Vaginal aspirate: Use 3 mL of sterile water for a vaginal lavage. Aspirate vagina and place contents into a test tube. Secure cap and initial test tube.

f. Place all swabs, slides, and aspirate in collection envelope.

6. Control samples

a. Blood: Use one purple-topped tube (serves as a control in blood typing) and one gray-topped tube (if drugs were suspected to be involved).

b. Saliva: Collect on a piece of clean gauze or let patient spit on filter paper. Let dry in labeled envelope.

c. Hair: Pubic, scalp hair, and hair from one or two other sites should be pulled or cut and placed in separate labeled containers.

7. With patient's permission, have photographs taken of any areas of trauma.

8. Reasons for slides, swabs, and aspirates: All these specimens are used to examine for presence of motile or nonmotile sperm. Slides are examined first by the criminology laboratory, then swabs, and then aspirates. Besides examining the slides and aspirate for the presence of motile or nonmotile sperm, an acid phosphatase test is performed on the swabs.

9. Chain of evidence: As findings are of importance in criminal prosecution, strict adherence to rape kit protocols are essential.

Laboratory Tests

1. Cultures: Gonorrhea cultures should be obtained from the endocervix, rectum, and pharynx, as appropriate, while *Chlamydia* cultures should be obtained from the endocervix and rectum. Do not use nonculture techniques of detection, as they have inadequate specificity for criminal prosecution.

2. Gram stain of any genital or anal discharge should be obtained.

3. Wet mount of vaginal secretions of female victim should be prepared and examined for evidence of *Trichomonas* or cervicitis.

4. Hepatitis B surface antigen and antibody in male victims should be checked.

5. A syphilis serologic examination should be obtained as a baseline test and should be repeated within 6 to 8 weeks.

6. A purple-topped tube should be used for control blood typing.

7. A urine or serum pregnancy test should be performed.

8. A complete blood count and urinalysis are recommended by some authorities.

9. Other serological testing: The practitioner may wish to discuss HIV and hepatitis B testing at this time or at a later date. This should be fully discussed with the victim.

10. An extra serum sample should be collected for possible future testing.

Therapy

1. Trauma: Treatment for significant trauma should precede collection of medicolegal information.

2. Tetanus toxoid is indicated for severe or penetrating trauma.

3. STD prophylaxis: Recommended to use empirically:
Ceftriaxone 250 mg IM or cefixime 400 mg orally; PLUS
Azithromycin 1 g orally single dose; OR
Doxycycline 100 mg orally two times a day for 7 days.

4. Prevention of pregnancy: The risk of pregnancy after a rape is approximately 1.5–4% (10% if on the day of ovulation). If the adolescent does not have an intrauterine device or is not taking oral contraceptives, pregnancy prophylaxis should be discussed. Use of Ovral as a postcoital contraceptive is effective, resulting in a 0–1.6% failure rate. The low dose of estrogen in Ovral makes nausea uncommon and would not mandate an abortion if unsuccessful. A second pregnancy test is indicated if menstruation does not occur within 30 days of therapy.

   Treatment: Ovral (50 µg ethinyl estradiol, 0.5 mg norgestrel), or any other contraceptive containing 50 mg ethinyl estradiol, two tablets at the time of examination, then two tablets 12 hours later. Ovral may be given at any time in the menstrual cycle; it is not effective if treatment is begun more than 72 hours after coitus. Diphenhydramine (Benadryl) 25 mg may be given in addition for expected nausea.

5. Sleep aids: These should be prescribed if indicated, but should be given in small quantities.

6. Psychological supports: The adolescent should be provided with psychological support, including the telephone numbers of rape hotlines or crisis centers. A follow-up appointment should also be scheduled with a physician or counselor. As stated earlier, the victim should be released to a caring friend or family member. In many cities, rape crisis centers will send a supportive individual to the emergency room if notified.

7. Medical follow-up: An appointment with a physician should be scheduled as indicated or 14–21 days after the alleged assault. A third visit may be scheduled at 8 to 12 weeks to repeat initial serologic studies, including tests for syphilis, hepatitis B, or HIV.

8. Written materials: Written materials regarding the rape experience should be given to the victim before leaving the hospital. A sample patient information sheet appears in Figure 81.4. Preferably, a booklet such as *Survivor* by the Los Angeles Commission on Assaults Against Women can be given to the victim. This publication discusses victims' rights, the rape experience, reporting rape, feelings about rape, and special reactions (the teenage victim, male victim, and the disabled victim). (*Survivor* is available from Los Angeles City Attorney, Victim-Witness Assistance Program, 1600 City Hall East, 200 N. Main Street, Los Angeles, CA 90012.

   Other resources of information include:

C. Henry Kempe National Center for Prevention and Treatment of Child Abuse and Neglect
1205 Oneida Street
Denver, CO 80220
(303-321-3963)

Child Help's National Child Abuse Hotline
P.O. Box 630
Hollywood, CA 90028
(1-800-4-A-CHILD)

National Center for Missing and Exploited Children
1835 K Street, NW, Suite 600
Washington, DC 20005
(800-843-5678)

National Coalition Against Sexual Assault
123 S. 7th Suite 500
Springfield, IL 62701
(217-753-4117)

PATIENT INFORMATION

Rape can be one of the most upsetting and frightening experiences that a man or woman ever faces.

Sexual assaults must be reported to the police, in accordance with Section [number inserted] of the State Penal Code. This report is confidential and need only include your name, address, type of crime, and extent of injuries.

We encourage you to sign a voluntary consent for the collection of evidence at the time of your examination. Only if you sign the consent may your medical record and the evidence be released to law enforcement officers.

We hope that you will cooperate with the police investigation. Most rapists will repeat their crime if not caught. Female victims have the right to request to make their report to a female police officer. If photographs of injuries are needed, females have the right to request a female photographer or a female chaperone. Male victims may request male officers.

Rape is legally considered a crime against the state. The city will pay for the examination to collect evidence (but not for tests or treatments). All cases that come to trial are prosecuted by the district attorney, so you will not need to have your own attorney.

Your examination includes tests for pregnancy (female victims) and venereal disease. You and the doctor will discuss any treatment to be given to prevent these conditions. It is important that you be tested again for exposure to venereal disease in 6 weeks. A positive result may take that long to appear.

For female victims: If, as a result of rape, you are receiving treatment to prevent pregnancy, you can be assured that the medication is safe and effective. The medicine is a low-dose hormone combination called Ovral. Two pills are taken shortly after your examination and two more pills are taken 12 hours later. It is okay to take the medicine with a little food. Your menstrual cycle may not be regular due to stress and the medication, and your period may be early or late. This is to be expected. However, if you do not have a period 30 days from now, we recommend that you see a doctor, or call [telephone number of clinic or referral center].

Rape is terrifying. You may feel ill or numb from the shock of the attack. Even with friends or helpful people present, being in an Emergency Room is difficult. Often a victim will feel very helpless and overwhelmed. Common reactions include disbelief, anger, confusion, and depression. A victim may be afraid of other people's reactions to the rape. Difficulties sleeping and stomach upset are common, as are fears of being alone. It takes time before you regain a sense of yourself.

For Teens

If you have been sexually assaulted, there are some things you need to know right away:
- Rape is any sexual activity forced upon you against your will.
- What happened was not your fault, whether you were assaulted by a stranger or by someone you know.
- It is important that you get medical care as soon as possible.
- It is wise that you let someone know what happened.
- Talking to someone you trust about your feelings is a good idea. It can help you feel better.
- You are not alone. It is estimated that one-third of all young people in the United States are sexually assaulted by the time they are 18. This could be by a stranger, acquaintance, date, or relative.

Perhaps the most difficult form of sexual abuse to deal with is incest. Nobody talks about it, but it can happen in any family. The offender can be a father, stepfather, uncle, or older brother. Usually the victim is a daughter. However, boys can be victims of incest, too. The most important things to remember are:

FIGURE 81.4.   Sample rape information sheet for patients.   *Figure continued on the following page.*

- You are not to blame for what happened.
- There are people who will believe you.
- There are people who want to help. You don't have to deal with these feelings alone. The rape hotline service can offer you support, advice on police and legal procedures, and counseling referrals. You can reach this help by calling [rape hotline number].

The staff of the [name of referral center] helps teenagers and young adults from the surrounding area. The doctor in the Emergency Room can help you get an appointment, or you can call [telephone number] during the day.

Information

Emergency Room Doctor's Name_____

Emergency Room Nurse's Name_____

Date Seen_____

Tests Done_____

Follow-up Blood Test_____

Treatment _____

FIGURE 81.4.   *continued*

National Committee for Prevention of Child Abuse
332 S. Michigan Avenue, Suite 1250
Chicago, IL 60604
(312-663-3520)

9. Areas to explore with the adolescent during the initial examination and follow-up include:
   a. Feelings during the assault
   b. Feelings and worries regarding the rape, medical examination, and the legal process
   c. Concerns regarding physical health, emotional reactions, sexuality, and unusual behaviors
   d. Feelings regarding the perpetrator, family, peers, school, and job

SEXUAL ABUSE AND INCEST

Although rape is a prevalent form of sexual abuse in all ages, incest is becoming increasingly recognized as a common form of sexual abuse in children and teenagers. Finkelhor (1984) defined sexual abuse as sexual contact with a child that occurs as a result of force or in a relationship where it is exploitative because of the existence of an age difference or a caregiving responsibility. Incest is defined as sexual intercourse between closely related persons: parent-child, siblings, or other blood relatives. Adolescents are more likely to be abused, either sexually, physically, or emotionally, than any other age group. Physicians can play an important role in detecting abuse and facilitating intervention.

Epidemiology

1. Prevalence or incidence
   a. The annual incidence of sexual abuse or incest in children and teenagers has been estimated at between 200 and 5,000 cases per 1 million population (Carper, 1979).
   b. Reported rates for child sexual abuse range from 6% to 62% for females and 3% to 31% for males (Watkins and Bentovim, 1992).

c. Retrospective surveys of college-aged females have identified a 20–30% rate of child-hood sexual victimization (Anderson, 1993; Finkelhor, 1979; Gagnon, 1965; Landis, 1956). Although these did not all involve incestuous experiences, 75–85% involved non-strangers. At least 70% involved genital contact or more severe abuse. In one study examining the prevalence of childhood sexual abuse experiences in a commu-nity sample of women, most of the abusers were young men, disclosure of the abuse was infrequent, and only 7% of all abuse was ever reported to authorities. The ages of greatest reported risk were 8–12 years, with the 11th year having the maximum abuse rate (Anderson, 1993).

d. Surveys of foster children, runaways, substance abusers, and prostitutes show an in-cestuous background in the 60–70% range (Summit, 1982). Eighty-four percent of juvenile delinquents are abuse victims.

e. An example of the reported increase in sexual abuse rates includes a 399% increase in sexual abuse reports between 1974 and 1984 in Los Angeles.

f. Teen clinics: A review of teens 15 or younger attending a teen family planning clinic found 7% of girls specifically stated that they had been sexually abused while an ad-ditional 19% described situations or exhibited symptoms consistent with a history of sexual abuse.

2. Demographics
   a. Twenty-eight percent of child abuse victims are between 12 and 17 years of age.
   b. The victim knows the offender in 80% of cases, and in more than 50% of cases, par-ents, parental substitutes, or relatives are the perpetrators.
   c. Ninety-five percent of offenders are male.
   d. Among adolescents, approximately two-thirds of the abuse is sexual and one-third is physical.
   e. The sexual abuse usually takes one of three forms (Lourie, 1977):
      — Abuse that is a continuation from childhood
      — Abuse that continues from childhood but is manifested in a new or more severe form
      — Abuse with its onset during adolescence, most commonly as a result of situational conflicts: Many adolescents fall into this third category.
   f. Abuse form: Twenty percent to 35% involve oral or anal penetration. Fifty-eight per-cent of males were sodomized, compared with 13% of females.
   g. Risk profile: Runtz and Brierz (1986) found the following characteristics in female college students with a prior history of sexual abuse as compared to controls: do-ing poorly in school, trouble with the law, undereating, lying to parents, and early sexual behavior. Contemporary patterns of divorce, remarriage, and cohabitation bring many children and young people in contact with multiple adults with whom they may share no emotional bond. This may contribute to the increasing prevalence of sexual abuse. Parental alcoholism and substance abuse may also contribute to the evolution of an environment in which young people may be sex-ually victimized.
   h. Barriers to disclosure include expected to be blamed (29%), embarrassment (25%), not wanting to upset anyone (24%), expected disbelief (23%), not bothered by abuse or denial (18%), wish to protect the abuser (14%), fear of abuser (11%), and want-ing to obey adults (3%) (Anderson, 1993).

Dynamics

Finkelhor and Browne (1985) have identified four trauma-causing dynamics in victims of sexual abuse:

1. Traumatic sexualization in a developmentally inappropriate and interpersonally dysfunctional fashion
2. Betrayal
3. Disempowerment, especially when threats or force are used and the child or adolescent is unable to reveal what is happening
4. Stigmatizations when negative messages surrounding the abusive acts are internalized by the abused individual

Summit (1982) identified characteristics of families with incest in the child sexual abuse accommodation syndrome:

1. Secrecy: Children or teenagers rarely tell anyone, especially when first molested; the victim typically feels too guilty or ashamed.
2. Helplessness: The victim feels obligated to and overpowered by the inherent authority. Threats are often used by the incestuous relative to keep the victim from discussing the abuse.
3. Entrapment and accommodation: The process of helplessness leads the victim to exaggerate his or her responsibility for the act. Self-esteem is lowered, and the victim takes on the responsibility for the act, as well as that of holding the family together.
4. Delayed, conflicting, and unconvincing disclosure: Most sexual abuse is never disclosed (Finkelhor, 1979). During adolescence, if disclosure occurs, it is often during a conflict or fight and is often dismissed by the family and others as an act of vengeance by the victim. Teenagers will often turn to drugs, promiscuity, runaway behavior, or suicide as a way of coping.
5. Retraction of complaint: Often the victim will retract his or her story because of guilt or ambivalent feelings or fear of the consequences of disclosure (family breakup, possible foster placement).

Legal Issues

Every state has mandatory reporting of child abuse and sexual abuse to a designated authority. The abuse does not need to be proven before being reported. In the role of mandated reporters, professionals are afforded legal immunity for such reports. Failure to report can result in most cases in a civil or criminal penalty.

One area of potential confusion is the issue of consenting sexual contact between two minors or one minor and an adult. The practitioner should consult with local legal and medical authorities regarding laws for a particular state. However, every practitioner should consider the following in making a decision:

1. How young is the adolescent? Adolescents who are sexually active under the age of 14 have a significant risk for a history of current or prior sexual abuse. This history should be explored even if the current relationship is consensual and nonabusive.
2. What is the age difference between the minor and the adult? Sexual activity between a 12-year-old and a 25-year-old is much different than that between a 17-year-old and a 19-year-old.
3. Does the sexual activity of the younger teen reflect inadequate parental monitoring and supervision?
4. What is the nature of the relationship between the two individuals? Is force or the threat of force being used?
5. With young people who have a history of sexual abuse but are over 18, are younger siblings still at home and in jeopardy?

A second area of concern is the potential breaking of confidentiality when abuse is reported in cases when the teen or family does not wish the incident reported. At present, society has determined that the public's right to protect the victim is more important than a patient's right of privacy. This leads to greater protection of abused individuals but less physician-patient confidentiality.

Diagnosis

The diagnosis of sexual or physical abuse should be considered in an adolescent in the following situations:

1. STD (including gonorrhea, syphilis, herpes, *Trichomonas,* and condylomata) in a prepubertal adolescent or any adolescent with no history of sexual intercourse.
2. Recurrent somatic complaints, especially involving the gastrointestinal, genitourinary, or pelvic areas.
3. Behavior indicators, including:
   a. School-aged child
      — Learning difficulties
      — Isolation from peers
      — Acting-out behavior
      — Sleep disturbances
      — Anxiety, phobias, or depression
   b. Adolescents
      — Substance abuse
      — Runaway behavior
      — School problems and truancy
      — Antisocial behavior
      — Anxiety or depression
      — Suicide attempt
      — Aversion to sex or sexual topics
      — Promiscuity or provocative dress
      — Early age at first sexual intercourse
      — Unusual aversive reaction to examination of abdomen or genitalia
      — Eating disorders
      — Posttraumatic stress disorder
      — Teenage pregnancy

As listed in Chapter 3, the HEADSS inventory is a helpful device to collect important psychosocial information regarding adolescents. In our experience at Childrens Hospital Los Angeles, adolescents who experience a significant problem in one of these areas are at risk for having a history of current or past abuse. In any teen with a problem in one of these areas, it is important to explore the possibility of abuse. The physician must make the adolescent aware that if abuse is disclosed, the professional is legally obligated to report this to a child protective agency. To introduce the terms of the concept of limited confidentiality, the physician may say "Generally, what you say in here stays in here, but there are some exceptions. Namely, if you tell me that you want to hurt yourself or someone else, or that you were sexually or physically abused, I may need to inform your parents or the appropriate agencies or both." The practitioner can ask for such information with a question like: "We have seen many teens your age who have been touched in an area or at a time when they did not want to be. Has this ever happened to you?" Or "Some of the teens with whom I have worked who have tried to hurt themselves [or whatever the problem behavior is] have told me that they have been touched in an area where they did not want to be or have been beaten by a relative or parent. Has this ever happened to you?"

Evaluation

Evaluation of the sexually abused adolescent is similar to that described earlier in this chapter for the management of the rape victim. However, evidence collection such as swabs for semen analysis and collection of clothing and debris would only be performed if sexual contact had occurred in the past 72 hours. In the prepubertal adolescent an internal pelvic examination should not be performed unless indicated by the presence of a foreign body or by trauma.

Bibliography

Adams JA, Ahmad M, Phillips P. Anogenital findings and hymenal diameter in children referred for sexual abuse examination. Adolesc Pediatr Gynecol 1988; 1:123.

American Academy of Pediatrics Committee on Adolescence. Sexual assault and the adolescent. Pediatrics 1994;94:761.

American College of Emergency Physicians. Management of the patient with the complaint of sexual assault. Ann Emerg Med 1995;25:728.

American School Health Association, Association for the Advancement of Health Education, & Society for Public Health Education. The National Adolescent Student Health Survey: a report on the health of America's youth. Oakland, California: Third Party Publishing Company, 1989.

Anderson SC, Griffith S, Bach CM, et al. Sexual abuse of adolescent males: an overview. Paper presented at the Third International Congress on Child Abuse and Neglect, Amsterdam, The Netherlands, April 1981.

Anderson J, Martin J, Mullen P, et al. Prevalence of childhood sexual abuse experiences in a community sample of women. Am Acad Child Adolesc Psychiatry 1993;32:5.

Bach CM, Anderson SC. Adolescent sexual abuse and assault. J Curr Adolesc Med 1980;2:10.

Bang L. Rape victims—assaults, injuries and treatment at a medical rape trauma service at Oslo Emergency Hospital. Scand J Prim Health Care 1993;11:15.

Boyer DK. Male prostitution: a cultural expression of male homosexuality. Dissert Abst Int 1986;47: 1377A (University Microfilms International No. DA 8613141, pp. 124).

Browne A, Finkelhor D. Impact of child sexual abuse: a review of the research. Psychol Bull 1986;99:66.

Burgess A, Holstrom L. Rape trauma syndrome. Am J Psychiatry 1974;131:981.

Carper JM. Emergencies in adolescents. Runaways and father-daughter incest. Pediatr Clin North Am 1979; 26:883.

Cavallin BJ. Treatment of sexually abused adolescents: views of a psychologist. Semin Adolesc Med 1987; 3:39.

Commmittee on Adolescence. Rape and the adolescent. Pediatrics 1983;72:738.

Committee on Adolescent Health Care. Adolescent acquaintance rape. ACOG committee opinion. Int J Gynaecol Obstet 1993;42:209.

Cunningham RM, Stiffman AR, Dore P, et al. The association of physical and sexual abuse with HIV risk behaviors in adolescence and young adulthood: implications for public health. Child Abuse Negl 1994; 18:233.

Davis TC, Peck GQ, Storment JM. Acquaintance rape and the high school student. J Adolesc Health 1993; 14:220.

Deighton JA, Najar HS, McPeek P. Identifying the sexually abused patient. Female Patient 1986;11:75.

Deisher RW, Bidwell RJ. Sexual abuse of male adolescents. Semin Adolesc Med 1987;3:47.

De Jong AR, Emmett GA, Hervada AA. Epidemiologic factors in sexual abuse of boys. Am J Dis Child 1982; 136:990.

DeKeseredy WS. Woman abuse in dating relationships: the relevance of social support theory. Journal of Family Violence 1988;3:1.

Dewdney D. Treatment of physically abused adolescents. Semin Adolesc Med 1987;3:55.

Dunn SF, Gilchrist VJ. Sexual assault. Prim Care 1993; 20:359.

Ellis GM. Acquaintance rape. Perspect Psychiatr Care 1994;30:11.

Endert CM, Daniel WA Jr. Intra-family sexual abuse of adolescents. Pediatr Ann 1986;15:767.

Enos WF, Beyer JC. Management of the rape victim. Am Fam Physician 1978;18:97.

Farber ED, Joseph JA. The maltreated adolescent: patterns of physical abuse. Child Abuse Negl 1985;9: 201.

Felman YM, Nikitas JA. Sexually transmitted disease and child sexual abuse. NY State J Med 1983;(April): 714.

Finkelhor D. Sexually victimized children. New York: Free Press, 1979.

Finkelhor D. Risk factors in the sexual victimization of children. Child Abuse Negl 1980;4:265.

Finkelhor D. Child sexual abuse: new theory and research. New York: Free Press, 1984.

Finkelhor D, Browne A. The traumatic impact of child sexual abuse: a conceptualization. Am J Orthopsychiatry 1985;55:530.

Furey EM. Sexual abuse of adults with mental retardation: who and where. Ment Retard 1994;32:173.

Fontana VJ. Detection and management of child sexual abuse. Medical Aspects of Human Sexuality 1988; (February):126.

Gagnon J. Female child victims of sex offenses. Social Problems 1965;13:176.

Gans JE, Blyth DA, Elster AB, et al. America's adolescents: how healthy are they? Chicago: American Medical Association, 1990.

Glaser JB, Hammerschlag MR, McCormack WM. Sexually transmitted diseases in victims of sexual assault. N Engl J Med 1986;315:625.

Golding JM. Sexual assault history and physical health in randomly selected Los Angeles women. Health Psychol 1994;13:130.

Gostin LO, Lazzarini Z, Alexander D, et al. HIV testing, counseling, and prophylaxis after sexual assault. JAMA 1994;271:1436.

Greydanus DE, Shaw RD, Kennedy EL. Examination of sexually abused adolescents. Semin Adolesc Med 1987;3:59.

Gross M. Incestuous rape: a cause for hysterical seizures in four adolescent girls. Am J Orthopsychiatry 1979; 49:704.

Guidelines for the interview and examination of alleged rape victims. A conjoint effort of the Committee on Evolving Trends in Society Affecting Life and the Advisory Panels of Obstetrics and Gynecology, Pathology, and Psychiatry of the Scientific Board of the California Medical Association. West J Med 1975;123:420.

Hammerschlag MR, Cummings M, Doraiswamy B, et al. Nonspecific vaginitis following sexual abuse in children. Pediatrics 1985;75:1028.

Hampton HL. Care of the woman who has been raped. N Engl J Med 1995;332:234.

Hanson KA, Gidycz CA. Evaluation of a sexual assault prevention program. J Consult Clin Psychol 1993; 61:1046.

Herman-Giddens ME, Frothingham TE. Prepubertal female genitalia: examination for evidence of sexual abuse. Pediatrics 1987;80:203.

Hicks DJ. Rape: sexual assault. Am J Obstet Gynecol 1980;137:931.

Hickson FC, Davies PM, Hunt AJ, et al. Gay men as victims of nonconsensual sex. Arch Sex Behav 1994; 23:281.

Irwin KL, Edlin BR, Wong L. Urban rape survivors: characteristics and prevalence of human immunodeficiency virus and other sexually transmitted infections. Multicenter Crack Cocaine and HIV Infection Study Team. Obstet Gynecol 1995;85:330.

Johnson RL, Shrier DK. Sexual victimization of boys: experience at an adolescent medicine clinic. J Adolesc Health Care 1985;6:372.

Kellogg ND, Huston RL. Unwanted sexual experiences in adolescents. Patterns of disclosure. Clin Pediatr 1995;34:306.

Kormos KC, Brooks CI. Acquaintance rape: attributions of victim blame by college students and prison inmates as a function of relationship status of victim and assailant. Psychol Rep 1994;74:545.

Lakey JF. The profile and treatment of male adolescent sex offenders. Adolescence 1994;29:755.

Landis J. Experiences of 500 children with sexual deviants. Psychiatr Q 1956;30(suppl):91.

Lefley HP, Scott CS, Llabre M, et al. Cultural beliefs about rape and victims' response in three ethnic groups. Am J Orthopsychiatry 1993;63:623.

Libow JA, Doty DW. An exploratory approach to self-blame and self-derogation by rape victims. Am J Orthopsychiatry 1979;49:670.

Lindon J, Nourse CA. A multi-dimensional model of groupwork for adolescent girls who have been sexually abused. Child Abuse Negl 1994;18:341.

Lourie I. The phenomenon of the abused adolescent. Victimology 1977;2:268.

Mann EB. Self-reported stresses of adolescent rape victims. J Adolesc Health Care 1981;2:29.

Martin CA, Warfield MC, Braen GR. Physician's management of the psychological aspects of rape. JAMA 1983;249:501.

McCormack A, Janus M, Burgess AW. Runaway youths and sexual victimization: gender differences in an adolescent population. Child Abuse Negl 1986;10: 387.

Munt LC. Sexual abuse of children and adolescents. J Curr Adolesc Med 1980;2:30.

Muram D. Child sexual abuse: genital tract findings in prepubertal girls. I. The unaided medical examination. Am J Obstet Gynecol 1989;160:328.

Neinstein LS, Goldenring J. Nonsexual transmission of sexually transmitted diseases: an infrequent occurrence. Pediatrics 1984;74:67.

Peipert JF, Domagalski LR. Epidemiology of adolescent sexual assault. Obstet Gynecol 1994;84:867.

Pokovny SF, Kozinetz CA. Configuration and other anatomic details of the prepubertal hymen. Adolesc Pediatr Gynecol 1988;1:97.

Rabkin JG. The epidemiology of forcible rape. Am J Orthopsychiatry 1979;49:634.

Rimza ME, Niggeman MS. Medical evaluation of sexually abused children: a review of 311 cases. Pediatrics 1982;69:8.

Rosenberg MS. Rape crisis syndrome. Medical Aspects of Human Sexuality 1986;20:65.

Rubinstein M, Yeager CA, Goodstein C. Sexually assaultive male juveniles: a follow-up. Am J Psychiatry 1993;150:262.

Runtz M, Brierz J. Adolescent "acting out" and childhood history of child abuse. J Interpersonal Violence 1986;1:326.

Schor DP. Sex and sexual abuse in developmentally disabled adolescents. Semin Adolesc Med 1987; 3:1.

Shaw JA, Campo-Bowen AE, Applegate B, et al. Young boys who commit serious sexual offenses: demographics, psychometrics, and phenomenology. Bull Am Acad Psychiatry Law 1993;21:399.

Shearer SL, Herbert CA. Long-term effects of unresolved sexual trauma. Am Fam Physician 1987;36:169.

Silber TJ. Ethical issues in the treatment of the sexually abused adolescent: a clinician's perspective. Semin Adolesc Med 1987;3:39.

Spencer MJ, Dunklee P. Sexual abuse of boys. Pediatrics 1986;78:133.

Struckman-Johnson C, Struckman-Johnson D. Men pressured and forced into sexual experience. Arch Sex Behav 1994;23:93.

Summit R. Beyond belief. The reluctant discovery of incest. In: Kirkpatrick M, ed. Women's sexual experience. New York: Plenum Press, 1982.

Symons PY, Groer MW, Kepler-Youngblood P. Prevalence and predictors of adolescent dating violence. J Child Adolesc Psychiatr Nurs 1994; 7:14.

Tipton AC. Child sexual abuse: physical examination techniques and interpretation of findings. Adolesc Pediatr Gynecol 1989;2:10.

Watkins B, Bentovim A The sexual abuse of male children and adolescents: a review of current research. J Child Psychol Psychiatry 1992;33:197.

Yeide HE Jr. Religious issues and the sexual abuse of adolescents. Semin Adolesc Med 1987;3:33.

Zoucha-Jansen JM, Coyne A. The effects of resistance strategies on rape [see comments]. Am J Public Health 1993;83:1633.

CHAPTER 82

Chronic Illness in the Adolescent

Lawrence S. Neinstein and Lonnie K. Zeltzer

Whereas for the healthy teenager the process of adolescence can be both frustrating and difficult, for the critically ill teenager it can be extremely debilitating, leading to great frustration on the part of the individual, his or her family, and the health-care provider. The adolescent, whose life is already in constant flux, is particularly vulnerable when disrupting illness occurs. The effect of an illness on the adolescent's development can often, in fact, far outweigh the impact of the illness itself. In addition, families with chronically ill adolescents are particularly prone to feelings of guilt, anger, and frustration, problems reflected in the fact that divorce rates are as much as 50% higher in these families. This chapter emphasizes the developmental effects and management of the chronically ill or hospitalized adolescent. It is beyond the scope of this book to discuss all the specific chronic conditions that can affect adolescents. The references at the end of this chapter address a number of the major chronic illnesses in this age group.

DEFINITION

The chronically ill adolescent may be defined as one who has either a permanent or a residual disability, who has a nonreversible pathological alteration, or who requires a long period of supervision, observation, care, and/or rehabilitation.

PREVALENCE

As many as 10% to 20% of teenagers have a chronic condition. However, accurate data on prevalence rates of chronic illnesses are difficult to obtain. Prevalence rates also change with time as previously untreatable conditions become more treatable. Gortmaker and Sappenfield (1984) noted that between 1967 and 1981 the percentage of children from birth to age 16 years in the United States with a major limitation of activity caused by a chronic condition increased from 1.1% to 2.0%. Estimates of prevalence rates of chronic conditions in children from birth to 20 years of age in the United States are included in Table 82.1.

EFFECTS OF CHRONIC ILLNESS ON THE ADOLESCENT

The effects of chronic illness can be best appreciated within the framework of the developmental tasks of the adolescent. The effects are also dependent on such factors as the age at onset and the course, visibility, and prognosis of the chronic illness. Recent research presents a less negative picture of the psychosocial implication of chronic illness. Wolman et al. (1994) examined adolescents with and without a chronic illness. They found that although adolescents with chronic conditions do less well than adolescents without chronic condi-

Table 82.1.   Number of Cases and Prevalence of Selected Chronic Conditions for Persons 10 to 24 Years of Age (United States, 1986–1988)

Chronic Conditions	Cases[a]	Prevalence (per 1000 Persons)
Deformities or orthopaedic impairments	4,874,000	90.8
Asthma	2,696,000	50.2
Hearing impairments	1,425,000	26.6
Visual impairments	1,003,000	18.7
Mental retardation	698,000	13.0
Arthritis	633,000	11.8
Speech impairments	561,000	10.5
Epilepsy	273,000	5.1
Diabetes mellitus	218,000	4.1
Paralysis of extremities (complete or partial)	97,000	1.8
Cerebral palsy	65,000[b]	1.2[b]
Cleft palate	46,000[b]	0.9[b]
Malignancies—all sites	21,000[b]	0.4[b]
Spina bifida	11,000[b]	0.2[b]
Multiple sclerosis	9,000[b]	0.2[b]

Reproduced with permission from Blum RW, Geber G. Chronically ill youth. In: McAnarney ER, Kreipe RE, Orr DP, Comerci GC, eds. Textbook of adolescent medicine. Philadelphia: WB Saunders, 1992.
[a]Based on total population of 10- to 24-year-old persons of 53,654,000.
[b]Does not meet standards of statistical reliability.

tions, having a disability is not the most influential factor in emotional well-being. Family connectedness is of fundamental importance for adolescents' emotional well-being. Bennett (1994) reviewed 60 studies of depressive symptoms among children and adolescents with chronic medical problems. Though the findings indicated that children and adolescents with a chronic medical problem are at slightly elevated risk of having depressive symptoms, most were not clinically depressed.

Effects on Adolescent Developmental Tasks

Independence-Dependence   The overwhelming medical requirements of a chronic illness can severely interrupt the movement toward independence that normally occurs during early and middle adolescence. With chronic illness thus prolonging dependence on parents and others, including physicians, the adolescent may become compliant and childlike or noncompliant and rebellious.

Body Image   As stressed in earlier chapters, adolescents are highly concerned with and self-conscious about their developing bodies. Delayed puberty or bodily malformations that occur with chronic illness can create an inferior self-image. This abnormal body image may lead to:

1. Lowered self-esteem
2. Segregation from peers
3. Increased absences from school and other activities
4. Increased anxieties over sexual function and sexual relations
5. Depression, anger, or both

Peer Group   Chronic illness may limit the teenager's activities, not only because of greater fatigue, but also because time must be spent at doctor's appointments and in the hospital. There may also be rejection by peers or fantasies of such rejection. These problems may lead to social segregation and a fear of peer involvement.

Identity   The adolescent with a chronic illness may have difficulties with his or her developing identity. Concerns with future vocation, financial resources, separation from parents, and sexual function may all lead to an identity crisis.

Chronic illness can profoundly affect an adolescent's developing sexuality. The sexual interests and activities of the chronically ill adolescent may parallel those of the healthy adolescent, but they are often ignored. The chronic illness may affect the adolescent's sexuality through:

1. Altered self-esteem
2. Specific organic alteration of the sexual response, caused, for example, by drug effects, body cast, or spinal cord injury
3. An illness that leads to decreased enjoyment of sexual pleasure, such as arthritis, which can cause pain

The female adolescent may not only suffer an increased health risk if she becomes pregnant, but she may also be at increased risk of becoming pregnant as she tries to prove her sexuality or fertility.

All these interruptions in the adolescent's normal developmental tasks can lead to noncompliance, social withdrawal, dependence, and, ultimately, out-of-control behavior, depression, and even suicide. The practitioner should keep in mind, however, that having a chronic illness does not guarantee distress. Kellerman et al. (1980) found no increase in anxiety or decrease in self-esteem in a group of teenagers with a chronic illness as compared with a healthy group of teenagers.

Modifying Factors

Age at Onset   The stage of development during which the chronic illness appears may have considerable bearing on the psychological impact of the illness on the adolescent.

1. Preadolescence: Chronic illness or disability that has begun at birth or in early childhood may lead to altered parental expectations of the developing adolescent. Lowered parentally perceived potential may lead to reduced self-expectations of the adolescent. These misconceptions have major implications for the setting and achievement of future goals for the adolescent.
2. Early adolescence: Chronic illness for the early adolescent may lead to many concerns about body image. Because the adolescent has yet to separate from his or her parents, there may be little struggle for independence.
3. Middle adolescence: This age may be the most devastating time for a chronic illness to strike. During this phase, the adolescent is intensely involved with separation, peer involvement, and sexual development. A chronic illness may thwart the adolescent's progress in these areas, in addition to conflicting with the high energy levels and feelings of omnipotence typical of middle adolescence. Noncompliance is a frequent problem during this period of life.
4. Late adolescence: Chronic illness starting in late adolescence usually causes less upheaval. At this stage, the teenager will have already gained more self-confidence and identity. Concerns are focused on how the disease may disrupt vocational and educational plans, as well as future serious relationships and the prospects for living independently.

Nature of the Illness

Another factor that may modify the adolescent's reaction is the type of illness, including its chronicity, course, visibility, side effects of any medication, amount of disruption of control, and prognosis. For example, a highly visible disease such as psoriasis may cause more emotional disruption than Hodgkin's disease. Illnesses that lead to a feeling of loss of control, such as that occurring with an amputation, can also have profound effects. This loss of self-mastery may occur in adolescents who fear a lack of control even while being individually well controlled—for example, adolescents with seizure disorders or diabetes mellitus. Bennett (1994), in reviewing studies among children and adolescents with chronic medical problems, found that certain disorders (e.g., asthma, recurrent abdominal pain, sickle cell anemia) are associated with a greater risk for depression than other disorders (e.g., cancer, cystic fibrosis, diabetes mellitus). Howe et al. (1993) found that adolescents with brain-based conditions had more behavior problems, less autonomous functioning, and poorer school achievement.

Number of Chronic Conditions

In an analysis of the National Health Interview Survey, children and adolescents who had multiple conditions of a chronic nature, even if few in number, had increased morbidity across a variety of measures (Newacheck et al., 1994).

BEHAVIORS OF THE CHRONICALLY ILL ADOLESCENT

To cope with difficulties and frustrations of chronic illness, the adolescent usually adopts one or more of the following coping mechanisms:

1. Insightful acceptance: Unusual in adolescents, especially during early and middle adolescence.
2. Denial: A common behavior among adolescents, often leading to noncompliance problems such as missed appointments and forgotten medications.
3. Regression: Also common in chronically ill adolescents. With regression, the teenager becomes more dependent on parents and other adults and exhibits increasingly childlike behavior. Wishing to remain in the hospital beyond the necessary period is an example of this behavior.
4. Projection: This coping mechanism allows feelings of rage, frustration, or guilt to be transferred onto parents or health-care providers. Projection is often observed on adolescent hospital wards, where anger is transferred to the staff.
5. Displacement: A similar coping mechanism to projection, but the anger is usually transferred to an object or an activity. Displacement is observed frequently on adolescent wards and is typified by behavior such as throwing of objects.
6. Acting out: Similar to displacement but less constructive. In frustration, the adolescent exhibits out-of-control behavior, necessitating disciplinary management.
7. Compensation: A highly useful technique in which an adolescent alters usual activities in response to the restrictions of the disease. For example, an adolescent who formerly achieved self-esteem through dancing switches to performing music for fulfillment.
8. Intellectualization: This behavioral mechanism separates the realities of the disease from the emotional impact. This method is frequently observed on adolescent hospital wards in teenagers who become highly involved in the technical aspects of their disease. Although intellectualization can be a positive mechanism, there needs to be some period during which the adolescent faces and ventilates his or her emotional concerns.

The adolescent with a chronic illness or disability likely uses many of the foregoing coping mechanisms with time and in different situations. Most adolescents who come from psychologically healthy and supportive families can cope amazingly well with a multitude of stressors and are able to use these situations as emotional growth experiences. It is not uncommon to observe regressed behavior in an adolescent during a period of acute distress, with a rapid regaining of maturational status almost immediately afterward (e.g., when a bone marrow aspiration needle is removed).

With maturation and experience in dealing with chronic illness and its treatment, many adolescents are able to use cognitive reframing of situations to render them less threatening and stressful. The adolescents will also have developed an array of coping mechanisms that have worked, and will reuse those mechanisms instead of any that have not worked. Exposure to multiple stresses of a similar nature permits stress inoculation and the ability to respond more rapidly and often more appropriately to familiar challenges.

For those adolescents who cannot consistently meet the challenges of chronic illness, breakdown of the coping mechanism may be manifested behaviorally by noncompliance with treatment, increased risk-taking behaviors, or overall withdrawal from developmental tasks as a manifestation of depression.

MANAGEMENT OF CHRONIC ILLNESS IN THE ADOLESCENT

General Principles

Obviously, care of the adolescent's medical condition is of great importance. However, consideration and exploration of the adolescent's psychological development and tasks—independence, peer-group involvement, body image, and sexual and vocational identity—are also essential. In addition, the impact of the illness on the needs of the family should be evaluated. Helpful principles include:

1. Education: Inform the adolescent of the nature of the disease and the limitations of treatment. The educational process must be directed at both patient and family and should be on a level they can understand. Technical terms must be eliminated or explained.
2. Ventilation: Allow the adolescent time to ventilate his or her feelings, fears, and hopes.
3. Social skills: Discuss the adolescent's social skills and talents.
4. Occupational goals: Explore occupational goals and alternatives with the adolescent.
5. Continuity of care: The chronically ill adolescent needs an advocate whom he or she can trust. At least one member of the health-care team should be permanent. Many adolescents with a chronic illness have no primary physician. In one survey, Carrol et al. (1983) found that 40% of a group of chronically ill teenagers had no primary-care physician; yet, many of the 90% who reported having a primary-care health concern (headaches, acne, enuresis, insomnia, anxiety, and school problems) would not discuss it with their specialist provider.
6. Patient involvement: The more an adolescent is involved with his or her own care, the greater the chance for compliance and a sense of self-control.
7. Involvement in peer support groups: This involvement allows for increased expression of concerns and anxieties. A number of support-group agencies are listed at the end of this chapter.
8. Self-help techniques: Training the adolescent in a variety of cognitive-behavioral techniques to manage stress and pain can enhance feelings of self-control and reduce perceived disease- and treatment-related stress. Examples of these strategies include hypnosis, relaxation and distraction techniques, guided imagery, and thought-stopping.
9. Multidisciplinary team: Many health-care professionals will be involved in the care of the chronically ill adolescent, including physicians, psychologists, social workers, nurses, occupational therapists, physical therapists, and nutritionists. Reliance on the skills of these

individuals, as well as communication in interdisciplinary conferences, can improve the care of the adolescent.

10. Consideration of sexual development: Chronically ill adolescents may feel asexual because of delayed development, protective parents, and avoidance of sexual topics by family and physicians. The health-care professional needs to address these concerns by discussion of sexual anatomy, function, and contraception as needed. Most important, the adolescent should feel comfortable expressing concerns about sexuality and fertility. Special education needs to be available to the mentally retarded teenager, who may be subject to exploitation, and to the teenager with a severe physical deformity that may hinder sexual function. References regarding sexuality and the disabled teenager are listed at the end of this chapter.

11. Limit setting: If compliance or behavior is a problem, then limits need to be considered, including discussion of the reasons for negative behavior.

12. Family involvement: Family support and guidance are crucial. Families must be coached to avoid the "overs": overprotection, overanxiety, and overattention.

13. Inpatient care: Inpatient hospital care is best handled in an environment conducive to the developmental needs of the adolescent.

The Hospitalized Adolescent

In the course of their sickness, many chronically ill adolescents will be hospitalized; conversely, many, if not most, hospitalized adolescents are chronically ill. There is considerable advantage in placing most adolescent patients on one or part of one ward. The adolescent inpatient ward provides an environment and staff oriented toward the developmental needs of the adolescent.

Environment and Setting

1. Separate ward: Allows for adolescents to interact together and for a staff expert in adolescents' needs to be involved in their care.

2. Rooms of two or four: Generally, roommates give supportive help during the adolescent's stay; however, avoid having three teenagers in one room because this can result in two-against-one problems.

3. Recreation room: The adolescent ward should include a recreation room that provides a variety of activities to enhance interaction, encourage peer involvement, and alleviate boredom. In the context of playing a game, the recreational therapist may be the first to discover a chronically ill adolescent's fears or anxieties. The activity program can also play an important role in pain management for those ill adolescents who require such intervention.

4. Full privacy for beds: Adolescents require privacy, so each bed should have full curtains to achieve this purpose when desired.

5. Interested staff: Caring for adolescents consumes much time and energy, so the staff should be chosen from among those who enjoy working with adolescents.

6. Relevant rules and regulations: Rules should be flexible, sensitive, and explicit in regard to the adolescent unit. Such rules can include patient and staff responsibilities, and regulations regarding guests, television, bedtime, the recreation room, and quiet times. Figure 82.1 lists a sample set of rules for an adolescent unit, along with a listing of patient rights and responsibilities.

7. Snacks: Adolescents are often hungry at times other than mealtimes, so some allowance should be made to provide snacks.

8. Other important areas include a treatment room, interview rooms, and educational areas.

Welcome to the adolescent unit. Our services have been especially designed for teenagers and young adults, and the staff is here to give you the best possible care. We encourage you to be a part of your own care, to know about your illness, and to ask questions whenever you're not sure about anything that is being said or done.

We know that being in a hospital is not easy and that you would rather be at home or somewhere else. Since it is necessary that you be here, we hope to make your stay as pleasant as possible, and we look forward to getting to know you as a friend.

1. The adolescent unit:
   The adolescent unit is a special part of the hospital set aside to care for young people who are age 12 years or older. It is located on the east wing of the 5th floor of the hospital and can be reached by the three elevators in the hospital's central area. The unit can have as many as 32 patients.

2. Who will be my doctor?
   You may have several different doctors who will see you regularly and help with your treatment. Other specialists may be part of the medical team. If you are confused as to who these people are, do not hesitate to ask.

3. Who is my nurse?
   You will have a nurse assigned to you on every shift. The nurse will take your temperature and blood pressure (called vital signs) and bring your medicines. Your nurses are familiar with your condition and will try to answer any questions you have during your hospital stay. With your help, they will do their best to make your stay comfortable.

4. Other staff members:
   The unit assistant answers the telephone at the nursing station, schedules your appointments, keeps medical records, and helps the nurse-in-charge. Other hospital people with a variety of duties may come into your room at times. These staff members have responsibilities such as cleaning your room, repairing equipment, providing food, or performing lab tests. You may also meet people from social services, physical therapy, occupational therapy, or respiratory therapy. They, too, will be happy to answer any questions about their work.

5. What are hospital rounds?
   Every day the doctors and nurses review the medical care of each patient. In the morning they will stop by your room to examine your medical record. Usually they will not stop to talk with you at that time, but will return later in the day.

   From time to time, other teams of physicians or staff make patient rounds and may come to your room to talk with you. These visits enable the entire staff to provide you with the best care.

6. My room:
   We have tried to make the rooms comfortable and pleasant. Each room has a telephone, television, bathroom, and closet. Next to each bed is a nightstand, and each patient has his or her own TV control and a buzzer to call the nurse. Drapes for the windows and around each bed are provided for your privacy. There are showers and a bathtub located near the center of the 5th floor.

7. When may I go home?
   The length of time you remain in the hospital is determined by your condition. Your doctor will discuss this with you and should be able to give you an idea of how long your stay will be.

FIGURE 82.1. Sample orientation sheet for an adolescent ward, used at Childrens Hospital of Los Angeles.

Figure continues through page 1182.

8. What clothing and personal things should I bring from home?
We provide pajamas, toothbrush, comb, and soap, though you may bring your own if you like. We do not usually supply items such as bathrobe, slippers, razor, deodorant, or cosmetics.

   You might want to bring street clothes along, since there may be times to wear them here or when you go home.

9. When can I have visitors?
Visiting hours are from 10:00 AM to 9:00 PM daily; however, parents may visit at any time. Ask your nurse about special arrangements for parents spending the night. Visitors under 12 years of age are not allowed on the unit. If you are able to leave the unit, you may see them in other visiting areas of the hospital such as the cafeteria or the main lobby. Because of space limitations, we must ask that you limit visitors in your room to two at a time.

10. Do I ever leave the unit?
Most of the time you will be on the unit, although you might go to other parts of the hospital for x-ray or other tests. If you would like to leave the unit, you must check with your nurse and sign out. You can go to the cafeteria, gift shop, or main lobby. There is a sign-out board at the nurse's station. Please sign in when you return. We must know where you are at all times.

11. Daily schedule:

7:30 AM	Vital signs (temperature, blood pressure, etc.)
8:00 AM	Breakfast
8:30 AM to 10:00 am	Doctors' rounds
12:00 noon	Lunch
5:30 PM	Dinner
8:30 PM	Snack
10:30 PM	In your own room, quiet hours
12:00 midnight	Lights (TV, radio) out

12. What may I have to eat?
You have the opportunity to select from a list of foods prepared in the kitchen, unless a special diet is ordered for you by your doctor. If your doctor has ordered a special diet, the dietitian will discuss it with you, and you can help write menus that you like by filling out a menu card. Snacks can also be provided on your trays to be saved for later, and a snack cart will be available every evening at 8:00 PM.

   On occasion, you may be able to have lunch or dinner in the cafeteria. Arrangements must be made with your nurse before 10:30 AM for lunch and before 4:30 PM for dinner. You do not have to pay for cafeteria meals, but all visitors do.

   You may bring in food from outside the hospital, so long as it is allowed on your diet.

13. Schoolwork:
If your doctor expects that your stay will be 2 weeks or longer, a hospital teacher is available to help you with your assignments. Please ask your nurse to call the teacher to be sure that the teacher knows you are here.

   Sometimes patients know that they will be entering the hospital for 2 weeks or longer. Before coming they can make arrangements with their classroom teachers and the hospital teacher. If you came to the hospital unexpectedly and will be staying for at least 2 weeks, the teacher will contact your home school for assignments.

   The teacher, from the Los Angeles City Schools, will help you do your work in classrooms on the 4th floor of the hospital, or in your hospital room if your condition requires it.

FIGURE 82.1.   *continued*

14. Special privileges:

The use of portable radios, tapes, blow dryers, and other such devices is permitted on the unit. Speakers/amplifiers must be left at home. For safety reasons, all electrical equipment must be checked by our engineering department. We want you to enjoy your music but please keep the volume down. The hospital does not accept responsibility for the safety of these items, so it is your responsibility to take care of them or leave them at home.

The telephone in your room may be used from 8:00 AM to 9:00 PM. Dial 9, listen for the tone, and then dial as you would normally. There is no charge for local calls. For long distance and other toll calls, an operator will automatically ask if you would like to make the call collect or have it billed to your home.

Telephones at the nurses' station are for the staff only. There are pay telephones across from the elevators for visitors' use.

Although we discourage smoking, patients who are accustomed to smoking may smoke cigarettes, with their doctor's permission, under the following conditions:
1. In the lobby across from the elevators
2. In the cafeteria on the ground floor
3. When confined to bed and if:
   a. The condition of the patient or the roommate is not affected by smoking
   b. The environment remains safe with regard to equipment in the room
   c. Agreeable to roommate
   d. Nursing personnel present in the room while cigarette is ignited and until extinguished

15. 5-East Activity Room:

When you walk onto the adolescent unit, the first room on the left is the activity room. This room is supervised by the Patient Activity Program staff, who plan and schedule a variety of activities. These activities include art projects, special guests, rap groups, buffet dinners, and medical education activities.

Always available in the room are Ping-Pong, Foosball, stereo, games, art supplies, and books and magazines. Family and friends are welcome to participate. The schedule of when the room is open is posted on the door.

16. Important reminders:
1. Sign out at the nurses' station when you leave the floor, and sign in when you return.
2. You should be in your room from 10:30 PM to 7:00 AM.
3. You should be on the unit from 10:00 PM to 10:00 AM unless you are scheduled for tests.
4. Ask questions when something is not clear to you. Part of our job is to keep you informed about what we are doing.

Patient Rights and Responsibilities

Every teenager and young adult who comes to our unit should receive the highest quality of care. To make that happen, you and the staff have certain rights and responsibilities.

You have the right to expect from us:

1. To be informed about our unit and its services:

We believe that it is important for you to understand as much as possible about your medical care because it is your body we are all concerned about. The staff will attempt to answer any questions you have concerning your illness. This includes what tests are being done and why, names of the doctors and nurses caring for you, information about your progress, and plans for your health care after leaving the hospital. We also realize that you have ideas and feelings about your illness and experience in the hospital. We would like you to feel free to discuss these with any of the staff.

FIGURE 82.1.   *continued*

2. To be respected as an individual:
This includes respect of your privacy by knocking on your door before entering your room, responding to your buzzer and to requests for medication as soon as possible, having medical students ask permission to interview you, having the staff consider your modesty during examinations, and sharing information about you only with those involved in your care. Along with rights come responsibilities. As examples, it is your responsibility:

1. To follow the policies of our unit and respect the facilities we provide for our patients. Our goal is to provide the best health care to you and others on our unit. Misusing our facilities or failing to follow the rules denies that goal for everyone.
2. To assist and participate in your medical care. As a member of your medical team, your responsibilities may include following doctors' orders, taking medications as scheduled, and being available when it is time for procedures or treatments.
3. To respect the hospital staff, and the rights of other patients. The hospital staff should be treated with respect. We are helping several people at the same time, and there will be times when the needs of other patients will have to be met first.
   It is your responsibility to be sure that the privacy of other patients is respected by you and your visitors. All patients have a right not to be disturbed by noise or by smoking in the room, and they have a right not to be put into an uncomfortable situation.

Childrens Hospital has a patient relations service. A person on that staff is available to patients and their families to hear their needs and concerns, and to speak on their behalf. To contact Patient Relations, call extension [number].

Figure 82.1. *continued*

Staffing

1. The staff should be chosen on the basis of interest and ability in working with adolescents.
2. The staff should include physicians, nurses, a psychologist, a social worker, a recreational therapist, a teacher, and a consultant nutritionist.
3. Staff meetings should include both continuing medical education and interdisciplinary case conferences.

In summary, the adolescent inpatient service can provide chronically ill teenagers with an environment that increases their independence, respects their privacy, and enhances their knowledge of their particular illness, while reinforcing behavior that encourages their continued growth.

BIBLIOGRAPHY

Adams JA, Weaver SJ. Self-esteem and perceived stress in young adolescents with chronic disease: unexpected findings. J Adolesc Health Care 1986;7:173.

Allen DA. Concerns of children with a chronic illness: a cognitive-developmental study of juvenile diabetes. Child Care Health Dev 1984;10:211.

American Academy of Pediatrics Committee on Children With Disabilities and Committee on Psychosocial Aspects of Child and Family Health. Psychosocial risks of chronic health conditions in childhood and adolescence. Pediatrics 1993;92:876.

Anderson CTM, Fanurik D, Zeltzer LK. Pain in adolescence. In: McAnarney ER, Kreipe RE, Orr DP, Comerci GD, eds. Textbook of adolescent medicine. Philadelphia: WB Saunders, 1992:140–145.

Barness LA. Adolescent nutritional determinants of chronic disease. Prog Clin Biol Res 1981;77:791.

Beales G. The child's view of chronic illness. Nurs Times 1983;79:50.

Bellamy GT, Wilcox B, Rose H, McDonnell J. Education and career preparation for youth with disabilities. J Adolesc Health Care 1985;6:125.

Bennett DS. Depression among children with chronic medical problems: a meta-analysis. J Pediatr Psychol 1994;19:149.

Blum R. Chronic illness and disabilities in childhood

and adolescence. Orlando, Florida: Grune & Stratton, 1984.

Bombardier CH, Divine GW, Jordan JS, et al. Minnesota Multiphasic Personality Inventory (MMPI) cluster groups among chronically ill patients: relationship to illness adjustment and treatment outcome. J Behav Med 1993;16:467.

Brent DA. A death in the family: the pediatrician's role. Pediatrics 1983;72:645.

Brook U, Rapaport A, Heim M. Care for chronically ill adolescents. World Health Forum 1994;15:233.

Carraccio CL, McCormick MC, Weller SC. Chronic disease: effect on health cognition and health locus of control. J Pediatr 1987;110:982.

Carrol G, Massarelli E, Opzoomer A, et al. Adolescents with chronic disease: are they receiving comprehensive health care? J Adolesc Health Care 1983;4:261.

Collins JG. Pediatrics: prevalence of selected chronic conditions—United States, 1986–88. Vital Health Stat [Series 10] 1993;182:1.

Coupey SM, Cohen MI. Special considerations for the health care of adolescents with chronic illnesses. Pediatr Clin North Am 1984;31:211.

Court JM. Issues of transition to adult care. J Paediatr Child Health 1993;29(suppl 1):S53.

Desguin BW, Holt IJ, McCarthy SM. Comprehensive care of the child with a chronic condition. II. Primary care management. Curr Probl Pediatr 1994;24:230.

Elkind D. Cognitive development and adolescent disabilities. J Adolesc Health Care 1985;6:84.

Frauman DA, Sypert NS. Sexuality in adolescents with chronic illness. Matern Child Nurs J 1979;4:371.

Geber G, Latts E. Race and ethnicity: issues for adolescents with chronic illnesses and disabilities: an annotated bibliography. Pediatrics 1993;91:1071.

Gortmaker SL, Sappenfield W. Chronic childhood disorders: prevalence and impact. Pediatr Clin North Am 1984;31:3.

Greydanus DE, ed. Caring for your adolescent. New York: Bantam Books, 1991.

Hauser ST, DiPlacido J, Jacobson AM, et al. Family coping with an adolescent's chronic illness: an approach and three studies. J Adolesc 1993;16:305.

Hofmann AD, Becker RD, Gabriel HP. The hospitalized adolescent: a guide to managing the ill and injured youth. New York: Free Press, 1976.

Howe GW, Feinstein C, Reiss D, et al. Adolescent adjustment to chronic physical disorders. I. Comparing neurological and non-neurological conditions. J Child Psychol Psychiatry 1993;34:1153.

Karon M. The physician and the adolescent with cancer. Pediatr Clin North Am 1973;20:965.

Kellerman J, Zeltzer L, Ellenberg L, Dash J, Rigler D. Psychological effects of illness in adolescence. I. Anxiety, self-esteem, and perception of control. J Pediatr 1980;97:126.

Kessell M, Resnick MD, Blum RW. Adventure, Etc.: a health promotion program for chronically ill and disabled youth. J Adolesc Health Care 1985;6:433.

Kramer JP, Ferrari M, Kline CS. The development and five-year experience of a day hospital for chronically ill adolescents (cost-effective ambulatory medical care/education for chronically ill adolescents). Del Med J 1994;66:271.

Lapham EV, Shevlin KM. The impact of chronic illness on psychosocial stages of human development. Washington, DC: Georgetown University Hospital and Medical Center, 1986.

Leichtman SR, Friedman SB. Social and psychological development of adolescents and the relationship to chronic illness. Med Clin North Am 1975;59:1319.

Lynch DJ, Funk JB, Fay LM. Helping the family with a chronically ill child. Am Fam Physician 1987;36:214.

Lynch EW, Lewis RB, Murphy DS. Educational services for children with chronic illnesses: perspectives of educators and families. Except Child 1993;59:210.

Magrab PR, Calcagno PL. Psychological impact of chronic pediatric conditions. In: Magrab PR, ed. Psychological management of pediatric problems; vol 1. Baltimore: University Park Press, 1978.

McAnarney ER. Social maturation: a challenge for handicapped and chronically ill adolescents. J Adolesc Health Care 1985;6:90.

Midence K. The effects of chronic illness on children and their families: an overview. Genet Soc Gen Psychol Monogr 1994;120:311.

Millstein SG, Adler NE, Irwin CE Jr. Conceptions of illness in young adolescents. Pediatrics 1981;68:834.

Neinstein LS, Katz B. Contraceptive use in the chronically ill adolescent female. I. J Adolesc Health Care 1986;7:123.

Newacheck PW, Stoddard JJ. Prevalence and impact of multiple childhood chronic illnesses. J Pediatr 1994;124:40.

Olson AL, Johansen SG, Powers LE, et al. Cognitive coping strategies of children with chronic illness. J Dev Behav Pediatr 1993;14:217.

Orr DP, Weller SC, Satterwhite B, Bless IB. Psychosocial implications of chronic illness in adolescence. J Pediatr 1984;104:152.

Pless IB, Roghmann KG. Chronic illness and its consequences: observations based on three epidemiologic surveys. J Pediatr 1971;79:351.

Sabbeth B. Understanding the impact of chronic childhood illness on families. Pediatr Clin North Am 1984;31:47.

Schulman JL. Coping with major disease: child, family, pediatrician. J Pediatr 1983;102:988.

Siegel DM. Adolescents and chronic illness. JAMA 1987;257:3396.

Sinnema G. The development of independence in chronically ill adolescents. Int J Adolesc Med Health 1986;2:1.

Smith MS, ed. Chronic disorders in adolescence. Boston: John Wright Publishing, 1983.

Spirito A, Stark LJ, Gil KM, et al. Coping with everyday and disease-related stressors by chronically ill children and adolescents. J Am Acad Child Adolesc Psychiatry 1995;34:283.

Stawski M, Auerbach JG, Barasch M, et al. Behavioral problems of adolescents with chronic physical illness: a comparison of parent-report and self-report measures. Eur Child Adolesc Psychiatry 1995;4:14.

Stetz KM, Lewis FM, Houck GM. Family goals as indicants of adaptation during chronic illness. Public Health Nurs 1994;11:385.

The self-image of adolescents with cystic fibrosis. J Adolesc Health 1995;16:204.

Turnbull AP, Turnbull HR III. Developing independence. J Adolesc Health Care 1985;6:108.

Waldman HB. Almost twenty million chronically ill children. ASDC J Dent Child 1994;61:129.

Weitzman M, Walker DK, Gortmaker S. Chronic illness, psychosocial problems, and school absences. Clin Pediatr 1986;25:137.

Wolfish MG, McLean, JA. Chronic illness in adolescents. Pediatr Clin North Am 1974;21:1043.

Wolman C, Resnick MD, Harris LJ, et al. Emotional well-being among adolescents with and without chronic conditions. J Adolesc Health 1994;15:199.

Wood PR, Zeltzer LK, Cox AD. Communicating with adolescents from culturally varied backgrounds: a model in the Mexican-American adolescents in South Texas. Semin Adolesc Med 1987;3(2):99.

Zeltzer LK. The adolescent with cancer. In: Kellerman J, ed. Psychological aspects of childhood cancer. Springfield, Illinois: Charles C Thomas, 1981.

Zeltzer L. Chronic illness and disability in adolescents. Int J Adolesc Med Health 1985;1(34):239.

Zeltzer LK, LeBaron S. The hypnotic treatment of children in pain. In: Routh D, Wolraich M, eds. Advances in developmental and behavioral pediatrics; vol 7. Greenwich, Connecticut: JAT Press, 1986.

Zeltzer L, Kellerman J, Ellenberg L, Dash J, Rigler D. Psychological effects of illness in adolescence. II. Impact of illness in adolescents: crucial issues and coping styles. J Pediatr 1980;97:132.

References for Specific Conditions
Asthma
American Academy of Pediatrics Committee on Children with Disabilities and Committee on Sports Medicine. The asthmatic child's participation in sports and physical education. Pediatrics 1984;74:155.

Balfour-Lynn L. Childhood asthma and puberty. Arch Dis Child 1985;60:231.

Balfour-Lynn L. Growth and childhood asthma. Arch Dis Child 1986;61:1049.

Becker MH, Radius SM, Rosenstock IM, Drachman RH, Shuberth K, Teets KC. Compliance with a medical regimen for asthma: a test of the health belief model. Public Health Rep 1978;93:268.

Bremberg SG, Kjellman NIM. Children with asthma: how do they get along at school? Acta Paediatr Scand 1985;74:833.

Brown CJ. Hospital management of chronic illness in adolescence: a developmental model. J Chronic Dis 1982;35:659.

Friberg S, Bevegard S, Graff-Lonnevig V. Asthma from childhood to adult age. Acta Paediatr Scand 1988;77:424.

Morikawa A, Mochizuki H, Shigeta M, et al. Age-related changes in bronchial hyperreactivity during the adolescent period. J Asthma 1994;31:445.

Neddenriep D, Schumacher M, Lemen R. Asthma in childhood. Curr Probl Pediatr 1989;19:327.

Pearlman DS. Bronchial asthma: a perspective from childhood to adulthood. Am J Dis Child 1984;138:459.

Slack MK, Brooks AJ. Medication management issues for adolescents with asthma. Am J Health Sys Pharm 1995;52:1417.

Taggart VS, Fulwood R. Youth health report card: asthma. Prev Med 1993;22:579.

Turner ES, Greenberger MD, Patterson R. Management of the pregnant asthmatic patient. Ann Intern Med 1980;6:905.

Cancer
Altman AJ. Chronic leukemias of childhood. Pediatr Clin North Am 1988;35:765.

Binger CM. Psychosocial intervention with the child cancer patient and family. Psychosomatics 1984;25:899.

Byrne J, Mulvihill JJ, Myers MH, et al. Effects of treatment on fertility in long-term survivors of childhood or adolescent cancer. N Engl J Med 1987;317:1315.

Clayton PE, Shalet SM, Price DA, Campbell RHA. Testicular damage after chemotherapy for childhood brain tumors. J Pediatr 1988;112:922.

Cohen DG, Klopovich P, eds. The adolescent with cancer. Semin Oncol Nurs 1986;2:73.

Copeland DR, Fletcher JM, Pfefferbaum-Levine B. Neuropsychological sequelae of childhood cancer in long-term survivors. Pediatrics 1985;75:745.

Dein RA, Mennuti MT, Kovach P. The reproductive potential of young men and women with Hodgkin's disease. Obstet Gynecol Surv 1984;39:474.

Easson WM. The seriously ill or dying adolescent. Postgrad Med 1985;78:183.

Finlay JL, Goins SC, Uteg R, et al. Progress in the management of childhood brain tumors. Hematol/Oncol Clin North Am 1987a;1:753.

Finlay JL, Uteg R, Giese WL. Brain tumors in children. II. Advances in neurosurgery and radiation oncology. Am J Pediatr Hematol Oncol 1987b;9:256.

Green DM, Zevon MA, Reese PA, et al. Factors that influence the further survival of patients who survive for five years after the diagnosis of cancer in childhood or adolescence. Med Pediatr Oncol 1994;22:91.

Jamison RN, Lewis S, Burish TG. Psychological impact of cancer on adolescents: self-image, locus of control, perception of illness, and knowledge of cancer. J Chronic Dis 1986;39:609.

Kaplan SL, Busner J, Weinhold C. Depressive symptoms in children and adolescents with cancer: a longitudinal study. J Am Acad Child Adolesc Psychiatry 1987;26:782.

Kashani J, Hakami N. Depression in children and adolescents with malignancy. Can J Psychiatry 1982;27:474.

Kellerman J, Katz ER. The adolescent with cancer: theoretical, clinical, and research issues. J Pediatr Psychiatry 1977;2:127.

Leikin S. The role of adolescents in decisions concerning their cancer therapy. Cancer 1993;71:3342.

Livesey EA, Brook CGD. Gonadal dysfunction after treatment of intracranial tumors. Arch Dis Child 1988;63:495.

Murphy SB. The lymphomas and lymphadenopathy. In: Nathan DG, Oski FA, eds. Hematology of infancy and childhood. Philadelphia: WB Saunders, 1987:1086–1117.

Nichols ML. Social support and coping in young adolescents with cancer. Ped Nurse 1995;21:235.

Nicholson HS, Byrne J. Fertility and pregnancy after treatment for cancer during childhood or adolescence. Cancer 1993;71:3392.

Nitschke R, Humphrey GB, Sexauer CL. Therapeutic choices made by patients with end-stage cancer. J Pediatr 1982;101:471.

Ochs J, Mulhern R. Late effects of antileukemic treatment. Pediatr Clin North Am 1988;35:815.

Patenaude AF, Rappeport JM. Surviving bone marrow transplantation: the patient in the other bed. Ann Intern Med 1982;97:915.

Peckham VC, Meadows AT, Bartel N, Marrero O. Educational late effects in long-term survivors of childhood acute lymphocytic leukemia. Pediatrics 1988;81:127.

Pfefferbaum-Levine B, Copeland DR, Fletcher JM. Neuropsychologic assessment of long-term survivors of childhood leukemia. Am J Pediatr Hematology Oncology 1984;6:123.

Poplack DG, Reaman G. Acute lymphoblastic leukemia in childhood. Pediatr Clin North Am 1988;35:903.

Rappaport R, Brauner R, Czernichow P, Renier TD, Zucker JM, Lemerle J. Effect of hypothalamic and pituitary irradiation on pubertal development in children with cranial tumors. J Clin Endocrinol Metab 1982;54:1164.

Ross JA, Severson RK, Robison LL, et al. Pediatric cancer in the United States: a preliminary report of a collaborative study of the Children's Cancer Group and the Pediatric Oncology Group. Cancer 1993;71:3415.

Sawyer M, Crettenden A, Toogood I. Psychological adjustment of families of children and adolescents treated for leukemia. Am J Pediatr Hematol Oncol 1986;8:200.

Shalet SM, Hann IM, Lendon M, Jones PHM, Beardwell CG. Testicular function after combination chemotherapy in childhood for acute lymphoblastic leukemia. Arch Dis Child 1981;56:275.

Sklar CA, Kim TH, Ramsay NK. Testicular function following bone marrow transplantation performed during or after puberty. Cancer 1984;53:1498.

Souhami RL. Care for the adolescent with cancer. Eur J Cancer 1993;29A:2215.

Susman E, Hersch S, Nannis E, et al. Conceptions of cancer: perspectives of child and adolescent patients and their families. J Pediatr Psychol 1982;7:253.

Tebbi C, ed. Major topics in adolescent oncology. Mt. Kisco, New York: Futura, 1987.

Teta MJ, Del Po MC, Kasl SV. Psychosocial consequences of childhood and adolescent cancer survival. J Chronic Dis 1986;39:751.

Wasserman AL, Thompson EI, Wilimas JA, Fairclough DL. The psychological status of survivors of childhood/adolescent Hodgkin's disease. Am J Dis Child 1987;141:626.

Zeltzer L, Kellerman J, Ellenberg L, Dash J. Hypnosis for reduction of vomiting associated with chemotherapy and disease in adolescents with cancer. J Adolesc Health Care 1983;4:77.

Zeltzer LK, LeBaron S, Zeltzer P. The adolescent with cancer. In: Blum R, ed. Chronic illness and disabilities in childhood and adolescence. Orlando, Florida: Grune & Stratton, 1984.

Cystic Fibrosis

Bartholomew LK, Parcel GS, Swank PR, et al. Measuring self-efficacy expectations for the self-management of cystic fibrosis. Chest 1993;103:1524.

Cohen LF, Di Sant'Agnese PA, Friedlander J. Cystic fibrosis and pregnancy: a national survey. Lancet 1980;2:842.

Cowen L, Corey M, Simmons R. Growing older with cystic fibrosis: psychologic adjustment of patients more than 16 years old. Psychosom Med 1984;46:363.

Dibble SL, Savedra MC. Cystic fibrosis in adolescence: a new challenge. Pediatr Nurs 1988;14:299.

Di Sant'Agnese PA, Davis PB. Cystic fibrosis in adults: 75 cases and a review of 232 cases in the literature. Am J Med 1979;66:121.

Fitzpatrick SB, Stokes DC, Rosenstein BJ, Terry P, Hubbard VS. Use of oral contraceptives in women with cystic fibrosis. Chest 1984;86:863.

Huang NH, Schidlow DV, Szatrowski TH, et al. Clinical features, survival rate, and prognostic factors in young adults with cystic fibrosis. Am J Med 1987;82:871.

Hymovich DP, Baker CD. The needs, concerns, and coping of parents of children with cystic fibrosis. Fam Relations 1985;34:91.

Landon C, Rosenfeld RG. Short stature and pubertal delay in male adolescents with cystic fibrosis: androgen treatment. Am J Dis Child 1984;138:388.

Logvinoff M-M, Fon GT, Taussig LM. Kyphosis and pulmonary function in cystic fibrosis. Clin Pediatr 1984;23:389.

Mador JA, Smith DH. The psychosocial adaptation of adolescents with cystic fibrosis: a review of the literature. J Adolesc Health Care 1989;10:136.

Mitchell-Heggs P, Mearns M, Batten JC. Cystic fibrosis in adolescents and adults. Q J Med 1976;45:479.

Moise JR, Drotar D, Doershuk CF, Stern RC. Correlates of psychosocial adjustment among young adults with cystic fibrosis. J Dev Behav Pediatr 1987;8:141.

Neinstein LS, Stewart D, Want C, Johnson I. Menstrual dysfunction in cystic fibrosis. J Adolesc Health Care 1983;4:153.

Palmer J, Dillon-Baker C, Tecklin JS, et al. Pregnancy in patients with cystic fibrosis. Ann Intern Med 1983; 99:596.

Patterson JM. Critical factors affecting family compliance with home treatment for children with cystic fibrosis. Fam Relations 1985;34:79.

Patton AC, Ventura JN, Savedra M. Stress and coping responses of adolescents with cystic fibrosis. Child Health Care 1986;14:153.

Pumariega AJ. The adolescent with cystic fibrosis: developmental issues. Child Health Care 1982;11:78.

Reiter EO, Stern RC, Root AW. The reproductive endocrine system in cystic fibrosis. I. Basal gonadotropin and sex steroid levels. Am J Dis Child 1981; 135:422.

Reiter EO, Stern RC, Root AW. The reproductive endocrine system in cystic fibrosis. II. Changes in gonadotropins and sex steroids following LHRH. Clin Endocrinol 1982;16:127.

Sawyer SM, Rosier MJ, Phelan PD, et al. The self-image of adolescents with cystic fibrosis. J Adolesc Health 1995;16:204.

Seale TW, Flux M, Rennert OM. Reproductive defects in patients of both sexes with cystic fibrosis: a review. Ann Clin Lab Sci 1985;15:512.

Simmons RJ, Corey M, Cowen L, Keenan N, Robertson J, Levison H. Emotional adjustment of early adolescents with cystic fibrosis. Psychosom Med 1985;47: 111.

Sinnema G, Bonarius JCJ, Stoop JW. Adolescents with cystic fibrosis in the Netherlands. Acta Paediatr Scand 1983;72:427.

Smith G. A patient's view of cystic fibrosis. J Adolesc Health Care 1986;7:134.

Smith MS, Gad MT, O'Grady L. Psychosocial functioning, life change, and clinical status in adolescents with cystic fibrosis. J Adolesc Health Care 1983;4:230.

Soutter VL, Kristidis P, Gruca MA. Chronic undernutrition/growth retardation in cystic fibrosis. Clin Gastroenterol 1986;15:137.

Steinhausen HC, Chindler HP. Psychosocial adaptation in children and adolescents with cystic fibrosis. J Dev Behav Pediatr 1981;2:74.

Stern RC, Boat TF, Doershuk CF, Tucker AS, Miller RB, Matthews LW. Cystic fibrosis diagnosed after age 13. Ann Intern Med 1977;87:188.

Strauss GD, Wellisch DK. Psychosocial adaptation in older cystic fibrosis patients. J Chronic Dis 1981;34: 141.

Thompson RJ Jr, Gil KM, Gustafson KE, et al. Stability and change in the psychological adjustment of mothers of children and adolescents with cystic fibrosis and sickle cell disease. J Pediatr Psychol 1994;19:171.

Diabetes Mellitus
Allen DA, Affleck G, Tennen H. Concerns of children with a chronic illness: a cognitive-developmental study of juvenile diabetes. Child Care Health Dev 1984;10:211.

Amiel SA, Sherwin RS, Simonson DC, Lauritano AA, Tamborlane WV. Impaired insulin action in puberty: a contributing factor to poor glycemic control in adolescents with diabetes. N Engl J Med 1986;315: 215.

Bacon GE, Ladu C, Shein HE, Rucknagel DL. Evaluation of glycosylated hemoglobin in the management of young patients with insulin-dependent diabetes mellitus. J Adolesc Health Care 1986;7:187.

Baker L, Lyen KR. The first hospitalization: cornerstone of juvenile diabetes management. Drug Ther 1981; 11:62.

Barglow P, Berndt DJ, Burns WJ. Neuroendocrine and psychological factors in childhood diabetes mellitus. J Am Acad Child Psychiatry 1986;25:785.

Bennett DL. The adolescent with diabetes mellitus. Pediatr Ann 1978;7:9.

Boehnert CE, Popkin MK. Psychological issues in treatment of severely noncompliant diabetics. Psychosomatics 1986;27:11.

Brand AH, Johnson JH, Johnson SB. Life stress and diabetic control in children and adolescents with insulin-dependent diabetes. J Pediatr Psychol 1986;11: 481.

Burns KL, Green P, Chase P. Psychosocial correlates of glycemic control as a function of age in youth with insulin-dependent diabetes. J Adolesc Health Care 1986;7:311.

Castells S, ed. Juvenile diabetes. Pediatr Clin North Am 1984;31:521.

Cohen HN, Paterson KR, Wallace AM. Dissociation of adrenarche and gonadarche in diabetes mellitus. Clin Endocrinol 1984;20:717.

Delamater AM, Kurtz SM, Bibb J. Stress and coping in relation to metabolic control of adolescents with type diabetes. J Dev Behav Pediatr 1987;8:136.

Fonagy P, Moran GS, Lindsay MKM, Kurtz AB, Brown R. Psychological adjustment and diabetic control. Arch Dis Child 1987;62:1009.

Gold MA, Gladstein J. Substance use among adolescents with diabetes mellitus: preliminary findings. J Adolesc Health 1993;14:80.

Golden MP, Gray DL. Diabetes mellitus in children and adolescents. In: Rakel RE, ed. Conn's current therapy 1991. Philadelphia: WB Saunders, 1991.

Hoare P, Mann H. Self-esteem and behavioural adjustment in children with epilepsy and children with diabetes. J Psychosom Res 1994;38:859.

Hoette SJ. The adolescent with diabetes mellitus. Nurs Clin North Am 1983;18:763.

Jackson RL. Growth and maturation of children with insulin dependent diabetes mellitus. Pediatr Clin North Am 1984;31:545.

Jacobson AM, Hauser ST, Wofsdorf JI. Psychologic predictors of compliance in children with recent onset of diabetes mellitus. J Pediatr 1987;110:805.

Jacobson AM, Hauser ST, Lavori P, et al. Family environment and glycemic control: a four-year prospective study of children and adolescents with insulin-dependent diabetes mellitus. Psychosom Med 1994; 56:401.

Johnson SB, Rosenbloom AL. Behavioral aspects of diabetes mellitus in childhood and adolescence. Psychiatr Clin North Am 1982;5:357.

Klusa Y, Habbick BF, Abernathy TJ. Diabetes in children: family responses and control. Psychosomatics 1983;24:367.

Kovacs M, Feinberg TL, Paulauskas S, Finkelstein R, Pollock M, Crouse-Novak M. Initial coping responses and psychosocial characteristics of children with insulin-dependent diabetes mellitus. J Pediatr 1985; 106:827.

Malone JI, Grizzard S, Espinoza LR. Risk factors for diabetic retinopathy in youth. Pediatrics 1984;73:756.

Meldman LS. Diabetes as experienced by adolescents. Adolescence 1987;22:433.

Miodovnik M, Lavin JP, Knowles HC. Spontaneous abortion among insulin-dependent diabetic women. Am J Obstet Gynecol 1984;150:372.

Orr DP. Psychosocial problems of diabetic teenagers. Medical Aspects of Human Sexuality 1986;20:86.

Orr DP, Eccles T, Lawlor R, Golden M. Surreptitious insulin administration in adolescents with insulin-dependent diabetes mellitus. JAMA 1986;256:3227.

Pollock M, Kovacs M, Charron-Prochownik D. Eating disorders and maladaptive dietary/insulin management among youths with childhood-onset insulin-dependent diabetes mellitus. J Am Acad Child Adolesc Psychiatry 1995;34:291.

Rosenbloom AL. Diabetes in childhood and adolescence. Pediatr Ann 1994;23:282.

Rosenbloom AL, Kohrman A, Sperling M. Classification and diagnosis of diabetes mellitus in children and adolescents. J Pediatr 1981;98:320.

Rother KI, Levitsky LL. Diabetes mellitus during adolescence. Endocrinol Metab Clin North Am 1993;22: 553.

Rudolf MC, Sherwin RS, Markowitz R, et al. Effect of intensive insulin treatment on linear growth in the young diabetic patient. J Pediatr 1982;101:333.

Ryan C, Vega A, Drash A. Cognitive deficits in adolescents who developed diabetes early in life. Pediatrics 1985;75:921.

Ryan C, Vega A, Longstreet C. Neuropsychological changes in adolescents with insulin-dependent diabetes. J Consult Clin Psychol 1984;52:335.

Schneider AJ. Starting insulin therapy in children with newly diagnosed diabetes: an outpatient approach. Am J Dis Child 1983;137:782.

Schriock EA, Winter RJ, Traisman HS. Diabetes mellitus and its effects on menarche. J Adolesc Health Care 1984;5:101.

Shaw NJ, McClure RJ, Kerr S, et al. Smoking in diabetic teenagers. Diabet Med 1993;10:275.

Skyler JS, ed. Childhood diabetes. Pediatr Ann 1987; 16:682.

Sperling MA. Outpatient management of diabetes mellitus. Pediatr Clin North Am 1987;34:919.

Tarnow JD, Silverman SW. The psychophysiologic aspects of stress in juvenile diabetes mellitus. Int J Psychiatry Med 1981;11(1):25.

Weissberg-Benchell J, Glasgow AM, Tynan WD, et al. Adolescent diabetes management and mismanagement. Diabetes Care 1995;18:77.

Wertlieb D, Hauser ST, Jacobson AM. Adaptation to diabetes: behavior symptoms and family context. J Pediatr Psychol 1986;11:463.

Disabled Adolescent

Bodzioch J, Roach JW, Schkade J. Promoting independence in adolescent paraplegics: a 2-week "camping" experience. J Pediatr Orthop 1986;6:198.

Breslau N. Psychiatric disorder in children with physical disabilities. J Am Acad Child Psychiatry 1985; 24:87.

Breslau N, Marshall IA. Psychological disturbance in children with physical disabilities: continuity and change in a 5-year follow-up. J Abnorm Child Psychol 1985;13:199.

Cleveland M. Family adaptation to traumatic spinal cord injury: response to crises. Family Relations 1980;29:558.

Gratz RR, Papalia-Finlay D. Psychosocial adaptation to wearing the Milwaukee brace for scoliosis: a pilot study of adolescent females and their mothers. J Adolesc Health Care 1984;5:237.

Hallum A. Disability and the transition to adulthood: issues for the disabled child, the family, and the pediatrician. Curr Probl Pediatr 1995;25:12.

Langley JD, Stanton WR, McGee RO, et al. Disability in late adolescence. I. Introduction, methods, and overview. Disabil Rehabil 1995;17:35.

Paxman JM. Health care for handicapped adolescents: international legislative and policy trends. J Adolesc Health Care 1982;3:103.

Stein R. Growing up with a physical difference. Child Health Care 1983;12:53.

Wallace HM, Biehl RF, Oglesby AC, et al, eds. Handicapped children and youth: a comprehensive community and clinical approach. New York: Human Sciences Press, 1987.

Sexuality and the Disabled Person

Barret M, Case N. Sexuality and the disabled. Toronto: Sex Information and Education Council of Canada, 1976.

Bernstein NR. Sexuality in mentally retarded adolescents. Med Aspects Hum Sexuality 1985;19:50.

Cass AS, Bloom BA, Luxenberg M. Sexual function in adults with myelomeningocele. J Urol 1986;136:425.

Chamberlain A, Rauh J, Passer A, McGrath M, Burket R. Issues in fertility control for mentally retarded female adolescents. I. Sexual activity, sexual abuse, and contraception. Pediatrics 1984;73:445.

Chipouras S, Cornelius D, Daniels S, Makas E. Who cares? A handbook on sex education and counseling services for disabled people. Washington, DC: Sex and Disability Project, 1979.

Eisenberg M. Sex and the handicapped: a selected bibliography. Cleveland: Veterans Administration Hospital, 1975.

Greydanus DE, Demarest DS, Sears JM. Sexuality of the chronically ill adolescent. Med Aspects Hum Sexuality 1985;19:36.

Mooney T, Cole T, Chilgren RA. Sexual options for paraplegics and quadriplegics. New York: Little, Brown, 1975.

Passer A, Rauh J, Chamberlain A, McGrath M, Burket R. Issues in fertility control for mentally retarded female adolescents. II. Parental attitudes toward sterilization. Pediatrics 1984;73:451.

Schultz JB, Adams DU. Family life education needs of mentally disabled adolescents. Adolescence 1987; 22:221.

Sexuality and the rheumatic diseases: an annotated bibliography, 1970–1982. Arlington, Virginia: Arthritis Information Clearinghouse (P.O. Box 9782, Arlington, VA 22209), 1982.

Walbroehl GS. Sexuality in the handicapped. Am Fam Physician 1987;36:129.

Epilepsy

Corbett JA, Trimble MR, Nichol TC. Behavioral and cognitive impairments in children with epilepsy: the long-term effects of anticonvulsants therapy. J Am Acad Child Psychiatry 1985;24:17.

Dalessio DJ. Seizure disorders and pregnancy. N Engl J Med 1985;312:559.

Diamantopoulos N, Crumrine PK. The effect of puberty on the course of epilepsy. Arch Neurol 1986; 43:873.

Golden NH, Bennett HS, Pollack MA, Schoenberg SK. Seizures in adolescence: a review of patients admitted in an adolescent service. J Adolesc Health Care 1985;6:25.

Hoare P, Mann H. Self-esteem and behavioural adjustment in children with epilepsy and children with diabetes. J Psychosom Res 1994;38:859.

Hodgman CH, McAnarney ER, Myers GJ, et al. Emotional complications of adolescent grand mal epilepsy. J Pediatr 1979;95:309.

O'Donohoe NV. What should the child with epilepsy be allowed to do? Arch Dis Child 1983;58:934.

Inflammatory Bowel Disease

Alperstein G, Daum F, Fisher SE. Linear growth following surgery in children and adolescents with Crohn's disease: relationship to pubertal status. J Pediatr Surg 1985;20:129.

Bruce T. Emotional sequelae of chronic inflammatory bowel disease in children and adolescents. Clin Gastroenterol 1986;15:89.

Daum F. Nutritional support for growth failure in children with inflamatory bowel disease. In: Balistreri WF, Vanderhoof JA, eds. Pediatric gastroenterology and nutrition. Aspen Seminars on Pediatric Disease;

vol 4. London: Chapman and Hall Medical, 1990: 237–243.

Daum F. The use of new drugs in the management of inflammatory bowel disease in children. In: Balistreri WF, Vanderhoof JA, eds. Pediatric gastroenterology and nutrition. Aspen Seminars on Pediatric Disease; vol 4. London: Chapman and Hall Medical, 1990:186–195.

Donaldson RM. Management of medical problems in pregnancy: inflammatory bowel disease. N Engl J Med 1985;312:1616.

Ferguson A. Crohn's disease in children and adolescents. J R Soc Med 1984;77:30.

Lake AM. Recognition and management of inflammatory bowel disease in children and adolescents. Curr Probl Pediatr 1988;18:377.

Lindquist BL, Jarnerot G, Wickbon G. Clinical and epidemiological aspects of Crohn's disease in children and adolescents. Scand J Gastroenterol 1984; 19:502.

Takacs LF, Kollman CE. An inflammatory bowel disease support group for teens and their parents. Gastroenterol Nurs 1994;17:11.

Wood B, Watkins JB, Boyle JT. Psychological functioning in children with Crohn's disease and ulcerative colitis: implications for models of psychobiological interaction. J Am Acad Child Adolesc Psychiatry 1987;26:774.

Renal Disease

Bosque M, Munian A, Bewick M. Growth after renal transplants. Arch Dis Child 1983;58:110.

Broyer M. Growth in children with renal insufficiency. Pediatr Clin North Am 1982;29:991.

Cameron JS. Lupus nephritis in childhood and adolescence. Pediatr Nephrol 1994;8:230.

Ferraris J, Saenger P, Levin L, et al. Delayed puberty in males with chronic renal failure. Kidney Int 1980; 18:344.

Hodson EM, Shaw PF, Evans RA, et al. Growth retardation and renal osteodystrophy in children with chronic renal failure. J Pediatr 1983;103:735.

Moquilner ME, Bauman A, De-Nour AK. The adjustment of children and parents to chronic hemodialysis. Psychosomatics 1988;29:289.

Price CA. Development maturity of adolescent and young adult patients on chronic hemodialysis: a comparative study. Journal of the American Association of Nephrology Nurses and Technicians 1982;9:17.

Rheumatological Conditions

Bradley LA. Psychological aspects of arthritis. Bull Rheum Dis 1985;35:1.

Karnreich H, Koster K, Hanson V. The rheumatic diseases in adolescence. Pediatr Clin North Am 1973; 20:911.

Leak AM. The management of arthritis in adolescence. Br J Rheumatol 1994;33:882.

Nashel DJ, Ulmer CC. Systemic lupus erythematosus: important considerations in the adolescent. J Adolesc Health Care 1982;2:273.

Silber TJ, Chatoor I, White P. Psychiatric manifestations of systemic lupus erythematosus in children and adolescents. Clin Pediatr 1984;23:331.

Spencer CH, Bernstein BH. Chronic disorders in adolescence. Boston: John Wright Publishing, 1983: 397–413.

Szer IS, Taylor E, Steere AC. The long-term course of Lyme arthritis in children. N Engl J Med 1991;325: 159.

Ungerer JA, Horgan B, Chaitow J, et al. Psychosocial functioning in children and young adults with juvenile arthritis. Pediatrics 1988;81:195.

Varni JW, Wilcox KT, Hanson V, Brik R. Chronic musculoskeletal pain and functional status in juvenile rheumatoid arthritis: an empirical model. Pain 1988;32:1.

Sickle Cell Anemia

Abbasi AA, Prasad AS, Ortega J, Congco E, Oberleas D. Gonadal function abnormalities in sickle cell anemia: studies in adult male patients. Ann Intern Med 1976;85:601.

Athale UH, Chintu C. The effect of sickle cell anaemia on adolescents and their growth and development: lessons from the sickle cell anaemia clinic. J Trop Pediatr 1994;40:246.

Daeschner CW III, Matustik MC, Carpentieri U, Haggard ME. Zinc and growth in patients with sickle cell disease. J Pediatr 1981;98:778.

Fowler MG, Whitt JK, Lallinger RR, et al. Neuropsychologic and academic functioning of children with sickle cell anemia. J Dev Behav Pediatr 1988;9:213.

Hurtig AL, White LS. Psychosocial adjustment in children and adolescents with sickle cell disease. J Pediatr Psychol 1986;11:411.

Kark JA, Posey DM, Schumacher HR, Ruehle CJ. Sickle-cell trait as a risk factor for sudden death in physical training. N Engl J Med 1987;317:781.

Kramer MS, Rooks Y, Pearson HA. Growth and development in children with sickle cell trait. N Engl J Med 1978;299:686.

Lemanek KL, Moore SL, Gresham FM, et al. Psychological adjustment of children with sickle cell anemia. J Pediatr Psychol 1986;11:397.

Midence K, Fuggle P, Davies SC. Psychosocial aspects of sickle cell disease (SCD) in childhood and adolescence: a review. Br J Clin Psychol 1993;32:271.

Milner PF, Jones BR, Dobler J. Outcome of pregnancy in sickle cell anemia and sickle cell-hemoglobin C disease. Am J Obstet Gynecol 1980;138:239.

Morgan SA, Jackson J. Psychological and social concomitants of sickle cell anemia in adolescents. J Pediatr Psychol 1986;11:429.

Platt OS, Rosenstock W, Espeland MA. Influence of sickle hemoglobinopathies on growth and development. N Engl J Med 1984;311:7.

Powars DR, Sandhu M, Niland-Weiss J. Pregnancy in sickle cell disease. Obstet Gynecol 1986;67:217.

Prasad AS, Cossack ZT. Zinc supplementation and growth in sickle cell disease. Ann Intern Med 1984; 100:367.

Samuels-Reid JH, Scott RB, Brown WE. Contraceptive practices and reproductive patterns in sickle cell disease. J Natl Med Assoc 1984;76:879.

Stevens MCG, Maude GH, Cupidore L, Jackson H, Hayes RJ, Serjeant GR. Prepubertal growth and skeletal maturation in children with sickle cell disease. Pediatrics 1986;78:124.

Vichinsky EP, Johnson R, Lubin BH. Multidisciplinary approach to pain management in sickle cell disease. Am J Pediatr Hematol Oncol 1982;4:328.

Wethers DL. Problems and complications in the adolescent with sickle cell disease. Am J Pediatr Hematol Oncol 1982;4:47.

Whitten CF, Fischhoff J. Psychosocial effects of sickle cell disease. Arch Intern Med 1974;133:681.

Yang YM, Cepeda M, Price C, et al. Depression in children and adolescents with sickle-cell disease. Arch Pediatr Adolesc Med 1994;148:457.

Spina Bifida

Appleton PL, Minchom PE, Ellis NC, et al. The self-concept of young people with spina bifida: a population-based study. Dev Med Child Neurol 1994;36: 198.

Blum RW. The adolescent with spina bifida. Clin Pediatr 1983;122:331.

Blum RW, Resnick M, Nelson R, St Germaine A. Family and peer issues among adolescents with spina bifida and cerebral palsy. Pediatrics 1991;88:280.

Cartright DB, Joseph AS, Grenier CE. A self-image profile analysis of spina bifida adolescents in Louisiana. J La State Med Soc 1993;145:394.

Castree B, Walker J. The young adult with spina bifida. Br Med J 1981;283:1040.

Loomis JW, Lindsey A, Javornisky JG, et al. Measures of cognition and adaptive behavior as predictors of adjustment outcomes in young adults with spina bifida. Eur J Pediatr Surg 1994;4(suppl 1):35.

McAndrew I. Adolescents and young people with spina bifida. Dev Med Child Neurol 1979;21:619.

Sandler AD, Worley G, Leroy EC, et al. Sexual knowledge and experience among young men with spina bifida. Eur J Pediatr Surg 1994;4(suppl 1):36.

Wolman C, Basco DE. Factors influencing self-esteem and self-consciousness in adolescents with spina bifida. J Adolesc Health 1994;15:543.

Spinal Cord Injury

Apple DF Jr, Anson CA, Hunter JD, et al. Spinal cord injury in youth. Clin Pediatr 1995;34:90.

LeBaron S, Currie D, Zeltzer LK. Coping with spinal cord injury in adolescents. In: Blum R, ed. Chronic illness and disabilities in childhood and adolescence. Orlando, Florida: Grune & Stratton, 1984.

Resources

Written Guides

Directory of National Information Sources on Disabilities
8455 Colesville Rd., Suite 935
Silver Spring, MD 20910
800-346-2742

Pocket Guide to Federal Help for Individuals with Disabilities (report No. E-87-22002)
Department of Education
Washington, DC 20202
"Resource Manual: Youth With Disabilities," by Smith-Lindall M, Blum RW, Leonard BJ.
    J Adolesc Health Care 1985;6:163. (Contains a comprehensive resource manual for
    youth with disabilities. Entire issue is devoted to this topic.)

Agencies

General

Administration on Developmental Disabilities
U.S. Department of Health and Human Services
200 Independence Ave. SW, Room 329D
Washington, DC 20201
202-690-5504

Clearinghouse on Disability Information
202-205-8241

Department of Education
Office of Special Education and Rehabilitation Services
Office of Special Education Programs
Rehabilitation Services Administration
National Institute on Disability and Rehabilitation Research
330 C St. SW
Washington, DC 20202
202-205-8241

Girl Scouts of the U.S.A.
Focus on Ability: Serving Girls With Special Needs
Scouting for Handicapped Girls Program
212-852-8000

March of Dimes Birth Defects Foundation
1275 Mamaroneck Ave.
White Plains, NY 10605
914-428-7100

National Center for Youth With Disabilities
University of Minnesota
Box 721
420 Delaware St. SE
Minneapolis, MN 55455
800-333-6293

(Information, policy, and resource center focusing on adolescents with chronic illnesses and disabilities and the issues surrounding their transition to adult life. Center also provides a national database containing comprehensive information about adolescents with chronic conditions, including journals, books, monographs, legislation, model programs, and educational materials. Also offers a network of professionals available for technical assistance.)

National Information Center for Children and Youth With Disabilities
800-659-0285

National Organization on Disability
910 16th St. NW, Suite 600
Washington, DC 20006-2903
202-293-5960

Parent Network/Federation for Children With Special Needs
95 Berkeley St., Suite 104
Boston, MA 02116
617-482-2915

Specific Conditions

American Cancer Society
1599 Clifton Rd. NE
Atlanta, GA 30329
800-ACS-2345
(Supports education and research in cancer prevention, diagnosis, and treatment.)

American Diabetes Association
1660 Duke St.
Alexandria, VA 22314
800-232-3472

American Foundation for the Blind
11 Penn Plaza
New York, NY 10001
800-232-5463

American Heart Association
7272 Greenville Ave.
Dallas, TX 75231-4596
800-242-8721
(Supports research and education to reduce death rates and disability from heart disease.)

Arthritis Foundation—American Juvenile Arthritis Organization
1314 Spring St.
Atlanta, GA 30309
800-283-7800
(A resource for educational material about the diagnosis and treatment of arthritis.)

Association for Retarded Citizens
500 East Border St., Suite 300
P.O. Box 1047
Arlington, TX 76010
800-433-5255

Asthma and Allergy Foundation of America
1125 15th St. NW, Suite 502
Washington, DC 20005
800-727-8462
(Provides information on support services and resource materials on asthma and allergy.)

Autism Society of America
7910 Woodmount Ave., Suite 650
Besthesda, MD 20814
800-328-8476

Candlelighters Childhood Cancer Foundation
7910 Woodmont Ave., Suite 460
Bethesda, MD 20814
800-366-2223

Children and Adults With Attention Deficit Disorders (CHADD)
499 Northwest 70th Ave., Suite 109
Plantation, FL 33317
800-233-4050

Children's Craniofacial Association
10210 Northcentral Expressway, Suite 230, LB37
Dallas, TX 75231
800-535-3643

Crohn's and Colitis Foundation of America
386 Park Ave. South
New York, NY 10016-8804
800-932-2423
(Information to patients and their families on inflammatory bowel disease.)

Cystic Fibrosis Foundation
6931 Arlington Rd.
Bethesda, MD 20814
800-344-4823
(Provides educational material to patients, parents, and health-care providers.)

Disabled Sports USA
451 Hungerford Dr., No. 100
Rockville, MD 20850
800-966-4647
(Sponsors a variety of sports and recreational activities through a network of community-based chapters.)

Epilepsy Foundation of America
4351 Garden City Dr.
Landover, MD 20785-2267
800-332-1000
(Provides educational material and resources to patients and their families.)

Independent Living Research Utilization (ILRU) Research and Training Center on Independent Living at The Institute of Rehabilitation and Research (TIRR)
2323 South Shepherd, Suite 1000
Houston, TX 77019
713-520-0232
(Provides resources on sexuality and the disabled person.)

Learning Disabilities Association of America
4156 Library Rd.
Pittsburgh, PA 15234
412-341-1515

Leukemia Society of America
600 3rd Ave., 4th Floor
New York, NY 10016
800-954-4572
(Sponsors programs of research, patient help, education, and community service.)

Lupus Foundation of America
4 Research Place, Suite 180
Rockville, MD 20850-3226
800-558-0121

Muscular Dystrophy Association, Inc.
3300 East Sunrise Dr.
Tucson, AZ 85718-3208
800-572-1717

National Alopecia Areata Foundation
710 "C" St., Suite 11
San Rafael, CA 94901
415-456-4644
(Provides information on hair loss and support for people with alopecia areata.)

National Association of the Deaf
814 Thayer Ave.
Silver Spring, MD 20910
301-587-1788

National Chronic Fatigue Syndrome Association
3521 Broadway, Suite 222
Kansas City, MO 64111
816-931-4777
(Organized to educate the public and health professionals about the nature of chronic fatigue syndrome.)

National Down Syndrome Society
666 Broadway, 8th Floor
New York, NY 10012-2317
800-221-4602

National Headache Foundation
5252 N. Western Ave.
Chicago, IL 60625
800-843-2256
(Committed to research, education, and service for the headache sufferer.)

National Head Injury Foundation
1776 Massachusetts Ave. NW, Suite 100
Washington, DC 20036-1904
800-444-6443
(Acts as an advocate for head-injured patients and support for their families.)

National Kidney Foundation
30 East 33rd St., 11th Floor
New York, NY 10016
800-622-9010
(Resource for information on kidney and urinary tract disease and organ donation.)

National Mental Health Association
1021 Prince St.
Alexandria, VA 22314-2971
800-969-6642
(Advocacy group concerned with all aspects of mental health and mental illnesses.)

National Multiple Sclerosis Society
733 3rd Ave., 6th floor
New York, NY 10017
800-344-4867
(A primary resource for information about multiple-sclerosis research, diagnosis, and treatments.)

National Neurofibromatosis Foundation
95 Pine St., 16th Floor
New York, NY 10005
800-323-7938

National Organization for Rare Disorders
P.O. Box 8923
New Fairfield, CT 06812-1783
800-999-6673

National Scoliosis Foundation
72 Mount Auburn St.
Watertown, MA 02172
617-926-0397

National Spinal Cord Injury Association
545 Concord Ave., Suite 29
Cambridge, MA 02138
800-962-9629 (Hotline only)

Sickle Cell Disease Association of America
200 Corporate Pointe, Suite 495
Culver City, CA 90203-7633
800-421-8453

Spina Bifida Association of America
4590 MacArthur Blvd. NW, No. 250
Washington, DC 20007-4226
800-621-3141

United Cerebral Palsy Association
1522 K St. NW, No. 1112
Washington, DC 20005
800-872-5827

SECTION XVI

Appendices

APPENDIX I
Reference Materials on Adolescence

General Adolescent Medicine

Adams GR, Montemayor R, Gullotta TP. Biology of adolescent behavior and development. Newbury Park, California: Sage Publications, 1989.

Adolescent health; vol 1. Washington, D.C.: U.S. Office of Technology Assessment, 1991.

Adolescent health; vol 2. Background and effectiveness of selected prevention and treatment services. Washington, D.C.: U.S. Office of Technology Assessment, 1991.

American Academy of Pediatrics. Guidelines for health supervision. Elk Grove Village, Illinois: The Academy: 1985. (Address: 141 Northwest Point Blvd., P.O. Box 927, Elk Grove Village, IL 60007.)

Baum A, Singer JE, eds. Issues in child health and adolescent health. Hillsdale, New Jersey: Lawrence Erlbaum Associates, 1982.

Bennett DL. Adolescent health care in Australia: an overview of needs and approaches to care. Glebe, Australia: Australian Medical Association, 1984.

Beunen GP. Adolescent growth and motor performance: a longitudinal study of Belgian boys. Champaign, Illinois: Human Kinetics Books, 1988.

Blum RW, ed. Chronic illness and disabilities in childhood and adolescence. Orlando, Florida: Grune & Stratton, 1984.

Braithwaite RL, Taylor SE, eds. Health issues in the black community. San Francisco: Jossey-Bass, 1992.

Brook CGD. All about adolescence. New York: John Wiley & Sons, 1985.

Castro-Magana M, Collipp PJ. Pediatric and adolescent endocrinology: case studies. New York: Medical Examination Publishing, 1983.

Coates TJ, Petersen AC, Perry C, eds. Promoting adolescent health: a dialog on research and practice. New York: Academic Press, 1982.

Dewhurst JS. Female puberty and its abnormalities. New York: Churchill Livingstone, 1984.

Elster AB, Kuznets NJ. AMA Guidelines for adolescent preventive services [GAPS]: Recommendations and rationale. Chicago: American Medical Association, 1994.

Farrow JA, ed. Adolescent medicine. Philadelphia: WB Saunders, 1990.

Feldman W, Rosser W, McGrath P. Primary medical care of children and adolescents. New York: Oxford University Press, 1987.

Felice ME, ed. Primary care: adolescent medicine. Philadelphia: WB Saunders, 1987:14:1.

Friedman SB, Fisher M, Schonberg K. Comprehensive adolescent health care. St. Louis: Quality Medical Publishers, 1992.

Gallagher R, Heald F, Garrell D. Medical care of the adolescent. New York: Appleton-Century-Crofts, 1976.

Gans JE, Elster DA, Elster AB, et al. America's adolescents: how healthy are they? Chicago: American Medical Association, 1990.

Golub S, ed. Health care of the female adolescent; vol 9. New York: Haworth Press, 1984. (Women and health.)

Green M, Haggerty RJ, eds. Ambulatory pediatrics; vol 3. Philadelphia: WB Saunders, 1984.

Hofmann AD, Greydanus DE, eds. Adolescent medicine. Norwalk, Connecticut: Appleton & Lange, 1989.

Holder AR. Legal issues in pediatrics and adolescent medicine. New Haven: Yale University, 1985.

Holmes KI, Mardh PA, Sparling PF, et al, eds. Sexually transmitted diseases. 2nd ed. New York: McGraw-Hill, 1990.

Kaufman M. Easy for you to say: questions and answers for teens living with chronic illness or disability. Toronto: Key Porter Books, 1995.

Kreipe R. Adolescent health: a primary care responsibility [Videotape]. Secaucus, New Jersey: Network for Continuing Medical Education, 1986.

Litt IF. Evaluation of the adolescent patient. Philadelphia: Hanley & Belfus, 1990.

Litt I, ed. Symposium on adolescent medicine. 1980; 27:1.

Mahan LK, Rees JM, eds. Nutrition in adolescence. St. Louis: CV Mosby, 1984.

McAnarney ER, et al, eds. Textbook of adolescent medicine. Philadelphia: WB Saunders, 1992.

McDonald RE, Avery DR, eds. Dentistry for the child and adolescent. St. Louis: CV Mosby, 1988.

Millar H, ed. Compendium of resource materials on adolescent health. (DHHS publication No. 81-5246.) Washington, D.C.: U.S. Department of Health and Human Services. 1981.

Millar H, ed. Adolescent health care: a guide for BCHS-supported programs and projects. (DHEW publication No. 79-5234.) Washington, D.C.: U.S. Department of Health, Education, and Welfare, 1979.

Montemayor R, Adams GR, Gullotta TP. From childhood to adolescence: a transitional period? Newbury Park, California: Sage Publications, 1990.

Morrissey JM, Hofmann AD, Thorpe JC. Consent and confidentiality in the health care of children and adolescents. New York: Free Press, 1986.

Morton CJ, Guendelman SR. New perspectives on monitoring child and adolescent health. Berkeley, California: University of California School of Public Health, 1985.

Ostrow DG, Sandholzen TA, Felman YM. STD in homosexual men: diagnosis, treatment, and research. New York: Plenum Books, 1983.

Paxman JM, Zuckerman RJ. Laws and policies affecting adolescent health. Geneva: World Health Organization, 1987.

Rees JM. Nutritional issues in adolescent health. Rockville, Maryland: Office of Maternal and Child Health, U.S. Department of Health and Human Services, 1988.

Reichert KE. Primary care of young adults: a practitioner's manual. Garden City, New York: Medical Examination Publishing, 1983.

Rickert VI. Adolescent nutrition: assessment and management. New York: Chapman & Hall, 1995.

Silber T, ed. Ethical issues in the treatment of children and adolescents. Thorofare, New Jersey: Slack, 1983.

Smith ME, ed. Chronic disorders in adolescence. Boston: John Wright Publishing, 1983.

Sommer BB. Puberty and adolescence. New York: Oxford University Press, 1978.

Sorenson RC. Adolescent sexuality in contemporary America. New York: World Publishing, 1973.

Strasburger VC, Greydanus DE, eds. Adolescent medicine: state of the art reviews [3 books per year]. Philadelphia: Hanley & Belfus.

Sugar M, ed. Female adolescent development. New York: Brunner/Mazel, 1993.

Tanner JM. Growth at adolescence. London: Blackwell Publishing, 1962.

Tebbi CK, ed. Major topics in adolescent oncology. Mount Kisco, New York: Futura Publishing, 1987.

WHO Technical Report. Young people's health: a challenge for society. (Series No. 731.) Geneva: World Health Organization, 1986.

Adolescent Gynecology

Brookman RR. Pediatric and adolescent gynecology: case studies. Garden City, New York: Medical Examination Publishing, 1980.

Carpenter SE, Rock JA. Pediatric and adolescent gynecology. New York: Raven Press, 1992.

Cowell CA, ed. Symposium on pediatric and adolescent gynecology. Pediatr Clin North Am 1981;28:1.

Dewhurst CJ. Dewhurst's practical paediatric and adolescent gynecology. 2nd ed. Boston: Butterworths Publications, 1989.

Emans SJH, Goldstein DP. Pediatric and adolescent gynecology. Boston: Little, Brown, 1990.

Friedman HL, Edstrom KG. Adolescent reproductive health: an approach to planning services and research. Geneva: World Health Organization, 1983.

Greydanus DE, Shearin RB. Adolescent sexuality and gynecology. Philadelphia: Lea & Febiger, 1990.

Hatcher RA, Guest F, Stewart F, et al. Contraceptive technology. 16th rev. ed. New York: Irvington Publishers, 1994.

Huffman JW. The gynecology of childhood and adolescence. Philadelphia: WB Saunders, 1981.

Kreutner K, Hollingsworth D. Adolescent obstetrics and gynecology. Chicago: Year Book Medical Publishers, 1978.

Lavery JP, San Filippo JS, eds. Pediatric and adolescent obstetrics and gynecology. New York: Springer-Verlag, 1985.

Mishell DR, Davajan V, Lobo A, eds. Infertility, contraception, and reproductive endocrinology. 3rd ed. Boston: Blackwell Scientific, 1991.

Neinstein LS. Issues in reproductive management. New York: Thieme, 1994.

Sanfilippo JS, ed. Pediatric and adolescent gynecology. Philadelphia: WB Saunders, 1994.

Speroff L, Glass RH, Kase NG. Clinical gynecologic endocrinology and infertility. Baltimore: Williams & Wilkins, 1994.

Strasburger VC, ed. Adolescent gynecology. Pediatr Clin North Am 1989;36.

Strasburger VC, ed. Basic adolescent gynecology. Baltimore: Urban & Schwarzenberg, 1990.

Yen S, Jaffe RB. Reproductive gynecology. Philadelphia: WB Saunders, 1991.

Psychosocial Concerns

Abelson J. Handbook of adolescent psychology. New York: John Wiley & Sons, 1980.

Aguilera DC. Crisis intervention: theory and methodology. St. Louis: Mosby–Year Book, 1994.

Allmond D, Buckman W, Gofman H. The family is the patient: an approach to behavioral pediatrics for children. St. Louis: CV Mosby, 1979.

Anderson EM, Clarke L. Disability in adolescence. London: Methuen, 1982.

Aten M, McAnarney E. Behavioral approach to the care of adolescents. St. Louis: CV Mosby, 1981.

Bell NJ, Bell RW, eds. Adolescent risk taking. Newbury Park, California: Sage Publications, 1993.

Berman AL. Adolescent suicide: assessment and intervention. Washington, D.C.: American Psychological Association, 1991.

Blos P. The adolescent passage: developmental issues. New York: International Universities Press, 1979.

Brooks-Gunn J, Petersen AC. Girls at puberty: biological and psychosocial perspectives. New York: Plenum Press, 1983.

Bruch H. Eating disorders: anorexia nervosa, obesity and the person within. New York: Basic Books, 1973.

Bruch H. The golden cage: the enigma of anorexia nervosa. New York: Vintage Books, 1979.

Brumberg JJ. Fasting girls: the emergence of anorexia nervosa as a modern disease. Cambridge, Massachusetts: Harvard University Press, 1988.

Canino IA. Culturally diverse children and adolescents: assessment, diagnosis, and treatment. New York: Guilford Press, 1994.

Cantwell DP, Carlson GA, eds. Affective disorders in childhood and adolescence: an update. New York: SP Medical and Scientific Books, 1983.

Carlson J, Lewis J. Counseling the adolescent: individual, family, and school interventions. Denver: Love Publishing, 1988.

Caissy GA. Early adolescence: understanding the 10- to 15-year-old. New York: Insight Books, 1994.

Chiles J. Teenage depression and suicide. New York: Chelsea House, 1986.

Christophersen ER, Levine MD. Development and behavior: older children and adolescents. Philadelphia: WB Saunders, 1992.

Clarke-Stewart A, Kock BK. Children: development through adolescence. New York: John Wiley & Sons, 1983.

Cohen RL, Dulcan MK. Basic handbook of training in child and adolescent psychiatry. Springfield, Illinois: Charles C Thomas, 1987.

Davis I. Adolescence: theoretical and helping perspectives. Hingham, Massachusetts: Kluwer Academic Publishers, 1985.

Davis JM. Suicidal youth: school-based intervention and prevention. San Francisco: Jossey-Bass, 1991.

Dusek J. Adolescent development and behavior. Englewood Cliffs, New Jersey: Prentice-Hall, 1987.

Elkind D. All grown up and no place to go: teenagers in crisis. Reading, Massachusetts: Addison-Wesley Publishing, 1984.

Elkind D. A sympathetic understanding of the child: birth to sixteen. 3rd ed. Boston: Allyn & Bacon, 1994.

Erikson E. Identity, youth, and crises. New York: WW Norton, 1968.

Farley GK, Eckhart L, Hebert FB. Handbook of child and adolescent psychiatric emergencies. Garden City, New York: Medical Examination Publishing, 1986.

Feinstein SC, ed. Adolescent psychiatry; vol 14. Chicago: University of Chicago Press, 1987.

Finkelhor D. Child sexual abuse: new theory and research. New York: Free Press, 1984.

Forgatch M, Patterson G. Parents and adolescents: living together. II. Family problem solving. Eugene, Oregon: Castalia Publishing, 1989.

Forisha-Kovach BE. The experience of adolescence: development in context. Glenview, Illinois: Scott, Foresman, 1983.

Frindler EL. Adolescent anger control: cognitive-behavioral techniques. New York: Pergamon Press, 1986.

Fritz GK. Child and adolescent mental health consultation in hospitals, schools, and courts. Washington, D.C.: American Psychiatric Press, 1993.

Fuhrmann BS. Adolescence, adolescents. Boston: Little, Brown, 1986.

Gallagher J, Harris HI. Emotional problems of adolescents. New York: Oxford University Press, 1976.

Garbarino J, Schellenbach CJ, Sebes JM. Troubled youth, troubled families. New York: Aldine Publishing, 1986.

Goethals GW. Experiencing youth: first person accounts. Lanham, Maryland: University Press of America, 1986.

Green WH. Child and adolescent clinical psychopharmacology. Baltimore: Williams & Wilkins, 1991.

Gunnar MR, Collins WA. Development during the transition to adolescence. Hillsdale, New Jersey: Lawrence Erlbaum Associates, 1987.

Haviland JM. Adolescent development in contemporary society. New York: Van Nostrand Reinhold, 1981.

Hawton K. Suicide and attempted suicide among children and adolescents. Beverly Hills, California: Sage Publications, 1986.

Hendee WR. The health of adolescents: understanding and facilitating biological, behavioral, and social development. San Francisco: Jossey-Bass, 1991.

Hill JP. Understanding early adolescence: a framework. Chapel Hill: University of North Carolina Center for Early Adolescence, 1980.

Hofmann A, Becker RD, Gabriel HP. The hospitalized adolescent: a guide to managing ill and injured youth. New York: Free Press, 1976.

Hoghughi M. Assessing child and adolescent disorders: a practice manual. Newbury Park, California: Sage Publications, 1992.

Holinger PC. Suicide and homicide among adolescents. New York: Guilford Press, 1994.

Indian adolescent mental health. Washington, D.C.: U.S. Office of Technology, 1990.

Irwin CE Jr. Adolescent social behavior and health. San Francisco: Jossey-Bass, 1987.

Jacobs J. Adolescent suicide. New York: Irvington Publishers, 1980.

Jessor R, Jessor SC. Problem behavior and psychosocial development: a longitudinal study of youth. New York: Academic Press, 1977.

Johnson JH. Life events as stressors in childhood and adolescence. Beverly Hills, California: Sage Publications, 1986.

Kaplan LJ. Adolescence: the farewell to childhood. New York: Simon & Schuster, 1984.

Kaplan LS. Coping with peer pressure. New York: Rosen Publishing Group, 1983.

Karoly P, Steffen JJ. Adolescent behavior disorders: foundations and contemporary concerns. Lexington, Massachusetts: Lexington Books, 1984.

Kimmel DC, Weiner IB. Adolescence: a development transition. Hillsdale, New Jersey: Lawrence Erlbaum Associates, 1985.

Kirk WG. Adolescent suicide: a school-based approach to assessment and intervention. Champaign, Illinois: Research Press, 1993.

Klerman GL. Suicide and depression among adolescents and young adults. Washington, D.C.: American Psychiatric Press, 1986.

Knopka G. Young girls: a portrait of adolescence. Englewood Cliffs, New Jersey: Prentice-Hall, 1976.

Kratochwill TR, Morris RJ, eds. Handbook of psychotherapy with children and adolescents. Boston: Allyn & Bacon, 1993.

Lerner RM, Foch TT. Biological, psychosocial interactions in early adolescents. Hillsdale, New Jersey: Lawrence Erlbaum Associates, 1987.

Leveton E. Adolescent crisis: family counseling approaches. New York: Springer Publishing, 1984.

Levine MD, McAnarney ER. Early adolescent transition. Lexington, Massachusetts: Lexington Books, 1988.

Lloyd MA. Adolescence. Cambridge, Massachusetts: Harper & Row, 1985.

Mann S. At twelve: portraits of young women. New York: Aperture, 1988.

Marohn RC, ed. Juvenile delinquents: psychodynamic assessment and hospital treatment. New York: Brunner/Mazel, 1980.

McKinney JP, Fitzgerald HE, Strommen EA. Developmental psychology: the adolescent and young adult. Homewood, Illinois: Dorsey Press, 1982.

Melton GB. Adolescent abortion: psychological and legal issues. Lincoln: University of Nebraska Press, 1986.

Miller D. The age between: adolescence and therapy. New York: Jason Aronson, 1983.

Miller D. Attack on the self: adolescent behavior disturbances and their treatment. Northvale, New Jersey: Jason Aronson, 1986.

Minuchin S, Rosman BL, Baker L. Psychosomatic families: anorexia nervosa in context. Cambridge, Massachusetts: Harvard University Press, 1978.

Mirkin MP, Koman SL. Handbook of adolescents and family therapy. New York: Gardner Press, 1985.

Mitchell JJ. The maturing of adolescence. Calgary, Alberta: Detselig Enterprises, 1986.

Moore S. Sexuality in adolescence. London: Routledge, 1993.

Moriarty A. The psychology of adolescent Satanism: a guide for parents, counselors, clergy, and teachers. Westport, Connecticut: Praeger, 1992.

Newman BM, Newman PR. Adolescent development. Columbus: Merrill Publishing, 1985.

Newton M. Adolescence: guiding youth through the perilous ordeal. New York: Norton, 1995.

Nielsen L. Adolescence: a contemporary view. Fort Worth: Holt, Rinehart and Winston, 1991.

Offer D, Ostroy E, Howard KI, eds. Patterns of adolescent self-imaging. San Francisco: Jossey-Bass, 1984.

Offer D, Sabshin M, Offer J. The psychological world of the teenager: a study of normal adolescent boys. New York: Basic Books, 1969.

Ollendick TH, Hersen M. Handbook of child and adolescent assessment. Boston: Allyn & Bacon, 1993.

Oster GD. Assessing adolescents. New York: Pergamon Press, 1988.

Pasnau RO. Psychosocial aspects of medical practice: children and adolescents. Menlo Park, California: Addison-Wesley Publishing, 1982.

Patterson G, Forgatch M. Parents and adolescents: living together. I. The basics. Castalia Publishing, 1987.

Pravada M, Koman S, eds. Adolescents and family therapy: a handbook of theory and practice. New York: Gardner Press, 1985.

Rahdert ER. The adolescent assessment/referral system manual. Rockville, Maryland: National Institute on Drug Abuse, U.S. Department of Health and Human Services, 1991.

Raphael R. The men from the boys: rites of passage in male America. Lincoln: University of Nebraska Press, 1988.

Reynolds WM, Johnston HF. Handbook of depression in children and adolescents. New York: Plenum Press, 1994.

Rice FP. The adolescent: development relationships and culture. Boston: Allyn & Bacon, 1987.

Robson B. My parents are divorced, too: what teenagers experience and how they cope. Toronto: Dorset Publishers, 1979.

Rutter M, Hersov L, eds. Child and adolescent psychiatry: modern approaches. 3rd ed. Oxford: Blackwell Scientific Publishers, 1994.

Santrock JW. Adolescence: an introduction. Dubuque, Iowa: WC Brown, 1984.

Sarafino EP, Armstrong JW. Child and adolescent development. St. Paul, Minnesota: West Publishing, 1986.

Schinke SP, Gilchrist LD. Life skills counseling with adolescents. Baltimore: University Park Press, 1984.

Shaw D. Make the most of a good thing: you! Boston: Atlantic Monthly Press, 1986.

Simmons RG, Blyth DA. Moving into adolescence: the impact of pubertal change and school context. New York: Aldine de Gruyter, 1987.

Sorenson RC. Adolescent sexuality in contemporary America. New York: World Publishing, 1973.

Stiffman AR. Ethnic issues in adolescent mental health. Newbury Park, California: Sage Publications, 1990.

Stone LJ. Childhood and adolescence: a psychology of the growing person. New York: Random House, 1984.

Sugar M. Female adolescent development. New York: Brunner/Mazel, 1993.

Van Hasselt VB, Hersen M. Handbook of adolescent psychology. New York: Pergamon Press, 1987.

Vargas LA, Koss-Chioino JD, eds. Working with culture: psychotherapeutic interventions with ethnic minority children and adolescents. San Francisco: Jossey-Bass, 1992.

Wallander JL, Siegel LJ, eds. Adolescent health problems: behavioral perspectives. New York: Guilford Press, 1995.

Wiener JM, ed. Textbook of child and adolescent psychiatry. Washington, D.C.: American Academy of Child and Adolescent Psychiatry and American Psychiatric Press, 1991.

Worden M. Adolescents and their families: an introduction to assessment and intervention. New York: Haworth Press, 1991.

Zarb JM. Cognitive-behavioral assessment and therapy with adolescents. New York: Brunner/Mazel, 1992.

Zimmerman JK, Asnis GM, eds. Treatment approaches with suicidal adolescents. New York: Wiley, 1995.

Zvirin S. The best years of their lives: a resource guide

for teenagers in crisis. Chicago: American Library Association, 1992.

For Parents

Ames LB, Ilg FL, Baker SM. Your ten- to fourteen-year-old. New York: Delacorte Press, 1988.

Blume J. Letters to Judy: what your kids wish they could tell you. New York: Putnam's Sons, 1986.

Brenton M. How to survive your child's rebellious teens: new solutions for troubled parents. Philadelphia: JB Lippincott, 1979.

Bruntman PH, Saris EM. How to live with your teenager: a survivor's handbook for parents. Pasadena, California: Birchtree Press, 1979.

Cassell C. Straight from the heart: how to talk to your teenagers about love and sex. New York: Simon & Schuster, 1987.

Cross W. Kids and booze: what you must know to help them. New York: Dutton Press, 1980.

Dinkmeyer D, McKay GD. The STEP approach to parenting your teenager. Circle Pines, Minnesota: American Guidance Service, 1983.

Dupont RL. Getting tough on gateway drugs: a guide for the family. Washington, D.C.: American Psychiatric Press, 1984.

Fairchild B, Hayward N. Now that you know what every parent should know about homosexuality. New York: Harcourt Brace Jovanovich, 1979.

Fine L. After all we've done for them: understanding adolescent behavior. Englewood Cliffs, New Jersey: Prentice-Hall, 1977.

Forrest GG. How to cope with a teenage drinker: new alternatives and hope for parents. New York: Atheneum, 1983.

Ginott HG. Between parent and teenager. New York: Macmillan, 1969.

Gould S. Teenagers: The continuing challenge. New York: Hawthorn Press, 1979.

Greydanus DE, ed. Caring for your adolescent: ages 12–21. (American Academy of Pediatrics.) New York: Bantam, 1991.

Harris SO. When growing up hurts too much: a parent's guide to knowing when and how to choose a therapist with your teenager. Lexington, Massachusetts: Lexington Books, 1990.

McCoy K. Coping with teenage depression. New York: Signet Press, 1982.

McCoy K, Wibbelsman C. Crisis-proof your teenager. New York: Bantam Books, 1991.

Melton D. Survival kit for parents of teenagers. New York: St. Martin's Press, 1980.

Nielsen L. How to motivate adolescents: a guide for parents, teachers, and counselors. Englewood Cliffs, New Jersey: Prentice-Hall, 1982.

Patterson G, Forgatch M. Parents and adolescents: living together. I. The basics. Castalia Publishing, 1987.

Rinzler CE. Your adolescent: an owner's manual. New York: Atheneum, 1981.

Rosenbaum J, Rosenbaum V. Living with teenagers. New York: Stein Day, 1980.

Silverstein C. A family matter: a parent's guide to homosexuality. New York: McGraw-Hill, 1978.

Slap GB, Jablow MM. Teenage health care. New York: Pocket Books, 1994.

Steinberg LD, Levine A. You and your adolescent: a parent's guide for ages 10 to 20. New York: Harper & Row, 1990.

Weisman B, Weisman M. What we told our kids about sex. San Diego: Harcourt Brace Jovanovich, 1987.

For Teenagers

American College of Obstetrics and Gynecology. Being a teenager: you and your sexuality. Washington, D.C.: The College, 1984. (600 Maryland Ave., S.W., Suite 300 East, Washington, DC 20024-2588.)

Bell R. Changing bodies, changing lives: a book for teens on sex and relationships. New York: Vintage Books, 1988.

Eagan AB. Why am I so miserable if these are the best years of my life? Philadelphia: JB Lippincott, 1976.

Frank DB. Deep blue funk and other stories: portraits of teenage parents. Chicago: Ounce of Prevention Fund, 1983.

Gordon S. When living hurts. New York: Union of American Hebrew Congregations, 1985.

Gordon S, Conant R. You: the teenage survival book. Harrisburg, Pennsylvania: Strawberry-Hill, 1975.

Kovar LC. Faces of the adolescent girl. Englewood Cliffs, New Jersey: Prentice-Hall, 1968

Leder JM. Dead serious: A book for teenagers about teenage suicide. New York: Atheneum, 1987.

Maderas L. Lynda Maderas' growing-up guide for girls. New York: Newmarket Press, 1986.

Maderas L. The what's happening to my body? book for boys. New York: Newmarket Press, 1987.

McCoy K. The teenage survival guide. New York: Simon & Schuster, 1981.

McCoy K. The teenage body book: guide to sexuality. New York: Wallaby, Pocket Books, 1983.

McCoy K. The teenage body book to dating. New York: Simon & Schuster, 1983.

McCoy K, Wibbelsman C. Growing and changing: a handbook for preteens. New York: Putnam, 1986.

McCoy K, Wibbelsman C. The new teenage body book. Los Angeles: Body Press, 1987.

Nonkin LJ. I wish my parents understood: a report on the teenage female. New York: Freundlich Books, 1985.

Rosenbaum A. The young people's Yellow Pages: a national sourcebook for youth. New York: Perigee, 1983.

Shaw D. Make the most of a good thing: you. Boston: Atlantic Monthly Press, 1986.

Simons J, Finlay B, Yang A. The adolescent and young adult fact book. Washington, D.C.: Children's Defense Fund, 1991.

Voss J, Gale J. A young woman's guide to sex. New York: Henry Holt, 1986.

Westheimer R, Kravetz N. First love: a young people's guide to sexual information. New York: Warner Books, 1985.

Relaxation Techniques

Benson H. Relaxation response. New York: William Morrow, 1975.

Brown B. New mind, new body. New York: Bantam Books, 1975.

Brown B. Stress and the art of biofeedback. New York: Bantam Books, 1978.

Haley J. Uncommon therapy: The psychiatric techniques of Milton Erickson. New York: WW Norton, 1973.

Jacobson E. Progressive relaxation. Chicago: Chicago Publishing, 1938.

Pelletier KR. Mind as healer, mind as slayer. New York: Delta Books, 1979.

Simonton OC, Matthew-Simonton S, Creighton J. Getting well again. New York: St. Martin's Press, 1978.

A syllabus on hypnosis and a handbook of therapeutic suggestions. American Society of Clinical Hypnosis, 1973.

Journals

Adolescence

Libra Publishers, 391 Willets Rd., Roslyn Heights, NY 11577. (Quarterly journal of current research in areas of social work and psychology.)

Adolescent and Pediatric Gynecology

Springer-Verlag, 175 Fifth Ave., New York, NY 10010. (Official quarterly publication of the North American Society for Pediatric and Adolescent Gynecology.)

Archives of Pediatrics and Adolescent Medicine

American Medical Association

Journal of Adolescent Health

Elsevier Science Publishing Co., 655 Avenue of the Americas, New York, NY 10010.

Journal of Adolescent Research

Sage Publications, Inc., 2455 Teller Rd. Newbury Park, CA 91320; 805-499-0721. (Official publication of the Society for Research on Adolescence.)

Journal of American College Health

Heldref Publications, 4000 Albemarle St., N.W., Washington, DC 20016. (Journal dedicated to the exchange of information related to health care issues in community colleges, colleges, and universities.)

Journal of Youth and Adolescence

Plenum Publishing Corp., 233 Spring St., New York, NY 10013. (Multidisciplinary quarterly research journal.)

Other Resources and Services

General Resources and Services
The Center for Early Adolescence
University of North Carolina
Suite 223
Carr Mill Mall
Carrboro, NC 27510
(Offers bibliographies and booklets on many areas concerning young adolescents, such as community services, parenting, and sexuality.)
Available from the center:
Understanding Early Adolescence: A Framework, by J. P. Hill
Understanding Families With Young Adolescents, by L. D. Steinberg
Schools for Young Adolescents: Adapting the Early Childhood Model, by S. Feeney
Resource Lists
"Adolescent Literature"
"Community Resources"
"Early Adolescence"
"Educating Young Adolescents"
"Parenting"
"Religion"
"Sex Education"

Abortion Services
Check telephone listings under:
Clergy counseling service
National Abortion Federation Hotline: 800-772-9100
National Organization for Women
Planned Parenthood

Counseling Services
Check telephone listings under:
Family Services Association
County department of health
Counseling clinics
Mental health clinics
United Fund

Hotline Services
Center for Disease Control and Prevention AIDS Hotline: 800-342-2437 (24 hours, 7 days)
Spanish: 800-344-7432 (8 AM to 2 AM, Eastern time, 7 days)

TTY: 800-243-7889 (Monday through Friday, 10 AM to 10 PM, Eastern time)
Teens AIDS: 800-440-8336 (staffed by teens for teens; Fridays and Saturdays, 6 PM to midnight, Eastern time)
Teens TAP (Teaching AIDS Prevention), an AIDS information line for teens (not a crisis line): 800-234-8336 (Monday through Friday, 4 PM to 8 PM, Central Standard time)
Gay and Lesbian Youth Hotline (not a crisis line): 800-347-8336 (Thursday through Saturday, 7 PM to 11:45 PM, Eastern time)
National Runaway Switchboard Hotline (for youth or parents: 800-231-6946) (24 hours)
Adolescent Crisis Intervention and Counseling (the "nine" line): 800-999-9999 (24 hours, 7 days)
Hit Home a national youth crisis line for suicide, abuse, pregnancy, depression, counseling, and intervention: 800-448-4663 (24 hours, 7 days)
National Child Abuse Hotline, for suspected child abuse reports and for referrals: 800-422-4453 (24 hours, 7 days)
National Herpes Hotline: 919-361-8488 (Monday through Friday 9 AM to 7 PM, Eastern time)
STD Hotline: 800-227-8922 (Monday through Friday, 8 AM to 11 PM, Eastern time)

Check local operator or directory for hotlines listed under:
Crisis Counseling
Counseling
Drug Abuse
Rape
Runaways
Suicide
Information also available from:
National Clearinghouse for Mental Health Information
5600 Fishers Lane Rd.
Rockville, MD 20857
301-433-4515
See also section in Appendix on "Adolescent Clinics," below

Alcohol and Drug Problems
Books
Barth RP. Preventing adolescent abuse: effective intervention strategies and techniques. Derezotes. Lexington, Massachusetts: Lexington Books, 1990.

Brounstein PJ, ed. Substance use and delinquency among inner city adolescent males. Washington, D.C.: Urban Institute Press, 1990.

Bukstein OG. Adolescent substance abuse: assessment, treatment, and prevention. New York: John Wiley & Sons, 1995.

Cox TC, Jacobs MR, LeBlanc AE, et al. Drugs and drug abuse: a reference text. Toronto: Addiction Research Foundation, 1983.

Davies J. The facts about adolescent drug abuse. London: Cassell, 1991.

Goplerud EN. Preventing adolescent drug use: from theory to practice. Rockville, Maryland: Office for Substance Abuse Prevention, U.S. Department of Health and Human Services, 1991.

Kaminer Y. Adolescent substance abuse: a comprehensive guide to theory and practice. New York: Plenum Medical, 1994.

Lawson GW, Lawson AW, eds. Adolescent substance abuse: etiology, treatment, prevention. Gaithersburg, Maryland: Aspen, 1992.

Litt IF, ed. Adolescent substance abuse. Columbus, Ohio: Ross Laboratories, 1983.

Rahdert E, Czechowicz D, eds. Adolescent drug abuse: clinical assessment and therapeutic interventions. Rockville, Maryland: National Institute on Drug Abuse, Division of Clinical and Services Research, U.S. Department of Health and Human Services, 1995.

Rogers PD, Werner MJ. Substance abuse. Philadelphia: WB Saunders, 1995.

Ross GR. Treating adolescent substance abuse: understanding the fundamental elements. Boston: Allyn & Bacon, 1994.

Organizations
Al-Anon Family Group Headquarters
    P.O. Box 862
    Midtown Station
    New York, NY 10018
    800-344-2666; or check local office
Alcohol and Drug Helpline
    800-821-4357
    (Provides referrals to local facilities where adolescents and adults can seek help for alcohol and drug problems.)
Alcohol Hotline
    800-252-6465 (800-ALCOHOL)
Alcoholics Anonymous
    Box 459
    Grand Central Annex
    New York, NY 10017
    212-686-1100; or check local office
American Council on Alcoholism
    800-527-5344
    (Provides treatment referrals, counseling, and advice for alcoholics and their families and friends.)
Boys Clubs of America
    771 First Ave.
    New York, NY 10017
    212-557-7755

Cocaine Anonymous World Services
    National Referral Information Line (not a hotline): 800-347-8998
    World Service Office: 310-559-5833
    National Cocaine Hotline: 800-262-2463 (800-COCAINE)
Narcotics Anonymous
    P.O. Box 9999
    Van Nuys, CA 94109
    818-780-3951
National Clearinghouse for Alcohol Information
    P.O. Box 2345
    Rockville, MD 20852
    301-468-2600
National Clearinghouse for Alcohol and Drug Information
    P.O. Box 2345
    Rockville, MD 20847-2345
    800-729-6686
National Council on Alcoholism
    12 West 21st St., Suite 700
    New York, NY 10010
    800-NCA-CALL
National Council on Alcoholism and Drug Dependence, Inc.
    800-622-2255
    (Provides information and referrals to local counseling.)
National Federation of Parents for Drug-Free Youth
    1423 North Jefferson
    Springfield, MO 65802
    417-836-3709
National Institute on Drug Abuse
    P.O. Box 2305
    Rockville, MD 20852
    800-662-4357
Parent Resources Institute for Drug Education (PRIDE)
    100 Edgewood Ave., Suite 1216
    Atlanta, GA 30303
    404-577-4500

Sexuality
Books
Chilman CS. Adolescent sexuality in a changing American society. New York: John Wiley & Sons, 1983.

Gordon S. Seduction lines heard around the world and answers you can give. Buffalo, New York: Prometheus Books, 1987.

Moore S. Sexuality in adolescence. New York: Routledge, 1993.

Planned Parenthood. Teen sexuality today: bibliography of selected resources. New York: Planned Parenthood Federation of America, 1986.

Rekers GA. Handbook of child and adolescent sexual problems. New York: Lexington Books, 1995.

Sex and America's teenagers. New York: Allan Guttmacher Institute, 1994.

Organizations
AIDS Information Line
    Centers for Disease Control and Prevention
    National HIV and AIDS Hotline
    800-342-AIDS

American Social Health Association
P.O. Box 13827
Research Triangle Park, NC 27709
919-361-8400

Center for Population Options
1025 Vermont Ave., NW, Suite 210
Washington, DC 20005
202-347-5700

International Planned Parenthood Federation
Western Hemisphere Regional Office
902 Broadway, 10th Floor
New York, NY 10010
212-995-8800

National Family Planning and Reproductive Health Association, Inc.
122 C St., NW, Suite 380
Washington, DC 20001
202-628-3535

National Sex and Drug Forums
330 Ellis St.
San Francisco, CA 94102

Planned Parenthood–World Population
810 7th Ave.
New York, NY 10019
800-230-7526

Sex Information and Education Council of the United States (SIECUS)
130 West 42nd St., Suite 2500
New York, NY 10036
212-819-9770

Society for Adolescent Medicine (SAM)
1916 Copper Oaks Circle
Blue Springs, MO 64015
816-224-8010

Sex Education Resources
MANUALS
Contact the following organizations for up-to-date educational manuals:
Planned Parenthood, national and local
Family Planning Federation
Local school district
National Clearinghouse for Family Planning Information, Rockville, Md.
U.S. Department of Health and Human Services (U.S. Government Printing Office)

Other Resources
Odin Books
1522 West Broadway
Vancouver, BC V6J 1W8
800-223-6346
(Education resource lists available on education curricula and reference lists on topics such as self-esteem, attention deficit disorder, depression, child abuse, eating disorders, and teen pregnancy.)

ETR Associates
P.O. Box 1830
Santa Cruz, CA 95061-1830
408-438-4081 or 800-321-4407

(Many pamphlets and books on AIDS, family life, sexual abuse, sexuality, drug abuse prevention, and reproductive health.)

POPLINE (POPulation information onLINE)
Johns Hopkins University
Population Information Program
111 Market Place, Suite 310
Baltimore, MD 21202-4024
410-659-6300
Online Service: National Library of Medicine, Bethesda, MD
800-638-8480 (for user ID and password)
(Citations and abstracts to the worldwide literature on population and family planning.)

Planned Parenthood-World Population
810 7th Ave.
New York, NY 10019
800-230-7526
(Many pamphlets, books, and videotapes on reproductive health care; also available is *Current Literature in Family Planning,* a monthly review of literature in family planning.)

Teenage Pregnancy
Books
Alan Guttmacher Institute. Eleven million teenagers: what can be done about the epidemic of adolescent pregnancy in the United States? New York: The Institute, 1976.

Alan Guttmacher Institute. Teenage pregnancy: the problem that hasn't gone away. New York: The Institute, 1981.

Alan Guttmacher Institute. Making choices evaluating the health risks and benefits of birth control methods. New York: The Institute, 1983.

Alan Guttmacher Institute. Teenage pregnancy in industrialized countries: a study. New Haven, Connecticut: Yale University Press, 1986.

Alan Guttmacher Institute. Sex and America's teenagers. New York: The Institute, 1994.

Allen JE, Bender D. Managing teenage pregnancy: access to abortion, contraception, and sex education. New York: Praeger Publishers, 1980.

Anastasiow NJ. The adolescent parent. Baltimore: Paul H. Brookes Publishing, 1982.

Battle SF. The black adolescent parent. New York: Haworth Press, 1987.

Bode J. Kids having kids: the unwed teenage parent. New York: Watts, 1980.

Card JJ. Handbook of adolescent sexuality and pregnancy: research and evaluation instruments. Newbury Park, California: Sage Publications, 1993.

Committee on Adolescence. Crises of adolescence: teenage pregnancy—impact on adolescent development. New York: Brunner/Mazel, 1986.

Corbett MA. The adolescent and pregnancy. Boston: Blackwell Scientific Publications, 1987.

Dickman IR. Teenage pregnancy: what can be done? New York: Public Affairs Committee, 1981.

Elster AB, Lamb ME. Adolescent fatherhood. Hillsdale, New Jersey: Lawrence Erlbaum Associates, 1986.

Evaluation of the Prevention of Early Teenage Pregnancy Project. Sacramento, California: Department of Health Services, 1981.

Foster S. Preventing teenage pregnancy: a public policy planning guide. Washington, D.C.: Council of State Policy and Planning Agencies, 1986.

Furstenberg FI, Brooks-Gunn J, Morgan SP. Adolescent mothers in later life. New York: Cambridge University Press, 1987.

Hardy JB, ed. Adolescent pregnancy in an urban environment: issues, programs, and evaluation. Washington, D.C.: Urban Institute Press; Baltimore: Urban & Schwarzenberg, 1991.

Humenick SS, Wilkerson NN, Paul NW. Adolescent pregnancy: nursing perspectives on prevention. White Plains, New York: March of Dimes Birth Defects Foundation, 1991.

Lancaster JB, Hamburg BA. School-age pregnancy and parenthood: biosocial dimensions. New York: Aldine De Gruyter Publishing, 1986.

Lawson A, Rhode DL. The politics of pregnancy: adolescent sexuality and public policy. New Haven: Yale University Press, 1993.

McAnarney ER. Premature adolescent pregnancy and parenthood. New York: Grune & Stratton, 1983.

Miller SH. Children as parents: final report on a study of childbearing and childrearing among 12- to 15-year-olds. New York: Child Welfare League of America, 1983.

Moore KA, Burt MR. Private crisis, public cost: policy perspectives on teenage childbearing. Washington, D.C.: Urban Institute Press, 1982.

National Research Council. Risking the future: adolescent sexuality, pregnancy, and childbearing. Washington, D.C.: National Academy Press, 1987.

Nickel PS, Delany H. Working with teen parents: a survey of promising approaches. Chicago: Family Resource Coalition, 1985.

Nutritional guide for pregnant and lactating adolescents. Sacramento: California State Department of Education, 1987.

Pittman K. Teenage pregnancy: an advocate's guide to the numbers. Washington, D.C.: Children's Defense Fund, 1988.

Robinson BE. Teenage fathers. Lexington, Massachusetts: Lexington Books, 1988.

Russel JK. Early teenage pregnancy. New York: Churchill Livingstone, 1982.

Scott KG, Field T, Robertson EF. Teenage parents and their offspring. New York: Grune & Stratton, 1981.

Smith PB, Mumford DM. Adolescent pregnancy: perspectives of the health professional. Boston: GK Hall, 1980.

Stuart IR, Wells CF, eds. Pregnancy in adolescence: needs, problems, and management. New York: Van Nostrand Reinhold, 1982.

Vinovskis M. An epidemic of adolescent pregnancy? some historical and policy considerations. New York: Oxford University Press, 1988.

Zabin LS, Hirsch MB. Evaluation of adolescent pregnancy prevention programs in the school context. Lexington, Massachusetts: Lexington Books, 1988.

Zabin LS. Adolescent sexual behavior and childbearing. Newbury Park, California: Sage Publications, 1993.

Zollar AC. Adolescent pregnancy and parenthood: an annotated guide. New York: Garland Publishing, 1990.

Teenage Pregnancy: A Challenge to Do Right by Each Other (by United Church Board, 1980)
United Church of Christ

Sexually Speaking—Who Am I? (grades 7–9); and *Youth Views Sexuality* (senior high)
(by Graded Press, 1973 and 1971, respectively)
The United Methodist Church

Education in Human Sexuality for Christians: Guidelines for Discussion and Planning
(by United States Catholic Conference, Publications Office, 1981)
The Roman Catholic Church

Relating
(by M.M. McCarty, William C. Brown Co., 1979)
The Roman Catholic Church

Course on Human Sexuality for Adolescents in Religious Schools, Youth Groups, and Camps
(by A. Daum and B. Strongin, New York Federation of Reform Synagogues, 1979)
Jewish

Adolescent Clinics

Alabama
Adolescent Health Training Program
Division of Adolescent Medicine
Department of Pediatrics
University of Alabama
1600 Seventh Ave. S., Suite 752
Birmingham, AL 35233
205-975-6573

California
Adolescent Clinic
Children's Hospital
3801 Sacramento St.
San Francisco, CA 94118
415-668-8211

Adolescent Clinic
University of California Medical Center
400 Parnassus Ave.
San Francisco, CA 94143
415-476-2184

Adolescent Clinic
Harbor-University of California at Los Angeles Medical Center
1000 W. Carson St.
Torrance, CA 90509
310-222-2321

Adolescent Medical Clinic
University of California at San Diego Medical Center
225 W. Dickinson St.
San Diego, CA 92103
619-543-5600

Adolescent Youth Clinic
  Stanford University
  750 Welch Rd., Suite 325
  Palo Alto, CA 94304
  415-725-8293
Teenage Health Center
  Childrens Hospital of Los Angeles
  4650 Sunset Blvd.
  Los Angeles, CA 90027
  213-669-2153
Teen Clinic
  Oakland Children's Hospital
  747 52nd St.
  Oakland, CA 94609
  510-428-3178
Teen Pregnancy Resource Center
  Valley Medical Center
  445 South Cedar
  Fresno, CA 93702
  209-453-4533
Youth Clinic
  San Francisco General Hospital
  1001 Potrero Ave.
  San Francisco, CA 94110
  415-206-8376

Colorado
Adolescent Clinic
  University of Colorado Medical Center
  Colorado Children's Hospital
  1056 E. 19th Ave.
  Denver, CO 80218
  303-861-6133

Connecticut
Adolescent Clinic
  Yale New Haven Hospital
  20 York St.
  New Haven, CT 06510
  203-785-4644
Adolescent Unit
  Bridgeport Hospital
  267 Grant St.
  Bridgeport, CT 06602
  203-384-3064
Department of Child and Adolescent Psychiatry
  Mt. Sinai Hospital
  500 Blue Hills Ave.
  Hartford, CT 06112
  203-286-4948
Fair Haven Clinic
  374 Grand Ave.
  New Haven, CT 06513
  203-777-7411
Young Adults Program
  St. Francis Hospital
  1000 Asylum Ave.
  Hartford, CT 06105
  203-548-5348

Delaware
Christiana Hospital
  4755 Ogletown Stanton Rd.
  Newark, Delaware 19718
  302-733-4107

District of Columbia
Adolescent Clinic
  Walter Reed Army Medical Center
  Georgia Avenue and 16th Street
  Washington, DC 20307-5001
  202-576-1107
Adolescent Medicine Associates
  Children's National Medical Center
  111 Michigan Ave., NW
  Washington, DC 20010
  202-884-3066
Adolescent Medicine Clinic
  Howard University Hospital
  2041 Georgia Ave., NW
  Washington, DC 20060
  202-865-1376
Child and Youth Ambulatory Services
  Georgetown University
  Children's Medical Center
  3800 Reservoir Rd., NW
  Washington, DC 20007
  202-687-KIDS

Florida
Miami Children's Hospital
  Division of Adolescent Medicine
  6125 SW 31st St.
  Miami, FL 33155
  305-662-8343

Hawaii
Adolescent Program
  Kapiolani Children's Medical Center
  1319 Punahou St.
  Honolulu, HI 96826
  808-949-3579

Illinois
Adolescent Family Center
  Rush Presbyterian Hospital
  1725 W. Harrison, Suite 407
  Professional Building
  Chicago, IL 60612
  312-942-6067
Adolescent Medicine
  Cook County Hospital
  700 S. Wood St.
  Chicago, IL 60612
  312-633-7438
Adolescent Medicine
  Department of Pediatrics
  Room 4671
  Loyola University

1701 South First Ave.
Maywood, IL 60153
708-327-9119

Indiana
Adolescent Clinic
Indiana University School of Medicine
720 Barnhill Dr.
Indianapolis, IN 46202
317-274-8812

Iowa
Adolescent Clinic
Department of Pediatrics
University of Iowa Hospitals and Clinics
200 Hawkins Dr.
Iowa City, IA 52242
319-356-2229

Kansas
Adolescent Medicine
University of Kansas Medical Center
3901 Rainbow Blvd.
Kansas City, KS 66160
913-588-5908

Kentucky
Pediatric Adolescent Medicine/Gynecology Clinic
Kosair Children's Hospital
P.O. Box 35070
Louisville, KY 40202
502-629-8836

Louisiana
Adolescent Medicine
Department of Pediatrics, slot 37
Tulane Medical Center
1430 Tulane Ave.
New Orleans, Louisiana 70112
504-584-2568

Maine
Teen and Young Adult Clinic
Eastern Maine Medical Center
Department of Pediatrics
417 State St.
Webber Building
Bangor, Maine 04401
207-973-7520

Maryland
Adolescent Clinic
The Johns Hopkins University Hospital
600 N. Wolfe St., Park 307
Baltimore, MD 21287
410-955-2910
Adolescent Clinic
nery County Health Department
gerford Dr.
e, MD 26850
-1600

Adolescent Clinic
University of Maryland Hospital
120 Penn St., 1st Floor
Baltimore, MD 21201
410-328-6495

Massachusetts
Adolescent Center
Boston City Hospital
818 Harrison Ave. ACC-2
Boston, MA 02118
617-534-4091
Adolescent Clinic
New England Medical Center
750 Washington St.
Boston, MA 02111
617-956-5312
Adolescent and Young Adult Medicine Clinic
Children's Hospital Medical Center
300 Longwood Ave.
Boston, MA 02115
617-735-6000

Michigan
Adolescent Clinic
Hurley Medical Center
1 Hurley Plaza
Flint, MI 48502
810-257-9773
Adolescent Medicine Clinic
Children's Hospital of Michigan
3901 Beaubien
Detroit, MI 48201
313-745-4045
Adolescent Medicine Program
Department of Pediatrics/Human Development
Michigan State University
College of Human Medicine
B-240 Life Sciences
East Lansing, MI 48824
517-353-5042
Division of Adolescent Medicine
Henry Ford Hospital
2799 W. Grand Blvd.
Detroit, MI 48202
313-876-3132
Internal Medicine Program
University Hospital
University of Michigan
3906 Taubman Center
Ann Arbor, MI 48109
313-936-5575

Minnesota
Adolescent Health Program
University of Minnesota Hospital and Clinic
Box 721 UMHC, Harvard Street at East River Rd.
Room D136 Mayo Bldg.
Minneapolis, MN 55455
612-626-2820

Mississippi
Adolescent Clinic
  University of Mississippi Medical Center
  2500 N. State St.
  Jackson, MS 39216
  601-984-2925

Missouri
Division of Adolescent Medicine
  Department of Pediatrics
  Children's Mercy Hospital
  24th Street at Gilham Road
  Kansas City, MO 64108
  816-234-3851

Nebraska
Omaha Children's Clinic
  12808 Augusta Ave.
  Omaha, NB 68144
  402-330-5690
Youth Village
  Children's Memorial Hospital
  8301 Dodge
  Omaha, NB 68114
  402-390-5537

Nevada
Adolescent Medicine
  Department of Pediatrics
  University of Nevada School of Medicine No. 200
  2040 West Charleston
  Las Vegas, NV 81902
  702-383-2741

New Jersey
Adolescent Clinic
  Department of Pediatrics
  Martland Hospital
  New Jersey Medical School
  150 Bergen St.
  Newark, NJ 07107
  201-982-5779
Adolescent Clinic
  Monmouth Medical Center
  Long Branch, NJ 07740
  201-222-5200, ext. 5048
Adolescent Services and Clinic
  Morristown Memorial Hospital
  100 Madison Ave.
  Morristown, NJ 07960
  201-540-5199

New Hampshire
Pediatric and Adolescent Medicine Clinic
  Dartmouth–Hitchcock Medical Center
  Lebanon, NH 03756
  603-650-5473

New Mexico
Adolescent Medicine
  University of New Mexico Medical Center

Albuquerque, NM 87131
  505-272-5551

New York
Adolescent Health Center
  The Door
  618 Avenue of the Americas
  New York, NY 10011
  212-941-9090
Adolescent Health Center
  Mount Sinai Medical Center
  19 E. 101st St.
  New York, NY 10029
  212-241-7570
Adolescent Medical Group
  601 Elmwood Ave.
  Rochester, NY 14642
  716-275-2964
Adolescent Medicine Program
  New York Medical College
  Munger Pavillion
  Valhalla, NY 10595
  914-285-7696
Adolescent Oncology Program
  Roswell Park Cancer Institute
  Calton and Elm St.
  Buffalo, NY 14263
  716-845-2333
Division of Adolescent Medicine
  Montefiore Hospital and Medical Center
  111 E. 210th St.
  Bronx, NY 10467
  212-920-6781
Division of Adolescent Medicine
  Schneider Children's Hospital of Long Island
  Jewish Medical Center
  269-01 76th Ave.
  New Hyde Park, NY 11042
  718-470-3270
Division of Adolescent Medicine Medical Program
  Brookdale Hospital Medical Center
  Linden Boulevard at Brookdale Plaza
  Brooklyn, NY 11212
  212-240-6451
Strong Adolescent Medical Group
  P.O. Box 690
  601 Elmwood Ave.
  Rochester, NY 14642
  716-275-2964

North Carolina
Ambulatory Care Center
  University of North Carolina
  CB No. 7735
  Chapel Hill, NC 27599-7735
  919-966-6669
Department of Pediatrics
  Duke Medical Center
  Box 3675
  Durham, NC 27710
  919-477-4297

Ohio
Adolescent Clinic
Cincinnati Children's Hospital
Elland & Bethesda
Cincinnati, OH 45229
513-559-4681
Adolescent Clinic
Cleveland Metropolitan General Hospital
2500 Metro Health Dr.
Cleveland, OH 44109
216-459-5721
Adolescent Clinic
University of Cincinnati
College of Medicine
Medical Science Bldg.
Department of Psychiatry
231 Bethesda Ave.
Cincinnati, OH 45267
513-558-1000

Oklahoma
Adolescent Medicine
Oklahoma City Children's Hospital of Okalahoma
P.O. Box 26901
940 NE 13th St.
Oklahoma City, OK 73190
405-271-6372
Adolescent Medicine Clinic
Children's Hospital of Oklahoma
940 NE 13th St., Room 4N456
Oklahoma City, OK 73104
405-271-6208

Pennsylvania
Adolescent Clinic
Children's Hospital of Philadelphia
3400 Spruce St., Silverstein 3
Philadelphia, PA 19104
215-662-3798

Rhode Island
Adolescent Medicine
Department of Pediatrics
Rhode Island Hospital
APC-585-A
593 Eddy St.
Providence, RI 02902
401-444-4712

South Carolina
Adolescent Program
Marshall I. Pickens Hospital
701 Grove Rd.
Greenville, SC 29605
803-242-8807

Texas
Adolescent Clinic
The University of Texas
6303 Harry Hines Blvd., Suite 101

Dallas, TX 75235
214-640-0300
Adolescent Medicine
University of Texas Medical Branch at Houston
P.O. Box 20708
Houston, TX 77225-0708
713-792-5330, ext. 3046
Teen Health Clinic
Baylor College of Medicine
6621 Fannin Blvd., 3-3340
Houston, TX 77030
713-770-3660
University of Texas Medical Branch at Galveston
Galveston, TX 77550
409-772-2254

Utah
Adolescent Medicine
University of Utah
50 North Media Dr.
Salt Lake City, UT 84132
801-581-3729

Virginia
Adolescent Health Service
Medical College of Virginia Hospitals
307 College St.
Richmond, VA 23298-0151
804-828-9449
Pediatric Endocrinology and Adolescent Medicine
Children's Hospital of the King's Daughters
601 Children's Lane
Norfolk, VA 23507
804-628-7237

Washington
Adolescent Clinic, Division of Adolescent Medicine
University of Washington
Seattle, WA 98105
206-543-8705

West Virginia
Adolescent Medicine
Department of Pediatrics
West Virginia University
Morgantown, WV 26506
304-293-1225

Wisconsin
Adolescent Clinic
Downtown Health Center
Milwaukee Children's Hospital
1700 Wells
Milwaukee, WI 53233
414-931-4105
Adolescent Section and Clinic
Marshfield Clinic
1000 North Oak Ave.
Marshfield, WI 54449
715-387-5511

Pediatric and Adolescent Department
  Beaumont Clinic LTD
  1821 South Webster Ave.
  Green Bay, WI 54301
  414-437-9051
Teenage and Young Adult Clinic
  Clinical Sciences Center
  600 Highland Ave.
  Madison, WI 53792
  608-263-6421

Canada
Adolescent Clinic
  British Columbia Children's Hospital
  3644 Slocan St.
  Vancouver, BC V5M 3E8
  604-434-3522
Adolescent Clinic
  Ste.-Justine Hospital
  3175 Chemin Cote Ste.-Catherine
  Montreal, Quebec H3T 1C5
  514-345-4722
Adolescent Medical Clinic
  Hospital for Sick Children
  555 University Ave.
  Toronto, Ontario M5G IX8
  416-813-5804
Adolescent Medicine and Gynecology Program
  Montreal Children's Hospital
  Gilman Pavilion
  1040 Atwater St.
  Montreal, Quebec H3Z 1X3
  514-934-4481
Child and Adolescent Service
  Allan Memorial Institute
  Royal Victoria Hospital
  3666 McTavish St.
  Montreal, Quebec H4A 3M6
  514-843-1619

Sleep Disorder Resources
Alabama
University of Alabama at Birmingham Sleep-Wake
    Disorders Center
  Center for Psychiatric Medicine
  1713 6th St. South
  Birmingham, AL 35233
  205-934-7110

Arizona
Sleep Disorder Center
  Good Samaritan Medical Center
  111 E. McDowell Rd.
  Phoenix, AZ 85006
  602-239-5815

California
North Valley Sleep Disorders Center
  11550 Indian Hills Rd., Suite 291

Mission Hills, CA 91345
  818-361-0996
Sleep Diagnostic Laboratory
  Veterans Administration
  3350 La Jolla Village Dr.
  San Diego, CA 92161
  619-552-8585 ext. 3369
Sleep Disorders Center
  University of California Irvine Medical Center
  101 City Dr. South
  Orange, CA 92668
  714-456-5105
Stanford Sleep Disorders Clinic
  401 Quarry Rd.
  Suite 3301 A
  Stanford, CA 94305
  415-723-6601
UCLA Sleep Disorders Center
  University of California Los Angeles
  710 Westwood Plaza
  Los Angeles, CA 90024
  310-206-8005

Florida
Sleep Disorders Clinic
  Mount Sinai Medical Center
  4300 Alton Rd.
  Miami Beach, FL 33140
  305-674-2613

Illinois
Sleep Disorders Center
  Northwestern Memorial Hospital
  233 East Erie, Suite 500
  Chicago, IL 60610
  312-908-7950
Sleep Disorders Center
  Rush Presbyterian–St. Luke's Medical Center
  1653 W. Congress Parkway
  Room 218, Rawson
  Chicago, IL 60612
  312-942-5440
Sleep Disorders Center
  University of Chicago (TS-301)
  5841 S. Maryland
  Chicago, IL 60637
  312-702-1780

Louisiana
Sleep Disorders Center
  Neurology
  Tulane Medical School
  New Orleans, LA 70112
  504-584-3592

Maryland
The Johns Hopkins Sleep Disorders Center
  Asthma and Allergy Bldg
  4th Floor
  5501 Hopkins Bay View Circle

Baltimore, MD 21224
410-550-0571

Massachusetts
Center for Pediatric Sleep Disorders
  The Children's Hospital
  300 Longwood Ave.
  Boston, MA 02115
  617-732-6750
Sleep Clinic
  Brigham and Women's Hospital
  221 Longwood Ave.
  Boston, MA 02115
  617-732-6753
Sleep Disorders Clinic
  Tufts-Newton Wellesley Hospital
  2014 Washington St.
  Newton, MA 02162
  617-243-6624
Sleep Laboratory
  Department of Neurology
  University of Massachusetts Medical Center
  Worcester, MA 01655
  508-856-3802

Michigan
Sleep Disorders Clinic
  New Center Pavilion
  2921 W. Grand Blvd.
  Detroit, MI 48202
  313-972-1800

Minnesota
Minnesota Regional Sleep Disorders Center
  Hennepin County Medical Center
  701 Park Ave. South
  Minneapolis, MN 55415
  612-347-6201

New Hampshire
Sleep Disorders Center
  Dartmouth-Hitchcock Medical Center
  1 Medical Center Dr.
  Lebanon, NH 03756
  603-650-5000

New Jersey
Sleep-Wake Studies and Consultants
  University of Medicine and Dentistry of New Jersey
  New Jersey Medical School
  30 Bergen St.
  Newark, NJ 07103
  210-982-4687

New York
Sleep Disorders Center
  Child's Hospital
  25 Hackett Blvd.
  Albany, NY 12208
  518-436-9253

Sleep Disorders Center
  University Hospital
  MR 120A
  State University of New York at Stony Brook
  Stony Brook, NY 11794-7139
  514-444-2916
Sleep-Wake Disorders Center
  Montefiore Medical Center
  111 E. 210th St.
  Bronx, NY 10467
  718-920-4841

Ohio
Sleep Disorders Center
  Mt. Sinai Medical Center
  1 Mt. Sinai Dr,
  Cleveland, OH 44106
  216-421-3700
Sleep Disorders Treatment and Research Center
  The Ohio State University
  473 W. 12th Ave.
  Columbus, OH 43210
  614-293-8260

Oklahoma
Sleep Disorders Center
  Presbyterian Hospital and Medical Center
  700 N. E 13th St.
  Oklahoma City, OK 73104
  405-271-6312

Pennsylvania
Sleep Disorders Center
  Department of Neurology
  Crozer Chester Medical Center
  Chester, PA 19103
  215-447-2688
Sleep Evaluation Center
  Western Psychiatric Institute and Clinic
  3811 O'Hara St.
  Pittsburgh, PA 15213
  412-624-2246
Sleep Research and Treatment Center
  Milton S. Hershey Medical Center
  P.O. Box 850
  Hershey, PA 17033
  717-531-8520

Tennessee
Sleep Disorders Center
  Baptist Memorial Hospital
  899 Madison Ave.
  Memphis, TN 38146
  901-227-5337

Texas
Sleep Disorders and Research Medicine
  Baylor College of Medicine
  One Baylor Plaza
  Houston, TX 77030
  713-798-4886

Virginia
Sleep Disorders Clinic
   University Of Virginia Medical Center
   P.O. Box 367-15
   Charlottesville, VA 22908
   804-982-0995

Organizations Involved in Adolescent Health
American Academy of Child and Adolescent Psychiatry
   (AACAP)
   3615 Wisconsin Ave, NW
   Washington, DC 20016
   202-966-7300
American Academy of Family Physicians (AAFP)
   8880 Ward Parkway
   Kansas City, MO 64114
   816-333-9700
American Academy of Pediatrics (AAP)
   141 Northwest Point Blvd.
   Elk Grove Village, IL 60009-0927
   708-228-5005
American College Health Association (ACHA)
   1300 Piccard Dr., Suite 200
   Rockville, MD 20850
   301-963-1100
American College of Obstetricians and Gynecologists
   (ACOG)
   Division of Program Services
   Department of Adolescent Health Care
   409 12th St., SW
   Washington, DC 20024-2188
   202-863-2579
American College of Physicians (ACP)
   Independence Mall West
   Sixth Street at Race
   Philadelphia, PA 19106-1572
   206-883-7252
American College of Preventive Medicine (ACPM)
   1015 15th St., NW, Suite 403
   Washington, DC 20005
   202-789-0033
American Dietetic Association (ADA)
   216 West Jackson Blvd., Suite 800
   Chicago, IL 60606-6995
   213-899-0040
American Medical Association (AMA)
   Department of Adolescent Health
   515 North State St.
   Chicago, IL 60610
   312-646-5570
American Nurses' Association (ANA)
   Council on Maternal-Child Nursing
   2420 Pershing Rd.
   Kansas City, MO 64108
   816-474-5720
American Osteopathic Association (AOA)
   142 East Ontario St.
   Chicago, IL 60611
   312-280-5800
American Psychiatric Association (APA)
   1400 K St., NW

Washington, DC 20005
   202-682-6093
American Psychological Association (APA)
   1200 17th St., NW
   Washington, DC 20036
   202-955-7673
American Public Health Association (APHA)
   1015 15th St., NW
   Washington, DC 20005
   202-789-5691
American School Health Association (ASHA)
   P.O. Box 708
   7263 State Route 43
   Kent, OH 44240
   216-678-1601
American Society for Adolescent Psychiatry (ASAP)
   4330 East West Highway, Suite 1117
   Bethesda, MD 20814
   301-718-6502
Association of State and Territorial Health Officials
   (ASTHO)
   6728 Old McLean Village Dr.
   McLean, VA 22101
   703-556-9222
Carnegie Council on Adolescent Development
   2400 N St., NW, 6th Floor
   Washington, DC 20037-1153
   202-429-7979
Centers for Disease Control and Prevention (CDC)
   National Centers for Chronic Disease Prevention
     and Health Promotion
   Division of Adolescent and School Helath (DASH)
   1600 Clifton Rd., NE, Mailstop K32
   Atlanta, GA 30333
   404-488-5324
Maternal and Child Health Bureau (MCHB)
   Health Resources and Services Administration (HRSA)
   U.S. Public Health Service (USPHS)
   Department of Health and Human Services (DHHS)
   5600 Fishers Lane, Room 9-05
   Rockville, MD 20857
   301-443-2170
National Association of Social Workers (NASW)
   7981 Eastern Ave.
   Silver Spring, MD 20910
   301-565-0333
National Coalition of Hispanic and Human Services
   Organizations (COSSMHO)
   1030 15th St., NW, Suite 1053
   Washington, DC 20005
   202-371-2100
National Institute on Alcohol Abuse and Alcoholism
   (NIAAA)
   Prevention Research Branch
   5600 Fishers Lane
   Room 13C-23
   Rockville, MD 20857
   301-443-1677
National Institute on Drug Abuse (NIDA)
   5600 Fishers Lane

Rockville, MD 20857
301-443-4060
National Medical Association (NMA)
1012 Tenth St., NW
Washington, DC 20001
202-347-1895
National Mental Health Association (NMHA)
1021 Prince St.
Alexandria, VA 22314-2971
703-684-7722
Office of Disease Prevention and Health Promotion
(ODPHP)
U.S. Public Health Service, Department of Health
and Human Services
330 C St., SW, Suite 2132
Washington, DC 20201
202-472-5660
The Robert Wood Johnson Foundation (RWJF)
College Road East, P.O. Box 2316
Princeton, NJ 08543
609-452-8701
Society for Adolescent Medicine (SAM)
1916 Copper Oaks Circle
Blue Springs, MO 64015
816-224-8010
Society for Research in Adolescence
122 W. Franklin, Suite 525
Minneapolis, MN 55404
612-870-9511
William T. Grant Foundation
515 Madison Ave.
New York, NY 10022-5403
212-752-0071

Sports Medicine Organizations
Academy for Sports Dentistry
University of Iowa Hospitals and Clinics
Department of Otolaryngology
Iowa City, IA 52242
American Academy of Orthopaedic Surgeons
6300 North River Rd.
Rosemont, IL 60018
708-823-7186
American Academy of Pediatrics
141 Northwest Point
Elk Grove Village, IL 60007
708-228-5005
American College Health Association
P.O. Box 28937
Baltimore, MD 21240-8936
410-859-1500
American College of Sports Medicine
P.O. Box 1440
Indianapolis, IN 46206
317-637-9200
American Council on Exercise
5820 Oberlin Dr., Suite 102
San Diego, CA 92121
619-535-8227

American Heart Association
7272 Greenville Ave.
Dallas, TX 75231-4596
800-242-8721
American Medical Association
Department of Adolescent Health
515 North State St.
Chicago, IL 60610
312-464-5000
American Medical Society for Sports Medicine
7611 Elmwood Ave., Suite 202
Middleton, WI 53562
608-831-4484
Cooper Institute for Aerobics Research
12330 Preston Rd.
Dallas, TX 75230
214-701-8001
National Athletic Trainers Association
2952 Stemmons Freeway
Dallas, TX 75247
214-637-6282
National Collegiate Athletic Association
6201 College Blvd.
Overland Park, KS 66211
913-339-1906
President's Council on Physical Fitness and Sports
701 Pennsylvania Ave., NW, Suite 250
Washington, DC 20004
202-272-3421

Statistical Resources
Alan Guttmacher Institute
111 Fifth Ave.
New York, NY 10003
212-254-5656
(Contraceptive data, pregnancy rates, and marital and
fertility patterns.)
Centers for Disease Control and Prevention
Reproductive Health Division
1600 Clifton Rd., NE
Atlanta, GA 30333
404-329-3311 or 329-3131
Institute for Social Research
426 Thompson St.
Ann Arbor, MI 48104
313-764-8363
National Center for Health Statistics
3700 East-West Highway
Hyattsville, MD 20782
301-436-8500
301-436-8954 (natality data)
301-436-8884 (mortality data)
National Institutes of Health
Demographic and Behavioral Sciences Branch
Center for Population Research
National Institute for Child Health and Human
Development
9000 Rockville Pike
Bethesda, MD 20205
301-496-1174

Internet sites

There is a wealth of information available over the Internet on adolescent medicine and general medical areas. These change rapidly and many are added every week. A net searcher such as WebCrawler, yahoo, or Lycos are helpful in finding sites. Some useful sites includes:

Society for Adolescent Medicine Home Page
http://cortex.ucha.edu/~sam/

Adolescent medicine listserver:
To subscribe send message to: LISTSERVE@UCONNVM.UCONN.EDU
Message should be: subscribe SAM-L
To unsubscribe, same as above but message is: unsubscribe SAM-L
To post a comment send message to: SAM-L@UCONNVM.UCONN.EDU
This message will be sent to all subscribers.

College Health listserver:
To subscribe send message to: LISTSERVE@UTKVM1.UTK.EDU
Message should be: subscribe SHS NAME
Name is your personal name, not a user or e-mail name
To unsubscribe, same as above but message is: unsubscribe SHS NAME
To receive a list of who's on, send a message to above address with entire message being: REVIEW SHS
To post a comment send message to: SHS@UTKVM1.UTK.EDU
This message will be sent to all subscribers.

The American Academy of Child & Adolescent Psychiatry Home Page
http://www.psych.med.umich.edu/web/aacap/

Alcohol & Drug Abuse Address Book
http://www.silcom.com/~paladin/alcnational.html

Archives of Pediatrics and Adolescent Medicine
http://www.ama-assn.org/journals/standing/ajdc/ajdchome.htm

Centers for Disease Control: CDC WONDER Searches and Queries
http://wonder.cdc.gov/rchtml/Convert/data/AdHoc.html

College and University Home Pages: Alphabetical listing of numerous colleges and universities
home pages including over 2450 entries
http://www.mit.edu:8001/people/cdemello/univ.html

Department of Health and Human Services
http://www.os.dhhs.gov

FedWorld Information Network: Entry to governmental web sites
http://www.fedworld.gov/

Health and medicine directory of sites
Subject areas include: Alternative Medicine, Disability, Diseases and Conditions, General Health, Mental Health, Nutrition, Professional Medicine, Sex and Health, Substance Abuse, U.S. and International Health Organizations
http://gnn.com/wic/wics/med.new.html

Kids Health Organization: Consultation to physicians concerning a wide range of adolescent health issues, including pubertal development, chronic complaints, and sexual health concerns, among others.
http://kidshealth.org/ai/service/adolescent.html

Internet Health Resources Company: Providing access to practical health and fitness information
Developed and maintained by Internet Health Resources Company
http://www.ihr.com/index.html

Morbidity and Mortality Weekly Report Serial Publications
http://www.cdc.gov/epo/mmwr/mmwr.html

National Center for Health Statistics
http://www.cdc.gov/nchswww/nchshome.htm

Pharmacy information network: Listing descriptions of various medications
http://pharminfo.com/drugdb/dbgn_mnuv.html

Index